Calculations for determining the amount of local anesthetic and/or vasoconstrictor in dental cartridges

Typical local anesthetic concentrations

Strength		mg/ml Equivalent
0.5%	=	5 mg/ml
1.5%	=	15 mg/ml
2.0%	=	20 mg/ml
3.0%	=	30 mg/ml
4.0%	=	40 mg/ml

Typical vasoconstrictor concentrations

Strength		mg/ml (or µg/ml) Equivalent
1:20,000	=	0.05 mg/ml (50 µg/ml)
1:50,000	=	0.02 mg/ml (20 µg/ml)
1:100,000	=	0.01 mg/ml (10 µg/ml)
1:200,000	=	0.005 mg/ml (5 µg/ml)

General calculation guidelines:

1) Convert % solution to mg/ml (or µg/ml) as shown above.
2) Multiply mg/ml (or µg/ml) × cartridge volume × number of cartridges = quantity of drug. *Note:* Cartridge volumes may vary between products.

Example: Two cartridges of a 2% lidocaine HCl and 1:100,000 epinephrine HCl solution were administered. The cartridge volume was 1.8 ml for each. What quantity of each drug was given?

Answer:
for lidocaine HCl: 20 mg × 1.8 ml × 2 cartridges = 72 mg
for epinephrine HCl: 0.01 mg/ml × 1.8 ml × 2 cartridges = 0.036 mg or 10 µg/ml × 1.8 ml × 2 cartridges = 36 µg

From Gage TW, Pickett FA: Mosby's Dental Drug Reference, ed 5, St. Louis, Mosby, 2001.

MOSBY'S

DENTAL

dictionary

MOSBY'S
DENTAL
dictionary

Thomas J. Zwemer, DDS, MSD, FACD, FICD

Vice President for Academic Affairs, Emeritus,
Professor of Orthodontics, Emeritus,
School of Dentistry, Medical College of Georgia,
Augusta, Georgia,
Diplomate, American Board of Orthodontics

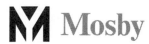 **Mosby**

An Affiliate of Elsevier Science

St. Louis   London   Philadelphia   Sydney   Toronto

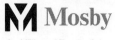

Mosby

An Affiliate of Elsevier Science

Publisher: John Schrefer
Acquisitions Editor: Penny Rudolph
Associate Developmental Editor: Angela Reiner
Project Manager: Linda McKinley
Production Editor: Julie Zipfel
Designer: Renée Duenow
Manufacturing Supervisor: Don Carlisle
Cover Design: Laura Eslinger

Printed in the United States of America
Composition by The Clarinda Co.
Lithography by Top Graphics
Printing/binding by RR Donnelly & Sons Co.

Mosby, Inc.
11830 Westline Industrial Drive
St. Louis, Missouri 63146

Library of Congress Cataloging in Publication Data

Mosby's dental dictionary / [edited by] Thomas J. Zwemer.—1st ed.
    p. cm.
  Includes bibliographical references.
  ISBN 0-8151-9888-4
  1. Dentistry—Dictionaries.   I. Zwemer, Thomas J.
  [DNLM: 1. Dictionaries, Dental.   WU 13 M894 1998]
RK27.M67   1998
617.6′003—dc21
DNLM/DLC
for Library of Congress   97-41342
                                                CIP

02 / 9   8   7   6

To
Those who are dental health professionals.
Those becoming dental health professionals.
Those wishing to communicate with dental health professionals.

Preface

Dentistry isn't just about teeth and gums anymore. It is about people—their values, their behavior, their health, and their priorities. No longer is a glossary of dental terms sufficient for dentists, their staffs, or their public. A much more inclusive compendium is necessary to cover the scope of dentistry as a health care profession.

Mosby's Dental Dictionary is a new work with a proud history. It stands on the shoulders of giants. The historic elegance of *Boucher's Current Dental Terminology* formed the core, and *Mosby's Medical, Nursing, and Allied Health Dictionary* and *Mosby's Dental Drug Reference* were the principal contemporary sources. The current literature and contemporary reference texts gave direction and validity to the terms that were included in this new reference work. The references listed in Acknowledgments were consulted to confirm clinical relevance and accuracy.

Production was an iterative process.

- Each entry in Boucher's 4th edition was checked against the international data base *Medline: 1992-1996* to establish current usage. Those words that did not appear on the *Medline* were either deleted or identified as (not current). "Not current" simply indicates that while the term has a recognized dental history, it has not appeared in any referred dental literature in the past 6 years.

- The entries in the National Library of Medicine *MESH* heading index, 1996, were matched with the word *dental*. Entries that showed concurrence with the word *dental* were included except for some vernacular entries.

- Each entry from Gage/Pickett: *Mosby's Dental Drug Reference* was abstracted using the format of that reference work and included in *Mosby's Dental Dictionary*.

- Matched entries from *MESH* that were not in Boucher's 4th edition were selected from *Mosby's Medical, Nursing, and Allied Health Dictionary* and included in this work.

- Those entries not found in *Mosby's Medical, Nursing, and Allied Health Dictionary* were located in the references acknowledged, particularly, the UMLS *Metathesarus* and abstracted for entry in *Mosby's Dental Dictionary*.

This work contains a rich source of reference materials in the nine appendices, none more so than the American Dental Association (ADA) *Code of Dental Procedures*, which is included under contract with the ADA.

The editor and publisher believe that this new dictionary will be a reliable and ready source of information for the student, the dental staff, the practicing dentist, and all of those associated with dental health care delivery.

The editor wishes to acknowledge and thank Jack D. Zwemer, BS, DDS, MS, PhD, for his strategic advice, wise counsel, and technical support.

Acknowledgments

Acknowledgment is made to the authors and publishers of the following publications used for reference sources by the author:

Accepted dental therapeutics, ed 3, 1977, American Dental Association.

Adopted terminology, 1961, American Academy of Pedodontics.

Adriani J: *The pharmacology of anesthetic drugs,* ed 4, Springfield, Ill, 1960, Thomas.

Aita JA: *Congenital facial anomalies with neurologic defects,* Springfield, Ill, 1969, Thomas.

Allen EV, Barker H: *Peripheral vascular diseases,* Philadelphia, 1962, Saunders.

American Academy of Maxillofacial Prosthetics, Workshop on nomenclature, Annual Meeting, 1971.

American jurisprudence, ed 2, Rochester, NY, 1979, Lawyers Cooperative.

American jurisprudence, Rochester, NY, 1991, Lawyers Cooperative.

Anderson GM: *Practical orthodontics,* ed 9, St Louis, 1960, Mosby.

Anderson KN, Anderson LE, Glanze WD: *Mosby's medical, nursing, and allied health dictionary,* ed 5, St Louis, 1998, Mosby.

Anderson WAD, ed: *Pathology,* ed 6, St Louis, 1972, Mosby.

Angle EH: *Angle system of regulation and retention of the teeth and treatment of fractures of the maxillae,* ed 7, Philadelphia, 1902, White Dental Manufacturing.

Archer WH: *Oral surgery: a step-by-step atlas of operative techniques,* ed 3, Philadelphia, 1961, Saunders.

Ash Major M: *A handbook of differential oral diagnosis,* St Louis, 1961, Mosby.

Avery JK: *Essentials of oral histology and embryology: a clinical approach,* St Louis, 1992, Mosby.

Bassett RW, Ingraham R, Koser JR: *An atlas of gold restorations,* Los Angeles, 1964, University of Southern California.

Behrman SJ: The implantation of magnets in the jaw to aid denture retention. *J Prosthet Dent* 10:807, 1960.

Bennett CR: *Monheim's general anesthesia in dental practice,* ed 4, St Louis, 1974, Mosby.

Bennett CR: *Monheim's local anesthesia and pain control in dental practice,* ed 5, St Louis, 1974, Mosby.

Bernier JL: *Management of oral disease,* ed 2, St Louis, 1959, Mosby.

Berry MF, Eisenson J: *Speech disorders: principles and practices of therapy,* New York, 1956, Appleton-Century-Crofts.

Bhaskar SN: *Synopsis of oral pathology,* ed 7, St Louis, 1986, Mosby.

Black HC: *Black's law dictionary,* St Paul, Minn, West.

Blackwell RE: *GV Black's operative dentistry,* ed 9, South Milwaukee, 1955, Medico-Dental.

Blakiston's Gould medical dictionary, ed 4, New York, 1979, McGraw-Hill.

Blass JL: *Motivating patients for more effective dental service,* Philadelphia, 1958, Lippincott.

Bodine RL Jr: Implant dentures: prosthodontic-favorable, *J Prosthet Dent* 10:1132, 1960.

Boucher CO, ed: *Swenson's complete dentures,* ed 6, St Louis, 1970, Mosby.

Boyd W: *A textbook of pathology,* ed 8, Philadelphia, 1970, Lea & Febiger.

Brand RW, Isselhard DE: *Anatomy of orofacial structures,* ed 6, St Louis, 1998, Mosby.

Brauer JD et al: *Dentistry for children,* ed 3, New York, 1952, McGraw-Hill.

Brodnitz FS: *Keep your voice healthy,* New York, 1953, Harper & Row.

Bureau of Health Manpower, Division of Dentistry. *Department of Health, Education, and Welfare: prepaid dental care: a glossary,* No (HRA) 76-20, Bethesda, Md, 1975, The Bureau.

Burnett GW, Scherp HW, Schuster GS: *Oral microbiology and infectious disease,* ed 4, Baltimore, 1976, Williams & Wilkins.

Carnahan CW: *The dentist and the law,* St Louis, 1955, Mosby.

CDT-2: a users manual, Chicago, 1993, American Dental Association.

CDT-1: a users manual, Chicago, 1991, American Dental Association.

Chusid JG, McDonald JJ: *Correlative neuroanatomy and functional neurology,* ed 11, Los Altos, Calif, 1962, Lange.

Clark JW, ed: *Clark's clinical dentistry,* Philadelphia, 1990, Lippincott.

Cohen MM: *Pediatric dentistry,* ed 2, St Louis, 1961, Mosby.

Cohen S, Burns RC: *Pathways of the pulp,* ed 7, St Louis, 1998, Mosby.

Collins VJ: *Principles of anesthesiology,* Philadelphia, 1966, Lea & Febiger.

Committee on Hospital Oral Surgery Service: *Oral surgery glossary,* 1971, American Society of Oral Surgeons.

Cooper HK: Integration of services in the treatment of cleft lip and cleft palate, *J Am Dent Assoc* 47:27, 1953.

Cooper HK: Oral aspects of rehabilitation, *J Am Coll Dent* 27:52, 1960.

Cooper HK et al: Psychological, orthodontic, and prosthetic approaches in rehabilitation of the cleft palate patient, *Dent Clin North Am* 4:381, 1960.

Cranin AN: Nomenclature, *J Implant Dent* 2:41, 1956.

Cranin AN: Some philosophic comments on the endosseous implant, *Dent Clin North Am* 14:173, 1970.

Cranin AN, Dennison TA: Blade and anchor construction technics, *J Am Dent Assoc* 83:833, 1971.

Cunnan N, ed: *Dun and Bradstreet's guide to your investments,* New York, 1987, Harper & Row.

Dawson PE: *Evaluation, diagnosis, and treatment of occlusal problems,* St Louis, 1974, Mosby.

Denton GB: *The vocabulary of dentistry and oral science,* Chicago, 1958, American Dental Association.

Donoff RB: *Manual of oral and maxillofacial surgery,* ed 3, St Louis, 1997, Mosby.

Dorland's American illustrated medical dictionary, ed 28, Philadelphia, 1994, Saunders.

English WB, English AC: *A comprehensive dictionary of psychological and psychoanalytical terms,* New York, 1958, McKay.

Etter E: *Glossary of words and phrases used in radiology and nuclear medicine,* Springfield, Ill, 1960, Thomas.

Facts about AIDS for the dental team, ed 3, Chicago, American Dental Association.

Fairbanks G: *Voice and articulation drill book,* New York, 1940, Harper & Row.

Finn SB, Volker JF, Cheraskin E: *Clinical pedodontics,* Philadelphia, 1957, Saunders.

Fischer B: *Orthodontics,* ed 2, Philadelphia, 1957, Saunders.

Gabel AB: *American textbook of operative dentistry,* ed 9, Philadelphia, 1954, Lea & Febiger.

Gage TW, Pickett FA: *Dental drug reference,* St Louis, 1997, Mosby.

Gellhorn E: *Physiological foundations of neurology and psychiatry,* Minneapolis, 1953, University of Minnesota Press.

Genco RJ, Goldman HM, Cohen DW: *Contemporary periodontics,* St Louis, 1990, Mosby.

Gilmore HW, Lund MR: *Operative dentistry,* ed 2, St Louis, 1973, Mosby.

Glasser O: *Medical physics,* Chicago, 1944, Mosby.

Glossary of dental prepayment terms, *J Am Dent Assoc* 98:601, 1979.

Glossary of terms used in dental radiology, 1964, American Academy of Oral Roentgenology.

Goaz PW, White SC: *Oral radiology,* ed 3, St Louis, 1994, Mosby.

Goldberg NL, Gershhoff A: The implant lower denture, *Dent Dig* 55:490, 1949.

Goldman HM, Cohen DW: *Periodontal therapy,* ed 4, St Louis, 1968, Mosby.

Goldman HM, Cohen DW: *An introduction to periodontia,* ed 4, St Louis, 1969, Mosby.

Goldman HM et al: *An introduction to periodontia,* ed 3, St Louis, 1966, Mosby.

Goldman HM et al: *Periodontal therapy,* ed 2, St Louis, 1960, Mosby.

Goodman LS, Gilman A: *The pharmacological basis of therapeutics,* ed 5, New York, 1975, Macmillan.

Gorlin RJ, ed: Summary of the workshop on ulcerative and bullous disorders of the orofacial region, *J Dent Res* 50:795, 1971.

Gorlin RJ, Goldman HM: *Oral pathology,* ed 6, St Louis, 1970, Mosby.

Gorlin RJ, Pindborg JJ: *Syndromes of the head and neck,* New York, 1964, McGraw-Hill.

Graber TM: *Orthodontics, principles and practice,* Philadelphia, 1961, Saunders.

Grant DA, Stern IB, Everett FG: *Orban's periodontics,* ed 4, St Louis, 1972, Mosby.

Gray GW, Wise CM: *Bases of speech,* ed 3, New York, 1958, Harper & Row.

Gregory WK: *Evolution emerging,* vol 1, New York, 1957, Macmillan.

Grossman LI: *Endodontic practice,* ed 7, Philadelphia, 1970, Lea & Febiger.

Gruebbel AO, ed: Symposium on practice administration, *Dent Clin North Am,* vol 5, March 1961.

Guide to dental materials and devices, ed 6, Chicago, 1972-1973, American Dental Association.

Healey HJ: *Endodontics,* St Louis, 1960, Mosby.

Heartwell CM Jr, Rahn AO: *Syllabus of complete dentures,* ed 2, Philadelphia, 1974, Lea & Febiger.

Henderson D, Steffel VL: *McCracken's partial denture construction,* ed 3, St Louis, 1969, Mosby.

Hickey JC, Zarb GA: *Boucher's prosthodontic treatment for edentulous patients,* ed 9, St Louis, 1985, Mosby.

Hine MK, ed: *Review of dentistry,* ed 5, St Louis, 1970, Mosby.

Hinsie LE, Campbell RJ: *Psychiatric dictionary,* New York, 1974, Oxford University Press.

Howard WW: *An atlas of operative dentistry,* St Louis, 1968, Mosby.

Ingle JI, Beveridge EE: *Endodontics,* ed 2, Philadelphia, 1976, Lea & Febiger.

Ingraham R, Koser JR, Quint H: *An atlas of gold foil and rubber dam,* Buena Park, Calif, 1961, Uni-Tro College Procedures.

Jablonski S: *Jabonski's dictionary of dentistry,* Malabar, Fla, 1972, Krieger.

Jermyn AC: Peri-implantoclasia—cause and treatment, *J Implant Dent* 5:25, 1958.

Johnston JF, Phillips RW, Dykema R: *Modern practice in crown and bridge prosthodontics,* Philadelphia, 1960, Saunders.

Kantner CE, West R: *Phonetics,* New York, 1941, Harper & Row.

Kazanjian VH, Converse JM: *The surgical treatment of facial injuries,* ed 2, Baltimore, 1959, Williams & Wilkins.

Kerr DA, Ash MM Jr, Millard HD: *Oral diagnosis,* ed 3, St Louis, 1970, Mosby.

Kilpatrick HC: *High speed and ultraspeed in dentistry,* Philadelphia, 1959, Saunders.

Kreps C, Wacht RF: *Financial administration,* Hinsdale, Ill, 1975, Dryden.

Kruger GO, ed: *Textbook of oral surgery,* ed 4, St Louis, 1974, Mosby.

Langley LL, Cheraskin E: *The physiological foundation of dental practice,* St Louis, 1956, Mosby.

Lehninger AL: *Biochemistry,* ed 2, 1975, New York, Worth.

Levy IR: *Textbook for dental assistants,* ed 2, Philadelphia, 1942, Lea & Febiger.

Loechler PS, Mueller MW: Successful implant dentures, *Northwest Dent* 31:134, 1952.

Longacre JJ, ed: *Craniofacial anomalies,* Philadelphia, 1968, Lippincott.

Lynch MA: *Burket's oral medicine: diagnosis and treatment,* ed 7, Philadelphia, 1977, Lippincott.

Mann WR, Easlick KA: *Practice administration for the dentist,* St Louis, 1955, Mosby.

Maurice CG: *Annotated glossary of terms used in endodontics,* St Louis, 1968, Mosby.

McCall JO: *Practical dental assisting,* Brooklyn, 1948, Dental Items of Interest.

McCoy JD, Shepard, EE: *Applied orthodontics,* ed 7, Philadelphia, 1956, Lea & Febiger.

McDonald RE, Avery DR: *Dentistry for the child and adolescent,* ed 6, St Louis, 1994, Mosby.

McGehee WHO, True HA, Inskipp EF: *A textbook of operative dentistry,* ed 4, New York, 1956, McGraw-Hill.

McGivney GP, Castleberry DJ: *McCracken's removable partial prosthodontics,* ed 9, St Louis, 1995, Mosby.

MEDLINE MSH96 (online database of MEDLARS), Bethesda, Md, 1996, National Library of Medicine.

The Merck manual, ed 15, Rahway, NJ, 1987, Merck Sharp and Dohme Research Laboratories.

MeSH: *Medical subject headings, annotated alphabetic list* (supplement to *Index Medicus*), Bethesda, Md, 1997, National Library of Medicine.

Metals handbook, Metals Park, Ohio, 1961, American Society for Metals.

Mitchell DF, Standish SM, Fast TB: *Oral diagnosis/oral medicine,* Philadelphia, 1971, Lea & Febiger.

Morrey LW, Nelsen RJ: *Dental science handbook,* Washington, DC, 1970, US Department of Health, Education, and Welfare.

Morrison GA: *In the dentist's office,* Philadelphia, 1959, Lippincott.

Moyers RE: *Handbook of orthodontics,* Chicago, 1958, Mosby.

Nagle RJ, Sears VH: *Dental prosthetics,* St Louis, 1959, Mosby.

National Bureau of Standards Handbook 59, *Permissible dose from external sources of ionizing radiation,* Washington, DC, 1954, US Government Printing Office.

National Dental Quality Assurance Advisory Committee: *Dental quality assurance terminology: a glossary,* Chicago, 1980, American Fund for Dental Health.

Nomenclature Committee, The Academy of Denture Prosthetics: *Glossary of prosthodontic terms,* ed 3, St Louis, 1968, Mosby.

Nomenclature Committee, American Association for Cleft Palate Rehabilitation. Proposed morphological classification of congenital cleft lip and cleft palate, *Cleft Palate Bull* 10:11, 1960.

Okeson JP: *Fundamentals of occlusion and temporomandibular disoders,* ed 4, St Louis, 1998, Mosby.

Orban B: Oral histology and embryology, ed 2, St Louis, 1949, Mosby.

Orban B, Wentz FM: *Atlas of clinical pathology of the oral mucous membrane,* St Louis, 1960, Mosby.

Orten JM, Neuhaus OW: *Human biochemistry,* ed 10, St Louis, 1982, Mosby.

Peterson LJ, et al: *Contemporary oral and maxillofacial surgery,* ed 3, St Louis, 1998, Mosby.

Peyton FA, Craig RG: *Restorative dental materials,* ed 4, St Louis, 1971, Mosby.

Phillips RW: *Skinner's science of dental materials,* ed 7, Philadelphia, 1973, Saunders.

Physicians' desk reference, ed 45, Oradell, NJ, Medical Economic.

Poppel MH, ed: Radiopaque diagnosis agents, *Ann NY Acad Sci* 78:705, 1959.

Proffit WR: *Contemporary orthodontics,* St Louis, 1996, Mosby.

Ramfjord SP, Ash M Jr: *Occlusion,* ed 2, Philadelphia, 1971, Saunders.

Robbins SL, Cotran RS: *Pathologic basis of disease,* ed 2, Philadelphia, 1979, Saunders.

Rosenstiel SF, Land MF, Fujimoto J: *Contemporary fixed prosthodontics,* ed 2, St. Louis, 1995, Mosby.

Salzmann JA: *Principles of orthodontics,* ed 3, Philadelphia, 1950, Saunders.

Salzmann JA: *Orthodontics: principles and prevention,* vol 1, Philadelphia, 1957, Lippincott.

Salzmann JA: *Orthodontics: practice and techniques,* vol 2, Philadelphia, 1957, Lippincott.

Sarnat BG: *The temporomandibular joint,* Springfield, Ill, 1951, Thomas.

Swuoouni V, Forrest EJ: *Orthodontics in dental practice,* St Louis, 1971, Mosby.

Schlyger SR, Yuodelis RA, Page RC: *Periodontal disease,* Philadelphia, 1977, Lea & Febiger.

Schroeter C: *Dentition of man,* Seattle, 1966, University of Washington Press.

Schwartz JR. *Inlays and abutments,* Brooklyn, 1952, Dental Items of Interest.

Schwarzrock LH, Schwarzrock SP: *Effective dental assisting,* ed 2, Dubuque, Iowa, 1959, Brown.

Selve H: *Stress of life,* New York, 1956, McGraw-Hill.

Selzer S: *Endodontology,* New York, 1971, McGraw-Hill.

Services for children with cleft lip and cleft palate, New York, 1955, American Public Health Association.

Shafer WG, Hine MK, Levy BM: A textbook of oral pathology, ed 3, Philadelphia, 1974, Saunders.

Sharry JJ: *Complete denture prosthodontics,* ed 2, New York, 1968, McGraw-Hill.

Shaw JH et al: *Textbook of oral biology,* Philadelphia, 1978, Saunders.

Shepard EE: *Technique and treatment with the twin-wire appliance,* St Louis, 1961, Mosby.

Sicher H, DuBrul EL: *Oral anatomy,* ed 5, St Louis, 1970, Mosby.

Slobody LB: *Survey of clinical pediatrics,* New York, 1959, McGraw-Hill.

Sodeman WA: *Pathologic physiology,* ed 2, Philadelphia, 1957, Saunders.

Sommer RF, Ostrander FD, Crowley MC: *Clinical endodontics,* ed 3, Philadelphia, 1966, Saunders.

Souder WH, Paffenbarger GC: *Physical properties of dental materials,* National Bureau of Standards Circular No. C433, Washington, DC, 1942, US Government Printing Office.

Stedman's medical dictionary, ed 25, Baltimore, 1990, Williams & Wilkins.

Stibbs GD: *Textbook of operative dentistry,* St Louis, 1967, Mosby.

Stibbs GD: *Cavity preparations,* Seattle, 1969, University of Washington Press.

Stinaff RK: *Dental practice administration,* ed 3, St Louis, 1968, Mosby.

Storch CB: *Fundamentals of clinical fluoroscopy,* New York, 1951, Grune & Stratton.

Sturdevant CM: *The art and science of operative dentistry,* ed 3, St Louis, 1994, Mosby.

Swidler G: *Handbook of drug interactions,* New York, 1971, Wiley.

Tarpley BW: *Technique and treatment with the labiolingual appliance,* St Louis, 1961, Mosby.

Terkla LG, Laney WR: *Partial dentures,* ed 3, St Louis, 1963, Mosby.

Thoma KH: *Oral surgery,* ed 5, St Louis, 1969, Mosby.

Thoma KH, Robinson HBB: *Oral and dental diagnosis,* ed 5, Philadelphia, 1960, Saunders.

Thurow RC: *Edgewise orthodontics,* ed 3, St Louis, 1973, Mosby.

Tiecke RW, Stuteville OH, Calandra JC: *Pathological physiology of oral disease,* St Louis, 1959, Mosby.

Tocchine JJ: *Restorative dentistry,* New York, 1967, McGraw-Hill.

Travis L: *Handbook of speech pathology,* New York, 1957, Appleton-Century-Crofts.

Tylman SD: *Theory and practice of crown and fixed partial prosthodontics (bridge),* ed 6, St Louis, 1970, Mosby.

UMLS: *Metathesaurus,* Bethesda, 1997, National Library of Medicine.

Van Riper C, Irwin JV: *Voice and articulation,* Englewood Cliffs, NJ, 1958, Prentice-Hill.

Weast RC, ed: *Handbook of chemistry and physics,* ed 56, Cleveland, 1975, CRC.

Webster's encyclopedic unabridged dictionary of the English language, New York, 1989, Portland House.

Webster's third new international dictionary of the English language (unabridged), Springfield, Mass, 1976, Merriam.

Weine FS: *Endodontic therapy,* ed 5, St Louis, 1996, Mosby.

Weinmann JP, Sicher H: *Bone and bones,* St Louis, 1955, Mosby.

West R, Ansberry M, Carr A: *The rehabilitation of speech,* New York, 1957, Harper & Row.

Wheeler RC: *A textbook of dental anatomy, physiology, and occlusion,* ed 5, Philadelphia, 1974, Saunders.

Windholz M: *The Merck index,* ed 9, Rahway, NJ, 1976, Merck.

Wuehrmann AH: *Radiation protection and dentistry,* St Louis, 1960, Mosby.

Wuehrmann AH, Manson-Hing LR: *Dental radiology,* ed 2, St Louis, 1969, Mosby.

Zwemer TJ: *Boucher's clinical dental terminology,* ed 4, St Louis, 1993, Mosby.

Contents

Pronunciation Guide

VOWELS

Symbols	Key words
/a/	hat
/ä/	father
/ā/	fate
/e/	flesh
/ē/	she
/er/	air, ferry
/i/	sit
/ī/	eye
/ir/	ear
/o/	proper
/ō/	nose
/ô/	saw
/oi/	boy
/o͞o/	move
/o͝o/	book
/ou/	out
/u/	cup, love
/ur/	fur, first
/ə/	(the neutral vowel, always unstressed, as in) ago, focus
/ər/	teacher, doctor
/œ/	as in (French) feu /fœ/; (German) schön /shœn/
/Y/	as in (French) tu /tY/; (German) grün /grYn/
/N/	This symbol does not represent a sound but indicates that the preceding vowel is a nasal, as in French bon /bôN/, or international /aNternäsyōnäl′/.

CONSONANTS

Symbols	Key words
/b/	book
/ch/	chew
/d/	day
/f/	fast
/g/	good
/h/	happy
/j/	gem
/k/	keep
/l/	late
/m/	make
/n/	no
/ng/	sing, drink
/ng·g/	finger
/p/	pair
/r/	ring
/s/	set
/sh/	shoe, lotion
/t/	tone
/th/	thin
/th/	than
/v/	very
/w/	work
/y/	yes
/z/	zeal
/zh/	azure, vision
/kh/	as in (Scottish) loch /lokh/; (German) Rorschach /rôr′shokh/
/kh/	as in (German) ich /ikh/ (or, approximated, as in English fish: /ish/, /rīsh/)
/nyə/	Occurring at the end of French words, this symbol is not truly a separate syllable but an /n/ with a slight /y/ (similar to the sound in "onion") plus a near-silent /ə/, as in Bois de Boulogne /boolō′nyə/

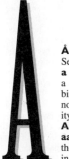

Å, symbol for **angstrom.** See also **unit, angstrom.**

a nativitate (nativ′itāt), a condition existing at birth or from infancy; denotes a congenital disability.

A point. See **point, A.**

aa, an abbreviation for the Greek term *ana,* used in prescription writing, meaning of each.

A-alpha fibers. See **fibers, nerve.**

ab (antecedente), beforehand; a notice given previously or a condition existing earlier.

abacterial (ab′aktir′ē·əl), nonbacterial; free from bacteria.

abandonment (of a patient), withdrawing a patient from treatment without giving reasonable notice or providing a competent replacement.

abatement (əbat′ment), a decrease in severity of pain or symptoms.

Abbé-Estlander operation (ab′ē·est′landər). See **operation, Abbé-Estlander.**

abdomen, the portion of the body between the thorax and the pelvis.

abduce (abdoōs′), to draw away; abduct. (not current)

abduct (abdukt′), to draw away from the median line or from a neighboring part or limb.

abduction (abduk′shən), the process of abducting; opposite of adduction.

aberrant (aber′ənt), a deviation from the usual or normal course, location, or action.

A-beta fibers. See **fibers, nerve.**

ablation, an amputation, an excision of any part of the body, or a removal of a growth or harmful substance.

abnormal, a departure from the norm, however defined; departure from the mean of a distribution (statistics); departure from the usual, from a state of integration or adjustment.

a. tooth mobility, excessive movement of a tooth within its socket as a result of changes in the supporting tissues caused by injury or disease.

abrade (əbrād′), to wear away by friction.

abrasion (əbrā′zhən), **1.** the abnormal wearing away of a substance or tissue by a mechanical process. **2.** the grinding or wearing away of tooth substance by mastication, incorrect brushing methods, bruxism, or similar causes.

a., dentifrice, the wearing away of the cementum and dentin of an exposed root by an abrasive-containing dentifrice.

abrasive (əbrā′siv), a substance used for grinding or polishing that will wear away a material or tissue.

a. disk. See **disk, abrasive.**

a. point, rotary. See **point, abrasive, rotary.**

a. strip. See **strip, abrasive.**

abscess (ab′ses), a localized accumulation of pus in a cavity formed by tissue disintegration.

a., alveolar. See **periapical abscess.**

a., apical. See **periapical abscess.**

a., dentoalveolar. See **periapical abscess.**

a., gingival, a superficial periodontal abscess occurring within the free gingival sulcus surrounding the tooth, frequently caused by the impaction of food. A hull of popcorn is a frequent culprit.

a., lateral. See **periodontal abscess.**

a., periapical, an abscess involving the apical region of the root, alveolus, and surrounding bone as a sequela of pulpal disease.

a., periodontal, an abscess involving the attachment tissues and alveolar bone as a sequela of periodontal disease.

a., pulpal, an abscess occurring within pulpal tissue.

absorb (absorb′, əbzôrb′) **1.** etymological: to suck up. **2.** incorporation or assimilation of a liquid or gas into tissue or cells.

absorbable gelatin sponge, *trade name:* Gelfoam; *drug class:* hemostatic; *action:* absorbs blood and provides area for clot formation; *uses:* hemostasis during and following surgery.

absorbefacient (absôr′bifā′shənt), caus-ing absorption, or an agent that promotes absorption.

absorbent (absôrb′ənt), a substance that causes absorption of diseased tissue; taking up by suction.

absorption (absôrp′shən), **1.** the pas-

A

sage of a substance into the interior of another by solution or penetration. **2.** the taking up of fluids or other substances by the skin, mucous surfaces, absorbent vessels, or dental materials. **3.** the process by which radiation imparts some or all of its energy to any material through which it passes.

a. coefficient, the ratio of the linear rate of change of intensity of roentgen rays in a given homogeneous material to the intensity at a given point within the same mass.

abstraction (abstrak′shən), indicates teeth or other maxillary and mandibular structures that are inferior to (below) their normal position; away from the occlusal plane.

abuse, the improper use of program benefits, resources, and/or services by either dentists, institutions, or patients.

abutment (əbut′mənt), a tooth, root, or implant used for support and retention of a fixed or removable prosthesis.

a., intermediate, an abutment located between the abutments that form the end of the prosthesis.

a., multiple, abutments splinted together as a unit to support and retain a fixed prosthesis.

a.c., the abbreviation for *ante cibum,* a Latin phrase used in prescription writing meaning "before eating."

acanthesthesia (əkan′thesthē′zē·ə), a form of paresthesia experienced as numbness, tingling, or "pins and needles."

acanthion (əkan′thēon), the tip of the anterior nasal spine.

acantholysis, the loosening, separation, or disassociation of individual prickle cells within the epithelium from their neighbor, often seen in conditions such as pemphigus vulgaris and keratosis follicularis.

acanthosis (ak′ənthō′sis), an increase in the number of cells in the prickle cell layer of stratified squamous epithelium, with thickening of the entire epithelial cell layer and a broadening and fusing of rete pegs.

acapnia (akap′nē·ə), a condition characterized by diminished carbon dioxide in the blood.

acarbia (akär′bē·ə), a condition in which the blood bicarbonate level is decreased.

acarbose, *trade name:* Precose; *drug class:* oligosaccharide, glucosidase enzyme inhibitor; *action:* inhibits α-glucosidase enzyme in the GI tract to slow the breakdown of carbohydrates to glucose; *uses:* a single drug or in combination with others when diet control is ineffective in controlling blood glucose levels.

acatalasemia (a′katələsē′mē·ə), a congenital lack of the enzyme catalase in blood and other tissues that leads to a progressive necrosis of the oral tissues (Takahara's disease).

accelerator (aksel′ərātər), **I.** that which increases rapidity of action or function. **2.** a catalyst or other substance that hastens a chemical reaction (for example, NaCl added to water and plaster to hasten the set).

a., platelet thrombin. See **factor, platelet 2.**

a., prothrombin conversion, I (factor V, labile factor, plasma accelerator globulin, proaccelerin, serum accelerator globulin), considered by some to be a factor in serum and plasma that catalyzes the conversion of inactive prothrombin to an active form.

a., prothrombin conversion, II (cothromboplastin, extrinsic thromboplastin, factor VII, serum prothrombin conversion accelerator [SPCA], stable factor), considered by some to be one of the factors in the blood that accelerates the conversion of active prothrombin to thrombin by thromboplastin. Vitamin K deficiency reduces the activity of this factor.

a., serum. See **factor V.**

accelerin. See **factor V.**

acceptability, overall assessment of the dental care available to a person or group; includes accessibility, cost, quality, results, convenience, and attitudes of dentists and patients.

acceptance, the act of a person to whom something is offered or tendered by another, whereby he receives that which is offered with the intention of retaining it. A contract is not valid without the acceptance of an offer by the party to whom the offer is made, either expressly or by conduct.

a., absolute, an express and positive agreement to pay a bill according to its text.

a., conditional, an agreement to pay a bill on the fulfillment of a condition.

a., implied, an acceptance interpreted by law from the acts or conduct of the patient.

access (ak'ses), **1.** means of approach. **2.** surgical preparation of hard or soft tissue to allow entrance to a treatment site and adequate space for visualization and instrumentation of the field.

a., cavity, a coronal opening required for effective cleaning, shaping, and filling of the pulp space.

a., computer, **1.** the process of transferring information into or out of a storage location. **2.** the time required to begin and complete the read and write functions of a specified piece of data.

a. flap, a periodontal surgical technique to provide visualization of the root in conjunction with curettage and root planning. Types of access flaps include supracrestal, subcrestal—full thickness, and partial thickness flaps.

a., form, the surgical removal of tooth structure sufficient for visualization and instrumentation of a restorative preparation.

accessory canal (akses'ōrē) See **canal, accessory root.**

accident, 1. an unusual, unforeseen event. **2.** an unusual or unexpected result attending the performance of a usual or necessary act or event. **3.** occurring without intent or happening by chance. The term does not have a precise legal definition but is generally used to indicate that an occurrence was not the result of negligence.

a., cerebrovascular (CVA), apoplexy resulting from hemorrhage into the brain or occlusion of the cerebral vessels resulting from embolism or thrombosis.

a., unavoidable, an accident not occasioned, either remotely or directly, by the want of such care or skill as the law holds every person bound to exercise; occurring without fault or negligence.

account, a basic storage unit in an accounting system. Individual accounts accept debit and credit entries that reflect the different types of transactions made by the practice.

a. book, a book in which the financial transactions of a business or profession are entered. Such books may be admitted as evidence.

a., open, a straightforward arrangement between the dentist and the patient for the handling of financial payments due the dentist and owed by the patient.

a., payable, a dollar amount owed to creditors for items of services purchased from them.

accountability, an obligation to periodically disclose appropriate information in adequate detail and consistent form to all contractually involved parties.

accreditation, a process of formal recognition of a school or institution attesting to the required ability and performance in an area of education, training, or practice.

accretions, (əkrē'shəns), an accumulation of foreign material such as mucinous plaque, materia alba, and calculus on teeth.

accrual, continually recurring short-term liabilities. Examples are accrued wages, taxes, and interest.

accrued interest, the interest accumulated on a bond since the last payment was made. The buyer of the bond pays the market price plus accumulated interest. Exceptions include bonds that are in default and income bonds.

accrued needs, the amount of treatment needed by an individual or a group at any given time. In dental plans, usually refers to conditions present at the time of enrollment. Synonym: accumulated needs.

acebutolol HCl, *trade names:* Monitan, Sectral; *drug class:* anithypertensive, selective β_1 blocker; *action:* produces fall in blood pressure without reflex tachycardia or significant reduction in heart rate; *uses:* mild-to-moderate hypertension and ventricular dysrhythmias.

acenesthesia (əsen'esthē'zē·ə), the loss, or lack, of the normal perception of one's own body; absence of the feelings of a physical existence, a symptom that is common with many psychiatric disorders.

acentric relation (āsen'trik). See **relation, jaw, eccentric.**

acetaminophen, *trade names:* Tylenol, Anacin-3; *drug class:* nonnarcotic analgesic; *action:* thought to block initiation of pain impulses by inhibition of prostaglandin synthesis; *uses:* mild-to-moderate pain, fever;

A

also used in combination with narcotic analgesics.

acetate (as'etāt), **1.** a salt of acetic acid. **2.** short for cellulose acetate, the film base for x-rays.

acetazolamide/acetazolaminde sodium, *trade names:* Dazamide, Acetazolam, Apo-Acetozolamide; *drug class:* diuretic; carbonic anhydrase inhibitor; *action:* inhibits carbonic anhydrase activity in proximal renal tubular cells to decrease reabsorption of water, sodium, potassium, bicarbonate; *uses:* open-angle glaucoma, epilepsy, drug-induced edema.

acetic acid, a clear, colorless, pungent liquid that is miscible with water, alcohol, glycerin, and ether and that constitutes 3% to 5% of vinegar.

acetohexamide, *trade names:* Dimelor, Dymelor; *drug class:* sulfonylurea; antidiabetic; *action:* causes functioning β-cells in the pancreas to release insulin, leading to a drop in blood glucose level; *uses:* stable adult-onset diabetes mellitus (type II).

acetone (as'ətōn), Dimethylketone; an organic solvent normally present in urine in small amounts but in increased amounts in individuals who have diabetes.

acetylcholine (as'ətilkō'lēn, əsē'til) **1.** an acetate ester of choline that serves as a neurohumoral agent in the transmission of an impulse in autonomic ganglia, parasympathetic postganglionic fibers, and somatic motor fibers. **2.** an ester of choline actively involved as a chemical mediator at the neuromuscular junction, at autonomic ganglia, and between parasympathetic nerve endings and visceral effectors.

acetylcysteine, *trade name:* Mucosil; *drug class:* mucolytic; *action:* decreases viscosity of pulmonary secretions by breaking disulfide links of mucoproteins; *uses:* acetaminophen toxicity, bronchitis, pneumonia, cystic fibrosis, emphysema, atelectasis tuberculosis, and complication of thoracic surgery.

achlorhydria (ā'klôrhī'drē· ə), the absence of free hydrochloric acid in the stomach, even with histamine stimulation.

achondroplasia (ākon'drōplā'zhə) (chondrodystrophia fetalis), a hereditary disturbance of endochondral bone formation transmitted as a

mendelian dominant factor and resulting in dwarfism. Malocclusion and prognathism may occur.

achromatopsia (əkrōm atōp'sē· ə), total color blindness.

Achromycin V, a proprietary name for the antibiotic tetracycline hydrochloride.

achylia, the absence or lack of hydrochloric acid and the enzyme pepsinogen in the stomach.

acid (as'id), a chemical substance that, in an aqueous solution, undergoes dissociation with the formation of hydrogen ions; pH levels range from 0 to 6.9.

a., acetic, the acid of vinegar, sometimes used as a solvent for the removal of calculus from a removable dental prosthesis. See also **solvent.**

a., ascorbic. See **vitamin C.**

a., carbolic. See **phenol.**

a., cevitamic. See **vitamin C.**

a. etching, treating the tooth enamel, generally with phosphoric acid, by removal of approximately 40 μm of rod cross-section to provide retention for resin sealant, restorative material, or orthodontic bracket.

a., folic. See **vitamin B complex.**

a., hydroxypropionic. See **acid, lactic.**

a., lactic (hydroxypropionic acid), a monobasic acid, $C_3H_6O_3$, formed as an end product in the intermediary metabolism of carbohydrates. The accumulation of lactic acid in the tissues is in part responsible for the lowering of pH levels during inflammatory states; that is, the drop in pH level is believed to hasten bone resorption in periodontitis because the minerals in the bone are stable within the matrix only at the normal tissue pH level of 7.4.

a., nicotinic (niacin, P.-P. factor, pyridine 3-carboxylic acid, vitamin P.-P.), **1.** one of the vitamins of the B complex group and its vitamer, niacinamide, specific for the treatment of pellagra. Niacinamide functions as a constituent of coenzyme I (DPN) and coenzyme II (TPN). Nicotinic acid is found in lean meats, liver, yeast, milk, and leafy green vegetables. **2.** an acid (C_5H_4N [COOH]) that forms part of the B complex group of vitamins. The body requires this acid as a cofactor in intermediary carbohydrate metabolism. This acid is a constituent of certain coenzymes that function in oxidative-reductive metabolic. systems. With niacinamide, nicotinic acid is a pellagra-preventive factor.

a., orthophosphoric. See **acid, phosphoric.**

a., pantothenic, 1. one of the B complex vitamins, the importance of which has not been established in human nutrition. Pantothenic acid is a constituent of coenzyme A and as such is presumed to be involved in adrenocortical function. 2. a vitamin of the B complex that is widely distributed in food and tissues and important for normal development in certain animals such as chickens and rats. Pantothenic acid deficiency in rats produces retrograde changes in alveolar and supporting bone.

a. phosphatase, an enzyme found in the kidneys, serum, semen, and prostate gland. Acid phosphatase is elevated in serum blood levels in individuals with prostate cancer and individuals who have recently experienced trauma.

a., phosphoric (H_3PO_4, orthophosphoric acid), the principal ingredient of silicate and zinc phosphate cement liquids.

a., pteroylglutamic. See **vitamin B complex.**

a. salt, a salt containing one or more replaceable hydrogen ions.

a., strong, an acid that is completely ionized in aqueous solution.

acid-base balance, in metabolism, the balance of acid to base necessary to keep the blood pH level normal (between 7.35 and 7.43).

acidemia (as'idē'mē- ə), a decreased pH level of the blood, irrespective of changes in the blood bicarbonate.

acidifier (əsid'ifi ər), a chemical ingredient (acetic acid) that maintains the required acidity of the fixer and stop-bath solutions in the photographic development process.

acidophilic (as'idōfil'ik), 1. readily stained with acid dyes. 2. Growing well in an acid medium.

acidosis (as'idō'sis), a pathologic disturbance of the acid-base balance of the body characterized by an excess of acid or inadequate base. Causes include acid ingestion, increased acid production such as seen in diabetes or starvation, or loss of base through the kidneys or intestine.

a., compensated, a condition of acidosis in which the body pH level is maintained within the normal range through compensatory mechanisms involving the kidneys or lungs.

a., respiratory, acidemia resulting from retention of an excess of CO_2 caused by hypoventilation.

a., uncompensated, acidosis in which compensatory mechanisms are unable to maintain the body pH level within the normal range.

Acinetobacter, a genus of nonmotile, aerobic bacteria of the family Neisseriacae that often occurs in clinical specimens.

Ackerman-Proffit orthogonal analysis, a taxonomy of malocclusion based on set theory or Boolean Algebra, which is organized using combinations and permutations of malocclusions within the three planes of space. See also **Appendix F.**

acne, an inflammatory, papulopustular skin eruption occurring most often in or near the sebaceous glands on the face, neck, shoulders, and upper back.

A. vulgaris, a common form of acne seen predominantly in adolescents and young adults. Acne vulgaris is probably an effect of the rise of androgenic hormones.

acoustic coupler, a connection between a phone line and a data set, or modem. The coupler makes use of an ordinary telephone and headset and requires no modification to the normal phone.

acquired centric relation (sen'trik). See **relation, centric** and **relation, jaw, eccentric.**

acquired immunodeficiency syndrome (AIDS), a disease caused by a retrovirus known as human immunodeficiency virus type 1 (HIV-1). A related but distinct retrovirous (HIV-2) has recently appeared in a limited number of patients in the United States. Patients are considered to have AIDS when one or more indicator diseases, as defined by the Centers for Disease Control (CDC), are present. The CDC has classified stages of the disease as follows:

Group 1 acute HIV infection: within one month of exposure, the first clinical evidence of HIV infection may appear as an acute retroviral syndrome. This is a mononucleosis-like syndrome with symptoms including fever, rash, diarrhea, lymphadenopathy, myalgia, arthralgia, and fatigue. Development of antibodies usually follows.

Group II asymptomatic HIV infection: most persons develop antibodies to the HIV within 6 to 12 weeks after exposure. Although individuals may remain asymptomatic for months or years, they can transmit the virus.

Group III persistent generalized lymphadenopathy (PGL): HIV-infected patients in this classification develop persistent generalized lymphadenopathy that lasts longer than 3 months.

Group IV HIV-associated diseases: patients in this group are clinically variable and have signs and symptoms of HIV infection other than or in addition to lymphadenopathy. Based on clinical findings, patients in Group IV may be assigned to one or more of the following subgroups: (A) constitutional disease, also known as *wasting syndrome.* This subgroup is characterized by fever that lasts more than one month, involuntary weight loss of greater than 10% for baseline, or diarrhea persisting more than one month, (B) neurological disease, (C) secondary infectious disease, (D) secondary cancers, and (E) other conditions resulting from HIV infections.

acridine, a dibenzopyridine compound used in the synthesis of dyes and drugs.

acroanesthesia (ak'rōanesthē'zē· ə), anesthesia of the extremities.

acrocephalia (akrōsefa'lē· ə), a deformity of the head characterized by an upward and forward bulge of the frontal bones and a flat occiput. Synonym: oxycephalia.

acrodermatitis, any eruption of the skin of the hands and feet caused by a parasitic mite, which is a member of the order Acarina.

acrodynia (akrōdīn'ē· ə) (erythredema polyneuropathy, Feer's syndrome, pink disease, Swift's syndrome, Selter's disease), a disease that occurs in infants and young children in which manifestations occur with the eruption of the primary teeth. Symptoms

include raw-beef hands and feet, superficial sensory loss, photophobia, tachycardia, muscular hypotonia, changes in temperament, stomatitis, periodontitis, and premature loss of teeth. The etiology has been related to mercury and deficiency of vitamin B_6 and essential fatty acids. See also **erythredema polyneuropathy.**

acroesthesia (akrōesthē'zē· ə), **1.** increased sensitivity. **2.** pain in the extremities.

acromegaly (akrəmeg'əlē), (Marie's disease), a condition caused by hyperfunction of the pituitary gland in adults. Characterized by enlargement of the skeletal extremities, including the feet, hands, mandible, and nose.

acrosclerosis (akrōsklerō'sis), a special form of scleroderma that affects the extremities, head, and face and is associated with Raynaud's phenomenon. There may be significant thickening of the periodontal membrane.

acrylic (əkril'ik), frequently improperly used as a noun. Should be used to modify nouns; for example, acrylic resin, acrylic resin denture, and acrylic resin tooth. See also **resin, acrylic; denture, acrylic resin;** and **tooth, acrylic resin.**

a. resin. See **resin, acrylic.**

ACTH (adrenocorticotropic hormone, adrenocorticotropin, adrenotropic hormone, codicotropic hormone, corticotropin), adrenocorticotropic hormone, produced by basophilic cells of the anterior lobe of the pituitary gland, which exerts a reciprocal regulating influence on the production of corticosteroids by the adrenal cortex.

actinic cheilitis (aktin'ik). See **cheilitis, actinic.**

Actinobacillus, a genus of nonmobile, gram-negative aerobic and facultatively anaerobic bacteria of the family Brucellaceae that is pathogenic to cattle, sheep, horses, and pigs.

Actinomyces viscosus, a species of *Actinomyces* occurring in high numbers in the dental plaque, cemental caries, and tonsillar crypts.

actinomycetemocomitans (aktinō-mīsē'temōcomitins), a microorganism found in and considered responsible for some periodontal infections.

actinomycetes (ak'tinōmīse'tēz), filamentous microorganisms that have been implicated in the formation of dental calculus and serve as a mode of attachment of dental calculus to the tooth surface. These microorganisms have also been found in pathologic lesions of the alveolar processes (actinomycosis).

actinomycosis (ak'tinōmīkō'sis) (lumpy jaw), an infection of humans and some animal species caused by species of *Actinomyces,* which are gram-positive, filamentous, microaerophilic microorganisms.

action potential, I. an electric impulse consisting of a self-propagating series of polarizations and depolarizations, transmitted across the cell membranes of a nerve fiber during the transmission of a nerve impulse and across the cell membranes of a muscle cell during contraction. **2.** the electrical potential developed in a muscle or nerve during activity.

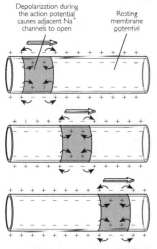

Depolarization during the action potential causes adjacent Na+ channels to open

Resting membrane potential

Action potential conduction.
(Thibodeau, 1996.)

activate (ak'tivāt), to adjust an appliance so it will exert effective force on the teeth and jaws.

activated resin. See **resin, autopolymer.**

activator (ak'tivātor), **I.** an alkali, sodium carbonate, which is a component of photographic developing solution that softens and swells the gelatin

of the film emulsion and provides the necessary alkaline medium for the developing agents to react with the sensitized silver halide crystals. **2.** a removable orthodontic appliance intended to function as a passive transmitter and sometimes stimulator of the forces of the perioral muscles. One in the myofunctional category of appliances also known by such names as *Andresen, Bimler, Monobloc,* and *Frankel.*

active, pertaining to the condition of an orthodontic appliance that has been adjusted to apply effective force to the teeth or jaws.

a. reciprocation. See **reciprocation, active.**

acuity (əkyōō'itē), sharpness; clearness; keenness.

a., auditory, the sensitivity of the auditory apparatus; sharpness of hearing. The ability to hear a given tone with respect to the degree of intensity required to produce a sensation that is just perceptible.

a., visual, sharpness, acuteness, clearness of vision. Visual acuity may be defective because of optical or neurologic dysfunction.

acupuncture, a method of producing analgesia or altering the function of a system of the body by inserting fine, wire-thin needles into the skin at specific sites on the body along a series of lines or channels called meridians. The needles may be twirled, energized electrically, or warmed. Acupuncture originated in the Far East and has gained increasing attention in the West since the early 1970's.

acute, a traumatic, pathologic, or physiologic phenomenon or process having a short and relatively severe course. Antonym: chronic.

a. phase reactions, a phrase that refers to abnormalities in the blood associated with acute and chronic inflammatory and necrotic processes and detected by a variety of tests, including erythrocyte sedimentation rate, C-reactive protein, serum hexosamine, serum mucoprotein, and serum nonglucosamine polysaccharides.

acyclovir (əsī'klōveer), an antiviral drug active against herpes viruses. Used as a 5% ointment, may be used systemically. Drug of choice in immunocompromised patients with candidiasis. *Trade name:* Zovirax.

a. sodium, trade names: Zovirax; *drug class:* antiviral; *action:* see **acyclovir topical;** *uses:* as above, plus herpes zoster and varicella (chickenpox).

a., topical, trade name: Zovirax; *drug class:* antiviral; *action:* interferes with viral DNA replication; *uses:* simple mucocutaneous herpes simplex, in immunocompromised patients with initial herpes genitalis.

ADA, 1. the abbreviation for *American Dental Association,* the national professional organization for dentists in the United States. **2.** the abbreviation for the *American Dairy Association.* **3.** the abbreviation for **adenosine deaminase,** an enzyme that breaks down toxic biological products. This failure causes a rare disease called *severe combined immunodeficiency.*

adamantinoma (adəman'tinō'mə). See **ameloblastoma.**

adamantoblastoma (adəman'tōblastō'mə). See **ameloblastoma.**

Adams' clasp, a retention clasp designed by C. Philip Adams to stabilize removable appliances by engaging the mesiobuccal and distobuccal surfaces of buccal teeth.

Adams-Stokes disease. See **disease, Adams-Stokes.** (not current)

adaptation, 1. an alteration that an organ or organism undergoes to adapt to its environment. **2.** a close approximation of a tissue flap, an appliance, or a restorative material to natural tissue. **3.** an accurate adjustment of a band or a shell to a tooth. **4.** a condition in reflex activity marked by a decline in the frequency of impulses when sensory stimuli are repeated several times.

adapter, band, an instrument used as an aid in fitting an orthodontic band to a tooth.

addict (ad'ikt), an individual who has developed physiologic or psychologic dependence on a chemical such as alcohol or other drugs.

addiction (ədik'shən), the state of being addicted. Although there is no universally accepted definition, addiction is generally considered a condition involving two factors: (1) a compulsive behavior pattern, and (2) an altered physiologic state that requires contin-

ued use of the drug to prevent withdrawal symptoms.

addictive (ədik'tiv), pertaining to a drug whose repeated use may produce addiction. Present federal regulations place greater emphasis on the broader designation of potential for abuse.

Addis test. See **test, Addis.** (not current)

Addison-Biermer anemia (ad'isun ber'mər). See **anemia, pernicious.**

Addison's disease. See **disease, Addison's.**

additive, an ingredient added to a food, drug, or other preparation to produce a desired result, such as color or consistency, unrelated to the primary purpose of the preparation.

adduct (ədukt'), to draw toward the center or midline.

adduction (əduk'shən), the process of bringing two objects toward each other; the opposite of abduction.

A-delta fibers. See **fiber, nerve.**

adenalgia (ad' ənal'jə), pain in a gland that usually results from inflammation (adenitis). (not current)

adenine, a component of the nucleic acids, DNA and RNA, and a constituent of cyclic AMP and the adenosine portion of AMP, ADP, and ATP.

adenitis (ad'ənī'tis), an inflammation of glandular tissue, often accompanied by pain (adenalgia).

adenoameloblastoma (ad'ənō-amel' ōblastō'mə), an epithelial neoplasm with a basic structure resembling enamel organs and glandular (adenomatous) tissue. It is generally benign.

adenocarcinoma (ad'ənōkarsinō'mə), any one of a large group of malignant, epithelial cell tumors of the glands. Specific tumors are diagnosed and named by the cell type of the tissue affected.

a., acinar cell, a malignant tumor whose cells appear as glandular tissue.

adenoid, 1. having a glandular appearance, particularly lymphoid. **2.** adenoids refer to the pharyngeal tonsil located on the posterior wall of the nasopharynx.

a. facies, an archaic term used to describe patients who exhibit a long, narrow face, short upper lip, openmouth breathing, and a hyperactive swallowing pattern.

adenoidectomy, the removal of the lymphoid tissue in the nasopharynx, usually in conjunction with the surgical removal of the tonsils.

adenoma (ad'ənō'mə), a benign epithelial neoplasm or tumor with a basic glandular (acinar) structure, suggesting derivation from glandular tissue.

a., acidophilic. See **oncocytoma.**

a., oxyphilic. See **oncocytoma.**

adenomatosis oris (ad'ənōmətō'sis), an enlargement of the mucous glands of the lip without secretion or inflammation. (not current)

adenopathy (ad'ənop'əthē), an enlargement or increase in size of glandular organs or tissues usually resulting from disease processes.

adenosine, a compound derived from nucleic acid, composed of adenine and a sugar, D-ribose. Adenosine is the major molecular component of nucleotides and the nucleic acids.

a. monophosphate (AMP), an ester, composed of adenine, D-ribose, and phosphoric acid, that affects energy release in work done by a muscle.

a. triphosphate (ATP), a compound consisting of the nucleotide adenosine attached through its ribose group to three phosphoric acid molecules. It stores energy in muscles, which is released when it is hydrolized to adenosine diphosphate.

adequacy, velopharyngeal, a functional closure of the velum to the postpharyngeal wall that restricts air and sound from entering the nasopharyngeal and nasal cavities.

ADH. See **hormone, antidiuretic.**

adhesion (adhē'zhən), **1.** the attraction of unlike molecules for one another. **2.** the molecular attraction existing between surfaces in close contact. **3.** the condition in which a material sticks to itself or another material. **4.** the abnormal joining of tissues, generally by fibrous connective tissue, to each other, that occurs after repair of an injury.

a., bacterial, microbial surface antigens that frequently exist in the form of filamentous projections and bind to specific receptors on epithelial cell membranes.

a., sublabial, the abnormal union of the sublabial mucosa of the upper lip to the alveolar process; usually pre-

sent in a unilateral or bilateral cleft of the lip.

adhesive, an intermediate material that causes two materials to stick together; a luting agent.

a. foil. See **foil, adhesive.**

adipose tissue, a connective tissue comprised of a collection of fat cells.

adjudicate, the final step in dental peer review at which the dental peer review committee renders a formal, nonlegal decision on a case.

adjunct (aj'ungkt), a drug or other substance that serves a supplemental purpose in therapy.

adjust (əjəst'), to make correspondent, comfortable, or to fit.

adjustment (əjəst'ment), a modification of a restoration or of a denture after insertion in the mouth.

a., occlusal, a grinding of the occluding surfaces of teeth to develop harmonious relationships between each other, their supporting structures, muscles of mastication, and temporomandibular joints.

adjuvant (áj'əvənt), in a prescription, an auxiliary active ingredient that supports the action of the basic drug. See also **basis.**

administration, to give, dispense, or apply medicines, drugs, or remedies to relieve or cure an illness.

a., buccal, to deliver a medication by application to the buccal mucosa.

a., inhalation, to deliver a medication by breathing it.

a., intranasal. See **administration, inhalation.**

a., oral, to deliver a medication by mouth.

a., rectal, to deliver a medication through the rectum.

a., sublingual, the placing of a drug under the tongue for dissolution and absorption through the mucous membrane.

a., topical, to deliver a medication by application to the skin.

administrative costs, the overhead expenses incurred in the operation of a dental benefits program, excluding costs of dental services provided.

administrative services only (ASO), an arrangement in which a third party, for a fee, processes claims and handles paperwork for a self-funded group. This frequently includes almost all insurance company services,

A

including actuarial services, underwriting, and benefit description, and excluding assumption of risk.

administrator, a person who manages or directs a dental benefits program on behalf of the program's sponsor. See also **third-party administrator** and **dental benefits organization.**

admission, the voluntary concession or admission that a fact or allegation is true.

a., hospital, 1. full stay. The formal acceptance by a hospital or other inpatient health care facility of a patient who is to be provided with room, board, and continuous nursing service in an area of the hospital or facility where patients generally reside at least overnight. 2. surgicenter with short stays. Day bed only with nursing; patient does not stay overnight. 3. outpatient admission. Pertains to a patient who enters the hospital but requires no bed; the patient enters for treatment and leaves after treatment.

adnexa (adnek'sə), conjoined anatomic parts, or tissues adjacent to or contained within a nearby space.

adolescence, the period of human development between the onset of puberty and adulthood. This period is generally marked by the appearance of secondary sex characteristics, usually from 11 to 13 years of age, and spans the teen years.

adrenal cortex, the greater portion of the adrenal gland fused with the gland's medulla and producing mineralocorticoids, androgens, and glucocorticoids, hormones essential to homeostasis. The outer cortex is normally a deep yellow; the inner part is dark red or brown.

adrenal corticoid. See **corticoid, adrenal.**

adrenal crisis. See **crisis, adrenal.**

adrenalectomy, the surgical removal of one or both of the adrenal glands or the resection of a portion of one or both of the adrenal glands.

Adrenalin (ədren'əlin), the trade name for epinephrine. See also **epinephrine.**

adrenaline (ədren'əlin), the British term for epinephrine.

adrenal steroids. See **corticoid, adrenal.**

adrenergic (ad'rinur'jik), 1. transmit-

ted by norepinephrine or activated by norepinephrine or the other sympathomimetic agents. 2. a term applied to nerve fibers that liberate epinephrine or norepinephrine at a synapse when a nerve impulse passes. 3. a drug that mimics the action of adrenergic nerves.

a. blocking agent. See **agent, adrenergic blocking.**

a. fibers. See **fibers, adrenergic.**

a. receptors. See **receptors, adrenergic.**

adrenic (adre'nik), pertaining to the adrenal gland.

adrenocortical insufficiency (ədre'nōkôr'tikəl). See **hypoadrenocorticalism.**

adrenocorticotropin (ədre'nōkôr'tikōtrō'pin). See **ACTH.**

adrenolytic (ədre'nōlit'ik), capable of impeding the action of epinephrine, levarterenol (norepinephrine), or both (sympatholytic).

a. agent. See **agent, adrenergic blocking.**

adrenotropic (ədre'nōtrōp'ik), having a special affinity for the adrenal gland.

adsorb, to attract molecules of a substance to the surface of another solid substance.

adsorbent, a substance that adsorbs, such as activated charcoal and clay.

adsorption, a natural process whereby molecules of a gas or liquid adhere to the surface of a solid.

adult, 1. a person who is fully developed and who has attained the intellectual capacity and the emotional and psychologic stability characteristic of a mature person. 2. a person who has reached full legal age.

adumbration (ad'əmbrā'shən), a geometric lack of sharpness of the x-ray shadow. See also **penumbra, geometric.**

advances, monies paid before the scheduled time of payment.

adverse drug effect, a harmful, unintended reaction to a drug administered at normal dosage.

adverse reaction, any harmful, unintended effect of a medication, diagnostic test, or therapeutic intervention.

adverse selection, a statistical condition within a group when there is a greater demand for dental services and/or more services necessary than the average expected for that group.

advertising, any paid form of nonpersonal presentation and promotion of ideas, goods, or services by an identified sponsor.

aeration (erā'shən), the passage of air or gases into liquid (for example, the passage of oxygen from pulmonary alveoli into the blood).

aerobiosis, life occurring in the presence of oxygen.

aerodontalgia (er'ōdontal'jə), pulpal pain with decreased barometric pressure. (not current)

aeroembolism (er'ō-em'bōlizəm) (air embolism), an obstruction of a blood vessel caused by the entrance of air into the bloodstream. (not current) See also **embolism.**

aerosinusitis (er'ōsī'nəsī'tis), the painful symptoms related to the maxillary sinus resulting from a change in barometric pressure. (not current)

aerosol (er'əsol'), **1.** the suspension of materials in a gas or vapor (for example, saliva vaporized in air-water spray from high-speed handpiece). **2.** a substance dispensed as constituent of gas or vapor suspension.

Aeromonas, a genus of bacteria usually found in water.

aesthetic factors. See **esthetic dentistry.**

affect (əfekt'), **1.** the feeling of pleasantness or unpleasantness produced by a stimulus. **2.** the emotional complex influencing a mental state. **3.** the feeling experienced in connection with an emotion.

afferent (af'ərənt), conveying from a periphery to a center.

a. impulse, an impulse that arises in the periphery and is carried into the central nervous system. An afferent nerve conducts the impulse from the site of origin to the central nervous system.

affiliation (əfilēā'shən), the incorporation or formation of a partnership by two or more dentists for the purpose of practicing the profession of dentistry.

afflux (af'ləks), the rush of blood to a body part.

affricative (əfrik'ətiv), a fricative speech sound initiated by a plosive.

aflatoxin, a group of carcinogenic and toxic factors produced by *Aspergillus flavus* food molds.

A:G ratio. See **ratio, A:G.**

agar (a'gär), **1.** a polysaccharide derived from seaweed. **2.** the basic constituent of a reversible hydrocolloid. See also **hydrocolloid, reversible.**

a., hydrocolloid, a reversible hydrocolloid made from agar-agar.

age, the period of time a person has existed since birth or an object since its beginning.

a. determination (by teeth), an estimate of age from the stage of tooth development and/or pattern of wear.

a. distribution, a grouping of the persons within a population on the basis of birth date.

a. factors, variables affected by time since birth.

a. hardening. See **hardening, age.**

a. of onset, the chronologic age of the patient at which the disease, affliction, or disability appeared.

aged, a state of having grown older or more mature than others of the population. See also **geriatrics.**

agenesis (ājen'əsis), the defective development or congenital absence of parts.

agent, 1. a person or product that causes action. **2.** a person authorized to act for, or in place of, another.

a., adrenergic blocking, a drug that blocks the action of the neurohormones norepinephrine and/or epinephrine or of adrenergic drugs to sympathetic neuroeffectors.

a., adrenolytic blocking, an uncertain term sometimes used in reference to adrenergic blocking agents.

a., anesthetic, a drug that produces local or general loss of sensation.

a., antiinflammatory, a drug that reduces inflammation.

a., bleaching, an agent used in the modification or removal of discoloration.

a., blocking, an agent that occupies or usurps the receptor site normally occupied by a drug or a biochemical intermediary (for example, acetylcholine or epinephrine).

a., chemotherapeutic, a chemical of natural or synthetic origin used for its specific action against disease, usually against infection.

a., cholinergic blocking, **1.** a drug that inhibits the action of acetylcholine or cholinergic drugs at the postganglionic cholinergic neuroeffectors. **2.** an anticholinergic agent.

a., ganglionic blocking, a drug that prevents passage of nerve impulses at the synapses between preganglionic and postganglionic neurons.

a., myoneural blocking, a drug that prevents transmission of nerve impulses at the junction of the nerve and the muscle.

a., oxidizing, an agent that provides oxygen in reaction with another substance or, in the broader and more definitive chemical sense, a chemical capable of accepting electrons and thereby decreasing the negative charge on an atom of the substance being oxidized.

a., polishing, an abrasive that produces a smooth, lustrous finish.

a., wetting, any agent that will reduce the surface tension of water. Generally used in investing wax patterns.

ageusia (əgyōō′sē-ə), a loss or impairment of the sense of taste.

agglutination (əglōō′tinā′shən), the aggregation or clumping together of cells as a result of their interaction with specific antibodies called agglutinins, commonly used in blood typing and in identifying or estimating the strength of immunoglobulins or immune sera.

agglutinin (əglōō′tinin), **1.** a specific kind of antibody whose interaction with antigens is manifested as agglutination. **2.** an antibody that agglutinates red blood cells or renders them agglutinable.

aging, in human development, the process of growing old. Physically, aging is marked by the reduction in the ability of cells to function normally or to produce new body cells at an optimal rate.

a. schedule, a report showing how long accounts receivable have been outstanding. It gives the percentage of receivables not past due and the percent past due by 1 month, 2 months, or other periods.

aglossia (əglos′ē-ə), a developmental anomaly in which a portion or all of the tongue is absent.

agnathia (ag·nath′ē-ə), an absence of the lower jaw.

agnosia (agnō′zē-ə), a loss of ability to recognize common objects (that is, a

loss of ability to understand the significance of sensory stimuli [for example, tactile, auditory, and visual] resulting from brain damage).

agonist (ag′onist), **1.** an organ, gland, muscle, or nerve center that is so connected physiologically with another that the two function simultaneously in forwarding a given process, such as when two muscles pull on the same skeletal member and receive a nervous excitation at the same time. Antonym: antagonist. **2.** a drug or other substance having a specific cellular affinity that produces a predictable response.

agony, **1.** severe pain or extreme suffering. **2.** the death struggle.

agoraphobia, an anxiety disorder characterized by a fear of being in an open, crowded, or public place where escape may be difficult or help may not be available if needed.

agranulocytopenia (āgran′yōōlōsītō-pē′nē-ə). (not current) See **agranulocytosis.**

agranulocytosis (āgran′yōōlōsītō′sis), a decrease in the number of granulocytes in peripheral blood resulting from bone marrow depression by drugs and chemicals or replacement by a neoplasm. Oral lesions are ulceronecrotic, involving the gingivae, tongue, buccal mucosa, or lips. Regional lymphadenopathy and lymphadenitis are prevalent.

agreement, the coming together in accord of two minds on a given proposition; a concord of understanding and intention with respect to the effect on relative rights and duties.

AH-26, an epoxy resin root canal sealer.

AHF, the abbreviation for **antihemophilic factor.** See also **factor VIII.**

aid, assistance; support.

a. in physiotherapy, an agent used by the patient to cleanse the teeth and oral tissues and provide pseudofunctional stimulation of the gingival tissues to maintain periodontal health.

a., speech therapy, a restoration, appliance, or electronic device used to improve speech.

a., visual, any model, drawing, or photograph used to help the patient understand proposed treatment.

AIDS, the abbreviation for **acquired immunodeficiency syndrome.**

AIDS-related complex (ARC). See acquired immunodeficiency syndrome.

air, the invisible, odorless, gaseous mixture that makes up the earth's atmosphere.

a. chamber. See **chamber, relief.**

a., complemental. See **volume, inspiratory reserve.**

a., functional residual. See **capacity, functional residual.**

a., minimal, the volume of air in the air sacs themselves (that is, part of the residual air).

a. reserve. See **volume, expiratory reserve.**

a., residual. See **volume, residual.**

a., supplemental. See **volume, expiratory reserve.**

a. syringe. See **syringe, air.**

a., tidal. See **volume, tidal.**

a. turbine handpiece. See **handpiece, air turbine.**

airborne contaminants, materials in the atmosphere that can affect the health of persons in the same or nearby environment. Also referred to as *air pollution.*

airway, 1. a clear passageway for air into and out of the lungs. **2.** a device for securing unobstructed respiration during general anesthesia or in states of unconsciousness.

a. obstruction, an abnormal condition of the respiratory pathway characterized by a mechanical impediment to the delivery or to the absorption of oxygen in the lungs, as in choking, bronchospasm, obstructive lung disease, or laryngospasm.

a. resistance, the ratio of pressure difference between the mouth, nose, or other airway opening and the alveoli to the simultaneously measured resulting volumetric gas flow rate.

ala (ā'lə), any winglike process (for example, the ala of the nose is the cutaneous-covered cartilaginous structure on the lateral aspect of the external naris).

alanine, a nonessential amino acid found in many proteins in the body. Alanine is metabolized in the liver to produce pryuvate and glutamate.

alarm reaction. See **reaction, alarm** and **syndrome, general adaptation.**

Albers-Schönberg disease (al'berz shœn'berg). See **osteopetrosis.**

Albright's syndrome. See **syndrome, Albright's.**

albumin (albyōō'min), the primary protein of plasma (4.5% g) that aids in maintaining capillary osmotic pressure.

albuminuria (albyōō'minur'ē·ə) (hyperproteinuria, proteinuria, proteuria), the presence of clinically detectable amounts of protein in the urine. Usually less than 100 mg/24 hr may be found normally by special methods. The usual protein is albumin, although globulins, Bence Jones protein, and fibrinogen may be present and may exceed albumin. The condition may be caused by prerenal or renal disease or by inflammation of the urinary tract.

albuterol, *trade names:* Proventil, Proventil Repetabs, Nova-Salmol, Ventodisk, Ventolin, Ventolin Rotacaps; *drug class:* adrenergic β_2-agonist; *action:* causes bronchodilation; *uses:* prevents exercise-induced asthma, bronchospasm.

alcohol (al'kōhol), a transparent, colorless liquid that is mobile and volatile. Alcohols are organic compounds formed from hydrocarbons by the substitution of hydroxyl radicals for the same number of hydrogen atoms.

a., absolute, alcohol containing no more than 1% H_2O.

alcoholism, the continued extreme dependence on excessive amounts of alcohol, accompanied by a cumulative pattern of deviant behaviors. The most frequent medical consequences of alcoholism are chronic gastritis, central nervous system depression, and cirrhosis of the liver, each of which can compromise the delivery of dental care.

aldehyde, any of a large category of organic compounds derived from a corresponding alcohol by the removal of two hydrogen atoms, as in the conversion of ethyl alcohol to acetaldehyde.

aldesleukin (interleukin-2, IL-2), *trade name:* Proleukin; *drug class:* antineoplastic; *action:* enhancement of lymphocyte mitogenesis and stimulation of IL-2–dependent cell lines; *uses:* metastatic renal cell carcinoma in adults.

alendronate sodium, *trade name:* Fosamax; *drug class:* amino biphosphonate; *action:* acts as a specific inhibitor of osteoclast-mediated bone resorption; *uses:* osteoporosis in postmenopausal women, Paget's disease of bone.

aldosterone (aldōs'tərōn) (electrocortin), an adrenal corticosteroid hormone that acts primarily to accelerate the exchange of potassium for sodium in the renal tubules and other cells. Aldosterone is a potent mineralocorticoid but also has some regulatory effect on carbohydrate metabolism.

aldosteronism, primary (aldōs'tərōnizəm), a hyperadrenal syndrome caused by abnormal elaboration of aldosterone and characterized by excessive loss of potassium and resultant muscle weakness. The symptoms suggest tetany. The condition is often associated with an adenoma or cortical hyperplasia of the adrenal glands.

alganesthesia (algan'esthē'zē-ə), the absence of a normal sense of pain.

algesia (aljē'zē-ə), sensitivity to pain; hyperesthesia; a sense of pain.

algesic (aljē'sik), painful.

algesimetry (aljesim'etrē), the measurement of response to painful stimuli.

algetic (aljet'ik), painful.

alginate (al'jināt), a salt of alginic acid (for example, sodium alginate), which, when mixed with water in accurate proportions, forms an irreversible hydrocolloid gel used for making impressions. See also **hydrocolloid, irreversible.**

algorithm, an explicit protocol with well-defined rules to be followed in solving a complex problem.

align (əlīn'), to move the teeth into their proper positions to conform to the line of occlusion.

alignment, tooth (əlīn'ment), the arrangement of the teeth in relationship to their supporting bone (alveolar process), adjacent teeth, and opposing dentition.

alkali (al'kəlī), a strong water-soluble base. A chemical substance that, in aqueous solution, undergoes dissociation, resulting in the formation of hydroxyl (OH) ions.

alkaline (al'kəlin), having the reductions of an alkali. A pH level of 7.1 to 14 designates an alkaline solution.

a. diet. See also **diet, alkaline.**

a. phosphatase, an enzyme present in bone, the kidneys, the intestine,

plasma, and teeth. It may be elevated in the serum in some diseases associated with bone, liver, and other tissues.

a. reserve. See **reserve, alkaline.**

alkaloid (al'kəloid), any one of the many nitrogen-containing organic bases derived from plants. The alkaloids are bitter and physiologically active. A number are useful therapeutic agents.

a., synthetic, a synthetically prepared compound having the chemical characteristics of the alkaloids.

alkalosis (alkəlō'sis), a disturbance of acid-base balance and water balance, characterized by an excess of alkali or a deficiency of acids.

a., compensated, a condition in which the blood bicarbonate is usually higher than normal, but in which the compensatory mechanisms have kept the pH level within normal range. See also **alkalosis, uncompensated.**

a., respiratory, alkalemia produced by hypoventilation. Plasma bicarbonate is therefore decreased in respiratory alkalosis but raised in metabolic alkalosis.

a., uncompensated, alkalemia usually accompanied by an increased blood bicarbonate.

allele (əlel') (allelomorph), one or more genes occupying the same location in a chromosome but differing because of a mutational change of one.

allelomorph (əle'lōmorf). (not current) See **allele.**

allergen (al'ərjin), a substance capable of producing an allergic response. Common allergens are pollens, dust, drugs, and foods.

allergy (al'ərjē), a hypersensitive reaction of the body to an allergen; an antigen-antibody reaction is manifested in several forms—anaphylaxis, asthma, hay fever, urticaria, angioedema, dermatitis, and stomatitis.

a., "spontaneous" clinical. See **atopy.**

allied health personnel, health professionals, other than physicians, dentists, clinical psychologists, pharmacists, and nurses, with education, training, and experience to serve as members of the health care delivery team.

allochiria (alōki'rē·ə), the tactile sensation experienced at the side opposite its origin.

allografts, the transplantation of tissue between genetically nonidentical individuals of the same species, also known as *homoplastic grafts,* or *homografts.*

alloplast (al'ōplast), a transplant (implant) consisting of material originating from a nonliving source that is surgically inserted to replace missing tissue.

alloplastic (al'ōplas'tik), nonbiologic material such as metal, ceramic, and plastic.

alloplasty (al'ōplas'tē), a plastic surgical procedure in which material not from the human body is used.

allopurinol, *trade names:* Lopurin, Zyloprim; *drug class:* antigout drug; *action:* inhibits the enzyme xanthine oxidase, reducing uric acid synthesis, *uses:* chronic gout, hyperuricemia associated with malignancies.

allowable benefits, any necessary, reasonable, and customary item of service or treatment covered in whole or in part under an insurance plan.

allowable charge, the maximum dollar amount on which benefit payment is based for each dental procedure.

allowable expenses, the dollar amounts allowable for each dental procedure covered by a dental insurance policy.

alloxan (əlok'sin), a substance, mesoxalylurea, capable of producing experimental diabetes by destroying the islet cells of the pancreas.

alloy (al'oi), **1.** metals that are mutually soluble in a liquid state. **2.** the product of the fusion of two or more metals.

a., amalgam, the alloy or product of the fusion of several metals, usually supplied as filings, that is mixed with mercury to produce dental amalgam.

a., cobalt-chromium (chrome-cobalt amalgam), base metal alloys. Used in dentistry for metallic denture bases and partial dentures.

a., dental amalgam. See **amalgam.**

a., dental gold, an alloy in which the principal ingredient is gold.

a., eutectic, any combination of metals, the melting point of which is lower than that of any of the individual metals of which it consists. One in which the components are mutually soluble in the solid state. A eutectic alloy has a nonhomogeneous grain structure and is therefore likely to be brittle and subject to tarnishing and corrosion.

a., nickel-chromium, a stainless steel.

alopecia (al'əpē'shə), normal or abnormal deficiency of hair. Baldness.

alpha-amylase, a starch-splitting enzyme used in the treatment of inflammatory conditions and edema of soft tissues associated with traumatic injury.

alphabet, international phonetic, a set of internationally agreed upon alphabetical symbols, one for each sound; supplements the existing alphabet to fill out needed representation of sounds.

alpha-estradiol (al'faestrədī'əl), an estrogenic steroid, prepared by dehydrogenation of estrone, which is one of the factors responsible for the maintenance of the epithelial integrity of the oral tissues. A deficiency results in epithelial desquamation.

alpha-hemihydrate (al'fəhemēhī'drāt), a physical form of the hemihydrate of calcium sulfate ($CaSO_4 \cdot H_2O$; dental artificial stone.

alpha-interferon. See **interferon, alpha.**

alphanumeric, pertaining to a character set that contains letters and numerals and usually other special characters.

alpha-tocopherol (al'fətōkōf'erôl). See **vitamin E.**

alprazolam, *trade names:* Xanax, Apo-Alpraz, Novo-Alprazol, Nu-Alpraz; *drug class:* benzodiazepine (Controlled Substance Schedule IV); *action:* produces CNS depression; *uses:* anxiety, panic disorders, anxiety with depressive symptoms.

alprostadil, *trade name:* Caverject; *drug class:* naturally occurring prostaglandin; *action:* induces erection by relaxation of trabecular smooth muscle and by dilation of cavernosal arteries; *uses:* treatment of erectile dysfunction caused by neurogenic, vasculogenic, psychogenetic, or mixed etiology.

alternate benefit, a provision in a dental plan contract that allows the third-party payer to determine the benefit based on an alternative procedure that is generally less expensive than the one provided or proposed.

alternate treatment, Contract provisions that authorize the insurance carrier to determine the amount of benefits payable, giving consideration to alternate procedures, services, or courses of treatment that may be performed to accomplish the desired result. The attending dentist and the patient have the option of which procedure to use, although payment for the procedure may be based on the alternate treatment principle.

alternative benefit plan, a plan, other than a traditional (fee-for-service, freedom of choice) indemnity or service corporation plan for reimbursing a participating dentist for providing treatment to an enrolled patient population.

alternative delivery system, an arrangement for the provision of dental services in other than the traditional (for example, licensed dentist providing treatment in a fee-for-service dental office) way.

alternative plan, a compromise plan of treatment deviating from the ideal plan in scope and financial investment.

altitude, pertaining to any location on earth with reference to a fixed surface point, which is usually sea level. The higher the altitude, the less the oxygen concentration and the greater the ultraviolet radiation, both of which can cause health problems.

altretamine, *trade name:* Hexalen; *drug class:* antineoplastic; *action:* products of metabolism interact with tissue macromolecules, including DNA, which may be responsible for cytotoxicity; *uses:* palliative treatment of recurrent, persistent ovarian cancer.

alumina (əlu'minə), aluminum oxide, an abrasive sometimes used as a polishing agent.

aluminum, a widely used metallic element and the third most abundant of all the elements. Aluminum is a principal component of many compounds used in antacids, antiseptics, astringents, and styptics. Aluminum hydroxychloride is the most commonly used agent in antiperspirants.

aluminum carbonate gel, *trade name:* Basajel; *drug class:* antacid;

action: neutralizes gastric acidity, binds phosphates in GI tract; *uses:* antacid, prevention of phosphate stones, phosphate binder in chronic renal failure.

aluminum hydroxide, *trade names:* AlternaGEL, Alu-Cap, Alu-Tab, Amphojel, Dialume; *drug class:* antacid; *action:* neutralizes gastric acidity, binds phosphates in GI tract; *uses:* antacid, hyperphosphatemia in chronic renal failure.

aluminum oxide, an aluminum compound found in many polishing agents.

Aluwax (al'ūwax), a commercially prepared wax wafer containing aluminum that is used to register jaw relationship. (not current)

alveolalgia (al'vēōlahl'jē-ə). See **socket, dry.**

alveolar (alvē'ōlär), pertaining to an alveolus.

a. bone loss. See **bone loss, periodontal.**

a. crest. See **crest, alveolar.**

a. process. See **process, alveolar.**

a. ridge. See **ridge, alveolar.**

a. r. augmentation, a surgical procedure to improve the shape and size of the alveolar ridge(s) in preparation to receive and retain a dental prosthesis.

alveolectomy (al'vē-əlek'təmē), the excision of a portion of the alveolar process to aid in the removal of teeth, modification of the contour after the removal of teeth, and preparation of the mouth for dentures.

alveolitis, in dentistry, the inflammation of a tooth socket.

alveololingual sulcus. See **sulcus, alveololingual.** (not current)

alveolus (alvēə'lus), 1. an air sac of the lungs formed by terminal dilations of the bronchioles. 2. the socket in the bone in which a tooth is attached by means of the periodontal ligament.

alveoplasty, the surgical shaping and smoothing of the margins of the tooth socket after extraction of the tooth, generally in preparation for the placement of a prosthesis.

Alzheimer's disease (Alois Alzheimer, German neurologist, b. 1854), a presenile dementia characterized by confusion, memory failure, disorientation, restlessness, agnosia, hallucinosis, speech disturbances, and the inability to carry out purposeful movement. The disease usually begins in later middle life with slight defects in memory and behavior which become progressively more severe. Also known as *primary progressive aphasia.*

amalgam (əmal′gəm) (dental amalgam alloy), an alloy, one of the constituents of which is mercury.

a. carrier. See **carrier, amalgam.**

a. carver. See **carver, amalgam.**

a. condenser. See **condenser, amalgam.**

a., copper, an alloy composed principally of copper and mercury. See also **amalgam.**

a., dental, an amalgam used for dental restorations and dies.

a. matrix. See **matrix, amalgam.**

a. plugger. See **condenser, amalgam.**

a., silver, a dental amalgam, the chief constituent of which is silver. The ADA composition specifications are as follows: silver, 65% minimum; tin, 25% minimum; copper, 6% maximum; zinc, 2% maximum.

a. squeeze cloth, a piece of linen used to hold plastic amalgam from which excess mercury is to be squeezed.

a. tattoo, a solitary discrete gray, blue, or black discoloration of tissue usually located in the gingiva, alveolar ridge, or buccal mucosa caused by minute amounts of dental amalgam that became embedded under the surface. The asymptomatic lesion is static and requires no treatment. If doubt exists about the lesion or if the lesion is unsightly, excisional biopsy is recommended.

amalgamation (əmal′gəmā′shən), the formation of an alloy by mixing mercury with another metal or other metals. See also **trituration.**

a. amalgamator (əmal′gəmātor), a mechanical device used to triturate the ingredients of dental amalgam into a plastic mass.

ambulatory care, health services provided on an outpatient basis to those who can visit a health care facility and return home the same day.

ambulatory surgery, surgical care provided to persons who do not require overnight nursing care.

amcinonide, *trade name:* Cyclocort; *drug class:* topical fluorinated corti-

costeroid, group II high potency; *action:* antipruritic, antiinflammatory; *uses:* psoriasis, eczema, contact dermatitis, pruritus.

ameloblast, an epithelial cell associated with the tooth bud which, during tooth formation, secretes the tooth enamel.

ameloblastic fibroma. See **fibroma, ameloblastic.**

ameloblastic sarcoma. See **sarcoma, ameloblastic.**

ameloblastoma (am′əl′ōblastō′mə) (adamantino blastoma, adamantinoma), an epithelial neoplasm with a basic structure resembling the enamel organ and suggesting derivation from ameloblastic cells. It is usually benign.

a., acanthomatous, an epithelial odontogenic tumor that differs from the simple ameloblastoma in that the central cells within the cell nests are squamous and may be keratinized rather than stellate. The peripheries of the cell nests are composed of ameloblastic cells. See also **ameloblastoma.**

amelogenesis imperfecta (am′əl′-ōjen′esis), a severe hypoplasia or agenesis of enamel that is inherited as a dominant characteristic.

amenorrhea (əmenôrrē′·ə), the absence or abnormal cessation of the menstrual cycle.

American Dental Association (ADA), a nonprofit professional association whose membership is made up of dentists in the United States. Its purpose is to assist its members in providing the highest professional and ethical care to the citizens of the United States and to serve as an advocate for the advancement of the profession.

American Dental Hygienists Association (ADHA), a nonprofit professional association of dental hygienists in the United States created to assist its members in providing the highest professional and ethical care to the citizens of the United States and to serve as an advocate for the advancement of the profession.

American Hospital Association (AHA), a nonprofit national organization of individuals, institutions, and organizations engaged in direct patient care. The Association works to promote the improvement of health care services.

American Medical Association (AMA), a nonprofit professional association of physicians in the United States, including all medical specialties. Its purpose is to provide the highest professional and ethical medical care to the citizens of the United States and to serve as an advocate for the advancement of the profession.

Americans with Disabilities Act, a federal law enacted on July 26, 1990, that defines a private dental office as a place of public accommodation, thereby requiring as of January 26, 1992, that dentists serve persons with disabilities.

amiloride HCl, *trade name:* Midamor; *drug class:* potassium-sparing diuretic; *action:* acts primarily on distal renal tubule, increasing the retention of potassium; *uses:* edema in chronic heart failure in combination with other diuretics, for hypertension, INH solution for cystic fibrosis.

amines, organic compounds that contain nitrogen.

amino acid, an organic acid in which one of the CH hydrogen atoms has been replaced by NH_2. Amino acids are the building blocks of proteins.

a. a., essential, amino acids that cannot be synthesized by the organism but are required by the organism. They must be supplied by the diet. Isoleucine, leucine, lysine, methionine, pheylalanine, threonine, tryptophan, and valine are essential for adults; these eight plus arginine and histidine are considered essential for infants and children.

a. a., nonessential, amino acids that can be synthesized by the organism and are not required in the diet.

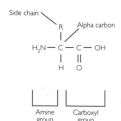

Basic structural formula for an amino acid.
(Thibodeau, 1996.)

aminocaproic acid (EACA), *trade name:* Amicar; *drug class:* hemostatic; *action:* inhibits fibrinolysis by inhibiting plasminogen activator substances; *uses:* hemorrhage from hyperfibrinolysis; adjunctive therapy in hemophilia; unapproved, hemorrhage following dental surgery in hemophilia.

aminoglutethimide, *trade name:* Cytadren; *drug class:* antineoplastic, adrenal steroid inhibitor; *action:* acts by inhibiting the enzymatic conversion of cholesterol to pregnenolone, thereby blocking synthesis of all adrenal steroids; *uses:* suppression of adrenal function in Cushing's syndrome, metastatic breast cancer, and adrenal cancer.

aminoglycosides, a group of bacteriocidal antibiotics obtained from *Streptomyces* that inhibit protein synthesis in bacterial ribosomes and are effective against aerobic gram-negative bacilli.

aminophylline (theophylline ethylenediamine), *trade names:* Paralon Phyllocontin; *drug class:* xanthine; *action:* relaxes smooth muscle of the respiratory system; *uses:* bronchial asthma, bronchospasm, Cheyne-Stokes respirations.

amiodarone HCl, *trade name:* Cordarone; *drug class:* antidysrhythmic (drug class III); *action:* prolongs action potential duration and effective refractory period; *uses:* documented life-threatening ventricular tachycardia.

amitriptyline HCl, *trade names:* Apo-Amitriptyline, Elavil, Emitrip, Endep, Enovil, Levate, Novotriptyn; *drug class:* tricyclic antidepressant; *action:* inhibits both norepinephrine and serotonin (5-HT); *uses:* major depression.

amlodipine besylate, *trade name:* Novasc; *drug class:* calcium channel blocker; *action:* inhibits calcium ion influx across cell membrane during cardiac depolarization; produces relaxation of coronary vascular smooth muscle and dilates coronary arteries, decreases SA/AV node conduction; *uses:* hypertension as a single agent or in combination with other antihypertensives, chronic stable angina pectoris, vasospastic angina.

ammeter (am'mēter), a contraction of amperemeter. An apparatus that measures the amperage of an electric current.

ammonia, a colorless aromatic gas consisting of nitrogen and hydrogen, produced by the decomposition of nitrogenous organic matter. Some of its many uses are as an aromatic stimulant, a detergent, and an emulsifier.

a. thiosulfate (əmō'nē·ə thiōsul'fāt), an ingredient of the photographic fixing solution that acts as a solvent for silver halides.

ammoniacal silver nitrate. See **silver nitrate, ammoniacal.**

ammonium chloride, the chlorine salt of the ammonium ion. Ammonium chloride is a popular deliquescent agent (that is, it attracts and absorbs water from the atmosphere).

amnesia (amnē'zē·ə), the lack or loss of memory.

amnesiac (amnē'zē·ak), a person affected by amnesia.

amnesic (amnē'zik). See **sedative.**

amnestic (amnes'tik), amnesic; causing amnesia.

amobarbital/amobarbital sodium, *trade name:* Amytal; *drug class:* barbiturate sedative-hypnotic (Controlled Substance Schedule II); *action:* nonselective depression of CNS ranging from sedation to hypnosis to anesthesia to coma, depending on dose administered; *uses:* sedation, preanesthetic sedation, insomnia, anticonvulsant, adjunct in psychiatry, hypnotic.

amorphous (ā'môrf, əmôrf), a substance having no specific space lattice, the molecules being distributed at random.

amortization, a generic term that includes various specific practices, such as depreciation, depletion, write off of intangibles, prepaid expenses, and deferred charges.

amoxapine, *trade name:* Asendin; *drug class:* tricyclic antidepressant; *action:* inhibits both norepinephrine and serotonin (5-HT) uptake in brain; *uses:* depression.

amoxicillin/clavulanate potassium, *trade names:* Augmentin, Clavulin; *drug class:* aminopenicillin with a β-lactamase inhibitor; *action:* interferes with cell wall replication of susceptible organisms; *uses:* sinus infections, pneumonia, otitis media, skin, urinary

tract infections; effective for strains of *E. coli, H. influenzae, S. pneumoniae,* and β-lactamase–producing organisms.

amoxicillin trihydrate, *trade names:* Amoxil, Apo-Amoxi, Novamoxin, Nu-Amoxi and others; *drug class:* aminopenicillin; *action:* interferes with cell wall replication of susceptible organisms; *uses:* sinus infections, pneumonia, otitis media, skin, urinary tract infections.

ampere (am'pēr) (Amp), a unit of measurement of the quantity of electric current, equal to a flow of 1 coulomb per second or the flow of 6.25 times 10^{18} electrons per second. The current produced by 1 volt acting through a resistance of 1 ohm.

amperemeter (am'permēt'er) (not current). See **ammeter.**

amphetamines, a group of nervous system stimulants that are subject to abuse because of their ability to reduce appetite and produce wakefulness and euphoria. Abuse of amphetamines may lead to compulsive behavior, paranoia, hallucinations, and suicidal tendencies.

amphotericin, an antibiotic and antifungal agent used extensively in the treatment of systemic mycoses.

a. B, topical, *trade name:* Fungizone; *drug class:* polyene antifungal; *action:* increases cell membrane permeability in susceptible organisms by binding to sterols; *uses:* cutaneous, mucocutaneous infections caused by Candida.

ampicillin, an acid-stable semisynthetic penicillin antibiotic with a broader spectrum of effectiveness than penicillin G.

amputation, pulp. See **pulpotomy.**

amputation, root, the removal of a root of a multirooted tooth.

amputation neuroma. See **neuroma, traumatic.**

amyloid, a starchlike protein-carbohydrate complex that is deposited abnormally in some tissues during certain chronic disease states, such as amyloidosis, rheumatoid arthritis, and tuberculosis.

amyloidosis (am'iloidō'sis), a condition in which amyloid, a glycoprotein, is deposited intercellularly in tissues and organs. Four types of amyloidosis are recognized, two of which, primary amyloidosis and amyloid tumor, frequently produce nodules in the tongue and gingiva.

a., primary, amyloidosis occurring without a known predisposing cause. Amyloid deposits are found in the tongue, lips, skeletal muscles, and other mesodermal structures. The disease may be manifested by polyneuropathy, purpura, hepatosplenomegaly, heart failure, and the nephrotic syndrome.

a., secondary, amyloidosis occurring secondary to chronic diseases such as tuberculosis, leprosy, rheumatoid arthritis, multiple myeloma, and prolonged bacterial infections. Amyloid deposits are found in parenchymal organs. The disease is usually manifested by proteinuria and hepatosplenomegaly.

amyotonia (ā′mī-ōtōnē·ə), an abnormal flaccidity or flabbiness of a muscle or group of muscles.

amyotrophic lateral sclerosis, a degenerative disease of the motor neurons, characterized by atrophy of the muscles of the hands, forearms, and legs, and spreading to involve most of the body. It is commonly known as *Lou Gehrig's disease.*

anabolic steroids, a group of compounds derived from testosterone or prepared synthetically to promote general body growth. Anabolic steroids are used in the treatment of aplastic anemia, anemias associated with renal failure, myeloid metaplasia, and leukemia. Anabolic steroids are subject to abuse to promote muscle mass in athletes.

anabolism (ənab′əlizəm), the constructive process by which substances are converted from simple to complex forms by living cells; constructive metabolism.

anaerobe (aner′ōb), a microorganism that can exist and grow only in the partial or complete absence of molecular oxygen.

analeptic (an əlep′tik), 1. an agent that acts to overcome depression of the central nervous system. 2. a strong central nervous system stimulant that is used to restore consciousness, especially from a drug-induced coma.

analgesia (an′əljē′zē·ə), insensibility to pain without loss of consciousness; a state in which painful stimuli are not perceived or interpreted as pain; usually induced by a drug, although

trauma or a disease process may produce a general or regional analgesia.

a., diagnostic, the administration of a local anesthetic to determine the location, source, or cause of pain.

a., endotracheal, an inhalation technique in which the anesthetic agent and respiratory gases are passed through a tube inserted in the trachea via either the nose or mouth.

a., infiltration, the arrest of the sensory responses of nerve endings at the surgical site by injections of an anesthetic at that site.

a., insufflation, the delivery of anesthetic gases or vapors directly to the airway of a patient while he or she is breathing room air. Insufflation is usually an open drop method.

a., intranasal, the delivery of an analgesic agent to the membrane of the nose by either topical application or insufflation.

a., nonnarcotic, drugs that relieve pain by action at the site of the pain. Generally, nonnarcotic analgesics do not produce tolerance or dependence.

a., patient-controlled, mechanisms by which the patient can administer and/or control the application of an analgesic agent to an area of the body. One such mechanism is the use of transcutaneous electric nerve stimulation (TENS) to control facial pain. The TENS unit is a variable controlled device designed to deliver a controlled electrical stimulus to the skin surface overlying a painful muscle.

a., regional, the reversible loss of pain sensation over an area of the body by blocking the afferent conduction of its innervation with a local anesthetic agent.

analgesic (anəljē′zik) (analgetic), 1. the property of a drug that enables it to raise the pain threshold. 2. an analgesic may be classified in one of two groups: an analgesic that blocks the sensory neural pathways of pain (for example, procaine and its derivatives) or an analgesic that acts directly on the thalamus to raise the pain threshold.

a., opioid, drugs that relieve pain by action on the central nervous system. Frequent use may lead to tolerance and dependence. See also **narcotic.**

analgetic (anəljet′ik). See **analgesic.**

analgia (anal′jē·ə), an absence of pain.

analysis (ənal′isis), a separation into component parts.

a., bite. See **analysis, occlusal.**

a., cephalometric (sef'əlōme'trik), the evaluation of the growth pattern or morphologic conoval of teeth, modification of the contour after the removal of teeth, and preparation of the mouth for dentures.

a., occlusal, a study of the relations of the occlusal surfaces of the opposing teeth and their functional harmony.

analyzing rod. See **rod, analyzing.**

anamnesis (an'amnē'sis), a past history of disease or injury based on the patient's memory or recall at the time of dental and/or medical interview and examination.

anaphylactic (an'əfilak'tik), pertaining to decreasing, rather than increasing, immunity.

a. hypersensitivity (Arthus' reaction), a local tissue response that is the result of an Ah-AB caused by repeated intradermal injections with one antigen, resulting in inflammation and necrosis.

anaphylactoid (an'əfilak'toid), resembling anaphylaxis; pertaining to a reaction, the symptoms of which resemble those of the anaphylactic produced by the injection of serum and other nonspecific proteins.

a. reaction. See **reaction, anaphylactoid.**

Anaphylactic hypersensitivity systemic manifestations

Conjunctivitis, angioedema
Rhinitis
Anaphylactic laryngeal edema (upper airway obstruction, stridor)
Shock
Asthma (lower airway obstruction, wheezing)
Gastrointestinal edema (vomiting)
Urticaria
Intestinal edema (diarrhea)
Angioedema

anaphylaxis (an'əfilak'sis), a violent allergic reaction characterized by sudden collapse, shock, or respiratory and circulatory failure after injection of an allergen.

anaplasia (an'əplā'zhə), a regressive change in cells toward a more primitive or embryonic cell type. Anaplasia is a prominent criterion of malignancy in tumors.

anasarca (an'əsar'kə) (dropsy), generalized edema.

anastomosis, the joining together of two blood vessels or other tubular structures to furnish a direct or indirect communication between the two structures.

a. grafts, the connection of two autogenous tubular structures as a part of reconstructive surgery.

anatomic (anətom'ik), pertaining to the anatomy of a structure.

a. crown. See **crown, anatomic.**

a. dead space, the actual capacity of the respiratory passages that extend from the nostrils to and including the terminal bronchioles.

a. form. See **form, anatomic.**

a. height of contour. See **contour, height of.**

a. impression. See **impression, anatomic.**

a. landmark. See **landmark, anatomic.**

a. teeth. See **tooth, anatomic.**

anatomy (ənat'ōmē), the science of the form, structure, and parts of animal organisms.

a., dental, the science of the structure of the teeth and the relationship of their parts. The study involves macroscopic and microscopic components.

a., radiographic, the images on a radiographic film of the combined anatomic structures through which the roentgen rays (x-rays) have passed.

ANB angle, a cephalometric measurement of the anterior-posterior relationship of the maxilla with the mandible.

anchorage, 1. the supporting base for orthodontic forces applied to stimulate tooth movement. 2. the area of application of the reciprocal forces generated when corrective forces are applied to teeth. Anchorage units may be one tooth or more or may be a portion of the neck or cranium.

a. bends, bends placed in an orthodontic wire to enhance the resistance to the anterior displacement of teeth during orthodontic treatment; primarily used in the Tweed and Begg techniques.

a., cervical, an extraoral anchorage based at the back of the neck.

a., cranial, an extraoral anchorage based at the back of the skull.

a., extraoral, an orthodontic anchorage based outside the mouth. Dental attachments are typically linked to a wire bow or hooks extending between the lips and attached elastically to a cap, a strap around the neck, or another extraoral device.

a., facial, an extraoral anchorage based on the face, usually the chin and forehead.

a., intermaxillary, an anchorage based in the opposite jaw.

a., intramaxillary, an anchorage based on teeth within the same jaw.

a., intraoral, an anchorage based within the mouth (intermaxillary, intramaxillary, or myofunctional).

a., occipital, a cranial anchorage based in the occipital area.

a., reciprocal, all anchorage is reciprocal; sometimes used to describe a force system in which the resistance units are similar.

a., simple, the use of a tooth as a resistance unit without tipping control.

a., stationary, the use of a tooth as an anchorage unit with tipping control.

Ancylostoma, a genus of Nematoda commonly known as *hookworm.*

Andresen appliance. See **appliance, Andresen.**

androgen (an′drōjen), any substance that possesses masculinizing qualities, such as testosterone.

anemia (ənē′mē·ə), a term indicating that the concentration of hemoglobin or the number of red blood cells is below the accepted normal value with respect to age and sex. In true anemia the total concentration of hemoglobin, or the total number of erythrocytes, is below normal regardless of concentration values. Symptoms, which may not be evident, include weakness, pallor, anorexia, and those related to the cause of the anemia.

a., Addison-Biermer. See **anemia, pernicious.**

a., aplastic, an anemia characterized by a decrease in all marrow elements, including platelets, red blood cells, and granulocytes.

a., Biermer's. See **anemia, pernicious.**

a., Cooley's. See **thalassemia major.**

a., displacement. See **anemia, myelophthisic.**

a., erythroblastic. See **thalassemia major.**

a., hemolytic, an anemia characterized by an increased rate of destruction of red blood cells, reticulocytosis, hyperbilirubinemia, and/or increased urinary and fecal urobilinogen, and, generally, splenic enlargement. Hereditary hemolytic anemias include congenital hemolytic jaundice, sickle cell anemia, oval cell anemia, and thalassemia. Acquired hemolytic anemias include paroxysmal nocturnal hemoglobinuria and those caused by immune mechanisms (erythroblastosis fetalis), transfusions of incompatible blood, infections, drugs, and poisons. Autoimmune hemolytic anemias are acquired hemolytic anemias associated with antibody-like substances that may not be true autoantibodies or even antibodies; they may be primary (idiopathic), or they may be secondary to lymphoma, lymphatic leukemia, disseminated lupus erythematosus, or sensitization to drugs and pollens.

a., hemorrhagic, a deficiency in red blood cells and/or hemoglobin resulting from excessive bleeding.

a., hyperchromic, an anemia in which the erythrocytes are larger than normal in size so that the content but not the concentration of hemoglobin is increased.

a., hypochromic, an anemia caused by impaired hemoglobin synthesis resulting from a deficiency of iron or pyridoxine and from chronic lead poisoning.

a., iron deficiency, an anemia resulting from a deficiency of iron, characterized by hypochromic microcytic erythrocytes and a normoblastic reaction of the bone marrow. Iron deficiency may result from an increased demand during growth or repeated pregnancies, chronic or recurrent hemorrhage such as from menstrual abnormalities, hemorrhoids, or peptic ulcer, a low intake of iron, or impaired absorption, as often occurs with chronic diarrhea.

a., macrocytic normochromic, an anemia related to a failure of nucleoprotein synthesis caused by a deficiency of vitamin B_{12}, folic acid, or related substances.

a., Mediterranean. See **thalassemia major.**

a., megaloblastic, an anemia characterized by hyperplastic bone marrow changes and maturation arrest resulting from a dietary deficiency, impaired storage and modification, or impaired use of one or more hematopoietic factors. Included are pernicious anemia, nutritional macrocytic anemias associated with gastrointestinal disturbances, anemias associated with impaired liver function (for example, macrocytic anemia of pregnancy), hypothyroidism, leukemia, and achrestic anemia.

a., microcytic hypochromic, an anemia in which the mean corpuscular volume (MCV), mean corpuscular hemoglobin (MCH) content, and mean corpuscular hemoglobin concentration (MCHC) are all low (for example, iron-deficiency anemia, hereditary leptocytosis, hemoglobin C anemia, and anemias resulting from pyridoxine deficiency and chronic lead poisoning).

a., myelophthisic (displacement anemia), an anemia resulting from displacement or crowding out of erythropoietic cells of the bone marrow by foreign tissue, as in leukemia, metastatic carcinoma, lymphoblastoma, multiple myeloma, osteoradionecrosis, and xanthomatosis.

a., normocytic normochromic, an anemia associated with disturbances of red cell formation and related to endocrine deficiencies, chronic inflammation, and carcinomatosis.

a., nutritional macrocytic, macrocytic normochromic anemia occurring as a result of a deficiency of substances necessary for deoxyribonucleic acid synthesis; for example, vitamin B_{12} and folic acid deficiency may result from a lack of intrinsic factors, sprue, or regional enteritis. Folic acid deficiency may occur in chronic alcoholism, as a result of a diet deficient in meats and vegetables, and in diseases causing intestinal malabsorption.

a., oval cell. See **elliptocytosis.**

a., pernicious (Addison-Biermer anemia), a macrocytic normochromic (megaloblastic) anemia associated with achlorhydria and a lack of a gastric intrinsic factor necessary for the binding and absorption of vitamin B_{12}, which is an erythrocyte maturing factor. In addition to hematologic findings, atrophic glossitis and gastrointestinal and nervous disorders occur.

a., physiologic, an anemia characterized by lowered blood values resulting from an increase in plasma volume that occurs most markedly during the sixth and seventh months of pregnancy.

a., sickle cell (drepanocythemia, sicklemia), a hereditary hemolytic anemia in which the presence of an abnormal hemoglobin (hemoglobin S) results in distorted, sickle-shaped erythrocytes. Manifestations include episodic crises of muscle, joint, and abdominal pain; neurologic symptoms; and leg ulcers. Sickle cell anemia occurs almost exclusively in African Americans. See also **trait, sickle cell.**

a., spherocytic. See **jaundice, congenital hemolytic.**

anergy (an'ərjē), in terms of hypersensitivity, an inability to react to specific antigens (that is, lack of reaction to intradermally injected antigens in measles, Hodgkin's sarcoma, and overwhelming tuberculosis).

anesthesia (an'esthē'zhə), the loss of feeling or sensation, especially loss of tactile sensibility, with or without loss of consciousness.

a., basal, a state of narcosis, induced before the administration of a general anesthetic, that permits the production of states of surgical anesthesia with greatly reduced amounts of general anesthetic agents.

a., block, an anesthesia induced by injecting the drug close to the nerve trunk, at some distance from the operative field. See also **anesthesia, infiltration.**

a., conduction, an anesthesia induced by injecting the drug close to the nerve trunk, at some distance from the operative field.

a., general, an irregular, reversible depression of the cells of the higher centers of the central nervous system that makes the patient unconscious and insensible to pain.

a., glove, an anesthesia with a distribution corresponding to the part of the skin covered by a glove.

a., infiltration, an anesthesia induced by injecting the anesthetic solution di-

A

rectly into or around the tissues to be anesthetized; used for operative procedures on the maxillary premolar, anterior teeth, and mandibular incisors. See also **anesthesia, block.**

a., intraosseous, an anesthesia produced by the injection of an anesthetic agent into the cancellous portion of a bone.

a., intrapulpal, the injection of a local anesthetic directly into pulpal tissue under pressure.

a., local (regional anesthesia), the loss of pain sensation over a specific area of the anatomy without loss of consciousness.

a., regional, a term used for local anesthesia. See also **anesthesia, local.**

a., topical, a form of local anesthesia whereby free nerve endings in accessible structures are rendered incapable of stimulation by applying a suitable solution directly to the surface of the area.

anesthesiologist (an'əsthē'zēol'əjist), a physician specializing in the administration of anesthetics.

anesthesiology, the branch of medicine concerned with the relief of pain and the administration of medication to relieve pain during surgery or other invasive procedures.

anesthetic (an'esthet'ik), a drug that produces loss of feeling or sensation generally or locally.

a. agent. See **agent, anesthetic.**

a., local, a drug that, when injected into the tissues and absorbed into a nerve, will temporarily interrupt its property of conduction.

a., topical, a drug applied to the surface of tissues that produces local insensibility to pain.

anesthetist (ənes'thətist), a person who administers anesthetics.

anesthetize (ənes'thətīz), to place under anesthesia.

aneurysm (an'yōōriz'əm), a localized dilation of an artery in which one or more layers of the vessel walls are distended.

a., arteriovenous. See **shunt, arteriovenous.**

angiitis, visceral (an'jēī'tis). See **disease, collagen.**

angina (anjī'nə), a spasmodic, choking pain. The term is sometimes applied to the disease producing the pain (for example, Ludwig's angina).

a., agranulocytic. See **agranulocytosis.**

a., Ludwig's, a cellulitis involving the submaxillary, sublingual, and submental spaces and characterized clinically by a firm swelling of the floor of the mouth, with elevation of the tongue.

a., monocytic, a "sore throat" associated with infectious mononucleosis.

a. pectoris, frequently a symptom of cardiovascular diseases; characterized by a severe, viselike pain behind the sternum that sometimes radiates to the arms, neck, or mandible. Symptoms may also include a sense of constriction or pressure of the chest. Angina pectoris is caused by exertion or excitement and is relieved by rest.

a., Vincent's, an incorrect term for involvement of the pharynx by the spread of acute necrotizing ulceromembranous gingivitis.

angioedema (an'jē-ō-ədē'mə). See **edema, angioneurotic.**

angiography, the radiographic visualization of the internal anatomy of the heart and blood vessels after the intravascular introduction of radiopaque contrast medium.

angioma (an'jēō'mə), a benign tumor of vascular nature. See also **hemangioma** and **lymphangioma.**

angioneurotic edema (an'jē-ōnurä'-tik). See **edema, angioneurotic.**

angle, the degree of divergence of two or more lines or planes that meet each other; the space between such lines. Measured in degrees of an arc.

a., bayonet former, a hoe-shaped, paired cutting instrument; biangled with the blade parallel with the axis of the shaft. The cutting edge is not perpendicular to the axis of the blade. Used to accentuate angles in an "invisible" class 3 cavity.

a., Bennett, the angle formed by the sagittal plane and the path of the advancing condyle during lateral mandibular movement, as viewed in the horizontal plane.

a. board, a device used to facilitate the establishment of reproducible angular relationships between a patient's head, the x-ray beam, and the x-ray film.

a., cavosurface, the angle in a prepared cavity, formed by the junction of the wall of the cavity with the surface of the tooth.

a., cranial base, the angle formed by a line representing the floor of the anterior cranial fossa intersecting a line representing the axis of the clivus of the base of the skull.

a., cusp, **1.** the angle made by the slopes of a cusp with the plane that passes through the tip of the cusp and is perpendicular to a line bisecting the cusp; measured mesiodistally or buccolingually. Half of the included angle between the buccolingual or mesiodistal cusp inclines. **2.** the angle made by the slopes of a cusp with a perpendicular line bisecting the cusp; measured mesiodistally or buccolingually.

a., facial, an anthropometric expression of the degree of protrusion of the lower face, assessed by measuring the inclination of the facial plane relative to a horizontal reference plane.

a., former, one of a series of paired, hoe-shaped cutting instruments having the cutting edge at an angle other than a right angle in relation to the axis of the blade.

a., Frankfort-mandibular incisor (FMIA), a measure of the mandibular incisor to the Frankfort horizontal plane.

a. incisal (insī′zal), the degree of slope between the axis-orbital plane and the palatal discluding skidway of the upper incisor.

a., i. guidance, the angle formed with the occlusal plane by drawing a line in the sagittal plane between the incisal edges of the maxillary and mandibular central incisors when the teeth are in centric occlusion.

a., i. guide, the inclination of the incisal guide on the articulator.

a., lateral incisal guide, the inclination of the incisal guide in the frontal plane.

a., line, an angle formed by the junction of the two walls along a line; designated by combining the names of the walls forming the angle.

a., occlusal rest, the angle formed by the occlusal rest with the upright minor connector.

a. of mandible, the gonial angle. The relation existing between the body of the mandible and the ramus of the mandible.

a., point, an angle formed by the junction of three walls at a common point; designated by combining the names of the walls forming the angle.

a., protrusive incisional guide, the inclination of the incisal guide in the sagittal plane.

a., rest. See **angle, occlusal rest.**

a., symphyseal, the angle of the chin, which may be protruding straight or receding, according to type.

Angle's classification modified, a classification of the different forms of malocclusion set up by Edward Hartley Angle, American orthodontist (1855-1930).

Class I, the normal anteroposterior relationship of the lower jaw to the upper jaw. The mesiobuccal cusp of the maxillary first permanent molar occludes in the buccal groove of the mandibular first permanent molar; special class I—mutilated.

Type I, all teeth in linguoversion.

Type II, narrow arches; labioversion of the maxillary anterior teeth and linguoversion of the mandibular lower anterior teeth.

Type III, linguoversion of the maxillary anterior teeth; bunched; lack of development in the proximal region.

Class II, the posterior relationship of the lower jaw to the upper jaw. The mesiobuccal cusp of the maxillary first permanent molar occludes mesial to the buccal groove of the mandibular first permanent molar.

Division 1, labioversion of the maxillary teeth.

Subdivision, signifies a unilateral condition.

Division 2, linguoversion of the maxillary central incisor teeth.

Subdivision, signifies a unilateral condition.

Class III, the anterior relationship of the lower jaw to the upper jaw, may have a subdivision. The mesiobuccal cusp of the maxillary first permanent molar occludes distal to the buccal groove of the mandibular first permanent molar.

Type I, good alignment general but arch relationship abnormal.

Type II, good alignment of the maxillary anterior teeth but linguoversion of the mandibular anterior teeth

Type III, an underdeveloped upper arch; linguoversion of maxillary anterior teeth; good mandibular alignment.

angstrom (Å) unit. See **unit, angstrom.**

angular cheilosis. See **cheilosis, angular.** (not current)

angulation (ang'yo͞olā'shən), the direction of the primary beam of radiation in relation to object and film.

a., horizontal, the angle measured within the occlusal plane at which the central ray of the x-ray beam is projected relative to a reference in the vertical or sagittal plane.

a., vertical, the angle measured within the vertical plane at which the central ray of the x-ray beam is projected relative to a reference in the horizontal or occlusal plane.

anhidrosis (an'hīdrō'sis), an abnormal deficiency in the production of sweat; may be associated with an odontia in ectodermal dysplasia.

anhidrotic ectodermal dysplasia. See **hypohidrotic ectodermal dysplasia.**

anhydremia (anhīdrē'mē-ə), a decrease in blood volume resulting from a decrease in the serum component of blood; occurs in shock or any condition in which blood fluid is passed into the tissue and results in hemoconcentration. (not current).

anion (an'ī-ən), a negatively charged ion.

anionic detergent (an'ī-on'ik). See **detergent, anionic.**

anirodia, the absence of the iris. Usually a congenital condition.

anisocytosis (ani'sōsītō'sis), an inequality in cell size, especially of red blood cells.

anisognathous (an'īsog'nathəs),a condition in which the maxillary and mandibular dental arches or jaws are of different sizes.

anisotropy, not having properties or characteristics that are the same in all directions.

ankyloglossia (ang'kilōglôs'ē-ə), tongue-tie; an abnormally short lingual frenum that limits movement of the tongue.

ankylosis (ang'kilō'sis), an abnormal fixation and immobility of a joint.

a., false, an inability to open the mouth because of trismus rather than disease of the joint.

a., fibrous, the fixation of a joint by fibrous tissue.

a. of tooth. See **tooth, ankylosed.**

anlage (on'lägə), the first cells in the embryo that form any distinct part or organ of the body.

anneal (anēl') (homogenizing heat treatment, softening heat treatment), the softening of a metal by controlled heating and cooling.

a. foil, a process of subjecting noncohesive foil to heat to volatilize a protective gaseous coating on its surface, thus leaving the surface clean, making it cohesive.

a. glass, a process of regulated heating and subsequent cooling to remove strain hardening or work hardening of glass.

a. metal, a process of regulated heating and subsequent cooling to remove strain hardening or work hardening of metal.

announcement, a communication, usually printed, that states office policies or practice limitations to the public and profession.

annual reports, statistical, fiscal, and descriptive yearly reports used to inform a constituency of the status of the institution or organization.

annual statement, the report of an insurer or carrier showing assets and liabilities, receipts and disbursements, and other information for a specified 12-month period (fiscal or calendar year).

annuity, a series of payments of a fixed amount for a number of years.

anochromasia (an'ōkrōmā'sē-ə), a variation in the staining quality of cells, particularly of degenerating red blood cells. (not current)

anociassociation (ənō'sē-əsōsē-ā'shən), the blocking of neuroses, fear, pain, and harmful influences or associations to prevent shock. (not current)

anode (an'ōd), the electrically positive terminal of a roentgen ray (x-ray) tube; a tungsten block embedded in a copper stem and set at an angle of 20 or 45 degrees to the cathode. The anode emits roentgen rays (x-rays) from the point of impact of the electronic stream from the cathode.

a., rotating, an anode that rotates during x-ray production to present a constantly different focal spot to the electron stream and to permit use of small focal spots or higher tube voltages without overheating the tube.

anode-film distance (not current). See **distance, target-film.**

anodontia (an'ōdon'tē-ə) (aplasia of dentition), the failure of teeth to form; may be partial or complete.

a., partial, the absence of parts of the dentition resulting from arrested tooth development.

a., total, a complete absence of teeth resulting from arrested tooth development.

anodyne (an'ōdīn), an agent or drug that relieves pain; milder than analgesia.

anomaly (ənom'əlē), an aberration or deviation from normal anatomic growth, development, or function.

a., dental, an abnormality in which a tooth or teeth have deviated from normal in form, function, or position.

a., dentofacial, a term indicating an oral or a dysgnathic anomaly.

a., dysgnathic, an anomaly that extends beyond the teeth and includes the maxillae, the mandible, or both.

a., eugnathic, an anomaly limited to the teeth and their immediate alveolar supports.

a., gestant. See **odontoma.**

a., maxillofacial, a distortion of normal development of the face and jaws; a dysgnathic anomaly.

a., oral, an abnormal structure other than of the teeth.

anophaxia (anōfax'ē-ə), a tendency for one eye to turn upward.

anophthalmos, a congenital absence of all tissues of the eyes.

anorexia (anōrek'sē-ə), the partial or complete loss of appetite for food.

a. nervosa, a psychoneurotic disorder characterized by a prolonged refusal to eat, resulting in emaciation, amenorrhea in women, emotional disturbance concerning body image, and an abnormal fear of becoming fat.

anoxemia (an'oksē'mē-ə), a deficient aeration of the blood; a total lack of oxygen content in the blood.

anoxia (anok'sē-ə), a condition of total lack of oxygen; a term frequently misused as a symptom of hypoxia.

anoxic hypoxia. See **hypoxia, anoxic.**

antagonist, 1. a drug that counteracts, blocks, or abolishes the action of another drug. **2.** a muscle that acts in opposition to the action of another muscle (for example, flexor vs. extensor). **3.** a tooth in one jaw that occludes with a tooth in the other jaw.

a., insulin, circulating hormonal and nonhormonal substances that stimulate glyconeogenesis (for example, 11-oxysteroids and S hormones).

a., narcotic, a narcotic drug that acts specifically to reverse depression of the central nervous system.

antagonistic reflex. See **reflex, antagonistic.**

ante cibum (an'tē-si'bəm). See **a.c.**

antegonial notch, the notch or concavity usually present at the junction between the ramus and body of the mandible, near the anterior margin of the masseter muscle attachment.

anterior, 1. situated in front of. **2.** a term used to denote the incisor and canine teeth or the forward region of the mouth. **3.** the forward position.

a. cranial base, the anterior cranial fossa, sometimes identified by related landmarks such as the sella turcica and nasion.

a. determinants of occlusion. See **occlusion, anterior determinants of cusp.**

a. guide. See **guide, anterior.**

a. nasal spine. See **spine, anterior nasal.**

a. palatal bar. See **connector, anterior palatal major.**

a. tooth arrangement. See **arrangement, tooth, anterior.**

anterior-posterior discrepancy, an anterior-posterior morphologic imbalance between the maxilla and mandible and consequently between structures attached to either.

anterocclusion, a malocclusion of the teeth, in which the mandibular teeth are in a position anterior to their normal position relative to the teeth in the maxillary arch. (not current)

anteversion, the tipping or tilting of teeth or other maxillary and mandibular structures too far forward (anterior) from the normal or generally accepted standard.

anthelmintic (an'thelmin'tik), a drug that acts against parasitic worms, especially intestinal worms.

anthrax (an'thraks), an infectious disease in herbivorous animals caused by a spore-forming *Bacillus* organism.

Primary lesions in human beings may be on the lips or cheeks.

anthrocyclanins, a group of floral pigments existing as glycosides that may be used as hemotoxylin substitutes.

anthropology, the science of human beings ranging from physical characteristics to cultural, social, and environmental aspects.

a., cultural, the study of the interpersonal and community mores of a society or isolate.

a., physical, the study of the physical attributes of a society or isolate.

anthropometry, the measurement of the human body and its parts.

antibiotic (antēbīot′ik), an organic substance produced by one of several microorganisms, especially certain molds, that is capable, in low concentration, of destroying or inhibiting the growth of certain other microorganisms.

Antibiotic: mode of action

Mode of action	Representative antibiotics
Inhibition of bacterial cell wall synthesis	Penicillins
	Cephalosporins
	Bacitracins
Alteration of membrane permeability	Polymyxin B
	Amphotericin B
	Nystatin
Inhibition of microbial DNA translation and transcription	Erythromycin
	Tetracyclines
	Streptomycin
	Lincomycin
	Kanamycin
	Chloramphenicol
Inhibition of essential metabolite synthesis	Paraaminosalicylic acid
	Sulfonamides

a., oral reactions to, manifestations on the oral mucous membrane of reactions to antibiotics; characterized by glossitis, angular cheilosis, and/or a hairy tongue. Reactions may result from imbalance of oral flora produced by the antibiotics or to hypersensitivity to the antibiotics.

a. prophylaxis, the use of an antibiotic to protect a patient from an anticipated bacterial invasion associated with a medical or dental invasive procedure, particularly patients with a compromised cardiovascular system.

a. therapy. See **therapy, antibiotic.**

antibody (an′tibodē), **1.** a specific substance that is produced by an animal as a reaction to the presence of an antigen and that reacts specifically with an antigen in some observable way. **2.** an immunoglobulin, essential to the immune system, produced by lymphoid tissue in response to bacteria, viruses, or other antigenic substances. Each antibody is identified by its action, agglutinins, bacterolysins, opsonins, and precipitins.

a., antinuclear, having an affinity for the cell nuclei.

a. formation, the response of the lymphatic system to the presence of foreign substances in the body such as bacteria, viruses, food substances, pollens, and other antigens.

a., monoclonal, produced by a clone or genetically homogeneous population of hybrid cells.

a., specificity, the lymphatic system produces antibodies specific to each antigen. Viruses have the capacity to alter an antigen's genetic makeup, thereby creating a mutant antigen that requires new antibodies to combat it.

anticholinergic (an′tikō′lənur′jik) (parasympatholytic, cholinolytic), a drug that acts to inhibit the effects of the neurohormone acetylcholine or to inhibit the cholinergic neuroeffects. A cholinergic blocking agent.

anticholinesterase (an′tikō′lines′terās), a drug or chemical that inhibits or inactivates the enzyme cholinesterase, resulting in the actions produced by the accumulation of acetylcholine at cholinergic sites.

anticoagulant (an′tīkō·ag′yələnt), a drug that delays or prevents coagulation of blood.

anticonvulsive (an′tikonvul′siv), relieving or preventing convulsion.

antidepressants, agents used to counteract or treat depression.

antidote (an′tidōt), a substance that acts to antagonize the toxic effects of a drug, especially in overdose, or of a poison.

antiemetic (an′tēimet′ik), a drug used to prevent, stop, or relieve nausea and emesis (vomiting).

antiepileptic drugs, agents that inhibit or control seizures associated with epilepsy.

antifibrinolytic agents, agents that decrease the breakdown of fibrin.

antiflux, a material that prevents and confines the flow of solder (for example, graphite).

antifungal agents, agents that inhibit, control, or kill fungi. The most common yeastlike fungus occuring in or near the oral cavity is *Candida albicans.*

antigen (an'tijən), a substance, usually a protein, that elicits the formation of antibodies that react with it when introduced parenterally into an individual or species to which it is foreign.

antigenic drift, the ability of viruses to alter their genetic makeup, thereby creating mutant antigens and thus bypassing the antibody barrier of the host.

antihemophilic factor (an'tīhē'mōfil'-ik). See **factor VII.**

antihistamine (an'tīhis'təmin), a drug that counteracts the release of histamine such as occurs in allergic reactions; also has topical anesthetic and sedative effects, as well as a drying effect on the nasal mucosa.

antihistaminic (an'tīhistəmin'ik), referring to a drug that acts to prevent or antagonize the pharmacologic effects of histamine released in the tissues.

antihypertensive drugs, agents that lower or reduce high blood pressure.

antihypnotic (an'tīhipnot'ik), preventing or hindering sleep. (not current)

antiinflammatory agents, compounds that counteract or reduce inflammation.

antiinflammatory agents, nonsteroidal, usually salicylates and salicylate-like substances that inhibit prostaglandin biosynthesis.

antiinflammatory agents, steroidal, a group of glucocorticoids used to reduce inflammation that is usually associated with joint pathology.

antileptic (an'tilep'tik), assisting, supporting, revulsive.

anti-Monson curve. See **curve, reverse.** (not current)

antinomy, a bluish crystalline metallic element occurring in nature both free and as salts. Antinomy compounds are used in the treatment of filariasis, leihmaniasis, and other parasitic diseases. Antinomy is also used as an emetic.

antineoplastic agent, a drug that prevents the development, maturation, or spread of neoplastic cells.

antiodontalgic, pertaining to a toothache remedy.

antioxidants, agents that reduce or prevent oxidation, such as occurs in the deterioration of fats, oils, and nonprecious metals.

antiphlogistic (an'tīflōjis'tik), an obsolete term for antiinflammatory or antipyretic.

antiplaque agents, compounds that inhibit, control, or kill organisms associated with dental plaque formation.

antipruritic (an'tīprŏŏrit'ik), relieving or preventing itching.

antipyretic (an'tīpīret'ik), a drug that reduces fever primarily through action on the hypothalamus, thereby resulting in increased heat dissipation through augmented peripheral blood flow and sweating.

antipyrine, an analgesic and antipyretic used in conjunction with salicylates.

antisepsis (an'tisep'sis), the prevention of infection of a body surface, usually skin or oral mucosa, through the application of an antimicrobial agent.

antiseptic (an'tisep'tik), an antimicrobial agent for application to a body surface, usually skin or oral mucosa, in an attempt to prevent or minimize infection at the area of application.

antisialic (an'tīsīal'ik), checking or that which checks salivary secretions.

antisialogogue (an'tīsīal'əgawg), a drug that reduces, slows, or prevents the flow of saliva. (not current)

antispasmodic (an'tīspazmod'ik) (antispastic), a drug that relieves muscle spasms.

antispastic. See **antispasmodic.**

antistreptolysin O (an'tīstreptol'əsin), an antibody against streptolysin O, a hemolysin produced by group A streptococci. A high titer is supporting evidence of rheumatic fever.

antitarter dentifrice, a toothpaste that contains antiplaque agents. (not current)

antithelmintics, agents used to destroy intestinal worms.

antithermic, reducing temperature. See also **antipyretic.**

antitussive (an'tītəs'iv), a drug that relieves or prevents cough.

antitoxin, a subgroup of antisera usually prepared from the serum of horses immunized against a particular toxin-producing organism, such as botulism antitoxin and diphtheria antitoxin given prophylactically to prevent those infections.

Antoni type tissue. See **tissue, Antoni types A and B.** (not current)

antrodynia (an′trōdĭ′nē·ə), pain in the maxillary antrum. (not current)

antrostomy (antros′təmē), a surgical opening into an antrum, either through the medial wall into the nose or through the lateral wall into the oral cavity.

antrum (an′trəm), a maxillary sinus. A cavity in the maxilla, lined by ciliated columnar epithelium, the inferior border of which approximates the apices of the roots of the maxillary posterior teeth.

a. of Highmore. See **sinus, maxillary.**

a., maxillary. See **sinus, maxillary.**

antuitrin S (antu′itrin) (not current). See **hormone, pregnancy.**

ANUG, the abbreviation for **acute necrotizing ulcerative gingivitis.** A distinct, recurrent periodontal disease primarily involving the interdental papillae, which undergo necrosis and ulceration.

anxiety, a condition of heightened and often disruptive tension accompanied by an ill-defined and distressing aura of impending harm or injury. Anxiety can disrupt physiologic functions through its effect on the autonomic nervous system. The patient may assume a tense posture, show excessive vigilance, move the hands and feet restlessly, and speak with a strained, uneven voice. The pupils may be widely dilated, giving the appearance of unrestrained fright, and the hands and face may perspire excessively. In extremely acute forms the patient may have generalized visceral reactions of respiratory, cardiac, vascular, and gastrointestinal dysfunction. The dentist must recognize the existence of anxiety, seek its etiology and relation to dental treatment, and determine ways that the patient's defenses against anxiety can be used to facilitate rather than inhibit treatment.

a. neurosis, an extreme manifestation of anxiety characterized by acute anxiety attacks (sympathetic overreactivity) and phobias, causing avoidance of the anxiety-provoking situations.

aorta, the main arterial trunk of the systemic circulation. Consists of four parts: the ascending aorta, the arch of the aorta, the thoracic portion of descending aorta, and the abdominal portion of the descending aorta.

aortic aneurysm, a localized dilatation or ballooning of the wall of the aorta caused by atherosclerosis, hypertension, or a combination.

aortic valve, a valve in the heart between the left ventricle and the aorta; also known as the *tricuspid valve.*

apathic (əpath′ik), without sensation or feeling.

apathism (ap′əthizm), the state of being slow in responding to stimuli.

Signs of anxiety

Appearance	Avoids focusing on feelings
↑ Muscle tension (rigidity)	Focuses on equipment or procedures
Skin blanches, pales	
↑ Perspiration, clammy skin	**Physiologic Signs Mediated through**
Fatigue	**Autonomic Nervous System**
↑ Small motor activity (e.g., restlessness, tremor)	↑ Heart rate
	↑ Rate or depth of respirations
Behavior	Rapid extreme shifts in body temperature, blood
↓ Attention span	pressure, menstrual flow
↓ Ability to follow directions	Diarrhea
↑ Acting out	Urinary urgency
↑ Somatizing	Dryness of mouth
↑ Immobility	↓ Appetite
	↑ Perspiration
Conversation	Dilation of pupils
↑ Number of questions	Signs of anxiety are dependent on the degree of
Constantly seeks reassurance	anxiety. Mild anxiety heightens the use of ca-
Frequently shifts topics of conversation	pacities, whereas severe and panic states se-
Describes fears with sense of helplessness	verely paralyze or overwork capacities.

apatite (ap'ətīt), the inorganic mineral substance of teeth and bone. See also **carbonate hydroxyapatite.**

A-P discrepancy. See **anterior-posterior discrepancy.**

APC. See **aspirin, phenacetin, caffeine.**

apertognathia (aper'tōnath'ē-ə), "open-bite" deformity. An occlusion characterized by a vertical separation between the maxillary and mandibular anterior teeth. Incorrectly called an *open bite.*

Apert's syndrome. See **syndrome, Apert's.**

aperture, an opening.

apex, the end of the root.

a. blunderbuss, an open or everted apex of a tooth, resembling the divergent form of the barrel of a blunderbuss rifle.

apexification (āpek'sifikāshən), the process of induced root development or apical closure of the root by hard tissue deposition.

apexigraph (āpek'sigraf), a device for determining the position of the apex of a tooth root.

APF, the abbreviation for **acidulated phosphate fluoride,** an agent used as a dental caries preventive and suggested by some for the control of plaque.

aphagia (əfā'jē·ə), the inability to swallow.

aphasia (əfā'zhə), a loss of power of expression through speech, writing, or signs of comprehension of spoken or written language resulting from disease or injury of the brain centers.

aphtha (af'thə) (aphthous stomatitis), **1.** a small ulcer on the mucous membrane. **2.** *pl.* **-hae** vesicles that undergo subsequent ulceration and are surrounded by a raised erythematous area.

a., Bednar's (bed'narz) (ptcrygoid ulcer), an ulcer on the soft palate near the greater palatine foramen; seen in newborns.

a., Mikulicz' (mik'ulich), a recurrent ulceration of the oral mucosa, resembling herpes. See also **periadenitis mucosa necrotica recurrens.**

a., recurrent. See **stomatitis, herpetic** and **ulcer, aphthous, recurrent.**

a., recurrent scarring. See **periadenitis mucosa necrotica recurrens.**

aphthosis, a clinical manifestation of apthae.

aphthous, characterized by aphthae or aphthosis.

a. fever, a fever associated with aphthosis.

a. pharyngitis, aphthosis of the pharynx.

a. stomatitis (af'thus). See **aphtha; stomatitis, aphthous;** and **stomatitis, herpetic.**

apical (ap'ikəl), pertaining to the end portion of the root.

a. curettage, surgical removal of diseased tissue surrounding a root apex.

a. fiber. See **fiber, apical.**

apicectomy (ap'isek'təmē). See **apicoectomy.**

apicoectomy (ap'ikŏck'təmē) (apicectomy, apiectomy, root amputation, root resection), the surgical removal of the apex or apical portion of a root.

apiectomy (ap'ēek'təmē) (not current). See **apicoectomy.**

aplasia (əplā'zhə), a lack of origin or development (for example, aplasia of dentition associated with ectodermal dysplasia).

a. of dentition. See **anodontia.**

apnea (apnē'·ə, ap'nē·ə), a temporary cessation of respiratory movements.

apneumatic (apnōōma'tik), free from air; used to describe something accomplished with the exclusion of air, such as an apneumatic operation. (not current)

apoplexy (ap'ōplek'sē), a stroke caused by acute vascular lesions of the brain.

apoptosis, cell reduction by fragmentation into membrane-bound particles that are phagacytosed by other cells.

apostematosa, cheilitis glandularis. See **cheilitis glandularis apostematosa.**

apothecaries' system. See **system, apothecaries'.** (not current)

apoxesis (ap'əksē'sis). See **curettage, apical.**

apparatus (ap'əra'tus), an arrangement of a number of parts that act together to perform some special function.

a., attachment, the tissues that invest and support the teeth for function: the cementum, periodontal ligament, and alveolar bone.

a., masticating, the structures involved in chewing (that is, the teeth,

A

mandibular musculature, mandible and its temporomandibular joints, accessory mandibular and facial musculature, and tongue), which are controlled by an exquisitely functioning neuromuscular mechanism. See also **system, stomatognathic.**

appellant (əpel′ənt), the party who, dissatisfied with the disposition of a case on the trial level, appeals to a higher court.

appendicitis, an inflammation of the vermiform appendix, usually acute, which if undiagnosed and not surgically removed, leads rapidly to perforation and peritonitis.

appendix, an accessory part of a main structure; in human anatomy, generally refers to the *vermiform appendix,* which is located at the junction of the small and large intestine.

appetite, a natural or instinctive desire for food.

appliance (əpli′əns), a device used to provide function or therapeutic effect. See also **restoration.**

a., Andresen removable orthodontic, an appliance intended to function as a passive transmitter and sometimes stimulator of the forces of the perioral muscles. One of the activator types of orthodontic appliances that induces or directs oral forces to contribute to improved tooth position and jaw relationship.

a., Begg fixed orthodontic, an appliance developed by P.R. Begg, based on a modified ribbon-arch attachment.

a., Bimler removable orthodontic, an activator-type appliance.

a., chin cup extraoral orthodontic, an extraoral traction appliance used to restrain the forward positioning of the mandible and/or the forward growth of the mandible.

a., Crozat removable orthodontic, a wrought wire appliance originally introduced by George Crozat in VXX.

a., edgewise fixed orthodontic, an orthodontic appliance, the last of those developed by E.H. Angle, characterized by attachment brackets with a rectangular slot for engagement of a round or rectangular arch wire.

a., extraoral orthodontic, a device that uses a portion of the face, neck, or back of the head as a base from which to deliver traction force to the teeth or jaws.

a., fixed orthodontic, an appliance that is cemented to the teeth or attached by an adhesive material.

a., fracture (biphase pin fixation, external pin fixation, Stader splint), any one of the various devices for extraoral reduction and fixation of fractures in which pins, clamps, or screws are placed in the fractured segments, the fractured parts aligned, and then the pins, clamps, or screws joined with metal bars or rigid plastic connectors (for example, the Stader splint or Roger-Anderson pin-fixation appliance).

a., Frankel removable orthodontic, an activator-type appliance developed by Rolf Frankel.

a., Hawley retaining orthodontic. See **retainer.**

a., hay rake fixed orthodontic, a device used to limit abnormal swallowing excursions of the tongue. In this manner, harmful effects of tongue thrusting are mitigated until the patient learns a new swallowing pattern.

a., intraoral orthodontic, a device placed inside the mouth to correct or alleviate a malocclusion.

a., Kloehn cervical extraoral orthodontic, the classical cervical extraoral traction appliance introduced by S.J. Kloehn. Uses a relatively light and flexible (0.045 inch; 1.15 mm) inner arch rigidly attached to a long outer bow.

a., labiolingual fixed orthodontic, an appliance using the maxillary and mandibular first permanent molars as anchorage, with labial arches 0.036 to 0.040 inch (0.090 to 0.10 cm) in diameter introduced into horizontal buccal tubes attached to the anchor bands and lingual arches of the same diameter fitted into vertical or horizontal tubes fastened to the lingual side of the anchor bands.

a., obturator. See **obturator.**

a., orthodontic, a device used for influencing tooth position. Orthodontic appliances may be classified as fixed or removable, active or retaining, and intraoral or extraoral.

a., pin and tube fixed orthodontic, a labial arch with vertical posts that insert into tubes attached to bands on the teeth.

a., prosthetic (archaic term; generally not used to refer to a prosthesis), a complete or partial denture for children when groups of teeth are lost or are congenitally missing. Used to maintain space or masticatory function or for esthetic reasons.

a., removable orthodontic, an appliance designed so that it can be removed and replaced by the patient.

a., retaining orthodontic, an orthodontic device used to hold the teeth in place, following orthodontic tooth movement, until the occlusion is stabilized.

a., straight-wire fixed orthodontic, a variation of the edgewise appliance in which an effort is made to obviate the need for many arch-wire adjustments by reorientation of the arch-wire slots. The first such modifications were introduced by E.H. Angle; L.M Andrews first proposed such variations in all planes of space.

a., therapeutic, a vehicle used to transport and retain some agent for therapeutic purposes (for example, a radium carrier).

a., twin-wire fixed orthodontic, an orthodontic appliance developed by J F Johnson, typically using a pair of 0.010-inch (0.25-mm) wires to form the midsection of the arch wire.

a., universal fixed orthodontic, an orthodontic appliance developed by S.R. Atkinson, combining some of the principles of edgewise and ribbon-arch appliances with very light arch wires.

application program, a standard and frequently used computer program tailored to medical and dental needs. It may be supplied to the user by the manufacturer, purchased from a software house, or written by the user.

applicator, a device for applying medication; usually a slender rod of glass or wood, used with a pledget of cotton on the end.

appointment, a mutually agreed-on time reserved for the patient to receive treatment.

a. book, a ledger or table of workdays divided into segments of time to enable the dentist to reserve specified lengths of time for patient treatment.

a. card, a small card given to the patient as a reminder of the time reserved for the appointment.

apposition (ap′əsish′ən), the condition of being placed or fitted together; juxtaposition; coaptation.

appropriate, 1. the determination that the service provided is suited for the condition. **2.** suitable for a particular person, group, community, condition, occasion, and/or place. **3.** Proper.

approved services, 1. all services provided in a dental plan. In some plans, authorization must be obtained before approved service is provided; other plans make exception for treatment of emergency needs; still others require no prior authorization for any treatment approved under the program. **2.** dental services that meet quality standards maintained in a dental plan.

approximal (approximating), contiguous; adjacent; next to each other.

approximating. See **approximal.**

apraclonidine, *trade name:* Iopidine; *drug class:* selective α_2-adrenergic agonist; *action:* reduces intraocular pressure; *uses:* control or prevention of increases in intraocular pressure related to laser surgery of eye.

apraxia (əprak′sē-ə), a loss of ability to execute a purposeful, goal-oriented, or skilled act resulting from selective damage to certain high-level brain centers, either sensory, motor, or both.

apron, a piece of clothing worn in front of the body for protection.

a. band, a labioincisal or gingival extension of an orthodontic band that aids in retention of the band and in proper positioning of the bracket.

a., lead, an apron made of materials containing metallic lead or lead compounds used to reduce radiation hazards.

a., lingual. See **connector, linguoplate major.**

a., rubber dam, a small strip of rubber dam, perforated to fit over an implant abutment that is used to inhibit introduction of cement into the peri-implant space.

aprotinin, a protease and kallikrein inhibitor useful in the treatment of pancreatitis.

aptitude, a natural ability. Usually refers to the quickness to learn, understand, or acquire a skill.

arachidonic acid, an essential fatty acid that is a component of lecithin and a basic material for the biosynthesis of some prostaglandins.

ARC, the abbreviation for **AIDS-related complex.** See also **acquired immunodeficiency syndrome.**

arc, reflex, a system of nerves used in a reflex or involuntary act, consisting primarily of an afferent nerve with sensory receptor, a nerve center, and an efferent nerve that stimulates the effector muscle or gland.

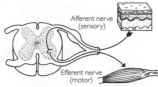

Simple reflex arc. (Modified from Ruby, 1984.)

arch(*pl.* **es),** a structure with a curved outline.

a., bar. See **bar, arch.**

a., basal. See **base, apical.**

a., dental, the composite structure of the dentition and alveolar ridge or the remains thereof after the loss of some or all of the natural teeth.

   a., d., contraction. See **contraction.**

a., dentulous dental, a dental arch containing natural teeth.

a., edentulous dental, a dental arch from which all natural teeth are missing. The residual alveolar ridge.

a. expansion. See **expansion.**

a. form. See **form, arch.**

a., high labial, a labial arch wire adapted so that it lies gingival to the anterior tooth crowns; it has auxiliary springs extending downward in contact with the teeth to be moved.

a. length, the length of a dental arch, usually measured through the points of contact between adjoining teeth.

   a. l., available, the space available for all teeth.

   a. l., deficiency, the difference between required and available arch length.

   a. l., required, the sum of the mesiodistal widths of all teeth.

a., ovoid, an arch that curves continuously from the molars on one side to the molars on the opposite side so that two such arches placed back to back describe an oval.

a., palatine (glossopalatine arch), the pillars of the fauces; the two arches of mucous membrane enclosing the muscles at the sides of the passage from the mouth to the pharynx.

a., partially edentulous dental, a dental arch from which one or more but not all teeth are missing.

a., passive lingual, an orthodontic appliance effective in maintaining space and preserving arch length when bilateral primary molars are prematurely lost.

a., pharyngeal, the branchial arches of the fetus.

a., removable lingual, an arch wire designed to fit the lingual surface of the teeth. It has two posts soldered on each end that fit snugly into the vertical tubes of the molar anchor bands.

a., stationary lingual, an arch wire designed to fit the lingual surface of the teeth and soldered to the anchor bands.

a., tapering, a dental arch that converges from molars to central incisors to such an extent that lines passing through the central grooves of the molars and premolars intersect within 1 inch (2.5 cm) anterior to the central incisors.

a., trapezoidal, an arch that has the same convergence as a tapering arch but to a lesser degree. The anterior teeth are somewhat square to abruptly rounded from canine tip to canine tip. The canines act as corners of the arch.

a., U-shaped, a dental arch in which there is little difference in diameter (width) between the first premolars and the last molars; the curve from canine to canine is abrupt, so a dental arch in the shape of a capital U is formed.

a. width, the width of a dental arch. The width, which varies in all diameters between the right and left opposites, is determined by direct measurement between the canines, between the first molars, and between the second premolars. These intercanine, interpremolar, and intermolar distances can be cited as arch width.

a. wire, a wire applied to two or more teeth through fixed attachments to cause or guide orthodontic tooth movement.

a. w., full, a wire extending from the molar region of one side of an arch to the other.

a. w., sectional, a wire extending to only a few teeth, usually on one side or in the anterior segment.

architecture, in medicine and dentistry, usually refers to the framework of a structure or system.

a., gingival. See **gingival architecture.**

archiving, the storage of older, rarely required data or patient information in a cheaper and/or more compact form.

arcus senilis (ar′kəs seni′lis), an opaque, grayish-white ring at the periphery of the cornea occurring in older adults.

area, region.

a., apical. See **base, apical.**

a., basal seat (denture-bearing area, denture-supporting area, stress-bearing area, stress-supporting area), the portion of the oral structures available to support a denture.

a., contact. See **point, contact.**

a., denture-bearing. See **area, basal seat.**

a., denture-supporting. See **area, basal seat.**

a., impression, the surface of the oral structures recorded in an impression.

a., pear-shaped. See **pad, retromolar.**

a., post dam. See **area, posterior palatal seal.**

a., posterior palatal seal, the soft tissues along the junction of the hard and soft palates on which compression, within the physiologic limits of the tissues, can be applied by a denture to aid in its retention.

a., postpalatal seal. See **area, posterior palatal seal.**

a., pressure, an area of excessive displacement of soft tissue by a prosthesis.

a., recipient, the portion of the body on which a skin, bone, tooth, or other graft is placed.

a., relief, the portion of the surface of the mouth under prosthesis on which pressures are reduced or eliminated.

a., rest (rest seat), the prepared surface of a tooth or fixed restoration into which the rest fits, giving support to a removable partial denture.

a., rugae (roo′jē) (rugae zone), that portion of the hard palate in which rugae are found.

a., saddle. See **area, basal seat.**

a., stress-bearing. See **area, basal seat.**

a., stress-supporting. See **area, basal seat.**

a., supporting, the areas of the maxillary and mandibular edentulous ridges best suited to carry the forces of mastication when the dentures are in use. See also **area, basal seat.**

arginine, one of the essential amino acids for infants and children. See also **amino acid.**

Argyll Robertson pupil (argil′). See **pupil, Argyll Robertson.**

argyria (arjir′ē-ə), a bluish color of the skin or mucous membranes produced by the deposition of silver salts in collagen fibers after prolonged use of silver salts.

a., local, a localized blue pigmentation of the oral mucosa from the deposition of silver amalgam in the submucosal connective tissue.

argyrosis (arjirō′sis), a pathologic bluish-black pigmentation in a tissue resulting from the deposition of an insoluble albuminate of silver.

ariboflavinosis (əri′bōflavinō′sis), a nutritional disease resulting from a deficiency of riboflavin (vitamin B_2); characterized by angular cheilosis, seborrheic dermatitis, a magenta tongue, and ocular disturbance. (not current)

Arkansas stone (ar′kansô). See **stone, Arkansas.**

arm, an extension or projection of a removable partial denture framework.

a., reciprocal, a clasp arm used on a removable partial denture to oppose any force arising from an opposing clasp arm on the same tooth. See also **arm, retention.**

a., retention, an extension or projection that is part of a removable partial denture and is used to aid in the retention and stabilization of the restoration. See also **retainer divet.**

a., truss. See **connector, minor.**

a., upright. See **connector, minor.**

armamentarium (ar′məmenta′rē-əm), the equipment and materials of a practitioner.

arrangement, the pattern into which a group of things is organized.

a., financial, an agreement between the dentist and patient on the method of handling the patient's account.

a., tooth, the placement of teeth on a denture or temporary base with definite objectives in mind.

arrhythmia (ərith′mē-ə), a variation from the normal rhythm of the heart.

arrow point tracer (not current). See **tracer, needle point.**

art, in medicine and dentistry, usually refers to the skill, craftsmanship, or facility in one's work.

arteriole (artē′rē-ōl), a minute arterial branch proximal to a capillary.

arteriosclerosis (artē′rē-ōsklerō′sis), a term applied to a group of diseases that affect the elasticity of the blood vessels. It may refer to atherosclerosis, hyperplastic arteriosclerosis, or Monckeberg's sclerosis. These degenerative processes generally affect only the tunica media and tunica intima. The effect is narrowing of the lumen of a blood vessel, causing rupture of the blood vessel or ischemia of an area of tissue that the vessel supplies.

arteriosclerotic heart disease (artē′-rē-ōsklerot′ik), See **disease, heart, arteriosclerotic.**

arteriovenous shunt (artē′rē-ōvē′nus). See **shunt, arteriovenous.**

arteritis, an inflammatory condition of the inner layers or the outer coat of one or more arteries. It may occur as a separate clinical entity or accompanying another disorder, such as rheumatoid arthritis, rheumatic fever, or systemic lupus erythematosus.

a., temporal (ar′terī′tis), an inflammation of the temporal artery that produces a nodular, tortuous swelling of the temporal artery accompanied by a burning, throbbing pain, initially in the teeth, temporomandibular joint, and eye, but ultimately localized over the artery. This disorder occurs primarily in persons over 55 years of age.

artery, a blood vessel through which the blood passes from the heart to the various structures of the body. There are three layers of tissue in every artery: the inner coat (tunica intima), composed of an inner endothelial lining, connective tissue, and an outer layer of elastic tissue (inner elastic membrane); the middle coat (tunica media), composed chiefly of muscle

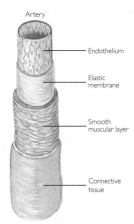

Artery cross-section. (Thibodeau, 1996).

tissue; and the outer coat (tunica adventitia), composed chiefly of connective tissue. The structure of the three layers varies with the location, size, and purpose of the blood vessel.

a. arthograms, an x-ray of a joint usually with the introduction of a contrast compound into the joint capsule. In dentistry, an arthogram usually involves the temporomandibular joint.

a., large, an elastic artery with an abundant supply of elastic tissue and a great reduction of smooth muscle. The tunica intima is thick, and the endothelial cells are round or polygonal. The tunica media is the thickest of the three layers. It contains few smooth muscle fibers, and its outer border has a special concentration of elastic fibers—the external elastic membrane. The tunica adventitia is relatively thin and ill defined and is continuous with the loose connective tissue surrounding the vessel.

a., medium-sized, most of the arteries in the body (for example, facial, maxillary, radial, ulnar, and popliteal). Thick muscular bands are found in the tunica media. Thin elastic fibers course circularly in the tunica media and run longitudinally in the tunica adventitia. The tunica adventitia is as thick as the tunica media, and its outer layer gradually blends with the connective tissue that supports the artery and surrounding structures.

arthralgia (arthral'jē-ə), pain in a joint or joints.

arthritis (ärthrī'tis), any of a number of types of inflammation of a joint or joints.

a., allergic, arthralgia, swelling, and stiffness of joints associated with food and drug allergies and serum sickness.

a., atrophic. See **arthritis, rheumatoid.**

a., bacterial. See **arthritis, infective.**

a., hypertrophic. See **osteoarthritis.**

a., infective (bacterial arthritis), a primary and secondary bacterial infection of the joints (for example, by staphylococcal, gonococcal, streptococcal, or pneumococcal organisms).

a., rheumatic (rōōmat'ik), an acute polyarticular and migratory arthritis of unknown cause but assumed to be related to group A streptococcal infection of the upper respiratory tract.

a., rheumatoid (rōō'mətoid), a chronic destructive inflammation of the joints of unknown origin, with associated constitutional manifestations. Chronic synovitis and regressive changes in the articular cartilage occur with pain, swelling, deformity, limitation of motion, and occasionally ankylosis of the joints. Variable systemic manifestations include weakness, loss of weight, anemia, leukopenia, splenomegaly, lymphadenopathy, and the formation of subcutaneous nodules. Small joints are principally affected. In most instances, onset is in the third or fourth decade of life.

a., senile, arthritis occurring in persons of advanced age.

a., specific infectious, arthritis caused by direct invasion and subsequent infection of joint structures by microorganisms from the bloodstream. Nearly all pathogenic bacteria have been isolated as etiologic agents.

a., traumatic, an acute or chronic inflammation of a joint as a result of acute or chronic injury.

Arthrobacter, a genus of a strictly aerobic gram-positive bacteria found in soil and present in dental caries.

arthroplasty (är'thrəplas'tē), the surgical correction of a joint abnormality.

a., gap. See **gap arthroplasty.**

a., interposition. See **interposition arthroplasty.**

arthroscope, an instrument to view the inside of a joint.

arthrostomy (arthros'təmē), the surgical formation of an opening into a joint.

articular cartilage. See **cartilage, articular.**

articulare, the point of intersection of the dorsal contour of the mandibular condyle and the temporal bone.

articulate, (artik'yōōlāt), **1.** to arrange or place in connected sequence. See also **arrangement, tooth. 2.** to connect by articulating strips, paper, or cloth coated with ink-containing or dye-containing wax, used for marking or locating occlusal contacts.

articulation (artik'yōōlā'shən), **1.** a joint. See also **joint. 2.** the relationship of cusps of teeth during jaw movement.

a., anatomic, a rigid or movable junction of a bony part.

a., articulator, the use of a device that incorporates artificial temporomandibular joints that permit the orientation of casts in a manner duplicating or simulating various positions or movements of the mandible.

a., balanced, the simultaneous contacting of the upper and lower teeth as they glide over each other when the mandible is moved from centric relation to the various eccentric relations. See also **occlusion, balanced.**

a., mandibular. See **articulation, temporomandibular.**

a., temporomandibular (temporomandibular joint, mandibular joint), **1.** the joint formed by the two condyles of the mandible. **2.** the bilateral articulation between the glenoid or mandibular fossae of the temporal bones and condyles (condyloid processes) of the mandible. The structures that make up the temporomandibular joint include the mandibular fossae of the temporal bones, articular disks, mandibular condyles, and articular tubercles of the zygomatic process of the temporal bone.

a., t., capsule, the ligamentous covering of the temporomandibular joint.

a., t., collagen disease, rheumatoid arthritis in which the joint may be so involved because of bone changes that the mandibular condyle is fused to the articular fossa in the base of the cranium.

a., t., hormonal disturbances, hormonal disorders that frequently affect growth patterns of the skeleton, involving the temporomandibular joint (for example, acromegaly).

a., t., neuromuscular disorders, neuromuscular disorders involving the temporomandibular joint, in which the patient is unable to maintain appropriate patterns of mandibular closure consistent with good dental occlusion. The natural teeth degenerate rapidly and are frequently lost prematurely; when dentures are substituted, they cause the residual tissues to deteriorate rapidly. In addition to the chronic masticatory disability, the deglutitive mechanism functions poorly because of incoordinated lip and tongue action.

a., t., pain-dysfunction syndrome. See **temporomandibular joint pain-dysfunction syndrome.**

articulator (artik′yo͞olātŏr), a mechanical device that represents the temporomandibular joints and jaw members to which maxillary and mandibular casts may be attached.

a., adjustable, an articulator that may be adjusted to permit movement of the casts into various recorded eccentric relationships.

artifact (ar′tifakt), a blemish or image in the radiograph that is not present in the roentgen image of the object.

artificial intelligence (A-I), a system that makes it possible for a machine to perform functions similar to human intelligence. Computer technology produces many systems and functions that mimic and surpass some human capabilities, such as chess.

artificial organs, devices used to support life because of the failure or limited capacity of the human organ. The most effective is the artificial kidney, which consists of a set of tubes that pass the blood through a dialysate solution where wastes are removed by osmosis and diffusion.

artificial respiration. See **respiration, artificial.**

artificial stone. See **stone, artificial.**

aryepiglottic (er′ē-ep′iglot′ik) (not current). See **arytenoepiglottic.**

arytenoepiglottic (er′ēte′nō-ep′iglot′-ik)

(aryepiglottic), pertaining to the arytenoid cartilage and the epiglottis.

asbestos, a group of fibrous impure magnesium silicate minerals. Inhalation of the fibers can lead to pulmonary fibrosis.

Ascaris, a genus of large parasitic intestinal roundworms such as *Ascaris lumbricoides.*

Aschheim-Zondek (AZ) test (ash′hīm tson′dek) (not current). See **test, pregnancy.**

ascites (əsī′tēz), an abnormal accumulation of serous fluid, containing large amounts of protein and electrolytes, in the peritoneal cavity. Ascites is a complication of cirrhosis, congestive heart failure, nephrosis, malignant neoplastic disease, and various fungal and parasitic diseases.

ascorbic acid (vitamin C), *trade name:* Generic; many brand names; *drug class:* Vitamin C, water-soluble vitamin; *action:* needed for wound healing, collagen synthesis, antioxidant, carbohydrate metabolism; *uses:* Vitamin C deficiency, scurvy, delayed wound and bone healing, chronic disease, urine acidification, before gastrectomy.

asepsis (əsep′sis), without infection; free of viable pathogenic microorganisms.

aseptic, not producing microorganisms or free from microorganisms.

asialia (ə′sēa′lē-ə). See **asialorrhea.**

asialorrhea (əsī′əlōrē′·ə) (asialia), a decrease in or lack of salivary flow. See also **hyposalivation.**

asjike (əsji′ke) (not current). See **beriberi.**

asparagine, a nonessential amino acid found in many proteins in the body.

aspartame, a low-calorie sweetening agent about 200 times as sweet as sucrose.

aspect, buccal, the facial surface or cheek side of posterior teeth.

aspergillosis, an infection caused by a fungus of the genus *Aspergillus.* Most commonly affects the ear but is capable of causing inflammatory, granlomatous lesions on or in any organ.

Aspergillus, a genus of fungi that is a common contaminant in the laboratory and a cause of nosocomial infection. See also aspergillosis.

asphyxia (asfik′sē-ə), a condition of suffocation resulting from restriction of oxygen intake and interference with the elimination of carbon dioxide.

aspirate (as'pirāt), **1.** to draw or breathe in. **2.** to remove materials by vacuum. **3.** a phonetic unit whose identifying characteristic is the sound generated by the passage of air through a relatively open channel; the sound of *h;* a sound followed by or combined with the sound of *h.*

aspiration (as'pirā'shən), **1.** the act of breathing or drawing in. **2.** the removal of fluids, gases, or solids from a cavity by means of a vacuum pump.

a. biopsy. See **biopsy, aspiration.**

a. pneumonia, pneumonia produced by aspiration of foreign material into the lungs.

aspirator (as'pirātor), an apparatus used for removal of fluids, gases, or solids from a cavity by vacuum.

aspirin, *trade name:* ASA, Aspirin, Ecotrin; *drug class:* nonnarcotic analgesic salicylate; *action:* inhibits prostaglandin synthesis, possesses analgesic, antiinflammatory, antipyretic properties; *uses:* mild to moderate pain or fever.

a. burn. See **burn, aspirin.**

aspirin, phenacetin, caffeine (APC, PAC), a pharmaceutical preparation used as an analgesic.

assault, an intentional, unlawful offer of bodily injury to another by force or unlawfully directing force toward another person to create a reasonable fear of imminent danger, coupled with the apparent ability to do the harm threatened if not prevented. A completed assault is a battery. In a medical setting, the unconsented touching of the body would be an assault and battery.

assertiveness, a form of behavior that is directed toward claiming one's rights without denying the rights of others.

assets, everything a business owns or that is owned. Cash, investments, money due, materials, and inventories are current assets. Buildings and equipment are fixed assets. Goodwill is an intangible asset.

assignment of benefits, a procedure whereby a beneficiary or patient authorizes the administrator of the program to forward payment for a cov-

ered procedure directly to the treating dentist.

assistant, an agent or employee.

a., dental, an auxiliary to the dentist. See also **certified dental assistant.**

association, a connection, union, joining, or combination of things.

astemizole, *trade name:* Hismanel; *drug class:* antihistamine, H_1-histamine antagonist; *action:* decreases allergic response by blocking pharmacologic effects of histamine; *uses:* rhinitis, allergy symptoms.

asthenia (asthē'nē-ə), the loss of vitality or strength; a condition of debility; weakness.

asthenic (asthēn'ik), a term describing an individual with a long, slender appearance who is thin and flat chested and has long limbs and a short trunk; comparable to the ectomorph in Sheldon's classification.

asthma (az'mə), paroxysmal wheezing and difficulty in breathing resulting from bronchospasms. Frequently has an allergic basis and occasionally an emotional origin.

a., cardiac, shortness of breath (paroxysmal dyspnea), sonorous rales, and expiratory wheezes that resemble bronchial asthma; related to cardiac failure.

astigmatism (əstig'mətizəm), a defective curvature of the refractive surfaces of the eye, resulting in a condition in which a ray of light is not focused sharply in the retina but is spread over a more or less diffuse area.

astringent (əstrin'jənt), styptic; an agent that checks the secretions of mucous membranes and contracts and hardens tissues, limiting the secretions of glands.

astrocytes, a large, star-shaped cell found in certain tissues of the nervous system.

astrocytoma, a primary tumor of the brain composed of astrocytes and characterized by slow growth, cyst formation, invasion of surrounding structures, and often, the development of a highly malignant glioblastoma within the primary tumor mass.

asymmetric (ā'sime'trik), unevenly arranged; out of balance; not the same on both sides; not a mirror image on both sides.

A

asynergy (āsin′ərjē), a lack of muscular coordination in special functions (for example, hand-to-mouth movements for feeding).

asystole (āsis′təlē), the faulty contraction of the ventricles of the heart, resulting in incomplete or imperfect systole.

ataractic (at′ərak′tik) (ataraxic, tranquilizer), one of a poorly defined group of drugs designed to produce ataraxia. The former concept, that the use of ataractics involved no mental or motor impairment, is subject to question.

ataraxia (at′ərak′sē·ə), a state of complete serenity without impairment of mental or physical functions. (not current)

ataxia (ətak′sē·ə), a muscular incoordination characterized by irregular muscle activity.

a., locomotor. See **tabes dorsalis.**

atelectasis (at′ilek′təsis), the complete or partial collapse of a lung.

atenolol, *trade name:* Nova-Atenol, Tenormin; *drug class:* antihypertensive, selective β_1 blocker; *action:* produces fall in blood pressure without reflex tachycardia or significant reduction in heart rate; *uses:* acute myocardial infaction, mild-to moderate hypertension, prophylaxis of angina pectoris.

atherosclerosis (ath′ərōsklərō′sis), a degenerative disease principally affecting the aorta and its major branches, the coronary artery, and the larger cerebral arteries. The arterial changes include narrowing of the lumen of the vessels; weakening of the arterioles, leading to rupture; an increased tendency toward development of atheromatous plaques; and thrombi. Atherosclerosis is a common cause of coronary thrombosis, congestive heart failure, aneurysms, hemorrhage, cerebral infarcts, and apoplexy.

athetosis (ath′ətō′sis), a neuromuscular impairment in which extensive twisting and swaying spasms of the skeletal musculature interfere with voluntary control of movement; the spasms are especially conspicuous and disconcerting during emotional stress and on initiation of conscious voluntary acts.

athiaminosis (əthī′əminō′sis). See **beri-beri.**

athletic (athlet′ik), pertaining to a bodily constitution characterized by a strong, muscular, robust appearance.

a. injuries, injuries sustained by persons while engaged in sports, more frequently while engaged in contact sports such as football.

atlantooccipital joint, one of a pair of condyloid joints formed by the articulation of the atlas of the vertebral column with the occipital bone of the skull.

atlas, the first cervical vertebra articulating above with the occipital bone and below with the axis (second cervical vertebra).

atmosphere (atm), the natural body of air, composed of approximately 20% oxygen, 78% nitrogen, and 2% carbon dioxide and other gases, that cover the surface of the earth.

atom (at′əm), the smallest part of an element capable of entering into a chemical reaction.

atomic (ətom′ik), pertaining to the atom.

a. energy. See **energy, atomic.**

a. mass number (symbol: A), the total number of nucleons (protons and neutrons) of which an atom is composed.

a. number (Z), 1. the number of electrons outside the nucleus of a neutral atom. 2. the number of protons in the nucleus.

a. structure theory, the theory that matter is composed of a vast number of particles, or atoms, bound together by a force of attraction of electrical charges.

a. weight, the weight of one atom of an element as compared with the weight of an atom of hydrogen.

atomizer (at′əmīzər), an apparatus for changing a jet of liquid into a spray.

atopy (ā′topē) (atopic hypersensitivity, "spontaneous" clinical allergy), a group of "allergic" disorders showing a marked familial distribution; although the susceptibility appears to be inherited, contact with the antigen must occur before hypersensitivity can develop. Disorders include asthma or hay fever resulting from pollens and gastrointestinal tract and skin reactions resulting from food.

atovaquone, *trade name:* Mepron; *drug class:* antipneumocystic; *action:* unknown, may inhibit synthesis of ATP and nucleic acids; *uses:* treatment of *Pneumocystis carinii* pneumonia in patients who are intolerant of trimethoprim-sulfamethoxazole.

atresia (ətrē′zē-ə), the congenital absence or occlusion of a normal opening of one or more ducts in an organ.

a., ***aural,*** the absence of closure of the auditory canal.

atrial fibrillation, a heart condition characterized by rapid random contractions of the atria at the rate of 130 to 150 ventricular beats per minute.

atrophy (at′rōfē), a progressive, acquired decrease in the size of a normally developed cell, tissue, or organ. Atrophy may result from a decrease in cell size, number of cells, or both.

a., ***adipose,*** atrophy resulting from a reduction in fatty tissue.

a., ***alveolar,*** a depletion of the size of the alveolar process of the jaws from disuse, overuse, or pathologic disturbance of the bone.

a., ***bone,*** **1.** bone resorption internally (in density) and externally (in form) (for example, of residual ridges). **2.** a loss of bone substance or volume. Atrophy of bone ordinarily occurs without a corresponding change in the volume or external dimensions of bone, but the mass of bone tissue may be reduced as much as 75%. The internal architecture of the bone gradually becomes attenuated and finally disappears. Atrophied bone is brittle and has a more spongy consistency than normal bone. In cross-section the cortex is thin, and the periosteal surface is smooth and unchanged, but the intramedullary substance is composed of a yellow, fatty, cancellous bone tissue. Bone atrophy may be systemic, regional, or local.

a., ***diffuse alveolar.*** See **periodontosis.**

a., ***facial,*** the failure of facial development. If it is bilateral, it may produce brachygnathia; unilateral types, although rare, are more common than the bilateral type. Causes include physical injury, neurovascular disease, and paralysis.

a., ***muscular,*** a wasting of muscle tissue, especially resulting from lack of use. There are numerous causes for simple atrophy of muscle, such as chronic malnutrition, immobilization, and denervation.

a. ***of disuse,*** atrophy resulting from a lack of function of a tissue, organ, or body part.

a., ***periodontal,*** the quantitative degenerative changes that occur in the attachment apparatus and supporting bone of a tooth as a result of disease or disuse. When a tooth loses its antagonist, osteoporotic changes in the supporting bone, an afunctional change in the direction of periodontal fibers, and a narrowing of the periodontal membrane space occur.

a., ***postmenopausal,*** a thinning of the oral mucosa after menopause.

a., ***pressure,*** the tissue destruction and reduction in size as a consequence of prolonged or continued pressure on a local area or group of cells.

a., p., ***by epithelial attachment,*** a theoretical type of atrophy. The theory, advanced to explain destruction of gingival fibers during gingival inflammation, states that gingival fiber degeneration is produced by pressure exerted by the proliferating pocket epithelium. It is now generally conceded that proteolytic substances produced in the tissues during inflammation are responsible for gingival fiber destruction; subsequently, the epithelium can proliferate apically.

a., ***senile,*** the atrophy or diminution of all tissues characteristic of advanced age.

atropine (at′rōpēn), an alkaloid that annuls parasympathetic effects and antagonizes the effects of pilocarpine. It acts directly on the effector cells, preventing the action but not the liberation of acetylcholine. It suppresses sweat and other glandular sections.

a. ***sulfate,*** *trade name:* Sal-Tropine; *drug class:* anticholinergic; *action:* inhibits muscarinic actions of acetylcholine at postganglionic parasympathetic neuroeffector sites; *uses:* reduction of salivary and bronchial secretions.

attached gingiva. See **gingiva, attached.**

A

attachment, 1. to fasten, connect, associate. **2.** a mechanical device for retention and stabilization of a dental prosthesis.

a., abnormal frenum (frē'nəm), aberrant insertions of labial, buccal, or lingual frena capable of initiating or perpetuating periodontal disease, such as creating diastemata between teeth, limiting lip or tongue movement.

a., epithelial, the continuation of the sulcular epithelium that is joined to the tooth structure.

a., gingival, the fibrous attachment of the gingival tissues to the teeth.

a., intracoronal (precision attachment, slotted attachment). See **intracoronal retainer.**

a., migration of epithelial, the apical progression of the epithelial attachment along the tooth root.

a., orthodontic, a device, secured to the crown of a tooth, that serves as a means of attaching the arch wire to the tooth.

a., parallel, a prefabricated device for attaching a denture base to an abutment tooth. Retention is provided by friction between the parallel walls of the two parts of the attachment.

a., precision. See **attachment, intracoronal.**

a., slotted. See **attachment, intracoronal.**

attack, heart. See **thrombosis, coronary.**

attending dentist's statement, a form used to report dental procedures to a third-party payer. The claim form was developed by the American Dental Association. Synonym: dental claim form.

attention, the element of cognitive functioning in which the mental focus is maintained on a specific issue, object, or activity. The length of time of such focus is called *attention span.*

attenuation (əten'ū-ā'shən), the process by which a beam of radiation is reduced in energy when passing through some material.

attitude, a person's mental set, opinion, or disposition.

attraction, the tendency of teeth or other maxillary or mandibular structures to become superior to (elevated above) the normal position.

attrition (ətrish'ən), the normal loss of tooth substance resulting from friction caused by physiologic forces.

attritional occlusion. See **occlusion, attritional.**

atypical (ātip'ikəl), pertaining to deviation from the basic or typical.

Au. See **unit, Angstrom.**

audiogram (ô'dē-əgram'), a graphic summary of the measurements of hearing loss showing the number of decibels lost at each frequency tested.

audiology (ôdē-əl'əjē), the study of the entire field of hearing, including the anatomy and function of the ear; impairment of hearing; and evaluation, education or reeducation, and treatment of persons with hearing loss.

audiometer (ôdē-om'ətər), a device for testing hearing; calibrated to register hearing loss in terms of decibels.

audit, 1. an examination of records or accounts to check accuracy. **2.** a post-treatment record review or clinical examination to verify information reported on claims.

a. of treatment, **1.** an administrative or professional review of a participating dentist's treatment recommendations (per audit). **2.** the review of reimbursement claims for service performed (postaudit).

augmentation (ôg'mentā'shən), **1.** assistance to respiration by the application of intermittent pressure on inspiration. **2.** an increase of the size beyond the existing size, such as an implant placed over the mandibular or maxillary ridges.

auranofin, *trade name:* Ridaura; *drug class:* gold salt; *action:* specific antiinflammatory action unknown; *uses:* rheumatoid arthritis.

Aureomycin (ô'rē-ōmī'sin), the trade name for chlortetracycline.

auricle (ô'rikul), **1.** pinna, the external part of the ear. **2.** atrium, the chamber of the heart that receives the blood: on the right, from the general circulation, and on the left, from the pulmonary circulation.

auricular fibrillation. See **fibrillation, auricular.**

auricular tags, rudimentary appendages of auricular tissue on the face along the line of union of the first branchial arch.

auriculotemporal syndrome. See **syndrome, auriculotemporal.**

aurothioglucose/gold sodium thiomalate, *trade name:* Solganal/Myochrysine; *drug class:* antiinflammatory gold compound; *action:* unknown; may decrease phagocytosis, lysosomal activity, prostaglandin synthesis; *uses:* rheumatoid arthritis; juvenile arthritis.

auscultation (ôskultā'shən), the examination procedure of listening for sounds produced by the body to detect or judge an abnormal condition.

autoclave (ô'tōklāv), an apparatus for effecting sterilization by steam under pressure.

autogenous bone graft. See **graft, autogenous bone.**

autograft. See **graft, autogenous.**

autoantibody, an immunoglobulin that reacts against a normal constituent in a person's body.

autoimmune, the development of an immune response to one's own tissues.

a. disease (ô'tō·imūn'). See **disease, autoimmune.**

automatic condenser. See **condenser, mechanical.**

automatic mallet (not current). See **condenser, mechanical.**

automation, the use of a machine designed to follow repeatedly and automatically a predetermined sequence of individual operations. Automation is used extensively in preparing tissue for microscopic examination.

automatism (ôtom'ətiz'əm), a tendency to take extra or superfluous doses of a drug when under its influence.

autonomic drugs, agents the act on the autonomic nervous system.

autonomic nervous system, the part of the nervous system that regulates involuntary vital function, including the activity of the cardiac muscle, the smooth muscle, and the glands. The autonomic nervous system has two parts: the sympathetic nervous system, which accelerates heart rate, constricts blood vessels, and raises blood pressure; and the parasympathetic nervous system, which slows heart rate, increases intestinal peristalsis and gland activity, and relaxes sphincters.

autopolymer (ô'tōpol'imər), a resin to which certain chemicals have been added to initiate and propagate polymerization without addition of heat.

a. resin. See **resin, autopolymer.**

autopolymerization (ô'tōpol'imərizā'shən) (coldcuring), the accomplishment of polymerization by chemical means without external application of heat or light.

autoprothrombin I (ô'tōprōthrom'bin) (not current). See **factor VII.**

autoprothrombin II (not current). See **factor IX.**

autopsy, a postmortem examination performed to confirm or determine the cause of death.

autoradiography (ô'tōrādēog'rəfē), **1.** a photographic recording of radiation from radioactive material, obtained by placing the surface of the radioactive material in close proximity to a photographic emulsion. **2.** the use of radioactive substances introduced into tissue followed by the placement of a photographic plate on the surface of the tissue preparation, usually employed in cytology and histology.

autosomal dominant disorders, genetic disorders that are transmitted by a dominant gene within an autosomal chromosome as opposed to a sex chromosome.

autosomal recessive disorders, genetic disorders carried by a recessive gene within an autosomal chromosome as opposed to a sex chromosome.

autotransformer, a transformer with a single winding, having a large number of connections, or taps. Used to deliver a precise voltage to the high-tension primary circuit. (not current)

autotransplant. See **graft, autogenous.**

auxiliary personnel, nonprofessional aides who assist the responsible professional in the provision of professional services. Dental hygienists are formally trained and may be licensed or certificated by state authorities. Dental assistants, laboratory technicians, and other auxiliaries may be formally trained.

auxilliary wires, orthodontic wires that support or augment the action of the main or primary arch wire in an orthodontic appliance. The Begg technique and the segmental technique make frequent and regular use of auxilliary wires.

AV, I. the abbreviation for **atrioventricular. 2.** the abbreviation for **auriculoventricular.**

availability, the supply in terms of type, volume, and location of health resources and services relative to the demands of a given individual or community.

average life (mean life), the average of the individual lives of all of the atoms of a particular radioactive substance; 1.443 times radioactive half-life. See also **half-life.**

avidin, a glycoprotein in nondenatured egg whites (raw) that binds biotin and prevents its absorption, causing biotin depletion.

avitaminosis (āvī'təminō'sis), a disease or condition resulting from a deficiency of one or more vitamins in the diet (for example, scurvy, which results from ascorbic acid deficiency, and beriberi, which results from a thiamine deficiency).

a., fat-soluble, a disease resulting from deficiency of the fat-soluble vitamins (that is, A, D, E, and K).

avoidance behavior, a conscious or unconscious defense mechanism by which a person tries to escape from unpleasant situations or feelings, such as anxiety and pain.

avoirdupois system. See **system, avoirdupois.**

avulse, to tear off forcibly, as when a tooth is lost in an accident.

avulsed tooth. See **tooth, evulsed.**

avulsion (əvul'shən). See **evulsion.**

a., nerve. See **evulsion, nerve.**

axial inclination (ak'sē-əl). See **inclination, axial.**

axial plane. See **plane, axial.**

axial wall plane. See **plane, axial wall.**

axilla, a pyramid-shaped space forming the underside of the shoulder between the upper part of the arm and the side of the chest.

axiopulpal (ak'sē-ōpəl'pəl), relating to the angle formed by the axial and pulpal walls of a prepared cavity.

axis (ak'sis), **I.** a straight line around which a body may rotate. **2.** the second cervical vertebra.

a., cephalometric. See **axis, Y.**

a., condylar, an imaginary line through the two manidibular condyles around which the mandible may rotate during a part of the opening movement.

a., c. determination, the location of the condylar axis by fixing a facebow rigidly to the lower teeth, having the patient open and close the jaws, and recording the most posteriosuperior points of pure rotation with tattoo ink on the outer skin. See also **face-bow** and **hinge-bow.**

a., condyle, one of three axes of the jaw condyles: (1) the hinge axis, an intercondyle imaginary line across the face through both condyles; whenever either condyle is chosen to be a rotator, it will display, (2) a vertical axis, and (3) a sagittal axis. The hinge axis is a moving center for the opening and closing movements. The vertical axis is a center for the horizontal components of orbital movements. The sagittal axis is the center for the vertical components of orbital movements.

a., hinge, -orbital plane, a craniofacial plane determined by three tattooed points. Two are located with one on each side of the face at the point of exit through the skin in front of the tragus of the imagined extended rearmost mandibular hinge axis. The third point is located on the right side of the nose at the level of the orbital rim just beneath the pupil when the patient is gazing directly forward. This plane corresponds to the anthropologic Frankfort plane.

a., horizontal. See **axis, hinge.**

a., long, an imaginary line passing longitudinally through the center of a body.

a., mandibular. See **axis, condylar.**

a. of preparation, the path taken by a restoration as it slides on or off of the preparation.

a., opening. See **axis, condylar.**

a., orbital movements of, movements projected on the axis-orbital plane in gathering the input data for an articulator.

a., sagittal, the imaginary line around which the working condyle rotates in the frontal plane during lateral mandibular movement. The sagittal and vertical axes function concurrently.

a. shift, the imprecise term used before the nine different directionalized laterotrusions were discovered and named.

a., vertical, the imaginary line around which the working condyle rotates in the horizontal plane during lateral mandibular movement. The sagittal and vertical axes function concurrently.

a., Y (cephalometric axis), the angle of a line connecting the sella turcica and the gnathion and related to a horizontal plane. An indicator of downward and forward growth of the mandible.

axon (ak'săn), an extension of a nerve cell body that conducts impulses away from the cell. Generally there is only one axon to a cell, and it may extend up to 3 feet (0.9 m) in length.

azatadine maleate, *trade name:* Optimine; *drug class:* antihistamine; *action:* decreases allergic response by blocking histamine; *uses:* allergy symptoms, rhinitis, chronic urticaria, pruritus.

azathioprine, *trade name:* Imuran; *drug class:* immunosuppressant; *action:* inhibits purine synthesis in cells, thereby preventing RNA and DNA synthesis; *uses:* renal transplants to prevent graft rejection, refractory rheumatoid arthritis, bone marrow transplants, glomerulonephritis.

azdiothymidine (AZT), a drug used to lengthen or extend the median incubation period of the human immunodeficiency virus. Brand name: Retrovir.

azelaic acid, *trade name:* Azelex; *drug class:* a naturally occurring straight-chain dicarboxylic acid; *action:* has antimicrobial activity against *Propionibacterium acnes* and *Staphylococcus epidermidis; use:* topical therapy of mild-to-moderate inflammatory acne vulgaris.

azithromycin, *trade name:* Zithromax; *drug class:* macrolide antibiotic; *action:* binds to 50S ribosomal subunits of susceptible bacteria and suppresses protein synthesis; similar spectrum of activity to erythromycin; *uses:* mild-to-moderate infections of the upper respiratory tract, lower respiratory tract, uncomplicated skin and skin structure infections.

AZT, the abbreviation for **azdiothymidine.** See also **azdiothymidine.**

B

B point. See **point, B.**

baby bottle tooth decay, a dental condition that occurs in children from 1 to 3 years of age as a result of being given a bottle at bedtime, resulting in prolonged exposure of the teeth to milk, formula, or juice with a high sugar content. Dental caries results from the breakdown of sugars to lactic acid and other decay-causing substances.

bacampicillin HCl, *trade names:* Penglobe, Spectrobid; *drug class:* aminopenicillin; *action:* interferes with cell-wall replication of susceptible organisms; *uses:* respiratory tract, skin, and urinary tract infections; effective for gram-positive cocci.

Bacillus, a genus of gram-positive, spore-producing bacteria in the family Bacillaceae, order Eubacteriales, including three that are pathogenic (the rest are saprophytic soil forms). Many microorganisms formerly classified as *Bacillus* are now classified in other genera.

B. anthracis, a species of gram-positive facultative anaerobes that causes anthrax. The spores of this organism, if inhaled, can cause a pulmonary form of anthrax; the spores can live for many years in animal products such as hides and wool and in the soil.

B. subtilis, a *Bacillus* species found in grass and hay. Some strains produce the antibiotic bacillomycin.

bacitracin (bas'itrā'sin), an antibiotic produced by a gram-positive, spore-forming organism of the *Bacillus licheniformis* group; usually administered topically.

b., topical, *trade names:* Baciguent, Bacitin; *drug class:* local antiinfective; *action:* interferes with bacterial cell-wall function by inhibiting protein synthesis; *uses:* topical for nonserious infections caused by staphylococci and streptococci.

back, the posterior or dorsal portion of the trunk of the body between the neck and the pelvis. The skeletal portion of the back includes the thoracic and lumbar vertebrae and both scapulae. The nerves that innervate the muscles of the back include some branches of the dorsal primary divisions of the spinal nerves, the lateral branches of the dorsal primary division of the middle and lower cervical nerves, and some branches of the ventral primary division of the spinal nerves.

b. pain, a pain in the lumbar, lumbosacral, or cervical regions of the back, varying in sharpness and intensity. Causes may include muscle strain or pressure on the root of a nerve.

b. pressure porosity. See **porosity, back pressure.** (not current)

back-action clasp. See **clasp, back-action.** (not current)

backing, a metal support used to attach a facing to a prosthesis.

baclofen, *trade name:* Lioresal; *drug class:* central-acting skeletal muscle relaxant; *action:* inhibits both monosynaptic and polysynaptic reflexes in the spinal cord; *uses:* treatment for skeletal muscle spasticity in multiple sclerosis and spinal cord injury.

bacteremia (bak′tirē′mē-ə), **1.** presence of bacteria in the bloodstream. It may be transient, intermittent, or continuous. Transient bacteremia may result from dental procedures such as root planing or tonsillectomy, or it may accompany the early phases of many infections. Continuous bacteremia is a feature of endocarditis. **2.** presence of bacteria in the blood (for example, as occurs during root planing of the tooth of a patient with rheumatism who has not been prophylactically premedicated with antibiotics).

bacteria, any of the small, unicellular microorganisms of the class *Schizomycetes.* The genera vary morphologically, being spheric (cocci), rod-shaped (bacilli), spiral (spirochetes), or comma-shaped (vibrios).

b., aerobic, bacteria that require the presence of oxygen to live and grow.

b., anaerobic, bacteria that can survive and grow without the presence of free oxygen in their immediate environment.

b., resident (oral), the microorganisms constant in the oral flora of an individual.

bacterial culture. See **culture, bacterial.**

bacterial toxin, any poisonous substance produced by a bacterium. Two general types of toxins are common: those formed within the cell (endotoxins) and those formed within the cell and excreted (exotoxins).

bacteriology, the scientific study of bacteria.

bacteriolytic action (baktēr′ē-ōlīt′ik), the breaking down of bacteria by an enzyme or other agent (for example, by antibacterial factors in saliva).

bacteriophage, any virus that causes lysis of host bacteria.

Bacteroides (bak′təroi′dēz), a genus of *Schizomycetes* made up of rod-shaped, highly pleomorphic, gram-negative, non–spore-forming obligate anaerobic bacteria sometimes associated with periodontitis.

B. endodontalis, a strain of *B. melaninogenicus* associated with pulpal infections.

B. forsythus, a recently identified anaerobic gram-negative species of *Bacteroides* found in periodontal pockets.

B. fragilis, the most common and virulent strain of a genus of obligate anerobic bacilli normally found in the mouth, upper respiratory system, colon, and genital tract.

B. gingivalis, a strain of *B. melaninogenicus* associated with acute periodontitis.

B. intermedius, a strain of *B. melaninogenicus* associated with acute necrotizing ulcerative gingivitis.

B. melaninogenicus, a small, gram-negative diplobacillus also known as *Bacterium melaninogenicum* found in the mouth and pharynx; an anaerobic organism sometimes associated with periodontitis.

bad-faith insurance practices, 1. the failure to deal with a beneficiary of a dental benefits plan fairly and in good faith. **2.** an activity that impairs the right of the beneficiary to receive the appropriate benefits of a dental benefits plan or receive them in a timely manner. Some examples of bad-faith insurance practices include evaluating claims based on standards significantly at variance with the standards of the community, failure to investigate a claim for benefits properly, and unreasonably and purposely delaying or withholding payment of a claim.

badge, film. See **film badge.**

bailment, the delivery of personal property by one person to another in trust for a specific purpose with an expressed or implied contract that after the purpose has been fulfilled the property shall be returned, duly accounted for, or kept until reclaimed.

balance, equilibrium or harmony. Frequently used as an adjective to describe occlusal equilibrium or facial esthetic harmony.

b., acid-base, in metabolism, the balance of acid to base necessary to keep the blood pH level normal (between 7.35 and 7.43).

b. billing, billing a patient for the difference between the dentist's actual charge and the amount reimbursed under the patient's dental benefits plan.

b. sheet, a condensed statement showing the nature and amount of a company's assets, liabilities, and capital on a given date. In dollar amounts the balance sheet shows the assets the company owns, the money it owes, and the ownership interest in the company of its stockholders.

balanced articulation. See **occlusion, balanced.**

balanced bite. See **occlusion, balanced.** (not current)

balanced occlusion. See **occlusion, balanced.**

balancing contacts, the contacts of teeth on the side opposite the bolus side. See also **contact, balancing.**

balancing occlusal surfaces. See **surfaces, occlusal, balancing.** (not current)

balancing side, the side opposite the working side of the dentition or denture.

balloon payment, a final payment larger than the preceding payments when a debt is not fully amortized.

balloon, sinus, a hollow rubber structure expandable with liquid or air that is used to support depressed fractures of the walls of the maxillary sinus.

balsam (bôl′səm), any of many viscous, sticky, aromatic fluids derived from plants; consists of resins plus oils.

BANA, an acronym for **benzol-arginine napthylamide.** See also **benzol-arginine naphthylamide.**

band, 1. a cord, tie, chain, or metal collar by which something is bound. **2.** a contrasting strip or strip of material running through or along the edge of a material.

b. adapter. See **adapter, band.**

b., adjustable orthodontic, a band provided with an adjusting screw to permit alteration in size.

b., apron. See **apron band.**

b., orthodontic, a thin metal ring, usually stainless steel, that secures orthodontic attachments to a tooth. The band, with orthodontic attachments welded or soldered to it, is closely adapted to fit the contours of the tooth and then is cemented into place.

b., pusher, an instrument used to adapt the metal band to the tooth.

b. remover, an instrument used to remove bands from the teeth.

b., rubber. See **elastic.**

b., slip, a band formed when a metal is placed under a load and one grain tends to slip or slide on another.

b., striated. See **striations, muscle.**

bandage, a strip of material wrapped about or applied to any body part.

b., Barton's, a figure-of-eight bandage passing below the mandible and around the cranial bone to give upward support to the mandible.

b., thyroid, a large bandage consisting principally of a towel applied around the neck that exerts moderate pressure to the anterolateral part of the neck.

bank plan, a financial arrangement made between the dentist, patient, and bank for financing dental accounts; the bank provides the capital for a rate of interest that enables the patient to pay the dental account over a longer period of time than would otherwise be possible—usually 12 to 18 months.

bankruptcy, the legal process by which a person, business, or corporation is declared to be insolvent and unable to pay creditors.

bar, a metal segment of greater length than width. See also **bar, connector.**

b., anterior palatal. See **connector, major, anterior palatal.**

b., arch, any one of several types of wires, bars, and splints conforming to the arch of the teeth and used for the treatment of fractures of the jaws and the stabilization of injured teeth (for example, *Erich, Jelenko, Niro, Winter*).

b., buccal, an orthodontic appliance auxiliary consisting of a rigid metal wire extending from the buccal side of the molar band anteriorly.

b. clasp. See **clasp, bar.**

b., connector, a connector of greater thickness and reduced width as compared with a platelike connector, which has greater width and is thinner.

b., fixable-removable cross arch. See **connector, cross arch bar splint.**

b., Gilson fixable-removable. See **connector, cross arch bar splint.**

b., Kennedy. See **connector, minor, secondary lingual bar.**

b., labial, a major connector located labial (or buccal) to the dental arch that joins bilateral parts of a mandibular removable partial denture.

b., lingual, a major connector located lingual to the dental arch that joins bilateral parts of a mandibular removable partial denture. See also **connector, major, lingual bar.**

b., palatal, a major connector that crosses the palate and unites bilateral parts of a maxillary removable partial denture. See also **connector, major.**

b., posterior palatal. See **connector, major, posterior palatal.**

b., secondary lingual. See **connector, minor, secondary lingual bar.**

barbiturate (bärbich' ōōrāt), a derivative of barbituric acid that acts as a sedative or hypnotic. Barbiturates are controlled substances that have addictive potentials.

barium (ber'ē· əm), a pale yellow, metallic element classified with the alkaline earths.

barium sulfate, a white, finely ground, tasteless powder that is insoluble in water, solvents, and solutions of acids and alkalis; used in radiography as a contrast medium because of its opacity to roentgen rays and as a protective barrier in plaster walls.

barrier, protective, material of a composition that greatly absorbs radiation (for example, lead or concrete).

barrier techniques, protocols used in infection control to prevent cross-contamination between health care worker and patient, between patient and health care worker, and between patients. Strict barrier techniques are recommended by the Centers for Disease Control and Prevention (CDC) and the American Dental Association (ADA) to prevent the transmission of hepatitis B virus and human immunodeficiency virus types 1 and 2. However, any number of bacterial, viral, and fungal microorganisms can be transferred through improper or inadequate infection-control procedures.

Bartonella, a genus of small gramnegative flagellated pleomorphic coccobacilli. Members of the genus are intracellular parasites that infect red blood cells and the epithelial cells of the lymph nodes, liver, and spleen. They are transmitted at night by the bite of a sandfly.

basal bone. See **bone, basal.**

basal metabolic rate (BMR) (basal metabolism), (bā'səl met'əbol'ik) the basal rate, or energy exchange, determined by means of a clinical test of oxygen consumption in a subject who has had a good night's rest, has fasted for 12 to 14 hours, and has been physically, mentally, and emotionally at rest for 30 minutes; usually indicated as a percentage of the normal calorie production per surface area, the normal values ranging between plus and minus 20%.

basal metabolism. See **basal metabolic rate.**

basal seat, the oral tissues and structures that support a denture.

b. s. area. See **area, basal seat.**

b. s. outline, an outline on the mucous membrane or on a cast of the entire area that is to be covered by a denture.

basal surface. See **surface, basal.**

base, 1. the foundation or support on which something rests; the point of attachment of a part; the principal ingredient of a material. **2.** a compound that yields hydroxyl ions in water solution and causes neutralization of acid to form a salt and water.

b., acrylic resin, a denture base made of an acrylic resin.

b., apical (basal arch), the portion of the jawbones that gives support to the teeth.

b., cement, a layer of insulated, sometimes medicated dental cement placed in the deep portions of a cavity preparation to protect the pulp, reduce the bulk of the metallic restoration, or eliminate undercuts in a tapered preparation.

b., denture, **1.** the part of a denture that fits the oral mucosa of the basal seat, restores the normal contours of the soft tissues of the dentulous mouth, and supports the artificial teeth. **2.** the portion of a denture that overlies the soft tissue, usually fabricated of resin or combinations of resins and metal.

b., extension (free-end), a unit of a removable prosthesis that extends anteriorly or posteriorly, terminating without end support by a natural tooth.

b., film, a thin, flexible, transparent sheet of cellulose acetate or similar material.

b., mandibular, the body of the mandible, on which the teeth and alveolar tissues are situated.

b., material, any substance from which a denture base may be made (for example, acrylic resin, vulcanite, polystyrene resin, metal).

b., metal, the basal surface of a denture constructed of metal (for example, aluminum, gold, cobalt-chromium), to which the teeth are attached.

b., plastic, a denture base, baseplate, or record base made of a plastic material.

b., record. See **baseplate.**

b., shellac, certain resinous materials adapted to maxillary or mandibular casts to form baseplates.

b., sprue. See **crucible former.**

b., temporary. See **baseplate.**

b., tinted denture, a denture base that simulates the coloring and shading of natural oral tissues.

b., trial. See **baseplate.**

Basedow's disease (bä′sədōz). See **goiter, exophthalmic.**

baseplate (record base, temporary base, trial base), a temporary form representing the base of a denture and used for making maxillomandibular (jaw) relation records, arranging artificial teeth, or facilitating trial placement in the mouth.

b., stabilized, a baseplate lined with plastic or other material to improve its adaptation and stability.

b. wax. See **wax, baseplate.**

basic metabolic rate. See **basal metabolic rate.**

basic services, frequently insurance companies split dental procedures into basic and major categories. Basic services usually consist of diagnostic, preventive, and routine restorative dental services. The plan may provide different deductibles, co-insurance, and maximums for basic versus major services as incentives to good dental care.

basion (bā′sē·on), the midline point at the anterior margin of the occipital foramen.

basis, the principal active ingredient in a prescription.

basophil (bā′səfil). See **leukocyte.**

basophilia (ba′sofil′ē·ə) (basophilic granular degeneration, basophilic stippling), an aggregate of blue-staining granules found in erythrocytes; seen in lead poisoning, leukemia, malaria, severe anemias, and certain toxemias.

basophilic line (basōfilik). See **line, basophilic.**

batch processing, data processing in which a number of similar input data items are grouped together and processed during a single machine run with the same program.

Battle's sign. See **sign, Battle's.**

bayonet, a binangled instrument, the nib or blade of which is generally parallel to the shaft; resembles a bayonet. See also **angle former, bayonet and condenser, bayonet.**

beading, the scribing of a shallow groove (less than 0.5 mm in width or depth) on a cast that outlines the major connector. It is used to transfer the design to the investment cast and ensure tissue contact of the major connector.

beam, a stream or approximately unidirectional emission of electromagnetic radiation or particles.

b., central, the center of the beam of roentgen rays emitted from the tube.

b., useful, the part of the primary radiation that passes through the aperture, cone, or other collimator.

beauty, the quality of an attribute that is pleasing to the senses or the mind.

beclomethasone dipropionate, *trade names:* oral—Beclovent, Vanceril; nasal—Vancenase AQ Nasal, Beconase AQ Nasal; *drug class:* corti-

B

costeroid, synthetic; *action:* prevents inflammation by depression of migration of polymorphonuclear leukocytes and fibroblasts and reversal of increased capillary permeability; *uses:* chronic asthma and rhinitis.

beeswax, a low-melting wax that is an ingredient of many dental waxes.

Begg's appliance. See **appliance, Begg's.**

behavior, the manner in which a person acts or performs; any or all of the activities of a person, including physical action learned and unlearned, deliberate or habitual.

b. management, techniques used to control or modify an action or performance of a subject. In dentistry, usually associated with the management of oral hygiene behavior, dietary behavior, or patient behavior under stress.

b. modification, alterations, changes, or transfers from a socially unacceptable and destructive act to a socially acceptable nondestructive one. In dentistry, usually associated with oral habits such as finger or thumb sucking, mouth breathing, nail biting, and smoking.

b. therapy, a kind of psychotherapy that attempts to modify observable, maladjusted patterns of behavior by the substitution of a new response or set of responses to a given stimulus.

behavioral medicine, a branch of clinical psychology that deals with behavior modification and may involve assertiveness training, aversion therapy, contingency management, operant conditioning, and systemic desensitization.

behavioral sciences, those sciences devoted to the study of human and animal behavior.

Behçet's syndrome. See **syndrome, Behçet's.**

belladonna alkaloids, *trade name:* Bellafoline; *drug class:* gastrointestinal anticholinergic; *action:* inhibits muscarinic actions of acetylcholine at postganglionic parasympathetic neuron effector sites; *uses:* treatment of peptic ulcer disease and irritable bowel syndrome in combination with other drugs.

Bell's palsy, sign, palsy test. See **palsy, Bell's; sign, Bell's; and palsy test, Bell's.**

Benadryl, trade name for diphenhydramine hydrochloride, an antihistamine with anticholinergic (drying) and sedative side effects.

benazepril, *trade name:* Lotensin; *drug class:* angiotensin-converting enzyme (ACE) inhibitor; *action:* selectively suppresses renin-angiotensin-aldosterone system; *uses:* treatment of hypertension, alone or in combination with thiazide diuretics.

Bence Jones protein. See **protein, Bence Jones.**

Benedict's test. See **test, Benedict's.**

beneficiary, 1. a person eligible for benefits under a dental plan. Synonyms include eligible individual, enrollee, member. **2.** a person who receives benefits under a dental benefit contract. See also **covered person; insured; member; and subscriber.**

benefit booklet, a booklet or pamphlet provided to the subscriber that contains a general explanation of the benefits and related provisions of the dental benefits program. Also known as a *summary plan description.*

benefit plan summary, the description or synopsis of employee benefits required by ERISA to be distributed to employees.

benefits, 1. the cash benefit paid for various procedures performed. **2.** the list of dental services or procedures covered by the insurance policy and referred to as the *schedule of benefits.* One synonym is coverage.

benign (benīn′), a neoplasm unable to metastasize.

Bennett angle, movement. See **angle, Bennett and movement, Bennett.**

benzathine penicillin G, a benzathine salt of natural penicillin that forms a slowly absorbable injectable antibiotic effective against penicillin-susceptible organisms.

benzocaine, a local anesthetic agent derived from aminobenzoic acid, used in many over-the-counter compounds for pruritus and pain. A minimum of 5% benzocaine is required for a compound to be effective.

b. (topical), trade names: 20% liquid—Anbesol Maximum Strength, Orajel Mouth Aid; 20% gel—Anbesol Maximum Strength, Hurricaine, Orajel Brace-Aid; 10%—Denture Orajel, Baby Orajel Nighttime; *drug class:* topical ester local anesthetic; *action:* inhibits conduction of nerve impulses from sensory nerves; *uses:* treatment of oral irritation, toothache, cold sores, canker sore, teething pain, and pain caused by dental prostheses or orthodontic appliances.

benzol-arginine naphthylamide, a bacterial enzyme that mimics the activity of trypsin. It is used as a marker of bacterial growth in dental plaque or as a marker for the diagnosis of periodontal disease involving *B. gingivalis, B. forsythus,* and *Treponema denticola.*

benzonatate, *trade name:* Tessalon; *drug class:* antitussive, nonnarcotic; *action:* inhibits cough reflex by anesthetizing stretch receptors in respiratory system; *uses:* nonproductive cough relief.

benzoyl peroxide, 1. a chemical incorporated into the polymer of resins to aid in the initiation of polymerization. **2.** an antibacterial, keratolytic drying agent prescribed in the treatment of acne.

benztropine mesylate, *trade names:* Apo-benzotropin, benztropine mesylate; *drug class:* anticholinergic, antidyskinetic; *action:* blocks central acetylcholine receptors; *use:* treatment of Parkinson's disease symptoms.

bepridil HCl, *trade names:* Vascor, Bepadin; *drug class:* calcium channel blocker; *action:* inhibits calcium ion influx across cell membrane during cardiac depolarization; *uses:* treatment of stable angina, alone or in combination with propranolol or nitrates.

beriberi (asjike, athiaminosis, endemic multiple neuritis, endemic polyneuritis, hinchazon, inchacao, kakke, loempe, panneuritis endemica, perneiras), a nutritional disease resulting from a deficiency of thiamine. Classically it is characterized by multiple neuritis, muscular atrophy, weakness, cardiovascular changes, and progressive edema.

beryllium, a steel-gray, lightweight metallic element. Alloys of beryllium are used in fluorescent powders. Inhalation of beryllium fumes or particles may cause the formation of granulomas in the lungs, skin, and subcutaneous tissues.

beta-hemihydrate (bā'tə hem'ihī'-drāt), the physical state of hemihydrate of calcium sulfate; plaster of paris. (not current)

betamethasone (valerate, betamethasone benzoate, betamethasone dipropionate), *trade names:* Uticort, Beben, and others; *drug class:* topical corticosteroid; *action:* interacts with steroid cytoplasmic receptors to induce antiinflammatory effects; possesses antipruritic, antiinflammatory actions; *uses:* treatment of psoriasis, eczema, contact dermatitis, pruritus, and oral ulcerative inflammatory lesions.

betatron (bā'tətron), a machine that produces high-speed electrons through magnetic induction.

betaxolol HCl, *trade name:* Kerlone; *drug class:* antihypertensive, selective beta$_1$-blocker; *action:* produces fall in blood pressure without reflex tachycardia or significant reduction in heart rate; *uses:* treatment of hypertension.

bethanechol chloride, *trade names:* Duvoid, Urecholine, Urebeth; *drug class:* cholinergic stimulant; *action:* stimulates muscarinic acetylcholine receptors directly; stimulates gastric motility; *uses:* treatment of postoperative or postpartum urinary retention and neurogenic atony of bladder with retention.

bevel, the inclination that one surface makes with another when not at right angles; in cavity preparation, a cut that produces an angle of more than 90° with a cavity wall.
b., cavosurface, the incline or slant of the cavosurface angle of a prepared cavity wall in relation to the plane of the enamel wall.
b., contra, blade placement toward the base of the periodontal pocket to separate the sulcular from the external epithelium. Also known as a *reverse,* or *internal, bevel.*
b., instrument, the sloping keen edge of a cutting instrument.
b., reverse. See **bevel, contra.**

BHN. See **number, Brinell hardness** and **test, Brinell hardness.**

bias, 1. a prejudiced or subjective attitude. **2.** in statistics, the systematic distortion of a statistic caused by a particular sampling process.

bicarbonate, a salt resulting from the incomplete neutralization of carbonic acid such as from passing excess carbon dioxide into a base solution.

Bicillin, trade name for penicillin G benzathine.

bicuspid (bīkus'pid). See **premolar.**

b.i.d., the abbreviation for *bis in die,* a Latin phrase meaning "twice a day."

Biermer's anemia (bēr'mərz). See **anemia, pernicious.**

bifid tongue (bi'fid). See **tongue, bifid.**

bifid uvula. See **uvula, bifid.**

bifidobacterium, a genus of anaerobic bacteria containing gram-positive rods of highly variable appearance. Pathogenicity for human beings or for animals has not been reported although these bacteria have been isolated from the feces of infants and older people.

bifurcation (bi'fərkā'shən), the division into two parts or branches such as any two roots of a tooth.

bilateral (bī lat'ərəl), pertaining to both sides.

bilharziasis (bil'hahrzī· əsis). See **schistosomiasis.**

biliary atresia, a congenital absence or underdevelopment of one or more of the biliary structures, causing jaundice and early liver damage.

bilirubinemia (bil'irōō'binē'mē-ə), the presence of bilirubin in the blood. It may result from obstruction inside or outside the liver or from increased hemolysis. The total serum bilirubin in an adult is 0.2 to 0.7 mg/100 ml.

bilirubinuria (bil'irōō'binu're-ə), the presence of bilirubin in the urine. More often, an excess of bilirubin in the urine resulting from excessive hemolysis.

billing, the procedure of preparing a financial statement.

bimaxillary (bīmak'silar'ē), pertaining to the right and left maxillae; sometimes incorrectly used to refer to the maxillae and mandible.

b. protrusion. See **protrusion, bimaxillary.**

bimeter (bī'mētər), a gnathodynamometer with a central bearing point adjustable to varying heights. See also **gnathodynamometer.**

Bimler's appliance. See **appliance, Bimler's.**

binangle (bin'ang·gəl), an instrument having two offsetting angles in its shank. The angles keep the cutting edge or the face of the nib within 3 mm of the axis of the shaft.

binder, a substance, usually sticky, that holds the solid particles in a mixture together, thus aiding in the preservation of the physical form of the mixture.

binding, a reversible combination of various drugs with body constituents such as plasma proteins.

binding site, the location on the surface of a cell or molecule where other cell fragments or molecules attach to initiate a chemical or physiologic action.

binocular loupe. See **loupe, binocular.**

biochemistry, the chemistry of living organisms and life processes.

biocompatible material, a substance that does not threaten, impede, or adversely affect living tissue.

biodegradability, the natural ability of a chemical substance to be broken down into less complex compounds with fewer carbon atoms by bacteria or other microorganisms.

bioethics, the study of social and moral issues raised in the field of biology, including medicine and dentistry.

biofeedback, the instrumented process or technique of learning voluntary control over automatically regulated body functions; useful in the treatment of bruxism, temporomandibular joint dysfunction, and pain and in facilitating anxiety control in the dental setting.

b., electromyographic (EMG), an instrumented process that helps patients learn control over muscle tension levels previously under automatic control; especially useful in treatment of dental disorders such as bruxism, temporomandibular joint dysfunction, tension headaches, and other disorders involving the muscles of mastication. In addition to neuromuscular education, electromyographic biofeedback is useful in treating dental phobias and anxiety and facilitating pain control by helping patients learn deep muscle relaxation techniques.

b., temperature, an instrumented learning process whereby a patient learns to control temperature of body parts. Training in self-controlled vasodilation (handwarming) technique has been found useful in treating migraine headaches and anxiety in dental patients.

bioflavonoids, naturally occurring flavone or coumarin derivatives having the activity of so-called vitamin P. Their use in controlling gingival bleeding remains controversial.

bioglass, a fused silica-containing aluminum oxide that presents a surface-reactive glass film compatible with connective and epithelial tissues. Bioglass is used as a surface coating in blade and endosteal implants.

biologic, pertaining to biology.

b. factors, the variables that influence life and living tissues.

b. science, the science that deals with life processes.

biology, the science of life or living matter in all its forms and phenomena.

biomass, the total quantity of living organisms in a particular volume of matter.

biomechanics (bī′ōməkan′iks). See **biophysics.**

biomedical engineering, a system of techniques in which knowledge of biologic processes is applied to solve practical medical problems and answer questions in biomedical research.

biometrics (bī′ōmet′riks), the science of the application of statistical methods to biologic facts.

bionator, a removable orthodontic appliance designed to correct functional and skeletal anteroposterior discrepancies between the maxilla and mandible.

biophysics (bī·ōfiz′iks), the science dealing with the forces that act on living cells of the body, the relationship between the biologic behavior of living structures and the physical influences to which they are subjected, and the physics of vital processes. Also known as *biomechanics.*

b., dental, the branch of biophysics that deals with the biologic behavior of oral structures as influenced by dental restorations.

biopsy (bī′opsē), the removal of a tissue specimen or other material from the living body for microscopic examination to aid in establishing a diagnosis.

b., aspiration, the procedure of obtaining a biopsy specimen by aspiration through a needle; used for diag-

nosing bone or deep soft tissue lesions. Also known as a *needle biopsy.*

b., excisional, the removal of an entire lesion, usually including a significant margin of contiguous normal tissue, for microscopic examination and diagnosis.

b., exploratory, exploration combined with biopsy to determine method and degree of local extension, usually of bone or deep soft tissue lesions.

b., incisional, the surgical removal of a selected mass of a lesion and adjacent normal tissue for microscopic examination and diagnosis.

b., needle. See **biopsy, aspiration.**

b., punch, biopsy material obtained by use of a punch.

biosynthesis, the formation of a chemical compound by enzymes.

biotechnology, 1. the study of the relationships between humans or other living organisms and machinery. **2.** the industrial application of the results of biologic research such as recombinant deoxyribonucleic acid (DNA) and gene splicing that permit the production of synthetic hormones or enzymes.

biotin (bī′ətin). See **vitamin, biotin.**

biotransformation, the chemical and physical changes produced in drugs after they enter the body (for example, hydrolysis, conjugation).

biperiden HCl, biperiden lactate, *trade name:* Akineton; *drug class:* anticholinergic; *action:* centrally acting competitive anticholinergic; *use:* treatment of Parkinson's disease symptoms.

bird face. See **brachygnathia; retrognathism.**

birth-control pills, oral contraceptives, usually a mixture of a steroid having progestational activity and an estrogen.

birth weight, the measured heaviness of a baby when born, the average of which is about 3500 g, or 7.5 lbs. A baby weighing less than 5 pounds is considered premature or underdeveloped.

bis-, a prefix meaning that two like or mirror-image moieties are joined together to form a chemical compound.

bisacodyl, *trade names:* Dulcolax, Fleet Bisacodyl, Bisacodyl Uniserts, Fleet Laxative; *drug class:* laxative, stimulant; *action:* acts directly on intestine by increasing motor activity; *uses:* short-term treatment of constipation, bowel or rectal preparation for surgery or examination.

biscuit, firing bakes, or stages (referred to as low, medium, and high), during the fusing of dental porcelain preceding the final, or glaze, bake.

bisexual, a person who engages in or desires sexual contact with persons of both sexes.

bismuth, (biz′məth), a reddish, crystalline, trivalent metallic element that in combination with other elements forms salts that are used in the production of many pharmaceutical compounds.

b. poisoning. See **bismuthosis.**

b. subsalicylate, trade names: Bisamatrol, Pepto-Bismol; *drug class:* antidiarrheal; *action:* mechanism of action unknown; *uses:* treatment of diarrhea, prevention of diarrhea when traveling.

bismuthia (bizmu′thē-ə), the discoloration of mucous membranes and skin from bismuth poisoning.

bismuthism. See **bismuthosis.**

bismuthosis (biz′məthō′sis), acute or chronic bismuth intoxication resulting from the ingestion or injection of bismuth salts. Possible manifestations include albuminuria, exfoliative dermatitis, gastrointestinal disturbances, and stomatitis. Also known as *bismuth poisoning,* or *bismuthism.* See also **stomatitis, bismuth.**

bisoprolol fumarate, *trade name:* Zebeta; *drug class:* antihypertensive, selective β_1-blocker; *action:* produces fall in blood pressure without reflex tachycardia or significant reduction in heart rate; *uses:* treatment of hypertension as a single agent or in combination.

bite, 1. the part of an artificial tooth on the lingual side between the shoulder and the incisal edge of the tooth. 2. an interocclusal record or relationship. See also **denture space; distance, interarch; record, interocclusal;** and **record, maxillomandibular.**

b. analysis. See **analysis, occlusal.**

b., balanced. See **occlusion, balanced.**

b. block, 1. in intraoral radiography, a film holder that the patient bites to provide stable retention of the film packet. 2. occlusion rim. See also **rim, occlusion.**

b., close. See **distance, small interarch.**

b., closed, 1. an abnormal overbite. 2. a decrease in the occlusal vertical dimension produced by factors such as tooth abrasion and loss or failure of eruption of supportive posterior teeth. See also **distance, reduced interarch.**

b. closing. See **dimension, vertical decrease.**

b., convenience. See **occlusion, acquired, eccentric.**

b., edge-to-edge, an occlusion in which the incisal edge of the maxillary incisors meets the incisal edge of the mandibular incisors. See also **occlusion, edge-to-edge.**

b. force, the interocclusal force produced in jaw closure, usually measured in grams or pounds.

b. fork. See **fork, face-bow.**

b. guard. See **guard, bite.**

b. g. splint. See **splint, acrylic resin bite-guard.**

b., human, a puncture or laceration of tissue caused by human teeth. The markings may be distinctive and useful in forensic pathology to determine the person responsible. Human bite wounds may become infected, requiring antibiotic treatment and tetanus toxoid injection.

b., locked. See **occlusion, locked.**

b. marks, distinctive tooth patterns in a wound that may have forensic or legal implications.

b., normal. See **occlusion, normal.**

b., open, a malformation in which the anterior teeth do not occlude in any mandibular position.

b. opening. See **dimension, vertical, increasing occlusal.**

b. o. bends, bends made in maxillary and mandibular light round wires mesial to the molar tubes in orthodontics.

b. plate. See **plate, bite.**

b. pressure, the pressure produced by jaw closure per unit of area, usually measured in grams per square millimeter. See also **pressure, occlusal.**

b. raising. See **dimension, vertical, increasing occlusal.**

b. record. See **path, generated occlusal.**

b. rest. See **position, rest, physiologic.**

b. rim. See **rim, occlusion.**

b., working. See **occlusion, working.**

biteplane (bīt′plān), a removable appliance that covers the occlusal surfaces of the teeth to prevent their articulation.

bite-wing film. See **film, bite-wing.**

bite-wing radiograph. See **radiograph, bite-wing.**

biting, cheek. See **habit.**

biting, lip. See **habit.**

biting, nail. See **habit.**

biting pressure. See **pressure, occlusal.**

biting strength. See **strength, biting.**

bitolterol mesylate, *trade name:* Tornalate; *drug class:* adrenergic β₂-agonist; *action:* causes bronchodilation; *uses:* treatment or prophylaxis of asthma, bronchitis, bronchospasm.

blade. (See specific instrument parts.)

blanching, gingival. See **gingival blanching.**

Blandin and Nuhn's gland. See **gland, Blandin and Nuhn's.**

blastomatoid lesion (blastō′matoid), an overzealous reactive process that because of tumescence has some features of neoplasia. Specific tissue elements, such as fibroblasts, endothelial cells, osteoblasts, osteoclastic giant cells, or nerves, predominate in a specific lesion to form granuloma pyogenicum, giant cell reparative granuloma, traumatic fibroma, tori, or traumatic neuroma.

Blastomyces brasiliensis (blastōmī′-sēz), a species of fungus not found in the United States that causes South American blastomycosis.

Blastomyces dermatitidis (dər′-məhtit′ idəs), a species of fungus causing North American blastomycosis.

blastomycosis (blastōmīkō′sis), an infection resulting from the fungus *Blastomyces dermatitidis* (North American blastomycosis) or *Blastomyces brasiliensis* (South American blastomycosis); characterized by chronic suppurative lesions. The disseminated form is usually fatal.

b., South American, a fungous infection that often begins when organisms enter the body through the oral mucosa, producing local ulcers, or through an extraction site, producing papillary lesions. Dissemination leads to granulomatous lesions of the lymph nodes, gastrointestinal tract, liver, and lungs and to microabscesses of the skin. The causative agent is *Blastomyces brasiliensis.*

bleaching, the use of a chemical oxidizing agent (sometimes in combination with heat) to lighten tooth discolorations. See also **agent, bleaching.**

bleeding, the flowing of blood.

b., gingival. See **gingival bleeding.**

b., occult, hemorrhage of such small proportions that the blood can be detected only by chemical test, microscope, or spectroscope.

b. points, a series of puncture points made through the gingival tissue; used as a guide for making the gingivectomy incision.

b. time, the time required for blood to stop flowing from a tiny wound. Normal bleeding time is from 2 to 6 minutes. Bleeding time is increased in disorders of platelet count, uremia, and ingestion of aspirin and other antiinflammatory medications.

blepharophimosis, a decrease in the size of the palpebral opening without a fusion of the eyelid margins.

blepharoptosis, a drooping of the upper eyelid.

blindness, color, defective color vision characterized by decreased ability to detect differences in color. See also **achromatopsia.**

b., c., blue-yellow, a color disability in which the spectrum is seen in reds and greens; a form of protanopia.

b., c., red-green, the more common form of color disability, in which the entire spectrum is constituted by yellows and blues; a form of protanopia.

blister, a vesicle or bulla, usually a consequence of a burn or friction.

Bloch-Sulzberger syndrome. See **syndrome, Bloch-Sulzberger.**

block, a mental obstacle that prohibits a patient from having favorable responses to the dentist and suggested treatment plans.

b., data, a physical unit of data that can be conveniently stored by a computer on an input or output device. The block is normally composed of one or more logical records or a portion of a logical record. Synonymous with physical record.

b., field, the reversible interruption of nerve conduction over terminal branches by infiltration of a suitable agent into the area.

B

b., nerve, the reversible interruption of conduction along a nerve trunk or its branches because of the absorption of a suitable agent. Also regional anesthesia secured by extraneural or paraneural injection in close proximity to the nerve whose conductivity is to be cut.

blocking, the process of obstructing or deadening, as a nerve.

b. agent. See **agent, blocking.**

blockout, elimination of undesirable undercut areas on a cast to be used in the fabrication of a removable denture. Also known as *waxout.*

blood, the fluid circulating through the heart, arteries, capillaries, and veins; carries nutrients and oxygen to body tissues.

b., bad, the lay term for syphilis.

b. calcium, the level of calcium in the blood plasma, generally regulated by parathyroid gland activity in conjunction with the degree of calcium ingestion, absorption, use, and excretion. Normal value is 8.5 to 11.5 mg/100 ml of blood serum.

b. cell count, an estimation of the number and types of circulating blood cells (for example, red blood cells [erythrocytic series], white blood cells, differential).

b. cells, any of the formed elements of the blood, including red cells (erythrocytes), white cells (leukocytes), and platelets (thrombocytes).

b. chemistry, the determination of the chemical constituents of blood by assay in a clinical laboratory as part of a diagnostic protocol.

b. circulation, the circuit of blood through the body from the heart through the arteries, arterioles, capillaries, venules, and veins and back to the heart.

b. clot. See **clot, blood.**

b. clotting, the conversion of blood from a free-flowing liquid to a semi-solid gel. Within seconds of injury to a blood vessel wall, platelets clump at the site. If normal amounts of calcium, platelets, and tissue factors are present, prothrombin will be converted to thrombin. Thrombin acts as a catalyst for the conversion of fibrinogen to a mesh of insoluble fibrin in which all the formed elements of blood are immobilized. Also called *blood coagulation.*

b. coagulation disorder, any disturbance in the normal clotting mechanism of the blood.

b., color index of, a figure gained by dividing the hemoglobin percentage by the red blood cell percentage. In most anemias the result is below 1, but in pernicious anemia it is characteristically above 1.

b. component transfusion, the administration of one or more elements of blood rather than the whole blood. May include red blood cells, platelets, and other elements.

b. disorders, hematologic dyscrasias that affect the component cells and plasma elements of the blood. Blood disorders are generally divided into two broad groups: those in which an increase in bulk occurs (for example, plethora, hydremia, polycythemia) and those in which a decrease in bulk occurs (for example, anhydremia, dehydration, anemia).

b. dyscrasias, pathologic conditions or disorders such as leukemia or hemophilia in which any of the constituents of the blood are abnormal or are present in abnormal quantity.

b. gas analysis, the study of gas dissolved in the liquid part of the blood. Blood gases include oxygen, carbon dioxide, and nitrogen, all components of inspired air.

b. groups, the division of blood into types on the basis of the compatibility of the erythrocytes and serum of one individual with the erythrocytes and serum of another individual. The groups are immunologically and genetically distinct.

b. pressure. See **pressure, blood.**

b. products, constituents of whole blood such as plasma or platelets that are used in replacement therapy.

b. sugar, the concentration of sugar (chiefly glucose—"true blood sugar") in the blood. It is usually kept within a narrow range by an interplay of many factors: glycogenolysis, glyconeogenesis, intestinal absorption, insulin, insulin antagonists, and other hormones. In the testing of total reducing substances, the normal range of concentration of fasting blood sugar is 80 to 120 mg/ml; in the testing of true blood sugar, the normal range of concentration is 70 to 100 mg/ml.

Blood products and their uses

Blood product	Uses
Red blood cells	Acute or chronic anemia, aplastic anemia, bone marrow failure, congestive heart failure, chronic renal failure, hepatic coma
Whole blood	Acute massive blood loss, hypovolemic shock
Platelets	Thrombocytopenia, platelet function abnormality
Fresh frozen plasma	Hypovolemia combined with hemorrhage because of deficiencies
Cryoprecipitate	Hemophilia, von Willebrand's disease, hypofibrinogenemia, factor XIII deficiency
Albumin	Shock caused by burns; maintains blood volume in patients with hypovolemia; hypoproteinemia
Leukocyte-poor red blood cells	Repeated febrile reaction; reaction from leukocyte antibodies and patients who are candidates for organ transplants

Adapted from Sheehy SB: *Emergency nursing principles and practice*, ed 3, St Louis, 1992, Mosby. Data courtesy Eastern Maine Medical Center, Bangor, Maine.

b. transfusion, the administration of whole blood or a component such as packed red cells to replace blood lost through trauma, surgery, or disease.

b. urea nitrogen (BUN), nitrogen in the form of urea in whole blood or serum. Its concentration is a gross measure of renal function. The upper limit of the normal range is 25 mg/100 ml.

b. vessel, any one of the network of muscular tubes that carry blood. The kinds of blood vessels are arteries, arterioles, capillaries, venules, and veins.
b., volume index of, the volume of red blood cells divided by the total volume of blood times 100 times the volume percent of packed red blood cells (hematocrit index). A value greater than 1 indicates an abnormally large number or size of erythrocytes.

blood-borne pathogens, pathogenic microorganisms that are present in human blood and cause disease in humans.

blood-brain barrier, an anatomic-physiologic feature of the brain thought to consist of walls of capillaries in the central nervous system and surrounding glial membranes. The blood-brain barrier prevents or slows the passage of some drugs, other chemical compounds, radioactive ions, and disease-causing organisms such as viruses from the blood into the nerve tissues of the central nervous system.

blower, chip. See **syringe, air, hand.**

blowpipe, a torch that employs gas-oxygen, or oxygen and acetylene, to melt metal in dental casting and soldering procedures.

blue, methylene (meth′ələn), **1.** a dye used to color bacteria for microscopic examination. **2.** an aniline dye often used as an antiseptic and topical analgesic in the treatment of lesions of the oral mucous membranes and skin.

blue nevus. See **nevus, blue.**

BMR. See **basal metabolic rate.**

board certification, the examination program that establishes the clinical proficiency of a dental specialist according to the procedures established by the individual specialty certification board under the rules and authority of the Council on Dental Education of the American Dental Association.

board certified, the status of a dental specialist such as an orthodontist who has become a board diplomate by successfully completing the certification program of the recognized certification board in that area of practice.

board diplomate, a dental specialist who has achieved certification by the recognized certifying board in that specialty, as attested by a diploma from the board.

board eligible, the status of a dental specialist whose educational qualifications have been verified by acceptance of an application for certification by the recognized certifying board. Board eligibility depends on advanced education in the specialty and timely progress toward completion of the certification procedure. Regular renewal is required to maintain eligibility until the examination is completed.

board qualified, an unrecognized term used variously and inaccurately to identify any of the stages from educational qualification to certification.

bodily movement. See **movement, body.**

body, any mass or collection of material.

b. burden, the activity of a radiopharmaceutical retained by the body at a specified time after administration.

b., Donovan's, an extracellular structure found in macrophages in lesions of granuloma inguinale.

b. fluid, any liquid portion of the body such as plasma, lymph, tears, saliva, and urine.

b., foreign, any object or material that is not normal for the area in which it is located.

b. height, the overall length of the body from the crown to the bottom of the feet, usually taken in the standing position. Body length refers to the overall length taken in the supine position.

b. image, a person's subjective concept of personal physical appearance. The loss of a limb, breast, or tooth may cause psychologic trauma because of unresolved conflict in the change of body image. A distorted body image may be a causal factor in anorexia nervosa and bulimia.

b., ketone, any of the compounds acetoacetic acid, betahydroxybutyric acid, and acetone that are formed in the liver and released in the blood. Elevated levels occur during excessive fat use such as in diabetes or starvation.

b., Lipschütz, any one of the eosinophilic oval structures in the nuclei of cells found in herpesvirus infection.

b., Schaumann's (shou´mänz), a round to oval cytoplasmic inclusion composed of concentric deposits of an amorphous material. Seen in the giant cells of sarcoidosis, in beryllium lesions, and sometimes in other giant cells.

b. temperature, the level of heat produced and sustained by body processes. Variations and changes in body temperature are major indicators of disease and other abnormalities.

b., Verocay, a component of Antoni type A tissue seen in neurilemoma. See also **neurilemoma.**

Boeck's disease (bərks). See **sarcoidosis.**

Boeck's sarcoid. See **sarcoidosis.**

Bogarad's syndrome. See **syndrome, auriculotemporal.**

Bohn's nodules. See **nodules, Bohn's.**

Boley gauge. See **gauge, Boley.**

Bolton analysis, a computation developed by Wayne Bolton for the evaluation of tooth size discrepancies between upper and lower arches.

Bolton-nasion plane. See **plane, Bolton-nasion.**

Bolton plane. See **plane, Bolton-nasion.**

Bolton point, triangle. See **point, Bolton** and **triangle, Bolton.**

bolus (bō´ləs), a mass of food ready to be swallowed or a mass passing through the intestines.

bond, the force that holds two or more units of matter together.

b., primary, a chemical bond that requires some change in structure of matter. Primary bonds are ionic, covalent, or metallic.

b., secondary, a physical bond (sometimes called van der Waals forces) that involves weak interatomic attractions such as variations in physical mass or location of electrical charge.

bonding, adhesion of orthodontic attachments to the teeth without use of an interposed band.

b., direct, individual placement of attachments on the teeth at the time of adhesion.

b., indirect, the positioning of attachments on a dental cast and transfer of them to the teeth en masse for adhesion by means of a molded matrix bone.

bone, 1. the material of the skeletons of most vertebrate animals; the tissue comprising bones. **2.** dense, hard, and slightly elastic connective tissue in which the fibers are impregnated with a form of calcium phosphate similar to hydroxyapatite. Bone tissue makes up the 206 bones of the human skeleton. **3.** any single element of the skeleton such as a rib or femur.

b., alveolar, the specialized bone structure that contains the alveoli or sockets of the teeth and supports the teeth.

b., a., architecture, the structural pattern of the alveolar bone and its subjacent latticework of supporting bone. The alveolar bone is thin and compact adjacent to the periodontal membrane.

The trabecular bone connects and reinforces the individual alveoli. The architecture of a bone is the result of functional stimuli to that bone; the stimuli vary according to type, intensity, and duration.

b., a., metabolism, the metabolic activity occurring within alveolar bone, which is generally slower than that occurring within metaphyseal bone but more rapid than that of diaphyseal bone.

b. apposition. See **bone deposition.**

b., basal, that part of the mandible and maxilla from which the alveolar process develops.

b., bundle, the bone forming the immediate bone attachment of the numerous bundles of collagen fibers of the periodontal ligament that have been incorporated into the bone.

b. bur, a drill designed to cut into bone.

b. calcium content, the amount of calcium stored in bone tissue. Plasma calcium is in constant exchange with the calcium of the extracellular fluid and bones. The parathyroid gland maintains the constancy of the calcium concentration in the plasma. The bones serve as a reservoir of calcium and phosphate to provide for the other needs of the body and supply minerals for deposition in the skeleton.

b., cancellous (spongiosa, spongy bone, supporting bone, trabecular bone), the bone that forms a trabecular network, surrounds marrow spaces that may contain either fatty or hematopoietic tissue, lies subjacent to the cortical bone, and makes up the main portion of a bone.

b., c., atrophy of disuse, wasting of bone tissue occurring with loss of function of a part (for example, a tooth). The supporting bone assumes an osteoporotic nature, and the marrow remains fatty or hematopoietic.

b. cells, osteoblasts, osteocytes, osteoclasts, and osteoprogenitor cells.

b. changes, mechanical factors, pressure and tension forces that play an important role in determining bone structure. Improperly controlled appliances can resorb bone faster than deposition can occur, causing mobile teeth and traumatic occlusion. Poor vascularity is a concomitant cause of undue pressure and tension and may inhibit repair and cause necrosis.

b. chips, small pieces of cancellous bone generally used to fill in bony defects and precipitate recalcification.

b., compact, hard, dense bone comprising the outer cortical layer and consisting of a variety of periosteal bone, endosteal bone, and haversian systems.

b. conduction. See **conduction, bone.**

b. crest, the most coronal portion of alveolar bone.

b. cyst, **1.** a vascular cyst eccentrically placed within a bone. **2.** ostitis fibrosa cystica, a parathyroid disorder characterized by cyst formation and the replacement of bone tissue with fibrous connective tissue.

b. density, the compactness of bone tissue. The demonstration of bone density by means of radiographs directly depends on the quantity of inorganic salts contained in the bone tissue.

b. deposition, the apposition or formation of new bone as a normal physiologic process.

b. development. See **bone, endochondral, formation; bone formation;** and **bone, membrane, formation.**

b., effect of external radiation to, damage to the bones of adults is most often seen after heavy and localized x-ray treatment.

b., endochondral (cn'dōkon'drəl), a bone that is developed in relation to antecedent cartilages (for example, long bones, mandible). See also **bone, membrane.**

b., e., formation, primarily a replacement of previously formed embryonic cartilage with an adult bony structure; a more complex bone formation than membrane bone. The actual replacement of cartilage by bone is only part of the process, however; much of the bone is laid down directly external to the embryonic cartilage. See also **bone, membrane, formation.**

b. formation, the deposition of an organic mucopolysaccharide matrix (osteoid) that is subsequently mineralized with calcium salts. See also **bone apposition** and **bone deposition.**

b. graft, autogenous. See **graft, autogenous bone.**

b. graft, donor site. See **donor site.**

b. graft, onlay. See **graft, onlay bone.**

b. graft, recipient site. See **recipient site.**

b. groove, osteotomy into or near the crest of the alveolar ridge for placement of an endosteal blade type of implant.

b. g., canted, an osteotomy sloped to avoid the mandibular canal or keep the implant infrastructure within the medullary confines.

b., internal reconstruction of, the formation of bone on the tensional side of the periodontal ligament with concurrent resorption from the marrow space; contralaterally, resorption of alveolar bone with apposition from the endosteum in the marrow space.

b., interproximal, the bone that forms the septa between the teeth; consists primarily of a spongiosa of supporting bone covered by a layer of cortical bone. See also **septum, interdental.**

b. involvement, changes in the alveolar and supporting bone occurring as a sequel to or accompanying inflammatory or dystrophic disease; usually of a resorptive nature.

b. lamella, bone having the appearance of layers of thin leaves or plates. This appearance is produced by lines representing periods of inactivity of bone formation.

b., malar (zygomatic bone), a quadrangular bone on each side of the face that unites the frontal and superior maxillary bones with the zygomatic process of the temporal bone. It forms the cheek prominence, a portion of the lateral wall and floor of the orbit, and parts of the temporal fossa and infratemporal fossa.

b., marble. See **osteopetrosis.**

b. marrow, the soft vascular tissue that fills bone cavities and cancellous bone spaces and consists primarily of fat cells, hematopoietic cells, and osteogenetic reticular cells.

b. m. transplant, the transplantation of bone marrow from healthy donors to stimulate production of formed blood cells. It is used in treatment of hematopoietic or lymphoreticular diseases such as aplastic anemia, leukemia, immune deficiency syndromes, and acute radiation syndrome.

b., membrane, a bone developed within a membrane but having no antecedent cartilage (for example, parietal, frontal, bones of upper face). See also **bone, endochondral.**

b., m., formation, membrane bone forms directly from the mesenchyme, first as a thin, flattened, irregular bony plate or membrane in the dermis and gradually expanding at its margins and becoming thickened by the deposition of successive layers of additional bone on the inner and outer surfaces. See also **bone, endochondral, formation.**

b. membranes, membrane structures associated with the growth, development, and repair of bone. They include the periosteum, a connective tissue layer adjacent to bone surfaces; periodontal membrane, a modified periosteum associated with tooth structure; and endosteum, a thin layer of connective tissue lining the walls of the bone marrow spaces.

b., microscopic appearance of, the composition of bone tissue as viewed under a microscope. Microscopically, bone is composed of osteocytes embedded within lacunae in a calcified intercellular matrix. Extending from the lacunae are minute canals called canaliculi, which communicate with canaliculi of adjacent lacunae. Through this system of canals, nutrient material reaches the osteocytes and provides avenues for the removal of waste products of metabolism. Bone is deposited in incremental layers (lamellae) around haversian canals, the lamellae toward the surface of the bone being more or less parallel to it.

b. mineral content, chemistry of, the hardness of bone results from its mineral content in the organic matrix. The minerals (commonly designated as bone salts) and the organic matrix make up the interstitial substance of bone. The bone salts consist essentially of hydroxyapatite ($Ca_{10}[PO_4]_6$ $[OH_2]$), carbon dioxide, and water, with small amounts of other ions.

b. onlay. See **graft, onlay bone.**

b., perichondrial, bone that is deposited in concentric layers around the long shaft of the bone in a manner similar to that of the growth of endochondral bone.

b., physical properties of, compact bone has the following physical char-

B

acteristics: specific gravity, 1.92 to 1.99; tensile strength, 13,000 to 17,000 psi; compressive strength, 18,000 to 24,000 psi; compressive strength parallel to the long axis, 7150 psi; compressive strength at right angles to the long axis, 10,800 psi. These physical characteristics make bone particularly suitable for carrying out its functions of weight bearing, leverage, and protection of vulnerable viscera.

b. rarefaction, a decreased density of bone such as a decrease in weight per unit of volume.

b. recession. See **recession, bone.**

b., resorption and repair of, an adaptive physiologic mechanism occurring as long as the individual retains the natural dentition. See also **resorption of bone.**

b., resting lines in, lines created by alternating periods of bone formation and rest, giving a tierlike appearance to lamellar bone.

b., reversal lines in, irregular lines containing concavities directed away from the bundle bone and serving as histologic indications that resorption has taken place up to that line from the marrow side.

b. sequestrum. See **sequestrum.**

b., sphenoid, an irregular, wedge-shaped bone located at the base of the skull in front of the temporal bone and the basilar portion of the occipital bone. It is composed of a cuboidal body hollowed out interiorly to form the sphenoidal air sinuses. Extending from the body laterally are two large wings and two small wings. Projecting below the body are two pterygoid processes. The lateral surfaces of the pterygoid processes give origin to the external pterygoid muscles, whereas the medial surfaces give origin to the internal pterygoid muscles.

b., spongy. See **bone, cancellous.**

b. support, the amount of alveolar and trabecular bone adjacent to a tooth that can provide attachment, investment, and support for the tooth.

b., supporting. See **bone, cancellous.**

b., s., atrophy of disuse. See **bone, cancellous, atrophy of disuse.**

b. surgery. See **surgery, osseous.**

b., thickened margin of, widening of the crest of the alveolus, primarily on the buccal and lingual aspects, varying from a thick ledge to a "beading" of the bone margin; results in a more or less bulbous contour of the gingival tissue overlying it.

b., trabecular. See **bone, cancellous.**

b. wax. See **wax, bone.**

b., woven, a character and pattern of bone resulting from the interweaving of broad bands of bone.

b., zygomatic. See **bone, malar.**

Bonwill-Hawley chart. See **chart, Hawley.**

Bonwill's triangle. See **triangle, Bonwill's.**

bony crater, a concave resorptive defect in the alveolar crest, usually occurring interdentally.

bony crepitus. See **crepitus, bony.**

borax, often a principal ingredient in casting fluxes. Used in gypsum products as a retardant for the setting reaction and a strengthener for hydrocolloids.

border, a circumferential margin or edge.

b., denture (denture edge, denture periphery), the limit, boundary, or circumferential margin of a denture base.

b., mandibular (mandibular plane), tangent to the lower border of the mandible. A line joining point gonion to point gnathion.

b. molding, the shaping of an impression material by the manipulation or action of the tissues to determine denture border position.

b. movement. See **movement, border.**

b. seal, the contact of the denture border with the underlying or adjacent tissues to prevent the passage of air or other substances.

b. structures, the oral structures that bound the borders of a denture.

b. tissues, movement, the action of the muscles and other structures adjacent to the borders of a denture.

bouton's terminaux. See **end-feet.**

Bowen's disease. See **carcinoma in situ.**

box, light. See **illuminator.**

boxing, the building up of vertical walls, usually in wax, around an impression to produce the desired size and form of the base of the cast.

b. strip. See **strip, boxing.**

brace, an orthotic device to support and hold any part of the body in the

B

correct position to allow function such as a leg brace that permits walking and standing. Sometimes used to describe orthodontic appliances.

brachycephalic (brak′isef′alik), descriptive term applied to a broad, round head having a cephalic index of more than 80.

brachydactyly, abnormal shortness of the fingers, usually associated with some congenital syndrome.

brachygnathia (bird-face, micrognathia) (brak′igna′thē·ə), marked underdevelopment of the mandible. See also **retrognathism.**

bracing, a resistance to the horizontal components of masticatory force.

bracket, a small metal attachment fixed to a band that serves as a means of fastening the arch wire to the band.

bradycardia (brad′ikär′dē·ə), abnormal slowness of the heart as evidenced by a slowing of the pulse rate (less than 50 beats per minute).

bradydiastole (brad′idī·as′tōle), abnormal prolongation of diastole.

bradykinin, one of a number of plasma kinins, a potent vasodilator; one of the physiologic mediators of an anaphylactic reaction.

bradypnea (brad′ipnē′·ə), abnormal slowness of breathing.

brain death, an irreversible form of unconsciousness characterized by a complete loss of brain function while the heart continues to beat.

brain, electrical activity of, electrical energy that can be observed as waves with electroencephalographic equipment. These rhythms and patterns have been organized into a system that imputes values for the state of health and disease. Electrical evidence of brain activity in the cerebral cortex reveals that different potential patterns are produced by different states of mental activity (for example, tension, mental work, sleep).

brainstem, the portion of the brain comprising the medulla oblongata, pons, and mesencephalon. It performs motor, sensory, and reflex functions.

branchial nerve. See **nerve, branchial.**

Branemark technique. See **osseointegration.**

breach of contract. See **contract, breach of.**

break-even point, the level of patient visits or net revenues at which the revenues for a period are equal to the expenses incurred in that period.

breath, air inhaled and exhaled in respiration.

b., bad (offensive). See **halitosis.**

breathing, mouth, the process of inspiration and expiration of air primarily through the oral cavity. It is commonly seen in nasal conditions such as deviated septum, hypertrophied adenoids, and allergies and may produce excessive drying of the oral mucosa with a tendency to gingival hyperplasia.

bregma (breg′mə), the point at which the sagittal and coronary sutures meet.

Breuer's reflex. See **reflex, Hering-Breuer.**

bridge, a colloquial expression for a fixed partial denture. See also **denture, partial, fixed.**

b., cantilever. See **denture, partial, fixed, cantilever.**

b., fixed. See **denture, partial, fixed.**

b., removable, a colloquial expression for a removable partial denture. See also **denture, partial, removable.**

b. splint. See **splint, fixed.**

Brill-Symmers disease. See **lymphoma, giant follicular.**

Brinell hardness number. See **number, Brinell hardness.**

Brinell hardness test. See **test, Brinell hardness.**

brittle, friable. Technically a brittle material is one in which the proportional limit and ultimate strength are close together in value. See also **ductility.**

broach, an instrument with numerous barbs protruding from a metal shaft. It is generally used to engage the dental pulp for extirpation.

b., barbed. See **broach.**

b. holder, an instrument similar to a pin vise used to hold a broach.

b., pathfinder. See **broach, smooth.**

b., smooth (pathfinder, pathfinder broach), an instrument used for locating the orifice of a root canal and exploring the canal to determine the accessibility of the root end.

Broders' classification. See **index, Broders'.**

bromine, a toxic, red-brown, liquid element of the halogen group.

Bromine is widely used in industry, photography, the manufacture of organic chemicals, and pharmaceuticals.

bromism (bro'mizəm), the toxic state induced by excessive exposure to or ingestion of bromine or bromine-containing compounds.

bromocriptine mesylate, *trade name:* Parlodel; *drug class:* dopamine receptor agonist, ovulation stimulant; *action:* inhibits prolactin release by activating postsynaptic dopamine receptors; *uses:* treatment of female infertility, Parkinson's disease, amenorrhea.

bromodeoxyuridine, a compound that competes with uridine for incorporation in ribonucleic acid.

brompheniramine maleate, *trade names:* Bromphen, Dehist, Veltane; *drug class:* antihistamine, H_1-receptor antagonist; *action:* acts on blood vessels and gastrointestinal (GI) and respiratory systems by competing with histamine for H_1-receptor sites; *uses:* treatment of allergy symptoms, rhinitis.

bromopnea (bramop'nē· ə). See **halitosis.**

bronchia (brong'kē· ə), bronchial tubes smaller than bronchi and larger than bronchioles.

bronchiarctia (brong'kē·ahrk'shē· ə), the stenosis of a bronchial tube.

bronchiectasis (brong'kē·ek'təsis), a chronic disease characterized by dilation of the bronchi and bronchioles, clinically recognizable by fetid breath and purulent matter; dilation of the bronchi, either local or general.

bronchiocele (brong'kē·ōsēl), a dilation or swelling of a branch smaller than a bronchus.

bronchiole (brong'kē·ōl), a terminal division of a bronchium.

bronchitis, an acute or chronic inflammation of the mucous membranes of the tracheobronchial tree.

bronchium (brong'kē· əm), one of the subdivisions of a bronchus.

bronchoalveolar, referring to both the bronchia and alveoli of the lungs.

bronchoconstriction (bron'kōkənstrik' shən), the reduction of the caliber of the bronchi.

bronchodilation (brong'kōdīlā'shən), the dilation of a bronchus; the operation of dilating a stenosed bronchus.

bronchodilator (brong'kōdīlā'tōr), a drug that dilates, or expands, the size of the lumina of the air passages of the lungs by relaxing the muscular walls.

bronchopneumonia, an acute inflammation of the lungs and bronchioles characterized by chills, fever, high pulse and respiratory rates, bronchial breathing, cough with purulent bloody sputum, severe chest pain, and abdominal distension.

bronchoscope, a curved flexible tube for visual examination of the bronchi.

bronchoscopy, the visual examination of the tracheobronchial tree using a standard rigid, tubular metal bronchoscope or a narrower, flexible, fiberoptic bronchoscope. Bronchoscopy is used to secure a biopsy, aspirate fluids, and diagnose such conditions as lung abscess, bronchial obstruction, and localized atelectasis.

bronchospasm (brong'kōspaz'əm), a spasmodic contraction of the muscular coat of the bronchial tubes such as occurs in asthma.

bronchostenosis (brong'kōstənō'sis), stenosis of the bronchi; bronchiarctia.

bronchus, one of the subdivision of the trachea serving to convey air to and from the lungs.

Brooke's tumor. See **epithelioma adenoides cysticum.**

brown pellicle. See **pellicle, brown.**

bruise, in medical terminology, a contusion; an injury made on the flesh by an instrument without breaking the skin.

bruit (brōō'ē), an extracardiac blowing sound heard at times over peripheral vessels; generally denotes cardiovascular disease.

brush, polishing, an instrument consisting of natural, synthetic, or wire bristles mounted on a mandrel or in a hub to fit on a lathe chuck; used to carry abrasive or polishing media to polish teeth, restorations, and prosthetic appliances.

brush, bristle polishing, a polishing brush with natural or synthetic bristles.

brush, wheel polishing, a polishing brush with bristles mounted similar to spokes of a wheel.

brush, wire polishing, a polishing brush with bristles of wire, usually steel or brass.

brushing. See **abrasion, denture.**

bruxism (bruk'sizəm), the involuntary gnashing, grinding, or clenching of teeth. Bruxism is usually an unconscious activity, whether the individual is awake or asleep; often associated with fatigue, anxiety, emotional stress, or fear, and frequently triggered by occlusal irregularities, usually resulting in abnormal wear patterns on the teeth, periodontal breakdown, and joint or neuromuscular problems.

BSP test. See **test, Bromsulphalein.**

bubo (byoo'bō), a lymph node that is enlarged as a result of an infection. The process may lead to suppuration; seen in primary syphilis, chancroid, plague, malaria, and other infectious processes.

buccal (buk'əl), pertaining to or adjacent to the cheek.

b. aspect. See **aspect, buccal.**

b. contour. See **contour, buccal.**

b. flange. See **flange, buccal.**

b. notch. See **notch, buccal.**

b. shelf. See **shelf, buccal.**

b. splint. See **splint, buccal.**

b. surface. See **surface, buccal.**

b. tube. See **tube, buccal.**

b. vestibule. See **vestibule, buccal.**

buccoclusion (buk'ōkloo'zhən), an occlusion in which the dental arch or group of teeth is buccal to the normal position.

buccolingual relationship. See **relationship, buccolingual.**

buccolingual stress. See **stress, buccolingual.**

buccoversion (buk'ōvər'zhən), any deviation from the normal line of occlusion toward the cheeks.

buck knife. See **knife, buck.**

buckling, the crowding of anterior teeth in the dental arch.

buclizine HCl, *trade name:* Bucladin-S; *drug class:* antihistamine, H_1-receptor antagonist; *action:* acts centrally by blocking chemoreceptor trigger zone; *uses:* treatment for motion sickness.

budesonide, *trade names:* Rhinocort Nasal Inhaler, Pulmicort; *drug class:* corticosteroid, synthetic; *action:* interacts with steroid cytoplasmic receptors to induce antiinflammatory effects; *uses:* management of symptoms of allergic rhinitis in adults and children; perennial nonallergic rhinitis in adults.

budget plan, a method of financing dental accounts in which arrange-ments are made for the patient to pay a series of small amounts on an account, usually over a period of 12 to 18 months.

buffer, any substance in a fluid that tends to lessen the change in hydrogen ion concentration that otherwise would be produced by adding acids or alkalis.

bug, an error in a computer program.

bulb, speech. See **aid, speech, prosthetic, pharyngeal section.**

bulimia, repeated secretive bouts of excessive eating followed by self-induced vomiting, purging, and anorexia, usually accompanied by feelings of guilt, depression, and self-disgust. Oral signs may include decalcification of the lingual aspect of the teeth.

bulla (bool'ə), a circumscribed, elevated lesion of the skin containing fluid and measuring more than 5 mm in diameter.

bumetanide, *trade name:* Bumex; *drug class:* loop diuretic; *action:* acts on the loop of Henle to decrease reabsorption of chloride and sodium with resultant diuresis; *uses:* treatment of edema in chronic heart disease, renal disease, pulmonary edema, ascites, and hypertension.

BUN. See **blood urea nitrogen.**

Bunnell test. See **test, Paul-Bunnell.**

bupivacaine HCl (local), *trade names:* Marcaine, Senorcaine; *drug class:* amide local anesthetic; *action:* inhibits ion fluxes across membranes, particularly sodium transport across cell membranes; decreases rise of depolarization phase of action potential; blocks nerve action potential; *uses:* local dental anesthesia, epidural anesthesia, peripheral nerve block, caudal anesthesia.

bupropion, *trade name:* Wellbutrin; *drug class:* antidepressant; *action:* weak uptake inhibitor of dopamine, serotonin, norepinephrine; mechanism unknown; *uses:* treatment of depression and anxiety disorders.

bur, a rotary cutting instrument of steel or tungsten carbide; supplied with cutting heads of various shapes.

b., carbide, a bur made of tungsten carbide; used at high rotational speeds.

b., crosscut, a bur with blades slot-ted perpendicularly to the axis of the bur.

b., end-cutting, a bur that has cutting blades only on the end of its head.

b., excavating, a bur used to remove dentin and debris from a cavity.

b., finishing, a bur with numerous fine-cutting blades placed close together; used to contour metallic restorations.

b., intramucosal insert base–preparing. See **insert, intramucosal.**

b., inverted cone, a bur with a head shaped like a truncated cone, the larger diameter being at the terminal (distal) end.

b., plug-finishing. See **bur, finishing.**

b., round, a bur with a sphere-shaped head.

b., straight fissure, a bur without crosscuts that has a cylindrical head.

b., tapered fissure, a bur having a long head with sides that converge from the shank to a blunt end.

burden of proof, in a legal proceeding, the duty to prove a fact or facts in dispute.

Burkitt's tumor (African lymphoma), a type of lymphosarcoma seen in African children. About half the patients have lesions in the jawbones. Recent evidence suggests a possible viral cause.

Burlew wheel, a trade name for an abrasive-impregnated, knife-edged, rubber polishing wheel; used on a mandrel in the dental handpiece to smooth metallic restorations and tooth surfaces.

B. w., high luster, Burlew wheel in which jeweler's rouge or iron peroxide is used as the abrasive agent.

B. w., midget (sulci Burlew wheel), a miniature form of Burlew wheel.

B. w., sulci. See **Burlew wheel, midget.**

burn, a lesion caused by contact of heat, radiation, friction, or chemicals with tissue. Thermal burns are classified as follows: first degree, manifested by erythema; second degree, manifested by formation of vesicles; third degree, manifested by necrosis of the mucosa or dermis; and fourth degree, manifested by charring into the submucous or subcutaneous layers of the body.

b., aspirin, an irregularly shaped, whitish area on the mucosa caused by the topical application of acetylsalicylic acid.

burnisher, an instrument shape with rounded edges used to burnish, polish, or work-harden metallic surfaces.

b., ball, a burnisher with a working point in the form of a ball.

b., beaver-tail. See **burnisher, straight.**

b., fishtail, a burnisher that slightly resembles a fish's tail in shape.

b., straight, a burnisher that resembles a beaver's tail in shape; the broad, flat blade is smoothly continuous with the shank, meeting it in a slight curve; the edges and the point are smoothly rounded.

burnishing, a process related to polishing and abrading; the metal is moved by mechanically distorting the normal space lattice. Commonly accomplished during the polishing of soft golds.

burnout, the elimination by heat of an invested pattern from a set investment to prepare the mold to receive casting metal.

b., high heat, the use of temperatures over 1100° F (593.5° C) to effect wax elimination and prepare the mold to receive casting metal.

b., inlay (wax), the elimination of wax from an invested inlay flask. See also **wax elimination.**

b., job, the condition of having no energy left to care, resulting from chronic, unrelieved job-related stress and characterized by physical and emotional exhaustion and sometimes by physical illness.

b., radiographic, excessive penetration of the x-ray beam of an object or part of an object, producing a totally black, or overexposed, area on the radiograph.

b., wax. See **burnout, inlay** and **wax elimination.**

business area, the area adjacent to the reception room in which the receptionist conducts the business affairs of the office and directly through which patients must pass to enter and leave the dental office.

business hours (office hours), those hours of the day during which professional, public, and other kinds of business are ordinarily conducted.

business office, the room reserved for the dentist in which the business of the dental practice is conducted.

buspirone HCl, *trade name:* BuSpar; *drug class:* antianxiety agent; *action:*

C

unknown, may inhibit 5-HT receptors or dopamine receptors; *use:* management and short-term relief of anxiety disorders.

busulfan, *trade name:* Myleran; *drug class:* antineoplastic; *action:* changes essential cellular ions to covalent bonding with resultant alkylation, which interferes with biologic function of deoxyribonucleic acid; *uses:* treatment of chronic myelocytic leukemia.

butoconazole nitrate, *trade name:* Femstat; *drug class:* antifungal; *action:* binds sterols in fungal cell membrane, which increases permeability; *use:* treatment of vulvovaginal infections caused by *Candida.*

butt, to place directly against the tissues covering the residual alveolar ridge; to bring any two square-ended surfaces into contact, as a butt joint.

button, the excess metal remaining from the casting and sprue; located at the end of the sprue, opposite the casting.

b., implant. See **insert, intramucosal.**

buttonhole approach, a method of surgical treatment of a periodontal abscess in which, after an incision is made in the fluctuant abscess, an additional attempt is made to curet the area adjoining the root and the fundus of the abscess through the destroyed portion of the alveolar plate or bone. (not current)

cachexia (kəkek'sē-ə), weakness, loss of weight, atrophy, and emaciation caused by severe or chronic disease.

c., hypophyseal. See **disease, Simmonds'.**

c., hypopituitary. See **disease, Simmonds'.**

cadaver, a dead body, most often used in reference to a body used for dissection and study.

cadaverine, a foul-smelling diamine formed by bacterial decarboxylation of lysine. It is poisonous and irritating to the skin.

cadmium, a bluish-white metallic element that resembles tin. Cadmium bromide, used in engraving, lithography, and photography, can cause severe gastrointestinal symptoms if ingested.

café-au-lait spots. See **spots, café-au-lait.**

cafeteria plan, employee benefits plan in which employees select their medical insurance coverage and other nontaxable fringe benefits from a list of options provided by the employer. Cafeteria plan participants may receive additional, taxable cash compensation if they select less expensive benefits.

caffeine (kafēn', kaf'ē·in), a white, odorless, bitter compound isolated from tea and coffee that is used as a stimulant of the central nervous system. See also **aspirin; phenacetin.**

Caffey's disease. See **hyperostosis, infantile cortical.** (not current)

calcific metamorphosis (of dental pulp), a frequently observed reaction to trauma, characterized by partial or complete obliteration of the pulp chamber and canal.

calcification (kal'sifikā'shən), the process whereby calcium salts are deposited in an organic matrix. The condition may be normal as in bone and tooth formation or pathologic in nature.

c., dystrophic, the pathologic deposition of calcium salts in necrotic or degenerated tissues.

c., metastatic, the pathologic deposition of calcium salts in previously undamaged tissues. This process is caused by an excessively high level of blood calcium such as in hyperparathyroidism.

calcifying epithelial odontogenic tumor (Pindborg tumor), an uncommon tumor arising from odontogenic epithelium characterized by focal areas of calcification. It has the same age, gender, and site distribution as the ameloblastoma.

calcination (kal'sinā'shən), a process of removing water by heat; used in the manufacture of plaster and stone from gypsum.

calcinosis (kal'sənō'sis), **l.** the deposition of calcium salts in various tissues because of hypercalcemia and tissue degeneration. **2.** the presence of calcification in or under the skin. The condition may occur in a localized (calcinosis circumscripta) or generalized (calcinosis universalis) form.

calcipotriene, *trade name:* Dovonex; *drug class:* vitamin D₃ derivative (synthetic); *action:* regulation of skin cell production and development; *use:* moderate plaque psoriasis.

calcitonin, *trade names:* Calcitonin, Calcimar, Miacalcin; *drug class:* synthetic polypeptide calcitonins; *action:* inhibits bone resorption, reduces osteoclast function, reduces serum calcium levels in hypercalcemia; *uses:* Paget's disease, postmenopausal osteoporosis, hypercalcemia.

calcitriol, *trade name:* Calcijex; *drug class:* vitamin D₃ hormone; *action:* increases intestinal absorption of calcium and phosphorus; *uses:* hypocalcemia in chronic renal dialysis and rickets, nutritional supplement.

calcium (kal′sē-əm), a basic element, with an atomic weight of 40.07, found in nearly all organized tissues. Essential for mineralization of bone and teeth. The normal level of calcium in the blood is 9 to 11.5 mg/100 ml. A deficiency of calcium in the diet or in use may lead to rickets or osteoporosis. Overexcretion in hyperparathyroidism leads to osteoporotic manifestations. See also **factor IV.**

c. binding protein. See **calmodulin.**

c., blood. See **blood calcium.**

c. carbonate, trade names: Maalox Antacid, Rolaids Calcium Rich, Tums E-X; *drug class:* antacid; *action:* neutralizes gastric acidity, supplies calcium; *uses:* antacid, calcium supplement.

c. carbonate and magnesium hydroxide, trade name: Rolaids; *drug class:* antacid; *action:* neutralizes gastric acidity; *use:* antacid.

c. channel blocker, a drug that inhibits the flow of calcium ions across the membranes of smooth muscle cells. The reduction of calcium flow relaxes smooth muscle tone and reduces the risk of muscle spasms. Calcium channel blockers are used in the prevention and treatment of coronary artery spasms.

c., dietary, the amount of absorbable calcium ingested daily.

c. fluoride, a compound that is used as a flux in the manufacture of some silicate cements.

c. hydroxide, a white powder that is mixed with water or another medium and used as a base material in cavity liners and for pulp capping.

c. oxalate, an insoluble sediment in the urine and urinary calculi.

c. phosphate, an odorless, tasteless white powder, the various forms of which are sometimes used as abrasives in dentifrices.

c. salts, calcium present in salivary fluid as phosphates and carbonates. They are believed to form dental calculus on their precipitation from saliva.

c. sulfate. See **alpha-hemihydrate; beta-hemihydrate; gypsum.**

c. tungstate, a chemical substance used in crystal form to coat screens; the screens fluoresce when struck by roentgen rays.

calculus, a concretion composed of calcium phosphate, calcium carbonate, magnesium phosphate, and other elements within an organic matrix composed of desquamated epithelium, mucin, microorganisms, and other debris.

c., dental, a salivary deposit of calcium phosphate and carbonate with organic matter on the teeth or a dental prosthesis.

c., serumal. See **calculus, subgingival.**

c., subgingival, calculus deposited on the tooth structure and found apical to the gingival margin within the confines of the gingival cervix, gingival pocket, or periodontal pocket. Usually darker, more pigmented, and denser than supragingival calculus.

c., supragingival, calculus deposited on the teeth occlusal or incisal to the gingival crest.

calibrated probe. See **probe, periodontal.**

calibration, the process of comparing a measurement instrument against a verified standard instrument. The US Bureau of Standards maintains the national calibration instruments for weights and measures.

c. of x-ray unit. See **unit, x-ray calibration.**

caliper, axis-orbital, a caliper used to record facial measurements and transfer them to an adjustable articulator. It consists of the following: (1) a hinge-bow, (2) a bite fork covered with compound, (3) an indicator of the axis-orbital plane, (4) an upright rod to hold the orbital indicator in place, (5) a

C

toggle to freeze the bow's base to the bite fork, and (6) a toggle to attach and allow adjustments for the support of the indicator. Synonym: hinge-bow transfer recorder.

Callahan's method. See **method, chloropercha.**

callus (kal'əs), the tissue near and about the broken fragments of a bone that becomes involved in the repair of the fracture through various stages of exudate, fibrosis, and new bone formation.

calmodulin, a calcium-binding protein that mediates a variety of biochemical and physiologic processes, including the contraction of muscles and the release of norepinephrine.

calorie, the amount of heat required to raise 1 g of water 1° C at atmospheric pressure, also called gram calorie or small calorie. A great calorie, or kilocalorie, consists of 1000 small calories. The kilocalorie is the unit used to denote the heat expenditure of an organism and the fuel or energy value of food.

calorimetry, the measurement of the amounts of heat radiated and absorbed.

Camper's line. See **line, Camper's.**

camphorated opium tincture, *trade name:* Paregoric; *drug class:* antidiarrheal; *action:* antiperistaltic and analgesic with activity related to morphine content; *use:* diarrhea.

camphorated parachlorophenol (par'əklōr'ōfē'nol), a mixture of 35% parachlorophenol and 65% camphor; used to treat root canals and periapical infections.

Campylobacter, a microorganism associated with progressive periodontal destruction and refractory forms of periodontitis.

canal, the portion of the root that contains the pulp tissue and is bounded by dentin.

c., accessory root, a lateral branching of the main root canal, usually occurring in the apical third of the root.

c., branching. See **canal, collateral pulp.**

c., collateral pulp (branching canal), a dental pulp canal branch that emerges from the root at a place other than the apex.

c., interdental (nutrient canal), the nutrient channels that pass upward through the body of the mandible. Seen as radiolucent lines on radiographs.

c., mandibular, a channel extending from the mandibular foramen on the medial surface of the ramus of the mandible to the mental foramen. It contains mandibular blood vessels (arteries and veins) and a portion of the mandibular branch of the trigeminal nerve.

c., nutrient. See **canal, interdental.**

c., pulp, the space in the radicular portion of the tooth occupied by the pulp.

c., root. See **canal, pulp.**

c., r., measurements, a technique employing the use of radiographs to determine the length of the root canal.

canaliculus (kan'əlik'yələs), a minute channel that extends from or to the lacunae of bone and cementum and contains filamentous processes of the cells that occupy the lacunae; interconnects with canaliculi extending from neighboring lacunae.

cancer (kan'sər), a malignant neoplasm. The term is sometimes incorrectly used to include all neoplasms, whether benign or malignant. *Carcinoma* and *sarcoma* are more limiting terms.

Cancer's seven warning signals

- Change in bowel or bladder habits
- A sore that will not heal
- Unusual bleeding or discharge
- Thickening or lump in breast or elsewhere
- Indigestion or difficulty swallowing
- Obvious change in a wart or mole
- Nagging cough or hoarseness

From American Cancer Society: *Cancer facts and figures 1990,* Atlanta, 1990, American Cancer Society.

cancrum oris (kang'krəm ō'ris). See **stomatitis, gangrenous.**

Candida albicans (kan'didə albəkanz), a budding, yeastlike fungus present in the normal flora of the mucous membrane of the female genital tract and human respiratory and gastrointestinal tracts (including the mouth) that is capable of assuming a pathogenic role in the production of oral and systemic moniliasis such as thrush and monilial infection.

candidiasis (kan'didī'·əsis), an infection by *Candida albicans*. See also **moniliasis; thrush.**

c., angular cheilitis, forms fissures or ulcers radiating from the angles of the mouth; often accompanied by white plaques. Usually observed in elderly patients, although when observed in a young person, it may be an indicator of HIV infection. Candidiasis of the esophagus, trachea, bronchi, or lungs is associated with group IV human immunodeficiency virus (HIV) infection. See also **acquired immunodeficiency syndrome; AIDS; ARC.**

c., erythematous (atrophic), forms smooth red patches on the hard or soft palate, buccal mucosa, or dorsal surface of the tongue.

c., hyperplastic, forms white plaques that cannot be removed by wiping or scraping.

c., pseudomembranous, forms loosely adherent (wipeable), yellowish-white plaques on the oral mucosal surface.

canine (kā'nīn) (cuspid), one of the four pointed teeth in human beings, situated one on each side of each jaw, distal to the lateral incisor; forms the keystone of the arch. The term *canine* is increasingly preferred to *cuspid.*

c. fossa. See **fossa, canine.**

c. guidance, a concept of occlusal function in which the canine teeth are assigned a major control role in the excursive movements of the mandible.

canker (kang'kər). See **herpes labialis.**

c. sore. See **sore, canker.**

cannabis, a psychoactive herb derived from the flowering tops of a variety of hemp, *Cannabis sativa.* It is the active ingredient of marijuana. Cannabis has no currently acceptable clinical use in the United States but has been employed in the treatment of glaucoma and as an antiemetic in some cancer patients to counter the nausea and vomiting associated with chemotherapy. Cannabis is controlled under Schedule I of the Comprehensive Drug Abuse Prevention and Control Act of 1970.

cannula (kan'yələ), a tube for insertion into the body; its caliber is usually occupied by a trocar during the act of insertion.

cantilever bridge. See **denture, partial, fixed, cantilever.** (not current)

cantilever partial denture. See **denture, partial, fixed, cantilever.** (not current)

cantle, a fragment, piece, portion. (not current)

capacity, legal qualification, competency, power, or fitness.

c., functional residual (normal capacity), the volume of gas in the lungs at resting expiratory level.

c., iron-binding, a measure of the binding capacity of iron in the serum; helps to differentiate the causes of hypoferremia. This capacity tends to increase in iron deficiency and diminishes in chronic diseases and during infection.

c., normal. See **capacity, functional residual.**

c., total lung (TLC), the volume of air in the lungs at the end of maximal inspiration.

c., vital (VC), the maximum volume of air that can be expired after maximal inspiration.

capillarity (kap'ĭler'ĭtē), the phenomenon by which a film of fluid is drawn and held between two closely approximating surfaces.

capillary (kap'iler'ē), the terminal vessels uniting the arterial with the venous systems of the body. Capillaries are organized into extensive branching reticular beds to provide a maximal surface for exchange of fluids, electrolytes, and metabolites between tissues and the vascular system. The capillary bed has the largest cross-sectional area of the entire vascular system.

c. attraction, the quality or state that, because of surface tension, causes elevation or depression of the surface of a liquid that is in contact with a solid. Considered to be one of the factors in retention of complete dentures.

capital budgeting, the process of planning expenditures on assets whose returns are expected to extend beyond 1 year.

capitation, 1. the practice of dentistry financed by a set fee per person per given period of time. A form of contracted dental care, usually by a corporation, institution, or other group. **2.** a system by which the contracting dentist, assuming the financial risk, is compensated at a fixed per-capita rate, usually on specific, predetermined dental services as appropriate and necessary to eligible subscribers. **3.** a dental benefits program in which a dentist or dentists contract with the program's sponsor or administrator to provide all or most of the dental services covered under the program to subscribers in return for payment on a per-capita basis.

c. fee, a predetermined per-person charge made by the carrier for benefits available under an insurance plan.

capitulum (kəpich'ələm), a small head. The term used by some European writers instead of *head* or *condyle.*

c. mandibulae. See **process, condyloid.**

capping, pulp, the covering of an exposed dental pulp with a material that protects it from external influences.

capping, direct pulp, application to the exposed pulp of a drug or material for the purpose of stimulating repair of the injured pulpal tissue.

capping, indirect pulp, a chemical (usually calcium hydroxide) placed over a layer of carious dentin remaining over the potentially exposed pulp to protect the pulp from external irritants.

capsaicin, *trade names:* Zostrix, Capzasin-P, Axsain; *drug class:* topical analgesic for selected pain syndromes; *action:* depletes and prevents reaccumulation of substance P in peripheral sensory neurons; *uses:* neuralgia associated with herpes zoster, rheumatoid arthritis, temporomandibular joint (TMJ) pain.

capsule, joint, a fibrous sac or ligament that encloses a joint and limits its motion. It is lined with synovial membrane.

capsule, temporomandibular joint. See **articulation, temporomandibular, capsule.**

captopril, *trade name:* Capoten; *drug class:* angiotensin-converting enzyme; *action:* dilation of arterial and venous vessels; *uses:* hypertension.

carat, a standard of fineness of gold, 24 carats being taken as expressing absolute purity.

carbamazepine, *trade names:* Apo-Carbamazepine, Epitol, Novo Carbamaz; *drug class:* anticonvulsant; *action:* inhibits nerve impulses by limiting influx of sodium ions across cell membrane in motor cortex; *uses:* tonic-clonic complex-partial, mixed seizures, a specific analgesic for trigeminal neuralgia, sometimes used in the treatment of herpes zoster.

carbenicillin, a semisynthetic penicillin that is acid resistant and rapidly absorbed from the small intestine and thus suitable for oral administration.

carbide bur. See **bur, carbide.**

carbohemia (kär'bōhē'mē-ə), an imperfect oxygenation of the blood.

carbohemoglobin (kär'bōhēmōglō'-bin), hemoglobin compounded with CO_2. (not current)

carbohydrates, a group of organic compounds with the class name saccharides, which are the aldehydic or ketonic derivatives of polyhydric alcohols. Carbohydrates such as sugar, starch, cellulose, and gum are generally synthesized by green plants. Carbohydrates constitute the main energy source in the diet and are classified as mono-, di-, tri-, and poly-saccharides.

carbohydrate tolerance. See **tolerance, carbohydrate.**

carbon, a nonmetallic tetravalent element that occurs in pure form in diamonds and graphite. It occurs as a component of all living tissue. Most of the study of organic chemistry focuses on the vast number of carbon compounds.

c. coated, a vitreous carbon coating to either an endosteal or blade implant to improve tissue compatability.

c. dioxide, a colorless, odorless gas produced by the complete oxidation of carbon. Carbon dioxide is a product of cell respiration and is carried by the blood to the lungs and exhaled. The acid-base balance of body fluids and tissues is affected by the level of carbon dioxide and its carbonate compounds.

c. markings, the markings made on the teeth when, with articulating paper interposed, the mandibular teeth are brought in contact with the maxillary teeth. (not current)

c. monoxide, a colorless, odorless, poisonous gas produced by the combustion of carbon or organic fuels in a limited oxygen supply. Carbon monoxide combines irreversibly with hemoglobin, preventing the formation of oxyhemoglobin and reducing the oxygen supply to the tissues.

Classes of carbohydrates

Chemical class name	Class members	Sources
Polysaccharides Multiple sugars, complex carbohydrates	Starch	Grains and grain products Cereal, bread, crackers, and other baked goods Pasta Rice, corn, bulgur Legumes Potatoes and other vegetables
	Glycogen	Animal tissues, liver and muscle meats
	Dietary fiber	Whole grains Fruits Vegetables Seeds, nuts, skins
Disaccharides Double sugars, simple carbohydrates	Sucrose	"Table" sugar: sugar cane, sugar beets Molasses
	Lactose	Milk
	Maltose	Starch digestion, intermediate Sweetener in food products Starch digestion, final
Monosaccharides Single sugars, simple carbohydrates	Glucose (dextrose)	Corn syrup (large use in processed foods)
	Fructose	Fruits, honey
	Galactose	Lactose (milk)

From Williams SW: *Basic nutrition and diet therapy,* ed 9, St Louis, 1997, Mosby.

carbonate, a mineral salt of carbonic acid.

   carbonate hydroxyapatite (kär'bə-nāt hīdrok'sē·ap'ətīt), the term indicating the composition and crystal structure of hard tissues.

carbonic acid, an unstable acid formed by dissolving carbon dioxide in water. It is the basis of carbonated beverages and contributes the negative ion to carbonate salts.

carcinogen, a substance or agent that causes the development or increases the incidence of cancer.

carcinoma (kär'sinō'mə), a malignant epithelial tumor. Also called *cancer.*

   c., adenoid cystic (cylindroma, adenocystic carcinoma, adenocystic basal cell carcinoma, basaloid mixed tumor), a pseudoadenomatous basal cell carcinoma originating from salivary glands, the cells of which resemble basal cells and form ductlike or cystlike structures. It grows slowly but is malignant.

   c., basal cell (basal cell epithelioma, rodent ulcer, turban tumor), an epithelial neoplasm with a basic structure resembling the basal cells of the epidermis. It develops from basal cells of the epidermis or from the outer cells of hair follicles or sebaceous glands, particularly the middle third of the face. It rarely, if ever, metastasizes but is locally invasive. It does not arise from oral mucosa.

   c., basosquamous, carcinoma that histologically exhibits both basal and squamous elements. It may occasionally be seen in the oral cavity; considered to have a greater tendency to metastasize than does basal cell carcinoma.

   c., epidermoid (squamous cell carcinoma), a malignant epithelial neoplasm with cells resembling those of the epidermis. The term *squamous cell carcinoma* is used for intraoral lesions of this nature.

   c., exophytic, a malignant epithelial neoplasm with marked outward growth similar to a wart or papilloma.

   c. in situ, a dysplastic epithelial disease involving the skin and mucous membranes and considered to be precancerous. Dyskeratosis is evident, but no invasion has yet occurred.

   c., intraepithelial. See **carcinoma in situ.**

   c., mucoepidermoid, a malignant epithelial tumor of the salivary gland;

characterized by acini with mucus-producing cells.

c., squamous cell. See **carcinoma, epidermoid.**

c., transitional cell, a malignant tumor arising from a transitional type of stratified epithelium.

cardia, the opening between the esophagus and the cardiac portion of the stomach; characterized by the absence of acid cells. Also an archaic term formerly used to describe the heart and the region surrounding it.

cardiac, relating to the heart.

c. arrest, a stopping of heart action; a complete cessation of heart function.

c. massage. See **massage, cardiac.**

c. output, the volume of blood put out by the heart per minute; the product of the stroke volume and the heart rate per minute.

c. pacemaker. See **pacemaker.**

cardioinhibitory (kär'dē-ōinhib'itōrē), restraining or inhibiting the movements of the heart.

cardiokinetic (kahr'dē-ōkinet'ik), exciting the heart; a remedy that excites the heart.

cardiology, the scientific study of the anatomy, normal function, and disorders of the heart.

cardiomyopathy, hypertrophic, a disease of the heart in which the heart is enlarged.

cardiopulmonary, pertaining to the heart and lungs.

c. resuscitation (CPR), a basic emergency procedure for life support, consisting of artificial respiration and manual external cardiac massage.

cardiovascular disease, any one of a number of abnormal conditions that involve dysfunction of the heart and blood vessels, including but not limited to systemic hypertension, atherosclerosis and coronary heart disease, and rheumatic heart disease.

cardiovascular system, the network of structures, including the heart and blood vessels, that convey the blood throughout the body.

care, as a legal term, the opposite of negligence.

c., reasonable, such care as an ordinarily prudent person would exercise under the conditions existing at the time that person is called on to act.

caregiver, a person providing treatment or support to a sick, disabled, or dependent individual.

caries (ker'ēz), in general medicine, the decay or death of a bone.

c., arrested dental, the state existing when the progress of the decay process has halted.

c., dental, an infectious disease with progressive destruction of tooth substance, beginning on the external surface by demineralization of enamel or exposed cementum.

c., healed dental. See **caries, dental, arrested.**

c., incipient dental, a decayed part of a tooth in which the lesion is just coming into existence.

c., proximal dental, decay occurring in the mesial or distal surface of a tooth.

c., rampant dental, a suddenly appearing, widespread, rapidly progressing type of caries.

c., recurrent dental, the extension of the carious process beyond the margin of a restoration.

c., residual dental (residual carious dentin), the decayed material left in a prepared cavity and over which a restoration is placed.

c., senile dental (senile decay), caries noted particularly in old age when supporting tissues have receded; occurs in cementum, usually on proximal surfaces of the teeth.

cariogenicity, the ability of a substance to induce or potentiate the formation of dental caries.

cariostatic agents, agents that inhibit or arrest dental caries formation. See also **flourides, sealants.** (not current)

carious (ker'ē-əs), pertaining to caries or decay.

c. dentin. See **wax, carious.**

carisoprodol, *trade names:* Soma, Vanasom; *drug class:* skeletal muscle relaxant, central acting; *action:* nonspecific central nervous system sedation; *uses:* adjunct for relief of muscle spasm in musculoskeletal conditions.

carnauba wax. See **wax, carnauba.**

Carnoy's solution. See **solution, Carnoy's.**

carotene (ker'ətin), an orange pigment found in carrots, leafy vegetables, and other foods that may be converted to vitamin A in the body.

carotenemia (ker'ətinē'mē-ə), excess carotene in the blood, producing a pigmentation of the skin and mucous membranes that resembles jaundice.

carotid (kərot′id), either one of the two main right and left arteries of the neck.

c. stenosis, the narrowing and hardening of the carotid artery.

carpal tunnel syndrome, an irritation and inflammation of the synovials surrounding the tendons controlling the fingers. Carpal tunnel syndrome is a disabling condition for persons who work with their hands, particularly those engaging in keyboard activities in music, typing, and data management.

carrier, I. a person harboring a specific infectious agent without clinical evidence of disease and who serves as a potential source or reservoir of infection for others. May be a healthy or convalescent carrier. **2.** the party of the dental plan contract who agrees to pay claims or provide service. Synonyms: insurer, underwriter, and administrative agent. See also **third party.**

c., amalgam, an instrument used to carry plastic amalgam to the prepared cavity or mold into which it is to be inserted.

c., foil. See **foil passer.**

carteolol, *trade name:* Cartrol; *drug class:* nonselective β-adrenergic blocker; *action:* competitively blocks stimulation of β-adrenegic receptors within vascular smooth muscle, decreases rate of sinoatrial (SA) node discharge, increases SA node recovery time; *use:* mild-to-moderate hypertension.

c. HCl, *trade name:* Ocupress; *drug class:* β-adrenergic blocker; *action:* nonselective β-adrenergic blocking agent, reduces production of aqueous humor by unknown mechanisms; *uses:* chronic open/angle glaucoma, ocular hypertension.

cartilage, a derivative of connective tissue arising from the mesenchyme. Typical hyaline cartilage is a flexible, rather elastic material with a semitransparent, glasslike appearance. Its ground substance, or matrix, is a complex protein (chondromucoid), through which is distributed a large network of connective tissue fibers. Distributed throughout the matrix are cartilage cells that are rounded and do not have the branching characteristics of bone cells. The cells are isolated in the matrix they have secreted and normally have no blood vessels. Therefore nutrients and metabolites are exchanged with the circulation by passage through the matrix.

c., articular, a thin layer of hyaline cartilage located on the joint surfaces of some bones. Not usually found on articular surfaces of temporomandibular joints, which are covered with an avascular fibrous tissue.

c., cricoid, the lowest cartilage of the larynx.

caruncle, submaxillary, the orifice of the sublingual (Wharton's) duct that opens into the mouth on a small papilla on either side of the lingual frenum.

carvedilol, *trade name:* Coreg; *drug class:* nonselective β-adrenergic blocking agent with α-blocking activity; *action:* produces fall in blood pressure without reflex tachycardia or significant reduction in heart rate, *use:* essential hypertension alone or with other antihypertensives.

carver (carving instrument), an instrument used to shape a plastic material such as wax or amalgam.

c., amalgam, an instrument used to shape plastic amalgam.

carving, shaping and forming with instruments.

case, the term often incorrectly used instead of the appropriate noun (for example, *patient, flask, denture, casting*). "Case" is not synonymous with "patient" because the latter is the human being affected with the disease.

c. charting, the recording of a patient's status of health or disease.

c. dismissal, the technique of illustrating to the patient the results of treatment, usually done during the last appointment of a series.

c. history. See **history, case.**

c. management, the monitoring and coordination of treatment rendered to patients with specific diagnoses or requiring high cost or extensive services.

c. presentation, explanation of dental needs to the patient.

c. summary, enumeration of all the services to be performed for an estimated amount of money.

case-control study, an investigation employing an epidemiologic approach in which previously existing incidents of a medical condition are used in lieu of gathering new information from a randomized population. Control is obtained by comparing known cases of the medical condition with a group of persons who have not developed the medical problem.

cash budget, a schedule showing cash flows (receipts, disbursements, net cash) for a firm over a specified period.

cash cycle, the length of time between the purchase of raw materials and the collection of accounts receivable generated in the sale of the final product.

cash flow, the reported net income of a corporation plus amounts charged off for depreciation, depletion, amortization, and extraordinary charges to reserves, which are bookkeeping deductions and not paid out in actual dollars and cents. A yardstick used in recent years to offer a better indication of the ability of a company to pay dividends and finance expansion from self-generated cash than the conventional reported net income figure.

cassette (kəset'), a light, tight container in which x-ray films are placed for exposure to x-rays; usually backed with lead to eliminate the effect of backscattered radiation.

c., cardboard (cardboard filmholder), a cardboard envelope of simple construction suitable for use in making radiographs on "direct exposure" or "no-screen" types of x-ray films.

c., screen-type, a cassette usually made of metal, with the exposure side of low–atomic number material such as Bakelite, aluminum, or magnesium and containing intensifying screens between which a "screen type" of film or films may be placed for exposure to x-rays.

cast, I. an object formed by pouring plastic or liquid material into a mold in which it hardens. **2.** to throw metal into an impression to form the casting.

c. bar splint. See **splint, cast bar.**

c., corrected master, a dental cast that has been modified by the correction of the edentulous ridge areas as registered in a supplemental, correctable impression.

c., dental, a positive likeness of a part or parts of the oral cavity reproduced in a durable hard material.

c., diagnostic, a positive likeness of dental structures for the purpose of study and treatment planning.

   c., d. implant, a cast made from a conventional mucosal impression on which the wax trial denture and surgical impression trays are made or selected.

c., gnathostatic, a cast of the teeth trimmed so that the occlusal plane is in its normal position in the mouth when the cast is set on a plane surface. Such casts are used in the gnathostatic technique of orthodontic diagnosis.

c., implant, a positive reproduction of the exposed bony surfaces made in a surgical bone impression and on which an implant frame is designed and fabricated.

c., investment. See **cast, refractory.**

c., keying of, the process of forming the base (or capital) of a cast so that it can be remounted accurately. Also referred to as the *split-cast method* of returning a cast to an articulator.

c., master, an accurate replica of the prepared tooth surfaces, residual ridge areas, or other parts of the dental arch reproduced from an impression from which a prosthesis is to be fabricated.

c., preextraction, a cast made before the extraction of teeth. See also **cast, diagnostic.**

c., preoperative. See **cast, diagnostic.**

c., record, a positive replica of the dentition and adjoining structures, used as a reference for conditions existing at a given time.

c., refractory, a cast made of materials that can withstand high temperatures without disintegrating and that, when used in partial denture casting techniques, expand to compensate for metal shrinkage.

c., study. See **cast, diagnostic.**

c., working, an accurate reproduction of a master cast; used in preliminary fitting of a casting to avoid injury to the master cast.

casting, I. a metallic object formed in a mold. **2.** forming a casting in a mold.

c. flask. See **flask, refractory.**

c. machine, a mechanical device used for throwing or forcing a molten metal into a refractory mold.

   c. m., air pressure, a casting machine that forces metal into the mold via compressed air.

c. m., centrifugal, a casting machine that forces the metal into the mold via centrifugal force.

c. m., vacuum, a casting machine in which the metal is cast by evacuation of gases from the mold. Atmospheric pressure actually forces metal into the mold.

c. model. See **cast, refractory.**

c. ring. See **flask, refractory.**

c. temperature. See **temperature, casting.**

c., vacuum, the casting of a metal in the presence of a vacuum. See also **casting machine, vacuum.**

c. wax. See **wax, casting.**

Castle's intrinsic factor. See **factor, Castle's intrinsic.**

castration, the surgical excision of one or both testicles or ovaries, usually to reduce the production and secretion of certain hormones that may stimulate the proliferation of malignant cells in women with breast cancer and men with prostate cancer. Surgically referred to as *orchidectomy* and *oophorectomy.*

c. anxiety, 1. the fantasized fear of injury to or loss of the genital organs. 2. a general threat to the body image of a person or the unrealistic fear of bodily injury or loss of power or control.

casualty insurance, insurance against loss caused by accidents; usually applied to property but may apply to bodily injury or death from accident.

catabolism (kətab′əliz′əm), the destructive processes (opposite of the anabolic-metabolic processes) by which complex substances are converted into more simple compounds. A proper relation between anabolism and catabolism is essential for the maintenance of bodily homeostasis and dynamic equilibrium.

c. of energy, dissipation of energy in living tissues as work or heat (one phase being metabolism, the other being anabolism).

c. of substance, destructive metabolism; the conversion of living tissues into a lower state of organization and ultimately into waste products.

catalase reaction (kat′əlās), the response of bubbling in the presence of hydrogen peroxide given by blood exudates or transudates.

catalysis (kətal′əsis), the increase in rate of a chemical reaction, induced by a substance called a catalyst, which takes no part in the reaction and remains unchanged.

catalyst (kat′əlist), a substance that induces an increased rate of a chemical reaction without entering into the reaction or being changed by the reaction.

catamenia (kat′əmē′nē·ə), menstruation. Frequently used to designate age at onset of menses.

cataract, an abnormal progressive condition of the lens of the eye, characterized by loss of transparency.

catatonia (kat′ətō′nē·ə), a form of schizophrenia characterized by alternating stupor and excitement. A patient's arms often retain any position in which they are placed.

catecholamine, any one of a group of sympathomimetic compounds composed of a catechol molecule and the aliphatic portion of amine. Some catecholamines (epinephrine and norepinephrine) are produced naturally by the body and function as key neurologic chemicals.

catechol-o-methyl transferase (COMT), an enzyme that deactivates epinephrine and norepinephrine.

catgut, sheep's intestine prepared as a suture and used for ligating vessels and closing soft tissue wounds.

catheter, a hollow, flexible tube that can be inserted into a vessel or cavity of the body to withdraw or instill fluids.

c., balloon-tip, a tube with a balloon at its tip that can be inflated or deflated without removal after insertion.

c., indwelling, a catheter left in place in the bladder; usually a type of balloon catheter.

catheterization, the process of introducing a hollow, flexible tube into a blood vessel or body cavity to withdraw or instill fluids.

cathode, a negative electrode from which electrons are emitted and to which positive ions are attracted. In x-ray tubes, the cathode usually consists of a helical tungsten filament, behind which a molybdenum reflector cup is located to focus the electron emission toward the target of the anode.

c. ray tube, a vacuum tube in which a beam of electrons is focused to a small point on a luminescent screen and can be varied in position to form a pattern.

cation (kat′īon), a positive ion carrying a charge of positive electricity, therefore attracted to the negatively charged cathode.

cationic detergent. See **detergent, cationic.**

cat-scratch disease. See **fever, cat-scratch.**

causalgia (kôzal′jə), a postextraction localized pain phenomenon usually characterized by a continuous burning sensation.

causality, a relationship between one event or action that precedes and initiates a second action or influences the direction, nature, or force of a second action. In scientific study, causality must be observable, predicatable, and reproducible and thus is difficult to prove.

cause of action, generally, a ground or reason for a legal action; a wrong subject to legal redress.

cause of death, the immediate or proximate agent or act that resulted in the loss of life.

caustic, the destruction of living tissue by chemical burning action.

cavernous sinus, one of a pair of irregularly shaped, bilateral venous channels located below the base of the brain between the sphenoid bone of the skull and the dura mater.

cavity, a carious lesion or hole in a tooth.

c., access. See **access cavity.**

c., axial surface, a cavity occurring in a tooth surface in which the general plane is parallel to the long axis of the tooth.

c. classification, carious lesions are classified according to the surfaces of a tooth on which they occur (for example, labial, buccal, occlusal), type of surface (that is, pit, fissure, or smooth surface), and numerical grouping (G.V. Black's classification).

c. classification, artificial (G.V. Black), classification of cavities.

　　Class 1—cavities beginning in structural defects of the teeth, as in pits and fissures.

　　Class 2—cavities in proximal surfaces of premolars and molars.

　　Class 3—cavities in proximal surfaces of canines and incisors that do not involve removal and restoration of the incisal angle.

　　Class 4—cavities in proximal surfaces of canines and incisors that require removal and restoration of the incisal angle.

　　Class 5—cavities in the gingival third (not pit cavities) of the labial, buccal, or lingual surfaces of the teeth.

　　Class 6—(not included in Black's classification) cavities on incisal edges and cusp tips of the teeth.

c., complex, a cavity that involves more than one surface of a tooth.

c. floor, the base-enclosing side of a prepared cavity. See also **cavity, prepared.**

c., gingival (gingival third cavity), a cavity occurring in the gingival third of the clinical crown of the tooth (G.V. Black's Class 5).

c. lining, material applied to the prepared cavity before the restoration is inserted to seal the dentinal tubules for protection of the pulp.

c. medication, a drug used to clean or treat a cavity before inserting a dressing, base, or restoration.

c., nasal (nasal fossa), two irregular spaces that are situated on either side of the midline of the face, extend from the cranial base to the roof of the mouth, and are separated from each other by a thin vertical septum. In radiographs the nasal cavity appears over the roots of the upper incisors as a large, structureless, radiolucent area.

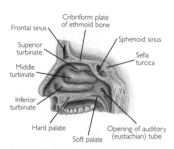

Frontal sinus
Superior turbinate
Middle turbinate
Inferior turbinate
Hard palate
Soft palate
Cribriform plate of ethmoid bone
Sphenoid sinus
Sella turcica
Opening of auditory (eustachian) tube

Nasal cavity. (Seidel, 1995.)

c., pit and fissure, a cavity that begins in minute faults in the enamel. Caused by imperfect closure of the enamel.

c. preparation, the orderly operating procedure required to remove diseased tissue and establish in a tooth

the biomechanically acceptable form necessary to receive and retain a restoration.

c., prepared, the form developed in a tooth to receive and retain a restoration.

   c., p., floor of, the flat bottom or enclosing base wall of a prepared cavity; on an axial plane it is called the *axial wall,* and on the horizontal plane it is called the *pulpal wall.*

   c., p., impression, a negative likeness of a tapered type of prepared cavity.

c., proximal, a cavity occurring on the mesial or distal surface of a tooth.

c., pulp, the space in a tooth bounded by the dentin; contains the dental pulp. The part of the pulp cavity within the coronal portion of the tooth is the *pulp chamber,* and the part found within the root is the *pulp canal,* or *root canal.*

c., simple, a cavity that involves only one surface of a tooth.

c., smooth surface, a cavity formed by decay beginning in surfaces of teeth that are without pits, fissures, or enamel faults.

c. toilet, G.V. Black's final step in cavity preparation. Consists of freeing all surfaces and angles of debris.

c. varnish. See **varnish, cavity.**

c. wall. See **wall, cavity.**

cavosurface angle. See **angle, cavosurface.**

cavosurface bevel. See **bevel, cavosurface.**

CBC, the abbreviation for **complete blood count,** a procedure in which all the blood cells are counted per cubic millimeter, including a differential counting of the white blood cells (leukocytes).

CDC, the acronym for the **Centers for Disease Control and Prevention.**

CD4 (T4) lymphocyte, an immunologically important white cell that is responsible for cell-mediated immunity. It is the cell invaded by the human immunodeficiency virus and in which the virus replicates itself.

CD-ROM, the acronym for **compact disk read only memory.** These disks are used to store program information (software) for computer programs. Information and instructions can be retrieved from these disks but information cannot be added or revised without destruction of the disk.

cecum, a cul-de-sac constituting the first part of the large intestine. It forms the junction between the ileum and the large intestine.

cefaclor, *trade names:* Ceclor, Ceclor CD; *drug class:* antibiotic second generation cephalosporin; *action:* inhibits bacterial cell wall synthesis; *uses:* eradication of gram-negative bacilli from the upper and lower respiratory tract and treatment of urinary tract and skin infections and otitis media.

cefadroxil, *trade names:* Duricef, Ultracef; *drug class:* first generation cephalosprin; *action:* inhibits bacterial cell wall synthesis, rendering cell wall osmotically unstable; *uses:* eradication of gram-negative bacilli from the upper and lower respiratory tract and treatment of urinary tract and skin infections and otitis media.

cefazolin sodium, *trade names:* Ancef, Kefzol, Zolicef; *drug class:* first generation cephalosporin; *action:* inhibits bacterial cell wall synthesis, rendering cell wall osmotically unstable; *uses:* eradication of gram-negative bacilli from the upper and lower respiratory tract and treatment of urinary tract, skin, bone, joint, biliary, and genital infections, endocarditis, surgical prophylaxis, and septicemia.

cefepime, *trade name:* Maxipime; *drug class:* fourth generation cephalosporin; *action:* inhibits cell wall synthesis in sensitive organisms and is bactericidal; *uses:* respiratory tract, urinary tract, and skin and other soft tissue infections associated with gram-negative organisms.

cefixime, *trade name:* Suprax; *drug class:* third generation cephalosporin; *action:* inhibits bacterial cell wall synthesis, rendering cell wall osmotically unstable; *uses:* uncomplicated urinary tract infections, pharyngitis and tonsillitis, otitis media, acute bronchitis, and acute exacerbations of chronic bronchitis.

cefpodoxime proxetil, *trade name:* Vantin; *drug class:* second generation cephalosporin; *action:* inhibits bacterial cell wall synthesis, rendering cell wall osmotically unstable; *uses:* upper and lower respiratory tract infections, pharyngitis and tonsillitis, gonorrhea, urinary tract infections, skin structure infections.

C

cefprozil monohydrate, *trade name:* Cefzil; *drug class:* second generation cephalosporin; *action:* inhibits bacterial cell wall synthesis, which renders cell wall osmotically unstable; *uses:* pharyngitis and tonsillitis, otitis media, secondary bacterial infection of acute bronchitis, skin and skin structure infections.

ceftibuten, *trade name:* Cedax; *drug class:* third generation cephalosporin; *action:* recently approved by the Food and Drug Administration, complete product information not available; *uses:* lower respiratory and urinary tract infections, gynecologic and enteric infections, pharyngitis, tonsillitis, and otitis media caused by susceptible organisms.

cefuroxime axetil, *trade name:* Ceftin; *drug class:* second generation cephalosporin; *action:* inhibits bacterial cell wall synthesis, rendering cell wall osmotically unstable; *uses:* eradication of gram-negative bacilli and gram-positive organisms; treatment of serious lower respiratory tract, urinary tract, skin, and gonococcal infections, septicemia, and meningitis.

cell, the basic unit of vital tissue. One of a large variety of microscopic protoplasmic masses that make up organized tissues. Each cell has a cell membrane, protoplasm, nucleus, and a variety of inclusion bodies. Each type of cell is a living unit with its own metabolic requirements, functions, permeability, ability to differentiate into other cells, reproducibility, and life expectancy.

c., connective tissue, the fibroblast, which for purposes of clarity is characterized by such terms as *perivascular connective tissue cell* or *young connective tissue cell.*

c. count, the number of cells contained in a unit volume, usually refers to red and/or white blood cells in a unit volume of blood.

c. culture, living cells that are maintained in vitro in artificial media of serum and nutrients for the study and growth of certain strains, experiments in controlling diseases, or study of the reaction to certain drugs or agents.

c. cycle, the sequence of events that occur during the growth and division of tissue cells.

c. death, the point in the process of dying at which vital functions have ceased at the cellular level. Cell death precludes the use of tissue or organs as transplant donors.

c., defense, a cell, mobilized within inflamed, irritated, or otherwise diseased tissue, that acts as a protective element to neutralize or wall off the foreign irritant. Defense cells include plasma cells, polymorphonuclear leukocytes, and the cells of the reticuloendothelial system.

c. differentiation, the development of the cells into the various basic cell units of tissue: the epithelial cell and the nerve cell, which arise from the ectodermal tissue layer of the embryo; and the blood, muscle, bone, cartilage, and other connective tissue cells, which arise from the mesodermal tissue of the embryo. The mature tissue cell has many intermediary, transitional forms that are sequential in their development from the primitive, less differentiated anlage cell forms. These intermediary forms are evident clinically in disease in blood dyscrasias, tumors, and inflammation and in health in the normal processes of growth, development, healing, and repair.

c., endosteal, a reticular cell that is modified and identified by its location; the endosteum is a condensation of the stroma of the bone marrow.

c., germ, a cell of an organism whose function is to reproduce an entity similar to the organism from which the germ cell originated. Germ cells are characteristically haploid.

c., giant, a large cell frequently having several nuclei.

c. homeostasis. See **homeostasis, cell.**

c., Langerhans', star-shaped cells of unknown function that appear to be permanent residents of the epithelium.

c. membrane, the outer covering of a cell. The membrane controls the exchange of materials between the cell and its environment.

c., mesenchymal, an embryonic connective tissue cell with an outstanding capacity for proliferation. Capable of further differentiation into reticular cells or osteoblasts. When persisting in the adult organism, the cells are usually arranged in loose connective

tissue along the small blood vessels or in reticular fibers. They are identified by their location and capacity to differentiate into other cell types, such as smooth muscle cells in the formation of new arteries, phagocytes in inflammatory processes, and bone cells in the formation of new bone tissue.

c., plasma, a cell of disputed origin (lymphatic versus undifferentiated mesenchymal cell) that is seen in chronic inflammation and certain disease states and tumors but not normally in the circulating blood. The cell is larger than a lymphocyte and has an eccentric nucleus with basophilic nuclear chromatin peripherally located similar to figures on a clock face. Currently the cells are believed to produce and carry antibodies.

c., reticular, a cell of reticular connective tissue, such as in the stroma of the bone marrow, that retains both osteogenic and hematopoietic potencies; it is identified by its location, morphology, potency, and direct origin from mesenchymal cells.

c., Sternberg-Reed, a giant tumor cell believed to be derived from reticular cells; it contains from one to many nuclei and is seen in Hodgkin's disease.

c., Tzanck, a degenerated epithelial cell caused by acantholysis and found in pemphigus.

c. wall. See **cell membrane.**

cellulitis (sel'yəli'tis), a diffuse inflammatory process that spreads along fascial planes and through tissue spaces without gross suppuration.

celluloid strip. See **strip, plastic.**

cellulose, oxidized (sel'yŏŏlōs), cellulose, in the form of cotton, gauze, or paper, that has been more or less completely oxidized.

cement, a material that produces a mechanical interlocking effect on hardening.

c., acrylic resin dental, a dental cement dispensed as a powder and a liquid that is mixed as is any other cement. The powder contains polymethyl methacrylate, a filler, plasticizer, and polymerization initiator. The liquid monomer is methyl methacrylate with an inhibitor and activator.

c., copper dental, a zinc phosphate cement to the powder of which has been added a copper oxide.

c., dental, any one of the materials used in dentistry as luting agents, bases, and temporary restorations. See also **cement, dental, acrylic resin; cement, dental, zinc oxide–eugenol; cement, silicate;** and **cement, zinc phosphate.**

  c., d. base, an insulating layer of cement placed in the deeper portion of a prepared cavity to insulate the pulp.

c. dressing, postoperative dressing applied after periodontal surgery.

  c. d., dental, Kirkland. See **dressing, Kirkland cement.**

c., Kryptex dental. See **cement, silicophosphate.**

c. line. See **line, cement.**

c., polycarboxylate, a dental cement used for cementation of cast restorations and orthodontic appliances and as bases. Prepared by mixing a zinc oxide powder with a liquid of polycarboxylic acid.

c. sealer, a compound used in filling a root canal; it is inserted in a plastic condition, solidifies after placement, and fills any irregularities in the surface of the canal.

c., silicate, a relatively hard, translucent restorative material used primarily in anterior teeth. Prepared by mixing a liquid and a powder. The powder is an acid-soluble glass prepared by the fusion of CaO, SiO, Al_2O_3, and other ingredients with a fluoride flux. The liquid is a buffered phosphoric acid solution.

c., silicious dental. See **cement, silicate.**

c., silicophosphate (Kryptex cement), a combination zinc phosphate and silicate cement. Less translucent, less irritating, and less soluble than silicate and stronger than zinc phosphate cement.

c., zinc oxide–eugenol dental, least irritating of the cements. The powder is essentially zinc oxide with strengtheners and accelerators. The liquid is basically eugenol.

c., zinc phosphate, a material used for cementation of inlays, crowns, bridges, and orthodontic appliances; occasionally used as a temporary restoration. Prepared by mixing a

C

powder and a liquid. The powders are composed primarily of zinc oxide and magnesium oxides. The principal constituents of the liquid are phosphoric acid, water, and buffer agents.

cemental line. See **line, cemental.** (not current)

cemental repair. See **repair, cemental.**

cemental spicule (spik′yo͞ol). See **spicule, cemental.** (not current)

cemental spike. See **spicule, cemental.** (not current)

cemental tear, a small portion of cementum forcibly separated, either partially or completely, from the underlying dentin of the root as a result of occlusal force; seen on the tension side in occlusal traumatism.

cementation (sē′mentā′shən), attachment of an appliance or a restoration to natural teeth or attachment of parts by means of a cement.

cementicle (səmen′tikəl), a calcified body sometimes found in the periodontal ligament of older individuals. Degenerated epithelial cells are presumed to form the nidus for this calcification. (not current)

cementifying fibroma. See **fibroma, cementifying.**

cementing line. See **line, cemental.**

cementoblast (səmen′tōblast), the cell that forms the organic matrix of cementum. Derived from the inner aspect of the central sac during the initial formation of cementum or from the mesenchymal cell of the periodontal membrane after completion of primary cementogenesis. The cementoblast, trapped within cellular cementum, becomes a cementocyte.

cementoclasia (səmen′tōklā′zhə), destruction of cementum by cementoclasts. (not current)

cementocyte (səmen′tōsīt), the cell found within lacunae of cellular cementum; possesses protoplasmic processes that course through the canaliculi of the cementum; derived from cementoblasts trapped within newly formed cementum.

cementoenamel junction. See **junction, cementoenamel.**

cementoid, the most recent uncalcified layer covering the surface of cementum.

cementoma (sēmentō′mə) (traumatic osteoclasia), an endontogenic tumor

associated with the apices of teeth. It may be present as a mass of fibrous connective tissue, fibrous connective tissue with spicules of cementum, or a calcified mass resembling cementum and having few cellular elements.

c., first-state. See **fibroma, periapical.**

cementopathia (simen′tōpath′ē·ə), the concept wherein necrotic, diseased cementum and lack of productivity of cementum are implicated in the causation of periodontitis and periodontosis. (not current)

cementoproximal, pertaining to the proximal surface apical to the cementoenamel junction of the clinical crown of a tooth. (not current)

cementum (simen′təm), a specialized, calcified connective tissue that covers the anatomic root of a tooth, giving attachment to the periodontal ligament.

c., acellular, cementum that contains no cementocytes.

c., cellular, the portion of the calcified substance covering the root surfaces of the teeth. It is bonelike and contains cementocytes embedded within lacunae, with protoplasmic processes of the cementocytes coursing through canaliculi that anastomose with canaliculi of adjacent lacunae. The lacunae are dispersed through a calcified matrix arranged in lamellar form. Cellular cementum is localized primarily at the apical portion of the root but may deposit over the acellular cementum or serve to repair areas of cemental resorption.

c., collagen fibrils of, fibrils that penetrate the cementum surface and are continuous with the periodontal fibers necessary for tooth support.

c., lamellar, cementum in which layers of appositional cementum are arranged in a sheaflike pattern, the layers of cementum being more or less parallel to the cemental surface and demarcated by incremental lines that represent periods of inactivity of cementum formation.

c., necrotic, nonvital cementum that is situated coronal to the bottom of the periodontal pocket.

c., secondary, the term used to describe all subsequent layers of cementum formed after the primary layer. It may be cellular or acellular.

center of rotation, a point or line around which all other points in a body move.

Centers for Disease Control and Prevention (CDC), the federal facility for disease eradication, epidemiology, and education; headquartered in Atlanta, Georgia.

central bearing, the application of forces between the maxilla and mandible at a single point located as near as possible to the center of the supporting areas of the upper and lower jaws. The purpose is to distribute the closing forces of the jaws evenly throughout the areas of the supporting structures during the registration and recording of maxillomandibular (jaw) relations and the correction of occlusal errors.

   c. b. device, a device that provides a central point of bearing or support between upper and lower occlusion rims. It consists of a contacting point attached to one occlusion rim and a plate on the other rim that provides the surface on which the bearing point rests or moves.

   c. b. point. See **point, central-bearing.**

central nervous system, that portion of the nervous system consisting of the brain and spinal cord. The portion of the nervous system beyond the brain and cord is known as the *peripheral nervous system.*

central occlusion. See **occlusion, centric.**

central processing unit (CPU), the central processor of the computer system, containing the internal memory unit (memory), arithmetic logic unit (ALU), and input/output control unit (I/O control).

central tendency, the tendency of a group of scores to cluster around a central representative score. The statistics most frequently used for measures of central tendency are the mean, median, and mode.

centric (sen'trik), (objectionable as a noun) an adjective that should be used in conjunction with a noun to describe jaw and tooth relationships. See also **position, centric; relation, centric; occlusion, centric;** and **occlusion, centric relation.**

   c. checkbite. See **record, occluding, centric relation.**

c. occlusion. See **occlusion, centric.**
c. position. See **position, centric.**
c. relation. See **relation, centric.**

centrifugal force (sentrif'oogəl). See **force, centrifugal.**

cephalexin, *trade names:* Ceporex, Keftab, Keflex; *drug class:* first generation cephalosporin; *action:* inhibits bacterial cell wall synthesis, rendering cell wall osmotically unstable; *uses:* eradication of gram-negative bacilli from the upper and lower respiratory tract, urinary tract, and skin, treatment of bone infections and otitis media.

cephalic index, an anthropometric value based on the ratio between the width and length of the head.

cephalogram (sef'əlōgram), a cephalometric radiograph. On tracings of these films, anatomic points, planes, and angles are drawn that assist in the evaluation of the patient's facial growth and development.

cephalometer (sef'əlom'ətər). See **cephalostat.**

   c., radiographic. See **cephalostat.**

cephalometric analysis. See **analysis, cephalometric.**

cephalometric landmark. See **landmark, cephalometric.**

cephalometric radiograph, a radiograph of the head made with precise reproducible relationships between x-ray source, subject, and film. The generally accepted distances between x-ray source and the center of the subject are 5 feet (152.4 cm) or 150 cm. The distance between subject and film is usually 12 cm but may be standardized at a different value or varied with patient size and recorded for each exposure. The two standard orientations are lateral (profile) and posteroanterior.

cephalometric skeletal analysis, an assessment of the facial type of a skeleton; the relationship of the parts to each other, to the skull, and to an estimated "normal."

cephalometric tracing, a tracing of selected structures from a cephalometric radiograph made on translucent drafting paper or film for purposes of measurement and evaluation.

cephalometrics (sef'əlōmet'riks), the scientific study of the measurements of the head.

cephalometry (sef'əlom'ətrē), the measurement of the bony structure of the head using reproducible lateral and anteroposterior radiograms.

cephalophore (sef′əlō′fōr), a cephalostat designed to take in-sequence–oriented facial photographs and gnathostatic models.

cephalosporins, semisynthetic derivatives of an antibiotic originally derived from the microorganism *Cephalosporium acremonium.* Cephalosporins are similar in structure to penicillins.

cephalostat (sef′əlōstat′), a head-positioning device that assures reproducibility of the relations between an x-ray beam, a patient's head, and an x-ray film in radiography.

cephradine, *trade name:* Velosef; *drug class:* first generation cephalosporin; *action:* inhibits bacterial cell wall synthesis, rendering cell wall osmotically unstable; *uses:* eradication of gram-negative bacilli and gram-positive organisms from serious respiratory tract, urinary tract, and skin infections and otitis media.

ceramics, the art of making dental restorations or parts of restorations from fused porcelain.

c., orthoclase. See **feldspar.**

cerebellum (ser′əbel′əm), a major division of the brain, behind the cerebrum and above the pons and fourth ventricle, consisting of a median lobe, two lateral lobes, and major connections through pairs of peduncles to the cerebrum, pons, and medulla oblongata. The cerebellum is intimately connected with the auditory vestibular apparatus and the proprioceptive system of the body and hence is involved in maintenance of body equilibrium, orientation in space, and muscular coordination and tonus.

cerebral arteries, arteries to the brain that supply the cerebrum.

cerebral cortex, a thin layer of gray matter on the surface of the cerebral hemisphere, folded into gyri with about two thirds of its area buried in fissures. The cerebral cortex integrates higher mental functions, general movement, visceral functions, perception, and behavioral reactions.

cerebral infarction, the blockage of the flow of blood to the cerebrum, causing or resulting in brain tissue death. Blockage may be caused by a thrombosis, an embolism, a vasospasm, or a rupture of a blood vessel.

cerebral ischemia, the reduction or loss of oxygen to the cerebrum; prolonged ischemia may lead to cerebral infarction.

cerebral palsy. See **palsy, cerebral.**

cerebrospinal fluid, the fluid that flows through and protects the four ventricles of the brain, subarachnoid space, and spinal canal.

cerebrum (ser′əbrəm, sərē′brəm), the largest portion of the brain. Operating at the highest functional level and occupying the upper part of the cranium, the cerebrum consists of two hemispheres united at the bottom by commissures of large bundles of nerve fibers. As with all parts of the nervous system, each part of the cerebrum has highly specific functions (for example, a specific outer cortical area controls voluntary chewing, whereas certain inner subcortical areas are involved in involuntary jaw posture).

cerium, a ductile, gray rare-earth element. Cerium oxalate is used as a sedative, an antiemetic, and an antitussive.

certificate holder, l. the person, usually the employee, who represents the family unit covered by the dental benefits program; other family members are referred to as *dependents.* **2.** generally refers to a subscriber of a traditional indemnity program. **3.** in reference to the program for dependents of active-duty military personnel, the certificate holder is called the sponsor. See also **subscriber.** Synonyms: subscriber, enrollee.

certificate of eligibility, an official identification card or similar document issued to program beneficiaries as evidence of entitlement to services.

certificate of insurance, a statement issued to a group member describing in general terms the policy provisions for eligibility, deductibles, coinsurance, allowances, and maximums. Used in lieu of issuing copies of the group or master contract to each individual employee member of an insured group.

certification, a process by which an individual, institution, or educational program is evaluated and recognized as meeting certain predetermined criteria and standards.

certified dental assistant, a person who has completed the Certification Board of the American Dental Assistant Association.

cervical (sur′vikəl), relating to the neck, or cervical line, of a tooth.

c. appliance. See **appliance, cervical.**

c. convergence. See **convergence, cervical.**

c. fibers. See **nerve fibers.**

c. line. See **junction, cementoenamel.**

c. vertebrae, one of the first seven segments of the vertebral column that define the neck.

cesium, an alkali metal element used in photoelectric cells and television cameras.

cetirizine HCl: *trade names:* Reactine, Zyrtec; *drug class:* antihistamine; *action:* competitive antagonist for peripheral H_1 receptors; *uses:* treatment of symptoms of seasonal allergic rhinitis, perennial allergic rhinitis, chronic urticaria.

Chagas' disease, a parasitic disease caused by *Trypanosoma cruzi* transmitted to humans by the bite of bloodsucking insects.

chalazion forceps (kəlā′zion). See **forceps, chalazion.**

chamber, an enclosed area.

c., air-equivalent ionization, a chamber in which the materials of the wall and electrodes produce ionization essentially similar to that produced in a free-air ionization chamber.

c., air-wall ionization, an ionization chamber with walls of material of low atomic number, having the same effective atomic number as atmospheric air.

c., extrapolation ionization, an ionization chamber with electrodes whose spacing can be adjusted and accurately determined to permit extrapolation of its reading to zero chamber volume.

c., free-air ionization, an ionization chamber in which a delimited beam of radiation passes between the electrodes without striking them or other internal parts of the equipment. The electric field is maintained perpendicular to the electrodes in the collecting region; as a result the ionized volume can be accurately determined from the dimensions of the collecting electrode

and limiting diaphragm. This is the basic standard instrument for dosimetry within the range of 5 to 400 kV.

c., ionization, an instrument for measuring the quantity of ionizing radiation, in terms of the charge of electricity associated with ions produced within a defined volume of air.

c., monitor ionization, an ionization chamber used for checking the constancy of performance of the roentgenray apparatus.

c., pocket ionization, a small, pocketsized ionization chamber used for monitoring radiation exposure of personnel. Before use it is given a charge, and the amount of discharge is a measure of the quantity of radiation received.

c., pulp (pulp cavity), the space occupied by the pulp.

c., relief, a recess in the impression surface of a denture created to reduce or eliminate pressure from the corresponding area of the mouth.

c., standard ionization. See **chamber, ionization, free-air.**

c., suction. See **chamber, relief.**

c., thimble ionization, a small cylindrical or spherical chamber, usually with walls of organic material.

c., thin-wall ionization, an ionization chamber having walls so thin that nearly all secondary corpuscular rays reaching them from external materials can penetrate them easily.

c., tissue-equivalent ionization, a chamber in which the walls, electrodes, and gas are selected to produce ionization essentially equivalent to the characteristics of the tissue under consideration.

chamfer (sham′fər), in extracoronal cavity preparations, a marginal finish that produces a curve from an axial wall to the cavosurface.

chancre (autochthonous ulcer) (shang′kər), the primary lesion of syphilis, located at the site of entrance of the spirochete into the body, that occurs about 3 weeks after contact; begins as a papule and develops into a clean-based shallow ulcer. Secondary infection may produce suppuration. Has the appearance of a buttonlike mass because of the contiguous induration and rolled border. Weeping characteristics also are present.

c. of lip, the primary lesion of syphilis that often appears as an ulcerated or crusted, indurated lesion with a brownish or copper-colored weeping base when located on the lip. The lesion is teeming with *Treponema pallidum.*

c., soft. See **chancroid.**

chancroid (shang′kroid) (soft chancre), a venereal disease caused by *Haemophilus ducreyi.* It is characterized by a soft chancre that is a necrotic draining ulcer similar to a chancre but without characteristic induration. A regional bubo may occur.

channel, a definite furrow, groove, or tubelike passage.

c., vascular, a blood or lymph vessel through which inflammatory infiltrate and periodontitis proceeds from a localized superficial area to involve the deeper structures of the periodontium.

character, one of a set of elementary symbols that may be arranged in groups to express information. They may include the decimal digits *0* to *9,* the letters *A* to *Z,* punctuation marks, operation symbols, and any other single symbol that a computer may read, store, or write.

characteristics, sex, 1. primary sex characteristics are those organs concerned with reproduction such as the gonads and genitalia. **2.** secondary sex characteristics include differences in voice range and timbre, muscularity, and distribution of hair and adipose tissue.

charcoal, a carbonized reduction of wood used as fuel and as an adsorptive substance to cleanse the air; it is used in some medical products.

Charcot's joint. See **joint, Charcot's.**

charges, the financial obligation made to a patient's account for services rendered, usually on a quoted fee for explicit services provided.

charlatan, a quack, a person who pretends to have skills or knowledge that he or she does not possess.

Charles' law. See **law, Charles'.** (not current)

chart, a sheet of paper or pasteboard that presents a graphic representation of a condition or state.

c., Bonwill-Hawley. See **chart, Hawley.**

c., dental, a diagrammatic chart of the teeth on which the findings from

the clinical and radiographic examinations are recorded.

c., Hawley (Bonwill-Hawley chart), graded outlines of dental arch sizes based on the mesiodistal diameters of the six anterior teeth.

c., health. See **chart, history.**

c., history, forms and records for obtaining a thorough medical and oral history combined with a complete record of findings that enable the practitioner to gather and have on hand the necessary records to render total patient care.

c., tooth. See **chart, dental.**

Charters' method. See **method, Charters'.**

charting, the tabulation of the progress of a disease; the compilation of a clinical record.

Chayes' attachment (shāz), believed to be the first internal precision attachment. See also **attachment, intracoronal.** (not current)

Cheadle's disease (chē′dəlz). See **scurvy, infantile.** (not current)

checkbite. See **record, interocclusal.**

c., centric. See **record, interocclusal, centric** and **record, maxillomandibular, centric.**

c., eccentric. See **record, interocclusal, eccentric.**

c., lateral. See **record, interocclusal.**

c., protrusive. See **record, interocclusal, protrusive.**

cheek, a fleshy prominence, especially the fleshy protuberances on each side of the face below the eye and between the ear and the nose and mouth.

c. biting, the chewing of one's cheek (buccal mucosa) because of malocclusion, oral habit, or lack of coordination in the chewing cycle.

cheilion (kīlē′ən), the corner of the mouth.

cheilitis (kīlī′tis), an inflammation of the lip.

c., actinic (solar cheilitis), crusting, desquamation, ulceration, atrophy, and inflammation of the lips, more especially the lower lip, caused by chronic exposure to the elements and actinic rays of sunlight.

c., cigarette paper, focal areas of inflammation of the lips caused by cigarette paper sticking to the surface and injury produced by efforts to remove it.

c., glandularis apostematosa, chronic diffuse nodular enlargement of the lower lip associated with purulent inflammatory hyperplasia of the mucous glands and ducts. Rare; unknown etiology.

c., solar. See **cheilitis, actinic.**

cheiloplasty (kī'ləplas'tē), corrective surgery or restoration of the lips.

cheilorrhaphy (kīlôr'əfē), surgical repair of a congenital cleft lip. (not current)

cheilosis (kīlō'sis), a noninflammatory condition of the lip usually characterized by chapping and fissuring. It is characteristic of either vitamin B complex deficiency of the mouth orifice or monilial infection.

c., angular, transverse fissuring at the angles of the mouth attributable to deficiencies of the B complex group of vitamins, loss of the vertical dimension, drooling of saliva, and superimposed monilial infection.

cheilotomy (kīlot'əmē), incision into or excision of a part of the lip.

chelating agents, chemical compounds used to bind or inactivate metal poisons in the body.

chelation (kēlā'shən), chemical reaction of a metallic ion (for example, calcium ion) with a suitable reactive compound (for example, ethylenediamine tetra-acetic acid) to form a compound in which the metal ion is tightly bound.

c. therapy, the use of a chelating agent to bind firmly and sequester metallic poisons.

chemamnesia (kem'amnē'zhə), reversible amnesia produced by a chemical or drug. (not current)

Chemclave, the brand name for chemical vapor sterilizer that uses a mixture of alcohols, ketones, formaldehyde, and water heated to approximately 127° C under a pressure of at least 20 pounds per square inch. American Dental Association accepted.

chemically induced, the initiation of a biologic action or response by the introduction of a chemical.

chemistry, the science dealing with the elements, their compounds, and the molecular structure and interactions of matter.

chemoreceptor (kē'mōrēsep'tər), a specialized sensory end organ adapted for excitation by chemical substances (for example, olfactory and gustatory receptors) or specialized sense organs of the carotid body that are sensitive to chemical changes in the bloodstream.

chemotaxis, a response involving movement that is positive (toward) or negative (away from) to a chemical stimulus.

c., leukocyte, the phagocytic activity of neutrophils and monocytes in response to chemical factors released by invading microorganisms.

chemotherapeutic agent. See **agent, chemotherapeutic.**

chenodiol, *trade name:* Chenix; *drug class:* anticholelithic; *action:* increases amount of bile acids in relation to cholesterol; *use:* dissolving gallstones.

cherubism (cher'əbiz'əm), **1.** a fibroosseous disease of the jaws of genetic nature. The swollen jaws and raised eyes give a cherubic appearance; multiple radiolucencies are evident on radiographic examination. **2.** a familial form of fibrous dysplasia characterized by unilateral or, more often, bilateral swelling of the jaws in children. See also **dysplasia, fibrous.**

chest pain, a physical complaint that requires immediate diagnosis and evaluation. Chest pain may be symptomatic of cardiac disease such as angina pectoris, myocardial infarction, or pericarditis or disease of the lungs and its linings. It also may be referred from the gastrointestinal tract or elsewhere. The differential diagnosis of chest pain is a crucial element of medical practice.

chewing, the movements of the mandible during mastication; controlled by neuromuscular action and limited by the anatomic structure of the temporomandibular joints.

c. cycle. See **cycle, chewing.**

c. force. See **force, chewing.**

chew-in technique, the method by which the dentist records a patient's occlusal paths in the wax patterns to be used in making restorations. In making the grooves and ridges in the wax patterns directly, the dentist asks the patient to make right-and-left and fore-and-aft sliding occlusal strokes to generate the paths of the opposite prominences. See also **path, generated occlusal.** (not current)

Cheyne-Stokes reflex. See **respiration, Cheyne-Stokes.** (not current)

Cheyne-Stokes respiration. See **respiration, Cheyne-Stokes.**

chickenpox. See **varicella.**

child, l. a person of either gender between the time of birth and adolescence, or puberty. **2.** in the law of negligence and in laws for the protection of children, a term used as the opposite of adult (generally under the age of puberty) without reference to parentage and distinction of gender.

c. abuse, the physical, sexual, or emotional maltreatment of a person under 18 years of age. Child abuse occurs predominantly with children under 3 years of age. Symptoms include bruises and contusions, medical record of repeated trauma, radiographic evidence of fractures, emotional distress, and failure to thrive.

c. neglect, a form of child abuse in which proper care is denied or withheld.

chin, the raised triangular extension of the anterior portion of the mandible below the lower lip. It is formed by the mental protuberance of the mandible.

c. cup. See **cup, chin.**

chip, a logic element containing electronic circuit components, both active and passive, embedded in a cohesive material of any shape.

c. blower. See **syringe, air, hand.**

chiropractic, a branch of the healing arts dealing with the nervous system and its relationship to the spinal column and interrelationship with other body systems in health and disease. The primary spinal and paraspinal structural derangements chiropractors are concerned with are known as *chiropractic subluxations.* Treatment is referred to as *chiropractic management* or *adjustment.*

chisel, an instrument modeled after a carpenter's chisel; intended for cutting or cleaving hard tissue. The cutting edge is beveled on one side only; the shank may be straight or angled.

c., contra-angle (binangle chisel), a chisel-shaped, binangled, paired cutting instrument whose blade meets the shank at an angle greater than 12°.

c., posterior. See **chisel, contra-angle.**

c., Wedelstaedt, a chisel with a blade that is continuous with the shank, has no constricting neck, curves rather than angles into the shank, and is available in varying widths.

chi square, a nonparametric statistic used with discrete data in the form of frequency count (nominal data) or percentages or proportions that can be reduced to frequencies. Used to determine differences between categories (for example, yes-no; visits dentist every 6 months, 1 year, 2 years, 5 years); compares the observed results with the expected results to determine significant differences. May be used with many categories of response.

Chlamydia, a genus of microorganisms that live as intercellular parasites and have a number of properties in

---

Signs of child abuse

Physical evidence of abuse or neglect, including previous injuries	Inappropriate response of caregiver such as an exaggerated or absent emotional response, refusal to sign for additional tests or agree to necessary treatment, excessive delay in seeking treatment, absence of the parents for questioning
Conflicting stories about the "accident" or injury from the parents or others	
Cause of injury blamed on sibling or other party	
An injury inconsistent with the history such as a concussion and broken arm from falling off a bed	
History inconsistent with child's developmental level such as a 6-month-old turning on the hot water	Inappropriate response of child such as little or no response to pain, fear of being touched, excessive or lack of separation anxiety, indiscriminate friendliness to strangers
A complaint other than the one associated with signs of abuse (for example, a chief complaint of a cold when evidence indicates first- and second-degree burns)	Child's report of physical or sexual abuse
	Previous reports of abuse in the family
	Repeated visits to emergency facilities with injuries

Modified from Wong DL: *Whaley & Wong's essentials of pediatric nursing,* ed 5, St Louis, 1997, Mosby.

common with gram-negative bacteria. Two species of *Chlamydia* organisms have been identified; both are pathogenic to humans.

C. psittaci, an organism that infests birds and causes a type of pneumonia in humans (psittacosis).

C. trachomatis, an organism that lives in the conjunctivae of the eye and the epithelium of the urethra and cervix and is responsible for conjunctivitis, lymphogranuloma venereum, and trachoma.

chloral hydrate, *trade names:* Aquachloror Supprettes, Novochlorhydrate; *drug class:* sedative-hypnotic, chloral derivative, controlled sustance schedule IV, schedule F; *action:* produces central nervous system depression; *uses:* sedation, treatment of insomnia, anesthesia adjunct.

chlorambucil, *trade name:* Leukeran; *drug class:* antineoplastic alkylating agent; *action:* inhibits enzymes that allow synthesis of amino acids in proteins; *uses:* chronic lymphocytic leukemia, Hodgkin's disease, breast carcinoma, ovarian carcinoma.

chloramine solution. See **solution.**

chloramphenicol, a broad-spectrum antibacterial and antirickettsial agent that should be reserved for serious infections in which other agents are ineffective.

chlordiazepoxide HCl, *trade names:* Librium, Novopoxide; *drug class:* benzodiazepine antianxiety; *action:* produces central nervous system depression; *uses:* short-term management of anxiety, acute alcohol withdrawal, preoperatively for relaxation.

chlorhexidine gluconate, *trade names:* Peridex, PerioGard; *drug class:* antiinfective oral rinse; *action:* absorbed by tooth surfaces, dental plaque, and oral mucosa; sustained reduction of plaque organisms; *uses:* as a rinse between dental visits as a part of treatment of gingivitis; unlabeled use—denture stomatitis.

chloride shift (klôr'īd). See **phenomenon, Hamburger's.**

chlorine, a yellowish-green gaseous element of the halogen group. Chlorine has a strong, distinctive odor that is irritating to the respiratory tract and is poisonous if ingested or inhaled. It occurs chiefly as a compound of sodium chloride. Chlorine is used as a bleach and disinfectant. Chlorine compounds are used in solvents, cleaning fluids, and chloroform and formerly in general use as an anesthetic.

chloroform, a nonflammable, volatile liquid that was the first inhalation anesthetic to be discovered. It is no longer in general use because of its inherent risk factors and low margin of safety.

chloroformization (klôr'əfôrm'izā'-shən), the administration of chloroform.

Chloromycetin, the brand name for chloramphenicol. See also **chloramphenicol.**

chloropercha (klôr'ōpər'chə), a solution obtained by mixing various amounts of chloroform with guttapercha.

c. method. See **method, chloropercha.**

chlorophyllin (klôr'əfəlin), any one of a number of products resulting from the reaction of certain decomposition products of chlorophyll with copper and other metallic ions.

chloroquine HCl/chloroquine phosphate, *trade names:* Aralen HCl, Aralen Phosphate; *drug class:* antimalarial; *action:* inhibits parasite replication; *uses:* malaria, rheumatoid arthritis, amebiasis.

chlorothiazide, *trade name:* Diuril; *drug class:* thiazide diuretic; *action:* acts on distal tubule by increasing excretion of water, sodium chloride, potassium; *uses:* edema and hypertension, diuresis.

chlorotrianisene, *trade name:* TACE; *drug class:* nonsteroidal synthetic estrogen; *action:* required for the development, maintenance, and adequate function of the female reproductive system, decreases release of gonadotropin-releasing hormone, inhibits ovulation, and helps maintain bone structure; *uses:* prostatic cancer, menopause, female hypogonadism, atrophic vaginitis.

chlorpheniramine maleate, *trade names:* Chlor-Trimeton, Novopheniram; *drug class:* antihistamine H_1-receptor antagonist; *action:* acts on blood vessels, gastrointestinal system, respiratory system by competing with histamine for H_1-receptor site; *uses:* relief of allergy symptoms, rhinitis.

chlorphensin carbamate, *trade name:* Maolate; *drug class:* skeletal muscle relaxant, central acting; *action:* unknown; may be related to sedative properties; does not directly relax muscle or depress nerve conduction; *use:* adjunct for relieving pain in acute, painful musculoskeletal conditions.

chlorpromazine HCl, *trade name:* Thorazine; *drug class:* antipsychotic; *action:* blocks neurotransmission at dopaminergic synapses in the cerebral cortex, hypothalamus, and limbic system; *uses:* psychotic disorders, mania, schizophrenia, anxiety, intractable hiccups, nausea, vomiting, preoperatively for relaxation, behavioral problems in children.

chlorpropamide, *trade names:* Apo-Chlorpromaide, Diabinese; *drug class:* antidiabetic, first generation sulfonylurea; *action:* causes functioning beta-cells in pancreas to release insulin, leading to drop in blood glucose levels; *uses:* stable adult-onset diabetes mellitus type II.

chlortetracycline (klōr'tetrəsī'klēn), (Aureomycin) a broad-spectrum antibiotic possessing bacteriostatic properties of some value in the treatment of disease produced by large viruses (the psittacosis and lymphogranuloma inguinale groups).

chlorthalidone, *trade names:* Novothalidone, Apo-Chlorthalidone, Thalitone; *drug class:* diuretic with thiazide-like effects; *action:* acts on distal tubule by increasing excretion of water, sodium, chloride, potassium; *uses:* edema, hypertension, diuresis, chronic heart disease.

chlorzoxazone, *trade names:* Paraflex, Parafon Forte DSC; *drug class:* skeletal muscle relaxant, central acting; *action:* depresses multisynaptic pathways in the spinal cord; *uses:* adjunct for relief of muscle spasm in musculoskeletal conditions.

choice of path of placement. See **placement, choice of path of.**

cholagogue (kō'ləgog), a substance that stimulates emptying of the gallbladder and flow of bile.

cholera, an acute bacterial infection of the small intestine characterized by severe diarrhea and vomiting, muscular cramps, dehydration, and depletion of electrolytes. The disease is spread by water and food that have been contaminated by feces of infected persons.

c. **toxin** (choleragen), an exotoxin produced by the cholera vibrio that stimulates the secretion of electrolytes and water into the small intestine, draining body fluids and weakening the patient.

c. **vaccine,** an active immunizing agent against cholera.

choleretic (kō'ləret'ik), a substance that stimulates production of bile by the liver.

cholestasis, the interruption in the flow of bile through any part of the biliary system from the liver to duodenum.

cholesteatoma, a cystic mass composed of epithelial cells and cholesterol that is found in the middle ear and occurs either as a congenital defect or as a serious complication of chronic otitis media.

cholesterol (kəles'tərôl), a lipid common to all animal, but not plant, cells. As a sterol, it contains the cyclopentanophenanthrene nucleus. High levels are found in nerve tissue, atheromas, gallstones, and cysts. Normally 140 to 220 mg are present in 100 ml of blood.

Cholesterol

Chemical structure of cholesterol.
(Thibodeau, 1996.)

cholestyramine, *trade names:* Questran, Cholybar; *drug class:* antilipemic; *action:* absorbs, combines with bile acids to form insoluble complex that is excreted through the feces; lowers cholesterol levels; *uses:* primary hypercholesterolemia, pruritus associated with biliary obstruction, diarrhea caused by excess bile acid, digitalis toxicity, xanthomas.

choline, a lipotropic or transmethylation factor found in most animal tissue either free or in combination as lecithin, acetylcholine, or as cytidine diphosphate. Its acetate form (acetylcholine) is essential for synaptic transmission. Administration of choline appears to improve memory and has shown some beneficial use in Alzheimer's disease.

c. salicylate, trade name: Arthropan; *drug class:* salicylate analgesic; *action:* inhibits prostaglandin synthesis by interfering with cyclooxygenase need for biosynthesis; *uses:* relief of mild-to-moderate pain from fever, arthritis, juvenile rheumatoid arthritis.

cholinergic (parasympathomimetic) (kō′linər′jik), producing or simulating the effects of acetylcholine.

c. blocking agent. See **agent, blocking, cholinergic.**

cholinesterase (kō′lines′tərās), an esterase that hydrolyzes acetylcholine. It is an enzyme that is widely distributed throughout the muscles, glands, and nerves of the body and converts acetylcholine into choline and acetic acid.

cholinolytic (kō′linōlit′ik). See **anticholinergic.**

chondrodysplasia punctata, an inherited form of dwarfism characterized by skin lesions, radiographic epiphyseal stippling, and a pug nose. Two types are most often seen: a benign type marked by mild asymmetric limb shortening that is transmitted by an autosomal dominant gene and a lethal type with marked proximal limb shortening that is transmitted by an autosomal recessive gene.

chondrodystrophia fetalis (kon′drōdistrō′fē·ə fētal′is) (not current). See **achondroplasia.**

chondroectodermal dysplasia (Ellis-van Creveld syndrome) (kon′drōek′təlur′məl displāzhə), a syndrome characterized by the following tetrad: (1) bilateral polydactyly; (2) chondrodysplasia of the long bones resulting in acromelic dwarfism; (3) anomalies of the teeth, nails, hair, and maxillary and mandibular region anteriorly; and (4) heart malformation.

chondroma (kondrō′mə), a benign tumor of cartilage. However, many chondrosarcomas arise in preexisting chondromas.

chondromyxosarcoma (kon′drōmik′-sōsahrkō′mə), chondrosarcoma that exhibits an appreciable amount of myxomatous degeneration. See also **chondrosarcoma.**

chondrosarcoma (kon′drōsärkō′mə), a malignant neoplasm composed of cartilage-like tissue.

chondrotin, a mucopolysaccharide present in the ground substance or matrix of connective tissue, particularly cartilage.

chorda tympani nerve, a nerve branching from the facial nerve that passes through the tympanic cavity to join the lingual branch of the mandibular nerve; it conveys taste sensation from the anterior two thirds of the tongue and carries parasympathetic preganglionic fibers to the submandibular and sublingual salivary glands.

chorea (kôrē′ə) (St. Vitus' dance), a disorder of the central nervous system resulting in purposeless, involuntary athetoid (writing) movements of the muscles of the face and extremities. It may be associated with or follow rheumatic fever (Sydenham's chorea), hysteria, senility, or infections or it may be a hereditary disorder (Huntington's chorea).

choriamnionitis, an inflammatory reaction in the amniotic membranes caused by bacteria or viruses in the amniotic fluid.

Christian's disease. See **disease, Hand-Schüller-Christian.**

Christmas disease. See **hemophilia B.**

chromatography, any one of several processes for separating and analyzing various gaseous or dissolved chemical materials according to differences in their absorbency with respect to a specific substance.

chromium, a hard, brittle, metallic element. Chromium strongly resists corrosion and is used extensively to plate other metals and as an alloy to harden steel. Stainless steels are more than 10% chromium.

chromium-cobalt-molybdenum, a stainless alloy used in interosseous implants for dental prostheses.

chromosome (krō′məsōm), one of a number of small, dark-staining, more or less rod-shaped bodies situated in the nucleus of a cell. At the time of cell division, chromosomes divide and distribute equally to the daughter cells. They contain genes arranged along their length. The number of chromosomes in the somatic cells of an individual is constant (the diploid number), whereas just half this number (the haploid number) appears in germ cells.

c. aberration, any rearrangement of chromosome parts as a result of breakage and reunion of broken ends.

chronic, characterized by a long, slow course, as opposed to acute.

chronology, the arrangement of events in a time sequence, usually from the beginning to the end of an event.

cicatrix (sik′ətriks) (scar), the result of healing by secondary intention; characterized microscopically by excessive collagenation of the granulation tissue.

cicatrization (sik′ətrizā′shən), the conversion of granulation tissue into scar tissue.

ciclopirox olamine (topical), *trade name:* Loprox; *drug class:* topical antifungal; *action:* interferes with fungal cell membrane; *uses:* tinea cruris, tinea corporis, tinea pedis, tinea versicolor, cutaneous candidiasis.

cimetidine, *trade names:* Tagamet, Apo-Cimetidine; *drug class:* H$_2$-histamine receptor antagonist; *action:* inhibits histamine at H$_2$-histamine receptor site in parietal cells, which inhibits gastric acid secretion; *uses:* short-term treatment of duodenal and gastric ulcers by the control of hyperacidity.

cineradiography (sin′irā′dēog′rəfē), the making of motion pictures by means of roentgen rays and image intensification. Studies are used for diagnosis and research purposes. Speech patterns can be studied during the process of phonation; the action of the tongue, jaws, and palate can be studied during mastication and deglutition.

cingulum (sing′gyələm), the portion of the incisor teeth and canines, occurring on the lingual or palatal aspects, that forms a convex protuberance at the cervical third of the anatomic crown. Represents the lingual or palatal developmental lobe of these teeth.

c. modification, the alteration of the lingual form of an anterior tooth to provide a definite seat for the support of a rest unit of a removable partial denture.

cinoxacin, *trade name:* Cinobac; *drug class:* urinary tract antibacterial; *ac-*

tion: interferes with deoxyribonucleic acid replication; *use:* urinary tract infections.

ciprofloxacin, *trade name:* Cipro; *drug class:* fluoroquinolone antiinfective; *action:* a broad-spectrum bactericidal agent that inhibits enzyme deoxyribonucleic acid (DNA) gyrase needed for replication of DNA; *uses:* adult urinary tract infection, uncomplicated gonorrhea, typhoid fever, effective against some periodontal organisms.

circulation, the movement of blood through blood vessels.

c., coronary, the circulation of blood within heart muscle.

c., peripheral, the passage of fluids, electrolytes, and metabolites through the walls of terminal vessels of the vascular tree into and out of the tissue spaces.

c., pulmonary, the circulation of venous blood from the right ventricle of the heart to the lungs and back to the left atrium of the heart.

c., systemic, the circulation of oxygenated blood from the left ventricle of the heart to the various tissues and of venous blood back to the right atrium of the heart.

circulatory system, the system for the circulation of blood, consisting of the heart, arteries, arterioles, capillaries, venules, and veins.

circumferential wiring. See **wiring, circumferential.**

cirrhosis, a chronic degenerative disease of the liver in which blood flow is restricted and metabolic and detoxification functions are impaired or destroyed. Cirrhosis is most commonly the result of chronic alcohol abuse.

cisapride, *trade name:* Propulsid; *drug class:* oral prokinetic; *action:* enhancement of acetylcholine release; *uses:* symptomatic treatment and prophylaxis of nocturnal heartburn caused by gastroesophageal reflux disease.

cisplatin, an antineoplastic prescribed in the treatment of a wide variety of neoplasms such as metastatic testicular, prostatic, and ovarian tumors.

citric acid, a white, crystalline, organic acid freely soluble in water and alcohol. It can be extracted from citrus fruits or through a fermentation of sugars. Citric acid is a key intermediary in metabolism. See also **citric acid cycle.**

c. a. cycle, a sequence of enzymatic reactions involving the metabolism of carbon chains of sugars, fatty acids, and amino acids to yield carbon dioxide, water, and high-energy phosphate bonds. Also called *Krebs' citric acid cycle* or *tricarboxylic acid cycle.*

citrin (sit′rin). See **factor, platelet 1.**

civil action, a noncriminal legal action.

civil law, a statutory law, as opposed to common law or judge-made law (such as case law). The dental practice act is a civil law.

claim, 1. in a juridic sense, a demand of some type made by one person or another. **2.** a request for payment under a dental benefits plan. **3.** a statement listing services rendered, the dates of services, and itemization of costs. Includes a statement signed by the beneficiary and treating dentist that services have been rendered. The completed form serves as the basis for payment of benefit.

c. form, the form used to file for benefits under a dental benefits program; includes sections for the patient and the dentist to complete.

claimant, a person who files a claim for benefits. May be the patient or the certificate holder.

claims payment fraud, the intentional manipulation or alteration of facts submitted by a treating dentist, resulting in a lower payment to the beneficiary or the treating dentist than would have been paid if the manipulation had not occurred.

claims reporting fraud, the intentional misrepresentation of material facts concerning treatment provided and charges made to cause a higher payment.

claims review, 1. in dental prepayment, the routine examination by a carrier or intermediary of the claim submitted to it for payment or predetermination of benefits; may include determination of eligibility, coverage of service, and plan liability. **2.** in quality assurance, examination by organizations of claims as part of a quality review or use review process.

clamp, a device used to effect compression or retention.

c., cervical. See **clamp, gingival.**

c., Ferrier 212 gingival, a purposely unbalanced gingival rubber dam clamp for retracting gingival tissue from the field of operation. It must be stabilized to position with modeling compound. Developed by W.I. Ferrier.

c., gingival (cervical clamp), a rubber dam clamp intended to retract gingival tissues.

c., Hatch gingival, an adjustable gingival rubber dam clamp.

c., root rubber dam, a clamp whose jaws are designed to fit on the root surfaces of a tooth; usually used for the retention of a rubber dam.

c., rubber dam (rubber dam retainer), a device made of spring metal and used to retain a rubber dam in place or improve the operating field by isolating it from the oral environment.

clarithromycin, *trade name:* Biaxin; *drug class:* macrolide antibiotic; *action:* binds to 50S ribosomal subunits of susceptible bacteria and suppresses protein synthesis; *uses:* treatment of mild-to-moderate infections of the upper and lower respiratory tracts, otitis media, acute maxillary sinusitis

Clarke-Fournier glossitis (fōōrnēā′). See **glossitis, interstitial sclerous.** (not current)

Clark's rule. See **rule, Clark's.**

clasp, an extracoronal direct retainer of a removable partial denture, usually consisting of two arms, a retentive arm and a reciprocal arm, joined by a body that may connect with an occlusal rest.

c., Adams, a formed wire clasp of modified arrowhead design using the buccomesial and distoproximal undercuts of a tooth for retention.

c., arm, clasp extensions, usually from minor connectors, that provide retention, reciprocation, or stabilization.

c., a., fatigue of, a situation in which the retentive arm of a clasp metal has undergone flexure at the same point repeatedly, and fracture has resulted. Tapering the clasp arm tends to distribute the flexure and reduce such tendency to fracture.

c., a., reciprocal, an arm of a clasp, usually at or occlusal to the height of contour, located in such a manner as to reciprocate any force arising from an opposing clasp arm on the same tooth.

C

c., a., retentive (retention terminal), a clasp arm that is flexible and engages the infrabulge area at the terminal end of the arm.

c., arrowhead, a wire clasp for retention of removable appliances whose active elements are in the shape of an arrowhead and engage the mesioproximal and distoproximal undercuts on the buccal aspects of adjacent teeth.

c., back-action, a clasp that originates on one surface of a tooth and traverses the suprabulge area to another surface, where it is supported by an occlusal rest; it then continues to encircle the tooth on the third surface, where it terminates in the infrabulge area beyond the opposite angle of the tooth surface where it originated.

c., bar, a clasp whose arms are bar-type extensions from major connectors or from within the denture base; the arms pass adjacent to the soft tissues and approach the point of contact on the tooth in a cervicoocclusal direction.

> *c., b., arm,* a clasp arm that originates from the denture base or from a major or minor connector. It consists of the arm that traverses but does not contact the gingival structures and a terminal end that approaches its contact with the tooth in a cervicoocclusal direction.

c., cast, a clasp made of an alloy that has been cast into the desired form and retains its crystalline structure.

c., circumferential, a clasp that encircles more than 180 degrees of a tooth, including opposite angles, tent of the clasp, at least one terminal being in the infrabulge area (cervical convergence).

> *c., c. arm,* a clasp arm that has its origin in a minor connector and follows the contour of the tooth approximately in a plane perpendicular to the path of placement of the removable partial denture.

c., combination, a clasp that employs a wrought wire retentive arm and a cast reciprocal or stabilizing arm. A clasp that employs a bar type of retentive arm and a cast reciprocal or stabilizing arm.

c., continuous, a secondary lingual bar.

c. design, the determination of the shape and construction of a clasp with its position outlined on the cast.

c., embrasure (embra'zhər), a clasp used where no edentulous space exists. It passes through the embrasure, using two occlusal rests, and clasps the two teeth with circumferential clasps that have a common body.

c. flexibility, the property of a clasp that enables it to be bent without breaking and to return to its original form. Factors that affect the flexibility of a retentive clasp arm are its length, diameter, cross-section form, structure, and the alloy of which it is made.

c. flexure. See **flexure, clasp.**

c., formed. See **clasp, wrought.**

c., mesiodistal, a type of clasp that embraces the distolingual and mesial surfaces of a tooth and takes its retention in either or both mesial and distal undercuts.

c., reciprocal, circumferential arm, an arm of a clasp located in such a manner as to reciprocate any force arising from an opposing clasp arm on the same tooth.

c., retentive circumferential arm (retention terminal), a circumferential clasp arm that is flexible and engages the infrabulge area at the terminal end of the arm.

c., Roach. See **clasp, bar.**

c., stabilizing circumferential arm, a circumferential clasp arm that is rigid and contacts the tooth at or occlusal to the surveyed height of contour.

c., stress-breaking action of, relief for the abutment teeth from all or part of torquing occlusal forces; partially achieved by having a retentive arm of maximum flexibility that will provide adequate retention.

c., wrought (formed clasp), a clasp made of an alloy that has been drawn into various forms of wire.

classification, the systematic arrangement according to characteristics of groups or classes.

c., Angle's. See **Angle's classification, modified.**

c., Broders'. See **index, Broders'.**

c., cavity. See **cavity, classification.**

c., Kennedy. See **Kennedy classification.**

c. of habits, a compilation of habits that may cause periodontal disease. Habit neuroses include lip biting, cheek biting, biting of foreign objects, and abnormal tongue pressure against the teeth. Occupational habits include thread biting, musician's habits, holding nails in the mouth, etc. Miscellaneous habits include thumb-sucking, pipe smoking, incorrect toothbrushing habits, cracking nuts with the teeth, and mouth breathing.

c. of motion, a classification system that identifies the extent of involvement of the body in completing a dental motor task.

Class 1, motions of the fingers only.

Class 2, motions of the fingers and wrist.

Class 3, motions of the fingers, wrist, and elbow.

Class 4, motions of the fingers, wrist, elbow, and upper arm.

Class 5, motions of the fingers, wrist, elbow, upper arm, and body.

c. of partial dentures, grouping of partially edentulous situations based on various conditions (for example, location of the edentulous space, location of remaining teeth, position of direct retainers, and ability of oral structures to support a partial denture).

c. of periodontal diseases, the division of periodontal diseases into three classes: (1) inflammation—gingival abrasion, gingivitis, marginal periodontitis; (2) dystrophy—disuse atrophy, occlusal traumatism, periodontosis; and (3) combinations of inflammatory and dystrophic diseases — periodontosis and periodontitis, and occlusal traumatism.

c. of pockets, the division of pockets into two classes: (1) suprabony-gingival and periodontal and (2) infrabony, according to the number of osseous walls (that is, three osseous walls, two osseous walls, one osseous wall).

clavicle, a long, curved, horizontal bone just above the first rib, forming the ventral portion of the shoulder girdle. It articulates medially with the sternum and laterally with the scapula.

cleansing, biomechanical, the process of cleaning and shaping a root canal with endodontic instrumentation in conjunction with irrigating solutions. (not current)

cleansing solution. See **solution, cleansing.**

clearance, l. a condition in which moving bodies may pass without hindrance. **2.** removal from the blood by the kidneys (for example, urea or insulin) or by the liver (for example, certain dyes).

c., interocclusal, the difference in the height of the face when the mandible is at rest and when the teeth are in occlusion. This is determined by measuring the amount of space between the upper and lower teeth when the mandible is in the position of physiologic rest. The difference between the rest vertical dimension and the occlusal vertical dimension of the face, as measured in the incisal area. See also **distance, interocclusal.**

c., occlusal, a condition in which the lower teeth may pass the upper teeth horizontally without contact or interference.

cleat, a fixed point of anchorage, usually in the form of a metal spur or loop embedded in the acrylic resin base of a Hawley retainer or soldered onto an arch wire, to which a rubber dam elastic or other device is attached during orthodontic tooth movement.

cleft, a longitudinal fissure of opening.

c., facial, fissures along the embryonal lines of the junction of the maxillary and lateral nasal processes; usually extend obliquely from the nasal ala to the outer border of the eye.

c., gingival, a cleft of the marginal gingiva; may be caused by many factors, such as incorrect toothbrushing, a breakthrough to the surface of pocket formation, or faulty tooth positions, and may resemble V-shaped notches.

c. lip, a congenital anomaly of the face caused by the failure of fusion between embryonic maxillary and medial nasal processes.

c., occult. See **submucous cleft.**

c., operated (postoperative cleft), a cleft that has been surgically repaired.

c. palate, a congenital anomaly of the oral cavity caused by the failure of fusion between the embryonic palatal shelves.

c. p. prosthesis. See **prosthesis, cleft palate.**

c., postoperative. See **cleft, operated.**

c., Stillman's, small fissures extending apically from the midline of the gingival margin in teeth subjected to trauma. Although these clefts may be found in traumatism, they are not necessarily diagnostic of occlusal trauma.

c., submucous. See **submucous cleft.**

c., **unoperated,** a cleft of the palate that has not been surgically repaired.

cleidocranial dysostosis. See **dysostosis, cleidocranial.**

clemastine fumarate, *trade names:* Tavist, Tavist-1; *drug class:* antihistamine, H_1-receptor antagonist; *action:* acts on blood vessels and gastrointestinal and respiratory systems by competing with histamine for H_1-receptor sites; *uses:* allergy symptoms, rhinitis, angioedema, urticaria.

clenching, the nonfunctional, forceful intermittent application of the mandibular teeth against the maxillary teeth.

cleoid (klē′oid), a carving instrument having a blade shaped like a pointed spade or claw, with cutting edges on both sides and tip.

clicking, a sound associated with dysfunction of the temporomandibular joint; also the sound made by poor fitting dentures.

clidinium bromide, *trade name:* Quarzan; *drug class:* gastrointestinal anticholinergic; *action:* inhibits muscarinic actions of acetylcholine at postganglionic parasympathetic neuroeffector sites; *use:* treatment of peptic ulcer disease in combination with other drugs.

climate, occlusal, the new occlusal relationship and environment produced by occlusal adjustment, orthodontic tooth movement, or a periodontal prosthesis.

clindamycin HCl/clindamycin palmitate HCl, *trade names:* Cleocin, Dalacin C.; *drug class:* lincomycin derivative antiinfective; *action:* binds to 50S subunit of bacterial ribosomes, suppresses protein synthesis; *uses:* infections caused by staphylococci, streptococci, pneumococci, topically for acne, bacterial vaginosis.

clinical, pertaining to a clinic or pertaining to direct patient care, or materials used in the direct care of patients.

c. clerkship, the assignment of medical and other health professionals to a tour of active learning in the direct care of patients.

c. crown. See **crown, clinical.**

c. crown: *clinical root ratio.* See **ratio, clinical crown:clinical root.**

c. diagnosis. See **diagnosis, clinical.**

c. medicine, that aspect of medicine that deals with direct patient care.

c. protocol, the detailed outline of the steps to be followed in the treatment of a patient.

c. trials, organized studies to provide large bodies of clinical data for statistically valid evaluation of treatment.

clinic, table, a display or demonstration of a topic, limited in scope, for transmitting information to a small number of persons at a time.

clinoidale (klinoid′al), the most superior point on the contour of the anterior clinoid.

clioquinol, an antifungal ointment or cream used topically to treat angular cheilitis. Brand name Vioform.

clobetasol propionate, *trade names:* Dermovate, Temovate, Temovate Emollient Cream; *drug class:* topical corticosteroid group I potency; *action:* possesses antipruritic and antiinflammatory actions; *uses:* psoriasis, exzema, contact dermatitis.

clocortolone pivalate, *trade name:* Cloderm; *drug class:* topical corticosteroid, group III medium potency; *action:* possesses antipruritic and antiinflammatory actions; *uses:* psoriasis, eczema, contact dermatitis, pruritus.

clofibrate, *trade names:* Abitrate, Atromid-S, Claripex, Novofibrate; *drug class:* antipherlipidemic; *action:* inhibits biosynthesis of VLDA and LDL, which are responsible for triglyceride development; increases excretion of neutral steroids; *use:* hyperlipidemia types III, IV, V.

clomiphene citrate, *trade names:* Clomid, Serophene, Milphene; *drug class:* nonsteroidal ovulatory stimulant; *action:* binds to estrogen receptors, resulting in increase of LH and FSH release from pituitary; *use:* female infertility.

clomipramine, *trade name:* Anafranil; *drug class:* tricylic antidepressant; *action:* inhibits both norephinepherine and serotinin (5-HT) uptake in brain; *uses:* obsessive-compulsive disorder, panic disorder, neurogenic pain.

clonazepam, *trade names:* Klonopin, Rivotril; *drug class:* anticonvulsant, benzodiazepine derivative, controlled substance schedule IV; *action:* inhibits spike wave formation; *uses:* akinetic myoclonic seizures.

clonidine HCl/clonidine transdermal, *trade names:* Catpres, Dixarit,

Catapres-TTS; *drug class:* antihypertensive, central α-adrenergic agonist; *action:* inhibits sympathetic vasomotor center in central nervous system; *uses:* hypertension, nicotine withdrawal, vascular headache.

clonus (klō'nəs), alternating muscular spasm and relaxation in rapid succession.

clorazepate dipotassium, *trade names:* Tranxene, Gen-Xene, Apo-Chlorazepate, Tranxene-SD; *drug class:* benzodiazepine, controlled substance schedule IV; *action:* produces central nervous system depression; *uses:* anxiety, acute alcohol withdrawal.

closed bite. See **bite, closed.**

closed panel, I. in a prepayment plan, a group of dentists sharing office facilities who provide stipulated services to an eligible group for a set premium. For beneficiaries of plans using closed panels, choice of dentists is limited to panel members. Dentists must accept any beneficiary as a patient. **2.** a closed panel dental benefits plan exists when patients eligible to receive benefits can receive them only if services are provided by dentists who have signed an agreement with the benefits plan to provide treatment to eligible patients. As a result of the dentist reimbursement methods characteristic of a closed panel plan, only a small percentage of practicing dentists in a given geographic area are typically contracted by the plan to provide dental services.

closed procedure, the reduction of a fracture of the maw or placement of an implant without surgical flap retraction.

Clostridium, a genus of spore-forming anaerobic bacteria of the Bacillaceae family.

C. bifermentans, found in gaseous gangrene.

C. botulinum, causes botulism.

C. perfringens, the main cause of gas gangrene in humans; also causes food poisoning, cellulitis, and wound infections.

C. tetani, causes tetanus.

closure, the act or condition of being brought together or closed up.

*c., **adjustive arcs of,*** arcs of jaw closure found in deflective malocclusion caused by an intercusping of the teeth

that does not coincide with a centrically related jaw closure.

*c., **arcs of mandibular,*** circular or elliptic arcs created by closure of the mandible.

*c., **centric path of,*** the path traversed by the mandible during closure when its associated neuromuscular mechanism is in a balanced state of tonus.

*c., **velopharyngeal,*** the closure of nasal air escape by the knee-action elevation of the soft palate and contraction of the posterior pharyngeal wall.

*c., **voluntary arcs of,*** a jaw closure direction consciously made by a patient.

clot, coagulated blood, plasma, or fibrin.

*c., **blood,*** a coagulum formed of blood of a semisolidified nature.

clotrimazole, *trade names:* Lotrimin, Canesten, Gyne-Lotrimin, Mycelex-7, Mycelex Troches; *drug class:* imidazole antiinfective; *action:* interferes with fungal DNA replication; *uses:* tinea pedis, tinea cruris, tinea corporis, tinea versicolor, and *Candida albicans* infection of the mouth, throat, vulva, and vagina.

clotting factors, chemical and cellular constituents of the blood responsible for the conversion of fibrinogen into a mesh of insoluble fibrin causing the blood to coagulate or clot.

cloxacillin sodium, *trade names:* Apo Cloxi, Cloxapen, Novo-cloxin, Tegopen; *drug class:* penicillinase-resistant penicillin; *action:* interferes with cell wall replication of susceptible organisms; *uses:* effective for gram-positive cocci when penicillinase-producing organisms are the confirmed pathogens.

clozapine, *trade name:* Clozaril; *drug class:* antipsychotic, atypical; *action:* interferes with binding of dopamine at D_1 and D_2 receptors; acts as adrenergic, cholinergic, histaminergic, and serotonergic antagonist; *uses:* management of psychotic symptoms in schizophrenic patients for whom other antipsychotics have failed.

clubbing (pulmonary osteoarthropathy), a deforming enlargement of the terminal phalanges of the fingers. It is usually acquired and may be associated with certain cardiac and pulmonary diseases.

cluster analysis, S complex statistical technique of data analysis of numeric scale scores that produces clusters of variables related to one another.

cluster headache. See **histamine headache.**

clutch, a device made for gripping the teeth in a dental arch, to which facebows or tracing devices may be attached rigidly enough to behave in space relations during the movements as if they were jaw outgrowths.

CMV, the abbreviation for **cytomegalovirus.** See also **cytomegalovirus.**

coagulating current. See **current, coagulating.**

coagulation time. See **time, coagulation.**

coal tar, an extract of coal used in combination with other compounds for the treatment of chronic skin diseases, such as eczema and psoriasis. Also a derivative of tobacco smoke that may act as an irritant and carcinogen.

coated tongue. See **tongue, coated.**

coating, enteric (enter′ik), a tablet covering that resists the action of the fluids and enzymes in the stomach but dissolves readily in the upper intestine.

coating material, a biologically acceptable, usually porous nonmetal applied over the surface of a metallic implant, with the expectation that tissue ingrowth will occur in the pores. Often a carbon polymer or ceramic substance.

cobalt-chromium alloy. See **alloy, cobalt-chromium.**

coccidioidomycosis, an infectious fungal disease caused by the inhalation of spores of the bacterium *Coccidioides immitis,* which is carried on windborne dust particles. Although endemic in the southeastern United States, coccidioidomycosis is considered among the opportunistic infections that are indicators of AIDS.

code, a system of recording information by symbols so that only selected people will know the meaning. Used also to conserve space.

c. of ethics, a series of principles used as a guide in assisting a dentist to fulfill the moral obligations of professional dental practice.

codeine (kō′dēn), a crystalline alkaloid, morphine methyl ether that is used as an analgesic and antitussive.

c./codeine sulfate/codeine phosphate, generic codeine; *drug class:* narcotic analgesic controlled substance schedule II, Canada N; *action:* depresses pain impulse transmission in central nervous system by interacting with opioid receptors; *uses:* mild-to-moderate pain, nonproductive cough.

coding, writing instructions for a computer either in machine language or nonmachine language.

Coecal (kō′kôl), the trade name for dental stone (hydrocal).

coefficient, absorption. See **absorption coefficient.**

coefficient of thermal expansion. See **expansion, thermal coefficient.**

coefficient, phenol, the ratio of potency of a given germicide to that of phenol under standard conditions.

coenzyme A (CoA), an important metabolite in the citric acid cycle. Although not a true enzyme, it plays a significant role in the transfer of acetyl groups and the metabolism of acids and amino acids.

cofactor V. See **factor VII.**

cognition (kognish′ən), the higher mental processes, including understanding, reasoning, knowledge, and intellectual capacity.

cognitive (kog′nitiv), pertaining to the mental processes of knowing, perceiving, or being aware; an expression of intellectual capacity.

cognovit note, a written authority of a debtor granting entry of a judgement against the debtor if the amount set forth in the note is not paid by the debtor when due. A cognovit note sets aside every defense that the maker of the note may otherwise have had.

cohere, to stick together, to unite, to form a solid mass.

cohesion, the ability of a material to adhere to itself.

cohesive, the capability to cohere or stick together to form a mass.

cohort, in statistics, a collection or sampling of individuals who share a common characteristic such as the same age or sex.

c. study, a scientific study that focuses on a specific subpopulation such as children born on a certain date in a specific environment.

coinsurance, l. a means of sharing, dividing, or splitting the cost of dental services between the dental plan and the insured patient. A common division is 80/20. This means the insurance company will pay 80% of the cost of the dental service, and the patient will pay 20%. Percentages vary and may be applied to scheduled or usual, customary, and reasonable fee plans. **2.** a provision of a dental benefits program by which the beneficiary shares in the cost of covered services, generally on a percentage basis. The percentage of a covered dental expense that a beneficiary must pay (after the deductible is paid). A typical coinsurance arrangement is one in which the third party pays 80% of the allowed benefit of the covered dental service and the beneficiary pays the remainder of the charged fee. Percentages vary and may apply to a table of allowance plans; usual, customary, and reasonable plans; and direct reimbursement programs.

c. clause, a provision in an insurance contract stipulating that the insurer will pay a specified share of dental expenses covered by the plan.

colchicine, generic colchicine; *drug class:* antigout agent, *action:* inhibits deposition of ureate crystals in soft tissues; *uses:* gout, gouty arthritis, arrest progression of neurologic disability in multiple sclerosis.

cold, clinical applications of, clinical uses of cold to treat cold injury such as frostbite, relieve pain in burn injury, relieve pain in severe and acute inflammation (pulpitis), and relieve pain and swelling in contusions, abrasions, and sprains. See also **heat, applied, and cold.**

cold-curing resin. See **resin, autopolymer.**

cold, physiologic effects of, in reference to application of cold to a local area, marked vasoconstriction followed by vasodilation and edema. In extreme exposure the effects include a significant drop in temperature on the surface and a lesser drop in deeper tissue layers, depending on the degree of cold and duration of application; decreased phagocytosis; a decrease in local metabolism; and analgesia to varying degrees of anesthesia of the part exposed to cold.

cold sore. See **sore, canker,** and **herpes labialis.**

cold welding. See **welding, cold.**

cold work, a deformation of the space lattice of metals by mechanical manipulation at room temperature. The process alters certain properties (for example, ductility).

colestipol HCl, *trade name:* Colestid; *drug class:* antihyperlipidemic; *action:* absorbs, combines with bile acids to form insoluble complex that is excreted through feces; loss of bile acids lowers cholesterol levels; *uses:* primary hypercholesterolemia, xanthomas, digitalis toxicity, pruritus caused by biliary obstruction, diarrhea caused by bile acids.

colic, a sharp visceral pain resulting from torsion, obstruction, or smooth muscle spasm of a hollow or tubular organ such as a ureter or an intestine.

colitis, an inflammatory condition of the large intestine. Most of the diseases of this group are of unknown origin.

collagen, an intercellular constituent of connective tissue and bone consisting of bundles of tiny reticular fibrils, most noticeable in the white, glistening, inelastic fibers of tendons, ligaments, and fascia.

collagenase, an enzyme capable of depolymerizing collagen, found in some microorganisms and believed to contribute to periodontal disease.

collapse, a state of extreme prostration and depression with failure of circulation; abnormal falling in of the walls of any part or organ; and, with reference to a lung, an airless or fatal state of all or part of the lung.

collar, the small part of the root of a tooth that is a part of an artificial tooth (denture).

collective bargaining, the negotiations between organized labor and employers on matters such as wages, hours, working conditions, and health and welfare programs.

collimation (kol'imā'shen), literally, making parallel. In radiology, *collimation* refers to the elimination of the peripheral (more divergent) portion of a useful x-ray beam by means of metal tubes, cones, or diaphragms interposed in the path of the beam. See also **diaphragm.**

collimator (kol′imātər), a diaphragm or system of diaphragms made of an absorbent material and designed to define the dimensions and direction of a beam of radiation.

collision tumor. See **tumor, collision.**

colloid (kol′oid), a suspension of particles in a dispersion medium. The particles generally range in size from 1 to 100 μm. Hydrocolloids and silicate cements are examples of dental colloids.

colon, the body of the large intestine between the cecum and rectum.

color blindness. See **blindness, color.**

coloring, extrinsic, coloring from without, as in the application of color to the external surface of a prosthesis. (not current)

coloring, intrinsic, coloring from within. The incorporation of pigment within the material of a prosthesis.

color, temper, the color produced by the thickening of the oxide coating on carbon steel as temperature is increased. Used as an indication of the degree of tempering.

coma (kō′mə), a state of unconsciousness from which the patient cannot be aroused, even by powerful stimulation. It is gradual in onset, prolonged, and not spontaneously reversible.

Coma: Glasgow scale scoring

Eyes Open
4 Spontaneously
3 On request
2 To pain stimuli (supraorbital or digital)
1 No opening

Best Verbal Response
5 Oriented to time, place, person
4 Engages in conversation, confused in content
3 Words spoken but conversation not sustained
2 Groans evoked by pain
1 No response

Best Motor Response
5 Obeys a command ("Hold out three fingers.")
4 Localizes a painful stimulus
3 Flexes either arm
2 Extends arm to painful stimulus
1 No response

From Phipps WJ et al: *Medical surgical nursing: concepts & clinical practice, ed 5,* St Louis, 1996, Mosby.

c., diabetic, unconsciousness accompanying severe diabetic acidosis. It may develop from omission of insulin, surgical complications, or disregard of dietary restrictions. Premonitory symptoms include weakness, anorexia, dry skin and mouth, drowsiness, abdominal pain, and fruity breath odor. Late symptoms are coma, air hunger, low blood pressure, tachycardia, dehydration, soft and sunken eyeballs, glycosuria, hyperglycemia, and a high level of ecetoacetic acid. See also **shock, insulin.**

combination clasp. See **clasp, combination.** (not current)

command, the portion of an instruction that specifies the operation to be performed. A term used with hardware operations.

comminution of food. See **food, comminution of.**

common deductible, a deductible amount that is common to the dental and another health insurance policy (usually a major medical policy). In a major medical policy with a $100 common deductible, once $100 of medical or dental expense has been incurred under either policy or both, no further deductible is required.

common law, Judge-made law, as contrasted with statutory law. That body of law originated in England and was in force at the time of the American Revolution; modified since that time on a case-by-case basis in the courts.

communicable disease, any disease transmitted from one person or animal to another directly or by vectors.

communicable period, the period of time when the infectious agent that causes a communicable disease may be transmitted to a susceptible host, such as in diseases that initially involve the mucous membrane (for example, diphtheria and scarlet fever). The period of communicability is from the time of exposure to the disease until termination of the carrier state, if one develops.

communication, the technique of conveying thoughts or ideas between two people or groups of people.

c., privileged, certain classes of communications between persons who stand in a confidential or fiduciary relationship to each other that the law will not permit to be divulged in court. Examples of confidential relationships are those of psychiatrist and patient and attorney and client. Confidentiality of communications depends on the law in each state.

community dentistry, a branch, discipline, or specialty of dentistry that deals with the community and its aggregate dental or oral health rather than that of the individual patient. Formal recognition of dentists engaged in community dentistry is through the American Board of Public Health Dentistry.

community health aides, paraprofessionals who assist in the treatment or support of patients (in their residential setting) within the patient's community environment.

compact, to form by uniting or condensing particles with the application of pressure (for example, the progressive insertion and welding of foil and the building up of plastic amalgam in a preparation).

compacter, a rotary instrument used in the McSpadden endodontic technique to condense the guttapercha cone into the root canal. (not current)

compaction, the act of compacting or the state of being compact.

compensating curve. See **curve, compensating.**

compensation, the monetary reward for rendering a service; insurance providing financial return to employees in the event of an injury that occurs during the performance of their duties and that prohibits work. Compulsory in many states.

c., unemployment, insurance covering the employee so that compensation may be provided for loss of income as a result of unemployment.

competence, a measure of the degree of a person's ability to cope with all aspects of the environment.

competent, having legal capacity, ability, or authority.

compiler, a computer program that translates a high-level language program into a corresponding machine instruction. The program that results from compiling is a translated and expanded version of the original program.

complaint, any ailment, problem, or symptom disclosed by the patient.

c., chief, the symptom or reason for which the patient seeks treatment. The most troublesome ailment, problem, or symptom.

complement, one of 11 complex, enzymatic serum proteins. In an antigen-antibody reaction, complement causes lysis. Complement is also involved in anaphlaxis and phagocytosis.

c. fixation, an immunologic reaction in which an antigen combines with an antibody and its complement, causing the complement factor to become inactive, or "fixed."

c.-fixation test (C-F test), a serologic test in which complement fixation is detected, indicating the presence of a particular antigen, the Wassermann test for syphilis is a C-F test, also used to detect amebiasis, Rocky Mountain spotted fever, tryanosomiasis, and typhus.

complemental air. See **volume, inspiratory reserve.**

complete blood count. See **count, blood, complete.**

complete denture. See **denture, complete.**

complex, a combination of a number of things; the sum or total of various things.

c., craniofacial, the bones and surrounding soft structure of the cranium and face.

c., dentofacial, referring to the dentition and surrounding structures.

compliance, 1. the fulfillment by the patient of the caregiver's prescribed course of treatment. **2.** the fulfillment of oversight criteria and/or standards of care necessary for licensure, certification, and accreditation.

complication, a disease or injury that develops during the treatment of an earlier disorder. An example is a bacterial infection acquired by a person weakened by a viral infection.

component(s), a part or element.

c., A. See **factor II.**

c. of force. See **force, component of.**

c. of partial denture. See **denture, partial, components of.**

c., salivary. See **lysozyme.**

c., thromboplastic cellular (TCC). See **factor, platelet, 3.**

composite odontoma. See **odontoma, composite.**

composite resin. See **resin, composite.**

compound, 1. a combination of elements held together in a well-defined pattern by chemical bonds. In pharmacy, a mixture of drugs. 2. a thermoplastic substance used as a nonelastic impression material.

c. A, B, E, F, S. See **corticoid, adrenal.**

c. cone, a compound in the form of a cone or pyramid; used for impressions of individual preparations.

c., impression (modeling compound). See **compound.**

c., intermetallic, a compound of two metals in which the metals are only partially soluble in one another; exhibits a homogeneous grain structure, but the atoms do not intermingle randomly in all proportions.

c., modeling. See **compound, impression.**

c. tracing stick, a compound dispensed in stick form.

c., tray, a compound similar to impression compound but with less flow and more viscosity when soft and more rigidity when chilled.

comprehensive dental care, the coordinated delivery of the total dental care required or requested by the patient.

comprehensive health care, the coordinated delivery of the total health care required or requested by the patient.

comprehensive orthodontic therapy, a coordinated approach to improvement of the overall anatomic and functional relationships of the dentofacial complex, as opposed to partial correction with more limited objectives such as cosmetic improvement. Usually but not necessarily uses fixed orthodontic attachments as a part of the treatment appliance. Includes treatment and adjunctive procedures, such as extractions, maxillofacial surgery, other dental services, nasopharyngeal surgery, and speech therapy, directed at malrelationships within the entire dentofacial complex. Optimal care requires periodic evaluation of patient needs, especially during the growing years. Treatment is most effective when begun in the deciduous or mixed dentition and accomplished in successive phases as the face matures. Active correction in the adult dentition can usually be accomplished in one phase.

compression, the act of pressing together or forcing into less space.

c. molding. See **molding, compression.**

c. of tissue. See **tissue, displaceability.**

compressive strength. See **strength, compressive.**

compromise (käm′prəmīz′), an arrangement arrived at, in or out of court, for settling a disagreement on terms considered by the parties to be fair.

compulsion (kəmpul′shən), a repetitive, stereotyped, and often trivial motor action, the performance of which is compelled even though the person does not wish to perform the act. Oral habits such as bruxism and clenching may become compulsions.

computed tomography (CT), a radiographic body scanning technique in which thin or narrow layer sections of the body can be imaged for diagnostic purposes. The technique uses a computer-linked x-ray machine to focus the x-rays on a particular section of the body to be viewed.

computer, a device capable of accepting data in the form of facts and figures, manipulating them in a prescribed way and supplying the results of these processes as meaningful information. This device usually consists of input and output devices, storage, arithmetic and logic units, and a control unit. Usually an automatic, stored-program machine is implied.

c.-aided design, the use of computers to assist a draftsman, architect, or artist in the creation of drawing, illustration, or visual art.

c., digital, a computer that operates on discrete data by performing arithmetic and logic processes on these data.

c. graphics, the use of computers to create illustrations or designs.

c. language, the vocabulary and syntax of a set of symbols that are used to instruct a computer what to do (for example, COBOL, FORTRAN, BASIC, and PASCAL).

c. literacy, a functional knowledge of the use and application of computers from word processing to data management.

c. output microfilm (COM), a system that allows a computer user to produce microfilm copies of computer output. The COM unit operates independently of the CPU and is therefore called an off-line device. Output from computer processing is recorded on magnetic tape, which is later removed from the computer's tape handler, mounted on the COM unit, and recorded on microfilm.

c. simulation, the use of computers to replicate a mechanical or biologic function.

concanavalin A, a hemagglutinin, isolated from the meal of the jack bean, that reacts with polyglucosans in the blood of mammals, causing agglutination. It has been used to stimulate T-cell production.

conceal, to hide; secrete; withhold from the knowledge of others.

Concise, the brand name for diacrylate resin adhesives used in composite restorations and for bonding orthodontic appliances to the enamel.

concrescence (känkres'əns), **1.** the union of two teeth after eruption by the fusion of their cementum surfaces. **2.** the fusion of teeth after their roots have formed. The union is effected by cementum. See also **fusion.**

condensation (kän'densā'shən), a commonly used term for the insertion and compression or compaction of dental materials into a prepared cavity. *Compaction* is a more accurate term than *condensation.* See also **compaction.**

condenser (känden'ser) (formerly called *plugger*), an instrument or device used to compact or condense a restorative material into a prepared cavity. Its working end is called the *nib,* or *point;* the end of the nib is termed the *face.* The face may be smooth or serrated.

c., amalgam (amalgam plugger), an instrument used to condense plastic amalgam.

c., automatic. See **condenser, mechanical.**

c., back-action, a condenser with the shank bent into a U shape so that the condensing force is a pulling motion rather than the usual pushing force.

c., bayonet, a condenser in which the offset of the nib and the approximately right-angled bends in the shank permit a better line of force for condensation of direct filling gold. There are many variations in angles, length, and diameter of the nib.

c., electromallet (McShirley's electromallet), an electromechanical device for compacting direct filling gold. Frequency of blows may be varied from 200 to 3600 strokes/min; the intensity of the blow is controlled electronically.

c., foil, a condenser used to compact direct filling gold.

c., foot, a foil condenser with the nib shaped like a foot.

c., hand, an instrument that compacts material, the force being applied by the muscular effort of the operator with or without supplementary force from a mallet in the hand of the assistant.

c., Hollenback. See **condenser, pneumatic.**

c., long-handled foil, a hand condenser of varied design for compacting gold foil.

c., mechanical (automatic mallet), a device to supply an automatically controlled blow for condensing restorative material. It may be spring-activated, pneumatic, or electronically controlled.

c., parallelogram, a condenser, the face of which is shaped like a rectangle or parallelogram.

c., pneumatic (Hollenback condenser), a pneumatic mechanical device developed by George M. Hollenback to supply a compacting force. The force is delivered by controlled pneumatic pressure. Blows are variable in intensity, with speed variable up to 300 strokes/min.

c. point. See **point, condenser.**

c., round, a condenser, the face of which has a circular outline.

c., stepping, the orderly movement of a condenser point over the surface of gold foil or amalgam during its placement and compaction.

condensing force. See **force, condensing.** (not current)

condensing osteitis. See **osteitis, condensing.**

condensor (spreader), an instrument used in filling a root canal to compress the filling material in a lateral direction.

conditioning, a form of learning based on the development of a response or set of responses to a stimulus or series of stimuli.

conduct, dishonorable, conduct that mars the character and lessens the reputation; conduct that is shameful, disgraceful, base. (not current)

conduction, the carrying of sound waves, heat, light, nerve impulses, and electricity.

c., air, the process of transmitting sound waves to the cochlea by way of the outer and middle ear. In normal hearing, practically all sounds are transmitted in this way, except those of the hearer's own voice, which are transmitted partly by bone conduction.

c., bone, the transmission of sound waves or vibrations to the cochlea by way of the bones of the cranium.

c., impulse, the conduction of an impulse along the nerve fiber, which is accompanied by an alteration of the electrical potential of the fiber tissue and an exchange of electrolytes across the nerve fiber membrane.

conductivity, the capacity for conduction; ability to convey.

c., electrical, the ability of a material to conduct electricity. Metals are usually good conductors, and nonmetals are poor conductors.

c., thermal, the ability of a material to transfer heat. Thermal conductivity is of great importance in dentistry, where a low thermal conductivity is desirable in restorative material and a high thermal conductivity is desirable when soft tissue is covered.

condylar (kän′dilər), pertaining to the mandibular condyle.

c. axis. See **axis, condylar.**

c. guide. See **guide, condylar.**

  c. g. inclination. See **guide, condylar, inclination.**

condyle (kän′dīl), the rounded surface at the articular end of a bone.

c. head, a redundant term; the word *condyle* means *head.* See also **condyle.**

c., lateral path, the path of the condyle in the glenoid fossa when a lateral mandibular movement is made.

c., mandibular, the articular process of the mandible; the condyloid process of the mandible.

c., neck of. See **process, condyloid, neck of.**

c., orbiting. See **orbiting condyle.**

c. path, the path traveled by the mandibular condyle in the temporomandibular joint during the various mandibular movements

c., protrusive path, the path of the condyle when the mandible is moved forward from its centric position.

c. rod. See **rod, condyle.**

c., rotating, the condyle on the side of the bolus formation, or the one that is braced and placed and rotated while the bolus is being chewed.

condylectomy (kän′dilek′tōmē), the surgical removal of a condyle.

condyloid process. See **process, condyloid.**

condyloplasty, a surgical procedure to alter the shape of the condyle to remove the effects of degenerative disease.

condylotomy (kän′dilot′ōmē), surgical division through, without removal of, a condyle; or removal of a portion, usually the articular surface, of a condyle.

cone, 1. a geometric shape with a circle for its base that tapers evenly to an apex. **2.** a solid substance, usually guttapercha or silver, having a tapered form similar in length and diameter to a root canal; used to fill the space once occupied by the pulp in the root of the tooth. **3.** an accessory device on a dental x-ray machine, designed to indicate the direction of the central axis of its x-ray beam and to serve as a guide in establishing a desired source-to-film distance.

c. distance, the distance between the focal spot and the outer end of the cone; usually expressed in inches or centimeters. Modern dental roentgenray units usually have cone distances of from 5 to 20 inches (12.5 to 50 cm).

c., long, a tubular "cone" designed to establish an extended anode-to-skin distance, usually within a range of from 12 to 20 inches (30 to 50 cm).

c., short, a conical or tubular "cone" having as one of its functions the establishment of an anode-to-skin distance of up to 9 inches (22.5 cm).

confidence interval, a statistical device used to determine the range within which an acceptable datum would fall. Confidence intervals are usually expressed in percentages, such as 95% or 99%.

confidential, an express or implied agreement that the dentist will not disclose the information received from a patient to anyone not directly involved in the care and treatment or not legally capable of requiring disclosure; generally an ethical rather than legally enforceable consideration in dentistry.

confidentiality, the nondisclosure of certain information except to another authorized person.

conflict of interest, the loss or perceived loss of objectivity by a caregiver who has or may be perceived as having a personal stake or investment in the outcome.

confusion, a mental state characterized by disorientation regarding time, place, or person that causes bewilderment, perplexity, lack of orderly thought, and the inability to act decisively or perform the activities associated with daily living.

congenital, a condition that is present at birth and usually developed in utero.

congestion. See **hyperemia.**

congestive heart failure, an abnormal condition characterized by circulatory congestion (retention of fluids) caused by cardiac or kidney disorders. This condition usually develops chronically in association with the retention of sodium and water by the kidneys. Acute congestive heart failure may result from myocardial infarction of the left ventricle.

conjugate, 1. to unite. **2.** the product of conjugation.

conjugation, in biochemistry, the union of a drug or toxic substance with a normal constituent of the body, such as glucuronic acid, to form an inactive product that is then eliminated.

conjunctiva, the mucous membrane lining the inner surfaces of the eye lids and anterior part of the sclera.

conjunctivitis, an inflammation of the conjunctiva, caused by bacterial or viral infection, allergy, or environmental factors. Also called *pinkeye.*

connective tissue. See **tissue, connective.**

connector, the part of a partial denture that unites its components.

c., anterior palatal major, a major connector uniting bilateral units of a maxillary removable partial denture. It is a thin metal plate that is located in the anterior palatal region.

c. bar. See **bar, connector.**

c., cross arch bar splint, a removable cross arch connector used to stabilize weakened abutments that support a fixed prosthesis by attachment to teeth on the opposite side of the dental arch. It can be removed by the dentist but not by the patient.

c., lingual bar major, a type of connector used to unite the right and left components of a mandibular removable partial denture and occupy a position lingual to the alveolar ridge.

c., linguoplate major, a major connector formed by the extension of a metal plate from the superior border of the regular lingual bar, across gingivae, and onto the cingulum of each anterior tooth.

c., major, a metal plate or bar (for example, lingual bar, linguoplate, palatal bar) used to join the units of one side of a removable partial denture to those located on the opposite side of the dental arch.

c., minor, the connecting link between the major connector or base of a removable partial denture and other units of the restoration, such as direct and indirect retainers and rests.

c., nonrigid, a connector used where retainers or pontics are united by a joint permitting limited movement. It may be a precision or a nonprecision type of connector.

c., posterior palatal major (posterior palatal bar), a major transpalatal connector located in the posterior palatal region. It is used when the anterior palatal bar alone is insufficient to provide the necessary rigidity.

c., rigid, a connector used where retainers or pontics are united by a soldered, cast, or welded joint.

c., saddle. See **connector, major.**

c., secondary lingual bar major (Kennedy bar), often called a continuous clasp or Kennedy bar. It rests on the cingulum area of the lower anterior teeth and serves principally as an indirect retainer and/or stabilizer for weakened anterior lower teeth.

c., subocclusal, a nonrigid connector positioned gingival to the occlusal plane.

consanguinity, a hereditary or "blood" relationship between persons, by having a common parent or ancestor.

conscious sedation, a state of sedation in which the patient remains aware of their person, surroundings, and conditions but without experiencing pain or anxiety.

consciousness, a state in which the individual is capable of rational response to questioning and has all protective reflexes intact, including the ability to maintain a patent airway.

consent, the concurrence of wills; permission.

c., express, consent directly given by voice or in writing.

c., implied, consent made evident by signs, actions, or facts, or by inaction or silence.

consideration, inducement to make a contract. It may be a benefit to the promisor or a loss or detriment to the promisee. Consideration must be regarded as such by both parties.

Consolidated Omnibus Budget Reconciliation Act (COBRA), legislation relative to mandated benefits for all types of employee benefits plans. The most significant aspects within this context are the requirements for continued coverage for employees and/or their dependents for 18 months who would otherwise lose coverage (30 months for dependents in the event of the employee's death).

consonant, a conventional speech sound produced, with or without laryngeal vibration, by certain successive contractions of the articulatory muscles that modify, interrupt, or obstruct the expired airstream to the extent that its pressure is raised.

c., semivowel (1, t), consonants that are like vowels both perceptually and physiologically.

constipation, a difficulty passing stools or an incomplete or infrequent passage of hard stools.

constitution, the general makeup of the body as determined by genetic, physiologic, and biochemical factors. An individual's constitution may be markedly influenced by environment.

constriction, an abnormal closing or reduction in the size of an opening or passage of the body.

construction, single denture, the making of one upper or lower denture as distinguished from a set of two complete dentures.

consultant, a professional or nonprofessional person who, by virtue of special knowledge of professional or nonprofessional aspects of a dental practice, is sought out for advice and training.

consultation, a meeting of persons to discuss or decide something.

c., patient, a meeting between the dentist, patient, and other interested persons for the purpose of discussing the patient's dental needs, proposing treatment, and making business arrangements.

c., professional, a joint deliberation by two or more dentists and/or physicians to determine the diagnosis, treatment, or prognosis for a particular patient.

consumer, one who may receive or is receiving dental service; the term is also used in health legislation and programs as a reference to someone who is never a practitioner or is not associated in any direct or indirect way with the supplying or provision of dental services.

contact, the act of touching or meeting.

c., balancing, the contact established between the upper and lower dentures at the side opposite the working side (anteroposteriorly or laterally) for the purpose of stabilizing the dentures.

c., deflective occlusal (cuspal interference), a condition of tooth contacts that diverts the mandible from a normal path of closure to centric jaw relation or causes a denture to slide or rotate on its basal seat. See also **contact, interceptive occlusal.**

c., faulty, imperfections in the contact between adjacent teeth. Often leads to food impaction between the teeth, with subsequent initiation or perpetuation of periodontal lesions.

c., initial, the first meeting of opposing teeth on elevation of the mandible toward the maxillae.

c., interceptive occlusal, an initial contact of teeth that interferes with the normal movement of the mandible. See also **contact, deflective occlusal.**

c., premature. See **deflective occlusal** and **contact, interceptive occlusal.**

c., working, a contact of the teeth made on the side of the dental arch toward which the mandible has been moved.

contaminated, made radioactive by the addition of minute quantities of radioactive material.

contamination, radioactive, the deposition of radioactive material in any place where it is not desired, and particularly where its presence may be harmful or may constitute a radiation hazard.

contingent (kuntin'jənt), dependent for effect on something that may or may not occur.

continuant, a speech sound in which the speech organs are held relatively fixed during the period of production.

continuing education, postgraduate study offered either in an institution of higher learning by groups with an organized dental program or by individuals who are especially qualified in certain areas. Required by some state licensing boards for license renewal. Credit accumulates for special qualifications to join special interest groups.

continuous bar retainer. See **retainer, continuous bar.** (not current)

continuous clasp. See **retainer, continuous bar.** (not current)

continuous loop wiring. See **wiring, continuous loop.** (not current)

contour, the external shape, form, or surface configuration of an object.
c., anatomic height of, a line encircling a tooth to designate its greatest convexity.
c., buccal, the shape of the buccal aspect of a posterior tooth. It normally has occlusocervical convexity, with its greatest prominence at the gingival third of the clinical buccal surface.
c., gingival, the shape of the natural or artificial gingiva as it approximates the natural or artificial tooth.
c., height of, the greatest convexity of a tooth viewed from a predetermined position.
c., proximal, the form of the mesial or distal surface of a tooth.
c., restoration, the restoration of a proper contour where surfaces of teeth have been destroyed because of disease processes or excessive wear.
c., surveyed height of, a line scribed or marked on a cast that designates the greatest convexity with respect to a selected path of denture placement and removal.
c., tooth, a shape of a tooth that is essential to a healthy gingival unit be-

cause it enables the bolus of food to be deflected from gingival margins during mastication.

contouring, occlusal, the correction, by grinding, of gross disharmonies of the occlusal tooth form (for example, uneven marginal ridges, plunger cusps, extruded teeth, malpositioned teeth) to establish a harmonious occlusion and protect the periodontium of the tooth.

contouring pliers. See **pliers, contouring.**

contra-angle (kän'trəang'gəl), more than one angle. An instrument having two or more offsetting angles of such degree that the end of the instrument is kept within 3 mm of the axis of the shaft.

contraception, a process or technique for the prevention of pregnancy by means of a medication, device, or method that blocks or alters one or more of the processes of reproduction in such a way that sexual union can occur without impregnation.

contract, 1. an agreement based on sufficient consideration between two or more competent parties to do or not to do something that is legal. 2. a legally enforceable agreement between two or more individuals or entities that confers rights and duties on the parties. Common types of contracts include (1) those contracts between a dental benefits organization and an individual dentist to provide dental treatment to members of an alternative benefits plan. These contracts define the dentist's duties both to beneficiaries of the dental benefits plan and the dental benefits organization, and usually define the manner in which the dentist will be reimbursed; and (2) contracts between a dental benefits organization and a group plan sponsor. These contracts typically describe the benefits of the group plan and the rates to be charged for those benefits.
c., breach of, the failure, without legal excuse, to perform an obligation or duty in a contract.
c. dentist, a practitioner who contractually agrees to provide services under special terms, conditions, and financial reimbursement arrangements.
c. dentistry, 1. providing dental care under a specific set of guidelines and

for a specific set of individuals under an accepted written agreement by the patient, dentist, and employer. **2.** the practice of dentistry whereby the dentist enters into a written agreement with either patients or an employer to provide dental care for a set group of people.

c., express, a contract that is an actual agreement between the parties, with the terms declared at the time of making, being stated in explicit language either orally or in writing.

c. fee schedule plan, a dental benefits plan in which participating dentists agree to accept a list of specific fees as the total fees for dental treatment provided.

c., implied, a contract not evidenced by explicit agreement of the parties but inferred by the law from the acts and circumstances surrounding the transactions.

c., open-end, **1.** a contract that permits periodic reevaluation of the dental plan during the contract year. If indicated by the reevaluation, dental services may be deleted or added to achieve a balance between the premium and cost of service provided. **2.** a contract that sets no dollar limits on the total services to be provided to beneficiaries but does list the particular services that will be included in the plan.

c. practice, dental practice in which an employer or third-party administrator contracts directly with a dentist or group of dentists to provide dental services for beneficiaries of a plan. See also **closed panel.**

c. term, the period of time, usually 12 months, for which a contract is written.

contraction, 1. a shortening, shrinkage, or reduction in length or size. **2.** a condition in which teeth or other maxillary and mandibular structures such as the dental arch are nearer than normal to the median plane.

c., concentric muscle, an unresisted ordinary shortening of muscle.

c., eccentric muscle, an increase in muscle tonus during lengthening of the muscle. Eccentric contraction occurs when muscles are used to oppose movement but not to stop it (for example, the action of the biceps in lowering the forearm gradually and in a controlled manner). Eccentric contractions are called *isotonic* because the muscle changes length.

c., isometric muscle, an increase in muscular tension without a change in muscle length, as in clenching the teeth.

c., isotonic muscle, an increase in muscular tension during movement without resistance (either lengthening or shortening), as in free opening and closing of the jaws.

c., metal, shrinkage associated with the congealing of a metal from its molten state to a solid after having been cast. See also **expansion, thermal.**

c., muscle, the development of tension in a muscle in response to a nerve stimulus.

  c., m., changes in striation bands, alterations in bands of striated muscle during contraction. Striated muscle is composed of a darker A band and a lighter I band. Both of these alternating bands develop tension during contraction but not to the same degree. In isometric contraction (clenched teeth), the sarcomere muscle unit remains unchanged in length, whereas the A band (the darker band) actually shortens and the I band (the lighter band) lengthens. When a muscle is passively stretched, such as when the mandible is opened by gravity, the A band lengthens relatively more than the I band, and during isotonic contraction, almost all the shortening is in the A segment. It is thus concluded that the contractile properties are not the same throughout the sarcomere, which is the unit of contractility. It is suggested that the darker A band has a greater concentration of contractile substance than the I band and that, in addition to contractile elements, the I band contains elastic noncontractile elements that constitute a series of elastic components throughout the fibril. Thus there is, throughout a fiber, an arrangement of dark, contractile components alternating with lighter, elastic components.

  c., m., chemical factors in, the chemical constituents and action involved in the contraction of muscle fibers. Muscle is a structure with working units built up largely from two proteins, actin and myosin, which appear to be organized into separate filaments running longitudinally through the muscle fibers. Neither type of filament runs continuously along the length of the fiber, although the effect is that of a continuous structure. The filaments are organized into a succession of groupings of one type of fiber. Each group is arranged in a regular palisade to overlap the next group of fibers, which are similarly arranged in palisades. This gives a banded appearance to the fiber. The thicker filaments contain myosin and are restricted to the A bands, where they give rise to a higher density and double refraction. The thinner filaments contain actin and extend to either side of the Z band, which is at the center of the I band. When the muscle contracts or is stretched, the two groups of filaments slide past each other like the alternating units of a sliding gate. The controlled sliding motion is presumably brought about through the mediation of oblique cross links between the filaments. These cross links are the structural expression of the biochemical interaction between actin and myosin. The chemical substance that initiates the interaction between these fibrils is adenosine triphosphate (ATP). The final effect of the interaction between ATP, myosin, and actin is to enable the two types of filaments to crawl past each other to create the shortened state of the muscle.

c., postural muscle, maintenance of muscular tension (usually isometric muscular contraction) sufficient to maintain posture.

c., smooth muscle, mechanism of, the mechanisms that regulate the functions of smooth muscle fibers. These regulatory mechanisms vary and are affected principally by two methods. First, the parasympathetic and sympathetic nerve fiber endings of the autonomic nervous system form a reticulum around the muscle cells before entering them. The action of these fibers is antagonistic; they act directly on the muscle cell, not on each other. Examples of the structures principally

under the control of the autonomic nerve mechanism are the blood vessels and the pilomotor fibers. Second, the selection response to rhythmic activity associated with the automaticity of a viscus or other organ depends on local or hormonal factors. An example of this mechanism is the function of the uterus under the control of the estrogenic hormone.

c., static muscle, contraction in which opposing muscles contract against each other and prevent movement. Fixation action of a muscle in a static contraction is termed *isometric* because it develops tension without changing length.

contractor, independent, one who, exercising an independent employment, contracts to do a piece of work according to the conditions of the contract and without being subject to control except as to the result of the work.

contracture, a permanent shortening, or contraction, of a muscle.

contraindication (kon′trə in′dikā′shən), any symptom or circumstance indicating the inappropriateness of a form of treatment otherwise advisable.

contrast, radiographic (radiographic image), the differences in photographic or film density produced on a radiograph by structural composition of the object radiographed or by varying amounts of radiation.

c. media, a radiopaque substance injected into the body to facilitate radiographic imaging of internal structures that otherwise are difficult to visualize on x-ray films.

c., radiographic, long-scale, an increased number of grays between the blacks and whites on a radiograph. Higher kilovoltages increase the scale of contrast.

c., radiographic, short-scale, a minimum number of grays between the blacks and whites on a radiograph. Lower kilovoltages decrease the scale of contrast.

contributory negligence. See **negligence, contributory.**

contributory plan, a method of payment for group insurance coverage in which part of the premium is paid by the employee and part is paid by the employer or union.

contributory program, a dental benefits program in which the enrollee shares in the monthly premium of the program with the program sponsor (usually the employer). Generally done through payroll deduction.

controlled clinical trial, a research strategy that calls for two samples: an experimental sample of patients receiving a pharmaceutical, and a second sample of control patients receiving a placebo. Neither the patient nor the researcher knows which is receiving the pharmaceutical and which the placebo.

controlled-release therapeutic systems, a drug or hormone delivery system that releases predetermined amounts of drug or hormone into the body over a specified period of time.

controlled substance, any drug as defined in the five categories of the federal Controlled Substances Act of 1970. The categories, or schedules, cover opium and its derivatives, hallucinogens, depressants, and stimulants.

control, stress, any method used to diminish or remove the stress load generated by occlusal contact, whether the contact is functional in origin or the result of a habit cycle.

contusion (kəntū′zhən), a bruise that is usually produced by impact from a blunt object and that does not cause a break in the skin.

convenience form. See **form, convenience.** (not current)

convergence, cervical, the angle formed between the cervicoaxial inclination of a tooth surface on one side and a diagnostic stylus of a dental cast surveyor in contact with the tooth at its height of contour. (not current)

conversion privilege, the right of an individual covered by a group dental insurance policy to continue having coverage on a direct payment basis when association with the insured group is terminated.

converter, rotary, a motor generator set or unit that, when operated by one type of current, produces another (for example, the conversion of alternating to direct current). (not current)

convertin. See **thromboplastin, extrinsic.**

coolant (kōō′lənt), air or liquid directed onto a tooth, tissue, or restoration to neutralize the heating effect of a rotary instrument.

Cooley's anemia. See **thalassemia major.**

Cooley's trait. See **thalassemia minor.**

Coolidge filament transformer, tube. See **transformer, Coolidge.**

coordination, harmonious functioning, such as muscles.

Classification of controlled substances

Classification	Description	Specific substances
Schedule I (Schedule H*)	Drugs that have high potential for abuse and no accepted medical use. Containers are marked C-I.	Heroin, LSD, peyote, marijuana.
Schedule II (Schedule F*)	Drugs that have high potential for abuse but have accepted medical use. Dependence may include strong physical and psychologic dependence. Containers are marked C-II.	Amobarbital, amphetamine, codeine, dextroamphetamine, meperidine, methadone, hydromorphone, morphine, opium, pentobarbital, phenazocine, methylphenidate, secobarbital.
Schedule III (Schedule F*)	Medically accepted drugs that may cause dependence but are less prone to abuse than drugs in Schedules I and II. Containers are marked C-III.	Codeine-containing medications, butabarbital, paregoric.
Schedule IV (Schedule F*)	Medically accepted drugs that may cause mild physical or psychologic dependence. Containers are marked C-IV	Chloral hydrate, chlordiazepoxide, diazepam, meprobamate, phenobarbital.
Schedule V	Medically accepted drugs with very limited potential for causing mild physical or psychologic dependence. Containers are marked C-V.	Drug mixtures containing small quantities of narcotics, such as over-the-counter cough syrups containing codeine.

*Canadian classification.
Adapted from Clark JF, Queerer SF, Karb VB: *Pharmacologic basis of nursing practice,* ed 5, St Louis, 1997, Mosby.

c. of benefits clause, **1.** a provision in an insurance contract that when a patient is covered under more than one group dental plan, benefits paid by all plans will be limited to 100% of the actual charges after each deductible has been satisfied. **2.** COB: A method of integrating benefits payable under more than one plan. Benefits from all sources should not exceed 100% of the total charges.

Copal resin, a mixed resin of diverse plant origin used in cavity varnishes. The effectiveness is questioned in protecting the pulp from the phosphoric acid in dental cements.

copayment, the beneficiary's share of the dentist's fee after the benefits plan has paid.

cope, the upper half of a flask in the casting art; hence also the upper, or cavity, side of a denture flask.

coping (thimble), a thin metal covering or cap over a prepared tooth.

c., parallel, a casting placed over an implant abutment to make it parallel to other casting or implant abutments.

c., transfer, a covering or cap, made of metal, acrylic resin, or other material, and used to position a die in an impression.

copolymer (kōpăl′imər), polymerization of two or more monomers that have slightly different chemical formulas. Used in dentistry to impart certain desirable physical properties such as flow.

copolymerization (kōpălimerizā′shən), the formation of a copolymer.

copper, a malleable, reddish-brown metallic element. Copper is a component of several important enzymes in the body and is essential to good health. Copper deficiency is rare because only 2 to 5 mg daily are necessary and are easily obtained in a normal diet.

coproporphyria (kop′rōpôr′fir′ē·ə), the presence of an abnormal concentration of coproporphyrin in the urine. Normal values range from 70 mg to 250 mg/day. An increased amount of coproporphyrin III occurs in the urine in clinical lead poisoning, exposure to lead without clinically apparent symptoms, infections, malignant disease, alcoholic cirrhosis, after ingestion of small amounts of ethanol, and normally in some individuals.

coproporphyrin, any of the nitrogenous organic substances normally excreted in the feces as a breakdown of bilirubin.

cord(s), a long, rounded organ or body.

c., spinal, the central nervous system cord contained in the vertebral column. The spinal cord is essential to the regulation and administration of various motor, sensory, and autonomic nerve activities of the body. Through its pathways it conducts impulses from the extremities, trunk, and neck to and from the higher centers and to consciousness. It thus provides for simple reflexes, has control over visceral activities, and participates in the conscious activities of the body.

c., vocal, the membranous structures in the throat that produce sound; the thyroarytenoid ligaments of the larynx. The inferior cords are called the *true vocal cords,* and the superior cords are called the *false vocal cords.*

core, the central part, A section of a mold, usually of plaster, made over assembled parts of a dental restoration or construction to record and maintain the relationships of the parts so that the parts can be reassembled in their original positions.

c., amalgam, the foundational replacement of the badly mutilated crown of a tooth whose purpose is to provide a rigid base for retention of a cast crown restoration. The core may be retained by undercuts, slots, pins, or the pulp chamber of an endodontically treated tooth.

c., cast, a metal casting, usually with a post in the canal or a root, designed to retain an artificial crown.

c., composite, composite resin buildup to provide retention for a cast crown restoration.

c., laboratory, a section of a mold, usually of plaster, made over assembled parts of a dental restoration or construction to record and maintain the relationships of the parts so that the parts can be reassembled in their original positions.

core-vent implant system, an ADA-provisionally accepted endosseous implant system using the criteria of osseous integration constructed of medical grade titanium alloy after the design of Branemark in which the apical portion that is able to be submerged is of a hollow-vented design. The superior part is machined to receive a variety of prosthodontic abutments.

corium, gingival (kō'rēəm), the most stable, inert, and mature phase of connective tissue elements of the gingiva lying between the periosteum and the lamina propria mucosae.

cornea, the transparent anterior part of the eye.

cornification, the conversion of epithelium to a hornlike substance. *Keratinization* is a more specific term implying the formation of true keratin.

coronal, pertaining to the crown portion of teeth.

coronary artery bypass, open-heart surgery in which a section of a blood vessel is grafted onto one or more of the coronary arteries to improve the blood supply to the muscles of the heart.

coronoidectomy (kor'ōnoidek'tōmē), the surgical removal of the coronoid process of the mandible.

coronoid process. See **process, coronoid.**

corporate dentistry, I. dental care provided for a specific group of employees within a single business under a contract arrangement or on a salaried basis, with costs borne by the corporation. **2.** a company-owned and operated dental care facility that provides services to employees and sometimes dependents.

corpus callosum, the largest commissure of the brain connecting the cerebral hemispheres.

corpuscle(s), any small body, mass, or organ.

c., blood, a formed element in the blood. See also **erythrocyte, leukocyte, lymphocyte, monocyte.**

c., Golgi's, a small, spindle-shaped proprioceptive endorgan located in tendons and activated by stretch.

c., Krause's, bulboid encapsulated nerve endings located in mucous membranes and activated by cold.

c., Meissner's, medium encapsulated nerve endings found in the skin and activated by light touch.

c., Merkel's, specialized sensory nerve endings located in the submucosa of the mouth and activated by light touch.

c., Pacini's, large sensory nerve endings, scattered widely in subcutaneous tissues, joints, and tendons and activated by deep pressure.

c., Ruffini's, specialized sensory nerve organs in the skin and mucous membranes for perceiving heat. Temperature variations of less than 5° C are not readily received by these end organs.

corrected master cast. See **cast, master, corrected.**

correction, occlusal, correction of malocclusion, by whatever means is employed, including the elimination of disharmony of occlusal contacts. (not current)

corrective, a prescription ingredient designed to compensate for or nullify specific undesirable effects of the principal pharmaceutical agent and the adjuvant.

correlation, a statistical procedure used to determine the degree to which two (or more) variables vary together. Correlation does not suggest a cause-effect relationship, but only the degree of parallelism or concomitance between the variables, the cause of which may be unknown. The Pearson product-moment correlation (r) is the most frequently used, and this coefficient is used unless another is specified.

c., coefficient number, the result of statistical computation that indicates the strength of the tendency of two or more variables to vary concomitantly. The coefficient is expressed in fractions (that is, $r = 80$), ranging from -1 to $+1$ and indicates the magnitude of the relationship between the variables. Perfect direct correspondence is expressed by $+1$; perfect inverse correspondence by -1; complete lack of correspondence by 0. Fractional values are not read as percents.

c., linear, a correlation in which the regression line, that line which best describes the relationship between the two variables, is a straight line, so that for any increase in the magnitude of one variable, there will be a proportional change in the magnitude of the other variable.

c., multiple, a complex correlation procedure in which scores on two or more variables are combined to predict scores on another variable called the *dependent variable.*

correspondence, written or typed communication between two individuals or groups of individuals.

corrosion, an electrolytic or chemical attack of a surface. Usually refers to the attack of a metal surface.

cortex, the outer layer of an organ or other structure.

c., adrenal, the outer layer of the adrenal gland, the site of secretion of the adrenocortical hormones.

c., cerebral, the outer gray matter of cerebrum, where many of the higher functions, such as volition, consciousness, conceptualization, and sensation, are carried out.

corticalosteotomy (kôr′tik·əlos′tēätōmē), an osteotomy through the cortex at the base of the dentoalveolar segment, which serves to weaken the resistance of the bone to the application of orthodontic forces. (not current)

corticoid, adrenal (kôr′tekoid), an adrenal corticosteroid hormone (for example, 11-dehydrocorticosterone [compound A], corticosterone [compound B], 11-deoxycorticosterone [cortexone, DOC], cortisone [compound E], cortisol [compound F], 11-desoxycortisol [substance S], aldosterone, androgen, progesterone, estrogen, and many other inactive steroids). See also **aldosterone, androgen, corticosterone, cortisone, estrogens, hydrocortisone,** and **progesterone.**

corticosteroid (kôr′tikōstir′oid). See **steroid, adrenocortical.**

corticosterone (Kendall's compound B) (kôr′tikōstir′on; kôr′tikōs′terōn), an adrenal corticosteroid hormone necessary for the maintenance of life in adrenalectomized animals; protects against stress, influences muscular efficiency, and influences carbohydrate and electrolyte metabolism.

corticotropin (kôr′tikōtrō′pin), a purified preparation of adrenocorticotropic hormone derived from the pituitary gland of animals. See also **ACTH.**

cortin, the general term for the hormonal secretions of the adrenal cortex. (not current)

cortisol. See **hydrocortisone.**

cortisone (17-hydroxy-11-dehydrocorticosterone, Kendall's compound E), a hormone produced by the adrenal cortex; a glucocorticoid, 17-hydroxy-11-dehydrocorticosterone; useful in the treatment of rheumatoid arthritis, lupus erythematosus, and some allergic conditions. Has marked antiinflammatory properties. Excess production or administration produces signs of hyperadrenocorticalism (Cushing's syndrome) with hyperlipemia and obesity hyperglycemia and edema.

c. acetate, *trade name:* Cortone; *drug class:* gluocorticoid, short acting; *action:* decreases inflammation by suppression of macrophage and leukocyte migration, reduces capillary permeability; *uses:* inflammation, severe allergy, adrenal insufficiency, collagen, and respiratory and dermatologic disorders.

Corynebacterium, a common genus of rod-shaped, curved bacilli. The most common parthogenic species are *Corynebacterium acnes,* commonly found in acne lesions, and *C. diphtheriae,* the cause of diphtheria.

cosmetic orthodontics, limited orthodontic therapy for the purpose of improving appearance, such as the closing of an unsightly diastema between central incisors that presents no other handicap.

cost-benefit analysis, the comparative study of the service or production costs of a service or item and its value to the subject.

cost containment, the features of a dental benefits program or of the administration of the program designed to reduce or eliminate certain charges to the plan.

cost-effective, the minimal expenditure of dollars, time, and other elements necessary to achieve the health care result deemed necessary and appropriate.

Costen's syndrome. See **syndrome, Costen's.**

cost sharing, the share of health expenses that a beneficiary must pay, including the deductibles, copayments, coinsurance, and charges over the amount reimbursed by the dental benefits plan.

cothromboplastin (kōthräm′bōplas′-tin). See **thromboplastin, extrinsic.** (not current)

cotton, absorbent, the fibers or hairs of the seed of cultivated varieties of *Gossypium herbaceum,* so prepared that the cotton readily absorbs liquid.

cotton pliers. See **pliers, cotton.**

cough, a sudden noisy expulsion of air from the lungs.

c., **gander,** the characteristic clanging, brassy cough of tracheal obstruction.

Council on Dental Therapeutics, an appointed Council within the Division of Scientific Affairs of the American Dental Association directed to study, evaluate, and disseminate information with regard to dental therapeutic agents, their adjuncts, and dental cosmetic agents that are offered to the public or profession.

counseling, the act of providing advice and guidance to a patient or the patient's family.

count, blood, complete, the determination of the number of red blood cells (erythrocytes), white blood cells, and platelets in an accurately measured volume of blood. It usually includes the quantity of hemoglobin per cubic millimeter of blood. A normal red blood count is 4 to 5.5 million cells/cubic mm of blood.

count, differential white blood cell, the determination of the number of each type of white blood cell in the peripheral blood. The relative count is obtained by counting the number of each type of cell in every 100 cells. The results are expressed in percentages. The normal figure for neutrophils is 60% to 70%, lymphocytes 20% to 35%, monocytes 2% to 8%, basophils 0% to 1%, and eosinophils 2% to 4%.

counter, a device for enumerating ionizing events.

c., **Geiger-Muller** (G-M counter, Geiger counter), a highly sensitive, gasfilled device that measures radiation.

c., **proportional,** a gas-filled radiation detection tube in which the pulse produced is proportional to the number of ions formed in the gas by the primary ionizing particle.

c., **scintillation,** the combination of phosphor, photomultiplier tube, and associated circuits for counting the light emissions that are produced in the phosphor.

counterdie, the reverse image of a die, usually made of a softer and lower fusing metal than the die. It is used to swage metal, wax, or other material over a die. See also **die.** (not current)

counterirritant, an irritant that blocks perception of pain by diverting attention to the sensation that it produces. (not current)

count, platelet, the determination of the number of platelets in a cubic millimeter of blood. The normal count is 200,000 to 500,000.

count, reticulocyte (retik'ūlōsĭt'), the number of reticulocytes in the circulating blood, giving some indication of bone marrow activity. The number is increased after acute blood loss and after recovery from anemia. The number is decreased in anemias associated with defective red cell or hemoglobin production (nutritional, endocrine, toxic, or displacement anemias). The normal range is 0.5% to 1.5% of the erythrocytes.

count, white blood cell, the determination of the number of white blood cells in an accurately measured volume of blood. The normal value is from 4000 to 9000 per cubic millimeter of blood.

coverage, 1. benefits available to an individual covered under a dental benefits plan. **2.** See **denture coverage.**

c. **year,** the 12-month period over which deductibles and maximum benefits apply for each person.

covered charges, the charges for services rendered or supplies furnished by a dentist that qualify as covered services and are paid for in whole or in part by the dental benefits program. May be subject to deductibles, copayments, coinsurance, annual or lifetime maximums, or table of allowances, as specified by the terms of the contract.

covered person, an individual who is eligible for benefits under a dental benefits program.

covered services, the services for which payment is provided under the terms of the dental benefits contract.

Coxiella, a genus of filterable bacteria of the order Rickettsiales.

C. burnetii, a species of *Coxiella* that causes Q fever in man.

Coxsackie A disease. See **herpangina.**

crack cocaine, a street drug made by chemically converting cocaine hydrochloride to a form that can be smoked. Smoking crack is a faster, more direct way of getting cocaine into the brain. The narcotic effect of smoking crack cocaine is faster and more intense than it is when injected, inhaled, or ingested. No medical application exists for crack cocaine.

cracked tooth syndrome, transient acute pain experienced occasionally while chewing. Difficult to locate and reproduce. Likely to occur among individuals who crack nuts and crush ice with their teeth, and among popcorn eaters. Usually a vertical crack or split in the tooth extends across a marginal ridge through the crown and into the root, involving the pulp. Visible by transilluminated light or with the use of disclosing dyes.

Crane-Kaplan pocket marker. See **pocket marker, Crane-Kaplan.** (not current)

cranial base, the bones forming the base of the skull. In cephalometric analysis, defined by the angle formed by a line drawn basion to point S (sella turcica) and from point S to point N (frontonasal suture).

cranial nerves, the twelve pairs of nerves, which emerge from the cranial cavity through various openings in the base of the skull, are as follows: olfactory, optic, oculomotor, trochlear, trigeminal, abducens, facial, acoustic, glossopharyngeal, vagus, accessory, and hypoglossal.

cranial prosthesis, an artificial replacement for a portion of the skull.

cranial sutures, the fibrous joints between the bones of the cranium, some of which are fused in adults.

craniofacial anomalies, congenital malformations of the skull and face, frequently associated with genetically transmitted syndromes.

craniofacial dysostosis (krā′nēōfā′- shəl dis′ōstō′sis). See **dysostosis, craniofacial.**

craniofacial templates, a series of cephalometric tracings of normal faces by age, sex, and race by which variations in the facial form of a patient can be determined and a treatment objective arranged.

craniometry (krā′nēäm′etrē), the study of the measurements of the skull.

craniopharyngioma (krā′nēōfərin′- jēō′mə), a tumor histologically identical to ameloblastoma that arises from remnants of the craniopharyngeal duct.

craniosynostosis, premature fusion of the cranial sutures resulting in a

malformed head, which may lead to an increase in intracranial pressure and consequential brain damage.

craniotabes (krā′nēōtā′bēz), a soft, yielding skull; shallow pitting and thinning of skull bones of infants as a result of congenital syphilis or rickets.

craniotomy, any surgical opening into the skull, performed to relieve intracranial pressure, to control bleeding, or to remove a tumor.

crater formation, the formation of interdental depressions in the gingival tissues and/or subjacent bone; often associated with the destructive effects of necrotizing ulcerative gingivitis.

crazing, the formation of small cracks on the surface of structures induced by release on internal stress.

c. of plastic teeth, minute cracks appearing on the surface of plastic teeth.

creatine kinase, an enzyme in muscle, brain, and other tissues that catalyzes the transfer of a phosphate group from adenosine triphosphate to creatine, producing adenosine diphosphate and phosphocreatine.

creatinine, a substance formed from the metabolism of creatine, commonly found in blood, urine, and muscle tissue.

creative, a term describing the ability or talent to think or act in a new or original way.

creditor, a person to whom a debt is owed by another person.

credit rating, the evaluation of any person's responsibility toward meeting financial obligations.

crenation (krinā′shən), a wrinkling of the surface of cells as a result of shrinkage in their volume.

c. of tongue, scalloping along the lingual periphery of the tongue caused by the tongue lying against the lingual surface of the mandibular teeth.

creosote, N.F. XI (wood creosote), a mixture of phenols obtained from wood tar and occasionally used to treat root canals.

crepitus (krep′itəs), a crackling sound such as that produced by the rubbing together of fragments of a fractured bone or by air moving in a tissue space.

c., bony, the crackling sound noted during auscultation; also the sensation noted during palpation when the fragments of a fractured bone are rubbed together.

crescent, sublingual, the crescent-shaped area on the floor of the mouth formed by the lingual wall of the mandible and the adjacent part of the floor of the mouth.

crest, a projecting ridge or structure.

c., alveolar. See **bone crest.**

c., gingival, the coronal margin of the gingival tissue.

crestal resorption, bone resorption at the border or crest of the dental alveolus. This bone loss follows tooth extraction and may result from periodontal infection or through the use of heavy orthodontic forces.

cretin, a thyroid-deficient dwarfed individual with mental subnormality.

cretinism (krē′tənizəm) (congenital hypothyroidism), **1.** a marked retardation of physical and mental development caused by congenital lack of secretion of thyrotropic hormone by the pituitary gland. Slow tooth eruption is one of the results. **2.** a thyroid deficiency that results in retardation of physical and mental development.

crevice, a narrow opening caused by a fissure or a crack.

c., gingival, the fissure between the free gingiva and enamel.

crib, Jackson, a removable orthodontic appliance retained in position by crib-shaped wires.

crib, lingual, an orthodontic appliance consisting of a wire framework suspended lingually to the maxillary incisor teeth; used to obstruct thumb and tongue habits.

cribriform, perforated (like a sieve).

c. plate, the aveolar bone that forms the tooth socket and to which the periodontal ligament is attached (radiographically the lamina dura).

crib splint. See **splint, crib.**

cricoid cartilage (krī′koid). See **cartilage, cricoid.**

cricoidynia (krī′koidīn′e·ə), pain in the cricoid cartilage. (not current)

cricothyrotomy (kri′kōthīrot′əmē), an incision between the cricoid and thyroid cartilages for the purpose of maintaining a patent airway.

cri-du-chat syndrome (krēdōōshat′). See **syndrome, cri-du-chat.**

criminology, the study of crime, the people who commit crimes, and the penal code used to deter crime and punish criminals.

crisis, adrenal, an acute adrenocortical insufficiency, with clinical manifestations of headache, nausea, vomiting, diarrhea, confusion, costovertebral angle pain, circulatory collapse, and coma. May occur in relation to stress of dental or medical procedures in patients with latent adrenal disease or in patients who have undergone prior ACTH or cortisone therapy, especially without control or termination of therapy.

crisis, thyroid, a complication occurring after thyroidectomy, or before or during other surgical procedures where even mild hyperthyroidism is present. It is characterized by tachycardia, a high temperature, nervousness, and occasionally delirium.

cristobalite (kristō′bəlīt), a form of crystalline silica used in dental casting investments because of its relatively high capacity for thermal expansion and resistance to breaking down by heat.

criteria, predetermined rules or guidelines for dental care, developed by dentists relying on professional expertise, prior experience, and the professional literature, with which aspects of actual instances of dental care may be compared. Explicit criteria are predetermined, specific, and measurable; implicit criteria are implied or understood but not directly expressed.

critical care. See **intensive care.**

cromolyn sodium, *trade names:* Intal, Nasalcrom, Rynacrom; *drug class:* antiasthmatic; *action:* stabilizes the membrane of the sensitized mast cell, preventing release of chemical mediators; *uses:* allergic rhinitis, severe perennial bronchial asthma, exercise-induced bronchospasm.

Crooke's tube. See **x-ray tube, Crooke's.** (not current)

cross arch bar splint. See **connector.**

cross arch bar splint connector. See **connector, cross arch bar splint.**

cross arch splinting. See **splinting, cross arch.**

cross-bite, an occlusion with the line of occlusion of the mandibular teeth anterior and/or buccal to the maxillary teeth. See also **occlusion, cross-bite.**

c.-b., anterior, primary or permanent maxillary incisors locked lingual to mandibular incisors.

c.-b., posterior, primary permanent maxillary posterior teeth in lingual position in relation to the mandibular teeth.

cross-examination, questioning of a witness by the party against whom he has been called and examined.

cross-infection, the transmission of a communicable disease from one person to another because of a poor barrier protection.

cross linkage. See **polymerization, cross.**

cross-resistance. See **resistance, cross-.**

cross-section form. See **clasp, flexibility of.**

cross-sectional study, the scientific method for the analysis of data gathered from two or more samples at one point in time.

cross-tolerance. See **tolerance, cross-.**

Crouzon's disease (krōō'zanz') See **dysostosis, craniofacial.**

Crouzon's syndrome. See **dysostosis, craniofacial.**

crowding, 1. more than filling the space provided or intended. In dentistry when the dental arch length is less than the mesial distal width of the teeth intended to occupy it **2.** malocclusion characterized by inadequate arch circumference to accommodate the teeth in proper alignment.

crown, that portion of a human tooth covered by enamel.

c., anatomic, that portion of dentin covered by enamel.

c. and bridge prosthodontics, the division of prosthodontics that deals with crown restorations and the fixed type of tooth-borne partial denture prosthesis. See also **prosthodontics, fixed.**

c., artificial, a dental prosthesis restoring the anatomy, function, and esthetics of part or all of the coronal portion of the natural tooth.

c., clinical, **1.** that portion of enamel visibly present in the oral cavity. **2.** the portion of a tooth that is occlusal to the deepest part of the gingival crevice.

c., complete, a restoration that reproduces the entire surface anatomy of the clinical crown and fits over a prepared tooth stump.

c., c. veneer, a restoration that reproduces the total clinical coronal surface contour of the tooth.

c., dowel, a restoration that replaces the entire coronal portion of a tooth and derives its retention from a dowel extending into a treated (filled) root canal.

c., extraalveolar clinical, the portion of a tooth that extends occlusally or incisally from the junction of the tooth root and the supporting bone.

c., faced. See **crown, veneered metal.**

c., full, restoration, an individual tooth prosthesis encompassing the entire prepared clinical crown. See also **crown, complete veneer.**

c., jacket. See **crown, complete.**

c. lengthening, a surgical procedure to remove marginal gingival tissues to expose more of the crown of the tooth to facilitate a reconstructive or operative procedure.

c., partial, a restoration that covers three or more, but not all, surfaces of a tooth.

c., porcelain-faced, an artificial crown that makes use of porcelain inlayed in or veneered onto the labial or buccal surface.

c.-root ratio, the relation of the clinical crown to the clinical roots of the teeth—an important consideration in diagnosis, prognosis, and treatment planning.

c., stainless steel, a preformed steel crown used for the restoration of badly broken-down primary teeth and first permanent molars. Also used as a temporary restoration of fractured permanent incisors.

c., three-quarter, a term frequently used to designate a partial veneer crown.

c., veneered metal, a complete crown that has one or more surfaces prepared for and covered by a tooth-colored substance such as porcelain or resin.

crown-rump length, the length of an embryo, fetus, or newborn as measured from the crown of the head to the prominence of the buttocks

Crozat appliance. See **appliance, Crozat.**

CRT, the abbreviation for **cathode-ray tube.**

crucible (krōō'sibal), a vessel or container that will withstand high heat and is used for melting or holding material.

c. crushing strength. See **strength, compressive.**

c. former (sprue base), the stand or base into which a sprued pattern is placed. It establishes the shape or form of the hollowed-out end of the investment in the casting ring, which will receive the molten metal on its course through the sprue hole. See also **sprue former.**

crust, a hard coating surface layer composed of coagulated tissue fluid and blood products mixed with epithelial and inflammatory cells covering a lesion formed by the rupture of a bulla, vesicle, or pustule.

cryolite (krī'ōlīt) (sodium aluminum fluoride [Na_3AlF_6]), a fluoride often used as a flux in the manufacture of silicate cements.

cryosurgery, the use of subfreezing temperature to destroy tissue. Cryosurgery is used to cause the edges of a detached retina to heal, to remove cataracts, and in the treatment of Parkinson's disease.

cryotherapy, a use of cryosurgery in the treatment of cutaneous tags, warts, actinic keratosis, and dermatofibromas. The agent is usually liquid nitrogen applied briefly with a sterile cotton-tipped applicator.

crystal(s), a naturally produced solid. The ultimate units of the substance from which it was formed are arranged systematically.

c. gold. See **gold, mat.**

c., platinocyanide, a chemical substance used in the manufacture of fluorescent screens. Barium platinocyanide was first used by Roentgen for this purpose.

c., silver halide, silver compounds, usually silver bromide and silver iodide, that are impregnated in the photographic emulsion of film. These compounds, when acted on by actinic rays, are disintegrated, with the formation of metallic silver in a finely divided state. The photographic image results when the film is subjected to processing.

crystallization, the production or formation of crystals, either by cooling a liquid or gas to a solid state or by cooling a solution until the solute precipitates as a crystalline deposit.

cubic centimeter (cc), a unit of volume sometimes used in prescription writing. For that purpose it may be considered identical with the milliliter (ml). See also **milliliter.**

cubital (kyoo'bitəl), pertaining to the forearm.

cubitus (kyoo'bitəs), the forearm.

cuboid (kyoo'boid) (cuboidal), resembling a cube in form.

cuboidal. See **cuboid.**

cue, a stimulus that determines or may prompt the nature of a person's response.

cultural characteristics. See **culture 2.**

cultural diversity, a population consisting of two or more cultural groups.

culture, 1. the growth of microorganisms or other living cells on artificial media. **2.** a set of learned values, beliefs, customs, and behavior that is shared by a group of interacting individuals.

c., bacterial, bacterial growth on or in an artificial medium. The medium used may be selective for a given type or genus of organism (for example, tomato juice agar for lactobacilli).

c., endodontic, the growth of microorganisms obtained from root canals or periapical tissues.

c., e. medium, a specific medium used for endodontic cultures.

c. medium, a substance, liquid or solid, used for cultivating bacteria.

cumulative, increasing in effect.

cup, chin, 1. an orthopedic device that directs a posterior and/or vertical force to the mandible, through the attachment of a cup fitting over the chin to a headcap. **2.** a drug used to cause muscle relaxation during anesthesia by blocking acetylcholine at the neuromuscular and synaptic junctions.

cure, 1. the successful treatment of a disease or wound. **2.** a procedure or reaction that changes a plastic material to a hard material (for example, vulcanization and polymerization). See also **process.**

curet, curette (kyooret'), a periodontal or surgical instrument having a sharp, spoon-shaped working blade; used for debridement. The periodontal curet, available in many sizes and shapes, is used for root and gingival curettage.

curettage (kyoo'rətäzh'), scraping or cleaning with a curet.

c., apical (apoxesis), curettement of diseased periapical tissue without excision of the root tip. See also **curettage, subgingival.**

c., infrabony pocket, enucleation, by means of suitable instrumentation, of the inflammatory soft tissue elements

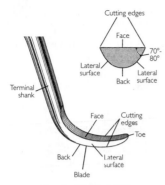

Curette. (Genco, 1990.)

lying within and surrounding the crest of an infrabony resorptive defect; also includes the debridement and planing of the root surface of the pocket.

c., root, debridement and planing to smoothness of the root surface of a tooth to eliminate accretions on the root and provide a suitable environment for the return of the gingival tissues to a state of health.

c., subgingival, the process of debridement of the epithelial attachment, the ulcerated and entire (pocket) epithelium, and subjacent inflamed and altered gingival corium; usually results in resolution of the inflammatory process and desirable shrinkage and repair of the edematous tissue.

curette. See **curet.**

curie (kyōō′rē), a measurement of radioactivity produced by the disintegration of unstable elements. The curie is that quantity of a radioactive nuclide in which the number of disintegrations per second is 3.700 times 10^{-10}. Since the curie is a relatively large unit, the millicurie (0.00 curie) and the microcurie (one millionth of a curie) are more often used. The curie is based on the number of nuclear disintegrations and not on the number or amount of radiations emitted.

curing, the act of polymerization.

c., denture. See **denture curing.**

current, a measure of the number of electrons per second that pass a given point on a conductor.

c., alternating, a current that alter-

nately changes its direction of flow. It usually consists of 60 complete cycles/sec.

c., coagulating, an electrical current, delivered by a needle, ball, or other variously shaped points, that coagulates tissue.

c. dental terminology (CDT), a listing of descriptive terms and identifying codes developed by the American Dental Association (ADA) for reporting dental services and procedures to dental benefits plans.

c., direct, an electrical current in which the electron flow is in only one direction.

c., galvanic, a direct current created by a battery.

c. procedural terminology (CPT), a listing of descriptive terms and identifying codes developed by the American Medical Association (AMA) for reporting practitioner services and procedures to medical plans and medicare.

c., saturation, the maximum current in a roentgen-ray tube that fully uses all electrons that are available at the cathode for the production of roentgen rays.

curriculum, a course of study; the linked series of academic courses leading to mastery of a discipline.

cursor, the pointer on the video screen that indicates the current position on the screen of the terminal.

curvature, occlusal. See **curve of occlusion.**

curve, a nonangular deviation from a straight line or surface.

c., alignment. See **alignment.**

c., anti-Monson. See **curve, reverse.**

c., compensating, the curvature of alignment of the occlusal surfaces of the teeth that is developed to compensate for the paths of the condyles as the mandible moves from centric to eccentric positions. A means of maintaining posterior tooth contacts on the molar teeth and providing balancing contacts on dentures when the mandible is protruded. Corresponds to the curve of Spee of natural teeth.

c., dose-effect, a curve relating the dose of radiation with the effect produced.

c., milled-in. See **path, milled-in.**

c., Monson, the curve of occlusion, described by Monson, in which each cusp and incisal edge touch or conform to a segment of the surface of a sphere 8 inches (20 cm) in diameter, with its center in the region of the glabella. See also **curve, compensating.**

c. of occlusion (occlusal curvature), **1.** a curved occlusal surface that makes simultaneous contact with the major portion of the incisal and occlusal prominences of the existing teeth. **2.** the curve of a dentition so which the occlusal surfaces of the teeth lie. See also **curve, reverse.**

c. of Spee, 1. an anatomic curvature of the occlusal alignment of teeth, beginning at the tip of the lower canine, following the buccal cusps of the natural premolars and molars, and continuing to the anterior border of the ramus, as described by von Spee. **2.** the curve of the occlusal surfaces of the arches in vertical dimension, brought about by a dipping downward of the mandibular premolars, with a corresponding adjustment of the upper premolars.

c. of Wilson, by-product term of the thinking that supported the theory that occlusion should be spherical. The curve in the lower arch is concave, whereas the one in the upper arch is convex.

c., reverse, a curve of occlusion that is convex upward when viewed in the frontal plane.

c., sine, the wave form of an alternating current, characterized by a rise from zero to maximum positive potential, then descending below zero to its maximum negative value, and then rising to its maximum positive potential, to fall to zero again.

c., survival, a curve obtained by plotting the number or percentage of organisms surviving at a given time against a given dose of radiation. A curve showing the percentage of individuals surviving at different intervals after a particular dosage of radiation.

Cushing's syndrome. See **syndrome, Cushing's.**

cusp, a notably pointed or rounded eminence on or near the masticating surface of a tooth.

c., angle. See **angle, cusp.**

c.-fossa relations, organic relations between a stamp cusp and its fossa.

c. height, the shortest distance between the deepest part of the central

fossa of a posterior tooth and a line connecting the points of the cusps of the tooth.

c., shoeing. See **restoration of cusps.**

cuspal interference. See **contact, deflective occlusal.**

cuspid. See **canine.**

cuspidor, a fixture provided on some dental operating units into which patients can expectorate. In current practice, most operating fields are kept clear of saliva by high volume suction saliva ejectors.

customary fee, the fee level determined by the administrator of a dental benefits plan from actual submitted fees for a specific dental procedure to establish the maximum benefit payable under a given plan for that specific procedure. See also **fee, usual** and **fee, reasonable.**

cuticle, the outer layer of the skin. Also, a layer that covers the free surface of an epithelial cell.

c., primary, 1. the transitory remnants of the enamel organ and oral epithelium covering the enamel of a tooth after eruption. Synonym: Nasmyth's membrane. **2.** believed to be the last substance formed by ameloblasts, mediating the attachment of ameloblasts to the enamel.

c., secondary, 1. the second cuticle formed when the ameloblasts are replaced by the oral epithelium. It then covers the primary cuticle on the enamel and is the only cuticle on the cementum. **2.** a keratinized pedicle found between the gingival epithelium and the surface of a tooth.

cuticula dentis (kyo͞otik'ūlə den'tis). See **cuticle, primary.**

cutting instrument. See **instrument, cutting.**

CVA. See **accident, cerebrovascular.**

cyanocobalamin (vitamin B_{12}), *trade names* (some): Alpha Redisol, Betalin-12, Cobex; *drug class:* Vitamin B_{12} water-soluble vitamin; *action:* needed for adequate nerve functioning, protein and carbohydrate metabolism, normal growth, red blood cell development, and cell reproduction; *uses:* vitamin B_{12} deficiency, pernicious anemia, hemolytic anemia, hemorrhage, and renal and hepatic diseases.

cyanosis (sīənō'sis), a characteristic bluish tinge or color of the skin and mucous membranes associated with reduction in hemoglobin brought about by inadequate respiratory change (5 gm/100 ml are necessary for color to be perceptible).

cyclamate, a noncaloric artificial sweetening agent used in conjunction with saccharin presently banned by the FDA because of its carcinogenic potential.

cycle, a succession of events.

c., chewing, a complete course of movement of the mandible during a single masticatory stroke.

c., masticating, three-dimensional patterns of mandibular movements formed during the chewing of food.

cyclic AMPcycloheximide, a cyclic nucleotide formed from adenosine triphosphate by the action of adrenyl cyclase. It is known as the "second messenger" and participates in the action of catecholamines, vasopressin, adrenocorticotropic hormone, and many other hormones.

cyclizine HCl/cyclizine lactate, *trade name:* Marezine; *drug class:* antiemetic, antihistaminic, anticholinergic; *action:* may act centrally to act on vomiting center, also antagonizes histamine peripherally; *uses:* motion sickness, prevention of postoperative vomiting.

cyclobenzaprine HCl, *trade name:* Cycoflex; *drug class:* skeletal muscle relaxant, centrally acting tricyclic; *action:* has actions similar to those of tricyclic antidepressants; *uses:* adjunct for relief of muscle spasm and pain in musculoskeletal conditions.

cyclophosphamide, *trade names:* Cytoxan, Neosar, Procytox; *drug class:* antineoplastic alkylating agent; *action:* alkylates DNA, RNA; inhibits enzymes that allow synthesis of amino acids in proteins; *uses:* Hodgkin's disease; lymphomas; leukemia; cancer of female reproductive tract, lung, prostate; multiple myeloma; neuroblastoma; retinoblastoma; Ewing's sarcoma.

cycloserine, *trade name:* Seromycin Pulvules; *drug class:* antitubercular; *action:* inhibits cell wall synthesis, analog of D-alanine; *uses:* pulmonary tuberculosis.

cyclosporine, *trade name:* Sandimmune; *drug class:* immunosuppressant; *action:* produces immunosuppression by inhibiting lymphocytes;

uses: to prevent rejection of tissues and/or organ transplants.

cyclothymia (sī′klōthī′mē·ə). See **psychosis, manic depressive.**

cyclotron (sī′kləträn), a device for accelerating charged particles to high energies by means of an alternating electrical field between electrodes placed in a constant magnetic field.

cylindroma (silindrō′mə), an adenocystic basal cell carcinoma of the salivary glands. A malignant tumor that may occur in the sublingual, submandibular, parotid, or labial salivary glands. See also **carcinoma, adenocystic.**

cyproheptadine HCl, *trade name:* Periactin; *drug class:* antihistamine H_1 receptor antagonist; *action:* acts on blood vessels, gastrointestinal and respiratory systems by competing with histamine for H_1-receptor site; *uses:* allergy symptoms, rhinitis, pruritus, cold urticaria.

cyst (sist), a pathologic space in bone or soft tissue containing fluid or semifluid material and, in the oral regions, almost always lined by epithelium.

c., aneurysmal bone, a nonmalignant osteolytic lesion expanding a long bone or within a vertebra in which the space, filled with blood, is networked with fibrous tissue containing multinucleated giant cells.

c., branchial (branchial cleft cyst), soft tissue cyst usually seen on the lateral side of the neck, arising from epithelial illusions within the cervical lymph nodes. Microscopic examination shows the epithelial lining of stratified squamous epithelium surrounded by lymphoid tissue.

c., calcifying and keratinizing odontogenic, a cyst arising from odontogenic epithelium, with abundant production of keratin-containing ghost cells and areas of dystrophic calcification. This lesion has no age or sex distribution.

c., dental. See **cyst, periodontal.**

c., dentigerous, an epithelium-lined sac filled with fluid or semifluid material that surrounds the crown of an unerupted tooth or odontoma.

c., dentoalveolar. See **cyst, periodontal.**

c., dermoid, an epithelium-lined sac with one or more skin appendages (hair follicles, sweat glands, sebaceous glands) in its wall. It may be found in the floor of the mouth. This lesion should not be confused with the teratomatous dermoid cyst of the ovary.

c., epidermoid, an epithelium-lined sac containing fluid; possesses characteristics of the epidermis but does not have the skin appendages seen in dermoid cysts.

c., eruption, a dentigerous cyst that causes a clinically evident bulging of the overlying alveolar ridge.

c., extravasation. See **cyst, traumatic.**

c., fissural, a cyst that arises from the enslaved epithelium in maxillary suture lines caused by fusion of the embryonic processes of the facial bones.

c., follicular, an odontogenic cyst that arises from the epithelium of the tooth bud and dental lamina. Follicular cysts include dentigerous, primordial, and multilocular cysts.

c., globulomaxillary, an epithelium-lined sac formed at the junction point of the globular (median nasal) and maxillary processes. It is seen as a pear-shaped radiolucency between the maxillary lateral incisor and canine, and it separates their roots.

c., hemorrhagic, an extravasation cyst or lesion; traumatic bone cyst or lesion. This is not a true cyst but is probably a defect in the bone produced by trauma and repair. It appears as a definite radiolucent area with a sharply marked radiopaque border. It contains air and is lined by a thin endosteum. See also **cyst, solitary bone.**

c., incisive canal. See **cyst, nasopalatine.**

c., indefinite bone. See **cyst, traumatic.**

c., lateral. See **cyst, periodontal.**

c., lateral follicular, a follicular cyst occurring on the lateral surface of a tooth, usually near the cementodentinoenamel junction. See also **cyst, follicular.**

c., median palatal, an epithelium-lined sac containing fluid; appears as a radiolucency in the midline of the palate. It is of developmental origin.

c., mucous (mucocele), an epithelium-lined sac containing mucus. Mucous cysts in the sinus may appear as spherical, radiopaque areas.

c., multilocular, a follicular cyst containing many loculi, or spaces, and not associated with a tooth.

c., nasoalveolar, a fluid-containing sac lined by epithelium and located at the ala of the nose. A developmental cyst, it may simulate a nasal or periapical abscess.

c., nasopalatine (nasopalatine duct), a cyst arising within the nasopalatine canal. Radiographically it may appear as a heart-shaped radiolucency between the maxillary central incisors. Histologically it may show mucous cells and nerve bundles in addition to a lining of stratified squamous or respiratory epithelium. The incisive canal cyst and the cyst of the papilla incisiva are the recognized subtypes.

c., odontogenic, an epithelium-lined sac produced from the tooth-forming tissues (for example, primordial, dentigerous, and periodontal cysts).

c., periapical. See **cyst, radicular.**

c., periodontal (dental root cyst, dentoalveolar cyst, lateral cyst, periapical cyst), an epithelium-lined sac containing fluid. Usually found at the apex of a pulp-involved tooth. Lateral types occur less frequently along the side of the root.

c., primordial, an epithelium-lined sac containing fluid and appearing as a radiolucency in the jaws. It is derived from an enamel organ before any hard tissue is formed.

c., radicular (periapical cyst, root end cyst), a cyst that has a fibrous connective tissue wall and a lining of stratified squamous epithelium and that is attached to the apex of the root of a tooth with a nonvital pulp or a defective root canal filling.

c., residual, an odontogenic cyst that remains within the jaw after the removal of the tooth with which it was associated. May be radicular or follicular.

c., root end. See **cyst, radicular.**

c., solitary bone, a pathologic bone space of disputed origin that may be either empty or filled with fluid. It may have a delicate connective tissue lining.

c., thyroglossal duct, an epithelium-lined sac containing fluid formed in portions of the incompletely involuted thyroglossal duct, which connects the primitive pharynx with the tongue in embryonic life. These cysts may appear in the midline at any region from the subhyoid to the base of the tongue.

c., traumatic (extravasation cyst, extravasation lesion, traumatic bone lesion), a radiolucent lesion appearing chiefly in the mandible as a well-defined area with a radiopaque border; clinically it appears as a cavity lined by extremely thin periosteum and filled with air. Assumed to be caused by injury to young spongy bone, hemorrhage resorption, and then walling off by cortical bone. See also **cyst, solitary bone.**

cystadenoma (sistad'ēnō'mə), an adenoma with the development of cystic spaces caused by dilation of acinar or ductal structures.

c., papillary, lymphomatosum (Warton's tumor), a benign salivary gland tumor that consists of numerous cystic spaces lined by a double layer of epithelium. A dense aggregate of lymphocytes containing germinal centers surrounds the cystic spaces.

cysteine, a nonessential amino acid found in many proteins in the body.

cystic fibrosis, an inherited disorder of the exocrine glands, causing those glands to produce abnormally thick secretions of mucus, elevation of sweat electrolytes, increased organic and enzymatic constituents of saliva, and overactivity of the autonomic nervous system.

cystostomy, creating a surgical opening into the urinary bladder or gall bladder.

cytochrome, one of a class of hemoproteins that act as electron transport. Cytochromes are classified as *a, b, c,* and *d.*

cytokine, a nonantibody protein such as lymphokine. Cytokines are released by a cell population on contact with a specific antigen. Cytokines act as intercellular mediators in the generation of immune response.

cytology (sītäl'əjē), the study of the anatomy, physiology, pathology, and chemistry of a cell.

c., exfoliative, the study of desquamated cells.

cytomegalic inclusion disease. See **disease, salivary gland.**

cytomegalovirus (CMV), a visceral disease virus, a member of the group of herpetoviruses having special affin-

ity for the salivary glands. Considered one of the indicator infections of AIDS.

cytoskeleton, the intracellular filaments that serve to support or stiffen cells.

cytosol, the totality of the intracellular substance exclusive of mitochondria and endoplasmic reticulum components.

cytozyme (sī'tōzĭm). See **thromboplastin.**

D

Dalton's law See **law, Dalton's.** (not current)

dam, a barrier to the passage of moisture or saliva.

d., post-. See **seal, posterior palatal.**

d., rubber, a thin sheet of latex rubber used to isolate a tooth or teeth and keep them dry during a dental procedure.

d., rubber punch, a hand-punch instrument with progressively larger openings, used to make a hole(s) in the rubber dam.

damages, compensation or indemnity that may be recovered in the courts by any person who has suffered loss, detriment, or injury to person, property, or rights through the unlawful act or negligence of another.

d., compensatory, a sum that compensates the injured party for injury only.

d., exemplary (punitive damages), damages awarded to the plaintiff over those that will barely compensate for property loss. Such compensation may be awarded when the wrong done to the plaintiff involved violence, malice, or fraud by the defendant. The object is to provide compensation for mental suffering or loss of pride. It may be employed as punishment of the defendant.

d., nominal, a trifling sum awarded to a plaintiff in an action in which there is no substantial loss or injury to be compensated but in which the law still recognizes a technical invasion of rights or a breach of the defendant's duty. Also awarded in cases in which, although there has been a real injury, the plaintiff's evidence is not sufficient to show its amount.

d., punitive. See **damages, exemplary.**

danazol, *trade name:* Danocrine; *drug class:* androgen, alpha-ethinyl testosterone derivative; *action:* decreases FSH and LH output; *uses:* endometriosis, prevention of hereditary angioedema, fibrocystic breast disease.

dantrolene sodium, *trade name:* Dantrium; *drug class:* skeletal muscle relaxant, direct acting; *action:* interferes with intracellular release of calcium necessary to initiate contraction; *uses:* spasticity in multiple sclerosis, stroke, spinal cord injury, cerebral palsy, malignant hyperthermia.

dapsone (DDS), *trade name:* Avlosulfon; *drug class:* leprostatic, antibacterial; *action:* bactericidal and bacteriostatic against *M. leprae;* may also be immunosuppressant; *uses:* Leprosy, dermatitis herpetiformis.

Darier's disease. See **disease, Darier's.**

darkroom, a completely lightproof room or cubicle that is used in the processing of photographic, medical, and dental films. See also **safe light.**

Darvon, the brand name for propoxyphene hydrochloride, a mild, centrally acting narcotic analgesic agent.

data, a collection of facts and figures, often called *raw data* to emphasize that they are unprocessed. Data are processed and interpreted to yield information.

d. base, an organized collection of data. A medical data base is all the information that exists in the practice at any time.

d. processing, the collection of data, processing of the data to obtain usable information, and communication of this usable information.

d. set, a hardware device that converts digital pulses (square waveform) into modulated frequencies (sinusoidal wave) for transmission, a process called modulation. It also converts modulated frequencies into voltage pulses, a process called *demodulation.* Synonym: modem.

daughter (decay product), a nuclide formed from the radioactive decay of another nuclide called the *parent.*

day care l. a specialized program or facility that provides care for children ages infant through preschool, usually within a group framework, either as a substitute for or extension of home care. **2.** a specialized program or facility that provides care for handicapped or dependent children or adults as a substitute for or extension of home care

day sheet, a form that permits systematic record keeping of treatment of patients and of monies received and spent.

Day's syndrome. See **syndrome, Riley-Day.**

DDC, the abbreviation for **dideoxycytidine.** See **dideoxycytidine.**

DDI, the abbreviation for **dideoxyinosine.** See **dideoxyinosine.**

dead, without life; destitute of life.

d. space. See **space;** **physiologic dead space;** and **anatomic dead space.**

deaf, without usable hearing.

deafen, to make deaf; to cause the loss of all usable hearing.

deafness (def′ness), a condition characterized by a partial or complete loss of hearing.

d., central, impaired hearing caused by interference with cerebral auditory pathways or in the auditory centers in the brain (for example, cerebrovascular accidents and other degenerative brain diseases). Hearing aids are of little benefit.

d., conduction. See **deafness, transmission.**

d., nerve, impaired hearing caused by pathologic conditions in the auditory nerve or the hair cells of the organ of Corti in the inner ear (for example, high-tone deafness, which comes with age; damage to the organ of Corti by noise; or a tumor of an auditory nerve). Hearing aids are usually of little benefit.

d., transmission *(conduction deafness),* impaired hearing caused by interference with passage of sound waves through the external ear (for example, interference caused by wax) or middle ear (for example, interference caused by otitis media, aerotitis media, or otosclerosis). May be characterized by greater interference with hearing of low tones. Hearing aids that amplify may be helpful.

deanesthesiant (de′·anəsthē′zē·ənt), anything that will arouse a patient from a state of anesthesia.

death (deth) **1.** cessation of life; the stoppage of life beyond the possibility of resuscitation. **2.** the cause or occasion of loss of life. **3.** the total absence of activity in the brain and central nervous system, the cardiovascular system, and the respiratory system as observed and declared by a physician or other legally authorized agent.

d., brain, in addition to the generally accepted definition of death, some states, either by statute or court decision, have added a "brain death" definition to the law, applicable where there has been an irreversible cessation of brain function.

d. certificate, the signed affidavit that life has ceased giving the time, place, and cause of death. Death certificates are required by law to be filed in the proper local or regional geopolitical office.

debility (dēbil'ĭtē), weakness; lack of strength; asthenia.

debridement (dabrēdmənt), the removal of foreign material and/or devitalized tissue from the vicinity of a wound.

d., epithelial (deepithelization). See **curettage, subgingival.**

debris (debrē'), foreign material or particles loosely attached to a surface.

d. of Malassez (maləsə'), the remnants of Hertwig's epithelial root sheath within the periodontal ligament.

debt, a sum of money due by agreement; the contract may or may not be express and does not necessarily set the precise amount to be paid.

debug, to locate and correct any errors in a computer program.

decalcification (dēkal'sifikā'shən), loss or removal of calcium salts from calcified tissues.

decarboxylation, a chemical reaction involving the removal of a molecule of carbon dioxide from carboxylic acid.

decay, to deteriorate, putrefy.

d., dental. See **caries, dental.**

d. product. See **daughter.**

d., radioactive, the disintegration of the nucleus of an unstable nuclide by the spontaneous emission of charged particles and/or photons.

d., senile. See **caries, dental, senile.**

deceleration, a decrease in the speed or velocity of an object or reaction.

decibel (des'ibel), a logarithmic ratio unit that indicates by what proportion one intensity level differs from another.

deciduous (dēsid'ū-əs), that which will be shed. Pertaining specifically to the first dentition of humans or animals.

d. dentition, teeth that will be shed.

d. teeth, the teeth constituting the first dentition.

decision making, the process of coming to a conclusion or making a judgment.

decision tree, an algorithm or a formal stepwise process used in coming to a conclusion or making a judgment.

declaration and provision for affairs, a systematic statement of the affairs and estate of a person, in which all assets and property are listed.

decompression, 1. a technique used to readapt an individual to normal atmospheric pressure after exposure to higher pressures, as in diving. **2.** the removal of pressure caused by gas or fluid in a body cavity such as the stomach or intestinal tract.

d., nerve, the release of pressure on a nerve trunk by surgical widening of the bony canal.

decontamination, the process of making a person, object, or environment free of microorganisms, radioactivity, or other contaminants.

deductible, 1. a stipulated sum the covered person must pay toward the cost of dental treatment before the benefits of the program go into effect. The deductible may be annual or payable only once and may vary in amount from program to program. **2.** the amount of dental expense for which the beneficiary is responsible before a third party will assume any liability for payment of benefits. Deductible may be an annual or one-time charge and may vary in amount from program to program. See also **family deductible.**

d. amount, that portion of dental care expense the insured must pay before the plan's benefits begin.

d. clause, a provision in an insurance contract stipulating that the insurer will pay only that amount that is in excess of a specified amount.

deep bite. See **overbite.**

deep sensibility. See **sensibility, deep.** (not current)

deepithelization (dē·ep'ithē'lizā'shən). See **debridement, epithelial.**

D

DEF rate. See **rate, DEF.** (not current)

defamation (defəma'sh ən), the act of detracting from the reputation of another. The offense of injuring a person's reputation by false and malicious statements.

default, 1. an omission of that which should be done. **2.** failure to fulfill an obligation or a promise.

defecation, the elimination of feces from the digestive tract through the rectum.

defect, 1. the absence of some legal requisite. **2.** an imperfection.

d., operative, the incomplete repair of bone after root resection or periapical curettage.

d., osseous, a concavity in the bone surrounding one or more teeth, resulting from periodontal disease.

d., speech, any deviation of speech that is outside the range of acceptable variation in a given environment.

defective, mentally, a mentally subnormal individual. A person in whom a basic nervous system defect may be assumed because of social and intellectual deficiencies (for example, persons afflicted with microcephaly, hydrocephalus, mongolism).

defendant, the party against whom relief or recovery is sought in a lawsuit.

defense, the reasons, in law or fact, offered by the defendant in a legal proceeding as to why the plaintiff should not prevail.

d. cell. See **cell, defense.**

d. mechanism, an unconscious, intrapsychic reaction that offers protection to the self from threatening or stressful situations. Defense mechanisms may be useful to diminish anxiety and facilitate coping behaviors, or may be harmful because of denying, displacing, isolating, or repressing anxiety and preventing useful coping responses.

defibrillation (defī'brilāshən) the arrest of fibrillation, usually that of the cardiac ventricles. An intense alternating current is briefly passed through the heart muscle, throwing it into a refractory state.

defibrillator (defī'brilā'tər), an apparatus for defibrillating the ventricles of the heart.

deficiency, a lack or defect.

d., ac-globulin. See parahemophilia.

d., dietary, an inadequate amount of food intake or an insufficiency of any of the food elements necessary for proper nutrition.

d., gingival hyperplasia in vitamin A, hyperplastic and hyperkeratotic gingival changes occurring with decreased ingestion, diminished absorption, faulty use, or overexcretion of vitamin A. For example, in diabetes, the liver often cannot effectively convert carotene to vitamin A.

d., mineral, a form of nutritional deficiency produced by the inadequate ingestion, absorption, use, and/or overexcretion of essential inorganic elements such as calcium, magnesium, and phosphorus.

d., nicotinic acid, a deficiency of nicotinic acid in the diet, resulting in acute erythematous stomatitis, papillary atrophy of the tongue, and ulcerative gingivitis.

d., plasma thromboplastic antecedent. See **hemophilia C.**

d., protein, a malnutritive state produced by inadequate ingestion, absorption, use, or overexcretion of essential protein elements. Degenerative lesions produced in the periodontium include osteoporosis of the alveolar and supporting bone and disappearance of fibroblasts and connective tissue fibers of the periodontal membrane.

d., PTA. See **hemophilia C.**

definition (image), the property of projected images relating to their sharpness, distinctness, or clarity of outline. Penumbra width is a measure of definition. See also **resolution.**

deflective occlusal contact. See **contact, deflective occlusal.**

deformation (dē'formā'shən), a distortion; a disfigurement.

d., elastic, the term used to describe the change in shape of an object under an applied load from which the object can recover or return to its original unloaded state when the load is removed.

d., inelastic, a deformation occurring when a material is stressed beyond its elastic limit.

d., permanent, a deformation occurring beyond the yield point so that the structure will not return to its original dimensions after removal of the applied force.

deformity, a distortion or disfigurement of a portion of the body; may be congenital, familial, hereditary, acquired, pathologic, or surgical.

d., gingival, a deviation from the normal gingival topographic and architectural pattern.

degeneration, ballooning, a condition seen in vesicles of viral origin, in which epithelial cells are washed from the vesicle wall. The cells swell and their nuclei undergo amitotic division, resulting in multinucleated giant cells that may be seen floating in vesicular fluid.

degeneration, basophilic granular (not current). See **basophilia.**

degenerative joint disease, a term to describe osteoarthritis. Osteoarthritis is a noninflammatory process as opposed to rheumatoid arthritis. Osteoarthritis occurs more frequently in women after the age of 40.

degloving, an intraoral surgical exposure of the bony mandibular anterior region. This procedure can be performed in the posterior region if necessary.

deglutition (di'glōotish'ən) (swallowing), a succession of muscular contractions from above downward or from front backward; propels food from the mouth toward the stomach. The action is generally initiated at the lips; it proceeds back through the oral cavity, and the food is moved automatically along the dorsum of the tongue. When the food is ready for swallowing, it is passed back through the fauces. Once the food is beyond the fauces and in the pharynx, the soft palate closes off the nasopharynx, and the hyoid bone and larynx are elevated upward and forward. This action keeps food out of the larynx and dilates the esophageal opening so that the food may be passed quickly toward the stomach by peristaltic contractions. The separation between the voluntary and involuntary characteristics of this wave of contractions is not sharply defined. At birth the process is already well established as a highly coordinated activity; that is, the swallowing reflex.

degradation (degrədā'shən), the reduction of a chemical compound to a less complex compound.

degrees of freedom (df), a statistic, based on the number of observations and groups in a study, that is necessary to determine statistical significance. One looks up the degrees of freedom and the significance level in a table of significance values to determine if the magnitude of the value obtained is significant. Used with the t-test, chi square, analysis of variance, and correlation.

dehiscence (dihis'əns), a fissural defect in the facial alveolar plate extending from the free margin apically.

dehiscent (dihis'ənt), opened wide; fissured.

d. mandibular canal, a condition caused by bone resorption that leaves the mandibular canal without a covering or roof of bone.

dehydration (dē'hidrā'shən), **1.** the removal of water (for example, from the body or tissue). **2.** a decrease in serum fluid coupled with the loss of interstitial fluid from the body. Dehydration is associated with disturbances in fluid and electrolyte balance.

d. of gingivae, the drying of gingival tissue, leading to a lowered tissue resistance, which can result in gingival inflammation; seen in mouth breathing.

delayed expansion. See **expansion, delayed.**

delict (delikt'), a wrong or an injury; an offense; a violation of public or private obligation.

delinquent (deling'kwent), pertaining to a debt or claim that is due and unpaid at the time due.

delirium (delir'ē-əm), a condition of mental excitement, confusion, and clouded sensorium, usually accompanied by hallucinations, illusions, and delusions; precipitated by toxic factors in diseases or drugs.

d. tremens, a delirious state marked by distressing delusions, illusions, and hallucinations, constant tremor, fumbling movements of the hands, insomnia, and great exhaustion.

delivery, a transfer of the possession of personal property from one person to another.

Delta Dental Plan, an active member organization of the Delta Dental Plans Association, formed and guided by state dental societies to provide prepaid dental care to the public on a group basis.

delusion, a persistent, aberrant belief or perception held inviolable by a person despite evidence to the contrary.

demand, in economics, refers to the buying of services or goods; in dental

D

care, generally denotes the active request for and purchase of dental care services.

demeclocycline HCl, *trade name:* Declomycin; *drug class:* tetracycline; *action:* inhibits protein synthesis, phosphorylation in microorganisms; *uses:* uncommon gram-positive and/ or gram-negative bacteria, protozoa.

dementia, a progressive, organic mental disorder characterized by chronic personality disintegration, confusion, disorientation, stupor, deterioration of intellectual capacity and function, and impairment or control of memory, judgment, and impulses (for example, senile psychosis, also associated with AIDS).

Demerol (dem'eräl), the trade name for meperidine hydrochloride.

demography, the study of human populations, particularly the size, distribution, and characteristics of members of population groups. Demographic techniques are employed in the long-term continuing study of the residents of Framingham, Massachusetts, by the National Institutes of Health.

demurrer (demer'ər), an admission of the facts charged by the opponent while maintaining that those facts are legally insufficient to establish liability.

denasality (dēnəsal'itē), the quality of the voice when the nasal passages are obstructed, preventing adequate nasal resonance during speech.

dendrite (den'drīt), **1.** fingerlike projections formed during the solidification of crystalline materials. **2.** a branched, treelike protoplasmic process of a neuron that carries nerve impulses toward the cell body. See also **axon.**

denervation (de'nervā'shən), the sectioning or removal of a nerve to interrupt the nerve supply to a part.

dens in dente (denz in den'tä) (dens invaginatus, gestant odontoma), an anomaly of the tooth found chiefly in upper lateral incisors; characterized by invagination of the enamel, giving a radiographic appearance that suggests a "tooth within a tooth."

dens invaginatus (denz invajinä'təs). See **dens in dente.**

Densite (den'sīt), the trade name for a form of alpha-hemihydrate with a low setting expansion and greater hardness; used for dies, models, and casts;

sometimes referred to as a *Class II stone.*

densitometer (den'sitom'ətər), an instrument for determining the degree of darkening of developed photographic or x-ray film, based on the use of a photoelectric cell to measure the light transmission through a given area of the film.

density, the concentration of matter, measured by mass per unit volume.

d., radiographic, the degree of darkening of exposed and processed photographic or x-ray film, expressed as the logarithm of the opacity of a given area of the film.

dental, relating to the teeth.

d. abutment. See **abutment.**

d. alloy. See **alloy.**

d. amalgam. See **amalgam.**

d. anxiety. See **anxiety.**

d. arch. See **arch, dental.**

d. articulator. See **articulator.**

d. assistant. See **assistant, dental.**

d. auxilliary. See **auxiliary personnel.**

d. benefits organization, any organization offering a dental benefits plan. Also known as *dental plan organization.*

d. benefits plan, entitles covered individuals to specified dental services in return for a fixed, periodic payment made in advance of treatment. Such plans often include the use of deductibles, coinsurance, and/or maximums to control the cost of the program to the purchaser.

d. benefits program, the specific dental benefits plan being offered to enrollees by the sponsor.

d. bonding. See **bonding.**

d. calculus. See **calculus.**

d. care, the treatment of the teeth and their supporting structures.

d. care for children. See **pedodontics.**

d. caries. See **caries, dental.**

  d. caries susceptible. See **susceptible.**

d. cavity lining. See **cavity lining.**

d. cement. See **cement, dental.**

d. chart. See **chart, dental.**

d. cementum. See **cementum.**

d. clinic. See **clinic.**

d. cooperative, a dental facility organized to provide dental services for the benefit of subscribers and not for profit. There is no discrimination as to who may subscribe, and each subscriber has equal rights and voice in the control of the cooperative. The operation of the cooperative usually rests with a lay board of directors elected by subscribers.

d. deposit. See **calculus.**

d. dysfunction. See **dysfunction, dental.**

d. enamel. See **enamel.**

   d. enamel hypoplastic. See **hypoplasia.**

d. engine. See **engine, dental.**

d. equipment. See **equipment.**

d. fissure. See **fissure.**

d. fistula. See **fistula.**

d. floss, waxed or plain thread of nylon or silk used to clean the interdental areas; an aid in oral physiotherapy.

d. geriatrics. See **geriatrics.**

d. granuloma. See **granuloma, dental.**

d. handpiece. See **handpiece.**

d. health services, the sum of the diagnostic, preventive, consultative, supportive, and therapeutic dental care offered by the dental profession or that portion provided a member of a dental health plan.

d. health surveys, the use of questionnaires and/or oral examinations of a target population to determine the need and/or demand for dental care or the opinions or attitudes of patients or consumers.

d. history. See **history.**

d. hygienist. See **hygienist, dental.**

d. identification, the process of establishing the unique characteristics of teeth and dental work of an individual, leading to the identification of an individual by comparison with the person's dental charts and records.

d. implant. See **implant.**

d. impression material. See **impression.**

d. instrument. See **instruments.**

d. insurance, a policy that insures against the expense of treatment and care of dental disease and accident to teeth.

d. jurisprudence, the application of the principles of law as they relate to the practice of dentistry. See also **jurisprudence, dental.**

d. laboratory technician. See **technician, dental laboratory.**

d. material. See **material, dental.**

d. model. See **model.**

d. occlusion. See **occlusion.**

d. papilla. See **papilla.**

d. pathology, that branch of dentistry that deals with all aspects of dental disease. See also **pathology.**

d. pin. See **pin.**

d. plan, any organized method for the financing of dental care.

d. plaque. See **plaque.**

d. porcelain. See **porcelain, dental.**

d. prepayment, a system for budgeting the cost of dental services in advance of their receipt.

d. prophylaxis. See **prophylaxis.**

d. prosthesis. See **prosthesis.**

d. prosthetic restoration. See **prosthesis, dental.**

d., public health, preferably called public health dentistry, this is a specialty of dentistry that deals with dental health on a community, regional, or national basis rather than on a provider-to-patient basis. However, some programs sponsored by public health dental agencies do provide for direct patient care for otherwise underserved populations. See also **community dentistry.**

d. pulp. See **pulp.**

   d. pulp capping. See **capping, pulp.**

   d. pulp cavity. See **cavity pulp.**

   d. pulp exposure. See **exposure.**

d. record, confidential documents containing the clinical and financial data of the dental patient, including the patient's identity, pertinent history, medical and dental conditions, services rendered, and charges and payments made.

d. research, the formal scientific study of issues related to dentistry.

d. review committee, a group of dentists and administrative personnel that reviews questionable dental claims and can suggest policy decisions regarding dental care.

d. scaling. See **scaling.**

d. sealant. See **sealant.**

d. senescence. See **senescence, dental.**

d. service corporation, a legally constituted, not-for-profit organization that negotiates and administers contracts for dental care. Delta Dental and Blue Cross/Blue Shield corporations are two such organizations.

d. service, hospital, **l.** the location of the dental facility within a hospital. **2.** the array of dental procedures offered within a hospital setting.

d. staff, the personnel employed or engaged by the dentist or the dentist's agent to conduct the assignable professional and management functions of the dental clinic, office, or practice.

d. stone. See **stone, dental.**
d. tape. See **tape, dental.**
d. technician. See **technician.**
d. unit. See **unit, dental.**

dentate (den'tāt), having teeth.

denticle (den'tikəl) (endolith, pulp nodule, pulpstone), a calcified body found in the pulp chamber of a tooth; it may be composed either of irregular dentin (true denticle) or an ectopic calcification of pulp tissue (false denticle).

dentifrice, a pharmaceutical compound used in conjunction with the toothbrush to clean and polish the teeth. Contains a mild abrasive, a detergent, a flavoring agent, a binder, and occasionally deodorants and various medicaments designed as caries preventives (for example, antiseptics).
d. abrasion. See **abrasion, dentifrice.**

dentigerous cyst. See **cyst.**

dentin (den'tin) (dentine), the portion of the tooth that lies subjacent to the enamel and cementum. Consists of an organic matrix on which mineral (calcific) salts are deposited; pierced by tubules containing filamentous protoplasmic processes of the odontoblasts that line the pulpal chamber and canal. It is of mesodermal origin.
d. bonding agent, a tissue compatible adhesive that adheres to dentin.
d., carious, dentin that is involved in or affected by the carious process.
d. dysplasia. See **dysplasia, dentinal.**
d. eburnation (ēburnā'shən), a change in carious teeth in which the softened and decalcified dentin assumes a hard, brown, polished appearance.
d., hereditary opalescent. See **dentinogenesis imperfecta.**
d., hyperesthesia of, an excessive sensibility of dentin.
d. irritation (tertiary dentin, reparative dentin), formed in response to an injury or irritant.
d., residual carious. See **caries, dental, residual.**
d., sclerotic. See **dentin, transparent.**
d., secondary, dentin formed or deposited on the walls of pulp chambers and canals subsequent to the complete formation of the tooth; caused by certain metabolic disturbances that result in irritation and stimulation of the odontoblasts to renewed activity.
d., transparent (sclerotic dentin), dentin formed as a defense mechanism in reaction to various stimuli. Dental tubules are obliterated by deposits of calcium salts that are harder and denser than normal dentin. This dentin appears transparent in ground sections.
d. wall, the portion of the wall of a prepared cavity that consists of dentin.

dentinal permeability, the degree to which fluids can pass through intact dentin.

dentine. See **dentin.**

dentinocemental junction (denti'nōsēmen'təl). See **junction, dentinocemental.**

dentinoenamel junction. See **junction, dentinoenamel.**

dentinogenesis imperfecta (den' tinō jen'əsis imperfek'tə) (hereditary opalescent dentin), **1.** a disturbance of the dentin of genetic origin; characterized by early calcification of the pulp chambers and root canals, marked attrition, and an opalescent hue to the teeth. **2.** a localized form of mesodermal dysplasia affecting the dentin of the tooth. It may be hereditary and may be associated with osteogenesis imperfecta. **3.** a hereditary condition associated with a defect in dentin formation; the enamel remains normal.

dentinoma (den'tinō'mə), an odontogenic tumor composed of regular or irregular dentin. (not current)

dentist, one who is educated, trained, and licensed to treat diseases and injuries of the teeth and oral cavity and to construct and insert restorations of and for the teeth, jaws, and mouth.

dentistry, the science and art of preventing, diagnosing, and treating diseases, injuries, and malformations of the teeth, jaws, and mouth and of replacing lost or absent teeth and associated structures.
d., forensic. See **jurisprudence, dental.**
d., four-handed, the technique of chairside operating in which four hands are kept busy working in the oral cavity simultaneously.
d., operative, the branch of oral health service concerned with operations to restore or reform the hard dental tissues (for example, operations necessitated by caries, trauma, and impaired function, and for improvement of appearance).

d., prosthetic. See **prosthodontics.**

d., psychosomatic, dentistry that concerns itself with the mind-body relationship.

d., washed-field, the constant flushing of the operative field with an irrigant (usually water) and the evacuation of the washing (debris) from the mouth by vacuum airstream. See also **technique, hydroflow.**

dentition (dentish′ən), the natural teeth in position in the dental arches.

d., artificial, artificial substitutes for the natural dentition. See also **denture.**

d., deciduous. See **dentition, primary.**

d., mixed, the complement of teeth in the jaws after the eruption of some of the permanent teeth but before all the deciduous teeth are absent.

d., natural, the natural teeth, as considered collectively, in the dental arches.

d., permanent (secondary dentition, permanent teeth), the 32 teeth of adulthood that either replace or are added to the complement of deciduous teeth.

d., primary, the teeth that erupt first and are usually replaced by the permanent teeth.

d., prognosis of, an evaluation by the dentist of the prospect of recovery from dental disease, combined with a forecast of the probability of maintaining the dentition and associated structures in function and health.

d., secondary. See **dentition, permanent.**

d., transitional, more commonly referred to as the *mixed dentition.* The transitional period usually begins with the eruption of the first permanent molars and ends with the exfoliation of the last primary tooth. In time span about 6 years from age 6 to 12.

dentoenamel junction. See **junction, dentinoenamel.**

dentofacial deformity, the malformation of the dentofacial complex with resultant disabling disharmony in size and/or form, as well as function. Includes malocclusion, cleft lip and palate, other skeletal deformities, and muscular dysfunctions.

dentofacial orthopedics, a more descriptive synonym for orthodontics; the adjustment of relationships between and among teeth and facial bones by the application of outside forces and/or the stimulation and redirection of functional forces within the craniofacial complex.

dentoform, a mock-up of the dentition and alveolar structures; used as a teaching aid or for display purposes.

dentulous (dent′yōōləs) (dentulism), having the natural teeth present in the mouth.

denture, an artificial substitute for missing natural teeth and adjacent tissues.

d., acrylic resin, a denture made of acrylic resin.

d., artificial. See **denture.**

d., basal surface of (impression surface of denture, foundation surface of denture), the part of a denture base that is shaped to conform to the basal seat for the denture.

d.-bearing area. See **area, basal seat.**

d., bilateral partial, a dental prosthesis that supplies teeth and associated structures on both sides of a semi-edentulous arch.

d. brush, a brush designed especially for cleaning dentures.

d. characterization, a modification of the form and color of the denture base and teeth to produce a more lifelike appearance.

d., complete (complete dental prosthesis), a dental prosthesis that replaces all of the natural dentition and associated structures of the maxillae or mandible.

  d., complete, lower, a prosthetic replacement of all the teeth in the mandibular dental arch.

  d., complete, upper, a prosthetic replacement of all the teeth in the maxillary dental arch.

d. coverage, the extent to which the oral tissue is covered by the denture base.

d. curing, the process by which the denture-base materials are hardened in a denture mold to the form of a denture. See also **process.**

d. design, a planned visualization of the form and extent of a denture.

d. dislodging force. See **force, denture dislodging.**

d., duplicate, a second denture intended to be a copy of the first denture.

d. edge. See **border, denture.**

d. esthetics. See **esthetics, denture.**

d., finish of, the final perfection of the form of the polished surfaces of a denture.

d. flange. See **flange.**

d. foundation, the portion of the oral structures that supports the complete or partial denture base under occlusal load. See also **area, basal seat.**

d. foundation, surface of. See **denture, basal surface of.**

d., full, improper term. See **denture, complete.**

d., heel of. See **distal end.**

d., immediate (immediate-insertion denture), a removable dental prosthesis constructed for placement immediately after removal of the remaining natural teeth.

d., implant, a denture that gains its support, stability, and retention from a substructure that is implanted under the soft tissues of the basal seat of the denture and is in contact with bone.

d., implant, substructure. See **substructure, implant.**

d., implant, superstructure. See **superstructure, implant.**

d., impression surface of. See **denture, basal surface of.**

d., interim, a dental prosthesis to be used for a short interval of time.

d. liner, a resin used to coat the tissue surface of a dental prosthesis to restore or improve the conformation of the prosthesis to the tissue; generally used to improve the retention of the denture.

d., maintenance of, an important part of prosthodontic treatment and a major factor in the longevity of the service that the restoration can be expected to give.

d., metal base, a denture with a base of gold, chrome-cobalt alloy, aluminum, or other metal.

d., model, wax. See **denture, trial.**

d. overlay, a complete denture that is supported by both tooth and mucosa. Remaining teeth are used to provide additional stability to the denture.

d. packing. See **packing, denture.**

d., partial (partial dental prosthesis), a prosthesis that replaces one or more, but less than all, of the natural teeth and associated structures.

d., partial, cantilever. See **denture, partial, fixed, cantilever.**

d., partial, cantilever fixed, a fixed dental prosthesis that has one or more abutments at one end of the fixed partial denture supporting pontic(s) at its other end.

d., partial, components of, the units that compose a removable partial denture (for example, the base, the artificial teeth, direct and indirect retainers, major and minor connectors).

d., partial, construction of, the science and technique of designing and constructing partial dentures.

d., partial, extension, a removable partial denture that is retained by natural teeth at one end of the denture base segments only; a portion of the functional load is carried by the residual ridge.

d., partial, fixed, a tooth-borne partial denture that is intended to be permanently attached to the teeth or roots that furnish support to the restoration.

d., partial, removable, a partial denture that can be readily placed in the mouth and removed by the wearer.

d., partial, temporary. See **denture, partial, treatment.**

d., partial, tissue-borne, a removable partial denture that is not supported entirely by the natural teeth.

d., partial, tooth-borne, a partial denture that is supported entirely by the teeth that bound the edentulous area covered by the base.

d., partial, tooth-borne/tissue-borne, a partial denture that gains support from both an abutment tooth or teeth and from the structures of an edentulous area covered by the base.

d., partial, treatment (temporary partial denture), a dental prosthesis used for the purpose of treating or conditioning the tissues that are called on to support and retain a denture base.

d., partial, unilateral, a dental prosthesis that restores lost or missing teeth on one side of the arch only.

d. periphery. See **border, denture.**

d., polished surface of, the portion of the surface of a denture that extends in an occlusal direction from the border of the denture and includes the palatal surface. It is the part of the denture base that is usually polished and includes the buccal and lingual surfaces of the teeth.

d. processing. See **processing, denture.**

d., provisional, a prosthetic appliance to be used for a short period of time for reasons of esthetics, function, or occlusal support; more commonly referred to as a temporary, interim, or transitional denture. A provisional denture is usually an immediate denture and is most often employed in the maxillary arch.

d. repair, the restoration of a broken or damaged dental prosthesis.

d. retention. See **retention, denture.**

d. sore mouth. See **mouth, denture-sore.**

d. space, the space between the residual ridges and between the cheeks and the tongue that is available for dentures. See also **distance, interarch.**

d. stability. See **stability, denture.**

d. supporting area. See **area, basal seat.**

d. supporting structure. See **structure, denture supporting.**

d., temporary, a denture intended to serve for a very short time in a temporary or emergency situation.

d., transitional, a removable partial denture that serves as a temporary prosthesis to which teeth will be added as more teeth are lost and that will be replaced after postextraction tissue changes have occurred. A transitional denture may become an interim denture when all the teeth have been removed from the dental arch.

d., trial (wax model denture), a temporary denture, usually made of wax on a baseplate, that is used for checking jaw relation records, occlusion, and the arrangement and observation of teeth for esthetics.

denturist, a person, other than a dentist, (usually a technician) who engages in the practice of dentistry, usually limited to complete and/or partial dentures. Such activity is outside the dental practice act of most states.

deoxyribonucleic acid probes, a nucleic acid fragment labeled with a radioisotope that is complementary to a sequence in another nucleic acid fragment that will bind to it and thus identify it. It is used as a diagnostic tool to identify the species of microbe

involved in an infectious process such as refractory periodontal disease.

dependency, the state of being dependent.

d., drug, a psychologic craving for, habituation to, or addiction to a chemical substance; the term replaces *drug addiction,* which emphasizes physiologic craving.

d., emotional, an emotional need manifested by a marked and habitual inclination to rely on another for comfort, support, guidance, and decision making; the tendency to seek help from others in making decisions or in carrying out difficult actions; the need to be mothered, loved, taken care of, emotionally supported. In extreme cases such persons lose their ability to function independently.

dependents, generally the spouse and children of a subscriber, as defined in a contract. Under some contracts, parents or other members of the family may be beneficiaries.

depletion, salt (dēplē'shən), a condition resulting from inadequate water intake, low intake of sodium and chlorides in the alimentary tract, and secretion of sweat and urine. The most significant of these losses are the gastrointestinal fluid losses resulting from vomiting, diarrhea, and fistulas.

depolarization (dēpō'larizā'shən), a neutralization of polarity; the breaking down of polarized semipermeable membranes, as in nerve or muscle cells in the induction of impulses.

deponent, one who gives under oath testimony reduced to writing.

deposit, bismuth. See **stomatitis, bismuth.**

deposit, calcareous. See **calculus.**

deposition (depōzi'shən), evidence given by a witness under interrogation, oral or written, and usually written down by an official person and intended to be used in the trial of an action in court.

depot (dē'pō), in physiology, the site of accumulation, deposit, or storage of body products not immediately or actively involved in metabolic processes (for example, a fat depot).

depreciation, normally, charges against earnings to write off the cost, less salvage value, of an asset over its estimated useful life. It is a bookkeeping entry and does not represent any cash outlay, nor are any funds earmarked for the purpose. Following are three classic methods of applying depreciation: straight line, sum of the year's digits, and double declining balance.

depressant (dēpres′ənt), a medicine that diminishes functional activity.

depression (dēpresh′ən), a decrease of functional activity.

    d., psychologic, a clinical syndrome of neurotic or psychotic proportions, consisting of lowering of mood tone (feelings of painful dejection), difficulty in thinking, and psychomotor retardation. As used by the layman, depression ordinarily refers only to the mood element, which would be more appropriately labeled dejection, sadness, gloominess, despair, or despondency. Many such patients lack motivation and concern for their oral health or dental needs.

derivative (dēriv′ətiv), a chemical substance that is the result of a chemical reaction.

dermatalgia (dermətal′jē·ə), pain, burning, and other sensations of the skin unaccompanied by any structural change; probably caused by some nervous disease or reflex influence. (not current)

dermataneuria (der′matənoo′rē·ə), a derangement of the nerve supply of the skin, causing disturbance of sensation. (not current)

dermatitis (dermətī′tis), an inflammation of the skin.

    d., allergic contact, the reaction of the skin to direct contact with a specific antigen. Poison ivy rash is a common example of an allergic contact dermatitis.

    d., atopic, atopic eczema characterized by the distinctive phenomena of atopy, a familial related allergic response associated with IgE antibody.

    d., contact, a delayed type of induced sensitivity (allergy) of the skin with varying degrees of erythema, edema, and vesiculation, resulting from cutaneous contact with a specific allergen. Contact dermatitis is an occupational hazard in dentistry.

    d. herpetiformis, dermatitis characterized by grouped, erythematous, papular, vesicular, pustular, or bullous lesions occurring in various combinations, often accompanied by vesico-

bullous and ulcerative lesions of the oral mucous membranes.

    d. infectiosa eczematoides *(Engman's disease),* a pustular eczematous eruption that frequently follows or occurs coincidentally with some pyogenic process.

    d., occupational, generally a contact dermatitis associated with allergens found in the workplace.

    d., radiation, an inflammation of the skin resulting from a high dose of radiation. The reaction varies with the quality and quantity of radiation used and is usually transitory.

dermatoglyphics, the study of the skin ridge patterns on fingers, toes, palms of hands, and soles of feet. The patterns are used as a basis of identification (fingerprinting).

dermatology, the study of the skin, including the anatomy, physiology, and pathology of the skin and the diagnosis and treatment of skin disorders.

dermatoma, a circumscribed thickening or hypertrophy of the skin. (not current)

dermatome, an instrument for cutting thin slices or layers of skin for grafting or for sequentially removing small lesions.

dermatomyositis (der′mətōmī′ōsī′ tis) (polymyositis, dermatomucosomyositis), a form of collagen disease related to scleroderma and lupus erythematosus. The skin lesions are diffuse erythematous desquamations or rashlike lesions. The skin symptoms are related to a variety of patterns of myositis.

dermatophyte, any of several fungi that cause parasitic skin disease in humans.

dermatosclerosis (der′mətōsklərō′ sis). See **scleroderma.**

dermatosis (der′mətō′sis), any disease of the skin. (not current)

dermoid cyst. See **cyst, dermoid.**

desaturation (dēsat′yərā′shən), the conversion of a saturated compound such as stearin into an unsaturated compound such as olein by the removal of hydrogen.

desensitization (dēsen′sitizā′shən), a condition of insusceptibility to infection or an allergen; established in experimental animals by the injection of an antigen that produces sensitization or an anaphylactic reaction. After recovery, a second injection of the antigen is made, bringing about no reaction and thus producing desensitization.

desiccate (des'ikāt), to dry by chemical or physical means; for example, electrocoagulation can produce desiccation in tissues.

desiccation (des'ikā'shən), excessive loss of moisture; the process of drying up. See also **electrocoagulation.**

design, to plan and/or delineate by drawing the outline of a proposed prosthesis.

designer drugs, synthetic organic compounds that are designed as analogs of illicit drugs, with the same narcotic or other dangerous effects.

desipramine HCl, *trade names:* Norpramin, Petrofane; *drug class:* antidepressant, tricyclic; *action:* inhibits both norepinephrine and serotonin (5-HT) uptake in the brain; *use:* depression.

desmins, α-amino acids, usually lysine and norleucine, condensed through their sidechains rather than through the α-amino and carboxyl groups. They copolymerize with vimentin to form constituents of connective tissue.

desmolysis (desmol'isis), the destruction and disintegration of connective tissue. Some authorities associate this desmolytic process with the destruction of connective tissue lying between the enamel and oral epithelium, which thus permits proliferation of the oral epithelium and fusion of enamel and oral epithelium.

desmopressin acetate, *trade name:* Stimate; *drug class:* synethetic antidiuretic hormone; *action:* promotes reabsorption of water by action on renal tubular epithelium; *uses:* primary nocturnal enuresis, hemophilia A with Factor VIII levels of less than 5%, von Willebrand's disease, and neurogenic diabetes insipidus.

desmosomes. See **epithelium, desmosomes of.**

desonide, *trade names:* DesOwen, Tridesilon; *drug class:* topical corticosteroid, group IV low potency; *action:* possesses antipruritic, antiinflammatory actions; *uses:* psoriasis, eczema, contact dermatitis, pruritus.

desoximetasone, *trade names:* Topicort, Topicort LP; *drug class:* topical corticosteroid group II potency (0.25%), group III potency (0.05%); *action:* interacts with steroid cytoplasmic receptors to induce antiinflammatory effects; *uses:* psoriasis, eczema, contact dermatitis, pruritus.

detector, radiation. See **radiation detector.**

detention, restraint; custody; confinement.

detergent (deter'jənt), a cleanser. Also applied in a more specific sense to chemicals that possess surface-active properties in water and whose solutions are therefore able to wet surfaces that are normally water repellent and thereby assist in the mechanical dispersion and emulsification of fatty or oily material and other substances that soil the surface.

d., anionic, a detergent in which the cleansing action resides in the anion. Soaps and many synthetic detergents are anionic.

d., cationic, a detergent in which the cleansing action resides in the cation. Many such detergents are strong germicides (for example, those that contain quaternary ammonium compounds).

d., nonionic, a cleanser that acts by depressing the surface tension of water but does not ionize.

d., synthetic, a cleanser, other than soap, that exerts its effect by lowering the surface tension of an aqueous cleansing mixture.

detoxicate (dētok'sikāt). See **detoxify.**

detoxify (detoxicate), to remove the toxic quality of a substance.

deuterium, a stable isotope of the hydrogen atom, used as a tracer. Also called *heavy hydrogen.*

d. oxide, heavy water, so named because it formed from an isotope of hydrogen, which has twice the weight of ordinary hydrogen.

developed countries, countries with an economic base built largely on manufacturing and technology rather than agriculture. Although the need for medical and dental care may not differ from undeveloped to developed countries, the effective demand does vary. Developed countries have the available health professionals, the economic base to support the purchase of health care, and an informed public.

developer, a chemical solution that converts the invisible (latent) image on a film into a visible one composed of minute grains of metallic silver.

developing countries, countries in transition from an agrarian economy to a manufacturing- and technology-based economy.

developing, time-temperature method, the procedure of developing dental films; a solution of fixed temperature is used, and the films are immersed in the solution for a specific length of time.

developing, visual method, the procedure of developing dental films by placing the films in the developing solution and holding them from time to time before a safelight. Correct development has occurred when the film becomes so dark that it is difficult to distinguish between tooth and bone structure.

development, the process by which an individual reaches maturity.

d. of film. See **film, processing.**

developmental biology, the study of life processes occuring during growth and maturation.

developmental disabilities (DD), pathologic conditions that have their origin in the embryology and growth and development of an individual. DDs usually appear clinical before 18 years of age. The limitations of physiologic or mental function usually persist throughout life.

deviation (dē′vē-ā′shən), turning from a regular course; deflection.

devital tooth. See **tooth, pulpless.** (not current)

dexamethasone/dexamethasone sodium phosphate, *trade name:* Decaderm; *drug class:* synthetic topical corticosteroid; *action:* interacts with steroid cytoplasmic receptors to induce antiinflammatory effects; *uses:* corticosteroid-responsive dermatoses; oral ulcerative inflammatory lesions.

dexamethasone/dexamethasone acetate/dexamethasone sodium phosphate, *trade names:* Decadron, Hexadrol, Oradexan; *drug class:* glucocorticoid, long-acting; *action:* decreases inflammation by suppression of macrophage and leukocyte migration, reduces capillary permeability; *uses:* inflammation, allergies, neoplasm, cerebral edema, shock, collagen disorders.

dexchlorpheniramine maleate, *trade names:* Dexchlor, Poladex TD; *drug class:* antihistamine; *action:* acts on blood vessels, gastrointestinal system, respiratory system by competing with histamine for H_1-receptor site; decreases allergic response by blocking histamine; *uses:* allergy symptoms, rhinitis, pruritus, contact dermatitis.

dextran (dek′stran) ($C_6H_{12}O_6$ l b_2 H_2O), a water-soluble polymer of glucose of high molecular weight. A purified form, having an average molecular weight of 75,000, dextran is used in 6% concentration in isotonic sodium chloride solution to expand plasma volume and maintain blood pressure in emergency treatment of hemorrhagic and traumatic shock.

dextro-, the prefix designating that an aqueous solution of a substance rotates the plane of polarized light to the right. See also **isomers, optical.**

dextroamphetamine sulfate, *trade names:* Dexedrine, Oxydress II; *drug class:* amphetamine Controlled Substance Schedule II; *action:* increases release of norepinephrine, dopamine in cerebral cortex to reticular activating system; *uses:* narcolepsy, attention deficit disorder with hyperactivity.

dextromethorphan hydrobromide, *trade names:* Benylin DM, Robitussin Pediatric, Vicks Formula 44; *drug class:* antitussive, nonnarcotic; *action:* depresses cough center in medulla; *use:* nonproductive cough.

dextrorotatory (dek′strōrō′tətor′ē), turning the plane of polarization, or rays of polarized light, to the right.

dextrose (dek′strōs), dextrorotatory glucose, a monosaccharide occurring as a white, crystalline powder; colorless and sweet.

diabetes (dī-əbē′tēz), a deficiency condition involving carbohydrate metabolism and characterized by the habitual discharge of an excessive amount of urine.

d., bronzed, the combination of hemochromatosis and diabetes mellitus. The skin takes on a bronzed appearance as a result of the deposition of an iron-containing pigment in the skin.

d., gestational, the term describing patients who acquire glucose intolerance when pregnant.

d. insipidus, **1.** a metabolic disturbance characterized by marked urinary excretion and great thirst but no elevation of sugar in the blood or urine. **2.** a pituitary dysfunction char-

Nutritional principles
in type I diabetes

1. Develop a basic daily meal plan that is relatively consistent in terms of:
   Total energy (calorie) intake
   Balance of energy-yielding nutrients (carbohydrates, fats, and proteins)
2. Provide for compensatory changes for nonbasal circumstances:
   Extra food for extra activity
   Extra insulin or activity for extra food
3. Avoid hyperglycemia by:
   Omitting rapidly absorbed simple sugars from regular meal planning
4. Avoid hypoglycemia by:
   Reasonably consistent meal timing
   Provision of snacks

From Skyler JS: Dietary planning in insulin-dependent diabetes mellitus, *Pediatr Ann* 12:652-657, 1983.

acterized by an insufficient output of the antidiuretic hormone and leading to polyuria and polydipsia.

d., juvenile, diabetes mellitus occurring in children and adolescents, usually of a more severe and rampant nature than diabetes mellitus in adults, with consequent difficulty of regulation.

d. mellitus, a metabolic disorder, caused primarily by a defect in the production of insulin by the islet cells of the pancreas, with resultant inability to use carbohydrates. Characterized by hyperglycemia, glycosuria, polyuria, hyperlipemia (caused by imperfect catabolism of fats), acidosis, ketonuria, and a lowered resistance to infection. Periodontal manifestations may include recurrent and multiple periodontal abscesses, osteoporotic changes in alveolar bone, fungating masses of granulation tissue protruding from periodontal pockets, a lowered resistance to infection, and delay in healing after periodontal therapy.

d. mellitus, insulin-dependent (IDDM), a Type I diabetes that includes patients requiring the administration of insulin to prevent ketosis. Previously called *juvenile-onset diabetes, brittle diabetes,* and *ketosis-prone diabetes.*

d. mellitus, non-insulin-dependent (NIDDM), a Type II diabetes that includes patients who can maintain proper blood sugar levels within the administration of insulin. Previously called *maturity-onset diabetes, adult-onset diabetes, ketosis-resistant diabetes,* and *stable diabetes.*

d., phlorizin, a condition of glycosuria caused by inhibition of phosphorylation of phlorizin. It is not related to an endocrine disturbance.

diabetic ketoacidosis (DKA), diabetic coma, an acute, life-threatening complication of uncontrolled diabetes mellitus in which urinary loss of water, potassium, ammonium, and sodium results in hypovolemia, electrolyte imbalance, extremely high blood glucose levels, and the breakdown of free fatty acids causing acidosis.

diadochokinesia (dī·ad'əkōkīnē'zə), the act or process of repeating at maximum speed a simple cyclical, reciprocating movement such as raising and lowering of the mandible or protrusion and retraction of the tongue.

diagnosis, the translation of data gathered by clinical and radiographic examination into an organized, classified definition of the conditions present.

d., clinical, the determination of the specific disease or diseases involved in producing symptoms and signs by examination of the patient and use of analogy.

d., differential, the process of identifying a condition by differentiating all pathologic processes that may produce similar lesions.

d., final, the diagnosis arrived at after all the data have been collected, analyzed, and subjected to logical thought. Treatment may be necessary in some instances before the final diagnosis is made.

d., laboratory, a diagnosis made from chemical, microscopic, microbiologic, immunologic, or pathologic study of secretions, discharges, blood, or tissue sections.

d., oral, the identification of the cause of a dental disease or abnormality.

d., radiographic, a limited term used to indicate those radiologic interpretations that cannot be verified or disproved by clinical examination.

d.-related group (DRG), a system of classifying hospital patients on the basis of diagnosis consisting of distinct groupings. A DRG assignment to a case is based on the patient's principal diagnosis, treatment procedures performed, age, gender, and discharge status.

Classification and characteristics of diabetes mellitus

Name	Previous synonyms	Characteristics
Type I: Insulin-dependent diabetes mellitus (IDDM)	Juvenile diabetes Juvenile-onset diabetes Ketosis-prone diabetes Brittle diabetes Idiopathic diabetes	Abrupt onset of symptoms Individual prone to ketoacidosis Insulin dependent Viral etiology, autoimmune basis, genetic importance being investigated Often affects young children Decrease in size and number of islet cells
Type II: Non-insulin-dependent diabetes mellitus (NIDDM)	Adult-onset diabetes Maturity-onset diabetes Stable diabetes Ketosis-resistant diabetes	Usually not insulin dependent Individual not ketosis prone (but individual may form ketones under stress) Several syndromes, both nonobese and obese Generally occurs in those over the age of 40 Strong familial pattern being investigated
Secondary diabetes	Same	Cause established or strongly suspected May be associated with pancreatic disease, hormonal diseases, drugs and chemical agents, genetic syndromes, or malnutrition
Impaired glucose tolerance (IGT)	Asymptomatic diabetes Chemical diabetes Borderline diabetes Subclinical diabetes Latent diabetes	Show abnormal response to oral glucose tolerance test May revert to normal, remain impaired, or progress to diabetes Many with IGT are obese
Gestational diabetes mellitus (GDM)	Same	Glucose intolerance first recognized during pregnancy Following pregnancy, glucose may normalize, remain impaired, or progress to diabetes mellitus
Statistical risk class: • Previously abnormal glucose level • Potential abnormal glucose tolerance	Latent diabetes Prediabetes Potential diabetes	Previous abnormality of oral glucose tolerance test or increased risk of developing diabetes because of genetic relationship with a diabetic

From McCance KL, Huether SE: *Pathophysiology: the biological basis for disease in adults and children*, St Louis, 1990, Mosby.

d., surgical, a surgical incision into a body part or the excision of a lesion for the purpose of determining the cause or nature of an illness.

diagnostic cast. See **cast, diagnostic.**

diagnostic equilibration, a measuring method of determining and recording on dentodes the amount and direction that interfering cusps deflect the closure direction of the mandible, as can be seen in mountings. (not current)

diagnostic error, a mistake in judgment regarding the cause of an illness.

diagnostic imaging, the use of radiographic, sonographic, and other technologies to create a graphic depiction of the body part(s) in question.

diagnostic services, those imaging and laboratory capabilities available for determining the cause of an illness.

dialysis (dī·al′isis), a type of filtration used to separate smaller molecules from larger ones contained in a solution. The molecular solution is placed on one side of a semipermeable membrane and water on the other side. The smaller molecules pass through the membrane into the water; the larger molecules are retained in the solution.

diamond, a crystalline carbon substance, the hardest natural substance known, used industrially and in dentistry for cutting and grinding.

diaphragm (dī′·əfram), **1.** a musculotendinous partition that separates the thorax and abdomen. **2.** a metal barrier plate, often of lead, pierced with a central aperture so arranged as to limit the emerging, or useful, beam of roentgen rays to the smallest practical diameter for making radiographic exposures. See also **collimation; collimator; distance, cone, long;** and **source-collimator distance.**

D

d., Potter-Bucky. See **grid, Potter-Bucky.**

diaphysis (dī·əfī'sis), the shaft of a long bone.

diarrhea, the frequent passage of loose, watery stools. The stool may also contain mucus, pus, blood, or excessive amounts of fat. Diarrhea is usually a symptom of some underlying disorder.

diarthrosis (dī'·arthrō'sis), a freely movable joint enclosed in a fluid-filled cavity and limited variously by muscles, ligaments, and bone. (not current)

diastema (dī'·əstē'mə), an abnormal space between two adjacent teeth in the same dental arch.

diastole (dī·as'təlē), **1.** the rhythmic period of relaxation and dilation of a chamber of the heart during which it fills with blood. **2.** the period after the contraction of the heart muscle, during which the aorta releases the potential energy stored in its elastic tissue. The energy is converted into kinetic energy and sustains the pressure necessary for steady flow of blood in the vessels. The pressure measured at this period is the lowest attained during the cardiac pumping cycle and is called the *diastolic pressure.* The normal pressure in the adult is approximately 120/80 mm Hg (systolic/diastolic) and increases with age from 128/85 at 45 years of age to 135/89 at 60 years of age.

diathermy (dī'·əther'mē), a generalized rise in tissue temperature produced by a high-frequency alternating current between two electrodes. The temperature rise is produced without causing tissue damage.

diathesis (dī·əth'ēsis), a tendency, based on body makeup; constitutional, hereditary, or acquired states of the body that cause a predisposition or susceptibility to diseases.

d., hemorrhagic, a condition that may be caused by defects in the coagulation mechanism, blood vessel wall, or both.

diazepam, *trade name:* Valium; *drug class:* benzodiazepine, anxiolytic Controlled Substance Schedule IV; *action:* produces CNS depression by acting on parts of the limbic system and the thalamus and hypothalamus, inducing a calming effect; *uses:* management of short-term anxiety disor-

ders and relief of symptoms of anxiety, short-term relief of skeletal muscle spasm, acute alcohol withdrawal.

Dick's test. See **test, Dick's.** (not current)

diclofenac, *trade names:* Cataflam, Voltaren; *drug class:* nonsteroidal antiinflammatory; *action:* inhibits prostaglandin synthesis; *uses:* acute and chronic rheumatoid arthritis, osteoarthritis, ankylosing spondylitis.

dicloxacillin sodium, *trade names:* Dycill, Dynapen, Pathocil; *drug class:* penicillinase-resistant penicillin; *action:* interferes with cell wall replication of susceptible organisms; *uses:* infections caused by penicillinase-producing *Staphylococcus.*

dicyclomine HCl, *trade names:* Antispas, Dibent; *drug class:* GI anticholinergic; *action:* inhibits muscarinic actions of acetylcholine at postganglionic parasympathetic neuroeffector sites; *uses:* peptic ulcer disease in combination with other drugs; infant colic.

didanosine, *trade name:* Videx; *drug class:* synthetic antiviral; *action:* converted by cellular enzymes that act as antimetabolite to inhibit HIV replication; *uses:* advanced HIV infections in adults and children who have been unable to use zidovudine or who have not responded to treatment with zidovudine.

dideoxycytidine, a dideoxynucleoside under study as an antiviral in the treatment of AIDS.

dideoxyinosine, a dideoxynucleoside under study as an antiviral in the treatment of AIDS. See also **didanosine.**

die, the positive reproduction of the form of a prepared tooth in any suitable hard substance, usually in metal or specially prepared (improved) artificial stone.

d. lubricant, a material applied to a die to serve as a separating medium so that the wax pattern will not adhere to the die but may be withdrawn from it without sticking.

d., stone, a positive likeness in artificial (dental) stone; used in the fabrication of a dental restoration.

d., waxing, a mold into which wax is forced for the production of standardized wax patterns.

dienestrol, *trade name:* Ortho Dienestrol; *drug class:* nonsteroidal synthetic estrogen; *action:* needed for adequate functioning of female reproductive system; affects release of pituitary gonadotropins, inhibits ovulation; *uses:* atrophic vaginitis, kraurosis vulvae.

diet, the food and drink consumed by a given person from day to day. Not all the diet is necessarily used by the body. For this reason, diet and nutrition must be differentiated.

d., alkaline, a diet that is basic in reaction; produced by the addition of alkaline salts, including sodium bicarbonate.

d., cariogenic, the intake of food that is heavy in refined carbohydrates and other food stuffs that support the growth of caries-producing bacteria.

d., lysine-poor, a diet deficient in lysine, an essential amino acid. All the essential amino acids must be present in the diet; should one or more be absent, proper use of the others cannot occur. Periodontal changes described in experimental animals with lysine deficiency include osteoporosis of supporting bone and disintegration and failure of replacement of periodontal fibers.

dietary analysis. See **analysis, dietary.**

dietary carbohydrates, the amount of simple and complex sugars consumed; the physical character of the diet. It may tend to produce or modify periodontal disease.

dietary fiber, a generic term for nodigestible chemical substances found in plant cell walls. Foods high in dietary fiber are fruits, green leafy vegetables, root vegetables, and whole grain cereals and bread.

dietetics, the science of applying nutritional principles to the planning and preparation of foods and the regulation of the diet in relation to both health and disease.

diethylpropion HCl, *trade names:* Tenuate Dospan, Ten-Tab; *drug class:* anorexant, amphetamine-like analog Controlled Substance Schedule IV; *action:* exact mechanism of appetite suppression is unknown, may have an effect on the satiety center of the hypothalamus; *use:* exogenous obesity.

diethylstilbestrol (dīeth'ilstilbes'trol), an estrogenic substance, $C_{18}H_{20}O_2$, that has an estrogenic activity considered to be greater than that of estrone. Useful in treating menopausal symp-

toms and occasionally used in the therapy of chronic desquamative gingivitis associated with artificial or natural menopause.

difenoxin HCl with atropine sulfate, *trade name:* Motofen; *drug class:* antidiarrheal Controlled Substance Schedule IV; *action:* inhibits gastric motility by acting on mucosal receptors responsible for peristalsis; *uses:* acute nonspecific and acute exacerbations of chronic functional diarrhea.

differential force, a term sometimes used to describe the design and application of an orthodontic appliance to distribute the reciprocal forces of the appliance over significantly different root areas with the objective of eliciting a differential response.

difficult eruption. See **teething.** (not current)

diffusibility (difyo͞oz'ibil'itē), capable of being diffused.

diffusion (difyo͞o'zhən), a property of ions or molecules of a solute that permits them to pass through a membrane or to intermingle by rapid or gradual permeation with the molecules of a solvent.

diflorasone diacetate, *trade names:* Florone, Maxiflor, Psorcon; *drug class:* topical corticosteroid group II high potency; *action:* possesses antipruritic, antiinflammatory actions; *uses:* psoriasis, eczema, contact dermatitis, pruritus.

diflunisal, *trade name:* Dolobid; *drug class:* salicylate derivative, nonsteroidal antiinflammatory; *action:* inhibits prostaglandin synthesis; *uses:* mild-to-moderate pain, symptoms of rheumatoid arthritis and osteoarthritis.

digestion, the conversion of food into absorbable substances in the GI tract.

digit, a single symbol or character representing a quantity.

d. sucking, an oral habit, usually referred to as *finger* or *thumb sucking,* that is not unusual in preschool children. Prolonged, persistent, or vigorous sucking into the transition dentition period can cause tooth displacement malocclusions.

digitalization (dij'italizā'shən), the administration of digitalis in sufficient amount by any of several types of dosage schedules to build up the concentration of digitalis glycosides in the body of a patient.

digitoxin, *trade names:* Crystodigin, Digitaline; *drug class:* cardia glycoside; *action:* inhibits the sodium-potassium ATPase, which makes more calcium available for contractile proteins; *uses:* congestive heart failure (CHF), atrial fibrillation, paroxysmal atrial flutter, atrial tachycardia.

digoxin, *trade names:* Lanoxicaps, lanoxin, Novadigoxin; *drug class:* cardiac glycoside; *action:* acts by inhibiting the sodium-potassium ATPase, which makes more calcium available for contractile proteins; *uses:* CHF, atrial fibrillation, atrial flutter, paroxysmal atrial tachycardia.

dihydrotachysterol (DHT), *trade names:* DHT Intensol, Hytakerol; *drug class:* vitamin D analog; *action:* increases intestinal absorption of calcium, increases renal tubular absorption of phosphate; *uses:* nutritional supplement, rickets, hypoparathyroidism, postoperative tetany.

dihydroxyaluminum sodium carbonate, *trade name:* Rolaids; *drug class:* antacid; *action:* neutralizes gastric acidity; *use:* antacid

dilaceration (dĭlas'er ā'shən), a severe angular distortion in the root of a tooth or at the junction of the root and crown. Dilaceration results from trauma during tooth development.

Dilantin enlargement. See **hyperplasia, gingival, Dilantin.**

Dilantin gingival hyperplasia. See **hyperplasia, gingival, Dilantin.**

Dilantin sodium (dĭlan'tin sō'dēəm), the trade name for diphenylhydantoin sodium.

dilation (dĭlā'shən), the act of stretching or dilating.

diltiazem HCl, *trade names:* Cardizem, Cardizem SR, Cardizem CD; *drug class:* calcium channel blocker; *action:* inhibits calcium ion influx across cell membrane during cardiac depolarization; produces relaxation of coronary vascular smooth muscle, dilates coronary arteries, slows SA/AV node conduction; *uses:* chronic stable angina pectoris, coronary artery spasm, hypertension.

diluent (dil'yōō ənt, dil'yōō ənt), an agent that dilutes the strength of a solution or mixture; medication that dilutes any one of the body fluids.

dilute (dĭlōōt', dīlōōt), to make weaker the strength of a solution or mixture.

dimenhydrinate, *trade names:* Calm-X, Dimentabs, Dinate, Dramamine; *drug class:* H_1-receptor antagonist; *actions:* acts on blood vessels and gastrointestinal and respiratory systems by competing with histamine for H_1-receptor site; decreases allergic response by blocking histamine; *uses:* motion sickness, nausea, vomiting.

dimension, vertical, l. a vertical measurement of the face between any two arbitrarily selected points that are conveniently located one above and one below the mouth, usually in the midline. **2.** the vertical height of the face with the teeth in occlusion or acting as stops. See also **relation, vertical.**

   d., v., decrease, a decrease of the vertical distance between the mandible and the maxillae by modifications of teeth or of the positions of teeth or occlusion rims, or through alveolar or residual ridge resorption.

   d., v., increase, an increase of the vertical distance between the mandible and the maxillae by modifications of teeth and the positions of teeth or occlusion rims.

   d., v., occlusal, the vertical dimension of the face when the teeth or occlusion rims are in contact in centric occlusion.

   d., v., rest, the vertical dimension of the face with the jaws in the rest relation.

   d., v., rest, decrease, may or may not accompany a decrease in occlusal vertical dimension. It may occur without a decrease in occlusal vertical dimension in patients with a preponderant activity of the jaw-closing musculature, as in chronic gum chewers or patients with muscular hypertension.

   d., v., rest, increase, may or may not accompany an increase in occlusal dimension. It sometimes occurs after the removal of remaining occlusal contacts, perhaps as a result of the removal of noxious reflex stimuli.

dimensional stability. See **stability, dimensional.**

dimethylbenzene (dīmeth'ilben'zēn). See **xylene.**

dimethyl sulfoxide, an antiinflammatory agent and organic solvent.

Dimitri's disease (demē′trēz) (not current). See **disease, Sturge-Weber-Dimitri.**

diphenhydramine HCl, *trade names:* Benadryl, Sominex Formula 3; *drug class:* antihistamine H_1-receptor antagonist; *action:* acts on blood vessels and gastrointestinal and respiratory systems by competing with histamine for H_1-receptor site; decreases allergic response by blocking histamine; *uses:* allergy symptoms, rhinitis, motion sickness, antiparkinsonism, nighttime sedation, infant colic, nonproductive cough.

diphenoxylate HCl with atropine sulfate, *trade names:* Lofrol, Logen, Lomotil, Lonox; *drug class:* antidiarrheal (opioid with atropine) Controlled Substance Schedule V; *action:* inhibits gastric motility by acting on muscosal receptors responsible for peristalsis; *use:* simple diarrhea.

diphenylhydantoin sodium (dī′fen′ ilhī′dan′tōin) (Dilantin sodium), a drug used for the control of convulsive grand mal and petit mal epileptic seizures; often associated with the production of a profuse gingival hyperplasia. (not current)

diphtheria (difthir′ē·ə), an acute disease caused by *Corynebacterium diphtheriae* and resulting in swelling of the pharynx and larynx with fever.

dipivefrin HCl, *trade name:* Propine; *drug class:* adrenergic agonist; *action:* converted to epinephrine with decreases aqueous production and increases outflow; *use:* open-angle glaucoma.

diplomate, a dental specialist who has achieved certification by the recognized certification board in that specialty, as attested by a diploma from the board.

diplopia (diplō′pē·ə), seeing a single object as two images. May occur after fracture of the bony orbital cavity as a result of displacement of the globe of the eye inferiorly.

dipyridamole, *trade name:* Persantine; *drug class:* platelet aggregation inhibitor; *action:* specific action unclear, inhibits ability of platelets to aggregate; *uses:* prevention of transient ischemic attacks (TIA), inhibition of platelet aggregation to prevent myocardial reinfarction, prevention of

coronary bypass graft occlusion with aspirin.

dipyrone, an analgesic, antiinflammatory, and antipyretic agent rarely used because of a high incidence of agranulocytosis.

direct (dīrekt′), relating to any restorative procedure performed directly on a tooth without the use of a die (for example, a wax pattern formed in the prepared cavity), silver amalgam, or one of the powdered, granular, or foil golds compacted into a prepared cavity.

d. **access storage device,** a device used for storage of direct access files. It could be magnetic disk or diskette units.

d. **billing,** a process whereby the dentist bills a patient directly for his or her fees.

d. **gold,** any of the forms of pure gold that may be compacted directly into a prepared cavity to form a restoration.

d. **pulp capping.** See **capping, pulp, direct.**

d. **reimbursement,** a self-funded program in which the individual is reimbursed based on a percentage of dollars spent for dental care provided, and which allows beneficiaries to seek treatment from the dentist of their choice.

d. **retainer.** See **retainer, direct.**

d. **retention.** See **retention, direct.**

director, a person elected by shareholders at the annual meeting to establish company policies. The directors appoint the president, vice presidents, and all other operating officers. Directors decide, among other matters, if and when dividends shall be paid.

directory, an organized list of names, organizations, or other data bases for ease of retrieval or reference currently used to describe the listing of files in a computer storage system.

dirithromycin, *trade name:* Dynabac; *drug class:* macrolide antibiotic; *action:* binds to 50S ribosomal subunits of susceptible bacteria to inhibit bacterial growth; *uses:* treatment of secondary bacterial infection of acute bronchitis, community-acquired pneumonia, streptococcal pharyngitis, and uncomplicated skin and skin structure infections.

disability, I. the lack of legal qualification to do a thing; legal incompetency.

2. the inability to function in the normal or usual manner; examples of an outcome measure are days missing from work or lessened productivity.

d., denial of, a symptom in which patients deny the existence of a disease or disability. A patient who is edentulous may insist he eats better, looks better, and speaks better than if he had teeth. Another may insist that filthy, carious, periodontally involved teeth are beautiful and healthy and enhance his appearance. Denial by these patients is a nonrealistic attempt to maintain their predisease status. These patients regard ill health and disability as an imperfection, a weakness, and even a disgrace.

disaccharide, a general term for simple carbohydrates (sugars) formed by the union of two monosaccharide molecules. Sucrose is the most common disaccharide sugar.

disarticulation (dis′artik′ūlā′shən), the amputation or separation of joint parts, as in hemimandibulectomy, with inclusion of the condyloid process of the mandible.

disc. See **disk.**

discharge, to release; liberate; annul; unburden. To cancel a contract; to make an agreement or contract null and void.

d. summary, the clinical notes written by the discharging physician or dentist at the time of releasing a patient from the hospital or clinic, outlining the course of treatment, the status at release, and the postdischarge expectations and instructions.

d., purulent. See **pus.**

disclosing solution, a material, usually some form of dye, applied to the teeth to stain bacterial and mucinous plaque on the tooth surface.

disclusion (disklōō′zhən), a separation of the occlusal surfaces of the teeth directly and simply by opening the jaws, or indirectly in excursions by the anterior teeth.

discoid (dis′koid), a carving instrument with a blade of circular form that has a cutting edge around the entire periphery.

discoloration, enamel. See **tetracycline.**

discoloration, gingival. See **gingival discoloration.** (not current)

discoplasty, the surgical shaping or

contouring of the meniscus of the temporomandibular joint.

discount, 1. an allowance or deduction made from a gross sum. **2.** the procedure of reducing the amount of a professional fee.

discrimination, legal, to treat unequally or unfairly on the basis of race, gender, national origin, religion, or handicap.

discrimination, tactile, the ability to perceive two simultaneous touch stimuli; two-point discrimination. When the distance between the two stimuli is diminished to the amount that only one stimulus is perceived, a value is determined for the two-point discrimination capacity of a special part. When patients are anesthetized by local agents, they have diminished tactile sense and frequently bite their lips rather severely without being aware of it. Thus patients should be instructed not to eat or chew until the "numbness" has completely gone and full tactile sense has returned.

disease(s) (dizēz′), a definite deviation from the normal state; characterized by a series of symptoms. Disease may be caused by developmental disturbances, genetic factors, metabolic factors, living agents, and physical, chemical, or radiant energy, or the cause may be unknown.

d., Adams-Stokes (Adams-Stokes syndrome), a disease characterized by a slow and perhaps irregular pulse, vertigo, syncope, occasional pseudoepileptic convulsions, and Cheyne-Stokes respiration.

d., adaptation (adaptation syndrome), metabolic disorders occurring as the result of adaptation or resistance to severe physical or psychologic stress. See also **syndrome, general adaptation.**

d., Addison's, chronic adrenocortical insufficiency caused by bilateral tuberculosis, aplasia, atrophy, or degeneration of the adrenal glands. Symptoms include severe weakness, weight loss, low blood pressure, digestive disturbances, hypoglycemia, lowered resistance to infection, and abnormal pigmentation (bronze color of the skin, with associated melanotic pigmentation of the oral mucous membranes, particularly of the gingival tissues).

d., adrenocortical, disorders of adrenocortical function, giving rise to Addison's disease, Cushing's syndrome, adrenogenital syndrome, and primary aldosteronism.

d., Albers-Schönberg. See **osteopetrosis.**

d., autoallergic. See **disease, autoimmune.**

d., autoimmune *(autoallergic disease, autoimmunization syndrome, chronic hypersensitivity disease),* any one of the diseases that are believed to be caused in part by reactions of hypersensitivity of the host tissue (antigens). Includes various hemolytic anemias, idiopathic thrombocytopenias, rheumatoid arthritis, systemic lupus erythematosus, glomerulonephritis, scleroderma, Hashimoto's thyroiditis, and Sjögren's syndrome.

d., Barlow's. See **scurvy, infantile.**

d., Basedow's. See **goiter, exophthalmic.**

d., Behçet's. See **syndrome,** Behçet's.

d., Besnier-Boeck-Schaumann. See **sarcoidosis.**

d., bleeder's. See **hemophilia.**

d., blood, a disease affecting the hematologic system (e.g., anemia, leukemia, agranulocytosis purpura, infectious mononucleosis). Such a disease often results in lesions of the oral structures, particularly of the mucosal surfaces.

d., Bowen's. See **carcinoma in situ.**

d., Brill-Symmers. See **lymphoblastoma, giant follicular.**

d., brittle bone. See **osteogenesis imperfecta.**

d., Caffey's. See **hyperostosis, infantile cortical.**

d., cardiac, a disease affecting the heart.

d., cat-scratch. See **fever, cat-scratch.**

d., Cheadle's. See **scurvy, infantile.**

d., Christmas. See **hemophilia B.**

d., chronic hypersensitivity. See **disease, autoimmune.**

d., collagen *(group disease, visceral angiitis),* collectively, a group of diseases affecting the collagenous connective tissue of several organs and systems. These diseases have in common similar biochemical structural alterations and include rheumatic fever, scleroderma, rheumatoid arthritis, systemic lupus erythematosus, periarteritis, and serum sickness.

d., combined system, pernicious anemia in which there is central nervous system damage associated with the hematologic findings.

d., communicable, any disease that may be transmitted directly or indirectly to a well person or animal from an infected person or animal. Any disease with the capacity for maintenance by natural modes of spread (for example, by contact, by airborne routes, through drinking water or food, by arthropod vectors).

d., congenital, any disease present at birth. More specifically, one that is acquired in utero.

d., Coxsackie A. See **herpangina.**

d., Crouzon's. See **dysostosis, craniofacial.**

d., Cushing's. See **syndrome, Cushing's.**

d., cytomegalic inclusion, generalized. See **disease, salivary gland.**

d., Darier's *(keratosis follicularis),* an apparently genetic dermatologic disease that also involves mucous membranes. The oral lesions are whitish papules of the gingiva, tongue, or palate. Darier's disease is characterized histologically by the presence of corps ronds.

d., deficiency, a disturbance produced by lack of nutritional or metabolic factors. Used chiefly in reference to avitaminosis.

d., degenerative joint. See **osteoarthritis.**

d., demyelinating, the diseases that have in common a loss of myelin sheath, with preservation of the axis cylinders (for example, multiple sclerosis, Schilder's disease).

d., dental, hereditary, heritable defects of the dentition without generalized disease include amelogenesis imperfecta, dentinogenesis imperfecta, dentinal dysplasia, localized and generalized hypoplasia of enamel, peg-shaped lateral incisors, familial dentigerous cysts, missing teeth, giantism, and fused primary mandibular incisors. Dental defects occurring with generalized disease include dentinogenesis imperfecta with osteogenesis imperfecta, missing teeth with ectodermal dysplasia, enamel hypoplasia with epidermolysis bullosa dystrophica, retarded eruption with cleidocranial dysostosis, missing lateral incisors with ptosis of the eyelids, missing premolars with premature whitening of the hair, and enamel hypoplasia in vitamin D-resistant rickets.

d., dermatologic, any one of the diseases affecting the skin; often accompanied by pathologic manifestations of various mucosal surfaces of the body (for example, the oral mucosa, genital mucosa, conjunctiva).

d., Engman's. See *Dermatitis infectiosa eczematoides.*

d., exanthematous, any one of a group of diseases caused by a number of viruses but having as a prominent feature a skin rash (for example, smallpox, chickenpox, cowpox, measles, rubella).

d., familial, a disease occurring in several members of the same family. Often used to mean members of the same generation and occasionally used synonymously with *hereditary disease*

d., Feer's. See **erythredema polyneuropathy** and **acrodynia.**

d., fibrocystic (mucoviscidosis), a hereditary defect of most of the exocrine glands in the body, including the salivary glands. The secretion of the affected mucous glands is abnormally viscous.

d., foot-and-mouth (aphthous fever, epidemic stomatitis, epizootic stomatitis), primarily a disease of animals caused by a filterable virus that may be transmitted to humans and that occasionally produces symptoms. The human form is characterized by fever, nausea, vomiting, malaise, and ulcerative stomatitis. Skin lesions consisting of vesicles may appear, usually on the palms of the hands and soles of the feet. Spontaneous regression usually occurs within 2 weeks.

d., Fordyce's. See **spots, Fordyce's.**

d., functional, a disease that has no observable or demonstrable cause.

d., Gaucher's, a constitutional defect in the metabolism of the cerebroside kerasin. This glycoprotein accumulates in the reticuloendothelial system and leads to splenomegaly, hepatomegaly, lymph node enlargement, and bone defects.

d., Graves'. See **goiter, exophthalmic.**

d., group. See **disease, collagen.**

d., Hand-Schüller-Christian (chronic disseminated histiocytosis X), a type of cholesterol lipoidosis characterized clinically by defects in membranous bones, exophthalmos, and diabetes insipidus.

d., Hansen's. See **leprosy.**

d., heart, any abnormal condition of the heart (organic, mechanical, or functional) that causes difficulty.

   d., h., arteriosclerotic, a variety of functional changes of the myocardium that result from arteriosclerosis.

   d., h., congenital, a defective formation of the heart or of the major vessels of the heart.

   d., h., rheumatic, scarring of the endocardium resulting from involvement in acute rheumatic fever. The process most often involves the mitral valve.

   d., h., thyrotoxic, cardiac failure occurring as the result of hyperthyroidism or its superimposition on existing organic heart disease. Thyrotoxicosis is an important cause of auricular fibrillation.

d., hemoglobin C, a disease resulting from an abnormal hemoglobin (hemoglobin C); occurs primarily in African Americans and causes a mild normochromic anemia, target cells, and vague, intermittent arthralgia.

d., hemolytic, of newborn, hemolysis caused by isoimmune reactions associated with Rh incompatibility or with blood transfusions in which there is an incompatibility of the ABO blood system. Several forms of the disease occur: erythroblastosis fetalis, congenital hemolytic disease, icterus gravis neonatorum, and hydrops fetalis.

d., hemophilioid, hemophilic states (conditions) that clinically resemble hemophilia (for example, parahemophila, hemophilia B [Christmas disease]).

d., hemorrhagic, of newborn, a hemorrhagic tendency in newborn infants occurring usually on the third or fourth day of life; believed to be caused by defects of prothrombin and factor VII, resulting from a deficiency of vitamin K.

d., hereditary, a disease transmitted from parent to offspring through genes. Three main types of mendelian heredity are recognized: dominant, recessive, and sex linked.

d., hidebound. See **scleroderma.**

d., Hodgkin's, a generally fatal lymphomatous disorder of unknown etiol-

D

ogy that has neoplastic and granulomatous characteristics. Chiefly involves the lymph nodes, but sometimes the spleen, liver, bone marrow, and other organs are involved. Three variants include Hodgkin's paragranuloma, Hodgkin's granuloma (classical or common type), and Hodgkin's sarcoma. All have in common the presence of Sternberg-Reed, or Dorothy Reed, cells and lymph node enlargement. Cervical lymph nodes are often the first to be affected. See also **cell, Sternberg-Reed.**

d., hypersensitivity. See **disease, autoimmune.**

d., iatrogenic, a disease arising as a result of the actions or words of a physician or dentist (for example, an obsession of having heart disease or bruxism as a result of a misunderstanding on the part of a patient).

d., idiopathic (id'ē-ōpath'ik), a disease in which the cause is not recognized or determined.

d., infectious, pathologic alterations induced in the tissues by the action of microorganisms and/or their toxins. Some of the infectious diseases involving the oral tissues are herpes zoster, herpetic gingivostomatitis, moniliasis, syphilis, and tuberculosis.

d., kissing. See **mononucleosis, infectious.**

d., Letterer-Siwe (se'veh) (acute disseminated histiocytosis X, nonlipid histiocytosis, nonlipid reticuloendotheliosis), a fatal febrile disease of unknown cause occurring in infants and children; characterized by focal granulomatous lesions of the lymph nodes, spleen, and bone marrow. Results in enlargement of the lymph nodes, spleen, and liver, defects of the flat and long bones, anemia, and sometimes purpura.

d., lipoid storage *(lipoidosis, reticuloendothelial granuloma),* any one of a group of diseases in which lipid substances accumulate in the fixed cells of the reticuloendothelial system. Included are Gaucher's disease, Niemann-Pick disease, and the Hand-Schüller-Christian complex. Other storage diseases include lipochondrodystrophy (gargoylism) and cerebral sphingolipidosis.

d., Lobstein's. See **osteogenesis imperfecta.**

d., Marie's. See **acromegaly.**

d., Mediterranean. See **thalassemia major.**

d., Mikulicz' (mik'yōōlich'ez), a benign hyperplasia of the lymph nodes of the parotid or other salivary glands and/or the lacrimal glands.

d., Moeller's. See **scurvy, infantile.**

d., molecule, a disease associated with genetically determined abnormalities of protein synthesis at the molecular level.

d., muscle, pathologic muscle tissue changes. Such changes reveal few structural alterations, and the highly differentiated contents of muscle fibers tend to react as a whole. The pathologic features that distinguish one muscle disease from another are the age and character of changes within a muscle, distribution of those changes within one or several muscles, presence of inflammatory cells and parasites, and coexistence of pathologic changes in other organs. Muscles undergo a number of degenerative changes. There are alterations in the striation in certain pathologic states, caused by cloudy swelling, granular degeneration, waxy or hyaline degeneration, and other cellular modifications, such as multiplication of the sarcolemmic nuclei and phagocytosis of muscle fibers.

d., neuromuscular, a condition in which various areas of the central nervous system are affected; results in dysfunction or degeneration of the musculature and disabilities of the organ.

d., Niemann-Pick (nē'man), a congenital, familial disorder occurring chiefly in Jewish female infants, terminating fatally before the third year, and characterized by the accumulation of the phospholipid sphingomyelin in the cells of the reticuloendothelial system.

d., oral, hereditary, heritable defects of oral and paraoral structures (excluding the dentition) without generalized defects; includes ankyloglossia, hereditary gingivofibromatosis, and possible cleft lip and cleft palate. Many oral and paraoral defects are associated with generalized defects (for example, Peutz-Jeghers, Franceschetti, Ehlers-Danlos, Pierre Robin, and Sturge-Weber syndromes; hemorrhagic telangiectasia; Crouzon's disease; sickle cell disease; acatalasemia; white spongy nevus; xeroderma pigmentosum; gargoylism; neurofibromatosis; familial amyloidosis; and achondroplasia).

d., oral manifestations of systemic, the lesions occurring within the stomatologic system in association with systemic diseases, often influenced by the local environmental factors within the oral cavity.

d., organic, a disease in which actual structural changes have occurred in the organs or tissues.

d., Osler's. See **erythremia.**

d., Owren's. See **parahemophilia.**

d., Paget's. See **osteitis deformans.**

d., periodic. See **disorders, periodic.**

d., periodontal, any disturbance of the periodontium or supporting structures of the teeth. Diseases affecting the periodontium include periodontitis, periodontosis, gingivitis, gingival enlargement, atrophy, and traumatism and may be loosely divided into two types: inflammatory and dystrophic. Etiologic factors may be local or systemic or may involve an interplay between the two.

  d., p., etiologic factors of, the local and systemic factors, singly or in combination, that initiate periodontal lesions.

  d., p., local factors of, the environmental conditions within the oral cavity that initiate, perpetuate, or alter the course of diseases of the periodontium (for example, calculus, diastemata between teeth, food impaction, prematurities in the centric path of closure, and tongue habits).

d., peripheral vascular, a disease of arteries, veins, and/or lymphatic vessels.

d., pink. See **acrodynia.**

d., Pott's, a spinal curvature (kyphosis) resulting from tuberculosis.

d. progression, the course of the disease within a patient/host from onset to resolution.

d., psychosomatic, a disease that appears to have been precipitated or prolonged by emotional stress; manifested largely through the autonomic nervous system. Various conditions may be included (for example, certain forms of asthma, dermatoses, migraine headache, hypertension, peptic ulcer, rheumatoid arthritis, and ulcerative colitis). Occlusal trauma associ-

ated with bruxism is often considered to be a disease of this type. See also **disorder, psychophysiologic, autonomic,** and **visceral.**

d., Quincke's. See **edema, angioneurotic.**

d., Recklinghausen's (von Recklinghausen's disease). See **hyperparathyroidism; osteitis; generalized fibrosa cystica;** and **neurofibromatosis.**

d., Rendu-Osler-Weber (ron'dōō). See **telangiectasia, hereditary hemorrhagic.**

d., rheumatic. See **rheumatism.**

d., rickettsial, a disease caused by microorganisms of the order Rickettsiales (for example, Rocky Mountain spotted fever, rickettsialpox, typhus, and Q fever).

d., Riga-Fede (re'gə-fā'də), an ulceration of the lingual frenum of infants caused by abrasion by natal or neonatal teeth.

d., Sainton's. See **dysostosis, cleidocranial.**

d., salivary gland (generalized cytomegalic inclusion), a generalized infection in infants caused by intrauterine or postnatal infection with a cytomegalovirus of the group of herpesviruses. Manifestations include jaundice, purpura, hemolytic anemia, vomiting, diarrhea, chronic eczema, and failure to gain weight.

d., Schuller's (shYl'erz). See **osteoporosis.**

d., Selter's. See **acrodynia.**

d., sex-linked, a hereditary disorder transmitted by the gene that also determines sex (for example, hemophilia).

d., sickle cell, a hematologic disorder caused by the presence of an abnormal hemoglobin (hemoglobin S) that permits the formation or results in the formation of sickle-shaped red blood cells. Two forms of the disease occur: sickle cell trait and sickle cell anemia. See also **anemia, sickle cell; trait, sickle cell.**

d., Simmonds' (pituitary cachexia, hypophyseal cachexia, hypopituitary cachexia), Panhypopituitarism resulting from destruction of the pituitary gland, usually from hemorrhage or infarction.

d., students'. See **mononucleosis, infectious.**

d., Sturge-Weber-Dimitri (encephalotrigeminal angiomatosis), a congenital condition characterized by venous angioma of the meninges and cerebral cortex and ipsilateral angiomatous lesions of the face and jaws.

d., subclinical, a latent, incipient, or mild form of a disease that does not produce known, clinically detectable manifestations. Abuse of the term occurs by including diseases deduced to be present only on the basis of borderline laboratory values.

d. susceptibility, the degree to which a patient and/or host is vulnerable to a disease.

d., Sutton's. See **periadenitis mucosa necrotica recurrens.**

d., Swift's. See **acrodynia.**

d., systemic, any disease involving the whole body.

d., Takahara's (ta′kəhar′əz), a form of rare progressive oral gangrene occurring in childhood and seen only in Japan. Apparently related to a congenital lack of enzyme catalase (acatalasemia). Characterized by a mild to severe form of a peculiar type of oral gangrene that may develop at the roots of the teeth or the tonsils. Loss of teeth occurs, with necrosis of the alveolar bone. Patients become symptom free after puberty.

d., transmissible, any disease capable of being transmitted from one individual to another; any disease capable of being maintained in successive passages through a susceptible host, usually under experimental conditions such as by injection. See also **disease, communicable.**

d. transmission, the method by which a disease is passed from one patient or host to another. The three most common methods of transmission are direct contact, aerosols, and vectors, such as insects.

d., Vaquez' (väkäz′). See **erythremia.**

d. vectors, intermediary hosts that carry the disease from one species to another, such as mosquitoes, ticks, and rabid animals.

d., von Recklinghausen's, of bone. See **hyperparathyroidism; osteitis fibrosa cystica, generalized.**

d., von Recklinghausen's, of skin. See **neurofibromatosis.**

d., Weil's (vilz) (epidemic jaundice), an acute febrile disease caused by *Leptospira icterohaemorrhagiae* or *L. canicola.* Manifestations include fever, petechial hemorrhage, myalgia, renal insufficiency, hepatic failure, and jaundice.

d., Werlhof's (verl′hofs). See **purpura, thrombocytopenic.**

disharmony, occlusal, a phenomenon in which contacts of opposing occlusal surfaces of teeth are not in harmony with other tooth contacts and with the anatomic and physiologic controls of the mandible. See also **contact, deflective occlusal; contact, interceptive occlusal;** and **malocclusion.**

disinfect (dis′infekt′), to destroy pathogenic microorganisms.

disinfectant (dis′infek′tənt), a chemical especially for use on instruments to destroy most pathogenic microorganisms.

disinfection, the process of destroying pathogenic organisms or of rendering them inert.

disintegration, induced nuclear, disintegration resulting from artificial bombardment of a material with high-energy particles such as alpha particles, deuterons, protons, neutrons, or gamma rays.

disintegration, nuclear, a spontaneous nuclear transformation (radioactivity) characterized by the emission of energy and/or mass from the nucleus. When numbers of nuclei are involved, the process is characterized by a definite half-life.

disk (disc), a thin, flat, circular object.

d., abrasive, a disk with abrasive particles attached to one or both of its surfaces or its edge.

d., diamond, a disk of steel with diamond chips bonded to its surface.

d., garnet, a disk with particles of garnet as the abrading medium.

d., Jo-dandy, the trade name for a separating disk. See also **disk, separating.**

d., lightning, a steel separating disk.

d., Merkel's. See **corpuscle, Merkel's.**

d. of temporomandibular joint, a plate of fibrous tissue that divides the temporomandibular joint into an upper and a lower cavity. The disk is attached to the articular capsule and moves forward with the condyle in free opening and protrusion.

d. pack, a set of circular magnetic surfaces mounted coaxially on a shaft for computer storage of files. Can be used for storage of serial or direct access files.

d., polishing, a disk with an extremely fine abrasive; used to finish and polish a surface.

d., safe-side, a separating disk with abrasive on one side only; the other side is smooth.

d., sandpaper, an abrasive disk with sandpaper as the abrading medium.

d., separating, a disk of steel or hard rubber.

d. storage, a storage device that uses magnetic recording on flat, rotating disks.

dislocation, the displacement of any part, especially a bone or bony articulation.

dislodgment, movement or removal of a prosthesis from its established position.

disopyramide, *trade name:* Norpace CR; *drug class:* antidysrhythmic (Class IA); *action:* prolongs action potential duration and effective refractory period; *uses:* PVCs, ventricular tachycardia, atrial flutter, fibrillation.

disorder(s), derangement of function.

d., coagulation, any one of the hemorrhagic diseases caused by a deficiency of plasma thromboplastin formation (deficiency of antihemophilic factor, plasma thromboplastic antecedent, Hageman factor, Stuart factor), deficiency of thrombin formation (deficiency of prothrombin, factor V, factor VII, Stuart factor), and deficiency of fibrin formation (afibrinogenemia, fibrinogenopenia).

d., periodic, a variety of disorders of unknown cause that have in common periodic recurrence of manifestations. Such disorders are usually benign, resist treatment, often begin in infancy, and occasionally have a hereditary pattern. Included are periodic sialorrhea, neutropenia, arthralgia, fever, purpura (anaphylactoid purpura), edema (angioneurotic edema), abdominalgia, and periodic parotitis (recurrent parotitis).

d., platelet, hemorrhagic disease caused by an abnormality of the blood platelets (for example, thrombocytopenia, thrombasthenia).

d., psychophysiologic, autonomic, and visceral, standard psychiatric nomenclature for what are commonly known as psychomotor disorders. The disorders are disturbances of visceral function, secondary to chronic attitude and long-continued reaction to stress. These disorders may occur in any organ innervated by the autonomic nervous system, since overactivity or underactivity of that system as a result of stress appears to trigger the disorder. See also **disease, psychosomatic.**

d., visual, disorders that may result from injury or disease to the eyeball and its adnexa, the retina, or the cornea (for example, contusions of the orbit and eyelids, opacities of the lens, corneal scars, vascular changes to the retina). These peripheral disorders are effective in causing partial or total loss of vision in one or both eyes. They are simple, concrete, and fundamental. One sees or one does not see, and gray visions are generally quantitative differences that affect the perception of light and shadow and color and form. Visual disorders may also result from injury or disease to the optic tract fibers, optic chiasma, cerebral pathways, and visual cortex in the occipital region of the cerebrum. These disorders are qualitative deviations from normal, and the symptoms include visual field defects such as tubular vision found in hysteria, complete blindness in one or both eyes as a result of optic nerve injury, and hemianopsia, in which vision may be lost in one half of the visual field of one or both eyes. Other visual disorders include night and day blindness, color blindness, and the serious visual agnosia that results from trauma, tumor, or vascular disorders in the visual cortex of the cerebrum.

disprove, to refute or to prove false by affirmative evidence to the contrary.

dissection, neck, the removal of the lymph nodes and contiguous tissues from a primary site in the mandibular and/or maxillofacial area as treatment of neoplastic cells that have involved the regional cervical lymphatic system.

disseminated intravascular coagulation (DIC), a grave coagulopathy resulting from the overstimulation of clotting and anticlotting processes in response to disease or injury, such as septicemia, acute hypotension, poisonous snake bites, neoplasms, and severe trauma.

dissolve, to terminate, cancel, annul, disintegrate. To release the obligation of anything, as to dissolve a partnership.

distal, away from the median sagittal plane of the face and following the curvature of the dental arch.

    d. end, the most posterior part of a removable dental restoration or denture flange.

distance, the measure of space intervening between two objects or two points of reference.

    d., anode-film. See **distance, target-film.**

    d., cone, the distance between the focal spot and the outer end of the cone; usually expressed in inches or centimeters. Modern dental roentgen-ray units usually have cone distances of from 5 to 20 inches (12.5 to 50 cm).

    d., focal-film. See **distance, target-film.**

    d., interarch (interridge distance), the vertical distance between the maxillary and mandibular arches under conditions of vertical relations that must be specified.

    d., interocclusal (interocclusal gap, free-way space), the distance between the occluding surfaces of the maxillary and mandibular teeth when the mandible is in its physiologic rest position. This can be determined by calculating the difference between the rest vertical dimension and the occlusal vertical dimension of the face.

    d., interridge. See **distance, interarch.**

    d., large interarch, a large distance between the maxillary and mandibular arches.

    d., long cone, long (extended) cone distance is usually 14 to 20 inches (35 to 50 cm). See also **cone, long.**

    d., object-film, the distance, usually expressed in centimeters or inches, between the object being radiographed and the cassette or film.

    d., short cone, a focal-skin distance of 9 inches (22.5 cm) or less; usually refers to the distance as determined by the cone supplied by the manufacturer in the basic x-ray unit.

    d., small interarch, a small distance between the maxillary and mandibular arches.

    d., target-film (anode-film distance, focal-film distance), the distance between the focal spot of the tube and the film; usually expressed in inches or centimeters.

distention, a state of dilation.

distoclusion, lower teeth occluding distal to their normal relationship to the uppers, as in an Angle Class II malocclusion.

    d., bilateral, distoclusion on both sides.

    d., unilateral, distoclusion on one side.

distomolar, a supernumerary (fourth) molar located posterior to the third molar.

distortion, 1. a deviation from the normal shape or condition. 2. a modification of the speech sound in some way so that the acoustic result only approximates the standard sound and is not accurate. 3. a twisting or deformation. A loss of accuracy in reproduction of cavity form.

    d., film-fault, an imperfection in the size or shape of a film image by either magnification, elongation, or foreshortening.

    d., horizontal, a disproportional change in size and shape of the image in the horizontal plane as a result of oblique horizontal angulation of the x-ray beam.

    d., magnification, a proportional enlargement of a radiographic image. It is always present to some degree in oral radiography but is minimized with extended focal-film distances.

    d., vertical (foreshortening), a disproportional change in size, either elongation or foreshortening, caused by incorrect vertical angulation or improper film placement.

distoversion, the placement of a tooth farther than normal from the median plane or midline.

distraction, the placement of teeth or other maxillary or mandibular structures farther than normal from the median plane.

disturbances, occlusal, derangements in the patterns of occlusion.

disulfiram, *trade name:* Antabuse; *drug class:* aldehyde dehydrogenase inhibitor; *action:* blocks oxidation of alcohol at acetaldehyde stage; *uses:* chronic alcoholism (as adjunct).

ditch *(ditching),* the undesirable loss of tooth substance in the region of a restoration margin (usually gingival).

ditching. See **ditch.**

diuretic (dī'yo͞oret'ik), **1.** a drug that increases the formation of urine. **2.** pertaining to the increased formation of urine.

diverticulitis, an inflammatory pouching of the intestinal wall.

dizziness, a sensation of faintness or an inability to maintain normal balance in a standing or seated position. A patient who experiences dizziness should be carefully lowered to a safe position on a bed, chair, or floor because of the danger of injury from falling. See also **syncope.**

DMF index rate. See **rate, DMF index.**

DNA, bacterial, the DNA specific to a bacterial strain.

DNA fingerprinting, the use of DNA analysis to identify a subject from blood or other suitable tissue.

DNA probe. See **deoxyribonucleic acid probes.**

DO cavity, a cavity on the distal and occlusal surfaces of a tooth. See also **cavity, Class 2.**

doctor, a learned person; one qualified in a science or art; one who has received the highest academic degree in a particular field.

documentation, the permanent record ing of information properly identified as to time, place, circumstances, and attribution.

docusate calcium/docusate potassium/docusate sodium, *trade names:* Colace, Correctol Extra Gentle, Sulfalax; *drug class:* laxative; *action:* increases water, fat penetration in intestine; allows for easier passage of stool; *uses:* stool softener.

dolichocephalic (dol'iko͞sefal'ik), pertaining to a long and narrow head (with a cephalic index below 75).

dolar (do͞'lôr), any kind of pain.

donor site, the portion of the body from which an organ or tissue is removed for transplant or grafting.

donor tissue, tissue contributed by the donor to be used in tissue or organ transplant.

Donovan body. See **body, Donovan.** (not current)

dopa, an amino acid derived from tyrosine that occurs naturally in plants and animals. It is a precursor of dopamine, epinephrine, and norepinephrine.

dopamine, a sympathomimetic catecholamine used in the treatment of shock, hypotension, and low cardiac output.

dope, a slang term denoting any drug taken temporarily or habitually without medical cause and that is intended to alter mood.

dornase alfa, *trade name:* Pulmozyme; *drug class:* recombinant human deoxyribonuclease (DNase); *action:* reduces sputum viscosity; *uses:* cystic fibrosis, reduces incidence of pulmonary infection, improves pulmonary function.

dorsal (dôr'səl), pertaining to the back or to the posterior part of an organ.

dorsum sellae (dôr'səm sel'ē), the most posterior point on the internal contour of sella turcica.

dosage (do͞'sij), the amount of a medicine or other agent administered for a given case or condition.

dose (dos), 1. the quantity of drug necessary to produce a desired effect. **2.** the total radiation delivered to a specified area or volume or to the whole body. See also **dose, radiation absorbed.**

d., absorbed (D), the amount of energy imparted by ionizing particles to unit mass of irradiated material at a place of interest. The unit of absorbed dose is the rad (100 ergs/Gm).

d., air, an x-ray dose delivered at a point in free air; expressed in roentgens. It consists only of the radiation of the primary beam and the radiation scattered from surrounding air; does not include backscatter from radiated matter (for example, tissue).

d., booster, the portion of an immunizing agent given at a later time to stimulate the effects of a previous dose of the same agent.

d., cumulative, the total accumulated dose resulting from a single or repeated exposure to radiation of the same region or of the whole body. If used in area monitoring, it represents the accumulated radiation exposure over a given period of time.

d., depth, the absorbed dose of radiation imparted to matter at a particular depth below the surface, usually expressed as "percentage depth dose." See also **dose, percentage depth.**

d. distribution, a representation of the variation of dose with position in any region of an irradiated object. The dose distribution may be measured using detectors small enough to avoid disturbing the distribution, or it may be calculated and expressed in mathematical form.

d., doubling, the amount of ionizing radiation, absorbed by the gonads of the average person in a population over a period of several generations, that will result in a doubling of the current rate of spontaneous mutations.

d. effect curve. See **curve, doseeffect.**

d. equivalent (DE), the product of absorbed dose and modifying factors, namely the quality factor (QF), distribution factor (DF), and any other necessary factors. The unit of dose equivalent is the rem (rads times qualifying factors).

d., erythema, the dose of radiation necessary to produce a temporary redness of the skin. This dose varies with the quality of radiation.

d., exit, the absorbed dose delivered by a beam of radiation at the surface through which the beam emerges from a phantom or patient.

d., exposure. See **exposure.**

d., fractionation, a dose given by a number of shorter exposures over a longer period than would be required if the dose was given by a continuous exposure in one session at the same dose rate.

d., gonadal, the dose of radiation absorbed by the gonads.

d., integral *(integral absorbed dose, volume dose),* the total energy absorbed by a part or object during exposure to radiation. The unit of integral dose is the gram rad (100 ergs).

d., lethal, 1. the amount of a drug that would prove fatal to the majority of persons. **2.** the amount of radiation that will be or may be sufficient to cause the death of an organism.

d., maintenance, the quantity of drug necessary to sustain a normal physiologic state or a desired blood or tissue level of drug.

d., maximum permissible (MPD), the maximum relative biologic effect dose that the body of a person or specific parts thereof shall be permitted to receive in a stated period of time. In most instances, for the roentgen rays used in dental radiography, it is satisfactory to consider the RBE dose in rems numerically equal to the absorbed dose in rads and the absorbed dose in rads numerically equal to the exposure dose in roentgens. See also **dose, weekly permissible.**

d., median effective (ED50), a dose that, under standard conditions, is effective in 50% of a randomly selected group of subjects.

d., median lethal (LD50), the amount of ionizing radiation required to kill, within a specified period, 50% of the individuals in a large group or population of animals or organisms.

d., minimum lethal (MLD), the minimal amount of a drug that will kill an experimental animal.

d., percentage depth, the ratio (expressed as a percentage) of the absorbed dose at a given depth in an irradiated body, to the absorbed dose at a fixed reference point on the central ray, usually the surface-absorbed dose.

d., priming, a quantity several times larger than the maintenance dose; used at the initiation of therapy to rapidly establish the desired blood and tissue levels of the drug.

d. protraction, a method of radiation administration delivered continuously over a relatively long period at a relatively low dosage rate.

d., radiation, the amount of energy absorbed per unit mass of tissue at a site of interest. Note: This definition limits the use of "dose" to conform with the 1962 recommendations of the International Commission on Radiological Units and Measurements (ICRUM). The following terms therefore become obsolete, but will be found in this dictionary under the general heading of **exposure: air dose, cumulative dose, exposure dose,** and **threshold dose.**

d., radiation-absorbed *(rad),* the unit of absorbed dose, with a value of 100 ergs per gram.

d. rate, the time rate at which radiation dose is applied, expressed in either roentgens per unit time or rads per unit time.

d., skin. See **dose, surfaceabsorbed.**

d., surface-absorbed, the absorbed dose delivered by a radiation beam at the point where the central ray passes through the superficial layer of the phantom or patient.

d., therapeutic, a quantity several times larger than the maintenance dose; used in vitamin therapy in which a marked deficiency exists.

d., threshold, the minimum dose that will produce a detectable degree of any given effect.

d., tissue, the dose absorbed by a tissue or the tissues in a region of interest.

d., tolerance. See **dose, maximum permissible.**

d., toxic, the amount of a drug that causes untoward symptoms in the majority of persons.

d., transit, a measure of the primary radiation transmitted through the patient and measured at a point on the central ray at some point beyond the patient.

d., U.S.P. See **dose, median effective (ED50); dose, lethal, median (LD50); dose, lethal, minimum (MLD);** and **drug, official.**

d., volume. See **dose, integral.**

d., weekly permissible, a dose of ionizing radiation accumulated in 1 week and of such magnitude that, in view of present knowledge, exposure at this weekly rate for an indefinite period of time is not expected to cause appreciable bodily injury during a person's lifetime.

dosimetry (dōsim'etrē), the accurate and systematic determination of the amount of radiation to which an animal or person has been exposed during a given period of time.

dovetail, a widened or fanned-out portion of a prepared cavity, usually established deliberately to increase the retention and resistance form.

d., lingual, a dovetail established as a step portion, with lingual approach, in some Class 3 and Class 4 preparations; used to supplement the retentions and resistance form.

d., occlusal, a dovetail established at the terminal of the occlusal step of a proximal cavity.

dowel, a post or pin, usually made of metal, fitted into a prepared root canal of a natural tooth to improve retention of a restoration.

downcoding, a practice of third-party payers in which the benefits code has been changed to a less complex and/or

lower cost procedure than was reported.

Down syndrome, a congenital condition characterized by varying degrees of mental retardation and multiple developmental defects. It is most commonly caused by the presence of an extra chromosome 21. It is also called *trisomy 21* and *trisomy G syndrome. Mongolism* is an archaic and discredited term.

downtime, the time interval during which a device is malfunctioning or inoperative.

doxazosin mesylate, *trade name:* Cardura; *drug class:* peripheral α-adrenergic blocker; action: peripheral blood vessels are dilated, peripheral resistance lowered, reduction in blood pressure reduced; *uses:* hypertension.

doxepin *(topical), trade name:* Zonalon; *drug class:* topical antipruritic (tricyclic antidepressant); *action:* antipruritic mechanism unknown; has antihistaminic activity; also produces drowsiness; *uses:* pruritus associated with eczema, atopic dermatitis, lichen simplex chronicus.

doxepin HCl, *trade name:* Sinequan; *drug class:* antidepressant, tricyclic; *action:* inhibits both norepinephrine and serotonin (5-HT) reuptake in synapses in brain; *uses:* major depression, anxiety.

doxycycline hyclate, *trade names:* Doryx, Doxy-Caps, Vibra-Tabs; *drug class:* tetracycline, broad-spectrum antiinfective; *action:* inhibits protein synthesis, phosphorylation in microorganisms; *uses:* Syphilis, *Chlamydia trachomatis,* gonorrhea, lymphogranuloma venereum, uncommon gram-negative and gram-positive organisms, necrotizing ulcerative gingivostomatitis.

drachm *(dram).* See **dram.**

draft. See **draw.**

drag, the lower, or cast, side of a denture mold or flask, to which the cope is fitted. The base of the cast is embedded in plaster or stone, with the remainder of the denture pattern exposed to be engaged by the plaster or stone in the cope (the upper part of the flask).

drain, any substance that provides a channel for release or discharge from a wound.

d., cigarette. See **drain, Penrose.**

d., Penrose (cigarette), a thin-walled rubber tube through which a piece of gauze has been pulled.

drainage, the placement or creation of a pathway from a deep lesion to the surface of the body to provide an avenue for the body to expel the byproducts of an infection or inflammation.

dram (drachm), a unit of weight that equals the eighth part of the apothecaries' ounce. Symbol ℨ.

draught (draft). See **draw.**

draw (draft, draught), the taper or divergence of the walls of a preparation for insertion of a cemented restoration.

drepanocythemia (drep'ənōsĭthē' mē-ə). See **anemia, sickle cell.** (not current)

dressing, Kirkland cement, a surgical dressing applied to the tissues after periodontal surgery; consists of zinc oxide, tannic acid, and powdered rosin, admixed with a liquid composed of lump rosin, sweet almond oil, and eugenol.

dressing, postoperative surgical, a surgical cement dressing applied to the teeth and tissues after surgical periodontal therapy. Possesses supportive, protective, hemostatic, analgesic, and other properties.

DRG, the abbreviation for **diagnosis-related group.**

drift. See **tooth, drifting.**

drill, a cutting instrument for boring holes by rotary motion.

d., bibevel, a drill with two flattened sides and the end cut in two beveled planes.

d., spear-point, a drill with a tri-beveled, or threeplaned, point.

d., twist, a drill with one or more deep spiral grooves that extend from the point to the smooth part of the shaft.

drilling, boring a hole with a rotary cutting instrument; used in reference to pinholes. (Objectionable as a term describing the general preparation of cavities with rotary instruments.)

drip, the continuous slow intravenous introduction of fluid containing nutrients or drugs.

droperidol, a butyrophenone drug used in neuroleptanalgesia and preanesthetic medication.

droplet spread, transmission of an infection through the projection of oral and nasal secretions by coughing, sneezing, or talking.

dropsy (dräp'sē). See **anasarca.**

drowning, asphyxiation because of submersion in a liquid.

drug(s), a substance used in the prevention, cure, or alleviation of disease or pain or as an aid in some diagnostic procedures.

d. abuse, an excessive or improper use of drugs, especially through self-administration for nonmedical purposes. This term has increased significance because of the enactment of the Comprehensive Drug Abuse Prevention and Control Act of 1970, which replaces the Harrison Narcotic Act.

d., antibiotic, chemical compounds obtained from certain living cells of lower plant forms, such as bacteria, yeasts, and molds, and from synthesis. They are antagonistic to certain pathogenic organisms and have a lethal effect on them.

d., antiseptic, a chemical compound used to reduce the number of microorganisms in the oral cavity.

d., autonomic, a drug that mimics or blocks the effects of stimulation of the autonomic nervous system.

d. combinations, the use of drugs together to enhance the properties of both to the benefit of the patient.

d., desensitizing, a pharmaceutical used to diminish or eliminate sensitivity of teeth to physical, chemical, thermal, or other irritants (for example, strontium chloride, silver nitrate [ammoniacal], sodium fluoride, formalin, zinc chloride).

d., endodontic, any one of the drugs used in treating the dental pulp and dental periapical tissues.

d. interaction, a modification of the effect of a drug when administered with another drug. The effect may be an increase or a decrease in the action of either substance, or it may be an adverse effect that is not normally associated with either drug.

d., nonofficial, a drug that is not listed in the United States Pharmacopeia (U.S.P.) or the National Formulary (N.F.).

d., official, a drug that is listed in the U.S.P. or N.F.

d., officinal (ofis'inəl), drugs that may be purchased without a prescription.

More commonly called *over-the-counter (OTC)* drugs.

d., over-the-counter (OTC), a drug that may be purchased without a prescription. Sometimes called a *nonlegend drug* because its label does not bear the prescription legend required on all drugs that may be dispensed only on prescription.

d., parasympathetic, belladonna alkaloids that inhibit glandular secretions of the nose, mouth, pharynx, and bronchi. This is the chief reason for using atropine and scopolamine for preanesthetic medication.

d., parasympatholytic (par'əsim'pə-thōlit'ik), a drug that blocks nerve impulses passing from parasympathetic nerve fibers to postganglionic neuroeffectors.

d., parasympathomimetic (par'ə-sim'pathōmimet'lk), a drug that has an effect similar to that produced when the parasympathetic nerves are stimulated.

d., proprietary, a drug that is patented or controlled by a private organization or manufacturer.

d. resistance, the capacity of a microorganism to build a tolerance to a drug.

d. stability, the length of time a drug will retain its properties without the loss of potency, usually referred to as *shelf life.*

d. therapy, the use of a drug in the treatment of a patient with a specific disease or illness.

dry field, the isolation of a surgical or operating field from body fluids such as saliva and blood. A dry field is essential in the placement of some sealants and restorative fillings.

Dry-foil, the trade name for tinfoil that is supplied with an adhesive powder or coating on one side.

dry heat, a method of sterilization of suitable instruments using a well-calibrated and time-controlled convection oven.

dry ice, solid carbon dioxide, with a temperature of about −140° F.

dry socket. See **socket, dry.**

dual choice (dual option), federal legislation that requires employers to give their employees the option to enroll in a local health maintenance organization rather than in the conventional employer-sponsored health program.

dual impression technique. See **technique, impression, dual.**

duct, a small passage.

d., nasopalatine. See **cyst, naso-palatine.**

d., Stensen's, the excretory duct of the parotid gland; it passes lateral to the masseter muscle and enters the oral cavity through the buccal tissues adjacent to the maxillary first and second molars.

d., Wharton's, the excretory duct of the submaxillary glands; opens into the oral cavity at the sublingual papillae of the mucous membrane of the floor of the mouth behind the lower incisor teeth.

ductility (daktil'itē), the property of a material that allows permanent deformation under tension without rupture. It is measured as a percentage increase in length on rupture compared with original length and is termed *percentage elongation,* or *elongation.*

Duke's test. See **test, Duke's.** (not current)

Dunlop file *(not current).* See **file, Hirschfeld-Dunlop.**

duodenal ulcer, a peptic ulcer located in the duodenum.

duodenum, the first, shortest, and most fixed portion of the small intestine. The duodenum courses from the pyloric valve of the stomach and terminates in a junction with the jejunum at the duodenojejunal flexure.

duplication, the procedure of accurately reproducing a cast or other object.

d. impression. See **duplication.**

duty, that which is due from a person; that which a person owes to another; an obligation.

dwarf, pituitary (pitū'iter'ē), an individual who is of small stature as a result of a deficiency of growth hormones. Such dwarfs usually are well proportioned.

dwarfism, deficient growth and development leading to small stature and often skeletal deformity. It may be associated with ovarian agenesis, pituitary insufficiency, mongolism, progeria, rickets, renal disease, dietary deficiency, achondroplasia, cleidocranial dysostosis, osteogenesis imperfecta, microcephaly, hydrocephaly, sexual precocity, and delayed adolescence.

dye, occlusal registration, a water-soluble dye used as an aid in locating occlusal contacts. A valuable aid in effecting the fine adjustments in the final phases of the selective grinding procedure. (not current)

dyes, treatment, the dyes used in medicine and dentistry in the treatment of diseased states, the most useful of which are the rosanilin dyes (for example, gentian violet, crystal violet) and the fluorescein dyes (for example, Mercurochrome), which possess antiseptic and protective properties. (not current)

dynamic relation. See **relation, dynamic.**

dyphylline, *trade names:* Dilor, Dyflex, Lufylin; *drug class:* Xanthine derivative; *action:* relaxes smooth muscle of respiratory system by blocking phosphodiesterase; *uses:* bronchial asthma, bronchospasm in chronic bronchitis, COPD, emphysema.

dysautonomia, familial (dis′ôtōnō′mēə). See **syndrome, Riley-Day.**

dyscrasia (diskrā′zhə), **1.** a morbid condition, especially one that involves an imbalance of component elements. **2.** an abnormal composition of the blood, such as found in leukemia and anemia.

dysdiadochokinesia (dis′dī·ədō′kō-kinē′zhə), a disturbance of musculoskeletal function. There is a disorganization in the reciprocal innervation of agonists and antagonists and a loss of the ability to stop one act in terms of rate, magnitude, and the direction of movement and immediately to follow it with another act diametrically opposite (for example, alternately elevating and depressing the mandible). Another example is observed in the inappropriate use of the tongue during mastication when it is necessary to change, reverse, and modify the energy and direction of movement. (not current)

dysentery, an inflammation of the intestine, especially of the colon, that may be caused by chemical irritants, bacteria, protozoa, or parasites. It is characterized by frequent and bloody stools and severe abdominal pain.

dysesthesia (dis′esthē′zhə), an impairment of the senses, especially of the sense of touch. Any sensation is not normally painful with dysesthesia.

dysfunction (disfunk′shən) (malfunction), any abnormality or impairment of function or the inability of a body, organ, or organ system to perform normally.

d., dental, an abnormal functioning or impairment of the functioning of the dental organ.

d., endocrine, an abnormality in the function of an endocrine gland, either by hypofunction or hyperfunction of the secretory elements of the gland.

dysgeusia, an abnormal or impaired sense of taste.

dysgnathia (disna′thēə), those abnormalities that extend beyond the teeth and include the maxilla, the mandible, or both. See also **anomaly, dysgnathic.**

dyskeratosis (dis′kerətō′sis), an irreversible alteration in the maturation of stratified squamous epithelium. Refers to an increase of abnormal mitosis, individual cell keratinization, epithelial pearls within the spinous layer, loss of polarity of the cells, hyperchromatism, nuclear atypia, and basilar hyperplasia.

dyslexia, an impairment of the ability to read. Dyslexic persons often reverse letters and words, cannot adequately distinguish the letter sequences in written words, and have difficulty determining left from right.

dysmenorrhea (dis′menərē′·ə), painful menstruation.

dysmetria (dismē′trē·ə), the loss of ability to gauge distance, speed, or power of movement associated with muscle function; for example, the patient is unable to control the force of closure and strikes the opposite occluding teeth with greater vigor than necessary.

dysostosis (disōstō′sis), defective ossification.

d., cleidocranial (klī′dōkrā′nē· əl) (Sainton's disease), a familial disease or congenital disorder characterized by failure to form, or retarded formation of, the clavicles; delayed closure of the sutures and fontanels; and delayed eruption of teeth, with formation of supernumerary teeth. Cleidocranial dysostosis is characterized by under-development of the maxillae, agenesis or aplasia of the clavicle, abnormalities in other skeletal bones and muscles, and irregularities of the dentition. The syndrome may be mutational or transmitted on an autosomal dominant basis.

d., craniofacial (Crouzon's disease, Crouzon's syndrome), a condition of unknown etiology that is similar to cleidocranial dysostosis but differs in that the clavicles are not affected. See also **dysostosis, cleidocranial.**

d., faciomandibular, a developmental disturbance of the cranial bones and hypoplasias of the upper part of the face. The mandibular body is underdeveloped, but the ramus is hyperplastic. The teeth are crowded and malposed.

d. multiplex. See **syndrome, Hurler's.**

dyspepsia, a vague feeling of epigastric discomfort, felt after eating. Dyspepsia is not a distinct condition but may be a sign of underlying intestinal disorder, such as peptic ulcer, gallbladder disease, or chronic appendicitis. The symptoms usually increase during periods of stress.

dysphagia (disfā'jē·ə), difficulty in swallowing. It may be caused by lesions in the mouth, pharynx, or larynx; neuromuscular disturbances; or mechanical obstruction of the esophagus (for example, dysphagia of Plummer-Vinson syndrome [sideropenic dysphagia], peritonsillar abscess, Ludwig's angina, and carcinoma of the tongue, pharynx, larynx).

dysphoria (disfor'ē·ə), a feeling of discomfort or restlessness. See also **euphoria.**

dysplasia (displā'zhə), **1.** developmental abnormality. See also **dysplasia, dentinal. 2.** reversible, regressive alteration in adult cells, seen as alterations in their size, shape, orientation, and functions; leads to change in tissue architecture and is related to chronic inflammation or protracted irritation. Abnormality of development. **3.** disharmony between component parts.

d., anteroposterior (anteroposterior facial dysplasia), an abnormal anteroposterior relationship of the maxillae and mandible to each other or to the cranial base.

d., craniofacial, a disharmony between the cranium and the face.

d., dentinal, a genetic disturbance of the dentin characterized by early calcification of the pulp chambers and root canals and by root resorption. It is differentiated from dentinogenesis imperfecta by the latter's characteristics of attrition and relative freedom from root resorption.

d., dentofacial, a disharmony between teeth and bones of the face (for example, crowding and spacing).

d., ectodermal, a disease of genetic origin characterized by failure to form ectodermal derivatives. Sweat glands and teeth may be missing (anhidrosis and anodontia, respectively), and there may be scant hair, faulty fingernails, and malformation of the iris.

d., fibroosseous. See **dysplasia, fibrous.**

d., fibrous (fibroosseous dysplasia), a metabolic disturbance characterized by replacement of the bone marrow with fibrous tissue and slow, progressive remolding and enlargement of the bone. It may be monostotic (limited to one bone) or polyostotic (present in many bones). Albright's syndrome shows polyostotic fibrous dysplasia and other symptoms. The monostotic lesions may be identical with ossifying fibroma or with osseous dysplasia. See also **osteofibroma** and **syndrome, Albright's.**

d., focal osseous. See **fibroma, periapical.**

d., polyostotic fibrous, fibrous dysplasia occurring in more than one bone. See also **dysplasia, fibrous; osteofibroma;** and **syndrome, Albright's.**

d., maxillomandibular, a disharmony between one jaw and the other.

d., osseous, a chronic reaction of the bone to injury characterized by replacement of the bone marrow with fibrous connective tissue, unilateral enlargement of the maxillae or mandible, and characteristic radiographic findings. It is similar to or identical with monostotic fibrous dysplasia and ossifying fibroma.

dyspnea (dispnē'·ə), difficult, labored, or gasping breathing; inspiration, expiration, or both may be involved.

dysrhythmia (disrith'mē·ə), disordered rhythm.

dystonia (distō'nē-ə), a disorder or lack of tonicity.

dystrophy (dis'trōfē), faulty nutrition. Often used to refer to the results of faulty nutrition; that is, wasting away. *d., muscular,* a chronic, degenerative, noncontagious, progressive disorder of unknown etiology manifested by weakness and wasting away of the voluntary muscles.

Eames' technique (mez). See **technique, Eames'.** (not current)

earnings report, a statement issued by a company showing its earnings or losses over a given period. The earnings report lists the income earned, expenses, and net result. Synonym: income statement.

eating disorders, a group of dysfunctional behaviors of nutrition, including anorexia, bulimia, or cravings for such nonfood items as ice, clay, or starch.

EBIT, the abbreviation for **earnings before interest and taxes.**

eburnation (ē'bernā'shən), an increase in bony density into an ivory-like mass. See also **osteitis, condensing** and **dentin eburnation.**

eccentric (eksen'trik), **I.** a deviation from the normal or conventional. **2.** away from the central or reference position.
e. checkbite. See **record, interocclusal, eccentric.**
e. jaw relation. See **relation, jaw, eccentric.**
e. occlusion. See **occlusion, eccentric.**
e. position. See **position, eccentric.**

ecchymosis (ek'imō'sis), a discoloration of mucous membranes caused by a diffuse extravasation of blood. Frequently called a *bruise.*

echocardiography, a diagnostic procedure for studying the structure and motion of the heart using ultrasonic waves that pass through the heart and are reflected backward, or echoed, when they pass from one type of tissue to another.

echoviruses (ECHO virus), an enteric pathogen associated with fever and mild respiratory disease; sometimes may produce an aseptic meningitis.

ecology, the study of the interaction between living organisms and their environment.

econazole nitrate (topical), *trade name:* Ecostatin; *drug class:* local antifungal; *action:* interferes with fungal cell membrane, which increases permeability, leaking of cell nutrients; *uses:* tinea pedis, tinea cruris, tinea corporis, tinea versicolor, cutaneous candidiasis.

economics, in dentistry, a broad term that covers all the business aspects of dental practice.

ecosystem, the sum total of all living and nonliving things that support the chain of life events within a particular area.

ectoderm, the outermost of the three primary cell layers of an embryo. The ectoderm gives rise to the nervous system, the organs of special sense, the epidermis, and epidermal tissues such as fingernails, hair, and skin glands.

ectodermal dysplasia, a developmental disturbance of tissues derived from the ectoderm (for example, hair, nails, sweat glands, and teeth). Dental findings are partial anodontia and microdontia.

ectomorph (ek'tōmorf), a constitutional body type (Sheldon's classification) characterized by long, fragile bones and a highly developed nervous system.

ectopia lentis, a displacement of the lens of the eye.

ectopic eruption. See **eruption, ectopic.**

ectropion (ektrō'pē-on), eversion, or rolling outward, of the eyelid margin.

eczema (ek'zēmə), an inflammatory skin disease characterized by vesiculation, inflammation, watery discharge, and the development of scales and crusts. The large variety of types can be distinguished according to location and etiology.

ED50. See **dose, median effective.**

edema (edē'mə), the accumulation of fluid in the tissues or in the peritoneal or pleural cavities. Primary factors favoring edema are increased capillary hydrostatic pressure (increased venous pressure), decreased osmotic pressure of plasma (hypoproteinemia), decreased tissue tension and lymphatic drainage, increased osmotic pressure of tissue fluids, and increased capillary permeability. Additional renal and hormonal factors are important. Clinical manifestations may consist of a steady weight gain or localized or generalized swelling.

e., angioneurotic (angioedema, giant urticaria, Quincke's disease), the spontaneous swelling of the lips, cheeks, eyelids, tongue, soft palate, pharynx, and glottis, frequently associated with allergy to foods or drugs and lasting from several hours to several days. Involvement of the glottis results in obstruction of the airway.

e., cardiac, edema caused by venous congestion in association with congestive heart failure; tends to appear first in such dependent parts as the legs.

e., dependent, edema that changes its position with the posture of dependent parts (for example, edema of the legs in progressive heart failure).

e. of glottis, a swelling caused by fluid accumulation in the soft tissues of the larynx. The condition, usually inflammatory, may result from an infection, injury, allergy, or inhalation of toxic substances.

e., periorbital, edematous swelling of the eyelids in association with local injury, allergic reactions, hypoproteinemia, trichinosis, and myxedema.

e., pitting, a persistent indentation of the skin when pressure is applied to an edematous area.

edentulate (ēden'tyo͞olāt). See **edentulous.** (not current)

edentulism (eden'tyo͞olizəm), the condition of being edentulous, without teeth.

edentulous (ēden'tyo͞oləs), without teeth; lacking teeth.

edge strength. See **strength, edge.**

edge-to-edge bite. See **occlusion, edge-to-edge.**

edge-to-edge occlusion. See **occlusion, edge-to-edge.**

edgewise appliance. See **appliance, edgewise.**

EDP, the abbreviation for **electronic data processing.**

Edtac, the trade name for a chelating agent used to soften calcified tissue.

education, the act or process of imparting or acquiring knowledge, skill, or judgment.

e., continuing, education that occurs after the completion of a course of study leading to a degree. Usually taken in short (1 to 2 days) courses covering a specific topic or procedure.

e., dental, the formal education necessary to become qualified to practice dentistry; typically 4 years of full-time study in an accredited school of dentistry.

e., predental, the formal education necessary to qualify for placement in a dental curriculum, typically 4 years of full-time study at the baccalaureate level.

e. of patient, effective communication between the dentist (and/or auxiliaries) and the patient concerning dentistry and the principles of treatment and prevention. The procedure of increasing the patient's knowledge of the oral cavity and its care to the point where the reasons for proposed dental services are understood.

educational status, the level of education and skill obtained within a discipline or profession, usually referred to as a generalist or specialist in a discipline.

effect, the result of an action.

e. of external radiation on bone. See **osteoradionecrosis.**

e. of function on bone. See **law, Wolff's.**

e., heel (anode heel effect), the variation of intensity over the cross-section of a useful x-ray beam, caused by the angle at which x-rays emerge from beneath the surface of the focal spot, which causes a differential attenuation of photons comprising the useful beam.

e., lysing, the disintegrating action on tissue components produced by the toxic and compressive products of inflammation. In gingival inflammation, lysis of the gingival fibers must occur before apical migration of the epithelial attachment can occur. In microbiology, the presence of complement in the antigen-antibody complex is necessary for bacterial lysis. Hemolysis occurs with coexistence of erythrocyte, antibody, and complement.

e., wedging, an effect produced by food impaction that forces the teeth apart.

effective half-life. See **life, radioactive.**

effectiveness, the degree to which action(s) achieves the intended health result under normal or usual circumstances.

effector (ēfek'tōr), **1.** a motor or secretory nerve ending in an organ, gland, or muscle; consequently called an *effector organ.* **2.** an on-the-job organ of the body that responds to stimulations asking for corrections. Antonym: receptor.

efferent (ef'ərənt), conveying away from a center toward the periphery.

efficiency, the operation of a dental practice in such a way that both business and professional services are performed in a minimal amount of time without sacrificing quality of work, sympathetic attitude, and kindliness.

eH, the symbol for oxidation-reduction potential, which is regarded as a significant factor in the protection of the body against anaerobic bacteria. The eH of living tissue of pH level 7.4 is about 0.12 volt.

Ehlers-Danlos syndrome (ā'lərz dan'los), a hereditary disorder of connective tissue, marked by hyperplasticity of skin, tissue fragility, and hypermotility of joints. Minor trauma may cause a gaping wound with little bleeding. Sprains, dislocations, and synovial effusions are common. See also **syndrome, Ehlers-Danlos.**

EIA, the abbreviation for **enzyme immunoassay;** better known as *ELISA* for enzyme-linked immunosorbent assay used to detect the presence of HIV antibody to HIV in the blood.

Eikenella corrodens, a gram-negative, rod-shaped facultatively anaerobic bacteria that is part of the normal flora of the oral cavity but may become an opportunistic pathogen in immunocompromised patients.

ejector, by common usage, a device used to remove debris and fluids by negative pressure. The correct term for such a device, however, is *aspirator.* See also **aspirator.**

e., saliva, a device (containing a removable tip) that is attached to a vacuum supply to remove saliva from a dental field of operation.

e., saliva, tip, a removable tip, made of metal, glass, rubber, plastic, or a combination of these, that is attached to a saliva ejector and bent to fit over lower teeth and reach the floor of the oral cavity.

elastic, referring to property of a solid substance that permits recovery of its shape after a deformation resulting from force application.

e. deformation. See **deformation, elastic.**

e. impression. See **impression, elastic.**

e., intermaxillary. See **elastic, maxillomandibular.**

e., intramaxillary, an elastic band used within either the maxillary or mandibular arch.

e. limit. See **limit, elastic.**

e., maxillomandibular, an elastic band used between the maxillary and mandibular dentitions.

e. memory, **1.** the property of a material such as wax that enables it, after being warmed, bent, and cooled, to return to its original form upon rewarming. **2.** a rubber plastic band used to apply force to the teeth.

elasticity, the quality or condition of being elastic.

e., modulus of (Young's modulus), a measurement of elasticity obtained by dividing stress below the proportional limit by its corresponding strain value. A measure of stiffness.

elastomer (ēlas'tōmer), a soft, rubberlike material; synthetic rubber. A rubber base impression material (for example, silicone, mercaptan).

elastosis (ē'lastō'sis), a degeneration of the elastic tissues; found particularly in the lips and associated with senile or actinic cheilitis.

e., senile, a dermatologic disease that results from degeneration of the elastic connective tissue.

elder abuse, the infliction of physical, sexual, or emotional trauma upon a senior citizen.

elderly, an adjective used to describe a person who is beyond middle age and approaching old age. It is politically correct to refer to those over 65 as *senior citizens.* See also **geriatric dentistry.**

electroanesthesia (ilek'trō-anesthē'zē-ə), local or general anesthesia induced by electric current.

electrocardiography, a method of recording electrical activity generated by the heart muscle.

electrochemistry, chemical reactions that elicit electrical potentials and/or electrical potentials that initiate chemical reactions.

electrocoagulation (ilek'trōkōag'yōōlā'shən), the use of electrically generated heat to destroy tissue by coagulation necrosis. Usually a platinum wire electrode or loop is used.

electroconvulsive therapy, the induction of a brief convulsion by passing an electric current through the brain for the treatment of affective disorders, especially in patients resistant to psychoactive drug therapy.

electrocortin (ilek'trōkōr'tin). See **aldosterone.** (not current)

electrode (ilek'trōd), an instrument with a point or a surface from which a current can be discharged into or received from the body of a patient or a solution.

electrodiagnosis, the diagnosis of disease or injury by applying electric stimulation to various nerves and muscles.

electroencephalograph (EEG) (ilek'trō·ensef'əlōgraf), an instrument for recording the electrical activity of the brain.

electrogalvanism (ilektrōgal'vənizəm) (galvanism), the flow of electric current between two different metals in an electrolyte solution. Dissimilar metals used in different intraoral restorations. (not current)

electrolyte (ilek'trōlīt), a solution that conducts electricity by means of its ions.

e. affinity, the attraction of the electrolytes in the body to the different fluid compartments of the intracellular and extracellular environments. Sodium is the predominant cation in the extracellular fluid; potassium is the predominant cation within the cells; chlorine and bicarbonate are the predominant anions in the plasma and interstitial fluids; and phosphates and proteins are the chief anions in the cells.

e. balance, fluid and. See **fluid and electrolyte balance.**

electrolyzer (ilek'trōlī'zər) (ionizer), an electric apparatus designed for use in a root canal to break down a treatment chemical into its various ions by direct current. See also **electrosterilizer.**

electromallet, McShirley's. See **condenser, electromallet.**

electromedication. See **electrosterilization.** (not current)

electrometer (ilektrom'ətər), an electrostatic instrument for measuring the potential difference between two points. In radiology, electrometers are used to measure changes in the potential of charged electrodes resulting from ionization occasioned by radiation.

electromyography (ilek'trōmi·og'r ə-fē), the detection, recording, and interpretation of electric voltage generated by the skeletal muscles.

electron (ilek'tron) (e), a negatively charged elementary particle constituent in every neutral atom, with a mass of 0.000549. (Particles with an equal but opposite charge are called *positrons.*)

e. beam. See **electron stream.**

e. stream (electron beam, cathode ray, cathode stream), a stream of electrons emitted from the negative electrode (cathode) in a roentgen-ray tube; their bombardment of the anode gives rise to the roentgen rays.

electronic, pertaining to the application of that branch of science that deals with the motion, emission, and behavior of currents of free electrons, especially in vacuum, gas, or phototubes and special conductors or semiconductors. Contrasted with electric, which pertains to the flow of large currents in wires only.

e. knife. See **knife, electronic.**

electrophoresis, the movement of charged suspended particles through a liquid medium in response to changes in an electric field.

electroplating, plating by electrolysis. Impressions are plated in dentistry to form metalized working dies.

electropolishing, the removal of a minute layer of metal by electrolysis to produce a bright surface.

electrosection, an incision created by electrosurgery, ideally by using a fully rectified, alternating high-frequency current and producing minimal cellular injury.

electrosterilization, medication of a prepared root canal by use of electrolysis of the medicament. (not current)

electrosterilizer, an electric apparatus designed for use in root canal treatment for the electrolysis of a halide, such as sodium iodide, to release iodine in the cleaned root canal for the purpose of destroying residual organisms. See also **electrolyzer.**

electrosurgery, the use of electrically generated energy from high-frequency alternating currents to cut or alter tissue within definite limits.

element, a simple substance that cannot be decomposed by chemical means and is made up of atoms that are alike in their peripheral electronic configuration and chemical properties but differ in their nuclei, atomic weights, and radioactive properties.

elephantiasis (el'əfənti'·əsis), a chronic disease caused by filariasis of the lymph channels with resultant inflammation and blockage. The term is also used for hypertrophy of tissues from other causes (for example, gingival elephantiasis).

e. gingivae. See **fibromatosis gingivae.**

elevator, an instrument used to raise or lift something.

e., dental, one of a variety of blades used for engaging teeth and/or roots to remove them from their alveoli.

e., malar, an instrument used to elevate or reposition the zygomatic bone.

e., periosteal, a thin blade used to lift periosteum from bone.

eligibility date, the date an individual and/or dependents become eligible for benefits under a dental benefits contract. Often referred to as *effective date.*

eligibility rules, conditions that define who may be entitled to dental benefits, when persons first become entitled to such benefits, and any provisions that determine how long an individual remains entitled to benefits.

eligible person. See **beneficiary.**

ELISA, the abbreviation for **enzyme-linked immunosorbent assay** used to detect the presence of HIV antibody to HIV in the blood.

elixir (ēlik'sər), a pleasantly flavored, sweetened hydroalcoholic solution of a drug intended for oral administration.

elliptocytosis (ēlip'tōsītō'sis) (ovalcytosis, oval cell anemia), a hereditary anomaly in which the red blood cells are elliptical, or oval shaped, and are predisposed to hemolysis.

elongation (i'longā'shən), the process or condition of increasing in length before breaking; indicates ductility (for example, a metal).

e., percent, **I.** the increase in length of a material after fracture in tension. **2.** a mechanical test usually employed to measure ductility.

emaciation, excessive leanness caused by disease or lack of nutrition.

embedded, referring to a tooth, root tip, or foreign body that is covered in bone.

embolism (em'bəliz'əm), the clogging of a vessel by matter, such as a clot, air, or oil, that is carried by the bloodstream to some point where the lumen of the vessel narrows. This is the opposite of thrombosis, in which the clotting mechanism is organized in situ.

e., air. See **aeroembolism.**

embolus (em'bələs), a blood clot or other material that travels in the bloodstream and then lodges in a vessel and obstructs circulation.

embrasure, an opening, as in a wall. The space between the curved proximal surfaces of the teeth.

e., buccal, an embrasure that opens toward the cheeks.

e. clasp. See **clasp, embrasure.**

e. hook, an extension of a removable partial denture into the embrasure above the contact area between two adjacent teeth, which resists movement in a cervical direction.

e., interdental, the spaces formed by the interproximal contours of adjoining teeth, beginning at the contact area and extending lingually, facially, occlusally, and apically.

e., labial, an embrasure that opens toward the lips.

e., lingual, an embrasure that opens toward the tongue.

e., occlusal, an embrasure that opens toward the occlusal surface or plane.

embryo, an organism in the earliest stages of development; in humans the stage between the time of implantation of the fertilized ovum until the end of the seventh or eighth week of gestation.

embryology, the study of the origin, growth, development, and function of an organism from fertilization to birth.

emergency, an unforeseen occurrence or combination of circumstances that calls for immediate action or remedy; pressing necessity; exigency.

e. medicine, a branch of medicine concerned with the diagnosis and treatment of conditions resulting from trauma or sudden illness.

e. treatment, treatment that must be rendered to the patient immediately because of acute infection or pain.

emesis (em'əsis, əmē'sis), the sudden expulsion of gastric contents through the esophagus into the pharynx. The act is partly voluntary and partly involuntary. See also **vomiting.**

emetic (imet'ik), a drug that induces vomiting.

emetine hydrochloride (em'ətēn), an alkaloid, $C_{29}H_{40}N_2O_4 \cdot 2HCl$, regarded as a protozoacide and formerly used in the treatment of periodontitis and amebic dysentery.

EMF, the abbreviation for **erythrocyte-maturing factor.**

eminence, retromylohyoid (em'in-ens, ret'rōmilōhī·oid), the distal end of the lingual flange of a lower denture. It occupies the retromylohyoid space. (not current)

eminenectomy (əm'inenek'tomē), the operative removal of the anterior articular surface of the glenoid fossa.

emollient (imōl'yənt), an agent that is soothing to the skin or mucous membrane; makes the skin softer or smoother.

emotiometabolic (ēmō'shē·ōmet'ə-bol'ik), modifying metabolism as a result of emotion. (not current)

emotion, a complex feeling or state (affect) accompanied by characteristic motor and glandular activities; feelings; mood.

emotional, description of a person experiencing an emotion; manifesting emotional behavior, rather than logical, rational behavior; a person who is easily or excessively given to emotion.

empathy, putting oneself into the psychologic frame of reference of another, so that the other person's feeling, thinking, and acting are understood and to some extent predictable. A desirable trust-building characteristic of a helping profession. It is embodied in the sincere statement, "I understand how you feel." Empathy is different from sympathy in that to be empathetic one understands how the person feels rather than actually experiencing those feelings as in sympathy.

emphysema (em'fisē'mə), **l.** a swelling caused by air in the tissue spaces. In the oral and facial regions it may be caused either by air introduced into a tooth socket or gingival crevice with the air syringe, or by blowing of the nose. **2.** a permanent dilation of the respiratory alveoli.

employee, a person who, under the direction and control of the employer, performs services for remuneration.

Employee Retirement Income Security Act (ERISA), a federal act, passed in 1974, that established new standards and reporting and disclosure requirements for employer-funded pension and health benefits programs. To date, self-funded health benefit plans operating under ERISA have been held to be exempt from state insurance laws. This exemption is currently under review.

employer-sponsored plan, a program supported totally or in part by an employer or group of employers to provide dental benefits for employees. The plan may be administered directly by the employer or another person or group under a contractual arrangement. Part of the cost may be borne by the employee.

employment, l. to be engaged in work for hire. **2.** to use a specific tool or technique in the accomplishment of a task.

empyema (em'pī·ē'mə, em'pē·ē'mə), the presence of pus in a cavity, hollow organ, or space (for example, the pleural cavity).

emulsifiers, an agent such as gum arabic or egg yolk used to suspend droplets of oil in a water-based solution. An agent to maintain any element or particle in suspension within a fluid medium.

emulsion (iməl'shən), a colloidal dispersion of one liquid in another. See also **suspension.**

e., double, a suspension of sensitive silver halide salts impregnated in gelatin and coated on both sides of a radiographic film base.

e., silver, a suspension of sensitive silver halide salts impregnated in gelatin and used for coating photographic plates and radiographic films.

e., single, a suspension of sensitive silver halide salts impregnated in gelatin and coated on only one side of a radiographic film base.

enalapril maleate, *trade names:* Vasotec, Vasotec IV; *drug class:* angiotensin-converting enzyme (ACE) inhibitor; *action:* selectively suppresses renin-angiotensin-aldosterone system; inhibits ACE; prevents conversion of angiotensin I to angiotensin II leading to dilation of arterial and venous vessels; *uses:* hypertension, heart failure adjunct.

enamel, I. the hard, glistening tissue covering the anatomic crown of the tooth. It is composed chiefly of hexagonal rods of hydroxyapatite, sheathed in an organic matrix (approximately 0.15%), and oriented with their long axis approximately at right angles to the surface. **2.** the outermost layer or covering of the coronal portion of the tooth that overlies and protects the dentin.

e., mottled. See **fluorosis, chronic endemic dental.**

e. pearl. See **pearl, enamel.**

enameloma. See **pearl, enamel.**

enanthem (enan'thəm). See **enanthema.**

enanthema (en'anthē'mə) (enanthem), lesions involving the mucous membrane.

encephalitis, an inflammatory condition of the brain.

encounter form, a document or record used to collect data about given elements of a patient visit to a dental office or similar site that can become part of a patient record or be used for management purposes or for quality review activities.

end-bulb. See **end-feet.**

end-feet (boutons terminaux, end-bulb), small, terminal enlargements of nerve fibers that are in contact with the dendrites or cell bodies of other nerve cells; the synaptic ending of a nerve fiber.

ending, a termination; the point at which something is concluded.

e., annulospiral, a nerve ending, associated with an intrafusal muscle fiber, that is stimulated by a stretch impulse resulting from the extension of a muscle. The ending is in the form of a gradual spiral around the length of the intrafusal muscle fiber in the muscle spindle and is connected to the coarse myelinated fibers.

e., flower spray, a sensory nerve ending that is attached to the distal end of an intrafusal muscle fiber and that is stimulated when the muscle fiber contracts, pulling on the nerve ending.

e., free nerve, the peripheral terminal of the sensory nerve.

endocarditis, bacterial, an inflammation of the heart valves and lining of the heart as a result of a bacterial infection.

endocarditis, subacute bacterial (SBE) (en'dōkardĭ'tis), a bacterial infection involving the endocardium that occurs primarily after bacteremia and the establishment of bacterial vegetation on an area of defective endocardium such as is found in patients with rheumatic or congenital heart disease.

endochondral bone. See **bone, endochondral.**

endocrine, refers to either the gland that secretes directly into the systemic circulation or the substance secreted.

e. diseases, an abnormal condition caused by some malfunction of an endocrine gland.

e. system, the interrelated nature of the physiologic function of endocrine glands.

endocrinology, the study of the anatomy, physiology, biochemistry, and pathology of the endocrine system and the treatment of endocrine problems.

endodontally involved (en'dōdon'tələ), pertaining to disease of the dental pulp and dental periapical tissues.

endodontia (en'dōdon'tē-ə) (not current). See **endodontology.**

endodontic implant, a metallic implant extending through the root canal into the periapical bone structure to increase support and retention of the tooth.

endodontics (en'dōdon'tiks), the branch of dental practice that applies the knowledge of endodontology.

endodontic techniques, procedures used in pulpless teeth or teeth that are to be made pulpless.

endodontist (en'dōdon'tist), a dentist who practices endodontics as a specialty.

endodontology (en'dōdontäl'ōjē) (endodontia, pulp canal therapy, root canal therapy), the division of dental science that deals with the etiology, diagnosis, prevention, and treatment of diseases of the dental pulp and their sequelae.

endolith (en'dōlith) (not current). See **denticle.**

endonuclease, an enzyme (nuclease) that cleaves polynucleotides at interior bonds, producing polynucleotide or oligonucleotide fragments.

endophthalmitis, an inflammation of the tissues of the eyeball.

endoplasmic reticulum, an extensive network of membrane-enclosed tubules in the cytoplasm of a cell.

end organ, the expanded termination of a nerve fiber in muscle, skin, mucous membrane, or other structure.

e. o., proprioceptor, sensory end organs, located chiefly in the muscles, tendons, and labyrinth, that provide information on the movements and position of the body. Four specific end organs are the muscle spindles; Golgi corpuscles, stimulated by tension; Pacini's corpuscles, stimulated by pressure; and bare nerve endings, stimulated by pain.

e. o., sensory, sensory nerve fibers that end peripherally as either unmyelinated fibers or special structures called *receptors.* Receptors are situated in the skin, mucous membranes, muscles, tendons, joints, and other structures and also in such special sense organs as those for vision, hearing, smell, and taste. The receptors are organized into a system that relates them to the environment: extroceptors, interoceptors, and proprioceptors.

endoscopy, the visualization of the interior of organs and cavities of the body with an illuminated flexible optical tube.

e., gastrointestinal, the visualization of the interior of the stomach and intestines with an illuminated flexible optical tube.

endosteal implants. See **implants, endosteal.**

endosteum (endos'tē-əm), a thin layer of connective tissue that lines the walls of the bone marrow cavities and haversian canals of compact bone and covers the trabeculae of cancellous bone. Endosteum has both osteogenic and hematopoietic potencies and, like the periosteum, takes an active part in the healing of fractures.

endothelioma (en'dōthē'lē-ō'mə). See **tumor, Ewing's.**

endothelium, the layer of simple squamous epithelial cells that line the heart, the blood and lymph vessels, and the serous cavities of the body.

endotoxin (en'dōtäk'sin), a nondiffusible lipid polysaccharide-polypeptide complex formed within bacteria (some gram-negative bacilli and others); when released from the destroyed bacterial cells, endotoxin is capable of producing a toxic manifestation within the host.

end-plate, the terminal fibers of the motor nerves to the voluntary muscles. The nerve endings lose their myelin sheaths as they enter the sheaths of striated muscle fibers, at which point they ramify across the muscle fiber like the roots of a tree.

e.-p., motor, the end-plate by which impulses from nerves are transmitted to the muscle fibers. It is a modification of the sarcolemma and is continuous with it. The end-plate potential generated by the nerve impulse activates the muscle impulse.

end section, the distal portion of a twin-wire labial arch wire, consisting of a tube in which the anterior section of the labial arch is engaged.

end-to-end bite, See occlusion, edge-to-edge.

end-to-end occlusion. See occlusion, edge-to-edge.

Endur, the brand name for a two-paste diacrylate resin adhesive used as a bonding agent in orthodontics.

enema, a procedure in which a solution is introduced into the rectum for cleansing or therapeutic purposes.

energy, the capacity for doing work.

e., atomic, energy that can be liberated by changes in the nucleus of an atom.

e., binding, energy represented by the difference in mass between the sum of the component parts and the actual mass of the nucleus of an atom.

e. dependence, the characteristic response of a radiation detector to a given range of radiation energies or wavelengths as compared with the response of a standard free-air chamber. Emulsions also show energy dependence.

e., excitation, energy required to change a system from its ground state to an excited state. With each excited state there is associated a different excitation energy. See also **excitation.**

e., ionizing, the average energy lost by ionizing radiation in producing an ion pair in a gas. (For air, ionizing energy is about 33 V.)

e., kinetic, energy possessed by a mass because of its motion.

e., nuclear. See **energy, atomic.**

e., photon (hv), electromagnetic energy in the form of photons, with a value in ergs equal to the product of their frequency in cycles per second and Planck's constant (E = hv).

e., potential, energy inherent in a mass because of its position with reference to other masses.

e., radiant, the energy of electromagnetic waves, such as radio waves, visible light, x-rays, and gamma rays.

enflurane, a nonflammable anesthetic gas belonging to the ether family, used for induction and maintenance of general anesthesia.

engine, dental, an electric motor that, by means of a continuous-cord drive over pulleys, activates a handpiece that holds a rotary instrument.

engineering, the organized application of the sciences of mathematics, physics, chemistry, and biology to the solving of problems.

e., dental, the application of physical, mechanical, and mathematical principles to dentistry.

Engman's disease (not current). See **dermatitis, infectiosa eczematoides.**

enkephalin, one of two pain-relieving pentapeptides produced in the body.

enlargement, an increase in size.

e., Dilantin. See **hyperplasia, gingival, Dilantin.**

e., idiopathic, gingival enlargement, of unknown causation, clinically characterized by a firm, rounded thickening of the gingival tissues and histologically characterized by connective tissue hyperplasia of the gingival corium.

enostosis (en'ōstō'sis), a bony growth located within a bone cavity or centrally from the cortical plate. See also **osteoma.**

enoxacin, *trade name:* Penetrex; *drug class:* Fluoroquinolone antiinfective; *action:* a broad-spectrum bactericidal agent that inhibits the enzyme DNA gyrase needed for replication of DNA; *uses:* uncomplicated urethral or cervical gonorrhea, uncomplicated and complicated urinary tract infections.

enrollee, an individual covered by a benefit plan. See **beneficiary.**

Entamoeba gingivalis (en'tǝmē'bǝ), a genus of protozoan amoeba found in the mouth; repeatedly, but not conclu-sively, associated with the initiation and/or perpetuation of periodontitis.

enteric coating (enter'ik). See **coating, enteric.**

enteritis, an inflammation of the mucosal lining of the small intestine.

Enterobacter cloacae, a common species of bacteria found in human and animal feces, dairy products, sewage, soil, and water. It is rarely the cause of disease.

Enterobacteriaceae, a family of aerobic and anaerobic bacteria that includes both normal and pathogenic enteric microorganisms such as *Escherichia, Klebsiella, Proteus,* and *Salmonella.*

enterococcus, any *Streptococcus* bacterium that inhabits the intestinal tract.

entropion (entrō'pē·on), the inversion, or infolding, of the eyelid margin.

enucleate (enōō'klē·āt), to remove a lesion in its entirety.

enunciation, an auxiliary function of teeth, particularly those in the anterior sector of the dental arch; the formation of sounds as in speech.

enuresis (enyōōrē'sis), involuntary urination (for example, during general anesthesia, at night).

environment (envī'rōnment), the aggregate of all the external conditions and influences affecting the life and development of an organism.

e., extracellular, the external, or interstitial, environment provided and maintained for the tissue cells.

e., oral, the aggregate of all oral conditions and influences.

environmental health, the total of various aspects of substances, forces, and conditions in and about a community that affect the health and well-being of the population.

environmental pollutants, substances and conditions, including noise, that adversely affect the health and well-being of the people within a community.

environmental pollution, the presence of substances and conditions that adversely affect the health and well-being of people within a community; usually substances in the air and water supply.

Environmental Protection Agency (EPA), a federal agency charged with the approval and overseeing of the use and disposal of hazardous materials. Workplace management of hazardous materials falls under the jurisdiction of the Occupational Safety and Health Administration (OSHA).

enzyme (en'zīm), a protein substance that acts as a catalyst to speed up metabolic and other processes involve organic materials. Some enzymes function within cells; others function in the extracellular fluids and tissue spaces and organs. They are active in all major tissue functions, such as cellular respiration, muscle contraction, digestive processes, and energy consumption, and are produced intracellularly.

e.-linked immunosorbent assay, a species-specific serologic laboratory procedure used to identify microorganisms infecting or inhabiting a tissue or organ system. Its dental use is in the identification of pathogens involved in periodontal disease.

eosinophil (o'-əsin' əfil). See **leukocyte, eosinophilic.**

eosinophilia (ē'-əsin'əfil'ē-ə), an absolute or relative increase in the normal number of eosinophils in the circulating blood. Various limits are given (for example, absolute eosinophilia if the total number exceeds $500/\text{mm}^3$ and relative if greater than 3% but total less than 500 mm^3. It may be associated with skin diseases, infestations, hay fever, asthma, angioneurotic edema, adrenocortical insufficiency, and Hodgkin's disease.

eosinophilic granuloma. See **granuloma, eosinophilic.**

EPA. See **Environmental Protection Agency.**

ephedrine sulfate, *trade name:* generic; *drug class:* adrenergic, mixed direct and indirect effects; *action:* causes increased contractility and heart rate by acting on β-receptors in heart; also acts on α-receptors, causing vasoconstriction in blood vessels; *uses:* shock, increased perfusion, hypotension, bronchodilation.

ephelis (efe'lis) (freckle), a circumscribed macular collection of pigment in the epidermis or oral mucosa. An increased amount of melanin pigment is seen in the region of the basal layer of cells.

epidemiology (ep'idē'mē-ol'əjē), the science of epidemics and epidemic diseases, which involve the total population rather than the individual. The aim of epidemiology is to determine those factors in the group environment that make the group more or less susceptible to disease.

epidermal cyst, a common, benign, variable, subcutaneous swelling lined by keratinizing epithelium and filled with a cheesy material composed of sebum and epithelial debris.

epidermis, the superficial, avascular layers of the skin.

epidermolysis bullosa (ep'idərmäl'isis), a disease of the skin characterized by bullae, vesicles, cysts, and, often, associated mandibular enlargement. See also **syndrome, Goldscheider's** and **syndrome, Weber-Cockayne.**

epiglottis (ep'iglot'is), an elastic cartilage, covered by mucous membrane, that forms the superior part of the larynx and guards the glottis during swallowing.

epilepsy (ep'ilep'sē), a group of neurologic disorders characterized by recurrent episodes of convulsive seizures, sensory disturbances, abnormal behavior, and loss of consciousness. Most epilepsy is of an unknown cause but may be associated with cerebral trauma, brain tumors, vascular disturbances, or chemical imbalance. Drugs used in the treatment of symptoms (for example, hydantoin sodium, diphenylhydantoin sodium) promote gingival hyperplasia.

epiloia (epiloi'yə). See **syndrome, Bourneville Pringle.**

epinephrine (ep'inef'rin), a hormone secreted by the adrenal medulla that stimulates hepatic glycogenolysis, causing an elevation in the blood sugar, vasodilation of blood vessels of the skeletal muscles, vasoconstriction of the arterioles of the skin and mucous membranes, relaxation of bronchiolar smooth muscles, and stimulation of heart action. Used in local anesthetics for its vasoconstrictive action.

e./e. bitartrate/e. HCl, trade names: EpiPen Jr., Bronkaid Mist, Primatene Mist; *drug class:* adrenergic agonist, catecholamine; *action:* β_1- and β_2-agonist causing increased levels of cAMP, producing bronchodilation and cardiac stimulation; *uses:* acute asthmatic attacks, hemostasis, bronchospasm, anaphylaxis, allergic reactions, cardiac arrest, vasopressor.

epiphysis (epif'isis), the terminal portion of a long bone. The epiphysis is separated from the diaphysis during growth by a cartilaginous zone that serves as a growth center. Once ossification unites the epiphysis with the diaphysis, growth is completed.

epispinal (epispī′nəl), located on the spinal column.

epistaxis (ep′istak′sis) (nosebleed), bleeding from the nose.

epithelial (ep′ithē′lē·əl), pertaining to the epithelium.

e. attachment. See **attachment, epithelial.**

e. cuff, attached, the attachment of the gingival epithelium to the enamel, including the close approximation of the free gingiva to the tooth.

e. cuff, implant, the band of tissue that is constricted around an implant abutment post.

e. inclusion, bits of epithelial tissue introduced into bone crypts during perforation osteotomies. See also **osteotomy, perforation.**

epithelioma (ep′ithē′lē·ō′mə), an epithelial cancer.

e. adenoides cysticum (Brooke's tumor, trichoepithelioma), a form of basal cell carcinoma believed to arise from the epithelium of hair follicles. Regarded as a less invasive form of basal cell carcinoma.

e., basal cell. See **carcinoma, basal cell.**

epithelium (ep′ithē′lē·əm), the structural arrangement of the various cellular components of epithelium characterized by two basic forms: medium suprapapillary width with medium-length rete pegs, and narrow suprapapillary width with long rete pegs.

e., basement membrane of. See **membrane, basement.**

e., desmosomes of, an electronmicroscopic finding of intercellular bridges that serve to attach adjacent epithelial cells to each other.

e., enamel, inner, the innermost layer of cells (ameloblasts) of the enamel organ that deposit the organic matrix of the enamel on the crown of the developing tooth. Also the innermost layer of Hertwig's epithelial root sheath.

e., enamel, outer, the outermost layer of cells of the enamel organ. It is separated from the inner enamel epithelium in the area of the developing crown by the stratum intermedium and stellate reticulum and lies immediately adjacent to the inner enamel epithelium in the area of the developing root.

e., enamel, reduced, combined enamel epithelium; the remains of the enamel organ after enamel formation is complete. After eruption of the tip of the crown, that part of the combined epithelium remaining on the enamel surface is called the *epithelial attachment.*

e., gingival, a stratified squamous epithelium consisting of a basal layer; it is keratinized or parakeratinized when comprising the attached gingiva.

e., hyperplastic, an increase in thickness, with alterations in structure, produced by proliferation of cellular elements of epithelium. The stratum spinosum epidermidis is usually the layer of cells that become thickened, resulting in acanthosis.

e., oral, the epithelial covering of the oral mucous membranes. Composed of stratified squamous epithelium of varying thickness and varying degrees of keratinization.

e., pocket, the epithelium that lines the gingival or periodontal pocket. Its most prominent characteristics are the presence of hyperplasia and ulceration, with exposure to the corium of the gingiva.

e., squamous, epithelium consisting of flat, scalelike cells.

e., stratified squamous, the variety of epithelium prevalent as the covering of the oral mucous membrane and of dermal surfaces; composed of layers of cells oriented parallel to the surface. The various layers of cells in order of ascent from basement membrane to surface are stratum germinativum, stratum spongiosum, stratum granulosum, stratum lucidum (in dermal epithelium), and stratum corneum. The gingival epithelium generally exhibits some degree of keratinization, variable from parakeratosis to hyperkeratosis.

e., sulcal, the stratified squamous epithelium forming the covering of the soft tissue wall of the gingival sulcus, or crevice. Extends from the gingival margin to the line of attachment of the epithelium to the tooth surface.

epithelization (ep′ithe′lizā′shən), the natural act of healing by secondary intention; the proliferation of new epithelium into an area devoid of it but which naturally is covered by it.

epizootic fever (not current), another name for foot and mouth disease in cloven-foot animals; also known as *aphthous fever;* caused by a type of coxsackievirus, uncommon in the United States. The disease in man is characterized by malaise, fever, headache, itchy skin, and a sensation of dry mouth despite heavy salivation. Vesicles appear in the mouth, around the lips, and on the hands and feet. Vesicles and ulcers of the mouth disappear within about 10 days.

epoxy resin (ĕpäk′sē). See **resin, epoxy.**

Epstein-Barr virus, a herpetovirus associated with Burkitt's lymphoma and reported in cases of infectious mononucleosis; more recently reported associated with AIDS.

Epstein's pearls. See **nodules, Bohn's.**

epulis (ep′yōō′lis), a tumor (tumescence) of the gingiva.

e., congenital of newborn, a raised or pedunculated lesion located on the anterior gingivae of the newborn. It is histologically similar to granular cell myoblastoma. See also **myoblastoma, granular cell.**

e. fissurata (inflammatory fibrous hyperplasia, redundant tissue), a curtainlike fold of excess tissue associated with the flange of a denture.

e., giant cell. See **granuloma, giant cell reparative, peripheral.**

e. granulomatosa, a tumorlike mass of red, easily bleeding, infected granulation tissue that occurs as a result of exuberant reparative phenomena. Seen arising from tooth sockets or is associated with exfoliating necrotic bone.

equilibration (ē′kwilibrā′shən), the act of placing a body in a state of equilibrium.

e., diagnostic. See **diagnostic equilibration.**

e., mandibular, the act or acts performed to place the mandible in a state of equilibrium.

e., occlusal, the modification of occlusal forms of teeth by grinding, with the intent of equalizing occlusal stress and of harmonizing cuspal relations in function.

e. of mounted casts, equilibration of the occlusion of mounted casts made of a patient for the purpose of observ-

ing and recording what must be done to adjust the natural occlusion.

equilibrator (ē′kwilibrā′tor), an instrument or device used in achieving or maintaining a state of equilibrium.

equilibrium (ē′kwilib′rēəm), a state of balance between two opposing forces or processes.

e., functional, the state of homeostasis within the oral cavity existing when biologic processes and local environmental factors, including the forces of mastication, are in a state of balance.

equipment, the nonexpendable items used by the dentist in the performance of professional duties.

equity, a free and reasonable claim or right; fairness; impartiality. The money value of a property or of an interest in a property in excess of claims or liens against it; a risk interest or ownership right in property.

equivalent, equal in force, value, measure, or effect; corresponding in function.

e., aluminum, the thickness of pure aluminum affording the same radiation attenuation, under specified conditions, as the material or materials being considered.

e., concrete, the thickness of concrete having a density of 2.35 g/cm^3 that would afford the same radiation attenuation, under specified conditions, as the material or materials being considered.

e., lead, the thickness of pure lead that would afford the same radiation attenuation, under specified conditions, as the material or materials being considered.

erbium, a rare-earth, metallic element with an atomic number of 68 and an atomic weight of 167.26.

erg, a unit of energy equal to the energy consumed by 1 dyne acting through 1 cm, which is equal to 10^{-7} joule.

ergoloid mesylate, *trade names:* Hydergine LC, Gerimal; *drug class:* ergot alkaloids; *action:* may increase cerebral metabolism and blood flow; *uses:* senile dementia, Alzheimer's dementia, primary progressive dementia.

ergotamine tartrate, *trade names:* Ergomar, Ergostat; *drug class:* α-adrenergic blocker; *action:* constricts by direct action vascular smooth muscle in peripheral and cranial blood vessels, relaxes uterine muscle; *uses:* vascular headache (migraine or histamine), cluster headache.

ergotoxine (er′gōtox′in), a potent alkaloid that paralyzes the motor and secretory nerves of the sympathetic system but has no effect on the inhibitory or parasympathetic nerves.

ERISA, the acronym for the Employee Retirement Income Security Act of 1974. See also **Employee Retirement Income Security Act.**

erosion (erō′zhən), the chemical or mechanicochemical destruction of tooth substance, the mechanism of which is incompletely known, that leads to the creation of concavities of many shapes at the cementoenamel junction of teeth. The surface of the cavity, unlike dental caries, is hard and smooth.

error, a violation of duty; a fault; a mistake in the proceedings of a court in matters of law or of fact.

e., legal, a mistaken judgment or incorrect belief as to the existence or effect of matters of fact, or a false or mistaken conception or application of the law.

e., numerical, the amount of loss or precision in a quantity; the difference between an accurate quantity and its calculated approximation. Errors occur in numerical methods; mistakes occur in programming, coding, data transcription, and operating; malfunctions occur in computers and are caused by physical limitations of the properties of materials.

e. of measurement, the deviation of an individual score or observation from its true value, caused by the unreliability of the instrument and the individual who is measuring.

e., sampling, any mistake in drawing a sample that keeps it from being unrepresentative; selection procedures that are biased; error introduced when a group is described on the basis of an unrepresentative sample.

e., variance, that part of the total variance caused by anything irrelevant to a study that cannot be experimentally controlled.

eruption (erup′shən), the migration of a tooth from within its follicle in the alveolar process of the maxilla or mandible into the oral cavity.

e., continuous, the normal occlusal progression of teeth noted throughout a lifetime.

e. cyst, a dentigerous cyst that causes a clinically evident bulging of the overlying alveolar ridge. See also **cysts, eruption.**

e., ectopic, the abnormal direction of tooth eruption, most common to mandibular first and third molars, which sometimes leads to abnormal resorption of the adjacent tooth.

e. hematoma, an eruption cyst that is blood-filled, visualized as a bluish purple area of elevated tissue of the overlying alveolar ridge.

e., passive, an increasing length of the clinical crown often seen with aging and in the absence of clinical evidence of inflammation. The stages of passive eruption are as follows: (1) the most apical limit of the epithelial attachment is at the cementoenamel junction; (2) the most apical limit of the attachment is on the cementum, with the base of the gingival sulcus still on the enamel surface; (3) the most apical limit of the epithelial attachment is on the cementum, with the base of the sulcus at the cementoenamel junction; and (4) both the base of the sulcus and the epithelial attachment are on the surface of the cementum.

e., surgical, the surgical removal of tissues covering an abnormally unerupted tooth to allow its natural progress into position.

eruptive gingivitis. See **gingivitis, eruptive.**

erysipelas, an infectious skin disease characterized by redness, swelling, vesicles, bullae, fever, pain, and lymphadenopathy. It is caused by a species of group A β-hemolytic streptococci.

erythema (er′ithē′mə), a patchy, circumscribed, or marginated macular redness of the skin or mucous membranes caused by hyperemia or inflammation.

e. multiforme complex, an acute, inflammatory dermatologic disease of uncertain etiology (although occasionally related to drug administration), characterized by erythematous macules, papules, vesicles, and bullae that appear on the skin and not infrequently on the oral mucosa. See also **syndrome, Stevens-Johnson.**

erythredema polyneuropathy (erith′re-dē′mə pol′inōōrop′əthē) (acrodynia, Feer's disease, pink disease, Selter's disease, Swift's disease), a disease of infancy believed to be caused by mercury poisoning. It is manifested by itching of the hands and feet, profuse sweating, hypertension, vasomotor disturbances, bruxism, and precocious shedding of the teeth.

erythremia (er′ithrē′mē-ə) (Osler's disease, polycythemia rubra, polycythemia vera, primary polycythemia, Vaquez' disease), a myeloproliferative disease characterized by a marked increase in the circulating red blood cell mass. Erythremia may represent a neoplastic growth of erythropoietic tissue. Neutrophilia, thrombocytopenia, and splenomegaly are common. Manifestations include plethora, vertigo, headache, and thrombosis.

erythroblastosis fetalis (erith′rō-blastō′sis fetal′is), an excessive destruction of red blood cells begun before or shortly after birth. It may be caused by an Rh factor reaction. The skin is yellow, and the teeth may be markedly discolored.

erythrityl tetranitrate, *trade name:* Cardilate; *drug class:* organic nitrate; *action:* causes relaxation of vascular smooth muscle; decreases preload/afterload, which is responsible for decreasing left ventricular end diastolic pressure; systemic vascular resistance; improved exercise tolerance; *uses:* chronic stable angina pectoris, prophylaxis of angina pain.

Erythrocin, the brand name for **erythromycin.**

erythrocyte (erith′rōsīt), red blood cell; a nonnucleated, circular, biconcave, discoid, hemoglobin-containing, oxygen-carrying formed element circulating in the blood.

e. count, the number of red blood cells per cubic millimeter of blood.

e. indices, the standard values of red blood cell numbers, morphologic characteristics, and behavior in comprehensive hematologic laboratory testing.

e.-maturing factor (EMF) (not current). See **vitamin, cyanocobalamin.**

e. sedimentation rate (ESR), the rate at which red blood cells settle in a pipette of unclotted blood, measured in millimeters per hour. It is used as an index of inflammation.

erythrocytosis (erith′rōsītō′sis) (secondary polycythemia), an increased circulating red blood cell mass resulting from compensatory effort to meet reduced oxygen content. May be seen in persons living at high altitudes, as well as in persons with emphysema, pulmonary insufficiency, and heart failure.

erythromycin, an antibiotic produced by a strain of *Streptomyces erythroeus,* effective against β-hemolytic streptococci (viridans group), and upper and lower respiratory tract, skin, and soft tissue infections of mild to moderate severity. Recommended by the American Heart Association and the American Dental Association for use in a regimen for prophylaxis against bacterial endocarditis in patients hypersensitive to penicillin.

e. base (et al), trade names: E-mycin, Ery-Tab (et al); *drug class:* macrolide antibiotic; *action:* binds to 50S ribosomal subunits of susceptible bacteria and suppresses protein synthesis; *uses:* infections caused by *Neisseria gonorrhoeae;* mild-to moderate respiratory tract, skin, soft tissue infections caused by *Streptococcus pneumoniae, Coryne-bacterium diphtheriae, Bordetella pertussis;* syphilis; Legionnaire's disease; *Haemophilus influenzae;* endocarditis prophylaxis.

erythroplasia of Queyrat (erith′rōplā′zhə əv kərat′), a form of intraepithelial carcinoma. The oral lesions are usually seen as plaques with a bright, velvety surface.

escharotic (es′kärot′ik), a caustic or corrosive agent that has the strength to burn tissue. (not current)

Escherichia coli, a species of coliform bacteria normally present in the intestines and common in water, milk, and soil.

esculin, a glucoside from horse-chestnut bark; used as a sunburn protective.

esophageal atresia, an abnormal esophagus that ends in a blind pouch or narrows to a thin cord and thus fails to provide a continuous passage to the stomach. It is usually a congenital anomaly.

esophageal stenosis, a narrowing or restriction of the lumen of the esophagus that slows or impedes the passage of fluid and foods from the mouth to the stomach.

esophagitis, an inflammation of the mucosal lining of the esophagus caused by infection or irritation of the mucosa by reflux of gastric juice from the stomach.

esophagus, the muscular canal, about 25 cm long, extending from the pharynx to the stomach.

E space, the net difference between the combined mesiodistal width of the primary canine, primary first molar, and the primary second molar and that of the permanent canine, first premolar, and second premolar. In the mandible the mean leeway space is 3.4 mm, and in the maxilla it is 1.9 mm. Synonym: leeway space.

essence (es′ens), an alcoholic solution of an essential oil.

essential oil. See **oil, essential.**

Essig-type splinting. See **splinting, Essig-type.** (not current)

estate, one's interest in land or other property.

e. planning, a detailed, written-out plan (usually arrived at with the advice of estate counselors), in which all the financial affairs of the dentist are clearly stated and provisions are made for alterations when changing conditions warrant it.

estazolam, *trade name:* ProSom; *drug class:* benzodiazepine, sedative-hypnotic, Controlled Substance Schedule IV in US; *action:* produces CNS depression by interaction with benzodiazepine receptor; *use:* insomnia.

ester (es′tər), any compound formed from alcohol and an acid.

esterase (es′tərās), an enzyme that catalyzes the hydrolysis of an ester into its alcohol and acid.

esterified estrogens, *trade names:* Estabs, Estratab, Menest; *drug class:* synthetic estrogen; *action:* required for development, maintenance, and adequate function of female reproductive system by increasing synthesis of DNA, RNA, and selected proteins; decreases release of gonadotropine-releasing hormone; inhibits ovulation and helps maintain bone structure; *uses:* menopause, breast cancer, prostatic cancer, hypogonadism, ovariectomy, primary ovarian failure.

esthetics (esthet′iks) (aesthetics), the branch of philosophy dealing with beauty, especially with the components thereof; that is, color and form.

e., dentistry, refers to those skills and techniques used to improve the art and symmetry of the teeth and face to improve the appearance as well as the function of the teeth, mouth, and face.

e., denture, the cosmetic effect, produced by a denture, that affects the desirable beauty, charm, character, and dignity of the individual.

e., denture base (gingival tissue esthetics), the esthetically proper tinting, contouring, and festooning of the gingival tissue portion of a denture base.

e., gingival tissue. See **esthetics, denture base.**

estimate, the anticipated fee for dental services to be performed.

Estlander's operation (not current). See **operation, Abbé-Estlander.**

estoppel (estäp′əl), a preclusion, in law, that prevents a person from alleging or denying a fact because of his or her own previous act or allegation.

estradiol benzoate (es′trədī′ōl ben′zōat), a topical steroid (B-estradiol-3-benzoate) with estrogenic activity, useful in the treatment of lesions produced by diminution of bodily production of estrogens. Experimental administration to aged laboratory mice has resulted in an increased downgrowth of epithelial attachment along the root surface of teeth and subsequent production of periodontal disease.

estradiol/estradiol cypionate/ estradiol valerate, *trade names:* Deladiol, Depogen, Estro-Cyp, Estra-LA; *drug class:* estrogen; *action:* increases synthesis of DNA, RNA, and selected proteins, decreases release of gonadotropin-releasing hormone, inhibits ovulation, and helps maintain bone structure; *uses:* menopause, breast cancer, prostatic cancer, atrophic vaginitis, kraurosis vulvae, hypogonadism, ovariectomy, primary ovarian failure.

estradiol transdermal system, *trade names:* Estraderm, Climara; *drug class:* estrogen; *action:* increases synthesis of DNA, RNA, and selected proteins; decreases release of gonadotropin-releasing hormone; inhibits ovulation and helps maintain bone structure;

uses: menopause, breast cancer, prostatic cancer, abnormal uterine bleeding, hypogonadism, ovariectomy, osteoporosis.

estrin (es'trin), the generic term for the ovarian estrogens estriol, estrone, and estradiol.

estrogens (es'trōjenz), the collective term for substances capable of producing estrus. The term also applies to the estrogenic hormones in women. Estriol is the principal estrogen found in the urine of pregnant women and in the placenta. Synthetic estrogens include diethylstilbestrol, hexestrol, and ethinyl estradiol.

etch, acid. See **acid etching.**

etching, a process used to decalcify the superficial layers of enamel as a step in the application of sealants or bonding agents in preventive dentistry and orthodontics. The agent of choice is phosphoric acid in concentrations of 30% to 40%.

ethacrynate sodium/ethacrynic acid, *trade name:* Edecrin Sodium; *drug class:* loop diuretic; *action:* acts on loop of Henle by increasing excretion of chloride, sodium; *uses:* pulmonary edema, edema in CHF, liver disease, nephrotic syndrome, ascites, hypertension.

ethambutal HCl, *trade name:* Myambutol; *drug class:* antitubercular; *action:* inhibits RNA synthesis, decreases tubercle bacilli replication; *uses:* pulmonary tuberculosis, as adjunct.

ethane, a constituent of natural and "bottled" gases.

ether, diethyl (ē'thər, dīeth'il) (ethyl ether, ether $[C_2H_5]_2O$), a volatile ether used as an anesthetic that causes excellent muscle relaxation with minimal effect on blood pressure, pulse rate, and respiration. It is irritating to the respiratory passages and produces nausea.

ether, divinyl (ē'thər, dīvī'nəl) (divinyl oxide $[CH_2:CH]_2O$), a highly volatile, unsaturated ether that is a rapid-acting anesthetic without the after-effect of nausea produced by diethyl ether.

etherization (e'therīzā'shun), Administration of ether to produce anesthesia.

ethics (eth'iks), **1.** the science of moral obligation; a system of moral principles, quality, or practice. **2.** the moral obligation to render to the patient the best possible quality of dental service and to maintain an honest relationship with other members of the profession and mankind in general.

e., dental. See **ethics, professional.**

e., professional, the principles and norms of proper professional conduct concerning the rights and duties of health professionals themselves and their conduct toward patients and fellow practitioners, including the actions taken in the care of patients and family members.

ethinyl estradiol, *trade names:* Estinyl; *drug class:* non-steroidal synthetic estrogen; *action:* affects release of pituitary gonad-otropins, inhibits ovulation, promotes adequate calcium use in bone structure; *uses:* menopause, prostatic cancer, breast cancer, postmenopausal osteoporosis.

ethionamide, *trade name:* Trecator SC; *drug class:* antitubercular; *action:* bacteriostatic against *Mycobacterium tuberculosis;* may inhibit protein synthesis; *uses:* pulmonary, extrapulmonary tuberculosis when other antitubercular drugs have failed.

ethnic group, a population of individuals organized around an assumption of common cultural origin.

ethosuximide, *trade name:* Zarontin; *drug class:* anticonvulsant; *action:* suppresses spike wave formation in absence seizures (petit mal); decreases amplitude, frequency, duration, spread of discharge in minor motor seizures; *uses:* absence seizures (PM).

ethotoin, *trade name:* Peganone; *drug class:* hydantoin derivative anticonvulsant; *action:* inhibits spread of seizure activity in motor cortex; *uses:* generalized tonic-clonic or complex-partial seizures.

ethyl chloride (eth'il klō'rīd) (C_2H_5Cl), a colorless liquid that boils between 12° and 13° C. It acts as a local, topical anesthetic of short duration through the superficial freezing produced by its rapid vaporization from the skin. Ethyl chloride is used occasionally in inhalation therapy as a rapid fleeting general anesthetic, comparable to nitrous oxide but somewhat more dangerous.

ethylene (eth'ilēn) (olefiant gas, CH_2CH_2), a colorless gas of slightly sweet odor and taste; used as an inhalation anesthetic.

e. oxide sterilization, a process that uses gas to sterilize instruments, equipment, and materials that would otherwise be damaged by heat or liquid chemicals. Effective at room temperature. Requires between 10 and 16 hours to be effective. Gas must penetrate the material. The gas is highly toxic and must be vented before opening the sealed sterilizing unit. Sterilized materials must also be well aerated before using.

etidocaine HCl (local), *trade names:* Duranest, Duranest MPF; *drug class:* amide, local anesthetic; *action:* inhibits ion fluxes across membranes, particularly sodium transport across cell membrane; decreases rise of depolarization phase of action potential; blocks nerve action potential; *uses:* local dental anesthetic, peripheral nerve block, caudal anesthetic, central neural block, vaginal block.

etidronate disodium, *trade name:* Didronel IV; *drug class:* antihypercalcemic; *action:* decreases bone resorption and new bone development (accretion); *uses:* Paget's disease, heterotopic ossification, hypercalemia of malignancy.

etiology (ē'tē·ol'əjē), **1.** causative factors. **2.** the factors implicated in the causation of disease. **3.** the study of the factors causing disease.

e., local factors, the environmental influences that may be implicated in the causation and/or perpetuation of a disease process.

e., systemic factors, generalized biologic factors that are implicated in the causation, modification, and/or perpetuation of a disease entity. Within the oral cavity, the actions of the systemic factors are modified by interaction with local factors.

etodolac, *trade name:* Lodine; *drug class:* nonsteroidal antiinflammatory; *action:* inhibits prostaglandin synthesis by interfering with cyclooxgenase, which is needed for biosynthesis; *uses:* mild-to-moderate pain, osteoarthritis.

Eubacterium, a genus of anaerobic, non-sporeforming, nonmotile bacteria containing straight or curved gram-positive rods that usually occur singly, in pairs, or in short chains. They usu-

ally metabolize carbohydrates and may be pathogenic.

eudaemonic (yōōdemon'ik), pertaining to a drug that brings about a feeling of normal well-being in a previously depressed patient. (not current)

eugenol (yōō'jenol), **1.** an allyl guaiacol obtainable from oil of cloves. Used with zinc oxide in a paste for temporary restorations, bases under restorations, and impression materials. Believed to have a palliative effect on dental pulp and possibly a limited germicidal effect. **2.** a colorless or pale yellow liquid obtained from clove oil; has a clove odor and pungent, spicy taste. Used as the liquid portion of zinc oxide and eugenol cements and in toothache medications.

eugnathia (yōōna'thē·ə), the normal or proper relationship of the jaws to each other.

euphoria (yōōfôr'ē·ə), a sense of well-being or normalcy. Pleasantly mild excitement.

euphoric (yōōfôr'ik), a substance that produces an exaggerated sense of well-being.

eupnea (yōōpnē'·ə), easy or normal respiration.

europium, a rare-earth metallic element with an atomic number of 63 and an atomic weight of 151.96.

eustachian tube, a tube, lined with mucous membrane, that joins the nasopharynx and the middle ear cavity, allowing equalization of the air pressure in the middle ear with atmospheric pressure. Also called the *auditory tube.*

eutaxia (yōōtak'se·ə), opposite of ataxia; muscular coordination in good order. (not current)

euthanasia, deliberately bringing about the death of a person who is suffering from an incurable disease or condition, also called *mercy killing.* Active euthanasia is illegal in most jurisdictions; passive euthanasia, or the withholding of some life support systems, has legal standing in some jurisdictions.

euthyroidism (yōōthī'roidizəm), a state of normal thyroid function.

evacuation system, a centralized vacuum system connected to each dental operating unit used to keep the oral cavity clear of water, saliva, blood, and debris, generally operating at a high volume, high velocity, and low pressure.

evaluation, to make a judgment or appraisal of a condition or situation. In dentistry, used to describe the clinical judgment of a patient's dental health or an appraisal of staff performance.

  e. studies, the control study of the comparative value of different treatment modalities or medications.

Evans blue, a diazo dye used for the determination of the blood volume on the basis of the dilution of a standard solution of the dye in the plasma after its intravenous injection.

evidence, proof presented at a trial by the parties through witnesses, records, documents, and concrete objects for the purpose of inducing the court or jury to believe their contentions.

  e., radiographic, the shadow images depicted in radiographs.

Evipal (e'vipäl), the trade name for **hexobarbital,** a rapid-acting barbiturate.

  e. sodium, the trade name for **hexobarbital sodium.** An ultrashort-acting barbiturate of the N-methyl type whose pharmacologic actions, from a clinical standpoint, are essentially similar to thiopental (Pentothal).

evoked potential, an electrical response in the brainstem or cerebral cortex that is elicited by a specific stimulus. This property of the brain may be used to monitor brain function during surgery.

evulsed tooth. See **tooth, evulsed.**

evulsion (avulsion), the sudden tearing out, or away, of tissue as a result of a traumatic episode.

  e., tooth, the displacement of a tooth from its alveolar housing; may be partial or complete.

  e., nerve, the operation of tearing a nerve from its central origin by traction.

Ewing's sarcoma. See **tumor, Ewing's.**

Ewing's tumor. See **tumor, Ewing's.**

examination, **I.** inspection; search; investigation; inquiry; scrutiny; testing. **2.** inspection and/or investigation of part or all of the body to measure and evaluate the state of health or disease. The examination may include visual inspection, percussion, palpation, auscultation, and measurement of mobility as well as various laboratory and radiographic procedures.

  e., anteroposterior extraoral radiographic, an examination in which the film is placed at the posterior direction with the rays passing from the anterior to the posterior direction to record images.

  e., bite-wing intraoral radiographic, radiography in which an intraoral radiograph records on a single film the shadow images of the outline, position, and mesiodistal extent of the crowns, necks, and coronal third of the roots of both the maxillary and mandibular teeth and alveolar crests.

  e., body section extraoral radiographic (tomogram), a radiographic procedure of various internal layers of the head and body accomplished by the synchronized movement of the roentgen-ray tube and film in parallel planes but in opposite directions from each other. Also known as *tomography, laminagraphy, planigraphy,* and *stratigraphy.*

  e., bregma-mentum extraoral radiographic, radiography in which the film is placed beneath the chin, with the rays directed downward through the junction of the coronal and sagittal sutures (bregma) to the chin (mentum).

  e., cephalometric extraoral radiographic. See **cephalometric radiography.**

  e., clinical, the visual and tactile scrutiny of the tissues of and surrounding the oral cavity.

  e., extraoral radiographic, an examination of the oral and paraoral structures by exposing films placed extraorally, in contrast to intraorally.

  e., extradental intraoral radiographic, an examination in which the film is placed between the teeth and the tissue of the cheek or lip for the exploration or localization of the internal structures of these tissues.

  e., gingival, the observation of the primary visual symptoms of periodontal disease, including color changes; changes in surface texture; deviations from normal contour and structure, tissue tone, and vitality; presence or absence of clefts; and the position of attachment.

  e., intraoral, an examination of all the structures contained within the oral cavity.

    e., intraoral radiographic, the examination of the oral and paraoral

E

E

structures by exposing films placed within the oral cavity.

e., lateral facial extraoral radiographic, an examination by means of a lateral head film.

e., lateral head extraoral radiographic, an examination in which the film is placed parallel to the sagittal plane of the head.

e., lateral jaw extraoral radiographic, an examination in which the film is placed adjacent to the mandible.

e., mental extraoral radiographic, an examination in which the film is placed beneath the chin, and the radiation is directed through the long axis of the lower central incisors while the mouth is open.

e., oblique occlusal intraoral radiographic, an exploratory examination of the maxillae or mandible using an occlusal type of film placed between the teeth. The rays are directed obliquely downward or upward (usually 60 degrees to 75 degrees in the vertical plane) and parallel to the sagittal plane.

e., panoramic extraoral radiographic, a curved single film radiography in which the beam source and film rotate in a synchronized manner about the head, exposing oral structures sequentially with simultaneous exposure of corresponding areas of the film.

e., periapical intraoral radiographic, the basic intraoral examination, showing all of a tooth and the surrounding periodontium.

e., posteroanterior extraoral radiographic, an examination in which the film is placed anteriorly, with the rays passing from the posterior to the anterior direction.

e., profile extraoral radiographic, a lateral head examination to show the profile of bone and soft tissue outline. It uses a decrease in milliampere seconds or an increase in target-film distance for recording the soft tissue image.

e., radiographic, **1.** the production of the number of radiographs necessary for the radiologic interpretation of the part or parts in question. **2.** the study and interpretation of radiographs of the mouth and associated structures.

e., stereoscopic extraoral radiographic, a radiographic examination used in conjunction with a stereoscope for localization. Exposures of two films are made, with identical placement of each film adjacent to the part in question and with a different angulation for each exposure.

e., temporomandibular extraoral radiographic, an examination in which the film is placed adjacent to the area to be examined, with the rays directed through a point that is 2.5 inches (6.25 cm) above the tragus of the opposite external ear with a vertical angulation of 15 degrees and a horizontal angulation of 5 degrees downward. Various other techniques and angulations are used, including laminagraphy, in examining this area.

e., true occlusal topographic intraoral radiographic, the radiography of the maxillae or mandible using an occlusal type of film placed between the teeth, with the rays directed at right angles to the plane of the film or through the long axis of the teeth adjacent to the part in question.

e., Waters extraoral radiographic, posteroanterior examination of the paranasal sinuses. The film is placed in contact with the nose and chin, with the rays directed at right angles to the plane of the film.

excavator, spoon (eks′kəvā′tŏr), a paired hand instrument intended primarily to remove carious material from a cavity.

excess, more than is necessary, useful, or specified.

e., marginal, a condition in which the restorative material extends beyond the prepared cavity margin.

e. overhang, gingival margin excess.

excipient (eksip′ē-ənt), an ingredient included in a pharmaceutical preparation for the purpose of improving its physical qualities. See also **binder; filler;** and **vehicle.**

excision (eksizh′ən), the act of cutting away or taking out.

e., local, an excision limited to the immediate area of the lesion in question.

e., radical, an excision involving not only the lesion in question but also anatomic parts remote from the site.

e., wide, an excision involving the lesion in question and immediately adjacent anatomic structures.

excitant (eksīt′ənt), an agent that stimulates the activity of an organ.

excitation (eksītā'shən), the addition of energy to a system, thereby transferring it from its ground state to an excited state.

exclusions, dental services not covered under a dental benefits program.

exclusive provider organization (EPO), a dental benefits plan that provides benefits only if care is rendered by institutional and professional providers with whom the plan contracts (with some exceptions for emergency and out-of-area services).

excursion, a trip; movement from a mean position.

e., lateral, the movement of the mandible from the centric position to a lateral or protusive position.

execute, to finish; accomplish; fulfill. To carry out according to certain terms.

exercise, the performance of any physical activity for the purpose of conditioning the body, improving health, or maintaining fitness or as a means of therapy for correcting a deformity or restoring the organs and bodily function to a state of health.

e. prosthesis. See **prosthesis, exercise.**
e., myotherapeutic. See **therapy, myofunctional.**

exertion, vigorous action, a great effort, a strong influence.

exfoliation (eksfō'lē-ā'shən) (shedding), the physiologic loss of the primary dentition.

exhalation (ekshəlā'shən), giving off or sending forth in the form of vapor; expiration.

exhaustion (egzôst'yən), the loss of vital and nervous power from fatigue or protracted disease.

exhibit (egzib'it), a paper, document, or object presented to a court during a trial or hearing as proof of facts, or as otherwise connected with the subject matter, and which, on being accepted, is marked for identification and considered a part of the case.

exocytosis, the appearance of migrating inflammatory cells in the epidermis.

exodontics (ek'sōdon'tiks), the science and practice of removing teeth from the oral cavity as performed by dentists.

exolever (eks'ole'vər), an instrument that uses the principles of leverage for extracting and removing teeth or roots of teeth from the oral cavity. (not current)

exophthalmos (ek'softhal'mōs), an abnormal protrusion of the eyeball. It is characteristic of toxic (exophthalmic) goiter.

exostosis (ek'səstō'sis) (hyperostosis), a bony growth projecting from a bony surface.

exotoxin (ek'sətok'sin), the toxic material formed by microorganisms and subsequently released into their surrounding environments.

expanded duty auxiliary, a person trained to carry out dental procedures more complex than the responsibilities usually delegated to dental auxiliaries.

expansile infrastructure endosteal implant, an intraosseous implant device designed to enlarge or open after its insertion into the bone to provide retention. (not current)

expansion, an increase in extent, size, volume, or scope.

e., delayed (secondary expansion), **1.** an expansion occurring in amalgam restorations as a result of moisture contamination. **2.** an expansion exhibited by amalgam that has been contaminated by moisture during trituration or insertion.

e., dental arch, the therapeutic increase in circumference of the dental arch by buccal and/or labial movement of the teeth.

e., hygroscopic, an expansion, caused by absorption of water during setting of an investment, used to compensate for the shrinkage of metal from the molten to the solid state.

e., secondary. See **expansion, delayed.**

e., setting, an expansion that occurs during the setting or hardening of materials such as amalgam and gypsum products.

e., thermal, an expansion caused by heat. Thermal expansion of the mold is one of the important factors in achieving adequate compensation for the contraction of cast metal when it solidifies.

e., thermal coefficient, a number indicating the amount of expansion caused by each degree of temperature change. The rate of change in restorative materials and tooth substance should be relatively the same.

experience rating, a determination of the premium rate for a particular group partially or wholly on the basis of that group's own experience. Age, sex, use, and costs of services provided determine the premium.

experiment, a trial or special observation made to confirm or disprove something doubtful; an act or operation undertaken to discover some unknown principle or effect or to test, establish, or illustrate some suggested or known truth.

expert, one who has special skill or knowledge in a particular subject, such as a science or art, whether acquired by experience or study; a specialist.

e. system, a computer program that follows a logical pathway or algorithm to a conclusion in a manner that mimics what an expert in the field would follow.

e. testimony, the sworn statements of a person with special knowledge about a subject under consideration by a court of law.

e. witness, a person who has special knowledge of a subject about which a court requests testimony to educate the court and the jury in the subject under consideration.

expiration, 1. the act of breathing forth or expelling air from the lungs. 2. a cessation; a termination; the expiration of a lease.

e. date, 1. the date on which a dental benefits contract expires. 2. the date an individual ceases to be eligible for benefits.

explanation of benefits, a written statement to a beneficiary, from a third-party payer, after a claim has been reported, indicating the benefits and charges covered or not covered by the dental benefits plan.

exploration, 1. an examination by touch, either with or without instruments. For example, a carious lesion is explored with a special explorer, but the mucobuccal fold may be explored with the finger. 2. the process of examination of a surface, with or without the use of instruments, to determine the condition or the surface depth of a defect or other similar diagnostic parameters.

explore, to investigate.

explorer, a dental instrument with a slender head that honed to a fine point, used to conduct a tactile exami-

nation and appraisal of pits and fissures, carious lesions, root surfaces, and margins of restoration.

explosion, a violent, noisy outbreak caused by a sudden release of energy.

exposure, uncovering; subjection to viewing or radiation.

e., accidental pulp, pulp exposure unintentionally created during instrumentation.

e., air, radiation exposure measured in a small mass of air under conditions of electronic equilibrium with the surrounding air, that is, excluding backscatter from irradiated parts or objects.

e., carious pulp, pulp exposure occasioned by extension of the carious process to the pulp chamber wall.

e., chronic, radiation exposure of long duration, either continuous (protraction exposure) or intermittent (fractionation exposure); usually referring to exposure of relatively low intensity.

e., cumulative, the total accumulated exposure resulting from repeated radiation exposures of the whole body or of a particular region.

e., double, two superimposed exposures on the same radiographic or photographic film.

e., entrance, exposure measured at the surface of an irradiated body, part, or object. It includes both primary radiation and backscatter from the irradiated underlying tissue or material.

e., erythema, the radiation exposure necessary to produce a temporary redness of the skin. The exposure required varies with the quality of the radiation to which the skin is exposed.

e., mechanical pulp. See **exposure, pulp, surgical.**

e., protraction, continuous exposure to radiation over a relatively long period at a low exposure rate.

e., pulp, an opening through the wall of the pulp chamber uncovering the dental pulp.

e., radiographic, a measure of the x or gamma radiation to which a person or object, or part of either, is exposed at a certain place, this measure being based on its ability to produce ionization. The unit of x- or γ-radiation exposure is the roentgen (R).

e. rate, output, exposure to radiation at a specified point per unit of time, usually expressed in roentgens per minute.

e., surface. See **exposure, entrance.**

e., surgical pulp (mechanical pulp exposure), pulp exposure created intentionally or unintentionally during instrumentation.

e., threshold, the minimum exposure that will produce a detectable degree of any given effect.

e. time, the time during which a person or object is exposed to radiation, expressed in one of the conventional units of time.

express, to state distinctly and explicitly and not leave to inference; to set forth in words.

exsufflation (ek'suffla'shən), forced discharge of the breath.

extension, 1. an enlargement in boundary, breadth, or depth. **2.** the process of increasing the angle between two skeletal levers having end-to-end articulation with each other; the opposite of flexion.

e. base. See **base, extension.**

e. for prevention, a principle of cavity preparation enunciated by G.V. Black in 1891. To prevent the recurrence of decay, he advocated extension of the preparation subgingivally, axially, and occlusally into an area that is readily polished and cleaned.

e., gingiva, attached, a gingival extension operation; a surgical technique designed to broaden the zone of attached gingiva by repositioning the mucogingival junction apically.

e., groove, the enlargement of a cavity preparation outline to include a developmental groove.

e. of benefits, an extension of eligibility for benefits for covered services, usually designed to ensure completion of treatment commenced before the expiration date. Duration is generally expressed in terms of days.

e., ridge, an intraoral surgical operation for deepening the labial, buccal, and/or lingual sulci.

extenuate, to lessen; to mitigate.

external oblique line (ōblēk'). See **line, external oblique.**

external pin fixation. See **appliance, fracture.**

external traction. See **traction, external.**

exteroceptors (ek'stərōsep'tōrs), sensory nerve end receptors that respond to external stimuli; located in the skin, mouth, eyes, ears, and nose.

extirpation, pulp (ek'stərpā'shən). See **pulpectomy.**

extracellular matrix, an amorphous or structured substance produced by cellular activity that lies within the tissue but outside of the cell.

extracoronal (ek'strəkôr'ōnəl), pertaining to that which is outside, or external to, the body of the coronal portion of a natural tooth.

e. retainer. See **retainer, extracoronal.**

extract, a concentrate obtained by treating a crude material, such as plant or animal tissue, with a solvent, evaporating part or all of the solvent from the resulting solution and standardizing the resulting product.

extraction, the removal of a tooth from the oral cavity by means of elevators and/or forceps.

e., serial, the extraction of selected primary teeth over a period of years (often ending with removal of the first premolar teeth) to relieve crowding of the dental arches during eruption of the lateral incisors, canines, and premolars.

extraoral, literally, outside of the mouth. Generally refers to an orthodontic appliance that extends outside the mouth to secure a firm base for force application within the mouth. See also **anchorage, extraoral.**

extraoral anchorage, orthodontic force applied from a base outside the mouth. See also **anchorage.**

extrapolate (ekstrap'ōlāt), to infer values beyond the observable range from an observed trend of variables; to project by inference into the unexplored.

extrasystole (ek'strəsis'tōlē), a heartbeat occurring before its normal time in the rhythm of the heart and followed by a compensatory pause.

extravasation (eksträv'əzā'shən), the escape of a body fluid out of its proper place (for example, blood into surrounding tissues after rupture of a vessel, urine into surrounding tissues after rupture of the bladder).

extremity, an arm or a leg; the arm may be identified as an upper extremity, and the leg as a lower extremity.

F

extrinsic coloring, Coloring from without (for example, coloring of the external surface of a prosthesis). (not current)

extroversion, a tendency of the teeth or other maxillary structures to become situated too far from the median plane.

extrude, to elevate; to move a tooth coronally.

extrusion, the movement of teeth beyond the natural occlusal plane that may be accompanied by a similar movement of investing tissues. See also **eruption, continuous.**

extubate (eks'tōōbāt), to remove a tube, usually an endotracheal anesthesia tube or a Levin gastric suction tube.

extubation (eks'tōōbā'shən), the removal of a tube used for intubation.

exudate (eks'ōōdāt), the outpouring of a fluid substance, such as exudated pus or tissue fluid.

e., gingival, the outpouring of an inflammatory exudate from the gingival tissues.

exudation (eks'ōōdā'shən). See **exudate.**

eye, one of a pair of organs of sight, contained in a bony orbit at the front of the skull.

eye-ear plane. See **plane, Frankfort horizontal.**

eyeglasses, transparent devices held in metal or plastic frames in front of the eyes to correct refractive errors or to protect the eyes from harmful electromagnetic waves or flying objects.

eyelids, a moveable fold of thin skin over the eye. The orbicularis oculi muscle and the oculomotor nerve control the opening and closing of the eyelid.

fabrication (fab'rikā'shən), the construction or making of a restoration.

face, the front of the head from the chin to the brow, including the skin and muscles and structures of the forehead, eyes, nose, mouth, cheeks, and jaw.

f. bow, a caliper-like device that is used to record the relationship of the maxillae to the temporomandibular joints (or opening axis of the mandible) and to orient the casts in this same relationship to the opening axis of an articulator.

f.-b., adjustable axis. See **facebow, kinematic.**

f.-b., kinematic *(hinge-bow),* a facebow attached to the mandible whose caliper ends (condyle rods) can be adjusted to permit the accurate location of the axis of rotation of the mandible.

f., changeable area of, the part of the face from the nose to the chin.

f. form. See **form, face.**

facet (fas'et), a flattened, highly polished wear pattern as noted on a tooth.

facial angle, an anthropomorphic expression of the degree of protrusion of the lower face, assessed by the measured inclination of the facial plane in relation to the Frankfort horizontal reference plane.

facial artery, one of a pair of tortuous arteries that arise from the external carotid arteries, divide into four cervical and five facial branches, and supply various organs and tissues in the head. The cervical branches of the facial artery are the ascending palatine, tonsillar, glandular, and submental. The facial branches are the inferior labial, superior labial, lateral nasal, angular, and muscular.

facial asymmetry, the variation in the configuration of one side of the face from the other when viewed in relation to a projected midsagittal line.

facial bones, the bones of the face, which include the frontal, nasal, maxillary, zygomatic, and mandibular bones.

facial cleft. See **cleft, facial.**

facial expression, the use of the facial muscles to communicate or to convey mood.

facial injuries, trauma to the face and its associated structures, most frequently from traffic accidents, contact sports, and domestic conflicts.

facial muscle, one of numerous muscles of the face, seldom remaining distinct over its entire length because of a tendency to merge with neighboring muscles at its termination or attachment. The five groups of facial muscles include the muscles of the scalp, the extrinsic muscles of the ear, the muscles of the nose, the muscles of the eyelid, and the muscles of the mouth. The platysma is one muscle of the facial group but is described with the muscles of the neck. Also called *muscles of expression.*

facial nerve, either of a pair of mixed sensory and motor cranial nerves that arise from the brainstem at the base of the pons and divide just in front of the ear into six branches, innervating the scalp, forehead, eyelids, muscles of facial expression, cheeks, and jaw. Also called the *seventh cranial nerve.*

facial neuralgia. See **neuralgia, trigeminal.**

facial pain. See **pain, facial.**

facial profile. See **profile, facial.**

facial tic, any repetitive spasmodic and involuntary contraction of groups of facial muscles.

facies (fā'shē·ēs), the features, general appearance, and expression of a face.

facilitation, the reinforcement of a lower level nerve stimulus by a higher level nerve stimulus. Thus a reflex that cannot be elicited by a subliminal impulse may be reinforced by an additional stimulus from a higher center. The combined effect of the two stimuli may cause a reflex response.

facsimile (faksim'ilē), a true copy that preserves all the markings and contents of the original.

fact, a thing done; an event or a circumstance; an actual occurrence.

factor(s), a constituent, element, cause, or agent that influences a process or system; a gene; a dietary substance.

f. I (fibrinogen, profibrin). See **fibrinogen.**

f. II (prothrombin, component A, prothrombase, prothrombin B, thrombogen, thrombozyme), considered to be the only essential precursor of thrombin.

f. III (thromboplastin [tissue], thrombokinase, cytozyme [platelet], thrombokinin [blood], thromboplastic protein). See **thromboplastin.**

f. IV (calcium, Ca^{++}), ionized and/or bound calcium, which is generally required for the coagulation of blood, although some early phases of coagulation and the thrombin-fibrinogen reaction can take place without calcium.

f. V (labile factor, proaccelerin, accelerin, acceleration factor, cofactor of thromboplastin, component A of prothrombin, plasma ac-globulin, plasma prothrombin conversion fac-

tor [PPCF], prothrombinase, prothrombin accelerator, prothrombin conversion accelerator I, thrombogen, thrombogene, proaccelerin-accelerin system), a factor apparently necessary for the formation of a prothrombin-converting substance in blood and tissue extracts, that is, intrinsic and extrinsic prothrombin activators. A deficiency results in parahemophilia (hypoproaccelerinemia).

f. VI, the term formerly used to indicate an intermediate product in the formation of thromboplastin and also used synonymously with accelerin and activated factor V. It has no designation at the present time.

f. VII (stable factor, serum prothrombin conversion accelerator [SPCA], proconvertin, autoprothrombin I, cofactor V, component B of prothrombin, cothromboplastin, kappa factor, precursor of serum prothrombin conversion accelerator [pro-SPCA], prothrombin conversion factor, prothrombin converting factor, prothrombin conversion accelerator II, proconvertin-convertin system, prothrombinogen, serozyme, stable factor), a factor that accelerates the conversion of prothrombin to thrombin in the presence of factors III, IV, and V; a serum factor necessary for the formation of extrinsic prothrombin activator.

f. VII deficiency, a deficiency associated with a lack of vitamin K. A deficiency may be congenital, or it may be acquired in liver disease, or from prothrombinopenic agents used in anticoagulation therapy; it results in a prolonged (quantitative) one-stage prothrombin time test.

f. VIII (antihemophilic factor [AHF], antihemophilic globulin, antihemophilic globulin A, antihemophilic factor A, plasma thromboplastin factor A [PTF-A], plasma thromboplastin factor [PTF], plasmokinin, platelet cofactor I, prothrombokinase, thrombocatalysin, thrombocytolysin, thrombokatilysin, thromboplastic plasma component [TPC], thromboplastinogen), a factor essential for the formation of blood thromboplastin. A deficiency results in classic hemophilia (hemophilia A); the clotting time is prolonged, and thromboplastin and prothrombin conversion is diminished.

f. IX *(Christmas factor, plasma thromboplastin component [PTC], antihemophilic factor B, antihemophilic globulin B, autoprothrombin II, beta prothromboplastin, plasma factor X, plasma thromboplastin factor B [PTF-B], platelet cofactor II),* a factor that is active in the formation of intrinsic blood thromboplastin. A deficiency results in Christmas disease (hemophilia B), which is caused by a decrease in the amount of thromboplastin formed.

f. X *(Stuart-Prower factor, Stuart factor, Prower factor),* a factor influencing the yield of intrinsic (plasma) thromboplastin. A deficiency results in a prolonged one-stage prothrombin time. Brain tissue or Russell's viper venom are used to test for thromboplastin deficiency.

f. XI *(plasma thromboplastin antecedent [PTA], antihemophilic factor C, PTA factor, plasma thromboplastin factor C [PTF-C]),* a factor related to intrinsic (plasma) thromboplastin activation, which occurs when blood is exposed to a foreign surface.

    f. XI deficiency, a deficiency caused by an autosomal recessive gene resulting in a hemorrhagic tendency. See also **hemophilia C.**

f. XII *(Hageman factor, antihemophilic factor D, clot-promoting factor, fifth plasma thromboplastin precursor, glass factor),* a factor whose absence results in a long clotting time and abnormal prothrombin consumption and thromboplastin generation tests when the tests are carried out in glass tubes. No abnormal bleeding tendency occurs with a deficiency of the factor.

f. XIII, a coagulation factor present in normal plasma that acts with calcium to produce an insoluble fibrin clot. Also called *fibrinase, fibrin stabilizing factor.*

    f. XIII deficiency, a deficiency caused by a deficiency of vitamin E.

f., acceleration. See **factor V.**

f., antihemophilic (AHF). See **factor VIII.**

f., antihemophilic A. See **factor VIII.**

f., antihemophilic B. See **factor IX.**

f., antihemophilic C. See **factor XI.**

f., antihemophilic D. See **factor XII.**

f., antipernicious. See **vitamin B$_{12}$.**

f. C *(contact factor, contact activation product, third thromboplastic factor),* a coagulation accelerator product formed by the interaction of active factor XII and factor XI.

f., Castle's intrinsic *(intrinsic factor),* a factor produced by the gastric mucosa and possibly the duodenal mucosa, and considered to be responsible for the absorption of vitamin B$_{12}$. See also **anemia, pernicious.**

f., Christmas. See **factor IX.**

f., clot-promoting. See **factor XII.**

f., clotting, "Trace" proteins (excluding calcium) present in normal blood in such small amounts (except fibrinogen) that their presence is usually established by deductive reasoning and by genetic and biochemical characteristics. They are associated with thromboplastic activity and the conversion of prothrombin to thrombin.

f., contact. See **factor C.**

f., environmental, local conditions that modify tissue response (for example, narrow interdental spaces, saddle areas, attachment of frenula, oblique ridges).

f., erythrocyte-maturation (EMF). See **vitamin B complex.**

f., etiologic, the element or influence that can be assigned as the cause or reason for a disease or lesion.

f., extrinsic. See **vitamin B complex.**

f., familial, a characteristic derived through heredity.

f., glass. See **factor XII.**

f., glucocorticoid. See **hormone, "S".**

f., Hageman. See **factor XII.**

f., Hr, blood factors that are reciprocally related to the Rh factors. They are present in agglutinogens when the corresponding Rh factor is absent from the gene.

f., hyperglycemic. See **glucagon.**

    f., hyperglycemic-glycogenolytic. See **glucagon.**

f., intrinsic. See **factor, Castle's intrinsic.**

f., kappa. See **factor VII.**

f., labile. See **factor V.**

f., local, includes dental and bacterial plaques, bacterial toxins and irritants, calculus, food impaction, and other surface and locally placed irritants that are capable of injuring the periodontium.

f., pellagra-preventive. See **acid, nicotinic.**

f., plasma prothrombin conversion (PPCF). See **factor V.**

f., plasma thromboplastin (PTF), substances with thromboplastic activity contributed by the plasma. Included are the antihemophilic factor, Christmas factor, plasma thromboplastin antecedent, and Hageman factor. See also **factor VIII.**

f., plasma thromboplastin, A (PTF-A). See **factor VIII.**

f., plasma thromboplastin, B (PTF-B). See **factor IX.**

f., plasma thromboplastin, C (PTF-C). See **factor XI.**

f., plasma thromboplastin, D (PTF-D), considered by some to be a fourth plasma substance with thromboplastic activity; not well characterized.

f., plasma, X. See **factor IX.**

f., platelet, a substance on or in the surface of blood platelet necessary for coagulation in the absence of extravascular thromboplastic substances.

f., p., 1 (platelet ac-globulin, citrin), either factor V or a factor with factor V activity; absorbed on platelets and accelerates conversion of prothrombin to thrombin.

f., p., 2 (platelet thrombin accelerator, platelet thromboplastic activity), a substance that accelerates the conversion of fibrinogen to fibrin.

f., p., 3 (thromboplastic cellular component [TCC], thromboplastinogenase, platelet activator), a substance associated with thromboplastin generation activity.

f., p., 4, an antiheparin factor.

f., prothrombin conversion. See **factor VII.**

f., prothrombin-converting. See **factor VII.**

f., Prower. See **factor X.**

f., psychosomatic, psychic, mental, or emotional factors that play a role in determining the initiation, course, and extent of a physical process, either directly or indirectly. Psychosomatic factors have been implicated in necrotizing ulcerative gingivitis (NUG), bruxism, clenching, and other oral habits.

f., PTA (plasma thromboplastin antecedent factor). See **factor XI.**

f., reparative, the ability of the tissues to heal or regenerate when they have been subjected to injury or disease.

f., Rh, agglutinogens of red blood cells responsible for isoimmune reactions such as occur in erythroblastosis fetalis and incompatible blood transfusions.

f., spreading, an enzyme that increases the permeability of ground substance.

f., stable. See **factor VII.**

f., Stuart. See **factor X.**

f., Stuart-Prower. See **factor X.**

f., third thromboplastic. See **factor C.**

faculty, 1. any normal physiologic function or natural ability of a living organism. **2.** an ability to do something specific, such as learn languages or to perceive and distinguish sensory stimuli. **3.** any mental ability or power. **4.** the group of people who teach within an institution of learning.

FAD, the abbreviation for **flavin-adenine dinucleotide.**

failure, a deficiency; an inefficiency as measured by some legal standard; an unsuccessful attempt.

f. to thrive, the abnormal retardation of the growth and development of an infant resulting from conditions that interfere with normal metabolism, appetite, and activity.

faint, a state of syncope, or swooning.

falsify, to forge; to give a false appearance to anything, as to falsify a record.

famciclovir, *trade name* Famvir; *drug class:* antiviral; *action:* converted to active metabolite, penciclovir triphosphate, which inhibits DNA viral synthesis and replication; *uses:* acute herpes zoster (shingles) infection.

family, 1. a body of persons who live in one house and under one head; a father, a mother, and a child or some children; a husband and wife living together. **2.** a group of people related by heredity, such as parents, children, and siblings. The term is sometimes broadened to include related by marriage or those living in the same household, who are emotionally attached, interact regularly, and share concerns for the growth and development of the group and its individual members. **3.** a group of persons who have a common surname, such as the Anderson family. **4.** a category of animals or plants situated on a taxonomic scale between order and genus. **5.** the legal definition varies, depending on the jurisdiction and purpose for which the term is defined.

f. counseling, a program that consists of providing information and professional guidance to members of a family concerning specific health matters.

f. deductible, a deductible that is satisfied by combined expenses of all covered family members. A plan with a $25 deductible may limit its application to a maximum of three deductibles, or $75, for the family, regardless of the number of family members.

f. dentistry, the branch of dentistry that is concerned with the diagnosis and treatment of dental problems in people of either sex and at any age. Family dentists were formerly known as *general practitioners,* and therefore family dentistry does not constitute one of the specialty areas of dentistry.

f. membership, a membership that includes spouses and/or dependents.

f. unit, an insured group member and dependents who are eligible for benefits under a dental care contract; an accounting unit.

famotidine, *trade names:* Pepcid, Pepcid IV; *drug class:* H_2 histamine receptor antagonist; *action:* inhibits histamine at H_2 receptor site in parietal cells, which inhibits gastric acid secretion; *uses:* short-term treatment of active duodenal ulcer, gastric ulcer, and heartburn.

fascia, the fibrous connective tissue of the body that may be separated from other specifically organized fibrous structures such as the tendons, the aponeuroses, and the ligaments. Fascia generally covers and separates muscles and muscle groups.

f. lata, the strong fascia that envelopes the muscles of the thigh.

fascitis (fəsī'tis), a tumorlike growth occurring in subcutaneous tissues in the mouth, usually in the cheek. A benign lesion sometimes mistaken for fibrosarcoma, fascitis consists of young fibroblasts and numerous capillaries. It grows rapidly and may regress spontaneously. (not current)

fasting, the act of abstaining from ingesting food for a specific period of time, usually for diagnostic, therapeutic, or religious purposes.

fat, I. a substance composed of lipids or fatty acids and occurring in various forms or consistencies ranging from oil to tallow. **2.** a type of connective tissue containing stored lipids.

f. embolism, a circulatory condition characterized by the blocking of an artery by an embolus of fat that enters the circulatory system after the fracture of a long bone, or less commonly, after traumatic injury to fatty tissue or to a fatty liver.

fatal outcome, a consequence that results in death. The course of a disease that results in the death of the patient.

fate, a synonym for the more modern term *biotransformation.* See also **biotransformation.**

fatigue, a condition of cells or organs under stress resulting in a diminution or loss of an individual's capacity to respond to stimulation.

f., muscle, a peripheral phenomenon caused by the failure of the muscle to contract when stimuli from the nervous system reach it. Occurs when muscle activity exceeds tissue substrate and oxygenation capacity.

fatty acid, any of several organic acids produced by the hydrolysis of neutral fats.

fauces (fô'sēz), the archway between the pharyngeal and oral cavities; formed by the tongue, anterior tonsillar pillars, and soft palate.

FDA, the abbreviation for the Food and Drug Administration. See also **Food and Drug Administration.**

fear, an emotion, generally considered negative and unpleasant, that is a reaction to a real or threatened danger; fright. Fear is distinguished from anxiety, which is a reaction to an unreal or imagined danger.

febrile, pertaining to or characterized by an elevated body temperature. A body temperature of over 100° F is commonly regarded as febrile.

feces, waste or excrement from the digestive tract that is formed in the intestine and expelled through the rectum. Feces consist of water, food residue, bacteria, and secretions of the intestines and liver.

Federal Tort Claims Act, a statute passed in 1946 that allows the federal government to be sued for the wrongful action or negligence of its employees. The act, for most purposes, eliminates the doctrine of governmental immunity, which formerly prohibited or limited the bringing of suit against the federal government.

Fede's disease. See **disease, Riga-Fede.** (not current)

fee, compensation for services rendered or to be rendered; payment for professional services.

f., customary, a fee is customary if it is in the range of the usual fees charged by dentists of similar training and experience for the same service within the specific and limited geographic area (that is, the socioeconomic area of a metropolitan area or of a county).

f.-for-service plan, a plan providing for payment to the dentist for each service performed rather than on the basis of salary or capitation fee.

f., reasonable, a fee is considered reasonable if, in the opinion of a responsible dental association's review committee, it is the usual and customary fee charged for services rendered, considering the special circumstances of the case in question.

f. schedule, **1.** a list of maximum dollar allowances for dental procedures that apply under a specific contract. **2.** a list of the charges established or agreed to by a dentist for specific dental services.

f., usual, the fee customarily charged for a given service by an individual dentist to a private patient.

feedback, the constant flow of sensory information back to the brain. When feedback mechanisms are deficient because of sensory deprivation, motor function becomes distorted, aberrant, and uncoordinated.

Feer's disease (ferz). See **erythredema polyneuropathy.**

felbamate, *trade name:* Felbatol; *drug class:* anticonvulsant; *action:* anticonvulsant action is unclear; *uses:* alone or as an adjunct therapy in partial seizures.

feldspar (feld'spär), a crystalline mineral of aluminum silicate with potassium, sodium, barium, or calcium— Na Al Si$_3$ O$_8$ or K Al Si$_3$ O$_8$. Feldspar melts over a range of 1100° to 2000° F (593.5° to 1093.5° C). An important constituent of dental porcelain.

f., orthoclase ceramic, a clay found in large quantity in the solid crust of the earth. It acts as a filler and imparts body to the fused dental porcelain.

felodipine, *trade names:* Plendil, Renedil; *drug class:* calcium channel blocker; *action:* inhibits calcium ion influx across cell membrane during cardiac depolarization; produces relaxation of coronary vascular smooth muscle; dilates coronary arteries; decreases SA/AV node conduction; *uses:* essential hypertension, alone or with other antihypertensives, chronic angina pectoris.

felony, a crime declared by statute to be more serious than a misdemeanor and deserving of a more severe penalty. Conviction usually requires imprisonment in a penitentiary for longer than one year.

fenestration (fenestrā'shən), an opening, a window, an interstice.

f. in alveolar plate, a round or oval defect or opening in the alveolar cortical plate of bone over the root surface.

fenfluramine HCl, *trade name:* Pondimin; *drug class:* nonamphetamine anorexiant, Controlled Substance Schedule IV; *action:* influences serotonin pathways in the central nervous system; anorexic mechanisms unknown; *use:* exogenous obesity.

fenoprofen calcium, *trade name:* Nalfon; *drug class:* nonsteroidal antiinflammatory; *action:* inhibits prostaglandin synthesis by interfering with cyclooxygenase needed for biosynthesis; *uses:* mild-to-moderate pain, osteoarthritis, rheumatoid arthritis, acute gout, dysmenorrhea.

fentanyl transdermal system, *trade name:* Duragesic 25, 50, 75, 100 Transdermal Patches; *drug class:* narcotic analgesic, Controlled Substance Schedule II; *action:* interacts with opioid receptors in the central nervous system to alter pain perception; *uses:* management of chronic pain when opioids are necessary.

fermentation, a chemical change that is brought about in a substance by the action of an enzyme or microorganism, especially the anaerobic conversion of foodstuffs to certain products such as acetic fermentation, alcoholic fermentation.

Ferrier's separator (fer'ē-ərz). See **separator, Ferrier's.** (not current)

ferrous fumarate/ferrous gluconate/ferrous sulfate, *trade names:* Femiron, Feostat; *drug class:* hematinic;

iron preparation; *action:* replaces iron stores needed for red blood cell development; *uses:* iron-deficiency anemia, prophylaxis for iron deficiency in pregnancy.

fertility, the ability to reproduce.

festoon(s) (festōōn'), a carving in the base material of a denture that simulates the contours of the natural tissues being replaced by the denture.

f., gingival, the distinct rounding and enlargement of the margins of the gingival tissue found in early gingival involvement.

f., McCall's, enlargements of the gingival margins that may be associated with occlusal trauma.

festooning (festōōn'ing), the process of carving the base material of a denture or denture pattern to simulate the contours of the natural tissues to be replaced by the denture.

fetal alcohol syndrome, a set of congenital psychologic, behavioral, cognitive, and physical abnormalities that tend to appear in infants whose mothers consumed alcoholic beverages during pregnancy. It is characterized by typical craniofacial and limb defects, cardiovascular defects, and retarded development.

fetor ex ore (fe'tor eks ō'rē). See **halitosis.**

fetor oris (fe'tor ō'ris). bad breath. See also **halitosis.**

fetus, the unborn offspring of any viviparous animal after it has attained the particular form of the species, more specifically, the human being in utero after the embryonic period and the beginning of the development of the major structural features, usually from the eighth week after fertilization until birth.

fever (pyrexia), elevation of the body temperature.

f., acute necrotizing ulcerative gingivitis (ANUG) and acute primary keratotic gingivostomatitis (APKG), a moderate-to-high elevation of temperature is not a symptom of ANUG; however, the presence of a significantly elevated temperature might suggest the presence of APKG, a viral disease accompanied by a bleeding and tender gingiva, marked halitosis, and lymphadenopathy.

f., aphthous. See **disease, foot-and-mouth.**

f., cat-scratch (benign inoculation lymphoreticulosis, cat-scratch disease), a granulomatous process that occurs at the site of a scratch or bite of a house cat. Local lesions occur at the site of injury, with a regional adenitis that is out of proportion to the primary lesion occurring within 1 to 3 weeks. Systemic symptoms of infection may occur. Diagnosis is confirmed by reaction to cat-scratch antigen or the antigen of lymphogranuloma venereum, which is a related form of disease.

f., hay, rhinitis and conjunctivitis resulting from allergy; frequently caused by allergy to pollens.

f. of unknown origin, the persistent elevation of body temperature without an identifiable cause.

f., rheumatic (rōōmat'ik), a severe, apparently infectious disease produced by hemolytic streptococci organisms or associated with their presence in the body; characterized by upper respiratory tract inflammation, cervical lymphadenopathy and lymphadenitis, polyarthritis, cardiac involvement, and subcutaneous nodules. The disease may be produced by an autoantibody reaction.

f., scarlet (scarlatina), an acute disease caused by a specific type of *Streptococcus* organism and characterized by a rash and strawberry tongue.

f., uveoparotid (Heerfordt's syndrome, uveoparotitis), **1.** a disease characterized by inflammation of the parotid gland and of the uveal regions of the eye. **2.** firm, nodular enlargement of the parotid glands, uveitis, and cutaneous lesions may be present. Considered to be a form of sarcoidosis. **3.** a syndrome consisting of sarcoidosis affecting the parotid glands, inflammation of the lacrimal glands, and inflammation of the uveal tract of the eye.

fiber(s), an elongated, threadlike structure of organic tissue.

f., A-alpha nerve, large-diameter nerve fibers that connect into the substantia gelatinosa of the dorsal horns of the spinal cord before synapsing with the central transmission of the dorsal horn. A-alpha fibers are associated with the "gate-control" theory of pain.

f., A-beta nerve, large-diameter nerve fibers that are mechanoreceptors for pressure occurring in both the pulp and periodontal ligament, which are necessary to operate the gate mechanism.

f., A-delta nerve, small-diameter nerve fibers that are mechanoreceptors for pain occurring in both the pulp and the periodontal ligament, which are necessary to operate the gate mechanism.

f., adrenergic, those nerve fibers, including most of the postganglionic sympathetic fibers, which transmit their impulses across synapses or neuroeffector junctions through the local release of the neurohormone more recently identified as *norepinephrine* and formerly designated *sympathin.*

f., alveolar, white collagenous fibers of the periodontal membrane (ligament) that extend from the alveolar bone to the intermediate plexus, where their terminations are interspersed with the terminations of the cemental group of fibers.

  f., a. crest, collagenous fibers of the periodontal membrane that extend from the cervical area of the tooth to the alveolar crest.

f., apical, the fibers of the periodontal ligament radiating apically from tooth to bone.

f., association, extensions of nerve cells that are neither efferent nor afferent neurons but that furnish a pathway of connection between them.

f., bundle, the gathering together of collagen fibers in a group, particularly the collagen fiber bundles of the periodontal membrane.

f., C nerve, small-diameter nerve fibers that are mechanoreceptors for pain occurring in both the pulp and the periodontal ligament, which are necessary to operate the gate mechanism.

f., cemental, the fibers of the periodontal membrane extending from the cementum to the zone of the intermediate plexus, where their terminations are interspersed with the terminations of the alveolar group of periodontal fibers.

f., circular, the fibers in the free gingiva that encircle the tooth in a ring-like fashion.

f., collagen, white fibers composed of collagen. The most conspicuous part of connective tissue, including the gingivae and periodontal membrane. Some fibers are distributed haphazardly throughout the connective tissue ground substance, and others are arranged in coarse bundles that exhibit a distinct orientation. Characterized by its hydroxyproline and hydroxylysine content.

f., crestal, one group of periodontal ligament fibers extending from the cervical area of the tooth to the alveolar crest.

f., dentogingival, the part of a fan shaped fiber system that emerges from the supraalveolar connective tissue; is composed of circular, dentogingival, dentoperiosteal, and transseptal fiber groups.

f., dentoperiosteal, a fiber system emerging from the supraalveolar part of the cementum of the tooth and passing outward beyond the alveolar crest

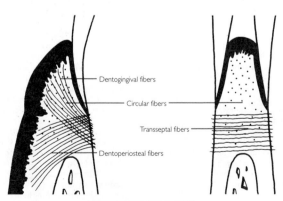

Dentogingival fibers

Circular fibers

Transseptal fibers

Dentoperiosteal fibers

Gingival fibers. (Genco, 1990.)

in an apical direction into the mucoperiosteum of the attached gingiva.

f., gingival, the group of fiber systems belonging to the gingival and supraalveolar connective tissue; is composed of circular, dentogingival, dentoperiosteal, and transseptal fiber groups.

f., horizontal, collagen fibers of the periodontal membrane that extend horizontally from the cementum to the alveolar bone.

f., nerve. See **fiber, nerve, myelinated** and **fiber, nerve, nonmedullated.**

f., myelinated nerve, a nerve fiber inside or outside the brain that is covered with an insulating medullary sheath along which are located nodes of Ranvier that facilitate as relay points the speed of nerve impulses over that of an equivalent nonmedullated fiber.

f., nonmedullated nerve, a nerve fiber not covered by an insulating medullary sheath that is thus exposed to other tissue fluids and their respective electric potentials. In nonmedullated fibers, the impulse is relayed from point to contiguous point. Most of the nonmedullated fibers are within the substance of the central nervous system, and the distances between the cells are short.

f., oblique, the group of collagen fibers in bundle arrangement in the periodontal ligament that are obliquely situated, with insertions in the cementum, and that extend more occlusally in the alveolus (approximately two thirds of the periodontal fibers fall into this group).

f., periodontal. See **ligament, periodontal.**

f., principal, the numerous bundles of collagenous tissue fibers arranged in groups that function as the mode of attachment of the tooth to the alveolus.

f., Sharpey's, collagenous fibers that become incorporated into the cementum.

f., transseptal, a part of the gingival fiber system that extends from the supraalveolar cementum of one tooth horizontally through the interdental attached gingiva above the septum of the alveolar bone to the cementum of the adjacent tooth.

fiberoptic light, a miniaturized light source that uses the property of flexible fiberglass strands to conduct light long distances with little or no distortion; used in intraoral application, such as a light attached directly to the dental handpiece.

fiberoptics, the technical process by which an internal organ or cavity can be viewed, using glass or plastic fibers to transmit light through a special tube designed to magnify and reflect an image of the surface of the internal region under observation.

fibrillation (fi′brilā′shən), a local quivering of muscle fibers.

f., atrial, a cardiac arrhythmia caused by disturbed spread of excitation through atrial musculature.

f., auricular (ôrik′yo͞olər), an uncoordinated, independent contraction of the heart that results in marked irregularity of heart action.

f., ventricular, an uncoordinated, independent contraction of the ventricular musculature resulting in cessation of cardiac output.

fibrinogen (fī′brin′əjən) (factor I, profibrin), a soluble plasma protein (globulin) that is acted on by thrombin to form fibrin. The normal level is 200 to 400 mg/100 ml in plasma. Coagulation is impaired if the concentration is less than 100 mg/100 ml. Another form of fibrinogen called *tissue fibrinogen,* which has the power of clotting the blood without the presence of thrombin, occurs in body tissues.

fibrinokinase (fī′brinōkī′nās) (fibrinolysokinase, lysokinase), an activator of plasminogen found in many animal tissues.

fibrinolysin (fī′brinol′isin). See **plasmin.**

fibrinolysis, the continual process of fibrin decomposition during the removal of small fibrin clots by the action of enzyme fibrinolysin.

fibrinolysokinase. See **fibrinokinase.**

fibroblast (fī′brōblast), a cell found within fibrous connective tissue, varying in shape from stellate (young) to fusiform and spindle shaped. Associated with the formation of collagen fibers and ground substance of connective tissue.

fibroblastoma (fī′brōblastō′mə), a tumor arising from an ordinary connective tissue cell or fibroblast. The tumor may be a fibroma or a fibrosarcoma.

f., neurogenic. See **neurofibroma.**

f., perineural. See **neurilemoma** and **neurofibroma.**

fibrocystic disease. See **disease, fibrocystic.**

fibroma (fĭbrō′mə), a benign mesenchymal tumor composed primarily of fibrous connective tissue.

f., ameloblastic, a mixed tumor of odontogenic origin characterized by the simultaneous proliferation of both the epithelial and mesenchymal components of the tooth germ without the production of hard structure.

f., calcifying. See **osteofibroma.**

f., cementifying, an intrabony lesion not associated with teeth, composed of a fibrous connective tissue stroma containing foci of calcified material resembling cementum; a rare odontogenic tumor composed of varying amounts of fibrous connective tissue with calcified material resembling cementum. Central lesion of the jaws.

f., irritation, a localized peripheral, tumorlike enlargement of connective tissue caused by prolonged local irritation and usually seen on the gingiva or buccal mucosa.

f., neurogenic. See **neurilemoma; neurofibroma.**

f., odontogenic, a central odontogenic tumor of the jaws, consisting of connective tissue in which small islands and strands of odontogenic epithelium are dispersed. A mesodermal odontogenic tumor composed of active dense or loose fibrous connective tissue; contains inactive islands of epithelium.

f., ossifying. See **osteofibroma.**

f., periapical (benign periapical fibroma, fibrous dysplasia, first-state cementoma, focal osseous dysplasia, traumatic osteoclasia), a benign connective tissue mass formed at the apex of a tooth with a normal pulp.

f., peripheral odontogenic, a fibrous connective tissue tumor associated with the gingival margin and believed to originate from the periodontium. Often contains areas of calcification. Localized form of fibromatosis gingivae.

f. with myxomatous degeneration. See **fibromyxoma.**

fibromatosis (fĭ′brōmətō′sis), a gingi-

val enlargement believed to be a hereditary condition that is manifested in the permanent dentition and characterized by a firm hyperplastic tissue that covers the teeth. Differentiation between this and diphenylhydantoin (Dilantin) hyperplasia is based on a history of drug ingestion.

f. gingivae (elephantiasis gingivae, idiopathic fibromatosis, idiopathic gingival hyperplasia), a generalized enlargement of the gingivae caused by fibrous hyperplasia. Idiopathic in nature and similar in appearance to Dilantin hyperplasia.

f., hereditary gingival, a condition possessing a familial attribute of distribution, in which there is gingival enlargement resulting from marked fibroplasia.

f., idiopathic. See **fibromatosis gingivae.**

fibromyalgia, a form of nonarticular rheumatism characterized by musculoskeletal aching and stiffness, fatigue, and poor sleep, as well as tenderness on palpation at various sites. Common sites of pain or stiffness are the lower back, neck, shoulder region, arms, hands, knees, hips, thighs, legs, and feet.

fibromyxoma (fĭ′brōmiksō′mə) (fibroma with myxomatous degeneration), a fibroma that has certain characteristics of a myxoma; a fibroma that has undergone myxomatous degeneration. Combination of both fibrous and myxomatous elements.

fibroosteoma (fĭ′brōäs′tēō′mə) (not current). See **osteofibroma.**

fibropapilloma (fĭ′brōpap′ilō′mə), a lesion that resembles a benign neoplasm and shows fibroblastic and epithelial proliferation. Such lesions occur in regions of cheek chewing or other trauma. Since they are not true neoplasms, they may be better designated as *irritation fibroses* or *fibrous hyperplasias.*

fibrosarcoma (fĭ′brōsarkō′mə), a malignant mesenchymal tumor, the basic cell type being a fibroblast. Most fibrosarcomas are locally infiltrative and persistent but do not metastasize.

f., odontogenic, an extremely rare, malignant form of odontogenic fibroma.

fibrosis (fĭbrō′sis), **1.** the process of forming fibrous tissue, usually by degeneration (for example, fibrosis of the pulp). The process occurs normally in the formation of scar tissue to replace normal tissue lost through injury or infection. **2.** an abnormal condition in which fibrous connective tissue spreads over or replaces normal smooth muscle or other normal organ tissue. Fibrosis is most common in the heart, lung, peritoneum, and kidney.

f., diffuse hereditary gingival, an uncommon form of severe gingival hyperplasia considered to be of genetic origin. The tissue is pink, firm, dense, and insensitive and has little tendency to bleed.

f., hereditary gingival, an uncommon form of severe gingival hyperplasia that may begin with the eruption of the deciduous or permanent teeth and is characterized by a firm, dense, pink gingival tissue with little tendency toward bleeding.

fiduciary (fidoo'shē·er'ē), a person who has a duty to act primarily for another's benefit, as a trustee. Also, pertaining to the good faith and confidence involved in such a relationship.

field, an area, region, or space.

f. block. See **block, field.**

f., operating, the area immediately surrounding and directly involved in a treatment procedure (for example, all the teeth included in a rubber dam application for the restoration of a single tooth or portions thereof).

f., radiation, the region in which radiant energy is being propagated.

file, 1. a metal tool of varying size and form with numerous ridges or teeth on its cutting surfaces; may be push-cut or pull-cut; used for smoothing or dressing down metals and other substances. **2.** a collection of records; an organized collection of information directed toward some purpose such as patient demographic data. The records in a file may or may not be sequenced according to a key contained in each record. **3.** To reduce by means of a file.

f.-access safeguards, methods of limiting certain users' access to particular data.

f., gold, a file designed for removing surplus gold from gold restorations; may be pull-cut or push-cut.

f., Hirschfeld-Dunlop, a kind of periodontal file used with a pull stroke for the removal of calculus; available in various angulations for approach to different surfaces of teeth.

f., root canal, a small metal hand instrument with tightly spiralled blades used to clean and shape the canal.

filing, the act of using a file to shape or smooth an object, usually metal.

filled resin. See resin, composite.

filling, a material used to fill a space. (Objectionable as a synonym for restoration.) See also **restoration.**

f., dental, a lay term for restoration. See **restoration, dental.**

f., "ditched," refers to the marginal failure of amalgam restorations caused by fracture of either the mater-

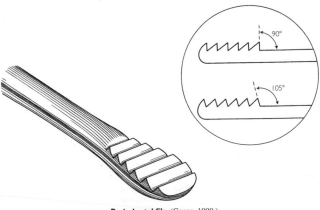

Periodontal file. (Genco, 1990.)

ial or the tooth structure itself in that area.

f. material. See **material, filling.**

f., postresection. See **filling, retrograde.**

f., retrograde (postresection filling, retrograde obturation), a filling placed in the apical portion of a tooth root to seal the apical portion of the root canal.

f., root canal, material placed in the root canal system to seal the space previously occupied by the dental pulp.

f. technique. See **technique, filling.**

f., treatment, a temporary filling, usually of a sedative nature, used to allay sensitive dentin before the final restoration of the cavity.

film, a thin, flexible, transparent sheet of cellulose acetate or similar material coated with a light-sensitive emulsion.

f. badge, a pack of x-ray-sensitive film used for the detection and approximate measurement of radiation exposure for personnel-monitoring purposes; the badge may contain two or three films of differing sensitivity, and it may contain a filter that shields part of the film from certain types of radiation.

f. base. See **base, film.**

f., bite-wing (interproximal film), a type of dental x-ray film that has a central tab or wing on which the teeth close to hold the film in position. See also **examination, radiographic.**

f. emulsion. See **emulsion, silver.**

f. fault, a defective result in a radiograph; usually caused by a chemical, physical, or electrical error in its production.

 f. f., black spots, spots caused by dust particles or developer on the films before development; also caused by outdated (expired) film.

 f. f., blurred, a fault caused by film movement during exposure, bent film during exposure, double exposures, or flowing of emulsion during processing in excessively warm solution

 f. f., dark, a fault caused by overexposure of the film to radiation, film fog from extended development, accidental exposure to light (light leaks in film packet or dark room), or an unsafe darkroom light.

 f. f., distorted. See **distortion, film-fault.**

f. f., dyschroic fog, a fogging of the radiograph, characterized by the appearance of a pink surface when the film is viewed by transmitted light and a green surface when the film is seen by reflected light. It usually is caused by an exhaustion of the acid content of the fixing solution (incomplete fixation).

f. f., fogged, a fault caused by stray radiation, use of expired film, or an unsafe darkroom light.

f. f., light, a fault caused by underexposure, underdevelopment (expired or diluted developing solution), development in temperatures that are too cold, or accidental use of a wrong film speed.

f. f., reticulation, a network of corrugations produced because of an excessive difference in temperature between any two of the three darkroom solutions.

f. f., stained, a fault caused by contaminated solutions, improper rinsing, exhausted solutions, improper washing, contamination by improper handling of the emulsions during or after processing, or film hangers containing dried fixer on the clips.

f. f., static electricity, an image in the emulsion that has the appearance of lightning. Caused by rapid opening of the film pocket or transfer of static electricity from the technician to the film.

f. f., white spots, a fault caused by air bubbles clinging to the emulsion during development or by fixing solution spotted on the emulsion before development.

f. hanger, an instrument or device for holding x-ray film during processing procedures.

f. holder, cardboard. See **cassette, cardboard.**

f. image, the shadow of a structure as depicted on a radiographic or photographic emulsion.

f., interproximal. See **film, bite-wing.**

f. mounting, the placement of radiographs in an orderly sequence on a suitable carrier for illumination and study.

f. on teeth, mucinous deposits on teeth, containing microorganisms, desquamated tissue elements, and blood cellular elements; usually thin and adherent.

f. packet, a small, lightproof, moisture-resistant, sealed paper or plastic envelope containing an x-ray film (or two x-ray films) and a lead-foil backing designed for use in making intraoral radiographs.

f. placement, the positioning of the x-ray film to receive the image cast by the roentgen rays.

f. processing, a chemical transformation of the latent image, produced in a film emulsion by exposure to radiation, into a stable image visible by transmitted light. The usual procedure is basically a selective reduction of affected silver halide salts to metallic silver grains (development), followed by the selective removal of unaffected silver halide (fixation), washing to remove the processing chemicals, and drying.

f. p., rapid, the use of high-speed chemicals or elevated temperatures to reduce processing time.

f. speed (film sensitivity), the amount of exposure to light or roentgen rays required to produce a given image density. It is expressed as the reciprocal of the exposure in roentgens necessary to produce a density of 1 above base and fog; films are classified on this basis in six speed groups, between each of which is a twofold increase in film speed.

f. thickness, refers to the thickness of a layer of material, particularly in reference to dental cements. In standardization tests, film thickness is the minimal thickness or layer obtained under a specific load.

f., x-ray. See **survey, radiographic.**

filter, a material placed in the useful beam to absorb preferentially the less energetic (less penetrating) radiations. See also **filtration.**

f., added, a filter added to the inherent filter.

f., compensating, a filter designed to shield less dense areas so that a more uniform image quality will be produced.

f., inherent, filtration introduced by the glass wall of the x-ray tube, any oil used for tube immersion, or any permanent tube enclosure in the path of useful beam.

f., total, the sum of inherent and added filters.

filtration, the use of absorbers for the selective attenuation of radiation of certain wavelengths from a useful primary beam of x-radiation.

f., built-in, filtration put into effect by nonremovable absorbers deliberately built into the tube head assembly to increase the inherent beam filtration.

f., external, the action of absorbers external to the tube-head assembly, consisting of added filtration plus the attenuating effect of materials of which any closed-end cone such as a pointer cone may be made. See also **filter, added.**

financial management, the management or control of the money or cash flow of a business or enterprise.

financial support, the funding of a project to assist in its accomplishment.

finasteride, *trade name:* Proscar; *drug class:* synthetic steroid; *action:* competitive inhibitor of 5-α-reductase, which converts testosterone to 5-α-dihydrotestosterone; *use:* symptomatic benign prostatic hyperplasia.

findings, radiographic (roentgenographic findings), the recorded radiographic evidence of normal and deviated anatomic structures.

fineness, a means of grading alloys with regard to gold content. The fineness of an alloy is designated in parts per thousand of pure gold, pure gold being 1000 fine.

finger, any one of the five digits of the hand.

f., clubbed, a condition seen in hypertrophic osteoarthropathy where the base angle between the base of the fingernail and adjacent dorsal surface of the terminal phalanx is obliterated and becomes 180 degrees or greater. The base of the nail projects downward, and the area of nail is increased.

f. positions, the positions of the fingers when operating; refers not only to the fingers grasping the instrument but also to the fingers used for rests, support, and holding the tissues out of the way.

f. rest, an integral part of instrumentation, in which the fingers of the working hand rest on the teeth, adjacent tissues, and fingers of the opposing hand to improve control of the working stroke of an instrument by providing a fulcrum for movement of the working fingers and instruments.

f. strut, a bar or similar component of the infrastructure of a subperiosteal or endosteal implant that projects from it, being attached only at one side.

f. sucking, the habit of sucking the finger (or thumb) for oral gratification. It is normal in infants and young children as a comforting device, especially when tired or hungry. If the habit persists beyond the eruption of the permanent teeth, it may cause a malocclusion of the anterior teeth.

finishing and polishing, the removal of excess restoration material from the margins and contours of a restoration, and polishing of the restoration.

finish line. See **line, finish.**

finish, satin, the degree of finish of a polished surface that has been made very smooth but is without a high sheen.

firmware, a special type of permanent program that takes the place of or accomplishes the function of traditional hardware components. Firmware is loaded into the equipment, either at the time it is manufactured or later, by the person installing the equipment or the person using the equipment.

first aid, the immediate care that is given to an injured or ill person before treatment by medically trained personnel.

first surgical stage (subperiosteal), the operation performed to obtain a direct bone impression.

fission (fish'ən), the splitting of a nucleus into two fragments. Fission may occur spontaneously or may be induced artificially. In addition to the fission fragments, particulate radiation energy and gamma rays are usually produced during fission.

f., nuclear, products, elements (nuclides) or compounds resulting from nuclear fission.

f. products, the nuclides produced by the fission of a heavy-element nuclide.

fissure, a deep groove or cleft; commonly the result of the imperfect fusion of the enamel or adjoining dental lobes.

f., gingival. See **cleft, gingival.**

f., pterygomaxillary, the most posterior point in the anterior contour of the maxillary tuberosity.

fissured tongue. See **tongue, fissured.**

fistula (fis'tyōōlə), an abnormal tract connecting two body surfaces or organs or leading from a pathologic or natural internal cavity to the surface. The tract may be lined with epithelium.

f., alveolar, a fistula communicating with the cavity of an alveolar abscess. More properly called *alveolar sinus.* See also **sinus, alveolar.**

f., arteriovenous. See **shunt, arteriovenous.**

f., branchial, a fistula associated with a branchial cyst; usually seen on the lateral surface of the neck.

f., dental. See **fistula, alveolar.**

f. of lip, a congenital malformation in which there is a deep pit or fistula on the mucosa of the lip; often bilateral and usually found on the lower lip.

f., oroantral, an opening between the maxillary sinus and the oral cavity, most often through a tooth socket. See also **fistula.**

f., orofacial, an opening between the cutaneous surface of the face and the oral cavity.

f., oronasal, an opening between the nasal cavity and the oral cavity.

f., salivary, an opening between a salivary duct and/or gland and the cutaneous surface or into the oral cavity through other than the normal anatomic pathway.

fit, an adaptation of any dental restoration. An adaptation of a denture to its basal seat, a clasp to a tooth, an inlay to a cavity preparation.

fix, to make firm, stable, immovable; to place in a desired position and hold there. In dentistry, to secure in position, usually by means of cementation, a prosthesis such as a crown or a fixed partial denture.

fixation, the act or result of fixing, such as being bound or limited in position or relationship.

f., biphase pin. See **appliance, fracture.**

f., elastic band, the stabilization of fractured segments of the jaws by means of intermaxillary or maxillomandibular elastic bands applied to splints or appliances.

f., external pin. See **appliance, fracture.**

f., intermaxillary. See **fixation, maxillomandibular.**

f., intraosseous, the reduction and stabilization of fractured bony parts by direct fixation to one another with surgical wires, screws, pins, and/or plates.

f., mandibulomaxillary. See **fixation, maxillomandibular.**

f., maxillomandibular (mandibulomaxillary fixation), a retention of fractures of the maxillae or mandible in the functional relations with the opposing dental arch through the use of elastic wire ligatures and interdental wiring and/or splints.

f., nasomandibular, mandibular immobilization, especially for edentulous jaws, using mandibulomaxillary splints, circummandibular wiring, and intraoral interosseous wiring through the nasal process of the maxillae.

f. of elements by the skeleton, the fixation of many elements for long periods of time in the bone matrix as a result of a special affinity of the elements for the matrix. Recent work with radioactive isotopes has firmly established the concept of the skeleton as a dynamic system. In addition to the changes in structure and distribution of the bone mineral mediated by cellular activity, every ionic grouping in the mineral is capable of replacement.

f., osseous, the immobilization of fractured bony segments.

f., radiographic, in film processing, the chemical removal of all the undeveloped salts of the film emulsion, so that only the developed (reduced) silver will remain as a permanent image.

f., restorative, the act of securing in position, usually by means of cementation, some treatment appliance such as a crown or fixed partial denture when willful removal of the restoration by the patient is not intended.

f., Roger-Anderson pin, an appliance used in extraoral fixation of mandibular fractures and prognathisms. See also **appliance, fracture.**

fixative, l. any substance used to bind, glue, or stabilize. **2.** any substance used to preserve gross or histologic specimens of tissue for later examination.

fixed costs, costs that do not change to meet fluctuations in enrollment or in use of services (for example, salaries, rent, business license fees, depreciation).

fixed fee schedule, a list of specified fees for services that will be paid to dentists participating in a dental plan.

fixed partial denture. See **denture, partial, fixed.**

fixed premium, a specified amount charged for insurance that is not changed by such factors as family size or initial year versus maintenance year of dental care coverage. Synonym: set premium.

flabby tissue. See **tissue, hyperplastic.**

flaccid (flak'sid), a relaxed or flabby state, as in a flail-like condition or paralysis of a muscle.

flag, l. any of various types of indicators used for identification. **2.** a character that signals the occurrence of some condition, such as the end of a word.

flagella, hairlike projections that extend from some unicellular organisms and aid in their movement.

flange (flanj), the part of the denture base that extends from the cervical ends of the teeth to the border of the denture.

f., buccal, the portion of the flange of a denture that occupies the buccal vestibule of the mouth and that extends distally from the buccal notch.

f., contour of, the topographic design of the flange of a denture.

f.-guide appliance, an appliance (prosthesis) with a lateral vertical extension designed to direct a resected mandible into centric occlusion.

f., labial, the portion of the flange of a denture that occupies the labial vestibule of the mouth.

f., lingual, the portion of the flange of a mandibular denture that occupies the space adjacent to the residual ridge and next to the tongue.

flap, a sheet of soft tissue partially or totally detached to gain access to structures underneath or to be used in repairing defects in an adjacent or a remote part of the body.

F

f., envelope, mucoperiosteal tissue retracted from a horizontal linear incision (as along the free gingival margin), with no vertical component of the incision.

f., lingual tongue, a flap used to repair a fistula of the hard palate, which combines the raising of a palatal flap to form the floor of the nose with a flap taken from the back or edge of the tongue to form the palatal surface.

f., mucoperiosteal, a flap of mucosal tissue, including the periosteum, reflected from a bone.

f., pedicle, a stalk-shaped flap.

f., sliding, a flap that is advanced from its original location in a direction away from its base, to close a defect.

f., V-Y, a flap in which the incision is shaped like a V and after closure like a Y, to lengthen a localized area of tissue. See also **flap, Y-V.**

f., Y-V, a flap in which the incision is shaped like a Y and after closure like a V, to shorten a localized area of tissue. See also **flap, V-Y.**

flash, excess material that is squeezed out of the mold (for example, during packing of a denture by compression technique).

flask, a metal case or tube used in investing procedures.

f., casting. See **flask, refractory.**

f. closure, the procedure of bringing the parts of a flask together to form a complete mold.

f., crown, a small, sectional, metal, boxlike case in which a sectional mold of plaster of paris or artificial stone is made for the purpose of compressing and curing plastics on small dental restorations.

f., denture, a sectional, metal, boxlike case in which a sectional mold of plaster of paris or artificial stone is made for the purpose of compressing and curing dentures or other resinous restorations.

f., final, closure, the last closure of a flask before curing and after trial packing the mold with a denture base material.

f., injection, a special flask designed to permit the filling of the mold after the flask is closed or to permit the addition of denture base material to that in the flask after the flask is closed.

f., refractory (casting flask, casting ring), a metal tube in which a refractory mold is made for casting metal dental restorations or appliances.

f., trial, closure, preliminary closures made for the purpose of eliminating excess denture base or other plastic material and of ensuring that the mold is completely filled.

flasking, the act of investing a pattern in a flask. The process of investing the cast and a wax denture in a flask preparatory to molding the denture base material into the form of the denture.

Flavobacterium, a genus of aerobic to facultatively anaerobic, nonspore-forming, motile, and nonmotile bacteria. These organisms characteristically produce yellow, orange, red, or yellow-brown pigments. They are found in soil and fresh and salt water. Some species are pathogenic.

flavonoids, a group of substances containing the plant pigment flavone. There is no known human requirement for them. They have a constriction effect on the capillary bed and decrease permeability of blood vessels. Some beneficial effects of flavonoids have been described in the treatment of bruises, contusions, and sprains. Synonym: bioflavonoid.

flavoxate HCl, *trade name:* Urispas; *drug class:* antispasmodic; *action:* relaxes smooth muscles in urinary tract; *uses:* relief of nocturia, incontinence, suprapubic pain, dysuria.

flecainide acetate, *trade name:* Tambocor; *drug class:* antidysrhythmic (Class IC); *action:* decreases conduction in all parts of the heart with greatest effect on His-Purkinje system; *uses:* life-threatening ventricular dysrhythmias, sustained supraventricular tachycardia.

flexibility, the property of elastic deformation under loading.

flexible benefits, a benefits program in which an employee has a choice of credits or dollars for distribution among various benefit options (for example, health and disability insurance, dental benefits, child care, pension benefits). See also **cafeteria plans** and **flexible spending account.**

flexible spending account, an employee reimbursement account primarily funded with employee-designated salary reductions. Funds are reimbursed to the employee for health care (medical and/or dental), dependent care, and/or legal expenses, and are considered a nontaxable benefit.

flexion (flek′shən), the bending of a joint between two skeletal members to decrease the angle between the members; opposite of extension.

f.-extension reflex. See **reflex, flexion-extension.**

flexure (flek′shər), the quality or state of being flexed.

f., clasp, the flexure of a retentive clasp arm to permit passage over the surveyed height of contour, thus permitting the seating or removal of the clasp.

floater, one or more spots that appear to drift in front of the eye, caused by a shadow cast on the retina by vitreous debris.

floor of cavity. See **cavity floor.**

floppy disk, a lightweight computer disk platter that is kept in a protective envelope and can be used for file information (storage). Synonym: diskette, flexible disk.

flora (flō′rə), the bacteria living in various parts of the alimentary canal.

f., fusospirochetal, the microorganisms *Fusobacterium fusiforme* and *Borrelia vincentii.* Present in most individuals as normal inhabitants of the oral cavity. Believed by some to be the primary and by others the secondary cause of acute necrotizing ulcerative gingivitis (ANUG).

f., oral, the microorganisms inhabiting the oral cavity of an individual. They are usually saprophytic in nature and live together in a symbiotic relationship. Some are potentially pathogenic, assuming a pathologic role when adverse local and/or systemic factors influence the symbiotic balance of the microorganic flora.

floss, dental, a waxed or unwaxed string or tape used to remove plaque from the interproximal and contact areas of the teeth. Its regular and proper use is essential to good oral hygiene and prevention of both dental caries and periodontal disease.

f. tape, a silk tape often incorporated with pumice and used to polish the proximal surfaces of teeth.

flossing, the mechanical cleansing of interproximal tooth surfaces with stringlike, waxed or unwaxed dental floss or tape.

flow, to move in a manner similar to a liquid stream.

f., dental material, the continued deformation or change in shape under a static load. As with waxes and amalgam.

f., traffic, the pattern of office personnel and patient movement from one area within the office to another.

flowchart, a graphic representation of a sequence of operations using symbols to represent the operations. Flowcharts often symbolize the most important steps of the process without detailing the algorithm of the way the work is to be performed.

flowmeter, a physical device for measuring the rate of flow of a gas or liquid.

fluconazole, *trade name:* Diflucan; *drug class:* antifungal; *action:* inhibits ergosterol biosynthesis; *uses:* oropharyngeal candidiasis, urinary candidiasis, cryptococcal meningitis, vaginal candidiasis.

fluctuation, a wavelike motion produced in soft tissues in response to palpation or percussion. Fluctuation is caused by a collection of fluids or exudates in the tissues.

flucytosine, *trade name:* Ancobon; *drug class:* antifungal; *action:* converted to fluorouracil after entering fungi, which inhibits DNA and RNA synthesis; *uses: Candida* infections.

fludrocortisone acetate, *trade name:* Florinef Acetate; *drug class:* glucocorticoid, mineralocorticoid; *action:* promotes increased reabsorption of sodium and loss of potassium from renal tubules; *uses:* adrenal insufficiency, salt-losing adrenogenital syndrome.

fluid (floo′id), a liquid or gaseous substance.

f., synovial, the small amount of fluid occurring in normal joints. Its principal function is to lubricate the joint surfaces and nourish the articular cartilage. Its content is approximately 95% water, with only 1% to 2% protein concentration.

f., total body, all the fluids contained in the body. There are two main types: the intracellular fluid, which is contained totally within the cells, and the extracellular fluid, which is contained entirely outside the cells.

f. wax. See **wax, fluid.**

flumazenil, *trade name:* Romazicon; *drug class:* benzodiazepine receptor antagonist; *action:* antagonizes actions of benziodiazepines on the central nervous system; *use:* reversal of sedative effects of benzodiazepines.

flunisolide, *trade name: Oral inh aerosol:* AcroBid, *drug class:* synthetic glucocorticoid; *action:* long-acting synthetic adrenocorticoid with antiinflammatory activity; *use:* rhinitis (seasonal or perennial).

fluocinonide, *trade names:* Licon, Lidex, Lidex-E; *drug class:* topical corticosteroid; *action:* interacts with steroid cytoplasmic receptors to induce antiinflammatory effects; possesses antipruritic, antiinflammatory actions; *uses:* psoriasis, eczema, contact dermatitis, pruritus, oral lichen planus lesions.

fluorescence (floōres'əns), the emission of radiation of a particular wavelength by certain substances as the result of absorption of radiation of a shorter wavelength.

fluorescent screen. See **screen, intensifying.**

fluoridate (flôr'idāt), to add fluoride to a water supply.

fluoridation, 1. the process of adding fluoride to a public water supply to reduce tooth decay. **2.** the use of a fluoride to reduce caries activity; may be by means of communal water supplies; oral hygiene preparations for home use; or topical applications for the purpose of prophylaxis.

fluoride, a salt of hydrofluoric acid, commonly sodium or stannous (tin).

fluorides, topical, salts of hydrofluoric acid (usually sodium or tin salts) that may be applied in solution to the enamel surface of the teeth to prevent dental decay.

fluoridization (flôr'idizā'shən), the topical application of a solution of a fluoride to teeth. See also **fluorides, topical.**

fluorine, an element of the halogen family and the most reactive of the nonmetals. Its atomic number is 9 and its atomic weight is 19. Small amounts of sodium fluoride added to the public water supply will reduce the incidence of dental caries, par-

ticularly among children. Excessive amounts of fluoride can mottle tooth enamel and cause osteosclerosis. Acute fluoride poisoning can cause death.

fluoroscope (floō'əskōp), a device consisting of a fluorescent screen mounted in a metal frame covered with lead glass. In the presence of a roentgen ray, the screen glows in direct proportion to the intensity of the remnant x-radiation, producing visual impressions of the densities traversed.

fluorosis (floōrō'sis), enamel hypoplasia caused by the ingestion of water containing excess fluoride during the time of enamel formation. General term for chronic fluoride poisoning. See also **fluorosis, chronic endemic dental.**

f., chronic endemic dental (mottled enamel), an enamel defect caused by excessive ingestion of fluoride in the water supply (usually 2 to 8 ppm) during the period of tooth calcification. Affected teeth appear chalky white on eruption and later turn brown.

fluorouracil (topical), *trade names:* Efudex, Fluoroplex; *drug class:* topical antineoplastic; *action:* inhibits synthesis of DNA and RNA in susceptible cells; *uses:* keratosis, basal cell carcinoma.

Fluothane, the trade name for halothane.

fluoxetine, *trade name:* Prozac; *drug class:* antidepressant; *action:* inhibits CNS neuron uptake of serotonin but not norepinephrine; *uses:* depressive disorders.

fluoxymesterone, *trade names:* Android-F, Halotestin; *drug class:* androgenic anabolic steroid, Controlled Substance Schedule III; *action:* increases weight by building body tissue; increases potassium, phosphorus, chloride, nitrogen levels; increases bone development; *uses:* impotence from testicular deficiency, hypogonadism, breast engorgement, palliative treatment of female breast cancer.

fluphenazine decanoate/fluphenazine enanthate/fluphenazine HCl, *trade names:* Decanoate, Moditen, Prolixin Enanthate; *drug class:* phenothiazine antipsychotic; *action:* blocks neurotransmission at dopaminergic synapses in the cerebral cortex, hypo-

F

thalamus, and limbic system; *uses:* psychotic disorders, schizophrenia.

flurandrenolide, *trade names:* Cordran, Cordran SP; *drug class:* topical corticosteroid, group III medium potency; *action:* possesses antipruritic, antiinflammatory actions; *uses:* corticosteroid-responsive dermatoses, pruritus.

flurazepam HCl, *trade name:* Dalmane; *drug class:* benzodiazepine, sedative-hypnotic, Controlled Substance Schedule IV; *action:* produces central nervous system depression by interaction with benzodiazepine receptor to facilitate action of inhibitory neurotransmitter γ-aminobutyric acid (GABA); *uses:* insomnia.

flurbiprofen, *trade name:* Ansaid; *drug class:* nonsteroidal antiinflammatory; *action:* inhibits prostaglandin synthesis by interfering with cyclooxygenase needed for biosynthesis; possesses analgesic, antiinflammatory, antipyretic properties; *uses:* acute, long-term treatment of rheumatoid arthritis, osteoarthritis.

f. sodium, *trade name:* Ocufen; *drug class:* nonsteroidal antiinflammatory ophthalmic; *action:* inhibits enzyme system necessary for biosynthesis of prostaglandins, inhibits miosis; *uses:* inhibition of intraoperative miosis, corneal edema.

flush, l. a blush or sudden reddening of the face and neck caused by vasodilation of small arteries and arterioles. **2.** a sudden, subjective feeling of heat. **3.** a sudden, rapid flow of water or other liquid.

flutamide, *trade name:* Eulexin; *drug class:* antineoplastic; *action:* interferes with testosterone at cellular level, inhibits androgen uptake; *uses:* metastatic prostatic carcinoma, stage D2 in combination with LHRH agonistic analogs (leuprolide).

fluticasone propionate, *trade name:* Cutivate (topical), Flonase (nasal spray); *drug class:* synthetic corticosteroid, medium potency; *action:* interacts with steroid cytoplasmic receptors to induce antiinflammatory effects; possesses antipruritic, antiinflammatory actions; *uses:* topical for inflammation of corticosteroid-responsive skin disorders; spray for seasonal and perennial allergic rhinitis.

flutter, a quick, irregular motion.

Fluvastatin sodium, *trade name:* Lescol; *drug class:* cholesterol-lowering agent; *action:* inhibits HMG-CoA reductase enzyme, which reduces cholesterol synthesis; *uses:* adjunct in primary hypocholesterolemia (types IIa and IIb).

fluvoxamine maleate, *trade name:* Luvox; *drug class:* antidepressant; *action:* selectively inhibits reuptake of serotonin in central nervous system neurons; *uses:* obsessive-compulsive disorder.

flux, any substance or mixture used to promote fusion, especially the fusion of metals or minerals. Used principally in dentistry as an inclusion in ceramic materials and in soldering and casting metals.

f., casting, a flux that increases fluidity of the metal and helps to prevent oxidation.

f., ceramic, a flux used in the manufacture of porcelain and silicate powders.

f., reducing, a flux that contains powdered charcoal to remove oxides.

f., soldering, a ceramic material such as borax, boric acid, or a combination, in paste, liquid, or granular form; used to keep metallic parts clean while they are being heated during a soldering procedure. It is a solvent for metallic oxides and will flow over the parts to be soldered at temperatures well below the fusion temperature of solder, but it becomes separated from the solid metal by the molten solder.

FMIA. See **angle, Frankfort-mandibular incisor.**

focal-film distance. See **distance, target-film.**

focal infection, the site or origin of an infectious process. Endodontically treated teeth have frequently been accused of being the source of septicemias, often without justification. See also **infection, focal.**

focal spot. See **spot, focal.**

focus group, a demographic target group of people used to gather opinions or data descriptive of the population represented by the sample selected.

fog (fogging). See **film fault, fogged.**

f., chemical. See **film fault.**

f., dyschroic. See **film fault, dyschroic fog.**

f., light. See **film fault.**

f., radiation, film darkening caused by radiation from sources other than intentional exposure to the primary beam; for example, film may be exposed to scatter radiation, or accidental exposure may occur if stored film is not protected from radiation.

foil, a very thin, flexible sheet of metal, usually gold, platinum, or tin.

f., adhesive, tinfoil that is covered on one side with powdered gum arabic or karaya gum.

f. assistant. See **foil holder.**

f., cohesive gold, a gold foil that has been annealed or whose surface is completely pure so that it will cohere or weld at room temperature.

f., corrugated gold, a gold foil made by burning gold-foil sheets between paper in the absence of air.

f. cylinder, a cylinder of gold foil formed by repeatedly folding a sheet of foil into a narrow ribbon, which is then rolled into cylindrical form.

f., gold (fibrous gold), pure gold that has been rolled and beaten from ingots into a very thin sheet. Thickness usually varies from 1/40,000 inch (No. 2 foil) to 1/20,000 inch (No. 4 foil). Classified as cohesive, semicohesive, or noncohesive. One of the oldest restorative materials, the most permanent if used properly, and the yardstick by which all others are measured. It is compacted or condensed into a retentive cavity form piece by piece, using this metal's property of cold welding.

f. holder (foil assistant), an instrument used to retain a foil pellet in place while it is being condensed or to retain a bulk of gold while additions to it are made.

f., noncohesive gold, a gold foil that will not cohere at room temperature because of the presence on its surface of a protecting or contaminating coating. If the coating is a volatile substance, such as ammonia, the foil may be rendered cohesive by heating or annealing it to remove the protection.

f. passer (foil carrier), a pointed or forked instrument used to carry pellets of gold foil through an annealing flame or from the annealing tray to the prepared cavity for compaction.

f. pellet. See **pellet, foil.**

f., platinized gold, a form rolled or hammered from a "sandwich" made of platinum placed between two sheets of gold; used in portions of foil restorations where greater hardness is desired.

f., platinum, pure platinum rolled into extremely thin sheets. A precious-metal foil whose high fusing point makes it suitable as a matrix for various soldering procedures; also suitable for providing the internal form of porcelain restorations during fabrication.

f., tin, a base-metal foil used as a separating material, or protective covering (for example, between the cast and denture base material during flasking and curing procedures).

fold, a doubling back of a tissue surface.

f., mucobuccal (mucobuccal reflection), the line of flexure of the oral mucous membrane as it passes from the mandible or maxillae to the cheek.

f., mucolabial, the line of flexure of the oral mucous membrane as it passes from the mandible or maxillae to the lip.

f., sublingual, the crescent-shaped area on the floor of the mouth following the inner wall of the mandible and tapering toward the molar regions. It is formed by the sublingual gland and the submaxillary duct beneath the mucous membrane of the alveololingual sulcus.

folder, usually a heavy paper envelope in which the patient's records are kept.

folic acid, vitamin B_9, a water-soluble B vitamin needed for erythropoiesis, increases red blood cell, white blood cell, and platelet formation in megaloblastic anemias. Folic acid functions as a coenzyme with vitamin B_{12} and C in the breakdown and utilization of proteins and in the formation of nucleic acids. It is prescribed for use during pregnancy, megaloblastic or macrocytic anemia caused by folic acid deficiency, liver disease, alcoholism, hemolysis, and intestinal obstruction.

follicular cyst, an odontogenic cyst that arises from the epithelium of a tooth bud and dental lamina.

follow-up, the process of monitoring the progress of a patient after a period of active treatment.

Fones' method. See **method, Fones'.** (not current)

food, ingested solids and liquids that supply the body with nutrients and energy.

f. additives, substances that are added to foods to prevent spoilage, improve appearance, enhance the flavor or texture, or increase the nutritional value.

f., comminution of (kom′inoo′shən), the reduction of food into small parts.

f. impaction. See **impaction, food.**

f., physical character of, the consistency, as the firmness, viscosity, or density, of food substances. Soft, adhesive, and nonabrasive foods tend to cling to the teeth, which may lead to calculus formation, whereas coarse foods leave little debris and create a frictional effect on the tissues, thus cleansing them.

Food and Drug Administration (FDA), an agency of the Department of Health and Human Services responsible for the enforcement of the Federal Food, Drug, and Cosmetic Act and other statutes assigned.

foot-and-mouth disease, a viral disease, common in farm animals outside the United States. It occasionally affects humans exposed to infected animals or animal products. Symptoms and signs in humans include headache, fever, and vesicles on tongue, oral mucous membranes, and hands and feet, lasting 7 to 10 days.

football, a popular American high school, collegiate, and professional team contact sport that may result in facial and dental injuries despite the use of protective headgear.

foramen (fôrā′mən), **1.** a natural opening in a bone or other structure. **2.** a natural opening in the root, usually at or near the apical end.

f., incisive (insī′siv) (nasopalatine foramen), **1.** the opening of the nasopalatine canal. **2.** the foramen, or opening, in the midline of the palate in the region where the premaxilla and maxillae join, which is situated palatal to the upper central incisors; contains nasopalatine vessels and nerve.

f. magnum, a passage in the occipital bone through which the spinal cord enters the spinal column.

f., mandibular, the opening on the medial aspect of the vertical ramus of the mandible approximately midway between the mandibular and gonial notches; may be located posterior to the middle of the ramus. It contains interior alveolar vessels and the inferior alveolar nerve.

f., mental, a circular opening on the lateral aspect of the body of the mandible either below the apex of the first premolar or below the apex of the second premolar, but usually between the first and second premolars inferior to their apices. The mental vessels and nerve pass through this foramen to supply the lip. In edentulous mandibles, the bone may have been resorbed, so that it is in such a position that the denture base will cover it.

f., nasopalatine. See **foramen, incisive.**

force, any application of energy, either internal or external to a structure; that which initiates, changes, or arrests motion.

f., centrifugal, a force that tends to recede from the center.

f., chewing, the degree of force applied by the muscles of mastication during the mastication of food.

f., component of, **1.** one of the factors from which a resultant force may be compounded or into which it may be resolved. **2.** one of the parts of a force into which it may be resolved.

f., condensing, **1.** the force required to compress gold-foil pellets, facilitating their cohesion, to fabricate or build up a gold-foil restoration. **2.** the force required to compact or condense a plastic material (for example, amalgam, wax).

f., constant, a continuous force or pressure applied to the teeth.

f., denture-dislodging, an influence that tends to displace a denture from its intended position on supporting structures.

f., denture-retaining, an influence that tends to maintain a denture in its intended position on its supporting structures.

f., electromotive, the difference in potential in a roentgen-ray tube between the cathode and anode; usually expressed in kilovolts.

f., intermittent, a force or pressure (applied to the teeth) that is alternated with a period of passiveness or rest.

f., line of, the direction of the power exerted on a body.

f., masticatory, the force applied by the muscles attached to the mandible during mastication.

f., occlusal (occlusal load), **1.** the result of muscular forces applied on opposing teeth. **2.** the force transmitted to the teeth and their supporting structures by tooth-to-tooth contact or through a bolus of food or other interposed substance.

f. and stress, pressure forcibly exerted on the teeth and on their investing and supporting tissues that is detrimental to tissue integrity. In occlusal trauma the production of lesions of the attachment apparatus depends on an interrelationship of the strength, duration, and frequency of the application of the force.

forced expiratory volume (FEV), the volume of air that can be forcibly expelled in a fixed time period after full inspiration.

forceps, 1. an instrument used for grasping or applying force to teeth, tissues, or other objects. **2.** an instrument used for grasping and holding tissues or specific structures. (Objectionable term in restorative dentistry because of its association with the extraction of teeth.)

f., bone, the force used for grasping or cutting bone.

f., chalazion, a thumb forceps with a flattened plate at the end of one arm and a matching ring on the other. Originally used for isolation of eyelid tumors. It is useful for isolation of lip and cheek lesions, such as a mucocele, to facilitate removal.

f., dental extracting, forceps used for grasping teeth.

f., hemostatic, an instrument for grasping blood vessels to control hemorrhage.

f., insertion. See **forceps, point.**

f., lock. See **forceps, point.**

f., mosquito, a small hemostatic forceps.

f., point (lock forceps, insertion forceps), a device used in filling root canals that securely holds the filling cones during their placement.

f., rubber dam clamp, forceps whose beaks are designed to engage holes in the rubber dam retainer to facilitate its placement, adjustment, or removal.

f., suture. See **needle holder.**

f., thumb, forceps used for grasping soft tissue; used especially during suturing.

f., tissue, a thumb forceps; an instrument with one or more fine teeth at the tip of each blade for controlling tissues during surgery, especially during suturing.

Fordyce's spots. See **spots, Fordyce's.**

forecasting, the attempt to predict the future on the basis of expert opinion, market research, trend projection, leading indicators, and other modalities.

forehead, that portion of the face directly above the orbits and extending posteriorly/superiorly to the hair line or crown of the head.

foreign body, any object or substance found in the body in an organ or tissue in which it does not belong under normal circumstances, such as a bolus of food in the trachea or a partical of dust in the eye. See also **body, foreign.**

forensic, pertaining to the law or to legal proceedings.

f. anthrolopgy, the use of anatomic structures and physical characteristics to identify a subject for legal purposes.

f. dentistry, the use of dental characteristics for the purpose of identifying a subject for legal purposes. See also **jurisprudence, dental.**

foreshortening. See **distortion, vertical.**

forging, working or shaping heated metal; hot-working a metal.

fork, face-bow, the part of the face-bow assembly used to attach an occlusion rim or transfer record of maxillary teeth to the face-bow proper.

form, the configuration, shape, or particular appearance of anything.

f., acquaintance, a registration sheet for new patients on which data (for example, the patient's name and address) are recorded and that contains a statement of the policies of the specific dentist's office and the responsibilities of the dentist to the patient.

f., anatomic, the natural shape of a part.

f., arch, the shape of the dental arch. See also **arch, dental.**

f., convenience, the modifications necessary, beyond basic outline form, to facilitate proper instrumentation for the preparation of the cavity or insertion of the restorative material; also the placing of starting points or slight undercuts to retain the first portions of restorative material while succeeding portions are placed.

f., face, the outline form of the face from an anterior frontal view.

f., functional, the shape that permits optimal performance.

f., message, a checklist form, by means of which auxiliary personnel can quickly make a record of telephone communications for the dentist to peruse later.

f., occlusal, the form of the occlusal surface of a tooth, a row of teeth, or dentition.

f., outline, the shape of the area of the tooth surface included within the cavosurface margins of a prepared cavity.

f., registration, a form used to gather personal data about a patient other than professional information.

f., resistance, the shape given to a prepared cavity to enable the restoration and remaining tooth structure to withstand masticatory stress.

f., retention, the provision made in a cavity preparation to prevent displacement of the restoration.

f., root, the shape of the root of the tooth; it is capable of being modified by such factors as resorption and cemental apposition.

f., tooth, the characteristics of the curves, lines, angles, and contours of various teeth that permit their identification and differentiation.

f., posterior tooth, the distinguishing contours of the occlusal surface of the various posterior teeth.

formaldehyde, a toxic, pungent water-soluble gas used in the aqueous form as a disinfectant, fixative, or tissue preservative.

formalin, a clear aqueous solution of formaldehyde. A 37% solution is used to fix and preserve tissues for histologic and pathologic study.

format, a predetermined computer arrangement of characters, fields, lines, page numbers, punctuation marks, and the like.

former, angle. See **angle former.**

former, crucible. See **sprue former.**

former, sprue. See **sprue former.**

formocresol, a compound consisting of formaldehyde, cresol, glycerin, and water used in vital pulpotomy of primary teeth and as a temporary intracanal medicament during root canal therapy. Brand name: Buckley's Formo Cresol.

fortified (fortə′fīd), containing additives more potent than the principal ingredient.

forward protrusion. See **protrusion, forward.**

foscarnet sodium/phosphonoformic acid, *trade name:* Foscavir; *drug class:* antiviral; *action:* antiviral activity is produced by selective inhibition at the pyrophosphate binding site on virus-specific DNA polymerases, inhibits replication of all known herpesviruses; *uses:* CMV retinitis in AIDS, acyclovir-resistant herpes zoster in HIV-infected patients.

Foshay's test. See **test, Foshay's.**

fosinopril, *trade name:* Monopril; *drug class:* angiotensin-converting enzyme (ACE) inhibitor; *action:* selectively suppresses renin-angiotensin-aldosterone system; *uses:* hypertension alone or in combination with thiazide diuretics.

fossa (fos′ə), a pit, hollow, or depression.

f., canine, the concavity, or depression, in the maxilla superior to the apex of the canine tooth.

f., depth of, the distance from the top of the shorter cusp downward into the bottom of the fossa.

f., nasal. See **cavity, nasal.**

foundation, 1. a charitable organization usually established to allocate private funds to worthy projects or to provide other services. **2.** in dentistry, any device or material added to a remaining tooth structure to enhance the stability and retention of an overlying cast restoration. May be a pin retainer of amalgam, plastic cement, or a casting.

four-handed dentistry. See **dentistry, four-handed.**

Fournier's glossitis (fŏŏrnē·āz′) (not current). See **glossitis, interstitial sclerous.**

Fox scissors. See **scissors, Fox.**

Fox's knife. See **knife, Goldman-Fox.** (not current)

fractionation, 1. the separation of a substance into its basic constituents.

2. the process of isolating a pure culture by secessive culturing of a small portion of a colony of bacteria. **3.** the process of isolating different components of living cells by centrifugation. **4.** the process of administering a dose of radiation in smaller units over a period of time to minimize tissue damage.

fracture, a break or rupture of a part. In the oral region, fracture is most frequently seen in teeth and bones.

f., avulsion, the loss of a section of bone.

f., blow-out, a fracture involving the orbital floor, its contents, and the superior wall of the maxillary antrum, in which orbital contents are incarcerated in the fracture area, producing diplopia.

f., cementum, the tearing of fragments of the cementum from the tooth root.

f., clasp, failure of a clasp arm because of stresses that have exceeded the elastic limit of the metal from which the arm was made.

f., closed reduction of, a reduction and fixation of fractured bones without making a surgical opening to the fracture site.

f., comminuted, a fracture in which the bone has several lines of fracture in the same region; a fracture in which the bone is crushed and splintered.

f., compound, a fracture in which the bony structures are exposed to an external environment.

f., craniofacial dysjunction (transverse facial fracture), a complex fracture in which the facial bones are separated from the cranial bones; a LeFort III fracture.

f., dislocation, a fracture of a bone near an articulation, with dislocation of the condyloid process.

f., fissured, a fracture that extends partially through a bone, with no displacement of the bony fragments.

f. fixation, to stabilize in close proximation the fractured fragments of bone to promote healing.

f., greenstick, a fracture in which the bone appears to be bent; usually only one cortex of the bone is broken.

f., Guérin's, a LeFort I fracture of the facial bones in which there is a bilateral horizontal fracture of the maxillae.

f., impacted, a fracture in which one fragment is driven into another portion of the same or an adjacent bone.

f., indirect, a fracture at a point distant from the primary area of injury caused by secondary forces.

f., intraarticular, a fracture of the articular surface of the condyloid process of a bone.

f., intracapsular, a fracture of the condyle of the mandible occurring within the confines of the capsule of the temporomandibular joint.

f., LeFort, a transverse fracture involving the orbital, malar, and nasal bones.

f., midfacial, fractures of the zygomatic, maxillary, nasal, and associated bones.

f., pyramidal, a fracture of the midfacial bones, with the principal fracture lines meeting at an apex in the area of the nasion; a LeFort II fracture.

f., root, a microscopic or macroscopic cleavage of the root in any direction.

f., simple, a linear fracture that is not in communication with the exterior.

f., stress, **1.** usually occuring from sudden, strong, violent, endogenous force, such as a simple fracture of the fibula in a runner. **2.** the fracture of metallic parts as a result of fatigue of prolonged or frequent stress.

f., transverse facial. See **fracture, craniofacial dysjunction.**

fragilitas ossium (frajil′ētəs os′ēəm). See **osteogenesis imperfecta.**

frail elderly, an older person (usually over the age of 75 years) who is afflicted with physical or mental disabilities that may interfere with the ability to independently perform activities of daily living.

frambesia (frambē′zē·ə) (not current). See **yaws.**

frame, a structure, usually rigid, designed to give support or attachment to a part, or to immobilize a part.

f., implant. See **substructure, implant.**

f., occluding, a device for relating casts to each other for the purpose of arranging teeth or for use in making an index of the occlusion of dentures; an articulator. See also **articulator.**

f., rubber dam. See **holder, rubber dam.**

framework, the skeletal metal portion of a removable partial denture around which and to which the remaining units are attached.

franchise dentistry, 1. the practice of dentistry under a trade name, the rights of which have been purchased from another dentist or dental practice. Under a franchise license agreement, the franchiser may use the trade name, marketing products, and treatment techniques for a sum of money, as long as certain rules and regulations of the franchise are adhered to. **2.** refers to a system for marketing a dental practice, usually under a trade name, where permitted by state laws. In return for a financial investment or other consideration, participating dentists may also receive the benefits of media advertising, a national referral system, and financial and management consultation.

Frankel appliance. See **appliance, Frankel.**

Frankfort horizontal plane. See **plane, Frankfort horizontal.**

Frankfort-mandibular incisor angle. See **angle, Frankfort-mandibular incisor.**

F-ratio (F-test), a value used in determining whether the difference between two variables is statistically significant or stable. A larger variance is divided by a smaller variance, both of which are the results of analysis of variance procedures. The value for F is looked up in a table that shows the probability of occurrence of a ratio of this size.

fraud, an intentional perversion of truth for the purpose of inducing another, in reliance on it, to part with something valuable or to surrender a legal right; deliberate deception; deceit; trickery.

fraudulent concealment, the deliberate attempt to withhold information or to conceal an act to avoid contractual responsibility. Fraudulent concealment as applied to health care providers arises when a treating doctor conceals from an aggrieved patient the fact that a previous treating doctor may have committed malpractice.

freckle. See **ephelis.**

freedom of choice, a provision in a dental benefits program that permits the insured to choose any licensed dentist to provide his or her dental care and receive full benefits under the program.

free-end. See **base, extension.**

free gingiva. See **gingiva, free.**

free gingival margin. See **margin, gingival, free.**

free mandibular movement. See **movement, mandibular, free.**

free radical, a compound with an unpaired electron or proton. It is unstable and reacts readily with other molecules.

free-way space. See **distance, interocclusal.**

freeze drying, the freezing of heat-sensitive liquid materials in a vacuum to preserve the characteristics of the substrate and remove the volume of water or liquid by sublimation.

Frei's test (frīz). See **test, Frei's.** (not current)

fremitus (frem'itəs), palpable vibrations of nonvascular origin that can be noted by placing the hand on the chest. See also **thrill.**

frenectomy (frenek'tōmē), **1.** the excision of a frenum. **2.** the surgical detachment and/or excision of a frenum from its attachment into the mucoperiosteal covering of the alveolar processes.

frenoplasty (frenōplas'tē), a correction of an abnormal frenum by repositioning it.

frenotomy (frənot'əmē), the cutting of a frenum; especially the release of tongue-tie, or ankyloglossia.

frenulum (fren'yələm). See **frenum.**

frenum (fre'nəm) (frenulum), a fold of mucous membrane attaching the cheeks and lips to the mandibular and maxillary mucosa and limiting the motions of the lips and cheeks.

f., abnormal (enlarged labial frenum), a labial frenum appearing to be unusually heavy, broad, or attached too near the crest of the ridge that may be an etiologic factor in the production, perpetuation, and/or modification of lesions of the marginal gingivae.

f., buccal, a fold or folds of mucous membrane connecting the residual alveolar ridge to the cheek in the premolar region. They exist in both the upper and lower jaws and separate the labial vestibule from the buccal vestibule.

f., enlarged labial. See **frenum, abnormal.**

f., labial, the fold of mucous membrane connecting the lip of the residual alveolar ridge near the midline of both the upper and lower ridges.

f., lingual, the vertical band of mucous membrane connecting the tongue with the floor of the mouth and the alveolar or residual alveolar ridge.

frequency, the number of cycles per second of a wave or other periodic phenomenon.

f. polygon, a graphic representation of a frequency distribution constructed by plotting each frequency above the score or midpoint of a class interval laid out on a base line and connecting the points so plotted by a straight line.

Frey's syndrome (frīz). See **syndrome, auriculotemporal.**

fricative (frik'ətiv), any speech sound made by forcing the airstream through such a narrow orifice or opening that audible high-frequency air currents or vibrations are set up.

friction, the resistance to movement as one object is moved across the other, usually creating heat.

Friedman splint (frēd'mən) (not current). See **splint, cast bar.**

Friedman's test (frēd'mənz). See **test, pregnancy.**

fringe benefits, benefits, other than wages or salary, provided by an employer for employees (for example, health insurance, vacation time, disability income).

frit (frit), a partly or wholly fused porcelain that is plunged into water while hot. The mass cracks and fractures, and from this "frit," dental porcelain powders are made.

Frohlich's syndrome (frä'liks). See **syndrome, Frohlich's.** (not current)

frontal bone, a single cranial bone that forms the front of the skull from above the orbits posteriorly to a junction with the parietal bones at the coronal suture.

frontal (PA) cephalometric radiograph, a cephalometric radiograph made with the subject facing the film (posteroanterior [PA] view); the axis between the ears is parallel to the film and perpendicular to the x-ray beam.

frontal lobe, the largest of five lobes constituting each of the two cerebral hemispheres. The frontal lobe lies beneath the frontal bone. The frontal lobe significantly influences personality and is associated with the higher mental activities, such as planning, judgment, and conceptualizing.

frontal sinus, one of a pair of small cavities in the frontal bone of the skull that communicates with the nasal cavity.

frozen sections, a histologic section of tissue that has been frozen by exposure to dry ice.

fructose, a yellowish-to-white, crystalline water-soluble levorotatory ketose monosaccharide that is sweeter than sucrose and is found in honey, several fruits, and combined in many disaccharides and polysaccharides. Also called *fruit sugar* and *levulose.*

fructose intolerance, an inherited disorder marked by an absence of enzymes needed to metabolize fructose. Symptoms include sweating, tremors, confusion, and digestive distress with vomiting, and failure of infants to grow.

fulcrum line. See **line, fulcrum.**

fulguration (fulgyərā'shən), the destruction of soft tissue by an electric spark that jumps the gap from an electrode to the tissue without the electrode touching the tissue. See also **electrocoagulation.**

function, the normal or special action of a part. As a noun, function has the following synonyms: role, capacity, task, use, purpose, service, activity, and direction. As a verb, it has the following synonyms: act, operate, work, perform, go, take effect, and serve. Use of the term to express intended purpose may be misleading.

f., auxiliary, a function that is supplementary or additional to the function for which the part or organ is primarily intended.

f., dental, normal, the correct action of opposing teeth in the process of mastication; sometimes referred to as *normal occlusion.*

f., group, the simultaneous contact of opposing teeth in a segment or group.

f., heavy (occlusal function), an increase in functional activities of the tooth, which may result in compensatory changes in the attachment apparatus (for example, a stronger periodontal ligament) with an increase in the number of fibers; a reinforcement of the supporting bone by formation of new bone; and the formation of cemental spikes, which are calcifications of the cemental fibers. Such changes take place so that the increased stress may be withstood without damage.

f., impaired, diminished, weakened, or less-than-optimal work or action.

f., insufficiency of, hypofunction of the tooth, which may lead to regressive changes in the attachment apparatus and supporting bone. The severity of lesions varies with the degree of hypofunction. See also **atrophy of disuse.**

f., muscle, the action of muscle, which is principally contraction.

f., occlusal. See **function, heavy.**

f., physiologic, the degree of activity that stimulates the physical structures but that is so limited as to stop short of irritation of those tissues.

f., skeletal, the role of the skeleton in relation to the maintenance of body functions. The bony skeleton welds together and protects the softer vital visceral organs, supports and maintains the body form, and accomplishes body movement for locomotion, respiration, manual skills, and the functions associated with mandibular motion.

f., subcortical, function controlled by all the structures of the brain except the outer cortical rim of the cerebrum; most of the nonconscious activities of a sensory and motor nature.

functional, 1. pertaining to the movements and actions of a part. **2.** of or pertaining to the functions of an organ, part, or prosthesis.

f. jaw orthopedics, the objectives of activator-type appliances.

fundoplication, a surgical procedure involving making tucks in the fundus of the stomach around the lower end of the esophagus. The operation is used in the treatment of gastric acid reflux into the esophagus.

fungal infection, an infection caused by a fungus or yeast organism.

fungate (fun'gāt), to produce fungus-like growths; to grow rapidly like a fungus.

fungus (fung'gəs), a class of vegetable organisms of a low order of development, including mushrooms, toad-stools, and molds. Many are saprophytic and/or pathogenic for humans (for example, *Candida albicans* and *Histoplasma, Trichophyton, Actinomyces,* and *Blastomyces* organisms. Oral and systemic moniliasis (thrush) is produced by overgrowth of *C. albicans,* which is a saprophytic resident in the oral cavity. When physiologic processes are sufficiently impaired, the organism may gain a foothold and assume a pathogenic role. Of the more than 100,000 identified species, 100 are common in humans and 10 are known pathogens.

furcation (fərkā'shən), the region of division of the root portion of a tooth.

f. defects, structural defects that occur in the region of the division of the root of a tooth into two, three, or four divisions. Generally, these defects constitute a communication channel between the pulp and the periodontal space.

f., root, the interradicular bone resorption in multirooted teeth caused by periodontal disease.

furnace, an apparatus in which to generate heat.

f., inlay, a furnace used for eliminating the wax from an inlay mold and establishing the proper condition and temperature of the investment to receive the molten casting gold.

f., porcelain, a furnace used for fusing, firing, or fusion.

furosemide, *trade names:* Lasix, Lasix Special; *drug class:* loop diuretic; *action:* acts on loop of Henle to decrease reabsorption of chloride and sodium and resultant diuresis; *uses:* pulmonary edema, edema in CHF, liver disease, ascites, hypertension.

fused teeth, teeth that are joined together during the formative process by one or more of the hard tissues: enamel, dentin, and/or cementum.

fusion, 1. the uniting or joining together of two or more entities. The fusion temperature of an alloy lies just below the lower limit of its melting range, which is particularly important in soldering operations because temperatures near or above fusion temperature will decrease ductility. See also **crescence** and **range, melting. 2.** The process of producing fused teeth.

f. of metal. See **metal, fusion of.**

f., nuclear, the union of atomic nuclei to form heavier nuclei, resulting in the release of enormous quantities of energy when certain light elements unite.

Fusobacterium, a genus of bacteria containing gram-negative, nonspore-forming, obligately anaerobic rods that produce butyric acid as a major metabolic product. These organisms are found in cavities of man and other animals; some species are pathogenic. *F. fusiforme* (fūzōbaktē′rēəm) (Vincent's bacillus), a microorganism that, along with *Borrelia vincentii,* is implicated in the causation of necrotizing ulcerative gingivitis. Although *F. fusiforme* and *B. vincentii* are inhabitants of the oral cavity, they may become pathogenic when tissue resistance is impaired.

F. nucleatum, a genus of schizomycetes, an anaerobic gram-negative bacterium often seen in necrotic tissue and implicated, but not conclusively, with other organisms in the causation and perpetuation of periodontal disease.

g. See **gram.**

gabapentin, *trade name:* Neurontin; *drug class:* anticonvulsant; *action:* anticonvulsant action is unclear; *use:* adjunctive therapy in adults with partial seizures.

gadolinium (Gd), a rare earth metallic element with an atomic number of 64 and an atomic weight of 157.25. Gadolinium is used as a phosphor to intensify x-ray screens.

gag, a surgical device for holding the mouth open.

g. reflex, a normal neural reflex elicited by touching the soft palate or posterior pharynx; the response is a symmetric elevation of the palate, a retraction of the tongue, and a contraction of the pharyngeal muscles. The reflex is used as a test of the integrity of the vagus and glossopharyngeal nerves.

gagging, an involuntary retching reflex that may be stimulated by something touching the posterior palate or throat region.

gait (gāt), a manner of walking; a cyclic loss and regaining of balance by a shift of the line of gravity in relationship to the center of gravity. A person's gait is as characteristic and as individual as a fingerprint.

g., cerebellar, an unsteady, irregular gait characterized by short steps and a lurching from one side to the other; most commonly seen in multiple sclerosis or other cerebellar diseases.

g., festinating, a gait characterized by rigidity, shuffling, and involuntary hastening. The upper part of the body advances ahead of the lower part. It is associated with paralysis agitans and postencephalitic Parkinson's syndrome.

g., sensor ataxic, an irregular, uncertain, stamping gait. The legs are kept far apart, and either the ground or the feet are watched, since there has been a loss of knowledge of the position of the lower limbs. This gait is caused by an interruption of the afferent nerve fibers and may be associated with tabes dorsalis and sometimes with multiple sclerosis and other lesions of the nervous system.

g., spastic (creeping palsy), a slow, shuffling gait in which the patient appears to be wading in water. Knee and hip movements are restricted. This gait may be associated with multiple sclerosis, syphilis, combined systemic disease, or other diseases affecting the spinal pyramidal tracts.

g., staggering, a reeling, tottering, and tipping gait in which the individual appears as if he may fall backward or lose his balance. A staggering gait is associated with alcohol and barbiturate intoxication.

g., waddling, an exaggerated alteration of lateral trunk movements, with an exaggerated elevation of the hip, suggesting the gait of a duck; characteristic of progressive muscular dystrophy.

galactin (gəlak′tin). See **hormone, lactogenic.**

galactosamine, a chondrosamine; a derivative of galactose, occurs in various mucopolysaccharides, notably of chondroitin sulfuric acid and B blood group substance.

galactose, a simple sugar found in the dextrorotatory form in lactose (milk sugar), nerve cell membranes, sugar beets, gums, seaweed, and, in the levorotatory form, in flaxseed mucilage. Galactose, a white crystalline substance, is less sweet and less soluble in water than glucose but is similar in other properties.

gallic acid, an astringent used topically, made from tannic acid or nutgalls, and chemically known as 3,4,5-trihydroxybenzoic acid.

gallium, a metallic element with an atomic number of 31 and an atomic weight of 69.72. Gallium is used in high temperature thermometers, and its radioisotopes are used in total-body scanning procedures.

galvanic current. See **current, galvanic.**

galvanic skin response (GSR), a reaction to certain stimuli as indicated by a change in the electric resistance of the skin. The GSR is used in some polygraph examinations.

galvanism. See **current, galvanic.**

galvanotherapy. See **ionization.**

gamma rays, an electromagnetic radiation of short wave-length emitted by the nucleus of an atom during a nuclear reaction. Composed of high-energy photons, gamma rays lack mass and an electric charge and travel at the speed of light.

ganciclovir, *trade names:* Cytovene, DHPG; *drug class:* antiviral; *action:* inhibits replication of most herpes viruses in vitro; in vivo by selective inhibition of human CMV DNA polymerase and by direct incorporation into viral DNA; *uses:* cytomegalovirus (CMV) retinitis in patients with AIDS.

ganglion(ia) (gang′glē·on), any collection or mass of nerve cells that serves as a center of nervous influence.

g., basal, a group of forebrain nuclei that, with the related structures of the brain, play an important role in the regulation of muscle tone and motor control. The cell groups of these ganglia and their respective nerve tracts are classified as the *extrapyramidal motor system* to differentiate them from the *pyramidal motor system,* which goes directly from the cerebral cortex to the lower motor neuron. Disease associated with the basal ganglia is manifested by three principal motor abnormalities: disturbance of muscle tone, derangement of movement, and loss of associated or automatic movement.

g., ciliary, a parasympathetic nerve ganglion in the posterior part of the orbit. The ciliary ganglion receives preganglionic fibers from the region of the oculomotor nucleus and sends postganglionic fibers via short ciliary nerves to (1) the constrictor muscle of the iris (constriction of pupil) and (2) circular fibers of the ciliary muscle (accommodation for vision).

g., otic, a ganglion located medial to the mandibular nerve just below the foramen ovale in the infratemporal fossa. It supplies the sensory and secretory fibers for the parotid gland. Its sensory fibers arise from the facial and glossopharyngeal nerves.

g., sphenopalatine, one of the four ganglia of the autonomic nervous system associated with the head and neck region. It is located deep in the pterygopalatine fossa and is intimately associated with the maxillary nerve. It lies distal and medial to the maxillary tuberosity. Its fibers supply the mucous membrane of the roof of the pharynx, tonsils, soft and hard palates, and nasal cavity. The mucous and serous secretions of all the mucous membranes in the oropharynx are also mediated by this ganglion.

g., submaxillary, a ganglion located on the medial side of the mandible between the lingual nerve and the submaxillary duct. The submaxillary ganglion is distributed to the sublingual and submaxillary glands. The sensory fibers arise from the lingual branch of the trigeminal nerve; that is, the chorda tympani of the facial nerve.

ganglionectomy, the excision of a ganglion.

ganglionitis, acute posterior (gang′-glē·ənī̄tis). See **herpes zoster.**

gangrene, the death of tissue en masse, usually the result of loss of blood supply, bacterial invasion, and subsequent putrefaction. For example, gangrene of the pulp is total death and necrosis of the pulp.

g., dry, a late complication of diabetes mellitus that is already complicated by arteriosclerosis in which the affected extremity becomes cold, dry, and shriveled and eventually turns black.

g., gas, necrosis accompanied by gas bubbles in soft tissue after trauma or surgery. It is caused by anaerobic microorganisms such as various species of *Clostridium,* particularly *C. perfringens.* If untreated, gas gangrene is rapidly fatal.

g., moist, a condition that may follow a crushing injury or an obstruction of blood flow by an embolism, tight bandages, or a tourniquet. This form of gangrene has an offensive odor, spreads rapidly, and may result in death in a few days. All types of gangrene require the removal of the necrotic tissue before healing can progress.

Gantrisin, the brand name for sulfisoxazole, an antibacterial sulfonamide, which is effective in the treatment of acute, recurrent, or chronic urinary tract infections, in the treatment of meningococcal meningitis, and in the treatment of acute otitis media.

gap arthroplasty, the surgical correction of ankylosis by creation of a space between the ankylosed part and the portion in which movement is desired.

gap, interocclusal. See **distance, interocclusal.**

Gardner-Diamond syndrome, a condition resulting from autoerythrocyte sensitization, marked by large, painful, transient ecchymoses that appear without apparent cause but often accompany emotional upsets, various collagen disorders, and abnormalities of protein metabolism. Treatment includes topical and systemic corticosteroids. Also called *autoerythrocyte sensitization syndrome.*

gargoylism. See **syndrome, Hurler's.**

GAS. See **syndrome, general adaptation.**

gas, a fluid with no definite volume or shape whose molecules are practically unrestricted by cohesive forces.

g., laughing. See **nitrous oxide.**

g., noble, a gas that will not oxidize; the inert gases (for example, helium, neon).

g., olefiant. See **ethylene.**

gasometer (gasäm'ətər), a calibrated instrument or vessel for measuring the volume of gases. Used in clinical and physiologic investigation for measuring respiratory volume.

gastric acid, hydrochloric acid secreted by the gastric glands in the stomach; aids in the preparation of food for digestion.

gastric intrinsic factor (GIF), a substance secreted by the gastric mucosa that is essential for the intestinal absorption of vitamin B_{12}; also known as *intrinsic factor.*

gastric juice, the digestive secretions of the gastric glands in the stomach, consisting chiefly of pepsin, hydrochloric acid, rennin, and mucin.

gastric mucosa, the lining of the stomach, which contains gastric glands.

gastrinoma, a gastrin-secreting tumor associated with the Zollinger-Ellison syndrome.

gastritis, an inflammation of the lining of the stomach that occurs both in an acute and a chronic form. Acute gastritis may be caused by aspirin or other antiinflammatory agents, corticosteroids, drugs, foods, condiments, and alcohol and chemical toxins. The symptoms are anorexia, nausea, vomiting, and discomfort after eating. Chronic gastritis is usually a sign of underlying disease, such as peptic ulcer or pernicious anemia.

g., atrophic, a chronic form of gastritis with atrophy of the mucous membrane and destruction of the peptic glands, sometimes associated with pernicious anemia or gastric carcinoma.

gastroenteritis, an inflammation of the stomach and intestines accompanying numerous gastrointestinal (GI) disorders. Symptoms are anorexia, nausea, vomiting, abdominal discomfort, and diarrhea.

gastroenterology, the study of diseases affecting the GI tract, including the esophagus, stomach, intestines, rectum, gallbladder, and bile duct.

gastroesophageal reflux, a backflow of the contents of the stomach into the esophagus that is often the result of incompetence of the lower esophageal sphincter. Gastric juices are acid and therefore produce burning pain in the esophagus.

G

gastrointestinal disease, any abnormal state or function of the GI system.

gastrointestinal system, the chain of organs of the GI tract, from the mouth to the anus.

gastroscopy, the visual inspection of the interior of the stomach by means of a flexible fiberoptic tube inserted through the mouth and passing the length of the esophagus into the stomach.

gastrostomy, the surgical creation of an artificial opening into the stomach through the abdominal wall, used to feed a patient who has cancer of the esophagus or other kind of barrier to oral feeding.

gate-keeper system, a managed-care concept used by some alternative benefit plans, in which enrollees elect a primary care dentist, usually a general practitioner or pediatric dentist, who is responsible for providing non-specialty care and managing referrals, as appropriate, for specialty and ancillary services.

Gaucher's cell, disease (gôshāz′). See **disease, Gaucher's.** (not current)

gauge, an instrument used to determine the dimensions or caliber of an object.

g., Boley, a vernier type of instrument used for measuring in the metric system. A Boley gauge is accurate to tenths of millimeters.

g., leaf, a device for measuring the distance between two objects. A leaf gauge consists of a series of thin strips of plastic or metal, each calibrated and arranged in a sequential fashion in ascending or descending thicknesses, usually expressed in millimeters or fractions of millimeters. In dentistry, the leaf gauge is used to measure interocclusal space or the magnitude of an interocclusal interference.

g., undercut, an attachment used in conjunction with a dental cast surveyor to measure the amount of infrabulge of a tooth in a horizontal plane.

gel (jel), a colloid in solid form, jelly-like in character. Hydrocolloid impression materials are examples of gels.

g. strength. See **strength, gel.**

g. time. See **time, gel.**

gelatin, a protein formed from collagen by boiling in water. Medically, gelatin is used as a hemostat, a plasma substitute, and a protein food adjunct in severe cases of malnutrition. Gelatin is used in the manufacture of capsules and suppositories. It is also used in the production of x-ray films as the medium for suspending the crystal salts on the surface of the acetate film.

gelation time (jelā′shən). See **time, gel.**

gemfibrozil, *trade name:* Lopid; *drug class:* antihyperlipidemic; *action:* reduces plasma triglycerides and very low density lipoproteins; *uses:* type IIb, IV, V hyperlipidemia.

gene, a fundamental unit of inheritance located in the chromosome. A gene determines and controls hereditarily transmitted characteristics.

g. locus. See **locus, gene.**

g., sex-linked, a gene located in a sex chromosome.

g. therapy, a procedure that involves injection of "health genes" into the bloodstream of a patient to cure or treat a hereditary disease or similar illness.

general practice, dental. See **family practice.**

generated path (chew-in). See **path, generated occlusal.**

generator, one who, or that which, begets, causes, or produces.

g., electric, a device that converts mechanical energy into electrical energy.

g., x-ray, a device that converts electrical energy into electromagnetic energy (photons).

genetic counseling, the process of advising a patient with a genetic disease, or child-bearing parents of a patient with a genetic disease, about the probabilities and risks of future genetic accidents in conception, and counseling such persons about future family planning.

genetic disease, a disease that is caused by a defect or anomaly in the genetic inheritance of the patient.

genetic effects of radiation (jə-net′ik), those changes produced in the individual's genes and chromosomes of all nucleated body cells, both somatic and gonadal. The more common meaning relates to the effect produced in the reproductive cells. Radiation received by the gonads before the end of the reproductive period has the potential to add to the number of undesirable genes present in the population.

genetic marker, any specific gene that produces a readily recognizable genetic trait that can be used in family and population studies or in linkage analysis.

genetics, the science that deals with the origin of the characteristics of an individual.

genial tubercle. See **tubercle, genial.**

genioplasty (jē'nē·ōplas'tē), a surgical procedure, performed either intraorally or extraorally, to correct deformities of the mandibular symphysis.

genome, the total gene complement of a set of chromosomes found in higher life forms.
   g., human, the complete set of genes in the chromosomes of each cell of a human being.

genotype (jē'nōtīp), the aggregate of ordered genes received by offspring from both parents; for example, a person with blood group AB is of genotype AB.

gentamicin sulfate (ophthalmic), *trade names:* Garamycin Ophthalmic, Gentak; *drug class:* aminoglycoside antiinfective ophthalmic; *action:* inhibits bacterial protein synthesis; *use:* infection of external eye.

gentian violet (jen'shən). See **violet, gentian.**

geographic tongue. See **tongue, geographic.**

geometric unsharpness, an impairment of image definition resulting from the geometric penumbra. See also **penumbra, geometric** and **x-ray beam.**

geometry of x-ray beam, the effect of various factors on the spatial distribution of radiation emerging from an x-ray generator or source. See also **law, inverse square; penumbra, geometric;** and **x-ray beam.**

gerbil, a small rodent used as a laboratory animal and/or household pet, native to Africa and Asia. The name applies to any of 13 genera of the subfamily Gerbillinae. They resemble kangaroo rats and can survive without drinking water.

geriatric assessment, the evaluation of the physical, mental, and emotional health of elderly patients.

geriatric dentistry, a branch of dentistry that deals with the special and unique dental problems of senior citizens.

geriatrics (jer'ē·at'riks), the department of medicine or dentistry that treats health problems peculiar to advanced age and the aging, including the clinical problems of senescence and senility.

germanium, a metallic element with some nonmetallic properties. Its atomic number is 32 and its atomic weight is 72.59.

germ cell, a sexual reproductive cell in any stage of development; that is, an ovum or spermatozoon or any of the preceding forms.

germicide (jur'misīd), a substance capable of killing a wide variety of microorganisms. More specifically, one capable of killing all microorganisms, except for spores, with which it is in contact for a standard period of time.

germination (jur'minā'shən), the division of a tooth bud that results in the formation of double, or twin, crowns on a single root with a single pulp canal.

gerodontics (jer'ōdän'tiks) (gerodontology), the branch of dentistry that deals with the diagnosis and treatment of the dental conditions of aging and aged persons.

gerodontology (jer'ōdäntol'ōjē). See **gerodontics.**

gestational age, the age of a fetus or newborn, usually expressed in weeks dating from the first day of the mother's last menstrual period.

giant cell, an abnormally large tissue cell. It often contains more than one nucleus and may appear as a merger of several normal cells.

giant follicular lymphoblastoma. See **lymphoblastoma, giant follicular.** (not current)

giantism (macrosomia), excessive growth resulting in a stature larger than the range that is normal for age and race.
   g., infantile, excessive growth occurring before adolescence.
   g., primary, excessive growth not attributable to a definite cause.

G

g., secondary, excessive growth secondary to a disorder of the adrenal, pineal, gonadal, or pituitary gland.

Giardia, a common genus of the flagellate protozoans. Many species of *Giardia* normally inhabit the digestive tract and cause inflammation in association with other factors that produce rapid proliferation of the organism.

giardiasis, an inflammatory, intestinal condition caused by overgrowth of the protozoan *Giardia lamblia.* The source of infection is usually contaminated water. Also called *traveler's diarrhea.*

GIF. See **gastric intrinsic factor.**

gift, 1. a voluntary transfer of personal property without condition. **2.** the abbreviation for **gamete intrafallopian transfer.**

Gigli's wire saw (jel′yəz). See **saw, Gigli's wire.** (not current)

Gillies' operation. See **operation, Gillies'.**

Gillmore needle. See **needle, Gillmore.**

Gilson fixable-removable bar. See **connector, cross arch bar splint.**

gingiva(e) (jin′jivə), the fibrous tissue covered by mucous membrane that immediately surrounds the teeth.

g., attached, the portion of the gingivae extending from the free gingival groove, which demarcates it from the free or marginal gingivae, to the mucogingival junction, which separates it from the alveolar mucosa. This tissue is firm, dense, stippled, and tightly bound down to the underlying periosteum, tooth, and bone.

  g., a., extension. See **extension, gingiva, attached.**

g., free, the unattached coronal portion of the gingiva that encircles the tooth to form the gingival sulcus.

g. hyperplasia. See **hyperplasia, gingival, Dilantin.**

g., interdental (*interproximal gingiva[e]*), the soft supporting tissue, consisting of prominent horizontal collagen fibers, that normally fills the space between two contacting teeth.

g., interproximal. See **gingiva, interdental.**

g., lymphatic drainage of, lymphatic drainage that follows the course of the gingival blood supply; that is, from the lymphatic vessels on the gingival side of the periosteum of the alveolar process to the lymphatic vessels in the periodontal membrane to vessels leaking into the alveolar bone.

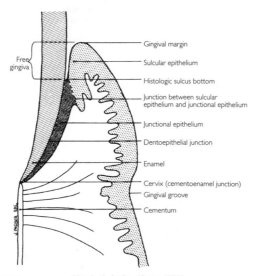

Gingival margin

Sulcular epithelium

Histologic sulcus bottom

Junction between sulcular epithelium and junctional epithelium

Junctional epithelium

Dentoepithelial junction

Enamel

Cervix (cementoenamel junction)

Gingival groove

Cementum

Free gingiva

Marginal gingiva. (Genco, 1990.)

g., marginal, the free gingiva at the labial, buccal, lingual, and palatal aspects of the teeth.

g., microscopic appearance of, stratified squamous epithelium that varies in degree of keratinization and overlies a corium of connective tissue with interspersed blood vessels and nerves. Rete pegs of epithelium project downward into the connective tissue corium, except from the base of sulcular epithelium. The gingival fiber apparatus is readily discerned.

gingival, pertaining to or in relation to the gingiva.

g. abrasion, the attrition (scraping or wearing away) of the gingival tissue by harsh irritants such as coarse foods or faulty toothbrushing.

g. anatomy, the gingiva, which is a dense connective tissue covered by keratinized mucosa except in the sulcus, where it is nonkeratinized. The margin is arcuate buccolingually with the peaks (papillae) interdentally. The sulcus depth normally is the apical limit to the free (unattached) gingiva, the attached gingiva extending from the free gingiva to the oral mucosa.

g. architecture, gingival form.

g. blanching, the lightening of gingival color resulting from stretching with diminution of blood supply; usually of a temporary nature.

g. bleeding, a prominent symptom of periodontal disease produced by ulceration of the sulcular epithelium and an inflammatory process.

g. blood supply, the vascular supply to the gingivae arises from the vessels that pass on the gingival side of the outer periosteum of bone and anastomoses with blood vessels of the periodontal membrane and intraalveolar blood vessels.

g. color, the color of the gingival tissues in health and in disease. It varies with the thickness and degree of keratinization of the epithelium, blood supply, pigmentation, and alterations produced by diseased processes affecting the gingival tissues. In health, often described as coral pink.

g. consistency, the visual and tactile characteristics of healthy gingival tissue. Visual consistency varies from a smooth velvet to an orange peel, either finely or coarsely grained. The tactile consistency of the gingival tissue should be firm and resilient.

g. crater, a concave depression in the gingival tissue. Especially seen in the area of the former apex of the interdental papilla as a result of the gingival destruction associated with necrotizing ulcerative gingivitis or when food impaction occurs against the tissue subjacent to the contact points of adjacent teeth.

g. crevicular fluid, an altered serum transudate found in the gingival sulcus. Irritation and inflammation of the gingival tissue increase the flow and alter the constituents of crevicular fluid.

g. discoloration, a change from the normal coloration of the gingivae; associated with inflammation, diminution of blood supply, and abnormal pigmentation.

g. hemorrhage, bleeding of the gum tissues; usually at the interpapillary crest, the gingival margin, or in the crevicular sulcus.

g. hormonal enlargement, an enlargement of the gingivae associated with hormonal imbalance during pregnancy or puberty.

g. mat, the gingival connective tissue composed of coarse, broad collagen fibers that serve to attach the gingivae to the teeth and to hold the free gingivae in close approximation to the teeth.

g. physiology, the gingivae encircle the teeth and serve as a protective mucosal covering for the underlying tissues; the gingival fiber apparatus serves as a barrier to apical migration of the epithelial attachment and binds the gingival tissues to the teeth. The normal topography permits the free flow of food away from the occlusal surfaces and from the cervical and interproximal areas of the teeth.

g. pigmentation, variations in gingival color may be correlated with the complexion of an individual or may be a reflection of pathologic influences, such as in the melanin pigmentation associated with hypoadrenocorticism (Addison's disease), nevi, and depositions of heavy metals.

g. pocket, a localized deepening of the gingival crevice of 2 mm or more.

g. position, the level of the gingival margin in relation to the tooth.

G

g. recession, the apical migration of the gingival crest

g. shrinkage, the reduction in size of gingival tissue, principally by diminution of edema, usually as a result of therapeutic elimination of subgingival deposits and curettement of the soft tissue wall of the pocket.

g. stippling, a series of small depressions characterizing the surface of healthy gingivae, varying from a smooth velvet to that of an orange peel.

g. sulcus, the space between the free gingiva and the tooth.

g. surface texture, the texture of the attached gingivae, which normally is stippled; in inflammatory conditions, the edema, cellular infiltration, and concomitant swelling cause loss of the surface stippling, and the gingivae take on a smooth, shiny, edematous appearance.

g. third, relating to the most apical one third of a given clinical crown or of an axial surface cavity or preparation.

g. topography, the form of the healthy gingival tissues. The marginal gingivae and the interdental papillae have a characteristic shape.

gingivectomy (jin'jĭvek'təmē), the surgical excision of unsupported gingival tissue to the level where it is attached, creating a new gingival margin apical in position to the old.

g. in edentulous area, the elimination of periodontal pockets surrounding abutment teeth; requires the removal of gingival tissue on the adjacent edentulous area.

gingivitis (jin'jĭvī'tis), any inflammation of the gingival tissue.

g. and malposed teeth, malposition may predispose the gingivae to inflammation by permitting food impaction or impingement, by providing irregular spaces in which calculus may be deposited, and by making cleaning difficult.

g., bacteria in, the causative organisms in gingival inflammation. The common chronic forms of gingivitis, from a bacterial standpoint, are nonspecific, with the exception of acute necrotizing ulcerative gingivitis, in which there is an apparent specificity of the bacterial flora: the fusospirochetal organisms.

g., bismuth, metallic poisoning caused by bismuth given for treatment of systemic disease; characterized by a dark, bluish line along the gingival margin.

g., chronic atrophic senile, gingival inflammation characterized by atrophy and areas of hyperkeratosis; found primarily in elderly women.

g., desquamative, an inflammation of the gingivae characterized by the tendency of the surface epithelium to desquamate. The disease is a clinical entity, not a pathologic entity. Desquamative gingivitis is most frequently associated with menopause but may be associated with any biologic stress.

g., eruptive (ērəp'tiv), gingival inflammation occurring at the time of eruption of the permanent teeth.

g., fusospirochetal. See **gingivitis, necrotizing ulcerative.**

g. gravidarum. See **gingivitis, pregnancy.**

g., hemorrhagic, gingivitis characterized by profuse bleeding, especially that associated with ascorbic acid deficiency.

g., herpetic, an inflammation of the gingivae caused by herpesvirus. See also **gingivostomatitis, herpetic.**

g., hormonal, gingivitis associated with endocrine imbalance, the endocrinopathy being modified, in most instances, by the influence of local environmental factors.

g., hyperplastic, gingivitis characterized by proliferation of the various tissue elements. May be accompanied by dense infiltration of inflammatory cells.

g., idiopathic, a gingival inflammation of unknown causation.

g., inflammatory cells in, since the gingival inflammatory process is usually chronic and progressive in nature, the inflammatory cells are, for the most part, lymphocytes, plasma cells, and some histiocytes. With acute exacerbations, polymorphonuclear leukocytes are also present.

g., marginal, an inflammation of the gingivae localized to the marginal gingivae and interdental papillae.

g., necrotizing ulcerative *(fusospirochetal gingivitis, NUG, trench mouth, ulcerative gingivitis, ulceromembranous gingivitis, Vincent's gingivitis, Vincent's infection),* an inflammation of the gingivae characterized by necrosis of the interdental papillae, ulceration of the gingival margins, the appearance of a pseudomembrane, pain, and a fetid odor.

g., n. u., inflammatory cells in, prevalent cellular infiltrate in necrotizing ulcerative gingivitis, including polymorphonuclear leukocytes, plasma cells, and lymphocytes. In the acute phase, polymorphonuclear leukocytes predominate.

g., nephritic (uremic gingivitis, uremic stomatitis), a membrane form of stomatitis and gingivitis associated with a failure of kidney function. Nephritic gingivitis is accompanied by pain, ammoniacal odor, and increased salivation.

g., pregnancy (gingivitis gravidarum, hormonal gingivitis), an enlargement of hyperplasia of the gingivae resulting from a hormonal imbalance during pregnancy.

g., puberty, an enlargement of the gingival tissues as a result of an exaggerated response to irritation resulting from hormonal changes.

g., scorbutic, gingivitis associated with vitamin C (ascorbic acid) deficiency.

g., ulcerative. See **gingivitis, necrotizing ulcerative.**

g., ulceromembranous. See **gingivitis, necrotizing ulcerative.**

g., uremic. See **gingivitis, nephritic.**

g., Vincent's. See **gingivitis, necrotizing ulcerative.**

gingivoplasty (jin'jivōplas'tē), the surgical contouring of the gingival tissues to secure the physiologic architectural form necessary for the maintenance of tissue health and integrity.

gingivosis (jin'jivō'sis), a noninflammatory degenerative condition of the gingivae. The term is applied to desquamative gingivitis. (not current)

gingivostomatitis (jin'jivōstō'məti'tis), an inflammation that involves the gingivae and the oral mucosa.

g., acute herpetic. See **stomatitis, herpetic, acute.**

g., herpetic, an inflammation of the gingivae and oral mucosa caused by primary invasion of herpesvirus. Herpetic gingivostomatitis occurs chiefly in childhood, one attack giving immunity to generalized stomatitis but not to isolated lesions (herpetic lesions).

The symptoms are red and swollen gingivae; red mucosa, which soon shows vesicles and ulcers; painful mouth; and elevated temperature. The course is about 14 days.

g., membranous, a disease, or group of diseases, in which false membranes form on the gingivae and oral mucosa; the membranes are a grayish white color and are surrounded by a narrow red margin. Detachment of the membrane leaves a raw, bleeding surface. One cause is mixed pyogenic infection, in which *Streptococcus viridans* and *Staphylococcus* organisms predominate.

g., white folded. See **nevus spongiosus albus mucosa.**

ginglymus (jing'glimas) (hinge joint), a joint that allows motion around an axis.

glabella (gləbel'ə), the most anterior point on the frontal bone.

gland(s), an organ producing a specific product or secretion.

g., accessory salivary, glands located at the posterior aspect of the dorsum of the tongue behind the vallate papillae and along the margins of the tongue; also located in the palate, labial mucosa, and buccal mucosa. The secretion is mucous.

g., Blandin and Nuhn's, minor anterior lingual salivary glands, partly serous and partly mucous. The duct of each gland opens on the inferior surface of the tongue.

g., ectopic sebaceous. See **spots, Fordyce's.**

g., endocrine, any one of the glands of internal secretion; a hormone-secreting gland (for example, the pituitary gland, thyroid gland, parathyroid glands, adrenal glands, ovaries, and testes).

g., parotid salivary, the largest of the salivary glands; situated between the ramus of the mandible in front, the mastoid process and sternocleidomastoideus behind, and the zygomatic arch above; irregularly wedge shaped, with the lateral surface flattened and the medial aspect more or less pointed toward the pharyngeal wall. Its secretion, which is serous, traverses Stensen's duct to empty into the mouth at the ductal orifice on the buccal mucosa opposite the upper molar teeth.

g., pituitary (hypophysis), an endocrine gland located at the base of the brain in the sella turcica. The pituitary gland is composed of two parts: the pars nervosa, which is an extension of the anterior part of the hypothalamus, and the pars intermedia, which is an epithelial evagination of secretory tissue from the stomodeum of the embryo. By its structural and functional relationships with the nervous system and the endocrine glands, it acts as a mediator of both the nervous system and the endocrine system.

g., salivary, glands in the mouth that secrete saliva. Three major groups of salivary glands contribute their secretions to form the whole saliva; accessory mucous glands found within oral mucosa contribute also in small part. The prime salivary glands are the parotid, submaxillary, and sublingual.

g., sublingual salivary, the smallest of the principal salivary glands. It lies below the mucous membranes of the floor of the mouth at the sides of the lingual frenum and is in contact with the sublingual depression on the inner side of the mandible. Its numerous ducts open directly into the mouth on the sides of the lingual frenum and/or join to form the duct of Bartholin (sublingual duct), which enters into the submaxillary duct (Wharton's duct). Its secretion is mucous in nature.

g., submaxillary salivary, a gland that has an irregular form and is situated in the submaxillary triangle, bordered anteriorly by the anterior belly of the digastricus and posteriorly by the stylomandibular ligament. Its mucoserous section is carried by Wharton's duct, whose orifice lies at the summit of a small papilla (submaxillary caruncle) at the side of the lingual frenum.

glass ionomer cement, a dental cement of low strength and toughness produced by mixing a powder prepared from a calcium aluminosilicate glass and a liquid prepared from an aqueous solution of prepared polyacrylic acid; used chiefly for small restorations on the proximal surfaces of anterior teeth and for restoration of eroded areas at the gingival margin.

glass, lead, lead-impregnated glass used in windows of control booths and in protective shields to protect radiologists and their assistants from primary and scattered radiation.

glaucoma, an abnormal condition of elevated pressure within the eye because of obstruction of the outflow of aqueous humor.

g., acute (closed-angle), a condition that occurs if the pupil in an eye with a narrow angle between the iris and cornea dilates markedly, causing the folded iris to block the exit of aqueous humor from the anterior chamber.

g., chronic (open-angle), a condition that is much more common than closed-angle glaucoma and is often bilateral. Open-angle glaucoma develops slowly and is genetically determined and progressive with age. The obstruction is believed to occur within the canal of Schlemm.

glaze, a critical stage in the final firing of dental porcelain when complete fusion takes place, with the formation of a thin, vitreous, glossy surface, or glaze.

glenoid, the fossae in the temporal bone in which condyles of the mandible articulate with the skull.

gliadin, a protein substance that is obtained from wheat and rye. Its solubility in diluted alcohol distinguishes gliadin from glutenin.

glide(s), 1. the passage of one object over another as guided by their contracting surfaces. **2.** the sounds *w, wh,* and *y,* which are voiced as bilabial and palatal glides, respectively. The rapid movement of the lips or tongue from a set position toward a neutral vowel (*u,* as in up).

g., mandibular, side-to-side, protrusive, intermediate movement of the mandible that occurs when the teeth or other occluding surfaces are in contact.

gliding occlusion. See **occlusion, gliding.** (not current)

glimepiride, *trade name:* Amaryl; *drug class:* oral antidiabetic; *action:* a sulfonylurea type action; *use:* non–insulin-dependent diabetes sometimes in combination with insulin support.

glioma, any of the largest group of primary tumors of the brain, composed of malignant glial cells.

glipizide, *trade name:* Glucotrol; *drug class:* oral antidiabetic (second generation); *action:* causes functioning β cells in pancrease to release insulin, leading to a drop in blood glucose levels; *use:* stable adult-onset diabetes mellitus (type II).

globin, a group of four globulin protein molecules that become bound by the iron in heme molecules to form hemoglobin or myoglobin.

globulin, a class of proteins. (not current)

g., antihemophilic. See **factor VIII.**

g., a. A. See **factor VIII.**

g., a. B. See **factor IX.**

glomerular disease, any of a group of diseases in which the glomerulus of the kidney is affected.

glomerular filtration rate, a kidney function test in which results can be determined from the amount of ultrafiltrate formed by plasma flowing through the glomeruli of the kidney. It may be calculated from insulin and creatinine clearance, serum creatinine, and blood urea nitrogen (BUN).

glomerulus, a tuft or cluster of blood vessels or nerve fibers, such as the cluster of blood vessels in the kidney that function as filters of the plasma portion of the blood.

glossalgia (glosal'jē·ə), painful sensations in the tongue.

glossectomy (glosek'təme), the surgical removal of the tongue, a portion of the tongue, or a lesion of the tongue.

glossitis (glosī'tis), an inflammation of the tongue.

g. areata exfoliativa. See **tongue, geographic.**

g., atrophic (bald tongue, smooth tongue), atrophy of the glossal papillae, resulting in a smooth tongue. The tongue may be pallid or erythematous and may appear small or enlarged. Atrophic glossitis may be associated with anemias, pellagra, vitamin B complex deficiencies, sprue, or other systemic diseases or may be local in origin. Because atrophy may be one phase, and circumscribed, painful, glossal excoriations may be another phase of one or more of the same systemic disease(s), much confusion in terminology has arisen (for example, Moeller's glossitis; Hunter's glossitis; slick, glazed, varnished, glossy, or

bald tongue; chronic superficial erythematous glossitis; glossodynia exfoliativa; beefy tongue; and pellagrous glossitis).

g., benign migratory. See **tongue, geographic.**

g., chronic superficial erythematous. See **glossitis, Moeller's.**

g., Clarke-Fournier. See **glossitis, interstitial sclerous.**

g., Hunter's. See **glossitis, Moeller's.**

g., interstitial sclerous (Clarke-Fournier glossitis), nodular, lobulated, indurated tongue associated with terminal syphilis.

g., median rhomboid, a developmental defect appearing as a red, slightly elevated area of the tongue just anterior to the foramen cecum. It is of no clinical significance and results from trapping of the median lobe of the tongue (tuberculum impar) at the surface during development.

g. migrans. See **tongue, geographic.**

g., Moeller's (chronic superficial erythematous glossitis, glossodynia exfoliativa, Hunter's glossitis, pellagrous glossitis), a chronic, superficial, irregular atrophy of the mucosa of the tongue. It may be caused by allergy, neural disturbance, or vitamin B complex deficiency. A smooth, red, painful tongue associated with pernicious anemia.

g., pellagrous. See **glossitis, Moeller's.**

glossodynia (glos'ōdīn'ē·ə), painful sensations in the tongue; a sensation of burning in the tongue; a sore tongue.

g. exfoliativa. See **glossitis, Moeller's.**

glossopyaryngeal nerve, either of a pair of the ninth cranial nerve essential to the sense of taste. The nerve has both sensory and motor fibers that pass from the tongue, parotid gland, and pharynx, communicates with the vagus nerve, and connects with a motor and sensory area of the brain. See also **nerve(s)**

glossoplasty (glos'ōplas'tē), a surgical procedure performed on the tongue.

glossoplegia (glos'ōplē'jē·ə), a paralysis of the tongue; may be unilateral or bilateral.

glossoptosis, a downward displacement of the tongue; a severe displacement may occlude the airway.

glossopyrosis (glos'ōpīrō'sis), a burning sensation of the tongue.

G

glossorrhaphy (glos'ôr'əfē), the suture of a wound of the tongue. (not current)

glossotomy (glosôt'ōmē), an excision or incision of the tongue.

glottal (glot'təl), pertaining to, or produced in or by, the glottis. The sound of *h* is a voiceless glottal fricative. The airstream on the exhalation phase moves unimpeded through the larynx, pharynx, and oral cavities.

glottidospasm (glotti'dōspazm). See **laryngospasm.** (not current)

glottis (glot'is), the vocal apparatus of the larynx, consisting of the true vocal cords (vocal folds) and the opening between them (rima glottidis).

gloves or surgical gloves, latex gloves used as an essential part of barrier protection in health care delivery.

glucagon (glōō'kəgon) (hyperglycemic factor, hyperglycemic-glycogenolytic factor [HGF]), a hormone from the α cells of the pancreas that raises the blood sugar by increasing hepatic glycogenolysis.

glucans, polyglucose compounds such as cellulose, starch, amylose, glycogen amylose, and callose.

glucocorticoids (glōō'kōkôr'təkoidz) (antiinflammatory hormone, 11-oxy-corticoids), adrenocortical steroid hormones that affect glycogenesis in the liver. They are antiinflammatory, are active in protection against stress, and affect carbohydrate and protein metabolism. Typical of the group are cortisol and cortisone.

glucokinase, a hexokinase or phosphotransferase that catalyzes the conversion of glucose to glucose 6-phosphate by ATP.

gluconeogenesis (glōō'kōnē'ōjen'esis), the formation of glycogen or glucose from noncarbohydrate sources (for example, the glycogenic amino acids, glycerol, lactate, and pyruvate) by pathways mainly involving the citric acid cycle and glycolysis.

glucose (glōō'kōs), a six-carbon (hexose) sugar that is the principal sugar in blood and serves as a major metabolic source of energy.

g. oxidase, an antibacterial flavoprotein enzyme obtained from *Penicillum notatum* and other fungi. It is antibacterial in the presence of glucose and oxygen.

g. tolerance test, a metabolic test that measures the ability of the body to metabolize carbohydrates. A patient is administered a standard dose of glu-

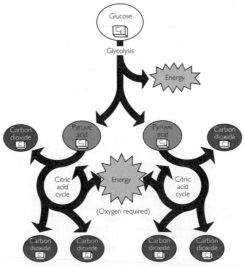

Catabolism of glucose. (Thibodeau, 1996.)

cose, and blood and urine samples are measured for glucose levels at periodic intervals following administration. The test is most often used to assist in the diagnosis of diabetes.

glucoside (gloo'kōsīd), a glycoside in which the sugar component is glucose.

glucuronidase, an enzyme that acts as a catalyst in the hydrolysis of various glucuronides with the liberation of glucuronic acid.

glutamic acid, a nonessential amino acid occurring widely in a number of proteins. Preparations of glutamic acid are used as aids for digestion.

glutaraldehyde, a germicidal agent used for the disinfection and sterilization of instruments or equipment that cannot be heat sterilized. An effective agent used in solution for "cold" sterilization.

glutathione, an enzyme whose deficiency is commonly associated with hemolytic anemia.

gluten, an insoluble protein constituent of wheat and other grains consisting of a mixture of gliadin, glutenin, and other proteins. Gluten provides the elastic qualities of bread dough.

glyburide, *trade names:* Apo-Glyburide, DiaBeta, Micronase; *drug class:* oral antidiabetic (2nd generation); *action:* causes functioning β cells in pancreas to release insulin, leading to a drop in blood glucose levels; *use:* stable adult-onset diabetes mellitus (type II).

glyceride (glis'erīd), an ester of glycerin with one or more aliphatic acids.

glycerin, a sweet, colorless, oily fluid that is a pharmaceutical grade of glycerol. Glycerin is used as a moistening agent for chapped skin, as an ingredient of suppositories for constipation, and as a sweetening agent and vehicle for drug preparation. It is also spelled **glycerine.**

glycerite (glis'erīt), a solution or suspension of a drug in glycerin.

Glycerol, an alcohol that is a component of fats. See also **glycerin.**

glycine, a nonessential amino acid occurring widely as a component of animal and plant proteins. Synthetically produced glycine is used in solutions for irrigation, in the treatment of various muscle diseases, and as an antacid and dietary supplement.

glycogen (glī'kōjen), a branched, homopolysaccharide of glucose held by α 1-4 and α 1-6 glucosidic bonds. Liver glycogen provides a ready source of blood glucose through glycogenolysis.

g. storage disease, any of a group of inherited disorders of glycogen metabolism. An enzyme deficiency causes glycogen to accumulate in abnormally large amounts in various parts of the body. The full taxonomy of glycogen storage diseases runs from Type I to Type VII.

glycogenesis (glī'kōjen'esis), the synthesis of glycogen from glucose.

glycogenolysis (glī'kōjēnol'isis), the formation of blood glucose by hydrolysis of stored liver glycogen.

glycolysis (glīkol'isis), **1.** oxidation of glucose or glycogen by cytoplasmic enzymes of the Embden-Meyerhof pathway to pyruvate and lactate. **2.** a series of enzymatically catalyzed reactions occurring within cells, by which glucose and other sugars are broken down to yield lactic acid or pyruvic acid, releasing energy in the form of adenosine triphosphate.

glycoprotein, any of the large group of conjugated proteins in which the nonprotein substance is a carbohydrate. These include the mucins, the mucoids, and the chondroproteins.

glycopyrrolate, *trade names:* Robinul, Robinul Forte; *drug class:* anticholinergic; *action:* inhibits acetylcholine at receptor sites in autonomic nervous system, which controls secretions, free acids in stomach; *uses:* decreased secretions before surgery, reversal of neuromuscular blockade, peptic ulcer disease, irritable bowel syndrome.

glycosaminoglycan. See **mucopolysaccharide.**

glycoside (glī'kōsīd), a compound that contains a sugar as part of the molecule.

glycosuria (glī'kōsoor'ē-ə), the presence of sugar in the urine. Glycosuria most commonly results from diabetes mellitus but may occur from a lowered renal threshold (renal glycosuria) in pregnancy, inorganic renal disease, and in patients taking adrenocorticosteroids.

Gm. See **gram.**

gnathic organ (nath'ik), a collective organ assembled about the upper and

G

lower dentolingual surface and used to pronounce the consonants *th, t, d, n, l,* and *r.* (not current)

gnathion (nā'thē·on), the lowest point in the lower border of the mandible at the median plane. It is a point on the bony border palpated from below and naturally lies posterior to the tegumental border of the chin.

gnathodynamometer (na'thōdī'nə-mom'ətər), an instrument used for measuring biting pressure.

  *g., **bimeter,*** a gnathodynamometer equipped with a central bearing point of adjustable height.

Gnathograph (nath'ōgraf), an articulator designed by McCollum. It resembles the Hanau instrument but differs chiefly by having a provision for increasing the intercondylar distance, an important determinant of groove directions in the occlusal surfaces of teeth. (not current)

Gnatholator, an articulator by Granger that has since been succeeded by an improved instrument called the Simulator (or Gnathosimulator).

gnathologic instrument, a term often used as a synonym for an articulator. Any dental instrument used for diagnosis and treatment, such as a probe for determining the depth of a periodontal pocket, is a gnathologic tool. (not current)

gnathology, the study of the functional and occlusal relationships of the teeth; sometimes also used to identify a specific philosophy of occlusal function.

gnathoschisis (nathōs'kisis). See **jaw, cleft.**

Gnathoscope, the name of an articulator designed by McCollum, with tiltable remnant hinge "axles" set in stirrup mounts that can be swiveled and turned so that the setting of each condylar element provides an approximate path of travel for the condyles of the patient. (not current)

gnathostatics (nath'ōstat'iks), a technique of orthodontic diagnosis based on relationships between the teeth and certain landmarks on the skull. See also **cast, gnathostatic.**

goal, the purpose toward which an endeavor is directed, such as the outcome of diagnostic, therapeutic, and educational management of a patient's health problem.

goiter (goi'ter), an enlargement of the thyroid gland.

  *g., **colloid** (endemic goiter, iodine deficiency goiter, simple goiter),* a visible enlargement of the thyroid gland without obvious signs of hypofunction or hyperfunction of the gland resulting from inadequate intake or to an increased demand for iodine.

  *g., **endemic.*** See **goiter, colloid.**

  *g., **exophthalmic,*** a disease of the thyroid gland consisting of hyperthyroidism, exophthalmos, and goiterous enlargement of the thyroid gland. A diffuse primary hyperplasia of the thyroid gland of obscure origin; may occur at any age. It produces nervousness, muscular weakness, heat intolerance, tremor, loss of weight, lid lag, and absence of winking and may lead to thyrotoxic heart disease and thyroid crisis.

  *g., **iodine deficiency.*** See **goiter, colloid.**

  *g., **nodular, nontoxic,*** recurrent episodes of hyperplasia and involution of colloid goiter, resulting in a multinodular goiter. Symptoms are related to pressure.

  *g., **simple.*** See **goiter, colloid.**

goitrogens (goi'trōjenz), agents such as thiouracil and related antithyroid compounds that are capable of producing goiter.

gold, a precious or noble metal; yellow, malleable, ductible, nonrusting; much used in dentistry in pure and alloyed forms.

  *g. **alloys,*** any alloy that contains gold; usually alloyed with copper, silver, platinum, palladium, and zinc. The alloying of gold enhances certain properties such as hardness, or creates a lower melting point for gold solder.

  *g. **compound,*** a drug containing gold salts, usually administered with other drugs in the treatment of rheumatoid arthritis. Various radioisotopes of gold have been used in diagnostic radiology and in the radiologic treatment of certain malignant neoplastic diseases.

  *g., **crystal.*** See **gold, mat.**

  *g., **fibrous.*** See **foil, gold.**

  *g. **file.*** See **file, gold.**

  *g. **foil.*** See **foil, gold.**

    *g. f. **cylinder.*** See **foil cylinder.**

    *g. f. **pellet.*** See **pellet, foil.**

  *g., **inlay,*** **l.** an alloy, principally gold, used for cast restorations. Desired physical properties may be obtained by selecting those with varying ingredients and/or proportions. Acceptable alloys are classified by the American Dental Association (ADA) specifications according to Brinell hardness: Type A—soft, Brinell 40 to 75; Type B—medium, Brinell 70 to 100; Type C—hard, Brinell 90 to 140. **2.** an intracoronal cast restoration of gold alloy fabricated outside the mouth and cemented into the prepared cavity.

g. knife. See **knife, gold.**

g., mat (crystal gold, sponge gold), a noncohesive form of pure gold prepared by electrodeposition. Sometimes used in the base of restorations and then veneered or overlaid with cohesive foil.

g., powdered, fine granules of pure gold, formed by atomizing the molten metal or by chemical precipitation. For clinical use, powdered gold is available either as clusters of the granules or as pellets of the powder contained in an envelope of gold foil.

g. saw. See **saw, gold.**

g. sodium thiosulfate, an antirheumatic used in the treatment of rheumatoid arthritis.

g., sponge. See **gold, mat.**

g., white, a gold alloy with a high palladium content. It has a higher fusion range, lower ductility, and greater hardness than a yellow gold alloy.

Goldent, the trade name for a direct gold restorative material. It consists basically of varying amounts of powdered gold contained in a wrapping or envelope of gold foil.

Goldman-Fox knife. See **knife, Goldman-Fox.** (not current)

Golgi apparatus, one of many small membranous structures found in most cells, composed of various elements associated with the formation of carbohydrate side chains of glycoproteins, mucopolysaccharides, and other substances. Also called **Golgi body, Golgi complex.**

Golgi's corpuscles (gol′jēz). See **corpuscle, Golgi's.**

gomphosis (gämfō′sis), a form of joint in which a conical body is fastened into a socket, as a tooth is fastened into the jaw.

gonad (gō′nad), an ovary or testis, the site of origin of eggs or spermatozoa.

gonadotrophin (gōnad′ōtrōf′in). See **gonadotropin.**

gonadotropin (gōnad′ōtrōp′in) (gonadotropic hormone), a gonad-stimulating hormone derived either from the pituitary gland (for example, follicle-stimulating hormone [FSH] and a luteinizing hormone [LH], which is also an interstitial cell stimulating hormone [ICSH]) or from the chorion (for example, chorionic gonadotropin, which is found in the urine of pregnant women).

g., chorionic. See **hormone, pregnancy.**

gonion (Go), the most posteroinferior point of the angle of the mandible near the lower border of the ramus.

good faith, honesty of intention. Generally, not a sufficient defense in a dental malpractice lawsuit.

good samaritan legislation, statutes enacted in some states protecting physicians, dentists, and some other health professionals from liability for aid rendered in emergency situations, unless there is a showing of willful wrong or gross negligence.

goodwill, the intangible assets of a firm established by the excess of the price paid for the going concern over its book value.

gothic arch tracer. See **tracer, needle point.**

gothic arch tracing. See **tracing, needle point.**

gout, a disease associated with an inborn error of uric acid metabolism that increases production or interferes with the excretion of uric acid. Excess uric acid is converted to sodium urate crystals that precipitate from the blood and become deposited in joints and other tissues. The great toe is a common site for the accumulation of urate crystals. This condition can be exceedingly painful with swelling of a joint and may be accompanied by chills and fever.

gr. See **grain.**

grace period, a specified time, after a plan's premium payment is due, in which the protection of the plan continues subject to actual receipt of premium within that time.

graft, a slip or portion of tissue used for implantation. See also **donor site; recipient site.**

g., allo-, a graft between genetically dissimilar members of the same species.

g., alloplast, a graft of an inert metal or plastic material.

g., auto-. See **graft, autogenous.**

g., autogenous, a graft taken from one portion of an individual's body and implanted into another portion of the individual's body.

g., a. bone, a bone graft taken from one part of a patient's body and transplanted to another part of the same patient's body.

g. donor site, the site from which graft material is taken.

g., filler, a graft used for the filling of defects, such as bone chips used to fill a cyst.

g., free, a graft of tissue completely detached from its original site and blood supply.

g., full-thickness, a skin graft consisting of the full thickness of the skin with none of the subcutaneous tissues.

g., hetero-. See **graft, heterogenous.**

g., heterogenous, a graft implanted from one species to another.

g., homo-. See **graft, homogenous.**

g., homogenous, a graft taken from a member of a species and implanted into the body of a member of the same species.

g., iliac, a bone graft whose donor site is the crest of the ilium. Various locations of the iliac crest duplicate areas of the mandible and curvatures of the midfacial skeleton.

g., iso-, a graft between individuals with identical or histocompatible antigens.

g., kiel, a denatured calf bone used to fill defects or restore facial contour.

g., mucosal, a split-thickness graft involving the mucosa.

g., onlay bone, a graft in which the grafted bone is applied laterally to the cortical bone of the recipient site, frequently to improve the contours of the chin or the malar eminence of the zygomatic bone.

g., pedicle, a stem or tube of tissue that remains attached near the donor site to nourish the graft during advancement of a skin graft.

g., split-thickness, a graft with varying thickness containing only mucosal elements and no subcutaneous tissue.

g., swaging, a procedure analogous to bone grafting. Also referred to as a *contiguous transplant,* which in-volves a greenstick fracture of bone bordering an infrabony defect and the displacement of bone to eliminate the osseous defect.

g., Thiersch's skin, a split-thickness skin graft containing cutaneous and some subcutaneous tissues, the line of cleavage through the rete peg layer.

grain (gr), I. a unit of weight equal to 0.0648 g. **2.** a crystal of an alloy.

g. boundary, the junction of two grains growing from different nuclei, impinging and causing discontinuity of the lattice structure. Important in corrosion and brittleness of metals.

g. growth. See **growth, grain.**

gram (Gm, g), the basic unit of mass of the metric system. Equivalent of 15.432 gr.

g.-negative, having the pink color of the counterstain used in Gram's method of staining microorganisms. Staining property is a common method of classifying bacteria. See also **Gram's stain.**

g.-positive, retaining the violet color of the stain used in Gram's method of staining microorganisms. Staining property is a common method of classifying bacteria. See also **Gram's stain.**

Gram's stain, also called *Gram's method.* A sequential process for staining microorganisms in which a violet stain is followed by a wash and then a counterstain of safranin. Gram-positive organisms appear violet or blue; gram-negative organisms appear rose pink.

gramicidin, an antibacterial agent generally used in conjunction with nystatin, a specific anticandidal agent, and neomycin, a complementary antibacterial agent, in the treatment of angular cheilosis. (not current)

granulation tissue, any soft, pink, fleshy projections that form during the healing process in a wound not healing by first intent. Granulation tissue consists of many capillaries surrounded by fibrous collagen. Overgrowth is termed *proud flesh.* Such tissue is evident at the opening to a fistulous tract.

granules, sulfur. See **actinomycosis.**

granulocyte, a type of leukocyte (white blood cell) characterized by the presence of cytoplasmic granules.

granulocytopenia (gran'yo͞olōsī'tōpē'-nē-ə), a deficiency in the number of granulocytic cells in the bloodstream.

granuloma (gran'yŏōlō'mə), a localized mass of granulation tissue characterized by an accumulation of macrophages, epithelioid macrophages, with or without lymphocytes, and giant cells into a discrete mass.

g., chronic *(chronic apical periodontitis),* chronic inflammatory tissue surrounding the apical foramina as a result of irritation from within the root canal system.

g., dental, a mass of granulation tissue surrounded by a fibrous capsule attached at the apex of a pulp-involved tooth. It produces a radiolucency that is fairly well demarcated.

g., eosinophilic (ē'ōsin'ōfil'ik), a granulomatous inflammatory disease of unknown etiology, usually monofocal in bone but sometimes affecting soft tissues. Sheets of histiocytes and masses of eosinophils characterize the lesion histologically.

g., giant cell reparative, an abnormal reparative reaction to an injury, characterized by fibroblastic proliferation with numerous giant cells. It may be peripheral (that is, on the gingiva, as in giant cell epulis) or central (that is, within the bone, producing a radiolucency). Most giant cell lesions of the jaws are reparative granulomas rather than neoplasms.

g. inguinale, a sexually transmitted disease characterized by ulcers of the skin and subcutaneous tissues of the groin and genitalia. It is caused by infection with *Calymmatobacterium granulomatis,* a small, gram-negative, rod-shaped bacillus.

g., pyrogenic, a tumorlike mass of granulation tissue produced in response to minor trauma in some individuals. It is highly vascular and bleeds readily.

g., reticuloendothelial. See **disease, lipoid storage.**

graphite, a soft carbon substance with a metallic black or gray sheen and a greasy feel. It is used in pencils, as a constituent of lubricants, and for making refractories such as crucibles in which to melt gold and other metals.

grasp, the manner in which an instrument is held.

g., finger, a modification of the palm and thumb grasp; it is more useful with modern, smaller handled instruments. The handle is held by the four flexed fingers rather than allowed to rest in the palm, and the thumb is used to secure a rest. Used when working indirectly on the upper arch.

g., instrument, a method of holding the instrument with the fingers in such a manner that freedom of action, control, tactile sensitivity, and maneuverability are secured. The most common grasp is the pen grasp.

g., palm-and-thumb, a grasp that is similar to the hold on a knife when one is whittling wood; the handle rests in the palm and is grasped by the four fingers, while the thumb rests on an adjoining object.

g., pen, a grasp in which the instrument is held somewhat as a pen is held, with the handle in contact with the bulbous portion of the thumb and index finger and the shank in contact with the radial side of the bulbous portion of the middle finger (not crossing the nail), while the handle rests against the phalanx of the index finger.

gratis, free, without reward or consideration.

Graves' disease. See **goiter, exophthalmic.**

gravity, specific, a number indicating the ratio of the weight of a substance to that of an equal volume of water.

grid, a device used to prevent as much scattered radiation as possible from reaching an x-ray film during the making of a radiograph. It consists essentially of a series of narrow lead strips closely spaced on their edges and separated by spacers of low-density material.

g., crossed, an arrangement of two parallel grids rotated in position at right angles to each other. See also **grid, parallel.**

g., focused, a grid in which the lead foils are placed at an angle so that they all point toward a focus at a specified distance.

g., moving, a grid that is moved continuously or oscillated throughout the making of a radiograph.

g., parallel, a grid in which the lead strips are oriented parallel to each other.

g., Potter-Bucky, a grid using the principle of the moving grid, with an oscillating movement.

G

G

g., stationary, a nonoscillating or nonmoving grid; the image of its strips will be visible on the radiograph for which it is used.

grinding-in, the process of correcting errors in the centric and eccentric occlusions of natural or artificial teeth.

grinding, selective, a modification of the occlusal forms of teeth by grinding at selected places to improve function.

griseofulvin microsize/griseofulvin ultramicrosize, *trade names:* Fulvicin U/F, Grifulvin V, Gris-PEG; *drug class:* antifungal; *action:* arrests fungal cell division at metaphase; binds to human keratin, making it resistant to disease; *uses:* mycotic infections: tinea corporis, tinea pedis, tinea cruris, tinea barbae, tinea capitis, tinea unguium if caused by *Epidermophyton, Microsporum, Trichophyton.*

groin, each of two areas where the abdomen joins the thighs.

groove, a linear channel or sulcus.

g., abutment, a transverse groove that may be cut in the bone across the alveolar ridge to furnish positive seating for the implant framework and to prevent tension of the tissue.

g., developmental, a fine depressed line in the enamel of a tooth that marks the union of the lobes of the crown in its development.

g., gingiva, free, the shallow line or depression on the surface of the gingiva at the junction of the free and attached gingivae.

g., interdental, a linear, vertical depression on the surface of the interdental papillae; functions as a sluiceway for the egress of food from the interproximal areas.

g., retention, a groove formed by opposing vertical constrictions in the preparation of a tooth that provides improved retention of the restoration.

ground, electrical, an electrical connection with the earth (or other ground).

g. state, the state of a nucleus, an atom, or a molecule when it has its lowest energy. All other states are termed *excited.*

grounded, pertaining to an arrangement whereby an electrical circuit or equipment such as an x-ray generator is connected by an electrical conductor with the earth or some similarly conducting body.

group, blood. See **blood groups.**

group function. See **function, group.**

group practice, the association of several health care providers to complement, facilitate, and extend their scope of health care delivery, not possible in a sole or single practice. See also **practice, group.**

group purchase, the purchase of dental services, either by postpayment or prepayment, by a large group of people.

growth, an increase in size.

g. and development, *growth* is defined as an increase in size; *development* is defined as a progression toward maturity. Thus the terms are used together to describe the complex physical, mental, and emotional processes associated with the "growing up" of children.

g. factor, one of about a hundred chemical messengers that induces cell growth by tissue type (for example, osteoinductive factor, epidermal growth factors).

g. failure, a lack of normal physical and psychologic development as a result of genetic, nutritional, pathologic, or psychosocial factors. See also **failure to thrive.**

g., grain, a phenomenon resulting from heat treatment of alloys. In excessive amounts, this growth produces undesirable physical properties.

g. hormone *(GH),* a single-chain peptide secreted by the anterior pituitary gland in response to growth hormone releasing factor (GHRF) from the hypothalamus. Growth hormone promotes protein synthesis in all cells, increased fat mobilization and use of fatty acids for energy, and decreased use of carbohydrates.

GTT. See **test, glucose tolerance.**

guaiacol, catecholmonomethyl ether, which is used as an expectorant and intestinal disinfectant.

guaifenesin, *trade names:* Anti-Tuss, Robitussin; *drug class:* expectorant; *action:* acts as an expectorant by stimulating mucosal reflex to increase production of less viscous lung mucus; *use:* dry, nonproductive cough.

guanabenz acetate, *trade names:* Wytensin; *drug class:* centrally acting antihypertensive; *action:* stimulates central α_2-adrenergic receptors resulting in decreased sympathetic outflow from the brain; *use:* hypertension.

guanadrel sulfate, *trade name:* Hylorel; *drug class:* antihypertensive; *action:* inhibits sympathetic vasoconstriction by inhibiting release of norephinephrine, depleting norepinephrine stores in adrenergic nerve endings; *use:* hypertension.

guanethidine sulfate, *trade name:* Ismelin; *drug class:* antihypertensive; *action:* inhibits norepinephrinc release, depleting norepinephrine stores in adrenergic nerve endings; *use:* moderate-to-severe hypertension.

guanfacine HCl, *trade name:* Tenex; *drug class:* antihypertensive; *action:* stimulates central α-adrenergic receptors, resulting in decreased sympathetic outflow from the brain; use: hypertension in individuals using a thiazide diuretic.

guanosine, a compound derived from a nucleic acid, composed of guanine and a sugar, D-ribose. Guanosine is a major molecular component of the nucleotides guanosine monophosphate and triphosphate and of DNA and RNA.

g. triphosphate (GTP), a high-energy nucleotide, similar to adenosine triphosphate, that functions in various metabolic reactions such as the activation of fatty acids and the formation of the peptide bond in protein synthesis.

guaranty, a contract that some certain and designated thing shall be done exactly as it is agreed to be done.

guard, bite, an acrylic resin appliance designed to cover the occlusal and incisal surfaces of the teeth of a dental arch to stabilize the teeth and/or provide a flat platform for the unobstructed excursive glides of the mandible. See also **plane, bite.**

guard, mouth, a resilient intraoral device worn during participation in contact sports to reduce the potential for injury to the teeth and associated tissue.

guard, night. See **guard, bite.**

guardian, a person appointed to take care of the person or property of another; one who legally has the care and management of the person or the property or both of a child until the child attains adulthood.

Guérin's fracture (gāranz'). See fracture, Guérin's.

guidance, a mechanical or other means for controlling the direction of movement of an object.

  g., condylar. See **guide, condylar.**

    g., c., inclination. See **guide, condylar, inclination.**

  g., developmental, comprehensive dentofacial orthopedic control over the growth of the jaws and eruption of the teeth, with the objective of optimizing the achievement of the genetic potential of the individual. Requires a combination of carefully timed active appliance therapy and supervisory examinations, including radiography and other diagnostic records, at various stages of development. May be required throughout the entire period of growth and maturation of the face, beginning at the earliest detection of a developing malformation.

  g., incisal, the influence on mandibular movements of the contacting surfaces of the mandibular and maxillary anterior teeth.

    g., angle. See **angle, incisal guidance.**

guide, a device for directing the motion of something.

  g., adjustable anterior, an anterior guide, the superior surface of which may be varied to provide desired separation of the casts in various eccentric relationships.

  g., anterior, the part of an articulator contacted by the incisal guide pin to maintain the selected separation of the upper and lower members of the articulator. The guide influences the changing relationships of mounted casts in eccentric movements. See also **guide, incisal.**

  g., condylar (condylar guidance), the mechanical device on an articulator; intended to produce guidance in articulator movement similar to that produced by the paths of the condyles in the temporomandibular joints.

    g., c., inclination (condylar guidance inclination), the angle of inclination of the condylar guide mechanism of an articulator in relation to the horizontal plane of the instrument.

G

g., incisal *(anterior guide),* the part of an articulator that maintains the incisal guide angle.

g., i., adjustment, occlusal adjustment that produces a minimum of overbite (vertical overlap) and a maximum of overjet (horizontal overlap), eliminates fremitus and racking effects on the anterior segment of teeth in the protrusive glide, and attains maximal incisive group function.

g., i., angle. See **angle, incisal guide.**

g. plane, a fixed or removable orthodontic appliance designed to deflect the functional path of the mandible and alter the positions of specific teeth.

guidelines, a set of standards, criteria, or specifications to be used or followed in the performance of certain tasks.

gum(s), the fibrous and mucosal covering of the alveolar process or ridges. See also **gingiva.**

g. pads, edentulous segments of the maxillae and mandible that correspond to the underlying primary teeth.

gumboil, an abscess of the gingiva and periosteum resulting from injury, infection, impacted food particles, or periapical infection. The gum is characteristically red, swollen, and tender. The abscess may rupture spontaneously, or it may require incision, as well as treatment of the underlying cause.

gumma (gum′ə), a granulomatous, gummy lesion of tertiary syphilis. The palate and tongue are sites of predilection in the oral region. A similar lesion occurring with tuberculosis is designated a *tuberculous gumma.*

Gunning's splint. See **splint, Gunning's.** (not current)

Gunn's syndrome. See **syndrome, Gunn's.** (not current)

gutta-percha (gut′əper′chə), the coagulated juice of various tropical trees that has certain rubberlike properties. Used for temporary sealing of dressings in cavities; also used in the form of cones for filling root canals and in the form of sticks for sealing cavities over treatment.

g.-p., baseplate, gutta-percha combined with fillers and coloring materials and rolled into sheets that are used as temporary bases for denture construction.

g.-p. points, fine, tapered cylinders of gutta-percha used, because of their radiopacity, for radiographic ascertainment of pocket depth and topography; used also as a root canal filling material.

g.-p., temporary stopping, gutta-percha mixed with zinc oxide and white wax. Used for temporary sealing of dressings in cavities.

gypsum (jip′səm), the dihydrate of calcium sulfate ($CaSO_4 \cdot 2H_2O$). α Hemihydrate and β hemihydrate are derived from gypsum. See also **plaster of paris.**

h II. See **hemophilia B.**

habit, the tendency toward an act that has become a repeated performance, relatively fixed, consistent, easy to perform, and almost automatic. Once learned, habits may occur without the intent of the person or may appear to be out of control and are difficult to change. In dentistry, habits such as bruxism, clenching, tongue thrusting, and lip and cheek biting may produce injury to the teeth, their attachment apparatus, oral mucosa, mandibular and temporomandibular musculature, and articulation.

habituation, a state in which an individual involuntarily tends to continue the use of a drug. Generally refers to the state in which an individual continues self-administration of a drug because of psychologic dependence without physical dependence.

Haemophilus, a genus of gram-negative pathogenic bacteria, frequently found in the respiratory tract of humans and other animals. *Haemophilus* species are generally sensitive to cephalosporins, tetracyclines, and sulfonamides.

H. influenzae, a small, gram-negative, nonmotile, parasitic bacterium that occurs in two forms, encapsulated and nonencapsulted, and in six types: A, B, C, D, E, and F. Almost all infections are caused by the encapsulated type B organisms. *H. influenzae* is found in the throats of 30% of healthy, normal people. It may cause destructive inflammation of the larynx, trachea, and bronchi in children and debilitated older people.

Hageman trait (häg'mən). See **factor XII.** (not current)

halazepam, *trade name:* Paxipam; *drug class:* benzodiazepine (Controlled Substance Schedule IV); *action:* produces central nervous system depression by interaction with benzodiazepine receptor to facilitate action of inhibitory neurotransmitter γ-aminobutyric acid; *use:* anxiety.

halcinonide, *trade names:* Halog-E, Halog; *drug class:* corticosteroid, synthetic topical; *action:* interacts with steroid cytoplasmic receptors to induce antiinflammatory actions; *use:* inflammation of corticosteroid-responsive dermatoses.

half-life, the time in which a radioactive substance will lose half of its activity through disintegration.

h.-l., biologic, the time in which a living tissue, organ, or individual eliminates, through biologic processes, half of a given amount of a substance that has been introduced into it.

h.-l., effective, the half-life of a radioactive isotope in a biologic organism, resulting from the combination of radioactive decay and biologic elimination.

h.-l., physical, the average time required for the decay of half the atoms in a given amount of a radioactive substance.

half-value layer (HVL), the thickness of a specified material (usually aluminum, copper, or lead) required to decrease the dosage rate of a beam of x-rays at a point of interest to half its initial value. A determination of the half-value layer of a given x-ray beam is used to denote the quality of the x-ray beam. The half-value layer will vary depending on kilovolt peak and the amount of filtration at the source.

halisteresis (həlis'tərē'sis), a theory of the method of bone resorption according to which bone salts can be re-

moved by a humoral mechanism and returned to the tissue fluids, leaving behind a decalcified bone matrix; osteolysis. This is not considered to be the mechanism under which resorption occurs in periodontal disease.

halitosis (hal'itō'sis) (bad breath, bromopnea, fetor ex ore, offensive breath), an offensive odor of the breath resulting from local and metabolic conditions (for example, poor oral hygiene, periodontal disease, sinusitis, tonsilitis, suppurative bronchopulmonary disease, acidosis, uremia).

Haller's plexus. See **plexus, Haller's.**

halobetasol propionate, *trade name:* Ultravate; *drug class:* topical corticosteroid, group VI potency; *action:* interacts with steroid cytoplasmic receptors to induce antiinflammatory effects, possesses antipruritic/antiinflammatory actions; *uses:* psoriasis, eczema, contact dermatitis, pruritus.

halogen (hal'ōjen), an element of a closely related group of elements consisting of fluorine, chlorine, bromine, and iodine.

haloperidol/haloperidol decanoate, *trade name:* Haldol; *drug class:* antipsychotic/butyrophenone; *action:* blocks neurotransmission at dopaminergic synapses in the cerebral cortex, hypothalamus, and limbic system; *uses:* psychotic disorders, control of tics and vocal utterances in Gilles de la Tourette syndrome, short-term treatment of hyperactive children showing excessive motor activity.

halothane (hal'ə-thān), a potent nonflammable and nonexplosive liquid anesthetic agent administered by inhalation. Common complications associated with other inhalation anesthetic agents are generally absent. Chemical name is 2-bromo-2-chloro-1, 1, 1-trifluoroethane.

hamartoma (ham'artō'mə), a localized error in the composition of the tissue elements of an organ. May be automatically manifested in three ways, either singly or in combination: abnormal quantity, abnormal structure, or degree of maturation of the tissue components.

Hamberger's schema. See **schema, Hamberger's.** (not current)

Hamburger's phenomenon. See **phenomenon, Hamburger's.** (not current)

hamster, any of four genera of small rodents widely used in research and commonly kept as pets. All hamsters are seed and plant feeders, store away their food, hibernate in winter, and breed throughout the year under laboratory conditions.

hamular notch. See **notch, pterygomaxillary.**

hamular process. See **process, hamular.**

hand condenser. See **condenser, hand.**

handicap, a disability that hinders effective function; may involve any combination of physical, emotional, or social factors.

handpiece, an instrument that is used to hold rotary instruments in the dental engine or condensing points in mechanical condensing units. It is connected by an arm, cable, belt, or tube to the source of power (e.g., motor, air, water).

h., air-turbine, a handpiece with a turbine powered by compressed air.

h., contra-angle, a binangled instrument for use with the dental engine; permits access to areas difficult or impossible to reach with a straight handpiece.

h., high-speed, a type of rotary or vibratory cutting tool that operates at speeds above 12,000 rpm. It is propelled by gears, a belt, or a turbine. Generally classified as an air turbine, a hydraulic turbine, or a high-speed handpiece on a conventional dental engine.

h., h.-s., ultra, a handpiece designed to permit rotational speeds of 100,000 to 300,000 rpm.

h., right-angle, a monangled instrument used with mechanical condensers to reach some operating areas.

h., straight, a handpiece whose axis is in line with the rotary instrument.

h., water-turbine, a handpiece with a turbine powered by water under pressure.

hand pressure. See **pressure, hand.**

Hand-Schüller-Christian disease (hand-shül' ər-kris' chan). See **disease, Hand-Schüller-Christian.**

Hansen's disease. See **leprosy.**

hapten, a nonproteinaceous substance that acts as an antigen by combining with particular bonding sites on an antibody. Unlike a true antigen, it does not induce the formation of antibodies. A hapten bonded to a carrier protein may induce an immune response. Also called *haptene.*

hard copy, readable output from a computer generated in a storable form such as printed on paper or on microfiche; contrasts with soft copy in which the data are displayed on a video terminal or presented in some other transitory form.

hardener, an ingredient (potassium alum) of the photographic and radiographic fixing solution that serves to harden the gelatin of the film to prevent softening and swelling of the gelatin.

hardening, the process of setting or becoming firm.

h., age, the precipitation of intermetallic compounds that alters certain physical properties in alloys; usually brought about through heat treatment.

h., precipitation. See **tempering.**

h. solution. See **solution, hardening.**

h., strain, an increase in proportional limit resulting from distortion of the space lattice and fracture of grain boundaries through cold working. Ductility is markedly reduced.

h., work, the hardening of a metal by cold work, such as repeated flexing.

hardness (of a substance), the ability of a material to resist an indenting type of load.

h., Mohs, relative scratch resistance of minerals based on an arbitrary scale: 10, diamond; 9, corundum; 8, topaz; 7, quartz; 6, orthoclase; 5, apatite; 4, fluorite; 3, calcite; 2, gypsum; and 1, talc.

h. (of x-rays), term used to indicate in a general way the quality of x radiation, with "hardness" being a function of the wavelength; the shorter the wavelength, the "harder" the x radiation.

h. tests. See **tests, hardness.**

hard of hearing, a term applied to persons whose hearing is impaired but who have enough hearing left for practical use.

hard palate. See **palate, hard.**

hardware, the mechanical, magnetic, electronic, and electric devices or components of a computer.

harelip (her'lip) (cheiloschisis, cleft lip, congenital cleft lip), a congenital nonunion or inadequacy of soft and hard tissues related to the lip. The deformity may be extensive enough to involve the nose, alveolar process, hard palate, and velum. The extent of the deformity varies among individuals. Various classifications have been established to identify the extent of a cleft. A rare midline cleft may occur in the lower lip at the embryonal junction of the two mandibular processes.

harmony, functional occlusal, an occlusal relationship of opposing teeth in all functional ranges and movements that will provide the greatest masticatory efficiency without causing undue strain or trauma on the supporting tissues.

harmony, occlusal, the nondisruptive relationship of an occlusion to all its factors (for example, the neuromuscular mechanism, temporomandibular joints, teeth and their supporting structures).

Hatch clamp. See **clamp, gingival, Hatch.** (not current)

hatchet, an angled cutting hand instrument in which the broad side of the blade is parallel with the angle(s) of the shank. Used to develop internal cavity form. May be bibeveled or single beveled like a chisel, in which case the instrument is paired with another.

haversian system. See **osteon.**

Hawley appliance, chart, retainer. (See under appropriate noun.)

Hawley retainer. See **retainer, Hawley.**

hay fever, an acute seasonal allergic rhinitis, stimulated by tree, grass, or weed pollens. Also called *allergic rhinitis.*

hay rake. See **appliance, hay rake.**

hazardous waste, any material, gas, liquid, or solid substance that has the potential to cause injury or illness; that in an unprotected state poses a risk to the environment, including plant and/or animal life.

hazard, radiation, the hazard that exists in any area in which a person is subject to radiation.

HDL, the abbreviation or acronym for **high-density lipoproteins.** HDL mol-

ecules are considered a protective factor in coronary heart disease.

head, steeple. See **oxycephalia.**

headache, pain in the cranial vault resulting from intracranial, extracranial, or psychogenic causes: intracranial vascular dilation; space-occupying lesions; diseases of the eyes, ears, and sinuses; extracranial vascular dilation; sustained muscular contraction; hysteria; certain habit patterns (clenching); and reaction to stress.

h., cluster. See **neuralgia, facial, atypical.**

h., lower-half. See **neuralgia, facial, atypical.**

h., migraine, a vascular type of headache, typically unilateral in the temporal, frontal, and retroorbital area, but may occur midface. It is described as throbbing, burning, pulsating, exploding, or pressure and may become generalized and persist for hours or days. Onset of pain is usually preceded by prodromal symptoms that may include visual disturbances, scotomas, vomiting, and nausea. A migraine headache is usually considered to be a psychophysiologic (psychosomatic) disorder.

headcap, the part of an extraoral orthodontic appliance that engages the back of the head, incorporating the skull as a source of resistance for tooth movement, and gives attachment to the intraoral element of the appliance.

h., plaster, a cap that is constructed of plaster-of-paris gauze and embodies points for applying fixation and traction appliances in the treatment of mandibular and maxillofacial injuries.

headgear, the apparatus encircling the head or neck and providing attachment for an intraoral appliance in use of extraoral anchorage.

h., radiologic, a device that is used to protect the head from injury by radiation.

health, a bodily state in which all parts are functioning properly. Also refers to the normal functioning of a part of the body. A state of normal functional equilibrium; homeostasis.

h. assessment, an evaluation of the health status of an individual by performing a physical examination after obtaining a health history. Various laboratory and functional tests may also be ordered to confirm a clinical impression or to screen for dysfunction.

h. behavior, an action taken by a person to maintain, attain, or regain good health and to prevent illness. Health behavior reflects a person's health beliefs.

h. care provider, any individual who provides health services to health care consumers (patients).

h. education, an educational program directed to the general public that attempts to improve, maintain, and safeguard the health of the community.

h. hazard, a danger to health resulting from exposure to environmental pollutants such as asbestos or ionizing radiation, or to a lifestyle influence such as cigarette smoking or chemical abuse.

h. maintenance organization (HMO), a legal entity that accepts responsibility and financial risk for providing specified services to a defined population during a defined period of time at a fixed price. An organized system of health care delivery that provides comprehensive care to enrollees through designated providers. Enrollees are generally assessed a monthly payment for health care services and may be required to remain in the program for a specified amount of time.

h., patient, the state of bodily soundness of the patient; the patient's absolute or relative freedom from physical and/or mental disease.

h. physics, the study of the effects of ionizing radiation on the body and the methods for protecting people from the undesirable effects of radiation.

h. policy, **1.** a statement of a decision regarding a goal in health care and a plan for achieving that goal; for example, to prevent an epidemic, a program for inoculating a population is developed and implemented. **2.** a field of study and practice in which the priorities and values underlying health resource allocation are determined.

h. professional, a person who by education, training, certification, and/or licensure is qualified to and is engaged in providing health care.

h. promotion, an educational program or effort directed at a targeted population to improve, maintain, and safeguard the health of that segment of society. See also **health education.**

h. resources, all materials, personnel, facilities, funds, and anything else that can be used for providing health care and services.

h. risk, a disease precursor associated with a higher than average morbidity or mortality. The disease precursors may include demographic variables, certain individual behaviors, familial and individual histories, and certain physiologic changes.

h. risk appraisal, a process of gathering, analyzing, and comparing an individual's prognostic characteristics of health with a standard age group, thereby predicting the likelihood that a person may develop prematurely a health problem associated with a high morbidity and mortality rate.

hearing disorders, any structural or functional impairment of the ability to detect and recognize sound.

hearing loss, a reduction in the acuity to detect and recognize sound.

hearsay, 1. the testimony given by a witness who relates not what is known personally but what others have stated. **2.** evidence that does not derive its value solely from the credit of the witness, but rests mainly on the veracity and competency of other persons and is admitted in court only in specified cases from necessity.

heart, artificial, a mechanical device that acts to pump blood to and from the body tissues during repair of the heart.

heart block, the condition in which the muscular interconnection between the auricle and ventricle is interrupted so that the auricle and ventricle beat independently of each other.

heartburn, a painful burning sensation in the esophagus just below the sternum. Heartburn is usually caused by the reflux of gastric contents into the esophagus, but it may be caused by gastric hyperacidity or peptic ulcer.

heart defect, a fault in the structural integrity of the heart.

h. d., congenital, structural errors in the heart formed during embryonic and fetal life.

heart disease, a disorder in the normal functioning of the heart.

h. d. risk factors, Hereditary, lifestyle, and environmental influences that increase one's chances of developing heart disease.

heart failure (hart' fālyər), a sudden, sometimes fatal, cessation of the heart's action.

h. f., acute, a rapid and marked impairment of the cardiac output.

h. f., backward, congestive heart failure in which the initiating factor is increased venous pressure resulting from ventricular failure to empty the atria.

h. f., congestive, a clinical syndrome resulting from chronic cardiac decompensation associated with left-sided and/or right-sided heart failure. Left-sided failure may result from rheumatic mitral valvular disease, aortic valvular disease, systemic hypertension, or arteriosclerotic disease. Manifestations include orthopnea, paroxysmal dyspnea, pulmonary edema, cough, and cardiac asthma. Right-sided failure results most commonly from pulmonary congestion and hypertension associated with left-sided failure but may result from anemia, myocarditis, beriberi, or dysrhythmia. Manifestations include peripheral pitting edema, ascites, cyanosis, oliguria, and hydrothorax.

h. f., forward, heart failure initiated by decreased cardiac output that leads to decrease blood supply to tissues, decreased excretion of salt (Na^+) and salt retention, elevated venous pressure, and edema.

heart massage. See **massage, cardiac.**

heart murmur, the sound of blood flowing back through a defective heart valve.

heart rate, the rate or tempo of heart contractions recorded in beats per minute.

heart sounds, a normal noise produced within the heart during the cardiac cycle that can be heard over the precordium and may reveal abnormalities in cardiac structure or function. The use of the stethoscope over the left side of the chest is a common clinical technique to assess heart function. The typical sounds are a rythmic *lub dup;* abnormal sounds include clicks, murmurs, rubs, snaps, and gallops.

heart surgery, any surgical procedure involving the heart, performed to correct acquired or congenital defects, to replace diseased valves, to open or bypass blocked vessels, or to graft a prosthesis or a transplant in place.

heart valves, one of the four structures within the heart that prevent backflow of blood by opening and closing with each heartbeat. The valves include two semilunar valves, the aortic and pulmonary; the mitral, or bicuspid, valve; and the tricuspid valve. The valves permit the flow of blood in only one direction, and any one of the valves may become defective, permitting the backflow associated with heart murmurs.

heat, the state of a body or of matter that is perceived as being opposite of cold and is characterized by elevation of temperature.

h., applied, the therapeutic application of wet or dry heat to increase circulation and produce hyperemia, accelerate the dissolution of infection and inflammation, increase absorption from tissue spaces, relieve pain, relieve muscle spasm and associated pain, and increase metabolism.

h., a., and cold, The most commonly employed physical agents in dental practice; they modify the physiologic processes and have both a systemic and a local effect. The principal effect on the tissues is mediated by the alteration in the circulatory mechanisms. Properly used, heat and cold have a salutary therapeutic result; improperly used, they may produce serious pathologic consequences.

h., a., contraindications, conditions that preclude the use of heat application: peripheral neuropathy, conditions in which maximum vasodilation and inflammation are already present, acute inflammatory conditions in which more swelling will cause acute pain and pulpitis, septicemia, and malignancies.

h., a., general physiologic effects, the physiologic effects of generally applied wet or dry heat; increase in body temperature, generalized vasodilation, rise in metabolism, decrease in blood pressure, increase in pulse rate and circulation, and increase in depth and rate of respiration.

h., a., local physiologic effects, the physiologic effects of locally applied wet or dry heat to the intraoral and/or extraoral tissues: increase in caliber and number of capillaries, increased absorption resulting from capillary dilation, increased lymph formation and flow, relief of pain, relief of spasm, increase of phagocytes, and a rise in local metabolism.

h. loss, metabolic causes, biologic factors that influence heat loss: redistribution of blood vasodilation and vasoconstriction, variations in blood volume, tendency of fat to insulate the body, and evaporation.

h., l., physical causes, physical factors that influence heat loss: radiation, convection, and conduction; evaporation from the lungs, skin, and mucous membranes; the raising of inspired air to body temperatures; and the production of urine and feces.

h. production, metabolic causes, chemical factors of the body that cause heat production: specific dynamic action of food, especially protein, that results in a rise of metabolism; a high environmental temperature that, by raising temperatures of the tissues, increases the velocity of reactions and thus increases heat production; and stimulation of the adrenal cortex and thyroid glands by the hormones of the pituitary glands.

h. treatment. See **treatment, heat.**

heavy function. See **function, heavy.**

hebephrenia (heb′efrē′nē-ə), a form of schizophrenia in which the individual behaves like a child (for example, inappropriate laughter and silliness).

heel effect. See **effect, heel.**

Heerfordt's syndrome. See **fever, uveoparotid.**

height of contour. See **contour, height of.**

Heimlich maneuver, an emergency procedure for dislodging a bolus of food or other obstruction from the trachea to prevent asphyxiation. The choking person is grasped from behind by the rescuer whose fist, thumb side in, is placed just below the victim's sternum and whose other hand is placed firmly over the fist. The res-

cuer then pulls the fist firmly and abruptly into the epigastrium, forcing the obstruction up the trachea.

Heimlich sign, a universal distress signal that a person is choking and unable to speak, made by grasping the throat with a thumb and index finger, thereby attracting the attention of others nearby.

Helicobacter, a genus of gram-negative, spiral-shaped bacteria that is pathogenic and has been isolated from the intestinal tract of mammals, including humans.

H. pylori, a newly classified spiral bacterium active as a human gastric pathogen. It is a gram-negative, urease-positive, curved or slightly spiral organism initially isolated in 1982 from patients with lesions of gastritis or peptic ulcers in Western Australia.

helium (hē′lē-əm), a colorless, odorless, tasteless gas; one of the inert gaseous elements. Symbol, **He;** atomic number, 2; atomic weight, 4.003. Used in medicine as a diluent for other gases.

Helsinki declaration (accords), a declaration signed by the representatives of 35 member nations of the Conference on Security and Cooperation in Europe in Helsinki, Finland, on August 1, 1975. The declared goals of the nonbinding document comprise four principal aspects of European security: economic cooperation, humanitarian issues, contact between East and West, and provision for a later follow-up conference. The principle and practice of informed consent in health care grew from the Helsinki accords.

hemangioameloblastoma (hēman′-jē-ō-əmel′ōblastō′mə), a neoplasm in the jaw that has characteristics of ameloblastoma and hemangioma. (not current)

hemangioendothelioma (hēman′jē-ō-en′dōthē′lē-ō′mə), a malignant tumor formed by proliferation of endothelium of the capillary vessels.

hemangiofibroma (hēman′jē-ō-fī-brō′mə), a benign neoplasm characterized by proliferation of blood channels in a dense mass of fibroblasts.

hemangioma (hēman′jē-ō′mə), **1.** a benign neoplasm characterized by blood vascular channels. A cavernous hemangioma consists of large vascular spaces. A capillary hemangioma consists of many small blood vessels. **2.** a benign tumor composed of newly formed blood vessels.

hemangiopericytoma (hēman'jē-ōper'isītō'mə), a vascular tumor composed of pericytes.

hemataerometer (hēm'atə'erom'ə-ter), a device for determining the pressure of the gases in the blood. (not current)

hematemesis (hēm'ətem'esis), vomiting of blood.

hematocrit (hēmat'ōcrit) (packed-cell volume), **l.** the percentage of the total blood volume composed of red blood cells (erythrocytes). Normal values are 42% to 45%. **2.** the percentage of the total volume of a blood sample that is taken up by the red blood cells. Normal values: children, 32% to 65%; adult men, 42% to 53%; adult women, 38% to 46%.

hematologic disorders, diseases of the blood and blood-forming tissues.

hematology, the scientific study of blood and blood-forming tissues.

h. tests, diagnostic tests of the blood and its constituent parts.

hematoma (he'mətō'mə), a mass of blood in the tissue as a result of trauma or other factors that cause the rupture of blood vessels.

h., subdural, a collection of extravasated blood trapped below the dural membranes of the brain causing pressure on the brain, resulting in pain and neural dysfunction. Subdural hematomas may be life threatening.

hematopoiesis, the normal formation and development of blood cells in the bone marrow.

hematosis (hēm'ətō'sis), oxygenation or aeration of the venous blood in the lungs.

hematoxylin, a dye or stain commonly used to treat tissue sections for microscopic examination, usually used in combination with eosin.

hematuria (hēm'ətoōr'ē-ə), blood in the urine.

h., gross, visible evidence of blood in the urine. It may occur from neoplasms of the kidney and bladder, hemorrhagic diathesis, hypertension with renal epistaxis, or acute glomerular nephritis.

h., microscopic, the demonstration of hematuria during the microscopic examination of centrifuged urine. It may

result from the same causes as gross hematuria or from toxicity of drugs, embolic glomerulitis, vascular diseases, or chronic glomerular nephritis.

heme, the pigmented, iron containing, nonprotein portion of the hemoglobin molecule.

hemiachromatosia, a state of being color blind in only one half of the visual field.

hemianesthesia (hem'ē-an'esthē'zhə), anesthesia or loss of tactile sensibility on one side of the body.

hemiatrophy (hem'ē-at'rōfē), atrophy of one half of the body, an organ, or a part (for example, facial hemiatrophy).

hemiglossectomy (hem'ēglôsek'tōmē), the surgical removal of half of the tongue.

hemihypertrophy (hem'ēhīper'trəfē), an excessive growth of half of the body, an organ, or a part (for example, facial hemihypertrophy).

hemiplegia (hēm'ēplē'jə), in medical jurisprudence, paralysis of one side of the body.

hemisection, the complete sectioning through the crown of a tooth into the furcation region.

hemocytes, a generic term referring to any cellular or formed element of the blood. Synonym: hematocyte.

hemodialysis, a procedure in which impurities or wastes are removed from the blood. This procedure is used in treating renal failure and various toxic conditions. The patient's blood is shunted from the body through a machine for diffusion and ultrafiltration and returned to the patient's circulation.

hemodynamics, the study of the physical aspects of blood circulation, including cardiac function and peripheral vascular physiology.

hemoglobin (hē'mōglō'bin), the oxygen-carrying red pigment of the red blood corpuscles. Hemoglobin is a reddish, crystallizable conjugated protein consisting of the protein globulin combined with the prosthetic group, heme.

h. A (HBA), a normal hemoglobin. Also called *adult hemoglobin.*

h. estimation, a determination of the hemoglobin content of the blood. By the Sahli method, 14 to 17 g/100 ml of blood is normal, and 15.1 Sahli units are taken as 100% for estimation of hemoglobin percentages.

H

hemoglobinopathy (hē'mōglō'binop'-əthē), any one of a group of genetically determined diseases involving abnormal hemoglobin (for example, sickle cell disease, in which hemoglobin S occurs, and hemoglobin C disease).

h., paroxysmal nocturnal, an acquired hemolytic anemia of unknown cause characterized by increased hemolysis during sleep, resulting in the presence of hemoglobin in the urine on awakening.

hemolysin (hēmol'isin), an antibody that causes hemolysis of red blood cells in vitro.

hemolysis, the breakdown of red blood cells and the release of hemoglobin that occurs normally at the end of the life span of a red blood cell.

hemophilia (hē'mōfil'ē-ə) (bleeder's disease), a sex-linked genetic disease manifested in males and characterized by severe hemorrhage.

h. A (classic hemophilia), a hemorrhagic diathesis resulting from a deficiency of antihemophilic globulin (AHG); inherited as a recessive sex-linked characteristic and characterized by recurrent bouts of bleeding from even trivial injury. The coagulation time is prolonged, but the bleeding time is normal.

h. B (Christmas disease, hemophilia II, hemophilioid state C), a hemorrhagic diathesis resulting from a deficiency of plasma thromboplastin component (FTC); transmitted as a sex-linked recessive characteristic and characterized clinically by the same manifestations as classic hemophilia. There is a delay in the generation of thromboplastin. The platelet count, bleeding time, tourniquet test, and thrombin and prothrombin times are normal.

h. C (plasma thromboplastin antecedent [PTA] deficiency, Rosenthal's syndrome), a hemophilia-like condition believed to result from a deficiency of plasma thromboplastin antecedent (PTA), transmitted as a simple autosomal dominant trait, and characterized by a moderate bleeding tendency after extraction of teeth or after tonsillectomy. Prothrombin consumption and thromboplastin generation are abnormal. See also **factor XI.**

h., classic. See **hemophilia A.**

h., vascular, a hereditary hemorrhagic disorder affecting both sexes and associated with a deficiency of antihemophilic globulin and vascular abnormalities characteristic of pseudohemophilia (von Willebrand's disease). The bleeding time is prolonged, and severity of bleeding varies considerably from among persons with this condition.

hemophilioid state A (hē'mōfil'ē-oid) (not current). See **parahemophilia.**

hemophilioid state C. See **hemophilia B.**

hemoptysis (hēmop'tĭsis), the expectoration of blood, by coughing, from the larynx or lower respiratory tract.

hemorrhage (hem'ərij), the escape of a large amount of blood from the blood vessels in a short period of time; excessive bleeding.

hemorrhagic bone cyst. See **cyst, hemorrhagic.**

hemorrhagic diathesis, an inherited predisposition to any one of a number of abnormalities characterized by excessive bleeding.

hemosiderin (hē'mōsid'ərin), an intracellular storage form of iron; the granules consist of an ill-defined complex of ferric hydroxides, polysaccharides, and proteins having an iron content of about 33% by weight. It appears as a dark yellow-brown pigment.

hemosiderosis, a focal or general increase in tissue iron stores without associated tissue damage.

hemostasis (hē'mōstā'sis), the arrest of an escape of blood.

hemostatic (hē'mōstatik), an agent used to reduce bleeding from minute vessels by hastening the clotting of blood or by the formation of an artificial clot.

Henderson's test. See **test, Henderson's.** (not current)

heparin/heparin calcium/heparin sodium, *trade names:* Hep Lock, Liquaemin Sodium; *drug class:* anticoagulant; *action:* acts in combination with antithrombin III (heparin cofactor) to inhibit thrombosis; inactivates factor Xa and inhibits conversion of prothrombin to thrombin; affects both intrinsic and extrinsic clotting pathways; *uses:* anticoagulant in thrombosis, embolism, coagulopathies, deep vein thrombosis, dialysis, maintenance of patency of indwelling IV lines.

heparinized lock system, an indwelling intravenous system developed by which multiple daily intravenous accesses can be accomplished and multiple penetrations of the veins can be avoided. The heparin chamber prevents the formation of a clot or thrombus at the needle site.

hepatitis (hep'ətī'tis), an inflammation of the liver.

h. C (HCV non-A, non-B hepatitis), a type of hepatitis transmitted largely by blood transfusion or percutaneous inoculation, such as with intravenous drug users sharing needles. The disease progresses to chronic hepatitis in up to 50% of the patients acutely infected.

h., chronic active, a subacute hepatitis with chronic portal inflammation with regional necrosis and fibrosis which may progress to nodular postnecrotic-cirrhosis

h. E (HEV, epidemic non-A, non-B hepatitis), a self-limited type of hepatitis that may occur after natural disasters because of fecal contaminated water or food. There is currently no serologic test available.

h., homologous serum (homologous serum jaundice, serum hepatitis, syringe jaundice, type B hepatitis), a viral hepatitis clinically difficult to distinguish from epidemic infectious hepatitis. It is transmitted by human serum (that is, through parenteral injection, transfusions, lacerations). The incubation period is 40 to 90 days or longer. Principal manifestations are jaundice, gastrointestinal symptoms, anorexia, and malaise.

h., infectious (IH, type A hepatitis), a viral hepatitis that is frequently epidemic in nature and has an incubation period of 1 to 4 or even 7 weeks. It is usually transmitted by the virus in fecal matter but may be transmitted by human serum (transfusions, lacerations, needle punctures).

h., serum. See **hepatitis, homologous serum.**

h., viral, **1.** hepatitis caused by any one of three immunologically unrelated viruses: h. A virus; h. B virus; and non-A, non-B virus **2.** Hepatitis caused by a viral infection, including

that by Epstein-Barr virus and cytomegalovirus.

hepatomegaly, abnormal, an enlargement of the liver that is usually a sign of liver disease. It is usually discovered by percussion and palpation as part of a physical examination. It may be caused by hepatitis, fatty infiltration, alcoholism, biliary obstruction, or malignancy.

Herbst appliance, the only fixed, tooth-borne, functional orthodontic appliance in which jaw position is influenced by a pin-and-tube spring-loaded appliance that is cemented or bonded to the teeth.

hereditary benign intraepithelial dyskeratosis, a hereditary disease seen in triracial isolates (whites, Indians, blacks) It involves the oral mucosa and may cause periodic seasonal keratoconjunctivitis.

hereditary opalescent dentin, a developmental disturbance in the formation of dentin, better known as dentiogenesis imperfecta. The teeth range from gray to brownish violet and are translucent or opalescent. The crowns fracture easily because of an abnormal dentinoenamel junction.

heredity (hered'itē), the inheritance of resemblance, physical qualities, or disease from a familial predecessor; the passage of characteristics from one generation to its progeny by genetic linkage.

Hering-Breuer reflex (her'ing broi' ər). See **reflex, Hering-Breuer.**

hermetic seal. See **seal, hermetic.**

hernia, the protrusion of an organ through an abnormal opening in the muscle wall of the cavity that surrounds it. A hernia may be congenital, may result from the failure of certain structures to close after birth, or may be acquired later in life because of obesity, muscular weakness, surgery, or illness.

h., hiatal, a protrusion of a portion of the stomach upward through the diaphragm. The condition occurs in about 40% of individuals and most people display few, if any, symptoms. The major difficulty is gastroesophageal reflux, which is the backflow of the acid contents of the stomach into the esophagus.

h., inguinal (direct), a protrusion of the intestines into an opening between the deep epigastric artery and the edge of the rectus muscle; (indirect) involves the internal inguinal ring and passes into the inguinal canal.

heroin, a highly addictive alkaloid prepared from morphine, previously used for cough relief. Use of heroin is prohibited by federal law because of its highly addictive properties and potential for abuse.

herpangina (her′panjĭnə) (Coxsackie A disease), a viral disease of children, usually occurring in summer, and characterized by sudden onset, fever (100° to 105° F; 38° to 40.5° C), sore throat, and oropharyngeal vesicles. Herpangina results from Coxsackie A viruses and is self-limiting.

herpes labialis (her′pēz lā′bē-al′is) (cold sore), a disease of the lips caused by herpesvirus and characterized by vesicles that rupture, leaving ulcers. The local lesions are often called *fever blisters* or *cold sores.* Herpes simplex of the lips.

herpes simplex (her′pēz sim′plex), an infection caused by the herpes simplex virus. Primary infection, occurring most often in children between 2 and 5 years of age, may result in apparent clinical disease or such manifestations as acute herpetic gingivostomatitis, keratoconjunctivitis, vulvovaginitis, or encephalitis. Recurrent manifestations may include herpes labialis (fever blisters or cold sores), dendritic corneal ulcers, or genital herpes simplex.

herpes zoster (her′pēz zäs′tər) (acute posterior ganglionitis, shingles), an acute viral disease involving the dorsal spinal root or cranial nerve and producing vesicular eruption in areas of the skin corresponding to the involved sensory nerve. Pain is a prominent feature and may persist, although skin lesions subside in 1 to 2 weeks.

herpetic lesion. See **lesion, herpetic.**

herpetic ulcer. See **ulcer, herpetic.** (not current)

heteresthesia (het′əresthē′zēə), a variation in the degree of cutaneous sensibility on adjoining areas of the body surface. (not current)

heterograft. See **graft, heterogenous.**

heterosexual, a person with a sexual attraction to or preference for persons of the opposite gender; having erotic attraction to, predisposition to, or sexual activity with a person of the opposite gender.

heterozygote, an organism whose somatic cells have two different allelomorphic genes on the same locus of each pair of chromosomes. It can produce two different types of gametes.

heterozygous (het′erōzī′gəs), a term indicating that genes lying at equivalent loci on chromosome pairs are different.

hexamethonium, a cholinergic blocking agent used to control bleeding and used in the treatment of peptic ulcers and hypertension. It produces ganglion blocking by occupying receptor sites.

hexosamine, the amine derivative (NH_2 replacing OH) of a hexose such as glucosamine.

HGF. See **glucagon.**

HIAA, the abbreviation for **Health Insurance Association of America.**

hiccup, an involuntary spasmodic contraction of the diaphragm that causes a beginning inspiration that is suddenly checked by closure of the glottis, thus producing a characteristic sound.

hidradenoma, a benign neoplasm derived from epithelial cells of sweat glands.

hidrocystoma, a cystic form of sweat gland adenoma. A hydrocystoma is produced by the cystic proliferation of apocrine secretory glands. It is not uncommon, occurring in adult life in no particular age group, with males and females equally affected. The most common site is around the eye. Hydrocystomas are cured by surgical removal.

hidrosis (hīdrō′sis), the secretion of sweat. (not current)

hierarchy, 1. any system of persons or things ranked one above the other. **2.** in psychology and psychiatry, an organization of habits or concepts in which simpler components are combined to form increasingly complex integrations.
h., Maslow's, a ranking of need, which man presumably fills successively in the order of the lowest to the highest, beginning with physiologic needs, love and belonging, self-esteem, and self-actualization. See **Maslow hierarchy.**

high labial arch. See **arch, high labial.**

high lip line. See **lip line, high.**

high-pull headgear, apparatus designed to give an upward pull on the face-bow.

high speed. See **speed, high.**

high-speed handpiece. See **handpiece, high-speed.**

hinchazon (hinch'əzon'). See **beriberi.**

hinge axis. See **axis, hinge.**

   h. a. determination. See **axis, condylar, determination.**

   h. a., orbital plane. See **axis, hinge, orbital plane.**

   h. a. point. See **point, hinge axis.**

hinge-bow, the kinematic face-bow used to determine the location of the hinge axis. The hinge-bow is a three-piece instrument with independently adjustable arms controlled by micrometer screws that lengthen or shorten them. Other micrometer screws raise or lower the caliper points to find the spots in or on the skin near the tragi where only rotary movements occur when the jaw is opened and closed at the rearmost point. See also **face-bow, kinematic.**

hinge movement. See **movement, hinge.**

hinge position. See **position, hinge.**

Hinton's test. See **test, Hinton's.** (not current)

hippocampus, a curved convoluted elevation of the floor of the inferior horn of the lateral ventricle of the brain. The hippocampus is composed of gray substance covered by a layer of white fibers, or the alveus, and functions as an important component of the limbic system.

hippus, respiratory (hip'əs), a dilation of the pupils occurring during inspiration and a contraction of the pupils occurring during expiration; often associated with pulsus paradoxus.

Hirschfeld-Dunlop file. See **file, Hirschfeld-Dunlop.** (not current)

Hirschfeld's method. See **point, Hirschfeld's silver.** (not current)

hirsutism (her'sootizəm), increased body or facial hair, which is especially noted in the female.

histamine, a compound found in all cells that is produced by the breakdown of histidine. Histamine is released in allergic, inflammatory reactions and causes dilation of capillaries, decreased blood pressure, increased secretion of gastric juice, and constriction of smooth muscles of the bronchi and uterus.

histidine, one of the essential amino acids for infants and children. See also **amino acid.**

histiocyte (his'tē·ōsīt'), a large phagocytic cell found in the interstices of the tissues; of reticuloendothelial origin.

histiocytosis, nonlipid (his'tē·ōsītō'sis). See **disease, Letterer-Siwe.**

   h., acute disseminated, X. See **disease, Letterer-Siwe.**

   h., chronic disseminated X. See **disease, Hand-Schüller-Christian.**

   h. X, a group of diseases characterized by abnormal histiocyte activity. Includes a chronic disseminated type (Hand-Schüller-Christian disease) and a chronic localized type (eosinophilic granuloma).

histoclasia, implant (his'tōklā'zē·ə), a condition of the tissues existing in the presence of an implant, in which the implant is not directly involved. It is a condition of the oral mucosal tissues, in which the pathology results from some external cause (for example, salivary calculus, attached prosthetic appliances).

histocompatibility, the compatibility of the antigens of donor and recipient of transplanted tissue.

   h. testing, the determination of the compatibility of the antigens of donor and recipient before tissue transplantation. Usually follows a blood typing protocol.

histocytoma, a tumor composed of histiocytes.

histogram, a bar graph; a graphic representation of a frequency distribution.

histology, microanatomy, which is the microscopic study of normal tissue and organs at the cellular level.

histopathology, the microscopic study of abnormal tissue and organs at the cellular level.

histoplasmosis (his'tōplazmō'sis), a disease caused by the fungus *Histoplasma capsulatum* and affecting the reticuloendothelial system. Ulceration of the oral mucosa may occur.

history, case, a detailed and concise compilation of all physical, dental, social, and mental factors relative and necessary to diagnosis, prognosis, and treatment.

histotoxic (histōtäk'sik), relating to poisoning of the respiratory enzyme system of the tissues.

HIV-1, the abbreviation for **human immunodeficiency virus type 1,** which is widely recognized as the etiologic agent of acquired immunodeficiency syndrome (AIDS). HIV-1 is characterized by its cytopathic effect and affinity for the T4-lymphocyte.

HIV-2, the abbreviation for **human immunodeficiency virus type 2,** which is related to HIV-1 but carries different antigenic components with differing nucleic acid composition. It shares serologic reactivity and sequence homology with the simian lentivirus SIV and infects only T4-lymphocytes expressing the CD4 phenotypic marker.

hives. See **urticaria.**

HIV-G. See **HIV gingivitis.**

HIV gingivitis (HIV-G), a distinct type of gingivitis found in HIV-infected patients, characterized by an intensely red linear erythemic band around the free gingiva that extends 2 to 3 mm apically into the attached gingiva. The involved gingiva tends to bleed spontaneously and may be present even in AIDS patients with good plaque control.

HIV-P. See **HIV periodontitis.**

HIV periodontitis (HIV-P), an aggressive form of periodontal disease with all of the characteristics of HIV-G combined with soft tissue ulceration and necrosis and rapid destruction of the periodontium and bone. The condition is very painful. HIV-P may resemble acute necrotizing ulcerative gingivitis (ANUG). However, ANUG is limited to the soft tissue, whereas HIV-P disease extends into the crestal bone.

HIV-wasting syndrome, a constitutional disease associated with AIDS, also known as the *slim disease.* Patients in this subgroup have a history of fever of more than 1 month, involuntary weight loss of more than 10%, and/or diarrhea persisting for more than 1 month.

hockey, a team contact sport played on ice skates or with roller blades. Since limited facial protection for the players exists (except for the goalie), there is opportunity for traumatic injury to the face and teeth.

Signs and symptoms of HIV-wasting syndrome

Chills and fever	Malaise
Night sweats	Fatigue
Dry, productive	Oral lesions cough
Dyspnea	Skin rashes
Lethargy	Abdominal discomfort
Confusion	Diarrhea
Stiff neck	Weight loss
Seizures	Lymphadenopathy
Headache	Progressive generalized edema

From Phipps WJ, Long BL, Woods NF, Cassmeyer VL: *Medical-surgical nursing: concepts and clinical practice,* ed 5, St Louis, 1995, Mosby.

Hodgkin's disease. See **disease, Hodgkin's.**

hoe, an angled instrument with the broad dimension of its blade perpendicular to the axis of the shank of the shaft.

hold, to possess by reason of a lawful title.

h. harmless clause, a contract provision in which one party to the contract promises to be responsible for liability incurred by the other party. Hold harmless clauses frequently appear in the following contexts: 1) Contracts between dental benefits organizations and an individual dentist often contain a promise by the dentist to reimburse the dental benefits organization for any liability the organization incurs because of dental treatment provided to beneficiaries of the organization's dental benefits plan. This may include a promise to pay the dental benefits organization's attorney fees and related costs, and 2) contracts between dental benefits organizations and a group plan sponsor may include a promise by the dental benefits organization to assume responsibility for disputes between a beneficiary of the group plan and an individual dentist when the dentist's charge exceeds the amount the organization pays for the service on behalf of the beneficiary. If the dentist takes action against the patient to recover the difference between the amount billed by the dentist and the amount paid by the organization, the dental benefits organization will take over the defense of the claim and will pay any judgments and court costs.

holder, an apparatus or instrument that is used to hold something.

h., broach. See **broach holder.**

h., clamp. See **holder, rubber dam clamp.**

h., matrix. See **retainer, matrix.**

h., rubber dam, an apparatus used to hold a rubber dam in place on the face and to secure the edges of the dam clear of the field of operation.

   h., r. d. clamp (clamp holder). See **forceps, rubber dam clamp.**

holistic health, a concept in which concern for health requires a perspective of the individual as an integrated system rather than a collection of parts and functions.

Hollenback condenser. See **condenser, pneumatic.**

hollow bulb, that portion of a prosthesis made hollow to minimize weight.

holograph, a writing completely in a person's handwriting, such as a deed, will, or letter. A holograph may have legal standing without witnesses.

holoprosencephaly, a congenital defect caused by the failure of the prosencephalon to divide into hemispheres during embryonic development. It is characterized by multiple midline facial defects, including cyclopia in severe cases.

homatropine hydrobromide *(optic), trade names:* AK-Homatropine, Isopto Homatropine; *drug class:* mydriatic (topical); *action:* blocks response of iris sphincter muscle and muscle of accommodation of ciliary body to cholinergic stimulation, resulting in dilation and paralysis of accommodation; *uses:* cycloplegic refraction, uveitis, mydriatic lens opacities.

home care, the physiotherapeutic measures employed by the patient for the maintenance of dental and periodontal health. Includes proper cleaning with a toothbrush, floss, or other device.

home health agency, an organization that provides health care in the home. Medicare certification for home health agency depends on the providing of skilled nursing services and of at least one additional therapeutic service, usually physical or occupational therapy.

homeless person, a person without a home, legal residence, or shelter either by choice or circumstances.

homeostasis (hō′mē-ōstā′sis), the term used to describe the tendency toward physiologic equilibrium (for example, acid-base balance, pH level of blood, blood sugar level).

h., cell, the tendency of biologic tissues and processes to maintain a constancy of environment consistent with their vitality and well being. For cells to maintain their stability or equilibrium, the cell membranes must be in continuous interaction with both the internal (intracellular) environment and the external (extracellular) environment. When the equilibrium of any component is disturbed, the interaction permits automatic readjustment by giving rise to stimuli that result in restoration of the equilibrium.

homicide, the killing of one human being by another. Legally there are differing degrees of homicide based on motive, opportunity, and circumstances.

Hominidae, the primate family, which includes humans.

homograft. See **graft, homogenous.**

homosexual, a person with a sexual attraction to or preference for persons of the same gender; having erotic attraction to, predisposition to, or sexual activity with a person of the same gender.

homovanillic acid, an acid that is produced by normal metabolism of dopamine and may be elevated in the urine in association with tumors of the adrenal gland.

homozygous (hōmōzī′gəs), a term indicating that genes lying at equivalent loci on chromosome pairs are the same.

hook, skin, a metallic instrument ending in a fine, sharp hook for handling soft tissues during surgery.

Hoover's sign. See **sign, Hoover's.**

HOP, the abbreviation for **high oxygen pressure.**

horizontal overlap. See **overlap, horizontal.**

horizontal plane. See **plane, horizontal.**

hormone(s) (hor′mōnz), the biochemical secretions of the endocrine glands that, in relatively small quantities, partially regulate the physiologic activity of the tissues, organs, organ systems, and other endocrine glands, and of the nervous system itself. The hormonal secretions are conducted and distributed throughout the body by the circulation of the bloodstream and tissue fluids.

h., adenohypophyseal, hormones secreted by the adenohypophysis. Includes seven distinct hormones: somatotropin (STH), thyrotropin (TSH), prolactin, follicle-stimulating hormone (FSH), luteinizing hormone (LH), melanocyte-stimulating hormone (MSH), and adrenocorticotropic hormone (ACTH).

h., adrenal medullary, hormones secreted by adrenal medulla, including two catecholamines: epinephrine and norepinephrine.

h., adrenocortical, steroid hormones secreted by the adrenal cortex that are biologically active in one or more of the following states: stress, inflammation, metabolism of carbohydrates, proteins, electrolytes, and water.

h., adrenocorticotropic. See **ACTH.**

h., adrenotropic. See **ACTH.**

h., androgenic. See **hormones, sex, male.**

h., anterior pituitary-like. See **hormone, pregnancy.**

h., antidiabetic. See **insulin.**

h., antidiuretic (ADH, vasopressin), a hormone of the posterior pituitary gland that encourages resorption of water by acting on the epithelial cells of the distal portion of the renal tubule. It raises blood pressure by its effect on the peripheral blood vessels and exerts an antidiuretic effect (antifacultative resorption of water in the renal tubules). An absence of antidiuretic hormone causes diabetes insipidus.

h., antiinflammatory. See **glucocorticoids.**

h., chorionic gonadotropic, a glycoprotein secreted by placental tissue early in normal pregnancy. This protein is also found in the urine or blood in association with chorioepitheliomas and some neoplastic diseases of the testes.

h., corticosteroid. See **steroid, adrenocortical.**

h., corticotropic, any one of the ovarian or adrenal hormones (for example, estradiol, estrone, estriol) that is capable of stimulating changes of a cyclic nature in the genital system. One of the ovarian or adrenal hormones capable of affecting the cyclic changes of the female genital system. See also **ACTH.**

h., female sex, hormones secreted by the ovary. They include two main types: the follicular, or estrogenic, hormones produced by the graafian follicle, and the progestational hormones from the corpus luteum.

h., follicle-stimulating, a pituitary tropic hormone that promotes the growth and maturation of the ovarian follicle and, with other gonadotropins, induces secretion of estrogens and possibly spermatogenesis.

h., gastrointestinal, hormones that regulate motor and secretory activity of the digestive organs; that is, gastrin, secretin, and cholecystokinin.

h., gonadotropic. See **gonadotropin.**

h., growth (somatotropic hormone, somatotropin), a growth, or somatotropic, hormone that is secreted by the anterior lobe of the pituitary gland and that exerts an influence on skeletal growth. As long as the growth apparatus is functional, it is responsive to the effects of the hormone.

h., ketogenic, the term used to describe a factor of the anterior pituitary hormone responsible for ketogenic effect. It is probably not an entity differing from known pituitary hormones.

h., lactogenic (galactin, mammotropin, prolactin), a pituitary hormone that stimulates lactation.

h., luteal. See **hormones, progestational.**

h., luteinizing, a pituitary hormone that causes ovulation and development of the corpus luteum from the mature graafian follicle. It is called an *interstitial cell and stimulating hormone* because of its action on the testis in maintaining spermatogenesis and because of its role in the development of accessory sex organs.

h., male sex (androgenic hormone, C-19 steroids), hormones found in the testes, urine, and blood. Included are testosterone found in the testes, androsterone excreted into the urine, and dehydro-3-epiandrosterone found in the blood.

h., melanocyte-stimulating (MSH, intermedin), a hormone of the middle lobe of the pituitary gland that increases melanin deposition by the melanocytes of the skin.

h., N. See **hormone, nitrogen** and **steroid, C-19 cortico-.**

h., neurohypophyseal, octapeptides of the neural lobe: oxytocin and vasopressin.

h., nitrogen (N hormone), C-19 corticosteroids that have androgenic and protein anabolic effects.

h., parathyroid, the secretory product of the parathyroid glands that promotes bone resorption and increases renal resorption of calcium and magnesium and diminishes that of phosphate. Excessive secretion of the parathyroid hormone produces generalized bone resorption, formation of fibrous marrow in the spongiosa, and, in young individuals, hypocalcification of the teeth.

h., pituitary, hormones of the anterior lobe of the pituitary gland, including the growth hormones (somatotropin 1, lactogenic hormone, prolactin, galactin, mammotropin) and pituitary tropins (gonadotropins, thyrotropic hormone, and ACTH). Whether or not a true diabetogenic pituitary hormone exists is a question. The melanocyte-stimulating hormone is secreted by the middle lobe of the pituitary gland, and vasopressin and oxytocin are secreted by the posterior lobe of the pituitary gland.

h., pregnancy (anterior pituitary-like hormone, antuitrin S, chorionic gonadotropin), a gonadotropic hormone found in the urine during pregnancy; it is a product of the very early placenta.

h., progestational (luteal hormone), hormones produced during the phase of the menstrual cycle just preceding menstruation. Includes progesterone, pregnanediol, and pregnenmolone.

h., proinflammatory. See **mineralocorticoids.**

h., "S" (glucocorticoid factor, sugar hormone), a factor in the secretions of the adrenal cortex related to the regulation of carbohydrate metabolism.

h., sex, steroid hormones that are produced by the testes and ovaries and that control secondary sex characteristics, the reproductive cycle, development of the accessory reproductive cycle, and development of the accessory reproductive organs. Also included are the gonadotropins produced by the pituitary gland.

h., somatotropic. See **hormone, growth.**

h., steroid, a group of biologically active organic compounds that are secreted by the adrenal cortex, testes, ovary, and placenta, and that have in common a cyclopentanoperhydrophenanthrene nucleus.

h., sugar. See **hormone, "S"** and **steroid, C-21 cortico-.**

h., testicular, hormones elaborated by the testes (chiefly testosterone) that promote the growth and function of the male genitalia and secondary sex characteristics and that have potent protein anabolic effects.

h., thyroid, hormonal variants, including thyroxin and triiodothyronine, derived from the thyroid gland. Thyroid hormone acts as a catalyst for oxidative processes of the body cell and thus regulates the rates of body metabolism and stimulates body growth and maturation.

h., t.-stimulating. See **hormone, thyrotropic.**

h., thyrotropic (TSH, thyroid stimulating hormone), a pituitary hormone that regulates the growth and activity of the thyroid gland.

horn, pulp, a small projection of vital pulp tissue directly under a cusp or developmental lobe.

hospital, an institution for the care of sick, wounded, infirm, or aged persons; generally incorporated as a nonprofit organization.

hostility, the tendency of an organism to threaten harm to another or to itself.

host site, an anatomic area surgically prepared to receive an implant or graft.

Howard's method. See **method, Howard's.**

Howe's silver nitrate. See **silver nitrate, ammoniacal.** (not current)

Howe's silver precipitation method. See **method, Howe's silver precipitation.**

h.s., the abbreviation for the Latin term *hora somni,* meaning "at bedtime."

human genome project, a federally sponsored research project to identify and map the entire human gene pool.

human immunodeficiency virus (HIV), a type of retrovirus that causes AIDS. Retroviruses produce the enzyme reverse transcriptase, which allows transcription of the viral genome onto the DNA of the host cell. It is transmitted through contact with an infected individual's blood, semen, cervical secretions, cerebrospinal fluid, or synovial fluid. HIV infects T-helper cells of the immune system and results in infection with a long incubation period, averaging 10 years.

human rights, the legal and moral rights of humans recognized by national and international laws.

humectant (hyo͞omek′tənt), a substance that prevents loss of moisture.

humidity, pertaining to the level of moisture in the atmosphere, the amount varying with the temperature. The percentage is usually represented in terms of relative humidity, with 100% being the point of air saturation or the level at which the air can absorb no additional water without an increase in temperature.

Hunter's glossitis (not current). See **glossitis, Moeller's.**

Huntington's chorea, a rare, abnormal hereditary condition characterized by chronic, progressive chorea and mental deterioration that terminates in dementia. The individual afflicted usually shows the first signs in the fourth decade of life and dies usually within 15 years. There is no known effective treatment but symptoms can be relieved with medications.

Hunt's syndrome. See **syndrome, Hunt's.**

hurt, to molest or restrain; not restricted to physical injuries; also includes mental pain, discomfort, or annoyance.

husband, a man who has a spouse.

Hutchinson-Gilford syndrome. See **syndrome, Hutchinson-Gilford.**

Hutchinson's incisors. See **incisors, Hutchinson's.**

Hutchinson triad. See **triad, Hutchinson.**

HVL. See **half-value layer.**

hyalinization (hī′əlin′izā′shən), the appearance of an acellular, avascular, homogeneous area in the periodontal ligament, in which compression of the ligament between bone and tooth occurs as a result of orthodontic forces.
  h. of periodontal ligament, a degenerative process resulting from long-continued occlusal trauma, in which the fibers become hyalinized into a homogeneous mass.

hyaluronic acid, a mucopolysaccharide that forms the gelatinous substance in the tissue spaces. Hyaluronic acid is the intercellular cementing substance found throughout the tissues of the body.

hyaluronidase (hī′əlo͞oron′ə-dās), an enzyme that produces hydrolysis of hyaluronic acid, the cementing substance of the tissues. Produced by certain pathogenic bacteria and also formed by sperm.

hybridization, crossbreeding; the process of breeding a hybrid, such as crossbreeding a horse with a donkey to produce a mule.

hydralazine HCl, *trade name:* Apresoline; *drug class:* antihypertensive, direct-acting peripheral vasodilator; *action:* vasodilates arteriolar smooth muscle by direct relaxation; *uses:* essential hypertension.

hydraulicity (hī′drăli′sitē), the ability of a material (cement) to set while in contact with moisture. (not current)

hydraulic pressure. See **pressure, hydraulic.**

hydremia (hī′drē′mē-ə), an increase in blood volume caused by an increase in serum volume. This may result from cardiac failure, renal insufficiency, pregnancy, or the intravenous administration of fluids.

hydroalcoholic (hī′drō-alkōhol′ik), containing both water and alcohol. See also **solution.**

Hydrocal (hī′drōkal), the trade name for a gypsum product, α-hemihydrate, known as artificial stone. It is used for making casts.

hydrocele, an accumulation of fluid in any saclike cavity or duct, specifically in the tunica vaginalis testis or along the spermatic cord.

hydrocephalus (hī′drōsef′ələs), an abnormal accumulation of cerebrospinal fluid in the cranial vault, resulting in a disproportionately large cranium.

hydrochloric acid, a compound consisting of hydrogen and chlorine. Hydrochloric acid is secreted in the stomach and is a major component of gastric juice.

hydrochlorothiazide, *trade names:* Esidrix, HydroDIURIL; *drug class:* thiazide diuretic; *action:* acts on distal tubule by increasing excretion of water, sodium, chloride, potassium;

H

uses: edema, hypertension, diuresis, CHF.

hydrocodone, a semisynthetic narcotic analgesic and antitussive with multiple actions similar to those of codeine. Hydrocodone is an ingredient in prescription analgesics and cough medicines.

h. bitartrate, trade name: Hycodan; *drug class:* narcotic analgesic, Controlled Substance Schedule III; *action:* interacts with opioid receptor in the central nervous system to alter pain perception; acts directly on cough center in medulla to suppress cough; *uses:* hyperactive and nonproductive cough; mild-to moderate pain.

hydrocolloid (hī'drōkol'oid), **1.** the materials listed as colloid solids with water; used in dentistry as elastic impression materials. Hydrocolloids can be reversible or irreversible. **2.** an agar-base impression material.

h., irreversible (alginate), a hydrocolloid whose physical condition is changed by a chemical action that is not reversible. It is an impression material that is elastic when set. See also **alginate.**

h., reversible (agar-agar type), a hydrocolloid whose physical condition is changed by temperature. The material is made fluid by heat and becomes an elastic solid on cooling.

hydrocortisone (hī'drōkôr'tisōn) (cortisol), a glucocorticosteroid secreted by the adrenal cortex in response to stimulation by ACTH. Hydrocortisone is antianabolic, stimulates gluconeogenesis, and probably acts on some cellular system in response to a need for adaptation to change (stress).

h. hydrocortisone acetate/hydrocortisone sodium phosphate/hydrocortisone sodium succinate/hydrocortisone cypionate, trade names: Cortef, Cortifoam, Cortenema; *drug class:* corticosteroid; *action:* decreases inflammation by suppression of macrophage and leukocyte migration; reduces capillary permeability and inhibits lysosomal enzymes; *uses:* severe inflammation, shock, adrenal insufficiency, ulcerative colitis, collagen disorders.

h. hydrocortisone acetate/hydrocortisone valerate, trade names: Acticort, Cortaid, Cort-Dome, Dermicort; *drug class:* topical corticosteroid; *action:*

interacts with steroid cytoplasmic receptors to induce antiinflammatory effects; possesses antipruritic, antiinflammatory actions; *uses:* psoriasis, eczema, contact dermatitis, pruritus.

hydrofluoric acid, a compound consisting of hydrogen and flourine. It is a very active, corrosive compound, used to etch glass and precious metals.

hydrogen (H), a gaseous, univalent element. Its atomic number is 1 and its atomic weight is 1.008. It is the simplest and lightest of the elements and is normally a colorless, odorless, highly flammable diatomic gas.

h. peroxide, an unstable compound of hydrogen and oxygen that is easily broken down into water and oxygen. A 3% solution is used as a mild antiseptic for the skin and mucous membranes; more concentrated solutions may be used as a bleach.

hydrolysis (hīdrol'isis), **1.** a reaction between the ions of salt and those of water to form an acid and a base, one or both of which is only slightly dissociated. A process whereby a large molecule is split by the addition of water. The end products divide the water, the hydroxyl group being attached to one and the hydrogen ion to the other. **2.** the splitting of a compound into two parts with the addition of the elements of water.

hydromorphone HCl, *trade names:* Dilaudid; *drug class:* synthetic narcotic analgesic (Controlled Substance Schedule II); *action:* inhibits ascending pain pathways in the central nervous system, increases pain threshold, alters pain perception; *uses:* moderate-to-severe pain.

hydrophilic (hī'drōfil'ik), having an affinity for water. Opposite of lipophilic. See also **ointment, hydrophilic.**

hydroquinone (hīdrōkwin'ōn), **1.** a reducing agent used as an inhibitor in resin monomers to prevent polymerization during storage. **2.** one of the two chemicals used as reducing agents in film-developing solutions. Hydroquinone is made from benzene (paradihydroxybenzene) and is sensitive to thermal changes. Above 70° F (21° C), the action of hydroquinone is rapid; below 60° F (15.5° C), hydroquinone becomes inactive. Its action is to control the contrast of the film.

hydrostatic pressure (hī'drōstat'ik). See **pressure, hydrostatic.**

hydrotherapy (hī'drōther'əpē), an empirical adjunct to oral physiotherapy where forced water irrigation is used to cleanse subgingival spaces, remove debris from interproximal spaces, and cleanse pockets.

hydroxide, an ionic compound that contains the OH⁻ ion, usually consisting of metals or the metal equivalent of the ammonium cation (NH_4-) that inactivates an acid.

hydroxyapatite (hīdrok'sē·ap'ətīt), a mineral compound of the general formula $3Ca_3(PO_4)_2 \cdot Ca(OH)_2$, which is the principal inorganic component of bone, teeth, and dental calculus.

hydroxychloroquine sulfate, *trade name:* Plaquenil Sulfate; *drug class:* antimalarial; *action:* inhibits parasite replications, transcription of DNA to RNA by forming complexes with DNA of parasite; *uses:* malaria, lupus erythematosus, rheumatoid arthritis.

hydroxyurea, *trade name:* Hydrea; *drug class:* antineoplastic; *action:* acts by inhibiting DNA synthesis without interfering with synthesis of RNA or protein; *uses:* melanoma, chronic myelocytic leukemia, recurrent or metastatic ovarian cancer.

hydroxyzine HCl/hydroxyzine pamoate, *trade names:* Atarax, Quiess, Visaject, Hyzine; *drug class:* antianxiety antihistamine; *action:* depresses subcortical levels of the central nervous system, antagonist for histamine H_1-receptors; *uses:* anxiety; preoperatively, postoperatively to prevent nausea, vomiting; to potentiate narcotic analgesics; sedation; pruritus.

hygiene (hī'jēn), the science of health and its preservation.

h., oral (mouth hygiene), the practice of personal maintenance of oral cleanliness.

h., radiation, the art and science of protecting human beings from injury by radiation. Since any amount of radiation is potentially harmful, the ideal objective is to prevent the exposure of any person without a definite medical purpose.

hygienist, dental, a person trained in an accredited school and licensed by the state where residing to provide health services, such as scaling and polishing teeth, health education and training, and radiography, under the direction of a licensed dentist.

hygroma (hīgrō'mə), a sac or cyst swollen with fluid.

h. colli cysticum (cystic hygroma, cystic lymphangioma), a cavernous lymphangioma involving the neck. It may be large, thereby impairing breathing and swallowing.

hygroscopic (hī'grōskop'ik), having the property of absorbing moisture. When applied to gypsum products in contact with free water during their set, the resultant expansion is implied. See also **expansion, hygroscopic.**

h. investment. See **investment, hygroscopic.**

hyoid bone, a single U-shaped bone suspended from the styloid processes of the temporal bone behind and lower border of the mandible in front by a system of muscle and ligament attachments.

hyoscyamine sulfate, *trade names:* Anaspaz, Levsin, Levsinex, Gastrosed; *drug class:* anticholinergic; *action:* inhibits muscarinic actions of acetylcholine at postganglionic parasympathetic neuroeffector sites; *uses:* treatment of peptic ulcer disease in combination with other drugs; other gastrointestinal disorders; other spastic disorders such as parkinsonism; also preoperatively to reduce secretions.

hypalgesia (hī'paljē'zē·ə), diminished sensitivity to pain that results from a raised pain threshold.

hyper- (hī'pər), a prefix signifying above, beyond, or excessive.

hyperadrenocorticism (hī'pərədrē'nōkor'tisizəm), adrenocortical hyperfunction resulting from neoplasia of the cortex or hyperplasia of the cortex secondary to an increase in ACTH. Manifestations include hyperglycemia, edema, hypertension, glycosuria, negative nitrogen balance, acne, and hirsutism. See also **syndrome, adrenogenital** and **syndrome, Cushing's.**

hyperalgesia (hī'pəraljē'zē·ə), a greater-than-normal sensitivity to pain that may result from a painful stimulus or a lowered pain threshold.

hyperalgia (hipəral'jē·ə), an abnormal sensitivity to pain.

hyperandrogenism, a state characterized or caused by an excessive secretion of androgens by the adrenal cortex, ovaries, or testes. The clinical significance in males is negligible, so the term is used most commonly with reference to the female. The common manifestations in women are hirsutism and virilism. Hyperandrogenism is often caused by either ovarian or adrenal diseases.

hyperbilirubinemia, greater than normal amounts of the bile pigment bilirubin in the blood, often characterized by jaundice, anorexia, and malaise. Hyperbilirubinemia is associated with liver disease and biliary obstruction, but it also occurs when there is excessive destruction of red blood cells, as in hemolytic anemia.

hypercalcemia (hī′pərkalsē′mē-ə) (hypercalcinemia), **1.** an elevated blood calcium level. **2.** an abnormal elevation of calcium in the blood. Causes include primary hyperparathyroidism, sarcoidosis, multiple myeloma, malignant neoplasms, prolonged androgen therapy, and massive doses of vitamin D. Symptoms suggestive of hypercalcemia are nausea, vomiting, constipation, polyuria, weight loss, muscular weakness, and polydipsia. The normal level of total serum calcium is 8.5 to 10.5 mg/100 ml.

hypercalcinuria. See **hypercalciuria.**

hypercalciuria (hī′pərkal′sēyoo̅′rē-ə) (hypercalcinuria), a condition in which there is an excessive increase in urinary calcium excretion. Major causes include primary hyperparathyroidism, hypervitaminosis D, excessive milk intake, metastatic malignancy, immobilization, and renal tubular acidosis. See also **hypercalcemia.**

hypercapnia (hī′pərkap′nē-ə), the presence of more than the normal amount of carbon dioxide in the blood tissues resulting from an increase of carbon dioxide in the inspired air or a decrease in elimination.

hypercementosis (hī′pərsē′mentō′sis), an excessive formation of cementum on the roots of one or more teeth.

hypercenesthesia (hī′pərsen′esthē′zhə), a feeling of exaggerated well-being such as is seen in general paralysis and sometimes in mania.

hyperchloremia (hī′pərklōrē′mē-ə), an excessive concentration of chloride in the plasma. Normal range is 98 to 100 mEq/L. It may occur in water depletion, dehydration, decreased bicar-

bonate concentration, or metabolic acidosis.

hypercholesterolemia, the presence of an abnormally large amount of cholesterol in the cells and plasma of the circulating blood.

hyperemia (hī′pərē′mē-ə) (congestion), an increased and excessive amount of blood in a tissue. The hyperemia may be active or passive.

h., **active,** hyperemia caused by an increased flow of blood to an area by active dilation of both the arterioles and capillaries. It is associated with neurogenic, hormonal, and metabolic function.

h., **passive,** hyperemia caused by a decreased outflow of blood from an area. It may be generalized, resulting from cardiac, renal, or pulmonary disorders, or it may be localized, as in the oral cavity, and caused by pressure from mechanical or physical obstruction or by pressure from a tumor, denture, filling, or salivary calculus.

hyperesthesia (hī′pəresthē′zhə), an excessive sensitivity of the skin or of a special sense.

hyperesthetic (hī′pəresthet′ik), pertaining to or affected with hyperesthesia.

hyperfunction, an increase in activity of a part or in the stresses applied to a part.

hypergammaglobulinemia (hī′pərgam′əglob′yəlinē′mē-ə), an excess of γ globulin in the blood. It occurs in chronic granulomatous inflammations, chronic bacterial infections, liver disease, multiple myeloma, lymphomas, and dysproteinemias.

hyperglobulinemia (hī′pərglob′yəlinē′mē-ə), an abnormally high concentration of globulins in the blood.

hyperglycemia (hī′pərglīsē′mē-ə), an increase in the concentration of sugar in the blood. It is a feature of diabetes mellitus.

hypergonadism (hī′pərgō′nadizəm), an excessive secretion of hormonal agents by the testes or ovaries. Gingival changes induced by the administration of estrogens and androgens include an increase in keratinization and hyperplasia of epithelial and connective tissue. (not current)

hyperhidrosis (hī′pərhīdrō′sis), excessive sweating, which may be generalized or localized.

h., *gustatory,* increased sweating in the preauricular region, forehead, or face associated with eating. See also **syndrome, auriculotemporal.**

h., *masticatory,* excessive sweating associated with chewing. The cause is traumatic injury producing anastomosis of the facial nerve with a sympathetic branch.

hyperkalemia (hī'pərkəlē'mē-ə), an abnormally elevated concentration of serum potassium. It may occur in renal failure, shock, and advanced dehydration, and in association with high intracellular potassium in Addison's disease. The normal adult range of serum potassium is 4.0 to 5.5 mEq/L.

hyperkeratosis (hī'pərker'ətō'sis), an excessive formation of keratin (for example, as seen in leukoplakia).

hyperlipidemia, an excess of lipids in the plasma, including the glycolipids, lipoproteins, and phospholipids.

hypermagnesemia (hī'pərmag'nesē'mē-ə), an excess of magnesium in the blood serum. Normal range is 1.5 to 2.5 mEq/L. It may result in respiratory failure and coma and may occur in untreated diabetic acidosis, renal failure, and severe dehydration.

hypernasality (hī'pərnāzal'itē), an excessive nasal resonance usually accompanied by emission of air through the nasal passageways.

hypernatremia (hī'pərnətrē'mē-ə), an abnormally elevated concentration of serum sodium. It may occur rarely in nephrosis, congestive heart failure, and Cushing's disease and after administration of adrenocorticotropic hormone (ACTH), cortisone, or deoxycorticosterone. Normal adult range of serum sodium is 135 to 145 mEq/L.

hyperocclusion (traumatic), premature tooth contact during mouth closure.

hyperostosis (hī'pərostō'sis), **1.** an excessive growth of bone, as in infantile cortical hyperostosis. **2.** hypertrophy of bone. See also **exostosis.**

h., *infantile cortical (Caffey's disease, Smyth's syndrome),* a disease of infants; of unknown etiology and characterized by tender, soft tissue swelling that is followed by hyperostosis of the cortex of the underlying bone. The mandible, clavicle, and ulna are most frequently affected.

hyperoxaluria, an excessive level of oxalic acid or oxalates, primarily calcium oxalate in the urine. The cause is usually an inherited deficiency of an enzyme needed to metabolize oxalic acid, which is present in many fruits and vegetables, or a disorder of fat absorption in the small intestine. An excess of oxalates may lead to the formation of renal calculi. Treatment may include pyridoxine, forced fluid, and a low-oxalate diet.

h., *primary,* an inherited deficiency of the enzyme that metabolizes oxalic acid, resulting in an excessive level of oxalic acid or oxalates in the urine.

hyperoxia (hī'pərok'sē-ə), an excess of oxygen in the system.

hyperparathyroidism (hī'pərper'ə-thī'roidizəm) (generalized osteitis fibrosa cystica, von Recklinghausen's disease of bone), **1.** increased parathyroid function resulting from primary hyperplasia, a functioning neoplasm of the parathyroid glands, or secondary hyperplasia related most often to chronic renal insufficiency. Manifestations are related to abnormalities of the bones, kidneys, and blood vessels. Skeletal changes are referred to as *generalized osteitis fibrosa cystica* or *von Recklinghausen's disease.* Brown tumors, which are essentially giant cell tumors, may develop generally, as well as in the jaws. Kidney changes include renal stones and nephrocalcinosis. Calcification of muscles in arteries occurs. Renal rickets is associated with secondary hyperparathyroidism in children with chronic renal disease. Laboratory findings include a high serum calcium level, low phosphorus level, and a normal or high alkaline phosphatase level. Renal impairment, such as occurs in secondary hyperparathyroidism, tends to nullify hypercalcemia because of an increased loss of calcium in the urine. **2.** an abnormal increase in activity of the parathyroid glands, causing loss of calcium from the bones and resulting in tenderness in bones, spontaneous fractures, muscular weakness, and osteitis fibrosa. **3.** excessive production of parathormone by the parathyroid gland (as in parathyroid hyperplasia and/or adenoma), resulting in increased renal excretion of phosphorus by lowering of the renal threshold for this substance.

The pathologic changes produced are osteoporotic or osteodystrophic in nature as a consequence of withdrawal of calcium and phosphorus from osseous tissues.

h., brown node of. See **node, brown, of hyperparathyroidism.**

hyperphosphatemia (hī′perfos′fətē′mē-ə), an increased concentration of inorganic phosphates in the blood serum. Hyperphosphatemia may occur in childhood and also in acromegaly, renal failure, and vitamin D intoxication. Normal adult range of serum inorganic phosphorus is 2.5 to 4.2 mg/100 ml.

hyperphosphaturia (hī′pərfos′fətōō′-rē-ə), an excessive excretion of phosphate in the urine.

hyperpigmentation, an unusual darkening of the skin. Causes include heredity, drugs, exposure to the sun, and adrenal insufficiency.

hyperpituitarism (hī′pərpitōō′iterizəm), a condition caused by excessive production of the hormones secreted by the pituitary gland. An excess of the growth hormone results in giantism or acromegaly; an excess of ACTH produces Cushing's syndrome.

hyperplasia (hī′pərplā′zhə), the abnormal multiplication or increase in the number of normal cells in normal arrangement in a tissue or organ, resulting in a thickening or enlargement of the tissue or organ.

h., denture (denture hypertrophy), an enlargement of tissue beneath a denture that is traumatizing the soft tissue.

h., Dilantin gingival (dilan′tin) (Dilantin enlargement), an enlargement of the gingivae caused by the use of diphenylhydantoin sodium (Dilantin sodium) in the treatment of epilepsy.

h., gingival, **1.** an enlargement of the gingival tissue resulting from proliferation of its cellular elements. Hereditary or inflammatory etiology may be involved. **2.** the proliferation of gingival epithelium to form elongated rete pegs and proliferation of fibroblasts with increased collagen formation in the underlying connective tissue; leads to nodular enlargement of the gingiva in diphenylhydantoin sodium therapy. **3.** gingival enlargement, primarily produced by proliferation of connective tissue elements; often accompanied by gingival inflammation as a result of trauma to the hyperplastic tissues and coincidental with or following the ingestion of diphenylhydantoin sodium.

h., idiopathic gingival. See **fibromatosis gingivae.**

h., inflammatory fibrous. See **epulis fissurata.**

h., inflammatory papillary (inflammatory papillomatosis, multiple papillomatosis, papillary hyperplasia), a condition of unknown etiology but associated with the presence of maxillary dentures. Characterized by numerous red papillary projections on the hard palate.

h., papillary, a growth in the midline of the hard palate, usually in the relief area of a denture; characterized by papillary, or raspberry, appearance.

hyperplastic tissue. See **tissue, hyperplastic.**

hyperpnea (hī′pərpnē′-ə), an abnormal increase in respiratory volume; an abnormal increase in the rate and depth of breathing.

hyperpotassemia (hī′pərpot′əsē′mē-ə). See **hyperkalemia.**

hyperproteinemia (hī′pərprō′tēne′inē-ə), an abnormal increase in serum and plasma proteins.

hyperproteinuria (hī′pərprō′tēnyə′rē-ə). See **albuminuria.**

hypersalivation. See **sialorrhea.**

hypersensitive, abnormally sensitive.

hypersensitiveness (hī′pərsen′sitiv′nes), a state of altered reactivity in which the body reacts more strongly than normal to a foreign agent.

hypersensitivity, 1. an adverse reaction to contact with specific substances in quantities that usually produce no reaction in normal individuals. **2.** usually, an allergic tendency. In general, a tendency to react with unusual violence to stimuli. **3.** a common complaint after periodontal therapy in which dentin may be exposed, resulting in pain in the teeth or sensitivity to heat, cold, and sweet substances.

h., atopic. See **atopy.**

h., bacterial, delayed inflammatory reaction resulting from previous sensitization of the host by an antigen.

h., delayed, hypersensitivity involving a latent period between the antigen introduction and the reaction; cellular reactions mediated by the T lymphocytes *h., immediate,* a humoral reaction, mediated by the circulating B lymphocytes, which causes any of three immediate responses: anaphylactic hypersensitivity, cytotoxic hypersensitivity, and immune system hypersensitivity.

hypersensitization, the process of rendering abnormally sensitive or the condition of being abnormally sensitive.

hypersplenism, a syndrome consisting of splenomegaly and a deficiency of one or more types of blood cells.

hypersthenuria (hī′pərstheny͞oo′rē·ə), urine with an abnormally high specific gravity. It is seen in uncontrolled diabetes mellitus and in severe dehydration.

hypersusceptibility (hī′pərsəsep′tibil′itē), a condition of abnormal susceptibility to poisons, infective agents, or agents that are entirely innocuous in the normal individual.

hypersympathicotonus (hī′pərsimpath′ikōtō′nəs), an increased tonicity of the sympathetic nervous system. (not current)

hypersystolic (hī′pərsistol′ik), characterized by hypersystole; having heartbeats of excessive force. (not current)

hypertarachia (hī′pərtərak′ē·ə), extreme irritability of the nervous system.

hypertelorism (hī′pərte′lərizəm), an excessive distance between paired organs. See also **syndrome, Greig's.**

hypertension (hī′pərten′shən), an abnormal elevation of systolic and/or diastolic arterial pressure. Systolic hypertension is generally related to emotional stress, sclerosis of the aorta and large arteries, or aortic insufficiency. Diastolic hypertension may result from obscure causes (essential), renal disease, or endocrine disorders.

h., essential, an elevated blood pressure of unknown etiology.

h., malignant, an elevated blood pressure characterized by a progressive course uncontrollable by medication.

h. portal, hypertension originating in the portal system as occurring in cirrhosis of the liver and other conditions caused by an obstruction of the portal vein.

h. pulmonary, Hypertension resulting from pulmonary or cardiac disease such as fibrosis of the lung or mitral stenosis.

hypertensive agents, agents that reduce or control blood pressure.

hyperthyroidism (Parry's disease), abnormalities of calorigenic mechanisms, body tissues, blood, and body fluids and of the circulatory, muscular, and nervous systems resulting from an excessive elaboration of thyroid hormone. Manifestations include increased sweating, increased appetite, intolerance to heat, weight loss, increased protein-bound iodine (PBI), early shedding of primary teeth and early eruption of permanent teeth, tachycardia, palpitation, tremors, nervousness, muscular weakness, diarrhea, increased excretion of calcium and phosphorus, hypocholesterolemia, creatinuria, and osteoporosis. May occur as the result of primary hyperplasia, hyperfunctioning nodular goiters, functional benign tumor, or adenoma of the thyroid gland. See also **goiter, exophthalmic.**

hypertonic (hī′pərton′ik), having an osmotic pressure greater than that of the solution with which it is compared.

hypertrichosis (hī′pərtrikō′sis), an excessive growth of hair on the body, possibly as a result of endocrine dysfunction, as in the hirsutism accompanying excessive adrenocortical function.

hypertrophy (hīper′trōfē), a morbid enlargement or overgrowth of an organ or part resulting from an increase in size of its constituent cells.

h., denture. See **hyperplasia, denture.**

h., muscle, hypertrophy denotes an increase in the size or number of constituent fibers of a muscle. Any other condition such as inflammation, tumor, and fatty infiltration that increases the size of a muscle is called *pseudohypertrophy.* True or physiologic hypertrophy results from excessive activity of muscle. Genetic and hormonal factors play a role in determining the size of muscles; for example, muscles in a male tend to be larger than in a female in the temporal and facial regions. The histologic characteristics of hypertrophied muscle are normal. The fibrils are slightly wider in diameter than is normal, and the only change might be a slight increase in vascularity.

hyperventilation, 1. an abnormally prolonged, rapid, and deep breathing; also the condition produced by overbreathing of oxygen at high pressures. It is marked by confusion, dizziness, numbness, and muscular cramps brought on by such breathing. **2.** Rapid, deep, forced breathing frequently resulting from anxiety. It results in a transient loss of carbon dioxide and respiratory alkalosis. Symptoms include anxiety, circumoral numbness, tingling sensation, faintness, and occasionally, carpopedal spasms, tetany, and syncope.

hypervitaminosis A (hi'pərvī'tə minō'sis), the effects of toxic doses of vitamin A. Manifestations include bone fragility, xeroderma, nausea, headache, and loss of hair.

hypervitaminosis D, the toxic effects of ingesting large amounts of vitamin D. Manifestations include symptoms resulting from hypercalcemia, impairment of renal function, and metastatic calcification.

hypervolemia, increased blood volume.

hypnalgia (hipnal'jē-ə), pain that recurs during sleep. (not current)

hypnic (hip'nik), inducing or pertaining to sleep.

hypno- (hip'nō), a combining form denoting a relationship to sleep.

hypnosis (hipnō'sis), a condition of artificially induced sleep or of a trance resembling sleep induced by drugs, psychologic means, or both. Generally creating a condition of heightened suggestibility in the subject.

hypnotic (hipnot'ik), **1.** a drug that induces sleep or depresses the central nervous system at a cortical level. **2.** causing sleep or a trance. See also **sedative.**

hypnotism (hip'nōtizəm), **1.** the method or practice of inducing sleep. **2.** in medical jurisprudence, a mental state rendering the patient susceptible to suggestion at the will and inducement of another.

hypnotize (hip'nōtīz), to put into a state of hypnosis in which there is a condition of heightened suggestibility.

hypo (hī'pō), an abbreviated form of the term *hyposulfite,* which is a

synonym of sodium thiosulfate ($Na_2S_2O_3$), a solution used in photography and radiography to fix and harden the manifest image. See also **fixation.**

hypo- (hī'pō), a prefix signifying beneath, under, or deficient.

hypoadrenocorticalism (hī'pōədrē' nōkor'tikəlizəm) (adrenocortical insufficiency, hypoadrenocorticism), acute or chronic adrenocortical hypofunction, as in Waterhouse-Friederichsen syndrome or Addison's disease. (not current)

hypoadrenocorticism (hī'pōədrēnō-kor'tisizəm). See **hypoadrenocorticalism.**

hypoalgesia (hī'pōaljē'zē-ə), a diminished sensation of pain resulting from a raised pain threshold.

hypocalcemia (hī'pōkalsē'mē-ə), an abnormally low concentration of calcium in the blood; may be associated with hypoparathyroidism, rickets, osteomalacia, renal rickets, pancreatic disease, sprue, obstructive jaundice, or tetany.

hypocalcification (hī'pōkalsifikā'shən), reduced calcification, especially of enamel. It produces opaque white spots that may be discolored later. See also **fluorosis.**

h., hereditary enamel, a hereditary anomaly of enamel formation affecting the primary and permanent dentition in which the enamel peels off after tooth eruption and exposes dentin, giving the teeth a yellow appearance.

hypocalciuria (hī'pōkal'sēyoo'rē-ə), a decrease in urinary calcium. Normal values vary considerably but are roughly related to calcium intake. Various values are given (for example, 100 to 200 mg/day on a normal diet, or 350 to 400 mg/day for calcium intake of 10 mg/kg of body weight in children). Hypocalciuria may occur in hypoparathyroidism, rickets, osteomalacia, metastatic carcinoma of the prostate, and renal failure. See also **test, Sulkowitch's.**

hypocapnia (hī'pōkap'nē-ə) (hypocarbia), a deficiency of carbon dioxide in the blood.

hypocarbia. See **hypocapnia.**

hypochloremia (hī'pōklərē'mē-ə), a decrease below normal of chloride concentration in the plasma. The normal range is 98 to 100 mEq/L. It may occur in adrenal insufficiency, persistent vomiting, renal failure, acute infections, and dehydration with sodium depletion.

hypochlorous acid, a greenish-yellow liquid derived from an aqueous solution of lime. An unstable compound that decomposes to hydrochloric acid and water, hypochlorous acid is used as a bleaching agent and disinfectant.

hypochondria (hī′pōkon′drē·ə) (hypochondriasis), anxiety about disease; a type of neurosis characterized by fear of disease or by simulated disease.

hypochondriasis (hī′pōkondrī′əsis). See **hypochondria.**

hypochromia (hīpōkro′mē·ə) (hypochromasia), a reduced staining quality of cells, particularly pale staining red blood cells associated with hemoglobin deficiency.

hypodermoclysis (hī′pōdərmok′lisis), a subcutaneous injection of fluid in large volume.

hypodontia (hīp′ōdon′shē·ə), fewer teeth than normal.

hypoesthesia (hī′pōesthē′zē·ə), a decreased sensitivity to touch or pressure.

hypoestrogenism (hī′pōes′trōjen′izəm), diminished production of estrogenic substances by the ovaries, such as that which occurs during menopause. May produce desquamative lesions on the oral mucous membranes. See also **gingivitis, desquamative.**

hypofibrinogenemia (hī′pōfibrin′ōjənē′mē·ə), a reduction of fibrinogen in the blood. Excessive bleeding may occur following trauma. The deficiency of fibrinogen may be congenital or may result from faulty synthesis associated with liver disease and defibrinogenation resulting from disorders of pregnancy involving the placenta and amniotic fluid. The normal range is 200 to 600 mg/100 ml of plasma. Clotting deficiencies do not occur until the concentration falls below 75 mg/100 ml.

hypogammaglobulinemia (hī′pōgam′əglob′yəlinē′mē·ə), a deficiency of gamma globulin, usually manifested by recurrent bacterial infections.

hypogeusia (hī′pōgo͞o′zē·ə), a decreased sense of taste.

hypoglossal nerve, either of a pair of cranial nerves, essential for swallowing and moving the tongue. Each nerve has four major branches, communicates with the vagus nerve, and connects to the nucleus XII in the brain. See nerve(s).

hypoglycemia (hī′pōglīsē′mē·ə), a condition existing when the concentration of blood sugar (true blood sugar) is 40 mg/100 ml or less. Symptoms may not occur even when the concentration is considerably less. Symptoms include nervousness, hunger, weakness, vertigo, and faintness. Hypoglycemia may occur in the fasting state and/or following the injection of insulin.

h., fasting, hypoglycemia occurring in the postabsorptive state; occurs in renal glycosuria, lactation, hepatic disease, and in central nervous system lesions.

h., insulin, hypoglycemia resulting from improper administration of insulin. If hypoglycemia is severe, convulsions, coma, and death may occur. See also **shock, insulin.**

h., mixed, hypoglycemia occurring during the fasting state and after the ingestion of carbohydrates; occurs in idiopathic spontaneous hypoglycemia of infancy, in anterior pituitary and adrenocortical insufficiency, and with tumors of the islet cells of the pancreas.

h., reactive, hypoglycemia occurring after the ingestion of carbohydrates with an excessive release of insulin, as in functional hyperinsulinism.

h., spontaneous, hypoglycemia that is functional (such as in renal glycosuria, lactation, and severe muscular exertion) or is caused by organic disease such as in hepatic disease and adrenocortical insufficiency.

hypoglycemic agents, a large heterogeneous group of drugs prescribed to decrease or control the amount of glucose circulating in the blood; used in the prevention and treatment of diabetes.

hypogonadism (hī′pōgō′nadizəm), a gonadal deficiency resulting from abnormalities of the testes and ovaries or to pituitary insufficiency. Manifestations include eunuchism, eunuchoidism, Fröhlich's syndrome, amenorrhea, and incomplete development or maintenance of secondary sex characteristics.

hypohidrotic ectodermal dysplasia (hī'pōhīdrot'ik ektōder'məl displā'zhə), a syndrome consisting of hypodontia, hypotrichosis, hypohidrosis, and other defects related to the development of ectodermal structures.

hypokalemia (hī'pōkəlē'mē·ə) (hypopotassemia), an abnormally low serum potassium level. Hypokalemia may occur in metabolic alkalosis, chronic diarrhea, Cushing's syndrome, primary aldosteronism, and excessive use of deoxycorticosterone, cortisone, or ACTH.

hypolarynx (hī'pōler'inks), the infraglottic compartment of the larynx that extends from the true vocal cords to the first tracheal ring.

hypolethal (hī'pōlē'thəl), not quite lethal; said of dosage.

hypomagnesemia (hī'pōmag'nesē'mē·ə), a deficiency of magnesium in the blood serum (normal values range from 1.5 to 2.5 mEq/L). It may be associated with chronic alcoholism, starvation, and prolonged diuresis in congestive heart failure. Manifestations include muscular twitching, convulsions, and coma.

hyponasality (hī'pōnāzal'itē), a lack of nasal resonance necessary to produce acceptable voice quality. The type of voice quality heard when the speaker's nose is occluded or when the speaker is suffering from a severe cold.

hyponatremia (hī'pōnətrē'mē·ə), an abnormally low concentration of sodium in the blood serum. It may develop in adrenocortical insufficiency and chronic renal disease or with extreme sweating.

hypoparathyroidism (hī'pōper'əthī'roidizəm), a decrease in parathyroid function, usually the result of surgical removal. Symptoms include tetany, irritability, and muscle weakness. The serum calcium is low, the blood phosphorus elevated, the blood magnesium reduced, and the alkaline phosphatase normal.

hypopharyngoscope (hī'pōfəring'gōskōp), an apparatus devised for bringing the lower part of the pharynx or hypopharynx into view.

hypopharynx (hī'pōfer'inks), the division of the pharynx that lies below the

upper edge of the epiglottis and opens into the larynx and esophagus.

hypophosphatasia (hī'pōfos'fətā'zhə), a familial disease in which the children may have very low serum alkaline phosphatase levels, total or partial aplasia of the cementum, and an abnormal periodontal ligament in the deciduous teeth; a decreased phosphatase level that has been linked to a premature loss of deciduous teeth in children. Examination reveals absence, hypoplasia, or dysplasia of cementum.

hypophosphatemia (hī'pōfos'fətē'mē·ə), an abnormally low concentration of serum phosphates. Blood phosphorus levels are low in sprue, celiac disease, and hyperparathyroidism and in association with an elevated alkaline phosphatase in vitamin D–resistant rickets and other diseases involving a renal tubular defect in resorption of phosphate.

hypophysis. See **gland, pituitary.**

hypopituitarism (hī'pōpitoo'iterizəm), a decrease in the hormonal secretions of the pituitary gland.

hypoplasia (hī'pōplā'zhə), the defective or incomplete development of any tissue or structure.

h., enamel, chronologic, a prenatal or postnatal systemic hypoplasia affecting amelogenesis occurring at the time of the systemic disorder.

h., enamel, hereditary (*hereditary brown tooth*), a hereditary anomaly of the enamel affecting the primary and permanent dentition in which a thin layer of hard enamel covering the yellow dentin gives the tooth a brown appearance.

h., mandibular, an abnormally small mandibular development (for example, in micrognathia or brachygnathia).

hypopnea (hīpop'nē·ə), abnormally shallow and rapid respirations.

hypopotassemia (hī'pōpot'əsē'mē·ə). See **hypokalemia.**

hypoproteinemia (hī'pōprō'tēnē'mē·ə), a decrease in serum and plasma proteins.

hypoprothrombinemia (hī'pōprōthrom'binē'mē·ə), a deficiency of prothrombin in the blood. It may be congenital or associated with vitamin K deficiency, large doses of salicylates, liver disease, or excessive anticoagulant. The normal level ranges from 70% to 120% plasma prothrombin concentration. There is little danger of hemorrhage if the prothrombin concentration is greater than 20% of normal.

hyposalivation (hī'pōsal'ivā'shən) (xerostomia), a decreased flow of saliva. It may be associated with dehydration, radiation therapy of the salivary gland regions, anxiety, the use of drugs such as atropine and antihistamines, vitamin deficiency, various forms of parotitis, and various syndromes (Sjögren's, Riley-Day, Plummer-Vinson, and Heerfordt's disease). See also **asialorrhea.**

hyposensitive (hī'pōsen'sitiv), less sensitive.

hyposthenuria (hī'pōsthenōō'rē·ə), a condition in which the urine has an abnormally low specific gravity. Hyposthenuria may occur in cases in which renal damage impairs concentrating power or when the kidneys are normal but lack hormonal stimulus for concentrations, as in diabetes insipidus.

hypotension (hī'pōten'shən), abnormally low tension, especially low blood pressure.

hypothalamus (hī'pōthal'əməs), a small extension of the brain that lies in the sella turcica in the cranium. The hypothalamus lies just at the superior level of the body of the sphenoid bone. It is intimately related structurally and functionally with the pituitary gland and is important in the central regulation of the endocrine glands, including the thyroid gland, pancreas, adrenal glands, and gonads. The most important visceral functions are under control of the hypothalamus because it functions in such close coordination with the endocrine glands. The control is mediated through its structural communication with the pituitary gland.

hypothermia, body temperature significantly below normal; that is, 98.6° F, 37° C.

hypothetical question, assumed or proved facts and circumstances, stated to constitute a specific situation or state of facts, on which the opinion of an expert is asked, in producing evidence at a trial.

hypothyroidism (hī'pōthī'roidizəm), diminished activity of the thyroid gland with decreased secretion of thyroxin, resulting in lowered basal metabolic rate, lethargy, sleepiness, dysmenorrhea in females, and a tendency toward obesity. Occasionally there is accompanying gingival hyperplasia. The condition is called *cretinism* in children and *myxedema* in adults.

hypotrichosis, a less-than-normal amount of hair on the head and/or body.

hypoventilation, an abnormal condition of the respiratory system, characterized by cyanosis, polycythemia, increased carbon dioxide arterial tension, and generalized decreased respiratory function. Hypoventilation occurs when the volume of air that enters the alveoli and takes part in gas exchanges is not adequate for the metabolic needs of the body.

hypoxanthine, a purine present in the muscles and other tissues, formed during purine catabolism by deamination of adenine.

hypoxanthine phosphoribosyltransferase, an enzyme present in human tissue that converts hypoxanthine and guanine to their respective 5 nucleotides, with 5-phosphoribose 1-diphosphate as the ribose-phosphate donor.

hypoxemia (hī'poksē'mē·ə), deficient oxygenation of the blood.

hypoxia (hīpok'sē·ə), low oxygen content or tension.

h., anemic, hypoxia brought about by a reduction of the oxygen-carrying capacity of the blood because of a decrease in the complete blood counts or an alteration of the hemoglobin constituents.

h., anoxic, hypoxia resulting from inadequate oxygen in inspired air or interference with gaseous exchange in the lungs.

h., histotoxic, hypoxia resulting from the inability of the tissue cells to use the oxygen that may be present in normal amount and tension.

h., metabolic, hypoxia resulting from an increased tissue demand for oxygen.

h., stagnant, hypoxia resulting from decreased circulation in an area.

hyrax appliance, a fixed orthodontic appliance used for the bilateral expansion of the maxillary posterior teeth and/or the bilateral expansion of the palate.

hysteresis (histerē'sis), a physical phenomenon whereby a material such as a reversible hydrocolloid passes from a solid to a gel state at one temperature and a gel to a solid state at another.

hysteria (hister'ē ə), **1.** a disease or disorder of the nervous system, more common in females than males, not originating in lesions and resulting from psychic rather than physical causes. **2.** a psychoneurosis characterized by lack of control over emotions or acts, exaggeration of sensory impression, and stimulation of disease or pain associated with disease. In some patients, trismus, neuralgia, and temporomandibular joint disturbance may be hysterical in origin.

I and D (surgical fistulation), the abbreviation for **incision and drainage,** which is the procedure of incising a fluctuant mucosal lesion to allow for the release of pressure and drainage of fluid exudate.

-ia, the Latin suffix that indicates a condition (for example, a disease) or a science, practice, or treatment.

iatrogenic (ī'-atrōjen'ik), originating as a result of professional care; for example, an iatrogenic dermatitis.

ibuprofen, *trade names:* Advil, Excedrin-IB, Midol-IB, Motrin IB; *drug class:* nonsteroidal antiinflammatory; *action:* inhibits prostaglandin synthesis by interfering with cyclooxygenase needed for biosynthesis; possesses analgesic, antiinflammatory, antipyretic properties; *uses:* rheumatoid arthritis, osteoarthritis, mild-to-moderate pain. Ibuprofen is useful for the temporary relief of minor aches and pains associated with the common cold, toothache, muscular aches, mi-

nor arthritic pain, and menstrual cramps and for the reduction of fever.

I cell disease, a congenital disease, also known as *mucolipidosis II.* It is characterized by shortness of stature, psychomotor retardation, coarse facial features, and gingival enlargement. The progressive gingival enlargement may delay tooth eruption and may impair closure of the mouth.

ichthyosis, any of several inherited dermatologic conditions in which the skin is dry, hyperkeratotic, and fissured, resembling fish scales. It usually appears at or shortly after birth and may be part of one of several rare syndromes. Some types respond temporarily to bath oils, topical retinoic acid, or propylene glycol. Also called *xeroderma.*

-ics, a suffix that indicates science, practice, or treatment. In dentistry the trend is from the use of *-ia* to the use of *-ics;* for example, in the year 1937, the term *orthodontics* began to replace the term *orthodontia.* In ancient Greek times, the adjectival ending *-ikos* was used without a following noun to indicate a practice, such as ethics. The ending *-ics,* unlike *-ia,* can indicate only a practice, not a condition. Preferred to *-ia.*

icterus (ik'terəs). See **jaundice.**

i., acholuric. See **jaundice, hemolytic, congenital.**

id, the part of the psyche functioning in the unconscious that is the source of instinctive energy, impulses, and drives. It is based on the pleasure principle and has strong tendencies toward self-preservation. The full taxonomy includes the id, the ego, and the superego.

identity, sameness; the fact that a subject, person, or thing before a court is the same as it is claimed to be.

idiopathic disease. See **disease, idiopathic.**

idiopathic enlargement (id'ē-ōpath'ik). See **enlargement, idiopathic.**

idiosyncrasy (id'ē-ōsing'krəsē), **1.** the tendency to react atypically or with unusual violence to a food, drug, or cosmetic. **2.** any characteristic that is peculiar to an individual.

idoxuridine-IDU (ophthalmic), *trade name:* Herplex; *drug class:* antiviral; *action:* inhibits viral replication by interfering with viral DNA synthesis; *uses:* herpes simplex keratitis, vaccinia virus keratitis, herpes simplex keratoconjunctivitis.

-id reaction. See **reaction, -id.**

IgA, the abbreviation for **immunoglobulin A.**

IgA deficiency, a selective lack of immunoglobulin A, which constitutes the most common type of immunoglobulin deficiency, appearing in about 1 in 400 individuals. Immunoglobulin A is a major protein antibody in the saliva and the mucous membranes of the intestines and bronchi. It protects against bacterial and viral infections. IgA deficiency is common in patients with rheumatoid arthritis and in patients with systemic lupus erythematosus.

IgE, the abbreviation for **immunoglobulin E.**

IgG, the abbreviation for **immunoglobulin G.**

IgM, the abbreviation for **immunoglobulin M.**

ignorance of law. See **law, ignorance of.**

ilium, the uppermost of the three bones that make up the innominate bone. The ilium forms part of the acetabulum. The iliac crest is a source of bone for mandibular and chin reconstruction and enhancement.

illegal, not authorized by law; illicit.

illuminator (light box), a source of light with uniform intensity for viewing radiographs.

illusion, a mistaken or erroneous perception of an object external to the individual. In some cases, the laws of physics explain the errors. In others, the explanation lies with the perceiver. Illusions should be distinguished from hallucinations, which are perceptions that lack external stimuli, and delusions, which are false beliefs. Illusions are seen in certain reactions to general anesthesia or intoxication.

illustration, a drawing or photograph used to help clarify the patient's concept of proposed treatment and conditions present.

image enhancement, the use of computer digital technology to improve the resolution of cathode ray images.

image, latent, the invisible image produced on photographic or radiographic film by the action of light or radiation before development.

imbalance, occlusal, an inharmonious relationship between the maxillary and mandibular teeth during closure or functional jaw movements. (not current)

imbedded. See **embedded.**

imbibition (im′bibish′ən), the absorption of liquid. Gel structures are particularly susceptible to imbibition.

imipramine HCl, *trade names:* Norfranil, Tipramine; *drug class:* tricyclic antidepressant; *action:* inhibits both norepinephrine and serotonin (5-HT) uptake in the brain; *uses:* depression, enuresis in children.

immediate denture. See **denture, immediate.**

immersion, the placing of a body or an object into water or other liquid so that it is completely covered by the liquid.

immobilization, to secure in a fixed relationship to prevent damage and to promote healing, such as the use of a splint or cast to maintain the fractured pieces of bone in proper relationship to each other for healing to occur.

immune reaction. See **reaction, immune.**

immune system, a biochemical complex that protects the body against pathogenic organisms and other foreign bodies. The system incorporates the humoral immune response, which produces antibodies to react with specific antigents, and the cell-mediated response, which uses T cells to mobilize tissue macrophages in the presence of a foreign body. The immune system also protects the body from invasion by creating local barriers and inflammation. The principal organs of the immune response system include the bone marrow, the thymus, and the lymphoid tissues.

immunity (imyoo′nitē), **1.** exemption from service or from duties that the law ordinarily requires other citizens to perform (for example, jury duty). **2.** the condition of an organism whereby it successfully resists or is not susceptible to injury or infection.

immunization, a process by which resistance to an infectious disease is induced or augmented.

immunoassay, a competitive-binding assay in which the binding protein is an antibody.

immunoblotting, immunologic methods for isolating and quantitatively measuring immunoreactive substances. When used with immune reagents such as monoclonal antibodies, the process is known generically as *western blot analysis.*

immunocompromised, an immune response that has been weakened by a disease or immunosuppressive agent.

immunodeficiency, a condition resulting from a defective immunologic mechanism. Primary immunodeficiency is caused by a defect in the immune system; secondary immunodeficiency is a result of another disease process such as HIV infection.

immunodiffusion, a technique for the identification and quantification of any of the immunoglobulins.

immunoelectrophoresis, a technique that combines eletrophoresis and immunodiffusion to separate and allow identification of complex proteins.

immunoglobulins (im′yōōnōglŏb′yŏŏ linz) (Ig), serum proteins (γ globulins) synthesized by plasma cells that act as antibodies and are important in the body's defense mechanisms against infection. Main classes are designated as IgG, IgA, and IgM.

immunohistochemistry, the demonstration of specific antigens in tissues by the use of markers that are either fluorescent dyes or enzymes, especially horseradish peroxidase. See also **peroxidase, horseradish.**

immunology, the study of the reaction of tissues of the immune system of the body to antigenic stimulation.

immunosuppressants, agents that lower or reduce immune response; useful in organ transplant surgery to prevent organ rejection. Corticosteroid hormones given in large amounts; cytotoxic drugs, including antimetabolites and alkylating agents; antilymphocytic serum; and irradiation may result in immunosuppression.

immunosuppression, l. the administration of agents that significantly interfere with the ability of the immune system to respond to antigenic stimulation by inhibiting cellular and humoral immunity. Immunosuppression may be deliberate, such as in preparation for bone marrow or other transplantation to prevent rejection by the host of the donor tissue. **2.** an abnormal condition of the immune system characterized by markedly inhibited ability to respond to antigenic stimuli.

immunotherapy, a special treatment of allergic responses that administers increasingly large doses of the offending allergens to gradually develop immunity.

impacted tooth. See **tooth, impacted.**

impaction, pressed closely together to be immovable

i., food, the impaction of food generally interproximally because of open contact areas, uneven marginal ridge height, or "plunger" cusps.

i., tooth, a situation in which an unerupted tooth is wedged against another tooth or teeth or otherwise located so that it cannot erupt normally.

Impact strength. See **strength, Impact.**

impaired function. See **function, impaired.**

impeachment of witness, the questioning of the veracity of a witness by means of evidence obtained for that purpose.

impetigo (im′pĕtī′gō), an inflammatory disease of the skin; characterized by pustules.

impingement, the striking or application of excessive pressure to a tissue by food or a prosthesis.

implant, a device, usually alloplastic, that is surgically inserted into or onto the jawbone. To be used as a prosthodontic abutment, it should remain quiescent and purely incidental to local tissue physiology.

i., abutment of, the portion of an implant that protrudes through the gingival tissues and is designed to support a prosthodontic appliance.

i., anchor endosteal, an implant with a narrow buccolingual wedge-shaped infrastructure that is designed to be placed deep into the bone. The outline of the implant appears similar to a nautical anchor, and there are a variety of sizes and shapes to satisfy many anatomic and prosthodontic needs. Endosteal anchor implants are cast of chromium-cobalt surgical alloy and annealed.

i., anterior subperiosteal, an implant placed in the anterior part of an edentulous mandible and designed to supply abutments in the two canine regions.

i., arms of anchor endosteal, the major portion of the implant infrastructure.

i., arthroplastic, a cast chrome-alloy glenoid fossa prosthesis available in right and left models.

i., blade endosteal, an implant with a narrow (buccolingually) wedge-shaped infrastructure bearing openings or vents through which tissue grows to obtain retention.

i., bone, See **graft, autogenous, bone; graft, iliac; graft, kiel; graft, onlay bone;** and **graft, swaging.**

i., ceramic endosteal, an endosteal implant of a variety of designs constructed of silicate or porcelain.

i., cervix of, that portion of an implant that connects the infrastructure with the abutment as it passes through the mucoperiosteum.

i., C.M. (crête manche) spiral endosteal, a narrow-diameter screw implant designed for thin ridges.

i., complete-arch blade endosteal, a blade type of implant designed to be inserted into a completely edentulous ridge as a single appliance bearing multiple abutments.

i., complete subperiosteal, an implant used for an entire edentulous jaw.

i., crown of anchor endosteal, the abutment part of an anchor implant.

i., endosseous. See **implant, endosteal.**

i., endosteal, an implant that is placed into the alveolar and/or basal bone and that protrudes through the mucoperiosteum.

i., endodontic endosteal, an implant with a threaded or nonthreaded pin that fits into a root canal and extends beyond the dental apex into the adjacent bone, thereby lengthening the clinical root.

i., fabricated, a custom-designed implant constructed for a specific operative site.

i., fixation screw of subperiosteal, screws, 5 to 7 mm long, that are made of the same surgical alloy as the implant and are used to affix the implant to the underlying bone.

i., flukes of anchor endosteal, the end portions of the arms that rise to the most superficial portion within the bone.

i., frame type of ramus endosteal, a prefabricated mandibular full-arch implant consisting of two posterior ramus implants: an anterior (symphyseal) endosteal component and a conjunction bar.

i., helicoid endosteal, a two-piece endosteal implant consisting of a helical steel spring that is inserted into bone as a female and a male that may be placed postoperatively and serves as the abutment.

i., infrastructure of, the part of an implant that is designed to give it retention.

i., intraperiosteal, an artificial appliance made to conform to the shape of a bone and placed beneath the outer, or fibrous, layer of the periosteum.

i., mandrel of needle endosteal, a hollow device available in full, half, and shallow depths into which needle implants fit. The mandrel, in turn, is used in the contraangle to drive the needle implant into place.

i., mesostructure, an intermediate superstructure. A series of splinted copings, each of which fits over an implant abutment or natural tooth and over which fits the completed prosthodontic appliance.

i., needle endosteal (pin endosteal), A smooth, thin shaft (self-perforating) that serves as an implant usually in conjunction with two others, the three being placed in bone in tripodal conformity.

i., oral. See **implant.**

i., polymer tooth replica, an acrylic resin implant, shaped like the tooth recently extracted, that is placed into the tooth's alveolus.

i., ramus endosteal, a blade type of implant designed for the anterior part of the ramus. See also **implant, endosteal, blade.**

i., seating instrument of anchor endosteal, arm type, a bayonet-shaped device designed to assist in seating an anchor implant by straddling its arms over a specially designed "seating notch."

i., seating instrument of anchor endosteal, crown type, a bayonet-shaped, double-ended device designed to assist in seating an anchor implant by cupping its crown or abutment.

i., seating instrument of endosteal, a device designed to be placed on a portion of an implant so that malleting on it will seat the implant into the bone. It usually has an angled or bayoneted shaft to enable it to protrude from the mouth in a more-or-less vertical direction.

i., shaft of anchor endosteal, the cervix of an anchor implant.

i., shoulder of blade endosteal, that unbroken surface of the wedge-shaped infrastructure that is widest and most superficial. This part is tapped during the seating of the implant.

i., single-tooth subperiosteal, an implant designed to replace a single missing tooth; usually unsupported by adjacent natural teeth.

i., spiral endosteal, a screw type of implant, either hollow or solid, usually consisting of abutment, cervix, and infrastructure.

i., stock, an implant, usually endosteal, that is available in manufactured form in uniform sizes and shapes.

i., strut of subperiosteal, a thin, strip like component of an infrastructure.

i., subperiosteal, an appliance consisting of an open-mesh frame designed to fit over the surface of the bone beneath the periosteum.

i., superstructure of, a completed prosthesis that is supported entirely or in part by an implant. It may be a removable or fixed prosthesis and may be a single crown or a complete arch splint.

i., two-piece, an implant, either endosteal or subperiosteal, having its infrastructure and abutment in separate parts. Generally, the abutment, which is threaded, is screwed to the infrastructure some weeks after its incision, so that healing has taken place.

implantation, tooth (not current). See **transplantation, tooth.**

implantodontology (implan′tōdontol′əjē), the study of the placement of a foreign material into or onto the jawbones to replace or support artificial dentition. (not current)

implantology, oral (im′plantol′əjē), the art and science of dentistry concerned with the surgical insertion of materials and devices into, onto, and about the jaws and oral cavity for purposes of oral maxillofacial or oral occlusal rehabilitation and/or cosmetic correction.

implied, inferred; conceded.

impression, an imprint or negative likeness of an object from which a positive reproduction may be made.

i., anatomic, an impression that records tissue shape without distortion.

i., area. See **area, impression.**

i., boxing of an. See **boxing.**

i., bridge, an impression made for the purpose of constructing or assembling a fixed restoration, fixed partial denture, or bridge.

i., cleft palate, an impression of the upper jaw of a patient with a cleft (incomplete closure, or union) in the palate.

i., closed mouth, an impression made while the mouth is closed and with the patient's muscular activity molding the borders.

i., complete denture, an impression (negative record) of an edentulous arch made for the purpose of constructing a complete denture.

i., composite, an impression consisting of two or more parts.

i., correctable, an impression whose surface is capable of alteration by the removal from or addition to some area of its surface or border.

i., dual. See **technique, impression, dual.**

i., duplicating. See **duplication.**

i., elastic, an impression made in a material that will permit registration of undercut areas by springing over projecting areas and then returning to its original position.

i., final (secondary impression), an impression used for making the master cast.

i., fluid wax, an impression of the functional form of subjacent structures made with selected waxes that are applied (brushed on) to the impression surface in fluid form.

i., functional, an impression of the supporting structures in their functional form. See also **structure, supporting, functional form of.**

i., hydrocolloid, an impression made of a hydrocolloid material.

i., lower. See **impression, mandibular.**

i., mandibular (lower impression), an impression of the mandibular jaw and related tissues and dental structures.

i., material. See **material, impression.**

i., maxillary (upper impression), an impression of the maxillary jaw and related tissues and dental structures.

i., mercaptan, an impression made of mercaptan (polysulfide), a rubber base elastic material.

i., partial denture, an impression of part or all of a partially edentulous arch made for the purpose of designing or constructing a partial denture.

i., pickup, an impression made with the superstructure frame in place on the abutments in the mouth after the implant has been surgically inserted and the mouth has healed. The superstructure frame is included in the impression material, and an accurate impression of the oral mucosal tissue over the implant is obtained.

i., preliminary (primary impression), an impression made for the purpose of diagnosis or the construction of a tray for making a final impression.

i., primary. See **impression, preliminary.**

i., secondary. See **impression, final.**

i., sectional, an impression that is made in sections.

i., silicone, a rubber base elastic impression using a material that contains a silicone. See also **silicone.**

i., snap. See **impression, preliminary.**

i., surface. See **denture foundation area** and **surface, basal.**

i., surgical bone, a negative likeness of the exposed bony surfaces necessary to support the implant substructure.

i. technique. See **technique, impression.**

i. tray. See **tray, impression.**

i., upper. See **impression, maxillary.**

impulse, a surge of electric current for a short time span; for example, in a 60-cycle AC current, there are 120 impulses per second. See also **impression, maxillary.**

i., muscle, a wave of excitation along a muscle fiber initiated at the neuromuscular endplate; accompanied by chemical and electrical changes at the surface of the muscle fiber and by activation of the contractile elements of the muscle fiber; detectable electronically (electromyographically); and followed by a transient refractory period.

i., nerve, a wave of excitation along a nerve fiber initiated by a stimulus; accompanied by chemical and electrical changes at the surface of the nerve fiber and followed by a transient refractory period during which further stimulation has no effect.

impulsive behavior, actions initiated without due consideration or thought as to the costs, results, or consequences.

IMZ implant system, an endosseous implant system provisionally accepted by the ADA.

inacidity, the absence of acidity. (not current)

inactivate, to render inactive; to destroy the activity of.

inactivator, a substance added to a culture medium to prevent the activity of an inoculant. Penicillinase is added to the culture medium to prevent the activity of penicillin that might be carried over from a root canal treatment.

inadequacy, velopharyngeal (vel'ōfə-rin'jē·əl), a lack of functional closure of the velum to the postpharyngeal wall.

inadmissible, that which cannot be admitted into evidence in a legal proceeding under the established rules of law.

inbreeding, the production of offspring by the mating of closely related individuals, organisms, or plants; self-fertilization is the most extreme form, which normally occurs in certain plants and lower animals. The practice provides a greater chance for recessive genes for both desirable and undesirable traits to become homozygous and to be expressed phenotypically.

incentive plan, a plan whereby the insurer pays an increasing share of the claim cost provided the covered individual visits the dentist as stipulated during each incentive period (usually a year) and receives the prescribed treatment.

incentive program, a dental benefits program that pays an increasing share of the treatment cost provided that the covered individual uses the benefits of the program during each incentive period (usually a year) and receives the treatment prescribed. For example, a 70% to 30% copayment program in the first year of coverage may become an 80% to 20% program in the second year if the subscriber visits the dentist in the first year as stipulated in the program. Most frequently, there is a corresponding percentage reduction in the program's copayment level if the covered individual fails to visit the dentist in a given year (but never below the initial copayment level).

inchacao (inchəkə'·ō) (not current). See **beriberi.**

in chief principal; directly obtained, evidence obtained from a witness on examination in court by the party producing the witness.

incidence, I. the number of times an event occurs. **2.** the number of new cases in a particular period of time. Incidence is often expressed as a ratio, in which the number of cases is the numerator and the population at risk is the denominator.

incipient (insip'ē·ent), beginning, initial, commencing.

incisal (insī'zəl), relating to the cutting edge of the anterior teeth, incisors, or canines.

 i. angle. See **angle, incisal.**

 i. guidance angle. See **angle, incisal guidance.**

 i. guide. See **guide, incisal.**

 i. guide pin. See **pin, incisal guide.**

 i. rest. See **rest, incisal.**

incision (insizh'ən), the act of cutting or biting.

 i. and drainage. See **I and D.**

 i. of food, the phase of the masticatory cycle, using the incisor teeth, that cuts or separates the bolus of food.

 i., preauricular, the incision of the soft tissue anterior to the external ear that permits access to the temporomandibular joint.

 i., relieving, a cut into the soft tissues adjacent to a wound to permit a tension-free closure.

 i., Risdon's, the incision of the soft tissues in the area of the mandibular angle that permits access to the lateral surface of the mandibular ramus, subcondylar neck, and condylar area.

incisive foramen. See **foramen, incisive.**

incisive papilla. See **papilla, incisive.**

incisor(s) (insī'zər), a cutting tooth, one of the four anterior teeth of either jaw.

 i., central, the first incisor.

 i., Hutchinson's, malformed teeth caused by the presence of congenital

syphilis during tooth development. The incisors usually are shorter than normal, show a single permanent notch on each incisal edge, and are screwdriver-shaped.

 i., lateral, the second incisor.

 i. point. See **point, incisor.**

inclination (in'klinā'shən), the angle of slope from a particular item of reference.

 i., axial, the alignment of a tooth in a vertical plane in relationship to its basal bone structure.

 i., lateral condylar, the direction of the lateral condyle path.

 i. of tooth. See **tooth, inclination of.**

inclusion cyst, an epidermal cyst formed of a mass of squamous epithelium cells with concentric layers of keratin.

income, the return in money from one's business, practice, or capital invested; gains, profit.

 i. tax, a tax upon an adjusted gross income (individual or corporate) imposed as a major source of governmental revenue at the state and federal levels.

incompatibility (in'kəmpat'ibil'itē), a term that refers to a disharmonious relationship among the ingredients of prescriptions and other drug mixtures.

 i., chemical, a situation in which two or more of the ingredients of a drug interact chemically, with resulting deterioration of the mixture.

incontinentia pigmenti. See **syndrome, Bloch-Sulzberger.**

incubation period, the lapsed time between exposure to an infectious agent and the onset of symptoms of a disease.

incubator (in'kyōōbātər), a laboratory container with controlled temperature for the cultivation of bacteria.

incurred claims, outstanding obligations of the insurer for dental services rendered to the insured.

indapamide, *trade name:* Lozol; *drug class:* diuretic, thiazide-like; *action:* acts on distal tubule by increasing excretion of water, sodium, chloride, potassium; *uses:* edema, hypertension.

indemnification schedule. See **table of allowances.**

indemnity benefit, a contract benefit that is paid to the insured to meet the cost of dental services received.

indemnity plan, 1. a plan that provides payment to the insured for the cost of dental care but makes no arrangement for providing care itself. **2.** a dental plan in which a third-party-payer provides payment of an amount for specific services regardless of the actual charges made by the provider. Payment may be made to enrollees or by assignment directly to dentists. Schedule of allowances, table of allowances, and reasonable and customary plans are examples of indemnity plans.

index, 1. the ratio of a measurable value to another. **2.** a core or mold used to record or maintain the relative position of a tooth or teeth to one another and/or to a cast. See also **splint.**

i., **Broders'** *(Broders' classification),* **1.** a system of grading of epidermoid carcinoma suggested by Broders. Tumors are graded from I to IV on the basis of cell differentiation. Grade I tumors are highly differentiated, with much keratin production; Grade IV tumors are poorly differentiated; the cells are highly anaplastic, with almost no keratin formation. **2.** the classification and grading of malignant neoplasms according to the proportion of malignant cells to normal cells in the lesion.

i., **cardiac,** the minute volume of blood per square meter of body surface.

i., **carpal,** the degree of ossification of the carpal bones noted in radiographs of the wrist; a method of determining the state of skeletal maturation.

i., **cephalic,** head shape and size.

i., **DEF,** a dental caries index applied to the primary dentition in somewhat the same manner as the DMF index is used for classifying permanent teeth. The letter *D* stands for decayed; *E* for extraction indicated because of caries; and *F* for filled. Missing primary teeth are ignored in this index because of the uncertainty in determining whether they were extracted because of advanced caries or exfoliated normally.

i., **DMF** *(decayed, missing, filled)* a technique for managing statistically the number of decayed, missing, or filled teeth in the mouth. Analysis may be based on the average number of DMF teeth (sometimes called DMFT) per person or the average number of DMF tooth surfaces (DMFS).

i., **gingiva and bone count** *(Dunning-Leach index),* an index that permits differential recording of both gingival and bone conditions to determine gingivitis and bone loss.

i., **gnathic,** the relationship of jaw size to head size.

i., **icterus.** See **test, Meulengracht's.**

i., **malocclusion,** a measure of the severity of a malocclusion, obtained by assigning values to a series of defined observations.

i., **measuring,** an expression of relationship of one measurable value to another, or a formula based on measurable values.

i., **oral hygiene, simplified** *(Greene-Vermillion index),* an index made up of two components, the debris index and the calculus index, which are based on numerical determination representing the amount of debris or calculus found on six preselected tooth surfaces.

i., **periodontal** *(Ramfjord index),* a thorough clinical examination of the periodontal status of six teeth: with an evaluation of the gingival condition, pocket depth, calculus and plaque deposits, attrition, mobility, and lack of contact.

i., **periodontal disease** *(Russell index),* an index that measures the condition of both the gingiva and the bone individually for each tooth and arrives at the average status for periodontal disease in a given mouth.

i., **PMA** *(Schour-Massler index),* an index used for recording the prevalence and severity of gingivitis in schoolchildren by noting and scoring three areas: the gingival papillae (P), the buccal or labial gingival margin (M), and the attached gingiva (A).

i., **Pont's,** the relation of the width of the four incisors to the width between the first premolars and the width between the first molars.

i., **Russell.** See **index, periodontal disease.**

i., **salivary Lactobacillus,** a count of the lactobacilli per milliliter of saliva; used as an indicator of present dental caries activity. The test is of questionable value in individual patients, although its use in large groups has led to valuable information on caries activity.

i., saturation, a number indicating the hemoglobin content of a person's red blood cells as compared with the normal content.

i., therapeutic, the ratio of toxic dose to effective dose.

i., ventilation, the index obtained by dividing the ventilation test by the vital capacity.

indication, that which serves as a guide or warning.

indicator diseases, opportunistic infectious diseases or neoplastic diseases that are associated with a primary immunodeficiency disease such as caused by the retrovirus HIV-I.

indirect method. See **method, indirect.**

indirect pulp capping. See **capping, pulp, indirect.**

indirect retention. See **retention, indirect.**

indium, a silvery metallic element with some nonmetallic chemical properties. Its atomic number is 49 and its atomic weight is 114.82. It is used in electronic semiconductors.

individuality, the aggregate of characteristics or traits that distinguish one person or thing from all others.

individual practice association (IPA), 1. the organization for the maintenance of the solo private practitioner as a lobbying force and vocal springboard. **2.** a legal entity organized and operated on behalf of individual participating dentists for the primary purpose of collectively entering into contracts to provide dental services to enrolled populations. Dentists may practice in their own offices and may provide care to patients not covered by the contract as well as to IPA patients

individual retirement account (IRA), a savings certificate exempt from income tax until the time of withdrawal. There are limits to the amount that can be saved annually under this plan, and there are conditions of withdrawal for maximal interest and tax advantage.

indomethacin/indomethacin sodium trihydrate, *trade names:* Indocin, Indocin SR, Indameth; *drug class:* nonsteroidal antiinflammatory; *action:* inhibits prostaglandin synthesis by interfering with cyclooxygenase needed for biosynthesis; possesses analgesic, antiinflamatory, antipyretic properties; *uses:* rheumatoid arthritis, osteoarthritis, ankylosing rheumatoid spondylitis, acute gouty arthritis.

induced, produced artificially.

induction, the act or process of inducing or causing to occur.

indurated, hardened.

i. tissue, soft tissue that is abnormally firm because of an influx of exudate or fibrous tissue elements.

industrial dentistry, 1. dentistry that is concerned with the dental health of the worker as it affects the working environment. **2.** dental service provided in the plant, usually restricted to emergency care.

inertia (inur'shə), according to Newton's law of inertia, the tendency of a body that is at rest to remain at rest and a body that is in motion to continue in motion with constant speed in the same straight line unless acted on by an outside force.

Infant, a child who is in the earliest stage of extrauterine life, a time extending from the first month after birth to approximately 12 months of age, when the baby is able to assume an erect posture; some extend the period to 24 months of age.

i. mortality, the statistical rate of infant death during the first year after live birth, expressed as the number of such births per 1000 live births in a specific geographic area. Neonatal mortality accounts for 70% of infant mortality.

infantilism (infan'tilism), a disturbance marked by mental retardation and retention of childhood characteristics into adult life. Teeth may be delayed in eruption or may be absent.

infarct (in'färkt), the death of a tissue caused by partial occlusion of a vessel or vessels supplying the area.

infection (infek'shən), an invasion of the tissues of the body by disease-producing microorganisms and the reaction of these tissues to the microorganisms and/or their toxins. The mere presence of microorganisms without reaction is no evidence of infection.

i. control, procedures and protocols designed to prevent or limit cross-contamination in the health care delivery environment.

i., focal, the process in which microorganisms located at a certain site, or focus, in the body are disseminated throughout the body to set up secondary sites, or foci, of infection in other tissues.

i., hemolytic streptococcal, 1. an infection usually caused by Group A hemolytic streptococci. Such infections include scarlet fever, streptococcal sore throat, cellulitis, and osteomyelitis. 2. an infection caused by streptococci that produce a toxic substance (hemolysin) that will lyse the erythrocytes and liberate hemoglobin from red blood cells.

i. resistance, the ability of an individual to fight off the detrimental effects of microorganisms and their toxic products. A complexity involving individual and interacting factors; for example, antibody formation, adequate nutrition, tissue tone, circulation, and emotional stability.

i. susceptibility, the degree of capability of being influenced by or involved in the pathologic processes produced by microorganisms and/or their toxins.

i., Vincent's. See **gingivitis, necrotizing ulcerative.**

infectious mononucleosis, a benign lymphadenosis caused by the Epstein-Barr virus and characterized by fever, sore throat, enlargement of lymph nodes and spleen, and prolonged weakness with a characteristic shift in the white blood cells during the course of the disease.

infertile, unable to produce offspring.

infiltrate (infil'trāt), material deposited by infiltration.

infiltration (in'filtrā'shən), an accumulation in a tissue of a substance not normal to it.

i., inflammatory, an influx or accumulation of inflammatory elements (cellular and exudative) in the interstices of the tissues as a result of tissue injury by physical, chemical, microbiologic, and other irritants. Cellular elements include lymphocytes, plasma cells, polymorphonuclear leukocytes, and/or the macrophages of reticuloendothelial origin.

i., local, the prevention of excitation of the free nerve endings by literally flooding the immediate area with a local anesthetic solution.

inflammation (in'fləmā'shən), the cellular and vascular response or reaction to injury. Inflammation is characterized by pain, redness, swelling, heat, and disturbance of function. It may be acute or chronic. The term is not synonymous with infection, which implies an inflammatory reaction initiated by invasion of living organisms.

i., gingival. See **gingivitis.**

i., granulomatous, a chronic inflammation in which there is formation of granulation tissue.

i., periodontal. See **periodontitis.**

inflation (inflā'shən), the act of distending with air or a gas.

influences, local environmental, factors or agents within the oral cavity that are responsible for the initiation, perpetuation, or modification of a pathologic state within the stomatognathic system.

influences, systemic environmental, systemic factors that may initiate, perpetuate, or modify disease processes within the stomatognathic system. Generally, the oral manifestations of systemic disease are modified by the influence of local environmental factors.

influenza, a highly contagious infection of the respiratory tract caused by a myxovirus and transmitted by airborne droplet infection. Symptoms include sore throat, cough, fever, muscular pains, and weakness. Fever and constitutional symptoms distinguish influenza from the common cold. Three main strains of influenza virus have been recognized: Type A, Type B, and Type C. New strains of the virus emerge at regular intervals and are named according to their geographic origin. Asian flu is a Type A influenza.

i.-virus vaccine, an active immunizing agent prescribed for immunization against influenza, generally recommended for at-risk populations such as the elderly.

information, a meaningful collection of data as perceived by its user.

i. retrieval, the methods and procedures for recovering specific information from stored data.

i. system, a computerized system with the capability of manipulating and processing data in different ways to facilitate their interpretation and use.

informed consent, an agreement by a patient, verbal or written, to have a procedure performed after being told in sufficient detail of possible risks.

infrabony pocket (in′frəbōnē). See **pocket, infrabony.**

infrabulge (in′frəbulj), the surface of the crown of a tooth cervical to the clasp guide line, survey line, or surveyed height of contour. (not current)

infraclusion (in′frəklōō′zhən) (infraversion), the position occupied by a tooth when it has failed to erupt sufficiently to reach the occlusal plane.

infracrestal pocket (in′frəkres′təl) (not current). See **pocket, infrabony.**

infradentale (in′frədenta′le), the most anterior point of the alveolar process of the mandible.

infraversion (in′frəver′zhən). See **infraclusion.**

infusion, I. the therapeutic introduction of a fluid such as saline solution into a vein. In contrast to injection, infusion suggests the introduction of a larger volume of a less concentrated solution over a more protracted period. **2.** a term used in pharmacy for a liquid extract prepared by steeping a plant substance in water.

Ingate. See **sprue.**

inhalant (inhā′lənt), a medicine to be inhaled.

inhalation (inhəlā′shən), the drawing of air or other vapor into the lungs.

i., endotracheal, the inhalation of an anesthetic mixture into the lungs through an endotracheal catheter at low or atmospheric pressure.

inhaler, nasal, a device that is placed over the nose to permit inhalation of anesthetic agents.

inhibition (in′hibish′ən), a neurologic phenomenon associated with the transmission of an impulse across a synapse. An impulse can be blocked from passing a synapse in a reflex situation by the firing of another, more dominant nerve. Inhibition can be achieved directly by preventing the passage of an impulse along an axon, or it can be achieved by liberation of a chemical substance at the nerve ending. This chemical inhibition is demonstrated by the sympathetic-parasympathetic control over smooth muscle activity in a blood vessel. Inhibition is the restraining of a function of a tissue or organ by some nervous

or hormone control. It is the opposite of excitation.

inhibitor of cholinesterase (inhib′itōr ko′lines′terās), a chemical that interferes with the activity of the enzyme cholinesterase.

inhouse, a computer located onsite, in the building where used, instead of being located remotely.

inion (in′ē·on), the most elevated point on the external occipital protuberance in the midsagittal plane.

initialize, to set counters, switches, and addresses to 0 or other starting values at the beginning of, or at prescribed points in, a computer routine.

initiator (inish′ē·ā′tor), a chemical agent added to a resin to initiate polymerization.

injection (injek′shən), the act of introducing a liquid into the body by means of a needle and syringe. Injections are designated according to the anatomic site involved. The most common injections are intraarterial, intradermal, intramuscular, intravenous, and subcutaneous.

i. molding. See **molding, injection.**

injury, the insult, harm, or hurt applied to tissues; may evoke dystrophic and/or inflammatory response from the affected part.

i., root, damage to the root, especially to the cementum, when an excessive force is placed on the tooth.

i., toothbrush, an insult or damage to the teeth and their investing structures produced by faulty toothbrushing.

inlay, a restoration of metal, fired porcelain, or plastic made to fit a tapered cavity preparation and fastened to or luted into it with a cementing medium.

i. furnace. See **furnace, inlay.**

i., setting, the procedure of fitting a casting to a preparation; adjusting the occlusal function and contact areas; securing the proper, clean dry field; cementing the cleaned, polished casting in an aseptic, dry prepared cavity; and completing the final finishing and polishing of the restoration.

i. wax. See **wax, inlay.**

innervation (in′ərvā′shən), the distribution or supply of nerves to a part.

i., reciprocal, the simultaneous excitation of one muscle with the inhibition of its antagonist. Rhythmic chewing is achieved efficiently when the masticatory muscles are reciprocally innervated, permitting alternate elevation and depression of the mandible in a smooth, coordinated sequence of actions.

inositol, an essential growth factor in tissue culture with no known human requirement. It has been used therapeutically in the management of diseases associated with the metabolism of fat.

in pais (in pā'), a legal transaction that has been accomplished without legal proceedings.

in potestate parentis (in pōtest'ət pəren'tis), under the authority of the parent.

input, computer, the data to be processed.

input/output control (I/O control), the portion of the central processor of some computer systems that contains electronics for supervising data flow between memory and the input/output devices connected to the CPU.

inquiry, a request for information from storage in a computer.

insert, intramucosal (in'trəmyo͞okō'səl) (mucosal insert, implant button), a nonreactive metal appliance that is affixed to the tissue-bone surface of a denture and offers added retentive qualities to the denture. An intramucosal insert consists of a base, cervix, and head. (not current)

insert, mucosal. See **insert, intramucosal.**

insertion (inser'shən), the act of implanting, placing, or introducing the needle into the tissues.

*i.***, path of,** the direction in which a prosthesis is inserted and removed.

insidious (insid'ē·ə), coming on in a stealthy manner.

insoluble, not susceptible to being dissolved.

insomnia, the chronic inability to sleep or to remain asleep throughout the night.

inspection, the visual examination of the body or portions thereof, which is an integral phase of the physical or dental examination procedure.

inspiration, the act of drawing air into the lungs.

inspirator (in'spirā'tōr), a form of inhaler or respirator. (not current)

inspirometer (inspirom'ətər), an instrument for measuring the force, frequency, or volume of inspirations.

institutionalize, to place a person in a health care or custodial facility for psychologic or physical treatment and/or for the protection of the person or society.

instruction, a set of characters, together with one or more addresses, that defines a computer operation and, as a unit, causes the computer to operate accordingly on the indicated quantities; a term associated with software operation.

i. **of partial denture patient.** See **denture, partial, instruction of patient.**

instrument(s), a tool or implement, especially one used for delicate or scientific work.

i., bibeveled cutting (bī'bevəld), an instrument in which both sides of the end of the blade are beveled to form the cutting edge, as in a hatchet.

i. blade, the part bearing a cutting edge; it begins at the terminal angle of the shank and ends at the cutting edge.

i., carving. See **carver.**

i., classification of, names, the classification of instruments by name to denote purpose (for example, excavator), to denote position or manner of use (for example, hand condenser), to describe the form of the point (for example, hatchet), or to describe the angle of the blade in relation to the handle.

i., cutting, an instrument used to cut, cleave, or plane the walls of a cavity preparation; the blade ends in a sharp, beveled edge. Unless otherwise specified, it refers to a hand instrument rather than to a rotary type.

i., diamond, a rotary abrasive instrument, wheel, or mounted point. Made of fine diamond chips bonded into a desired form; used to reduce tooth structure.

i., double-plane, an instrument with the curve of the blade in a plane perpendicular to that of the angles of the shank.

i., formula name of, a method of naming and describing dental hand instruments. Measurements are in the metric system. The working point is described first, and then the formula is given in three (or sometimes four) units. The first figure denotes the width of the blade in tenths of millimeters, the second shows the length of the blade in millimeters, and the third indicates the angle of the blade in relation to the shaft in centigrades or hundredths of a circle. Whenever it is necessary to describe the angle of the cutting edge of a blade with its shaft, the number is entered in brackets as the second number of the formula. Paired instruments are also designated as right or left. In lateral cutting instruments the one used to cut from right to left is termed *right;* in direct cutting instruments with right and left bevels, the one having the bevel on the right side of the blade as it is held with the cutting edge down and pointing away from the observer is termed *right.*

i. grasp. See **grasp, instrument.**

i., **hand,** an instrument used principally with hand force.

i., **holding,** an instrument used to support gold foil while a foil restoration is inserted.

i., **McCall's,** periodontal instruments designed by John Opple McCall, used for gingival curettage and for removing accretions from the tooth surfaces.

i. nib, the counterpart of the blade in the condensing instrument; the end of the nib is the face.

i., **parts,** handle or shaft, blade or nib, and shank.

i., **plastic,** an instrument used to manipulate a plastic restorative material.

i., **rotary cutting,** a power-activated instrument used in a dental handpiece, such as a bur, mounted diamond point, mounted carborundum point, wheel stone, or disk.

i., **single-beveled cutting,** an instrument in which one side of the end of the blade is beveled to form the cutting edge, as in a wood chisel.

i., **screwdriver,** an instrument made of surgical alloy; it may have a screw

holder at its tip that is designed to drive screws into the bone.

i. shaft/handle, the part that is grasped by the operator's hand while using the instrument.

i. shank, the part that connects the shaft and the blade or nib.

i. sharpening. See **sharpening, instrument.**

i., single-plane, an instrument with all its angles and curves in one plane; when the instrument lies on a flat surface, the cutting edge and the blade will parallel the surface.

i. stop, a device, usually metal, that can be placed on a reamer or file to mark the measurement of the root.

instrumentation (in′stro͞omentā′ shən), the use of, or work done by, instruments in the treatment of a patient.

insufficiency, adrenocortical (ədrē′ nōkŏr′tikəl). See **hypoadrenocorticalism.**

insufficiency, functional, the inadequacy of usage of stimulation to a part of the body, often resulting in atrophic tissue changes.

insufflation (in′səflā′shən), the act of blowing a powder, vapor, gas, or air into a cavity such as the lungs.

i., endotracheal, the forcing of an anesthetic mixture into the lungs through an endotracheal catheter under pressure.

i., mouth-to-mouth, the oldest recorded procedure for artificially ventilating the lungs. The lungs are inflated by blowing into the mouth, and expiration either is passive or is assisted by compressing the thorax. Adequate ventilation is produced, and the procedure should be used when other techniques are not applicable; for example, in thoracic injury. Auxiliary airway tubes are available for use

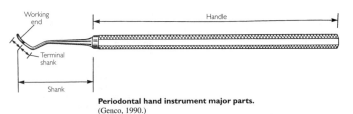

Periodontal hand instrument major parts.
(Genco, 1990.)

when mouth-to-mouth insufflation is required. Such tubes maintain the airway and prevent the tongue from obstructing the glottis.

insufflator (in′səflā′tōr), an instrument used in insufflation.

insulator, thermal, a material having a low thermal conductivity.

insulin (antidiabetic hormone), a hormone produced by the β cells of the islets of Langerhans in the pancreas. It promotes a decrease in blood sugar. Its action may be influenced by the pituitary growth hormone, adrenocorticotropic hormone; hormones of the adrenal cortex; epinephrine; glucagon; and thyroid hormone.

insulin (obtained from beef or pork, or human recombinant technology), *trade names:* Velosulin, Humulin R, Novolin R, Lente Insulin; *drug class:* exogenous insulin, antidiabetic; *action:* decreases blood glucose; important in regulation of fat and protein metabolism; *uses:* ketoacidosis; Type I, Type II diabetes mellitus; hyperkalemia; hyperalimentation.

i. resistance, a complication of diabetes mellitus characterized by a need for more than 200 units of insulin per day to control hyperglycemia and ketosis. The cause is associated with insulin binding by high levels of antibody.

i. shock. See **shock, insulin.**

insurance, a contract, or policy, whereby, for a stipulated consideration, or premium, one party (the insurer or underwriter) promises to compensate the other (the insured or assured) for loss on a specified subject (insurable interest) by specified perils, or risks.

i. benefits, the contractual pay-out agreed to by the carrier for the policy holder.

i. carriers, organizations that for a contractual fee, underwrite the payment of losses or costs incurred by the policy holder within the conditions of the policy.

i., group, insurance covering a group of persons, usually employees of a single employer or members of a union local, under one contract for the benefit of the members of the group.

i., guaranteed renewable, a policy that is renewable at the option of the insured until a stated time, such as the 70th birthday of the insured. See also **noncancellable insurance.**

i., health, insurance that provides financial return when the dentist is unable to practice because of prolonged illness.

i., liability, insurance protecting the dentist from financial loss resulting from liability suits.

i., life, a protective contract providing for compensation to the beneficiaries of the insured.

i., malpractice, in dentistry, insurance covering accidents or catastrophes that may occur during the performance of professional duties.

i., retirement, life insurance that carries, as an additional benefit, payments to the insured when he or she reaches a specific age.

insured, a person covered by an insurance program. See also **beneficiary.**

insurer, an organization that bears the financial risk for the cost of defined categories or services for a defined group of beneficiaries. See also **third party.**

intake, the substance or quantities thereof taken in and used by the body.

integral endosseous implant system, an endosseous implant system provisionally accepted by the ADA.

intelligence, mental potential or capacity; an individual's total repertoire of those problem-solving and cognitive discrimination responses that are usual and expected at a given age level and in the large population unit; that which is measured by an intelligence test.

i., dental, quotient, an estimated appraisal of a patient's knowledge and appreciation of dental services.

i. quotient (IQ), an estimate of intelligence level; an index determined by dividing the mental age in months by the chronologic age in months and multiplying the result by 100. Thus, the IQ of a child of 100 months with a mental age of 110 months would be 110.

intensifying screen. See **screen, intensifying.**

intensity of an x-ray beam, the amount of energy in an x-ray beam per unit volume or area.

intensity, radiation, the energy flowing through a unit area perpendicular to the beam per unit of time. It is expressed in *ergs per square centimeter* or in *watts per square centimeter.*

intensive care, the constant, complex, detailed health care as provided in various acute life-threatening conditions, such as multiple trauma, severe burns, and myocardial infarction, and after certain kinds of surgery.

interaction, according to Newton's law of interaction, the phenomenon in which every force is accompanied by an equal and opposite force. For every force there are two bodies—one to exert the force and one to receive it. Furthermore, whenever there is one force, another force must also be involved. If there is force to the right on one body, there is force to the left on another. Since the one force acts as long as the other, the impulses are equal. The total momentum of the two interacting bodies cannot change. Continuous interaction is demonstrated between the food that is masticated and the force applied to the food.

interalveolar space (in'təralvē'ōlər). See **distance, interarch.**

interarch distance. See **distance, interarch.**

interceptive occlusal contact (not current). See **contact, interceptive occlusal.**

interceptive orthodontics, an extension of preventive orthodontics that may include minor local tooth movement in an otherwise normally developing dentition.

intercondylar distance (in'tərkon'dilər), the distance between the vertical axes of a pair of condyles.

intercuspation (in'tərkəspā'shən), the cusp-to-fossa relationship of the upper and lower posterior teeth to each other.

interdental (in'tərden'təl), situated between the proximal surfaces of adjacent teeth.

i. canal. See **canal, interdental.**
i. embrasure. See **embrasure, interdental.**
i. septum. See **septum, interdental.**
i. splint. See **splint, interdental.**

interdigitation (in'tərdij'itā'shən). See **intercuspation.**

interface (in'tərfās), the surface, such as a plane surface, formed between the walls of a prepared cavity or extracoronal preparation and a restoration. It forms a common boundary between the tooth structure and the restorative material.

i., computer, a common boundary (connection) between automatic data processing systems or parts of a system.

interfacial surface tension. See **tension, interfacial surface.**

interference, cuspal. See **contact, deflective occlusal.**

i., occlusal, any tooth-to-tooth contact that interferes with jaw movement.

interincisal angle, the A-P angle made by the intersection of the long axis of the maxillary central incisor with the mandibular central incisor. Statistically a normal angle is about 130 degrees. A more acute angle may indicate a proclined incisor, and a more obtuse angle may indicate a retracted incisor.

interferon, a small class of glycoproteins capable of exerting antiviral activity in homologous cells through metabolic processes involving synthesis of RNA.

i. alpha, formed by leukocytes in response to viral infection and/or by stimulation with double-stranded RNA. These protein products are used as antineoplastic agents. Specifically used as an antineoplastic agent for the treatment of Kaposi's sarcoma in AIDS patients. See also **interferon alfa-2a.**

i. alfa-2a/interferon alfa-2b/interferon alfa-n1/interferon alfa-n3, trade names: Roferon-A, Intron-A, Alferon N; drug class: biologic response modifier; action: antiviral action inhibits viral replication by reprogramming virus; antitumor action suppresses cell proliferation; immunomodulating action phagocytizes target cells; uses: hairy cell leukemia in persons older than 18 years, metastatic melanoma, AIDS, Kaposi's sarcoma, bladder carcinoma, lymphomas, malignant myeloma, mycosis fungoides.

i. beta, formed by fibroblasts by similar stimulation as the α form.

i. gamma, formed by lymphocytes in response to mitogenic stimulation. See also **interferon gamma-1b.**

i. gamma-1b, trade name: Actimmune; drug class: biologic response modifier; action: species-specific protein synthesized in response to viruses, enhances antibody-dependent cellular cytotoxicity, enhances natural killer cell activity; *uses:* serious infections associated with chronic granulomatous disease.

interim denture. See **denture, interim.**

interleukin-1 (IL-1), a protein with numerous immune system functions, including activation of resting T cells, and endothelial and macrophage cells, mediation of inflammation, and stimulation of synthesis of lymphokines, collagen, and collagenases. It can also induce fever, sleep, and nonspecific resistance to infection. A number of interleukin proteins with varying immune response properties exist. They are identified by numbers of 1 through 8.

interleukin-2, a hormone produced by T helper and suppressor lymphocytes that functions to control the expansion and reactivity of T lymphocytes. Used to boost the immune system in HIV-positive patients.

intermaxillary, between the maxillae and mandible.

i. anchorage. See **anchorage, intermaxillary.**

i. elastic. See **elastic, maxillomandibular.**

i. fixation. See **fixation, maxillomandibular.**

i. relation. See **relation, maxillomandibular.**

i. traction. See **traction, maxillomandibular.**

intermedin (intərmed'in). See **hormone, melanocyte stimulating.**

intern, a dental or medical college graduate serving and residing for 12 months in a hospital, usually during the first year after receiving a D.D.S., D.M.D., or M.D. degree.

internal medicine, the branch of medicine concerned with the study of the physiology and pathology of the internal organs and with the medical diagnosis and treatment of diseases and disorders of these organs.

International Classification of Diseases (ICD), diagnostic codes designed for the classification of morbidity and mortality information for statistical purposes, for the indexing of hospital records by disease and operations, and for data storage and retrieval.

interneurons, combinations or groups of neurons between sensory and motor neurons, which govern coordinated activity.

interocclusal (in'tərəklyōō'səl), between the occlusal surfaces of the maxillary and mandibular teeth.

i. clearance. See **clearance, interocclusal.**

i. contacts, tooth contact between maxillary and mandibular teeth in closure.

i. distance, the distance between the maxillary and mandibular teeth when the mandible is in the rest position or other defined position of the mandible to maxillary. See also **distance, interocclusal.**

i. gap. See **distance, interocclusal.**

i. record. See **record, interocclusal.**

i. rest space. See **distance, interocclusal.**

interoceptors (inter'ōsep'tōrz), those sensory nerve end receptors lining the mucous membrane of the respiratory and digestive tracts. They are similar to exteroceptors but differ from them essentially in their location, which is in the viscera.

interphase, the metabolic stage in the cell cycle during which the cell is not dividing.

interpolate (inter'pōlāt), to insert intermediate terms in a series according to the trend of the series; to calculate intermediate values according to observed values.

interposition arthroplasty (arthrōplastē), the surgical correction of ankylosis by the separating of the immobile fragment from the mobilized fragment and the interpositioning of a substance, such as fascia, cartilage, metal, or plastic, between them. See also **ankylosis.**

interpretation, the translation of radiographic changes seen by the dentist into real variations in the object radiographed for diagnostic purposes.

i., radiographic (radiologic interpretation, roentgenographic interpretation), an opinion formed from the study of a radiograph.

i., radiologic. See **interpretation, radiographic.**

interproximal, between the proximal surfaces of adjoining teeth.

interradicular alveoloplasty (in'tər·rədik'yələr alvē'əlōplas'tē) (intraseptal alveoloplasty), the removal of the interradicular bone and the collapsing of the cortical plates to a more normal alveolar contour. (not current) See also **alveolectomy.**

interradicular osseous defect, radiographic evidence of a discontinuity in the bony image in the area between the roots of a multirooted tooth.

interridge distance. See **distance, interarch.**

intervention studies, epidemiologic investigations designed to test a hypothesized cause and effect relation by modifying the supposed causal factor (s) in the study population.

interview, a question-and answer conference, at which time the parties concerned state the principles and facts regarding their relationship. In dental practice, this usually refers to the relationship between dentist and employee, and between dentist and patient.

intolerance, the inability to endure or withstand.

intraarterial, situated within an artery or arteries.

intracellular (in′trəsel′yoolər), situated or occurring within a cell or cells.

intracoronal (in′trəkôrō′nəl), pertaining to the inside of the coronal portion of a natural tooth.

i. attachment. See **attachment, intracoronal.**

i. retainer. See **retainer, intracoronal.**

intracranial pressure, pressure that occurs within the cranium, trauma to the head, inflammation, or infection of the linings of the brain may cause an increase in pressure within the cranium, which is painful, dysfunctional, and may become life-threatening.

intramaxillary anchorage. See **anchorage, intramaxillary.**

intramaxillary elastic. See **elastic, intramaxillary.** (not current)

intramucosal insert. See **insert, intramucosal.**

intramuscular (in′trəmus′kyoolər), situated in the substance of a muscle.

intraocular pressure, the internal pressure of the eye, regulated by resistance to the flow of aqueous humor through the fine sieve of the trabecular meshwork. Obstruction within the trabecular meshwork will cause an increase in the intraocular pressure. High persistent intraocular pressure may lead to blindness.

intraoral (in′trə·ôr′əl), within the mouth.

i. tracing. See **tracing, intraoral.**

intraosseous fixation (in′trə·os′ē·əs). See **fixation, intraosseous.** (not current)

intrapulmonary (in′trəpul′məner′ē), situated in the substance of a lung.

intravenous (in′trəvē′nəs), in, into, or from within a vein or veins.

intraversion, indicating teeth or other maxillary structures that are too near the medial plane.

intrinsic coloring, coloring from within; the incorporation of pigment within the material of a prosthesis. (not current)

intrude, to move a tooth apically.

intrusion, a depression; an inward projection.

intubate (in′toobāt), to treat by intubation.

intubation (in′toobā′shən), the insertion of a tube; especially the introduction of a tube into the larynx through the glottis for the introduction of an anesthetic gas or oxygen.

intubator (in′toobātōr), an instrument used in intubation.

inulin, a frutose-derived substance used as a diagnostic aid in tests of kidney function, specifically glomerular filtration. Inulin is not metabolized or absorbed by the body but is readily filtered through the kidney.

inunction (inungk′shən), the local application of a drug in an oily or semisolid vehicle, such as an ointment, or the preparation that is thus applied. (not current)

invagination of enamel (not current). See **dens in dente.**

i., epithelial, the downgrowth of epithelium along the cervical tract of an implant.

inventory, an itemized compilation of materials on hand.

i., equipment, a detailed listing of all the nonexpendable items owned by the dentist and used in the practice of the profession.

i., materials, a detailed listing of expendable supplies that are on hand in the practice. This is a constantly fluctuating list, depending on the quantity of the various materials presently on hand.

inverse-square law. See **law, inverse-square.**

inversion, the state of being upside down.

invest (invest'), to surround, envelop, or embed in an investment material; for example, a gypsum product.

investing (invest'ing), the process of covering or enveloping an object wholly or in part.

i., vacuum, the investing of a pattern within a vacuum to form a mold.

investment (invest'ment), the material used to enclose or surround a pattern of a dental restoration for casting or molding or to maintain the relations of metal parts during soldering.

i., casting, the material from which the casting mold is made in fabrication of gold or cobalt-chromium castings.

i., gypsum-bonded casting, a casting investment that can be bonded by α-hemihydrate, a derivative of gypsum, because the fusion temperatures of the metal alloys to be cast in it are relatively low. All gold alloy investments and some low-fusing cobalt-chromium alloy investments are gypsum bonded.

i., hygroscopic, an investment specially designed for use with the hygroscopic investing techniques.

i., phosphate-bonded casting, a casting investment that is bonded by a phosphate and a metallic oxide that react to form a hard mass; generally used for high-fusing alloys.

i., refractory, an investment material that can withstand the high temperatures used in soldering or casting.

i., sectional, a mold made in sections.

i., silica-bonded casting, a casting investment that is bonded by a silica gel that reverts to cristobalite in heating and is generally used for high-fusing alloys.

i., soldering, a quartz investment, preferably one with a very low thermal expansion, used for the investment of appliances during the soldering procedure.

involucrum (in'vəlo͞okrəm), a covering; usually a covering of new bone around a sequestrum.

involuntary, performed independently of the will.

involute (in'vəlo͞ot), to decrease normally, in size and functional activity, an organ whose role in the body economy is temporary or confined to certain periods of life. Involute should be distinguished from atrophy, which means to waste away from abnormal causes.

involvement, the state of becoming involved.

i., bifurcation (bī'fərkā'shən), the extension of pocket formation into the interradicular area of multirooted teeth in periodontitis.

i., pulp, a condition wherein consideration of the vitality or health of the dental pulp is a factor.

i., trifurcation. See **involvement, bifurcation.**

iodine, a halogen element that is nonmetallic in nature; atomic weight is 126.91. As a nutritional element, iodine is vital to the production of thyroxin by the thyroid gland. In radioactive form, iodine is used as a diagnostic substance to determine the ability of the thyroid gland to take up iodine. In tincture form, iodine is used as a locally applied antiseptic, germicide, and disclosing solution.

i., protein-bound (PBI), iodine bound to protein, mainly thyroxin in the plasma. The thyroid hormone is precipitated by protein-denaturing agents, and, in general, the amount of iodine in a protein precipitate indicates the amount of thyroid hormone present and is thus an index of thyroid activity. Various values are given for thyroid function: hypothyroidism, 0 to 3.5 μg/ml of protein-bound iodine; euthyroidism, 3.5 to 8 μg/ml; hyperthyroidism, values higher than 8 μg/ml.

iodism (iodine poisoning, iodine stomatitis), acute or chronic intoxication caused by the ingestion or absorption of iodides. Manifestations of acute poisoning include abdominal pain, nausea, vomiting, hypersalivation, conjunctivitis, and collapse. Chronic manifestations include hypersalivation, fever, acute rhinitis, swelling and tenderness of the salivary glands, and dermatitis and stomatitis in hypersensitive individuals. Iodism is a toxic condition that sometimes follows the use of preparations containing iodine.

iodophor (ī·ō'dəfôr), a loose chemical compound of iodine with certain organic compounds; for example, polyvinylpyrrolidone.

ion (ī'ən, ī'on), an atomic particle, atom, or chemical radical bearing an electrical charge, either negative or positive.

i. exchange chromatography, the process of separating and analyzing different substances according to their affinities for chemically stable but very reactive synthetic exchangers, which are composed largely of polystyrene and cellulose. The process uses an absorbent containing ionizing groups and accommodates the exchange of ions between a solution of substances to be analyzed and the absorbent. Ion exchange chromatography is often used to separate components of nucleic acids and proteins.

i. pair, two particles of opposite charge, usually the electron and the positive atomic residue resulting after the interaction of ionizing radiation with the orbital electrons of atoms. The average energy required to produce an ion pair is approximately 33 (or 34) electron volts.

i.-selective electrode, a potentiometric electrode that develops a potential in the presence of one ion (or class of ions), but not in the presence of a similar concentration of other ions.

ionization (ī'ənizā'shən), the process or the result of a process by which a neutral atom or molecule acquires either a positive or negative charge.

i., air-equivalent, chamber. See **chamber, ionization, air-equivalent.**

i. chamber. See **chamber, ionization.**

i. density, the number of ion pairs per unit volume.

i path (ionization track), the trail of ion pairs produced by ionizing radiation in its passage through matter.

i. potential, the potential necessary to separate one electron from an atom, resulting in the formation of an ion pair.

ionizer. See **electrolyzer.**

iontophoresis (īən'tōfōrē'sis), application, by means of an appropriate electrode, of a galvanic current to an ionizable agent in contact with a surface to hasten the movement into the tissue of the ion of opposite charge to that of the electrode. See also **ionization.**

ipratropium bromide, *trade name:* Atrovent; *drug class:* anticholinergic

bronchodilator; *action:* inhibits interaction of acetylcholine at receptor sites on the bronchial smooth muscle, resulting in bronchodilation; *uses:* bronchodilation during bronchospasm in those with chronic obstructive pulmonary disease, bronchitis, emphysema, asthma; not for rapid bronchodilation; maintenance treatment only.

IQ. See **intelligence quotient.**

iridium, a silvery-bluish metallic element. Its atomic number is 77 and its atomic weight is 192.2.

iris, a circular, contractile disc suspended in aqueous humor between the cornea and the crystalline lens of the eye and perforated by a circular pupil. The iris regulates the amount of light passing into the chambers of the eye.

iron, a common metallic element essential for the synthesis of hemoglobin. Its atomic number is 26 and its atomic weight is 55.85. Normal blood levels of iron range between 60 and 190 micrograms.

irradiation (irā'dē·ā'shən), **1.** the exposure of material to roentgen or other radiation. (One speaks of "radiation therapy" but of "irradiation of the patient.") **2.** the exposure to radiation.

irresuscitable (ir'rəsəs'itəbəl), beyond the possibility of being revived. (not current)

irreversibility (ir'rəvor'sibil'itē), the quality of being incapable of being revived.

irreversible (ir'rəver'sibəl), incapable of being reversed or returned to the original state.

i. hydrocolloid. See **hydrocolloid, irreversible.**

irrigation (ir'igā'shən), the technique of using a solution to wash or flush debris from the root canal or from a wound.

irritability, the quality of being irritable or of responding to a stimulus.

irritant, 1. an agent that causes an irritation or stimulation. **2.** an agent that is toxic, bacterial, physical, or chemical, and that is capable of inducing functional derangements or organic lesions of the tissues.

i., chemical, a chemical agent that causes irritation. The primary agents that have a etiologic relationship to periodontal disease are plaque and calculus. Other agents that serve as a medium for the growth of microorganisms include food debris, sloughed cells, and necrotic material.

irritation, the act of stimulating. Any condition of functional derangement and nervous irritability.

i. of gingival tissues. See **impingement.**

i., mechanical, tissue damage, injury, or insult by physical forces directed against the tissue; for example, tissue irritation produced by faulty toothbrushing.

i. from overstimulation. See **impingement.**

ischemia (iskē′mē·ə), a focal deficiency of blood to a part of the body or simply a local anemia. It results from encroachment of the lumen of an artery or the capillaries supplying the affected area. The reduction in the lumen may be caused by allergic hypersensitivity, degeneration of the tunica intima (atherosclerosis), inflammation, physical pressure, pharmacologic and toxic agents, and/or neurogenic disorders.

isobar (i′səbär), in radiochemistry, one of two or more different nuclides having the same mass number.

isoelectric focusing, the ordering and concentration of substances according to their isoelectric points.

isoelectric point, the pH at which a molecule containing two or more ionizable groups is electrically neutral.

isoetharine HCl/isoetharine mesylate, *trade names:* Bronkosol, Bronkometer, Dispos-a-Med; *drug class:* adrenergic β_2-agonist; *action:* causes bronchodilation by β_2 stimulation, resulting in increased levels of cAMP and causing relaxation of bronchial smooth muscle with very little effect on heart rate; *uses:* bronchospasm, asthma.

isolation of a tooth, a technique to protect a tooth against contamination from oral fluids during a surgical or restorative procedure, usually through the application of a rubber dam or the use of cotton rolls.

isoleucine, one of the essential amino acids occurring in most dietary proteins. Isoleucine is essential for proper growth in infants and for nitrogen balance in adults. See also **amino acid.**

isomers (i′sōmərz), **1.** organic compounds having the same empirical formula; that is, the same number of

the same atoms, but different structural formulas and therefore different physical and chemical properties. **2.** one of several nuclides having the same number of neutrons and protons but capable of existing, for a measurable time, in different quantum states with different energies and radioactive properties. The isomer of higher energy commonly decays to one with lower energy by a process known as *isomeric transition.*

i., optical, two isomers whose structures, dextro- and levo-, differ only in a spatial arrangement that makes them mirror images. This occurs only when there is an asymmetric carbon atom; that is, one attached to four different substituents. The pharmacologic activity often resides very largely in one of the two forms.

i., stereo-, molecules that differ only in the spatial arrangement of the atoms. This term includes optical isomers.

isometric muscle contraction (i′sōmet′rik). See **contraction, muscle, isometric.**

isoniazid (INH), *trade names:* Laniazid, Nydrazid; *drug class:* antitubercular; *action:* bactericidal interference with lipid, nucleic acid biosynthesis; *uses:* treatment and prevention of tuberculosis.

isoproterenol HCl/isoproterenol sulfate, *trade names:* Isuprel, Vapo-Iso, Aerolone; *drug class:* adrenergic β_1- and β_2-agonist; *action:* relaxes bronchial smooth muscle and dilates trachea and main bronchi by increasing levels of cAMP, which relaxes smooth muscles; causes increased contractility and heart rate; *uses:* bronchospasm, asthma, heart block, bradycardia, shock.

isosorbide dinitrate, *trade names:* Iso-Bid, Isotrate, Dilatrate-SR, Isordil; *drug class:* nitrate antianginal; *action:* decreases preload/afterload, which is responsible for decreasing left ventricular end-distolic pressure, systemic vascular resistance; *uses:* chronic stable angina pectoris, prophylaxis of angina pain.

isosorbide mononitrate, *trade name:* ISMO; *drug class:* antianginal, organic nitrate; *action:* decreases preload/afterload, which is responsible for decreasing left ventricular end-diastolic pressure, systemic vascular resistance; arterial and venous dilation; *use:* prevention of angia pectoris caused by coronary artery disease.

isosthenuria (ī'sosthenoo'rē·ə), the excretion of urine with fixed specific gravity. It may occur in terminal renal disease when the specific gravity reaches that of the glomerular filtrate, 1.010.

isotone (ī'sətōn), one of several different nuclides having the same number of neutrons in their nuclei, but different mass numbers. (not current)

isotonic (ī'səton'ik), the equivalent in osmotic pressure. Specifically used in reference to a solution whose osmotic pressure is equal to that of a body fluid, such as blood plasma or tears, to which the solution is compared.
i. muscle contraction. See **contraction, muscle, isotonic.**

isotope (ī'sətōp), one of several nuclides having the same number of protons in their nuclei, and hence having the same atomic number but differing in the number of neutrons, and therefore in the mass number. The isotopes of a particular element have virtually identical chemical properties.
i., stable, a nonradioactive isotope of an element.

isotretinoin, *trade name:* Accutane; *drug class:* retinoic acid isomer, vitamin A derivative; *action:* decreases sebum secretion, improves cystic acne; *uses:* severe recalcitrant cystic acne.

isoxsuprine HCl, *trade name:* Vasodilan; *drug class:* peripheral vasodilator; *action:* α-adrenoreceptor antagonist with β-adrenoreceptor-stimulating properties; may also act directly on vascular smooth muscle; causes cardiac stimulation, uterine relaxation; *uses:* symptoms of cerebrovascular insufficiency, peripheral vascular disease including arteriosclerosis obliterans, Raynoud's disease.

Isradipine, *trade name:* DynaCirc; *drug class:* calcium channel blocker; *action:* inhibits calcium ion influx across cell membrane during cardiac depolarization; produces relaxation of coronary vascular smooth muscle, peripheral vascular smooth muscle; increases myocardial oxygen delivery

in patients with vasospastic angina; *use:* essential hypertension.

itraconazole, *trade name:* Sporanox; *drug class:* antifungal, systemic; *action:* inhibits cytochrome P-450 enzyme's blocking synthesis of essential membrane sterols in fungal organism; *uses:* blastomycosis, histoplasmosis.

Ivalon sponge, a polyvinyl alcohol sponge.

Ivy loop wiring. See **wiring, Ivy loop.**

Ivy's test. See **test, Ivy's.**

jacket. See **crown, complete, veneer, acrylic resin** and **crown, veneer, porcelain.**

jackscrew, a threaded device used in appliances for separation or approximation of teeth or jaw segments.

Jackson's sign. See **sign, Jackson's.**

Janet's test. See **test, Janet's.**

jaundice (jôn'dis, jän'dis), a condition characterized by an abnormal accumulation of bilirubin (red bile pigment) in the blood and manifested by a yellowish discoloration of the skin, mucous membranes, and cornea. Seen in hemolytic anemias, biliary obstruction, hepatitis, cholangiolitis, and cirrhosis of the liver. Oral mucous membranes may be pigmented.
j., acholuric, jaundice without bile in the urine.
j., congenital hemolytic (acholuric icterus, spherocytic anemia, hereditary spherocytosis), a familial hemolytic anemia transmitted as a mendelian dominant. The intrinsic defects of the red blood cells include a spheroidal shape, which allows them to be trapped by the spleen, and increased mechanical fragility.
j., epidemic. See **disease, Weil's.**
j., hemolytic (prehepatic jaundice), excess bile pigments in the blood resulting from increased destruction of erythrocytes.

j., hepatic. See **jaundice, hepatocellular.**

j., hepatocellular *(hepatic jaundice, infective jaundice, medical jaundice, toxic jaundice),* jaundice resulting from disease of liver cells by infectious agents or toxins, decreasing the ability of the liver to handle the bile pigments that are continually produced by the destruction of red blood cells.

j., homologous serum. See **hepatitis, homologous serum.**

j., infective. See **jaundice, hepatocellular.**

j., latent, increased bilirubin in the blood without clinical signs of jaundice.

j., medical. See **jaundice, hepatocellular.**

j., obstructive *(posthepatic jaundice),* extrahepatic and intrahepatic obstruction of the biliary tract, resulting in retrograde retention of bile pigments and jaundice.

j., posthepatic. See **jaundice, obstructive.**

j., prehepatic. See **jaundice, hemolytic.**

j., regurgitating, jaundice resulting from reentry of conjugated bilirubin into the blood as a result of obstruction of the biliary tract or hepatocellular damage and failure to excrete conjugated bilirubin from liver cells.

j., retention, an increase in bilirubin in the blood from hemolysis; failure of the liver cells to conjugate bilirubin or remove free bilirubin.

j., surgical, extrahepatic obstruction of the biliary tract.

j., syringe. See **hepatitis, homologous serum.**

j., toxic. See **jaundice, hepatocellular.**

jaw, a common name for either the maxillae or the mandible; the meaning is usually extended to include their soft tissue covering.

j., cleft *(gnathoschisis).* See **palate, cleft.**

j. cyst, an abnormal bladder-like sac within the jaw. For the types that may occur in either the maxilla or mandible associated with or not associated with the dentition and its formation; see also **cyst.**

j. fracture, a break in the continuity of the bone of the maxilla or mandible. See also **fracture.**

j.-to-jaw relationship. See **relation, jaw.**

j., lumpy. See **actinomycosis.**

j. movement. See **movement, jaw.**

j., phossy. See **poisoning, phosphorus.**

j. reflex. See **reflex, jaw.**

j. relation. See **relation, jaw.**

JCAHO, an acronym for the **Joint Commission on Accreditation of Healthcare Organizations.**

jealousy, resentment against a rival or competitor. Jealousy may be a significant barrier to functional interpersonal relationships within any group.

jejunum, the middle or intermediate of the three portions of the small intestine, connecting proximally with the duodenum and distally with the ileum. The jejunum has a slightly larger diameter, a deeper color, and a thicker wall than the ileum and contains heavy, circular folds that are absent in the lower part of the ileum.

jelly, petroleum. See **petrolatum.**

job satisfaction, the state of finding fulfillment in one's work.

Johnston's method. See **method, chloropercha.**

joint(s), the junction of union between two or more bones or cartilages of the skeleton.

j., Charcot's (sharcōz´), a manifestation of late syphilis in which there is degeneration, hypertrophy, hypermobility, and loss of contour of a joint, usually a weight-bearing joint. It is most common in tabes dorsalis.

j. diarthrosis (diarth´rōsis), a joint that moves freely in contact. The adjacent bone surfaces are typically covered by a film of cartilage and are bound by stout connective tissues, frequently enclosing a liquid-filled joint cavity.

j. disease, any inflammatory, infectious, or functional disorder within a joint.

j., hinge. See **ginglymus.**

j. mice, cartilaginous material present in the synovial spaces of a joint.

j. prosthesis, the addition to or replacement of a member(s) or of structural elements within a joint to improve and enhance the function of the joint. Principal joint prostheses include hip replacement and knee replacement. Less common is a joint prosthesis for the TMJ.

j. synarthrosis (sin'arthrō'sis) *(junctura fibrosa, fibrous joint),* a joint in which the bony elements are connected by thin intervening layers of cartilage, connective tissue, or direct contact of bone to bone such as the rigid unions in the adult skull.

j., temporomandibular. See **articulation, temporomandibular.**

Joint Commission on Accreditation of Health Care Organizations (JCAHO), formerly the Joint Commission on Accreditation of Hospitals. The JCAHO conducts accreditation programs for most of the health care facilities in the United States. The American Dental Association is a corporate member of the JCAHO. Hospitals and clinics are surveyed on a regular basis for compliance with the standards and criteria for accreditation.

Joint Commission on Accreditation of Hospitals. See **Joint Commission on Accreditation of Healthcare Organizations.**

Jones protein. See **protein, Bence Jones.**

Jorgensen's drug administration principles, principles employed in the selection and administration of intravenous sedative agents that have a wide margin of safety and predictable effects and which, in combination, can elevate the pain threshold, produce euphoria, have an antisialogogue effect, and promote an amnesic response. The principles include the sequence and rate of administration while monitoring patient response signs.

judgment, 1. a legal finding. **2.** the ability to discriminate between or among two or more states or conditions.

junction (jəngk'shən), a place of coming together or union.

j., cementoenamel (cervical line), the junction of the enamel of the crown and the cementum of the root of a tooth. The area above the junction corresponds to the anatomic crown of the tooth; the area apical to the junction constitutes the anatomic root of the tooth.

j., dentinocemental, the line of union or apposition of the cementum and dentin of a tooth.

j., dentinoenamel (dentoenamel junction), the interface of enamel and dentin of the tooth crown, conforming in a general way to the shape of the crown.

j., dentoenamel. See **junction, dentinoenamel.**

j., dentogingival, the junction between the gingival attachment, a nonkeratinized epithelium, and the tooth surface.

j., mucogingival, the scalloped linear area denoting the approximation or separation of the gingivae and alveolar mucosa.

jurisprudence, the philosophy of law.

j., dental (forensic dentistry), **1.** the science that teaches the application of every branch of dental knowledge to the purposes of the law; this also includes the elucidation of doubtful legal questions. **2.** the state laws and codes covering the legal limitations of the practice of the profession of dentistry.

j., medical, the science that applies the principles and practice of the different branches of medicine in the elucidation of doubtful questions in a court of justice. Synonym: forensic medicine.

jury, a certain number of citizens selected according to law and sworn to inquire of certain matters of fact and to declare the truth on evidence submitted to them.

just, right; according to law and justice.

justice, the constant and perpetual disposition to render every man his due. Also, the conformity of one's actions and will to the law.

juvenile periodontitis, a distinct form of periodontal disease that may present with symptoms such as localized or generalized inflammatory changes in the periodontium of prepubertal children. The disease is characterized by severe pocketing and rapid destruction of alveolar bone. Several subtypes of the disease are recognized (formerly called "periodontosis").

juxtaposition, adjacent situation; apposition or contact.

Kahn's test. See **test, Kahn's.** (not current)

kakke (käk'kā). See **beriberi.**

kallikrein, a group of enzymes (plasma, tissue, pancreatic, urinary, submandibular kallikrein) that can convert kininogen to bradykinin or kallidin; trypsin and plasmin can also affect the conversion.

k.-kinin system, a proposed hormonal system that functions within the kidney, with the enzyme kallikrein in the renal cortex mediating production of bradykinin, which acts as a vasodilator peptide.

kanamycin, an aminoglycoside antibiotic that acts by inhibiting the synthesis of protein in susceptible organisms. Kanamycin requires close clinical supervision because of its potential toxicity and adverse side effects to the auditory and vestibular branches of the eighth cranial nerve and to the renal tubules.

kaolin (kā'əlin), a fine, pure-white clay (hydrated aluminum silicate) used in porcelain teeth.

Kaposi's sarcoma. See **sarcoma, Kaposi's.**

Kazanjian's operation (kəzan'jē-ənz). See **operation, Kazanjian's.**

Kazanjian's procedure. See **operation, Kazanjian's.**

keloid (kē'loid), a dense, proliferative growth on the skin (hypertrophy of scar tissue) that appears to be an abnormal reaction to trauma, especially burns. Keloids tend to recur after excision and occur more frequently in blacks than in whites.

keloplasty (kē'lōplas'tē), the excision of scar tissue in the skin.

Kendall's compound B. See **corticosterone.**

Kendall's compound E. See **cortisone.**

Kennedy bar. See **connector, minor, secondary lingual bar.**

Kennedy classification, a method of classifying partially edentulous conditions and partial dentures; based on the location of the edentulous spaces in relation to the remaining teeth. (not current)

keratin (ker'ətin), an insoluble sulfur-containing protein with a high content of the amino acids tyrosine and leucine; the main component of epidermis, hair, nails, keratinized epithelium. It contains a relatively large amount of sulfur, is insoluble in the gastric juices, and is sometimes used for coating enteric pills that are intended to be dissolved only in the intestine.

keratinization (ker'ətin'izāshən), the process of becoming keratinized.

keratinocytes, a cell of the living epidermis and certain oral epithelium that produces keratin in the process of differentiating into the dead and fully kertinized cells of the stratum corneum.

keratitis, any inflammation of the cornea.

keratoacanthoma (ker'ətō·ak'anthō'mə), a rapidly growing papular lesion with a superficial crater filled with keratin.

keratoconjunctivitis sicca (ker'ah-to-kon-junk'tivi'tis sik'ah) See syndrome, Sjögren's.

keratocyst (kerə'tōsist), a homified cyst.

keratohyalin granules (ker'ətōhī'əlin), basophilic granules (0.2 to 4.5 micron) found in cells of the stratum granulosum that are presumed to play a role in keratinization.

keratolytic agents, agents that loosen or remove the horny outer layer of the skin.

keratoplasty, corneal transplantation.

keratosis (ker'ətō'sis), **I.** a horny or cornified growth (for example, wart, callosity). **2.** a condition characterized by cornification, or hyperkeratinization, of the tissues.

k., actinic, an overgrowth of the horny layer of the epidermis caused by excessive exposure to the sun.

k. blennorrhagia, a skin condition found in Reiter's syndrome characterized by pustules and crusting; once incorrectly associated with gonorrhea; more recently considered a genetic disorder occuring mostly in men between the ages of 20 and 25.

k., chronic senile, keratosis of the lips in elderly individuals. These lesions should be considered precancerous.

k., focal, localized areas of increased cornification (hyperkeratinization). Such lesions are seen particularly on the lips.

k. follicularis. See **disease, Darier's.**

k., seborrheic (basal cell papilloma, verruca senilis), benign, pigmented, superficial epithelial tumors that clinically appear to be pasted on the skin of the trunk, arms, or face. Characterized histologically by marked hyperkeratosis, with keratin cyst formation, acanthosis of basal cells, and melanin pigmentation, all above the level of the adjacent epidermis.

k., senile, small, firm lesions occurring principally on the face and back of the hands in elderly people or those exposed to the sun. There is hyperkeratosis with irregular and atypical proliferation of the cells of the rete Malpighi. The condition is one of premalignancy with tendency toward epidermoid carcinoma. See also **leukoplakia.**

ketamine, a parenterally administered anesthetic that produces catatonia, profound analgesia, increased sympathetic activity, and little relaxation of skeletal muscles.

ketoacidosis (kē'tō·as'idō'sis), a form of acidosis characterized by an increased accumulation of ketone bodies (acetoacetic acid, β-hydroxybutyric acid, acetone) in the blood (for example, the acidosis of uncontrolled diabetes mellitus).

ketoconazole, a broad-spectrum synthetic antifungal agent applied to the skin to inhibit the growth of dermatophytes and yeasts, effective in *Candida* infections and in the treatment of seborrheic dermatitis; *trade name:* Nizoral; *drug class:* imidazole antifungal; *action:* alters cell membranes and inhibits several fungal enzymes; *uses:* systemic candidiasis, chronic mucocutaneous candidiasis, candiduria, coccidioidomycosis, histoplasmosis, chromomycosis, paracoccidioidomycosis, tinea pedis.

ketone, an organic chemical compound characterized by having in its structure a carbonyl, or keto group attached to two alkyl groups. It is produced by oxidation of secondary alcohols.

k. body. See **body, ketone.**

ketoprofen, *trade name:* Orudis, Oruvail, Actron; *drug class:* nonsteroidal antiinflammatory; *action:* inhibits prostaglandin synthesis by interfering with cyclooxygenase needed for biosynthesis; possesses analgesic, antiinflammatory, antipyretic properties; *uses:* osteoarthritis, rheumatoid arthritis, dysmenorrhea.

ketorolac/ketorolac tromethamine injection, *trade name:* Toradol; *drug class:* nonsteroidal antiinflammatory; *action:* inhibits prostaglandin synthesis by interfering with cyclooxygenase needed for biosynthesis; possesses analgesic, antiinflammatory, antipyretic properties; *use:* acute mild-to-moderate pain, not for chronic pain use.

ketosis. See **ketoacidosis.**

kev, the abbreviation for 1000 electron volts.

keyway, the slot into which the male portion of precision attachments fits.

kg. See **kilogram.**

KHN, the abbreviation for **Knoop hardness number.** See also **test, Knoop hardness.**

kidney, one of a pair of bean-shaped urinary organs in the dorsal part of the abdomen, one on each side of the vertebral column. The kidneys produce and eliminate urine through a complex filtration network and reabsorption system comprising more than 2 million nephrons. More than 2500 pints of blood pass through the kidneys every day.

killer cell, a lymphocyte that develops in the bone marrow and lacks the characteristic surface markers of the B and T lymphocytes. Killer or null cells represent a small proportion of the lymphocyte population. Stimulated by the presence of antibody, null cells can attach certain cellular targets directly and are known as "natural killer cells."

kilo- (kil'ō), the prefix that means 1000.

kilocalorie, one thousand calories, a unit of measure of the energy value in foodstuffs.

kilogram (kil'əgram) **(kg),** 1000 Gm, or equivalent to about 2.2 pounds avoirdupois.

kilovolt (kil'əvōlt) **(kv),** the unit of electrical potential equal to 1000 volts.

K

k. peak (kvp), the crest value of the potential wave in kilovolts in an alternating current cycle. When only half of the wave is used, the value refers to that of the useful half of the wave.

kilovoltage (kil'əvōl'tij), the electrical potential difference between the anode and cathode of an x-ray tube.

k., constant potential, the potential of a constant voltage generator, in constant potential kilovolts (kvcp).

k., equivalent (effective kilovoltage), the kilovoltage of monoenergetic radiation having the same half-value layer (HVL) as the heterogeneous beam produced by a peak kilovoltage in question.

k., peak, the crest value of the potential wave, in peak kilovolts (kvp).

kinanesthesia (kin'anesthē'zē·ə), a loss of the power to perceive the sensation of movement resulting from derangement of deep sensibility. (not current)

kinematic face-bow (kinəmat'ik). See **face-bow, kinematic.**

kinesiology (kinē'sē·ol'əjē), the study of human motion that attempts to explain the manner in which movements of the body occur. The principles of kinesiology may be used to describe the laws of articulation and the several theories of mandibular movement.

kinetics, the study of the forces that produce, arrest, or modify the motions of the body. Kinetics is the application of Newton's first and third laws of inertia to body dynamics. The reaction forces of the muscles contribute to the equilibrium and motion of the body.

kinin, one of a number of widely differing substances having pronounced and dramatic physiologic effects. Some are formed in blood by proteolysis secondary to some pathologic process. Kinins stimulate visceral smooth muscle but relax vascular smooth muscle, thus producing vasodilation.

kink, a bend or twist.

Kirkland cement dressing, knife. See **knife, Kirkland.** (not current)

Kirschner wire. See **wire, Kirschner.**

Kirstein's method. See **method, Kirstein's.**

kissing disease, a vernacular term for infectious mononucleosis, a viral infection frequently occurring in teenagers and young adults. See also **infectious mononucleosis.**

Klebsiella, a genus of diplococcal bacteria that appear as small, plump rods with rounded ends. Several respiratory diseases, including bronchitis, sinusitis, and some forms of pneumonia are caused by infection of species of *Klebsiella.*

K. pneumoniae, a species of bacteria, also called *Friedlander's bacillus,* found in soil, water, cereal grains, and the intestinal tract of humans and other animals. It is associated with several pathologic conditions, including pneumonia.

Klinefelter's syndrome, a syndrome of gonadal defects, appearing in males with an extra X chromosome in at least one cell line. Characteristics are small, firm testes, long legs, gynecomastia, poor social adaptation, subnormal intelligence, chronic pulmonary disease, and varicose veins.

Kline's test. See **test, Kline's.**

Kloehn headgear, an extraoral orthodontic appliance consisting of a face-bow and a cervical strap used to retract maxillary teeth or to reinforce the anchorage during tooth retraction.

knee, a joint complex that connects the thigh with the lower leg. It consists of three condyloid joints, 12 ligaments, 13 bursae, and the patella.

knife, an instrument used for cutting that consists of a sharp-edged blade provided with a handle.

k., buck, a periodontal knife possessing spear-shaped cutting points; used for interdental incision during gingivectomy.

k., electronic, an electrosurgical scalpel used to incise or shave tissue.

k., gold, an instrument sometimes contraangled, with a blade or cutting edge; used to trim excess metal and develop contour in foil restorations.

k., Goldman-Fox, any of a group of surgical instruments designed for the incision and contouring of gingival tissue.

k., Kirkland, a heart-shaped knife, sharp on all edges, used for the primary gingivectomy incision.

k., Merrifield's, a knife that has a long, narrow, triangular blade in a shank; used for gingivectomy incisions.

K

Knoop hardness test. See **test, Knoop hardness.**

Kobayashi ties, orthodontic ligature ties used to fix an orthodontic arch wire to the brackets attached to the teeth; also provides attachment for the use of inter- and intramaxillary elastic traction.

Koeber's saw. See **saw, Koeber's.**

koilocytosis, a histologic feature of the mucosal changes associated with the intraoral use of smokeless tobacco. The spinous cells of the squamous epithelium present with pyknotic, irregularly shaped nuclei surrounded by a perinuclear clear zone.

Koplik's spots. See **spots, Koplik's.**

Kramer-Rhodes periodontal collection system, a plaque-scoring and record-keeping system used to monitor plaque accumulation and to motivate patients to improve oral hygiene. It is based upon a surface-by-surface, tooth-by-tooth assessment using a 0-3 scale. 0 means no plaque is present, 3 means there is full surface, heavy plaque accumulation. (not current)

Krause's corpuscles. See **corpuscle, Krause's.** (not current)

Kryptex. See **cement, silicophosphate.** (not current)

krypton, one of the inert gases, present in small amounts in the atmosphere with an atomic number of 36 and an atomic weight of 83.80.

KS. See **Kaposi's sarcoma.**

Kurer anchor system, an endodontic post system with parallel sides, threaded and made of stainless material.

Kustner's test (kist′nərz). See **test, skin, indirect.** (not current)

kv. See **kilovolt.**

kvcp. See **kilovoltage, constant potential.**

kvp. See **kilovolt peak.**

kyphosis (kĭfō′sis) (humpback), an abnormal curvature of the spine with the convexity backward.

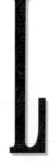

label (lā′bəl), **1.** the portion of the prescription in which the directions for use are stated. **2.** one or more characters used to identify an item of data. Synonym: key. See also **signa.**

labetatol, *trade names:* Normodyne, Trandate; *drug class:* nonselective adrenergic β-blocker and α-blocker; *action:* produces falls in BP without reflex tachycardia or significant reduction in heart rate through mixture of α-blocking and β-blocking effects; elevated plasma renins are reduced; *use:* mild- to-severe hypertension.

labial (lā′bē-əl), of or pertaining to a lip.

l. notch. See **notch, labial.**

labile (lā′bīl), unstable, as labile fever.

labioversion (lā′bē-ōver′zhən), any deviation of a tooth toward the lips from the line of occlusion.

labium superius oris (lā′bē-əm sōōpē′rē-əs ō′ris), the point of the upper lip lying in the midsagittal plane and a line drawn across the boundary of the mucous surface tangent to the curves. (not current)

laboratory, dental, the room in which the dentist or auxiliaries perform technical procedures related to dental treatment but not done directly in the patient's mouth.

laceration, a wound produced by tearing; the process of tearing.

laches (latch′iz), negligence; inexcusable delay; a failure to claim or enforce a claim or right at a proper time. (not current)

lacquer, a resin dissolved in a volatile solvent used to create a protective coating on the surface of an object.

lacrimal apparatus, a network of structures of the eye that secrete tears and drain them from the surface of the eyeball. The parts include the lacrimal glands, the lacrimal ducts, the lacrimal sacs, and the nasolacrimal ducts.

lacrimation, gustatory. See **syndrome, auriculotemporal.**

lactalbumin, a simple, highly nutritious protein found in milk. Lactalbumin is similar to serum albumin.

lactate dehydrogenase, an enzyme found in the cytoplasm of almost all body tissues, where its main function is to catalyze the oxidation of L-lactate to pyruvate.

Lactobacillus acidophilus, a species of the genus *Lactobacillus* of the family Lactobacillaceae characterized by gram-positive rods found in cultured buttermilk and in the gastrointestinal tract of persons on a high milk, lactose-, or dextrin-containing diet. *L. acidophilus* preparations may be effective in the treatment of some recurrent aphthous ulcers and for the prevention of candidiasis secondary to tetracycline and/or steroid therapy.

Lactobacillus casei, a species of *Lactobacillus* found in milk and cheese.

lactoferrin, an iron binding protein found in the specific granules of neutrophils where it apparently exerts an antimicrobial activity by withholding iron from ingested bacteria and fungi. It also occurs in many secretions and exudates such as milk, tears, mucus, saliva, and bile.

lactoflavin (lak′tōflāvin). See **vitamin B₂.** (not current)

lactone, an organic anhydride formed from a hyroxyacid by the loss of water between an −OH and a −COOH group.

lactoperoxidase, a peroxidase enzyme obtained from milk

lactose, a disaccharide found in the milk of all mammals. Lactose is used as a component of formulas for infants, it is also used as a laxative and a diuretic.

lacuna (ləkōō′nə), a term used in anatomic nomenclature to designate a small hollow cavity or pit.

l., absorption (Howship's lacuna), an area (pit) of bone resorption, usually irregular in outline, and often containing osteoclasts.

l., osteocyte, a hollow cavity within bone, containing osteocytes, from which canaliculi, containing protoplasmic processes of the osteocytes, radiate.

lambda (lam′də), **1.** the eleventh letter of the Greek alphabet. **2.** the point in the skull at which the sagittal and lambdoid sutures meet. The strap of a rubber dam holder placed at this level will hold its position without slipping up or down.

lameila, cemental (ləmel′ə), the arrangement and deposition of cementum in incremental layers more or less parallel to the root configuration.

lamina (lam′inə), a flat, thin plate.

l. dura, a radiographic term denoting the plate of compact bone (alveolar bone) that lies adjacent to the periodontal membrane.

l. propria, the zone of connective tissue subjacent to the epithelium of a mucous membrane.

laminagraphy (lam′ināg′rəfē), body section radiography.

laminate veneer restorations, a conservative esthetic restoration of anterior teeth to mask discoloration, restore malformed teeth, close diastemas, and correct minor tooth alignment. The materials of choice are acrylic veneers, processed composite resin veneers, and/or porcelain veneers that are bonded directly to a properly prepared tooth.

laminectomy, the excision of a vertebral lamina, commonly used to denote the removal of the posterior arch.

laminin, a large polypeptide glycoprotein component of the basement membrane.

lamivudine (3TC), *trade name:* Epivir; *drug class:* antiviral, nucleoside analog; *action:* inhibition of HIV reverse transcriptase; also inhibits RNA- and DNA-dependent DNA polymerase; *use:* used in combination with zidovudine for the treatment of HIV infection.

lamotrigine, *trade name:* Lamictal; *drug class:* antiepileptic; *action:* may be result of blockage of voltage-dependent sodium channels with inhibition of excitatory amino acids; *uses:* adjunctive treatment of refractive partial seizures in adults.

lamp, mouth, a device to produce light or illumination directly in the oral cavity and to transilluminate the dental tissues.

lance, to cut open with a lancet; to incise.

lancinating, pertaining to a stabbing pain (for example, the pain occurring in tic douloureux).

landmark, an anatomic structure used as a guide for anatomic relationships.

l., cephalometric (sef'əlōmet'rik), one of the points located on oriented head radiographs from which lines, planes, and angles may be constructed to analyze the configuration and relationship of elements of the craniofacial skeleton.

Langerhans cells, the cells of the pancreas that produce insulin.

language, a defined set of characters that is used to form symbols and words and the rules and connections for combining these into meaningful communications.

l., machine, a language designed for interpretation and use by a computer system without translation. Synonym: machine code.

lansoprazole, *trade name;* Prevacid; *drug class:* antisecretory, proton pump inhibitor; *action:* suppresses gastric secretion by inhibiting hydrogen/potassium ATPase enzyme system in gastric parietal cell; *uses:* short-term treatment for healing and symptomatic relief of active duodenal ulcer and erosive esophagitis.

lanthanum, a rare earth metallic element. Its atomic number is 57 and its atomic weight is 138.91

laparotomy, any surgical incision into the peritoneal cavity, usually performed under general or regional anesthesia, often on an exploratory basis.

large intestine, the portion of the digestive tract comprising the cecum; the appendix; the ascending, transverse, and descending colons; the rectum. The ileocecal valve separates the cecum from the ileum.

laryngectomy, the surgical removal of the larynx, performed to treat cancer of the larynx.

laryngismus (lar'injiz'məs), a spasm of the larynx. (not current)

laryngitis, an inflammation of the mucous membrane lining the larynx, accompanied by edema of the vocal cords with hoarseness or loss of voice.

laryngopharyngeal (ləring'gōfərin'jē-əl), related jointly to the larynx and the pharynx.

laryngopharynx (ləring'gōfer'ingks), the lower portion of the pharynx, which extends from the corner of the hyoid bone or the vestibule of the lar-

ynx to the lower border of the cricoid cartilage.

laryngoscope (ləring'gōskōp), a hollow tube equipped with electrical lighting, used to examine or operate upon the interior of the larynx through the mouth.

laryngoscopy, the use of a laryngoscope to view the larynx.

laryngospasm (ləring'gōspaᴄəm), the spasmodic closure of the larynx, sometimes noted during the induction phase of general anesthesia or during the recovery period.

larynx, the organ of voice that is part of the air passage connecting the pharynx with the trachea. It accounts for the large bump in the neck called the *Adam's apple.*

laser, a high-energy coordinated light source used in surgery, including for the experimental removal of the hard tissues of the teeth.

last will and testament, the legal document describing the desires of a person for the distribution of that person's worldly goods after death.

latent image. See **image, latent.**

latent period. See **period, latent.**

lateral (lat'ərəl), a position either to the right or the left of the midsagittal plane.

l. checkbite. See **record, interocclusal.**

l. condylar inclination. See **inclination, lateral condylar.**

l. condyle path. See **path, lateral condyle.**

l. excursion. See **excursion, lateral.**

l. movement. See **movement, lateral.**

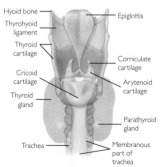

Hyoid bone — Epiglottis
Thyrohyoid ligament
Thyroid cartilage
Cricoid cartilage
Corniculate cartilage
Arytenoid cartilage
Thyroid gland
Parathyroid gland
Trachea — Membranous part of trachea

Anatomy of the larynx. (Thibodeau, 1996.)

L

l. protrusion. See **protrusion, lateral.**

laterodetrusion (lat′ərōdētroo′zhən), a noun that describes precisely the directions in which the muscles thrust a condyle outward and downward in the side shift preparatory to handling a large bolus of food. (not current)

lateroprotrusive (lat′ərōprōtroo′siv), pertaining to a movement direction of the jaw that has both sideward and forward components of movement. (not current)

lateroretrusive (lat′ərōrētroo′siv), pertaining to a movement direction in cusp or condyle thrusts that has both lateral and backward components of movement.

laterotrusion (lat′ərōtroo′zhən), the outward thrust given by the muscles to the rotating condyle or the condyle on the bolus side.

l., precurrent, laterotrusion in which the working side condyle is rotated as it is thrust laterally.

latex (lā′teks), natural rubber.

latitude (lat′itood″), the range between the minimum and maximum film exposures to radiation that yield images of structures whose photographic density differences are discernible under normal viewing conditions. Latitude chiefly varies directly with kilovoltage and inversely with contrast. See also **contrast.**

lattice, space (lat′is), an arrangement of atoms in a definite relationship to each other, forming a lattice.

lavage (ləväzh′), irrigation, or washing out, as in oral lavage.

law(s), l. that which is laid down or established. An enforceable rule of conduct. **2.** that which must be obeyed and followed by citizens, subject to sanctions or legal consequences. The term is also used in opposition to fact; for example, in a lawsuit, questions of law are to be decided by the court, whereas the jury decides questions in fact.

l., Charles', the principle that states that all gases expand equally upon heating and contract equally upon cooling.

l., Dalton's, the principle that states that the pressure of a mixture of gases equals the sum of the partial pressures of the constituent gases.

l., ignorance of, a want of knowledge or acquaintance with the laws of the land insofar as they apply to the act, relation, duty, or matter under consideration.

l., inverse-square, the principle that states that the strength of x radiation from a point source varies inversely as the square of the distance.

l., moral, the aggregate of those rules and principles of ethics that relate to right and wrong conduct and prescribe the standards to which the actions of persons should conform in their dealings with each other.

l., neurologic. See **law of specific energy.**

l. of specific energy (neurologic law), the principle that states, in essence, that sensory quality is perceived according to the nerve that is excited, not according to the object that excites. If pressure placed on the eyeballs stimulates the retina, light is perceived, not pressure; similarly, electrical stimulation will produce sensations of smell, taste, touch, or pain in accordance with the nerve stimulated but not a sensation of electricity as such. The special as well as the general senses maintain this principle.

l., Pascal's, the principle that states that pressure applied to a liquid at any point is transmitted equally in all directions.

l., Wolff's, the principle that states that all changes in the function of bone are attended by definite alterations in its internal structure.

l., written, law or laws created by express legislation or enactment, as distinguished from unwritten or common law, which includes all law or laws from any other legal source.

lay, nonprofessional.

layer, Beilby's (bil′bēz), an amorphous layer formed on the surface of metals by a disorientation of the crystalline structure during polishing. (not current)

LD50. See **dose, lethal, median.**

LD50 time. See **time, median lethal.**

lead, a common soft, blue-gray, metallic element. Its atomic number is 82 and its atomic weight is 207. In its metallic form, lead is used as a protective shielding against x-rays. Lead is poisonous, a characteristic that has led to a reduction in the use of lead compound as pigments for paints and inks.

l. apron. See **apron, lead.**

l. glass. See **glass, lead.**

l. poisoning. See **plumbism.**

leadership, the ability to influence others to achieve individual and group goals. Kinds of leadership include authoritarian, democratic, participative, and permissive.

leaf gauge. See **gauge, leaf.**

learning, the process of acquiring knowledge or some skill by means of study, practice, and/or experience.

l. disability, the inability to learn at a rate comparable to most members of a peer group. Some learning disorders have been traced to nutritional and behavioral causes, others stem from trauma or disease, and still others have genetic origins.

lease, 1. a conveyance of lands or tenements to a person for life, for a stated number of years, or at will, in consideration of rent or some other recompense. **2.** any agreement that gives rise to a landlord and tenant relationship.

least expensive alternative treatment (LEAT), a limitation in a dental benefits plan that will only allow benefits for the least expensive treatment. Also referred to as *least expensive professionally acceptable alternative treatment (LEPAAT).*

lecithin (les'ithin) (phosphatidylcholine), a class of phosphatides containing glycerol, phosphate, choline, and fatty acids. Lecithins are widely distributed in cells and possess both metabolic and structural functions in membranes. Dipalmityl lecithin is an important surface-active agent in the lungs.

ledger sheet, an accounting form for keeping track of debits, expenditures, credits, and charges.

Leede's test. See **test, capillary resistance.** (not current)

leeway space, the arch circumference difference between the primary canine, first primary and second primary molars, and the permanent canine and the first and second premolars. According to Black's means, the maxillary arch leeway space is 1.9 mm, and the mandibular arch leeway space is 3.4 mm.

LeFort fracture. See **fracture, LeFort.**

left justified, data are left-justified when the left-most digit or character occupies the left-most position of the space allotted for those data.

legal, 1. in compliance with the law. **2.** not forbidden by law.

Legionella, a genus of areobic, motile, non-acid–fast, nonencapsulated, gram-negative bacilli that have a non-fermentative metabolism. They are water-dwelling and air-borne spread, and are pathogenic for man.

L. pneumonia, a form of pneumonia caused by a gram-negative bacillus identified as *Legionella pneumophila.* It was discovered after an outbreak of the disease among veterans attending a 1976 convention of the American Legion.

L. pneumophila, a small, gram-negative, rod-shaped bacterium that is the causative agent of Legionnaires' disease.

Legionnaires' disease, an acute bacterial pneumonia caused by infection with *L. pneumophila* and characterized by an influenza-like illness followed within a week by high fever, chills, muscle aches, and headache. Contaminated air conditioning cooling towers and stagnant water supplies, including water vaporizers and water sonicators, may be a source of organisms.

legislation, the act of making or forming law, or the laws and/or statutes formed by the legislative process.

leiomyoma (lī'ōmīō'mə), a benign tumor derived from smooth muscle.

leiomyosarcoma, a malignant neoplasm of muscle that contains spindle cells of unstriated muscle.

leishmaniasis, an infection with any species of protozoan of the genus *Leishmania.*

length, the longest measure of an object, or the measurement between the two ends.

l., muscle, the variable end-to-end measurement of a muscle. The physical changes in muscle observed in the isotonic and isometric states of contraction are related to the alteration in the striated bands of muscle.

l.-of-stay, the expected length of time, usually a median, for which institutionalized patients in a hospital or other health care facility of similar age and diagnosis or condition would be expected to remain.

l., *tooth*, the distance along the long axis of the tooth from the apex of the root to the tip, or incisal edge, of the tooth.

lens, crystalline, the lens of the eye.

lenses, curved, transparent pieces of plastic or glass that are shaped, molded, or ground to refract light in a specific way, as in eyeglasses, microscopes, or cameras.

lentula (lentōō′lə), a flexible spiral-wire instrument used in a handpiece to apply paste filling materials in root canals. (not current)

leontiasis ossea (lē′ôntī′əsis os′ē·ə), an enlargement of the bones of the face, leading to a lionlike appearance. Osseous encroachment may cause obliteration of sinuses, blindness, and malocclusion.

leproma, a nodular lesion of leprosy seen on the skin, mucous membranes (including those of the eyes), upper respiratory tract, tongue, and palate.

leprosy (lep′rōsē) (Hansen's disease), a chronic granulomatous infection caused by *Mycobacterium leprae.* It may exist in lepromatous (contagious), tuberculoid (noncontagious), and intermediate forms.

leptocytosis, hereditary (lep′tōsītō′sis). See **thalassemia.** (not current)

Leptothrix (lep′tōthriks), a filamentous microorganism, apparently not directly capable of pathogenicity, that may act as a nidus for the formation of dental calculus and its attachment to the tooth structure. Some investigators have associated this organism with the presence of periodontitis in human beings.

Lesch-Nyhan syndrome, a hereditary disorder of purine metabolism, characterized by mental retardation, self-mutilation of the fingers and lips by biting, impaired renal function, and abnormal physical development. It is transmitted as a recessive, sex-linked trait.

lesion (lē′zhən), any pathologic disturbance of a tissue, with loss of continuity, enlargement, and/or function.

l., *extravasation.* See **cyst, traumatic.**

l., *herpetic,* a vesicle and/or ulceration of the mucosa caused by the herpes virus.

l., *herpetiform,* a painful ulceration of the oral mucosa with a red center and yellow border; occurs as a solitary lesion or in groups and appears similar to those lesions caused by herpes virus. The term *herpetiform* is used as a clinical designation unless the viral cause has actually been demonstrated.

l., *indefinite bone.* See **cyst, extravasation.**

l., *traumatic bone.* See **cyst, traumatic.**

Lesser's triangle. See **triangle, Lesser's.** (not current)

LET. See **transfer, linear energy.**

Letterer-Siwe disease. See **disease, Letterer-Siwe.** (not current)

leucine, one of the essential amino acids. See also **amino acid.**

leucovorin calcium (citrovorum factor/folinic acid), *trade name:* Wellcovorin; *drug class:* folic acid antagonist antidote, antineoplastic adjunct; *action:* chemically reduced derivative of folic acid, converted to tetrahydrofolate; counteracts folic acid antagonists; *uses:* megaloblastic or macrocytic anemia caused by folic acid deficiency, overdose of folic acid antagonist, methotrexate toxicity caused by pyrimethamine or trimethoprim, or in colorectal cancer with fluorouracil.

leukemia (lōōkē′mē·ə), a usually fatal disease of the blood-forming tissues characterized by the abnormal proliferation of leukocytes and their precursors and attended by fatigue, weakness, fever, lymphadenopathy, splenomegaly, and a tendency toward profuse tissue hemorrhage. Oral lesions include gingival enlargement, severe gingivitis, and necrosis. Lymphatic, monocytic, and myelogenous leukemias are the chief types.

l., *aleukemia,* a phase of the leukemic state marked by proliferation of leukocytes within the blood-forming tissues, but without an increase in the white blood cell count: relatively few precursor cells are found in the blood smear until the phase passes and the blood becomes flooded with white cells. Oral lesions, when present, are ulceronecrotic and hypertrophic.

l., *lymphatic (lymphoid leukemia),* a hyperplasia, of undetermined origin, affecting lymphoid tissue. Predominating cells are lymphocytes and lymphoblasts. Generally assumes a more chronic course than other forms of leukemia but may be acute. Oral lesions include swollen and hyperplastic gingivae, ulceronecrotic lesions, and marked tendency to gingival hemorrhage.

l., monocytic, a form of leukemia characterized by an abnormal increase in the number of monocytes. Manifestations include progressive weakness, anorexia, lymphadenopathy, hepatomegaly, splenomegaly, and secondary anemia. Oral lesions may be ulceronecrotic and hemorrhagic.

l., myelogenous, leukemia in which the leukocytes are of bone marrow origin (for example, polymorphonuclear leukocytes, myelocytes, myeloblasts). Oral manifestations may include gingival enlargement and necrosis.

leukocyte (loo'kōsīt), 1. a white blood cell. 2. a white blood cell; a nucleated ameboid mass of protoplasm circulating in the blood. See also **lymphocyte** and **monocyte.**

l., basophilic, a basophil; a leukocyte that has coarse granules stainable with basic dyes and a bent lobed nucleus.

l. count, the number of leukocytes in a cubic millimeter of blood. Normal values range from 5000 to 10,000/mm³.

l., eosinophilic, an eosinophil; a leukocyte that has coarse granules stainable with eosin and a bilobed nucleus.

l., immature, one of several forms of leukocyte usually found in disease (for example, myelocytes, myeloblasts, lymphoblasts).

l., polymorphonuclear, 1. a neutrophil; a white blood cell with finely granular cytoplasm, an irregularly lobulated nucleus, and the appearance of a microphage. It is found in the tissues during acute inflammatory processes and in the superficial surface aspects of a lesion during subacute or chronic inflammation. It is the predominating leukocyte of the blood. Blood levels may be increased during acute inflammatory states and myelogenous leukemia, and decreased in agranulocytosis (malignant neutropenia). 2. a neutrophil; a polymorph; a leukocyte that has fine granules stainable with neutral dyes and an irregularly lobed nucleus.

leukocytosis (loo'kōsītō'sis), an increase in the normal number of white blood cells; may be a defensive reaction, as in inflammation, or may result from a disturbance in white blood cell formation, as in leukemia. Various limits are given; for example, leukocytosis in the adult is indicated when there are more than 10,000 white blood cells per cubic millimeter. See also eosinophilia; lymphocytosis; neutrophilia.

leukoedema (loo'kō-ede'mə), an innocuous oral condition characterized by a filmy, opalescent, white covering of the buccal mucosa consisting of a thickened layer of parakeratotic cells. It is most commonly associated with mechanical and chemical irritation.

leukopenia (loo'kōpē'nē-ə), a decrease in the normal number of white blood cells in the circulating blood. Various lower limits are given; for example, leukopenia signifies less than 4000 white blood cells per cubic millimeter. See also **lymphocytopenia; neutropenia.**

leukoplakia (loo'kōpla'kē-ə), 1. a white plaque formed on the oral mucous membrane from surface epithelial cells. It is leathery, opaque, and somewhat thickened. Excluded from this are the white lesions of lichen planus, white sponge nevus, burns, thrush, and other clinically recognizable entities. Histologically, hyperkeratosis, acanthosis, and subepithelial and perivascular infiltrate of round cells may be seen. Dyskeratosis may be present. Leukoplakia lesions may progress to malignancy, with cellular atypicism, dyskeratosis, epithelial pearl formation, and infiltration of malignant cells into connective tissue corium. 2. a premalignant surface lesion of the mucous membrane characterized by hyperkertosis and dyskeratosis of the stratified squamous epithelium. See also **dyskeratosis; hyperkeratosis.**

l., hairy, a white lesion appearing on the tongue, occasionally on the buccal mucosa, of patients with AIDS; the lesion appears raised, with a corrugated or "hairy" surface as a result of keratin projections.

leukotaxine (loo'kōtak'sin), a substance that appears when tissue is injured and can be removed from inflammatory exudates. Increases capillary permeability and the diapedesis of leukocytes. (not current)

lev-. See **levo-.**

levamisole HCl, *trade name:* Ergamisol; *drug class:* immunomodulator; *action:* may increase the action of macrophages, monocytes, and T cells, which will restore immune function; *uses:* Dukes' stage C colon cancer, given with fluoruracil after surgical resection.

levarterenol, the official (USP) drug name for norepinephrine. The British (BP) name is noradrenaline. In contrast to epinephrine, levarterenol produces its pressor effect primarily through vasoconstriction in certain areas rather than by cardiac excitatory action. See also **norepinephrine.** (not current)

level (lev'əl), to reduce the curve of Spee by intrusion and/or extrusion of the teeth in an arch.

leveling arch wire, an arch wire used to align teeth in the same plane.

lever (lev'er), a bar or rigid body that is capable of turning about one joint or axis and in which are two or more other points where forces are applied. There are three classes of levers, and each has its own most effective use.

l. leverage (lev'ərij), the mechanical advantage gained by the use of a lever. A factor in the magnification of stresses generated by an extension-base partial denture.

l., second-class, a lever in which the force arm is longer than the work-producing arm; thus the work produced is always greater than the energy used, with a resultant high efficiency.

l., third-class, a lever in which the axis is at one end, the load at the other end, and the effort is exerted in between, as in a treadle.

levo- (lev), a prefix applied to the name of optical isomers that rotate the plane of polarized light to the left.

levobunolol hydrochloride, *trade name:* Akbeta, Betagan C Cap BID, Betagan C Cap QD, Betagan Standard; *drug class:* β-adrenergic blocker; *action:* reduces production of aqueous humor by unknown mechanisms; *uses:* chronic open-angle glaucoma, ocular hypertension.

levocabastine HCl, *trade name:* Livostin; *drug class:* antihistamine, H_1-receptor antagonist; *action:* selective antagonist for histamine at H_1 receptors; little or no systemic absorption; intended for topical effect; *uses:* temporary relief of seasonal allergic conjunctivitis.

levodopa, *trade names:* Larodopa, Dopar; *class drug:* antiparkinson agent; *action:* levodopa is decarboxylated to dopamine, which can interact with dopamine receptors; *uses:* parkinsonisn or parkinsonian symptoms.

levodopa-carbidopa, *trade names:* Sinemet, Sinemet CR; *drug class:* antiparkinson agent; *action:* decarboxylation of levodopa to periphery is inhibited by carbidopa; more levodopa is made available for transport to brain and conversion to dopamine in the brain; *uses:* treatment of idiopathic, symptomatic, or postencephalitic parkinsonism.

levomethadyl acetate HCl, *trade name:* ORLAAM; *drug class:* synthetic opioid; *action:* mimics the action of opioid analgesics by interacting with CNS opioid receptors; *use:* management of opioid dependence.

levonorgestrel implant, *trade name:* Norplant System; *drug class:* contraceptive system; *action:* as a progestin, transforms proliferative endometrium into secretory endometrium; inhibits secretion of pituitary gonadotropins, which prevents follicular maturation and ovulation; *use:* prevention of pregnancy.

levothyroxine sodium, *trade names:* Levo-T, Synthroid; *drug class:* thyroid hormone; *action:* increases metabolic rate, with increase in cardiac output, O_2 consumption, body temperature, blood volume, growth/development at cellular level; *uses:* hypothroidism, myxedema coma, thyroid hormone replacement, cretinism.

Leydig cells, cells of the interstitial tissue of the testes that secrete testosterone.

liabilities, all the claims against a corporation. Liabilities include accounts and wages and salaries payable, dividends declared payable, accrued taxes payable, and fixed or long-term liabilities such as mortgage bonds, debentures, and bank loans.

l., current, short-term debts and obligations that must be paid within a period of 1 year.

liability (līəbil′itē), the state of being bound by law or justice to do something or to make something good; legal responsibility.

libel (lī′bəl), **1.** that which is written and published, calculated to injure the character of another by ridicule or contempt. **2.** defamation expressed by print, writing, pictures, or signs.

library, a place established to contain books, manuscripts, and other material for reading, study, viewing, listening, or reference, usually consisting of organized stacks and files to contain reference materials as well as places to read, copy, view, or listen to the selected material.

license, permission, accorded by a competent authority, granting the right to perform some act or acts that without such authorization would be contrary to law.

licensure, the granting of permission by a competent authority (usually a government agency) to an organization or individual to engage in a practice or activity that would otherwise be illegal. Licensure is usually granted on the basis of education and examination rather than performance. It is usually permanent, but a periodic fee, demonstration of competence, or continuing education may be required. Licensure may be revoked by the granting agency for incompetence, criminal acts, or other reasons stipulated in the statutes or rules governing the specific area of licensure.

l., dental, the permission to practice dentistry in a specific geopolitical area, granted by a government agency.

lichen planus (lī′kən plā′nəs), **1.** a disease of unknown etiology affecting the skin and oral mucous membranes, either alone or concomitantly. The oral lesions are most common on the buccal mucous membrane, where they appear as a lacy pattern or bilateral network of raised white or bluish-white, porcelain-like fine lines or a series of small, similarly appearing dots. The lesions are painless. On the tongue the lesions may appear as flat white plaques resembling leukoplakia. **2.** a dermatologic disease affecting the skin and mucous membranes; of unknown etiology but often associated with nervousness, fatigue, emotional depression, and allergy and considered to be a manifestation of quinacrine (Atabrine) therapy. Oral lesions often appear as white or blue-white striae forming an interweaving lacelike network of lines of epithelial thickening. Associated with the striated network; bullous or erosive lesions may be found. Histologically, varying degrees of hyperkeratosis and epithelial acanthosis may be found, with formation of sawtooth-shaped rete pegs of epithelium projecting into connective tissue corium. Subjacent to the epithelium is a bandlike infiltrate of round cells with perivascular accumulation of leukocytes. Treatment is symptomatic.

l. p., oral. See **lichen planus.**

lidocaine HCl (cardiac), *trade names:* Lidopen, Xylocaine, Xylocard; *drug class:* antidysrhythmic (Class IB); *action:* increases electrical stimulation threshold of ventricle and His-Purkinje system, which stabilizes cardiac membrane and decreases automaticity and excitability of ventricles; *uses:* ventricular tachycardia, ventricular dysrhythmias during cardiac surgery, cardiac catheterization.

lidocaine HCl (local), *trade names:* Dalcaine, Dilocaine, Lidoject, Octocain, Xylocaine, Xylocaine-MPF; *drug class:* amide local anesthetic; *action:* inhibits ion fluxes across membranes, particularly sodium transport across cell membrane; decreases rise of depolarization phase of action potential; blocks nerve action potential; *uses:* local dental anesthesia, peripheral nerve block; caudal anesthesia; epidural, spinal, surgical anesthesia.

lidocaine HCl (topical) *generic name:* Xylocaine Viscous; *drug class:* topically acting local anesthetic, amide; *action:* inhibits nerve impulses from sensory nerves, which produces anesthesia; *uses:* topical anesthesia of inflamed or irritated mucous membranes; to reduce gag reflex in dental radiologic examination or in dental impressions.

lien (lē-in), a qualified right of property that a creditor has in specific property of the debtor as security for the debt or for performance of some act.

life, effective half-. See **half-life, effective.**

life expectancy, the probable number of years a person will live after a given age, as determined by the mortality rate in a specific geographic area. This number may be individually qualified by the person's condition, race, sex, age, and other demographic factors.

life, radioactive. See **half-life.**

ligament (lig'əment), any tough, fibrous connective tissue band that connects bones or supports viscera. Some of the ligaments are distinct fibrous structures; others are folds of fascia or of indurated peritoneum; still others are the relics of unused fetal organs.

l., biologic width of periodontal, the width of the periodontal ligament in normal, functioning teeth. It varies with the age of the individual and the functional demands made on the tooth. In normalcy, the periodontal ligament is about 0.25 and 0.1 mm in width, narrowest at the center of the alveolus and widest at the margin and apex.

l., periodontal (PDL), the mode of attachment of the tooth to the alveolus. The ligament consists of numerous bundles of collagenous tissue (principal fibers) arranged in groups, between which is loose connective tissue, together with blood vessels, lymph vessels, and nerves. It functions as the investing and supportive mechanism for the tooth.

l., sphenomandibular, the ligament extending from the spine of the sphenoid bone to the mandibular lingula.

l., stylohyoid, a fibroelastic cord attached superior to the styloid process of the sphenoid bone.

l., stylomandibular, a ligament extending from the styloid process of the temporal bone and attached to the mandibular gonial angle.

l., temporomandibular, a triangular-shaped fibrous band extending from the lateral aspects of the root of the zygomatic process of the temporal bone to the mandibular subcondylar neck.

ligand, I. a molecule, ion, or group bound to the central atom of a chemical compound such as the oxygen molecule in hemoglobin, which is bound to the central iron atom. **2.** an organic molecule attached to a specific site on a surface or to a tracer element.

ligate (lī'gāt), to tie or bind with a ligature or suture.

ligation (līgā'shən), the binding together of tissue or teeth with wire, string, or thread for stabilization and immobilization.

l., surgical, the exposure of an unerupted tooth with placement of a metal ligature around its cervix. The free ends of the ligature are fixed to a fine, precious-metal chain, which in turn is fixed to an orthodontic appliance for the purpose of placing traction on the unerupted tooth to cause its eruption.

ligature (lig'əchər), I. a cord, thread, or fine wire tied around teeth for the purpose of holding a rubber dam in place on retained teeth with fractured roots or split crowns or on teeth that have been replanted. **2.** a wire or threadlike substance used to tie a tooth to an orthodontic appliance or to another tooth.

l., grass-line, a ligature composed of the fibers of a grass-cloth plant (ramie); used for minor tooth movement. It depends for its activation in movement on the property of shrinkage of the ligature when it is wet by the saliva of the patient.

l., steel, a form of ligature, available as steel filaments in several useful diameters.

light, I. electromagnetic radiation of the wavelength and frequency that stimulate visual receptor cells in the retina to produce nerve impulses that are perceived as vision. **2.** visible light ranges from 400 to 800 nm.

l. box. See **illuminator.**

l., operating, a light with a strong beam that may be directed for concentrated illumination of a part being operated on.

l. pen, a pointerlike device available with some computer terminals. A light pen selects data displayed on the screen by being pointed at any desired item.

l. touch. See **touch, light.**

lighting, the arrangement of a light source to create a certain effect. The lighting of a dental operatory is done to achieve a sufficient level of lighting to reduce eye strain in shifting from one field of vision to another and to achieve a light intensity across the spectrum to mimic natural light.

limbic system, a group of structures within the rhinencephalon of the brain that are associated with various emotions and feelings, such as anger, fear, sexual arousal, pleasure, and sadness. Unless the limbic system is modulated by other cortical areas, periodic attacks of uncontrollable rage may occur in some individuals. The function of the system is poorly understood.

limit, restriction.

l., elastic (proportional limit), the greatest stress to which a material may be subjected and still be capable of returning to its original dimensions when the forces are released.

l., proportional. See **limit, elastic.**

limitations, restrictive conditions stated in a dental benefits contract, such as age, length of time covered, and waiting periods, which affect an individual's or group's coverage. The contract may also exclude certain benefits or services, or it may limit the extent or condition under which certain services are provided. See also **exclusions.**

limited treatment, treatment directed at a limited objective; not involving the entire dentition. It may be directed at the only existing problem, or at only one aspect of a larger problem in which a decision is made to defer more comprehensive therapy.

lincomycin, *trade names:* Lincocin, Lincorex; *drug class:* antibacterial; *action:* binds to 50S subunit of bacterial ribosomes; suppresses protein synthesis; *uses:* infections caused by group A β-hemolytic streptococci, pneumococci, staphylococci (respiratory tract, skin, soft tissue, urinary tract infections; osteomyelitis; septicemia), and anaerobes. Lincomycin should be reserved for pencillin-allergic patients. Close clinical supervision is required because severe colitis has been associated with lincomycin therapy. Brand name: Lincocin.

lindane, γ-benzene hexachloride prescribed in the treatment of pediculosis and scabies.

line, a boundary; demarcation.

l. angle. See **angle, line.**

l., basophilic, a group of microscopic sections of bone that stains darkly with hematoxylin. Represents periods of bone inactivity.

l., Camper's, the line running from the inferior border of the ala of the nose to the superior border of the tragus of the ear.

l., cement, the line of cement exposed at the margin of an inlay or crown.

l., cemental (cementing line), a basophilic line distinguishing adjacent lamellae of bone; represents periods of inactivity of bone formation and resorption.

l., cementing. See **line, cemental.**

l., cervical. See **junction, cemento-enamel.**

l., cross arch fulcrum. See **line, fulcrum, cross arch.**

l., external oblique, a ridge of osseous structure on the body of the mandible extending from the anterolateral border to the mandibular ramus, passing downward and forward, after covering the buccocervical portion of the third molar, and ending by blending into the molar teeth.

l., finish, in cavity preparations, a minimal line of demarcation at the wall of the preparation at the cavosurface angle; usually results from a slice made by an abrasive disk.

l. focus, a principle employed in the design of x-ray tubes, by which the effective focal spot is sharply reduced relative to the actual (larger) focal spot desirable to deal with the heat generated. It involves focusing the cathode stream, in the pattern of a thin rectangle, onto an anode truncated at about 20 degrees to the transverse axis of the tube. See also **spot, focal, effective.**

l., fulcrum, any imaginary line around which a removable partial denture tends to rotate.

l., f., anteroposterior, an imaginary line of rotation extending through the rest and other support areas along the same side of a removable partial denture.

l., f., cross arch, an imaginary line through the tooth-supported rest areas nearest to soft tissue-supported areas and around which the partial denture will tend to rotate when forces are applied to the soft tissue-supported areas.

l., lead, a bluish-black patch on the gingival tissues, usually about 1 mm from the gingival crest. Caused by the deposition of fine granules of lead sulfide in the tissues. A sign of lead absorption in lead poisoning (plumbism).

l., median, the intersection of the midsagittal plane with the maxillary and mandibular dental arches. The center line divides the central body surface into right and left.

l., mercurial, a linear area of abnormal pigmentation of the gingival tissues associated with mercury poisoning. Seen along the gingival margin, it has been variously described as bluish, brownish, dirty reddish, or purplish in coloration.

l. of credit, an arrangement whereby a financial institution (bank or insurance company) commits itself to lend up to a specified maximum amount of funds during a specified period. Sometimes the interest rate on the loan is specified; at other times it is not. Sometimes a commitment fee is imposed for obtaining the line of credit.

l. of draw, the direction or plane of withdrawal or seating of a removable or cemented restoration.

l. of force. See **force, line of.**

l. of occlusion, the alignment of the occluding surfaces of the teeth in the horizontal plane. See also **plane, occlusal line.**

l. printer, a fast printing device. A line printer prints on paper each line of characters in one operation, rather than character by character.

l., protrusive, one of the three tracings made on each of the six projection planes of a jaw motion data recorder.

l., survey, a line produced on the various portions of a dental cast by a surveyor, scriber, or marker. It designates the greatest height of contour in relation to the orientation of the cast to the vertical scriber.

l., vibrating, the imaginary line across the posterior part of the palate marking the division between the movable and relatively immovable tissues of the palate.

linea alba buccalis, a normal variation in the buccal mucosa that appears as a white line beginning at the corners of the mouth and extending posteriorly at the level of the occlusal plane.

linear energy transfer (LET), the linear rate of loss of energy by an ionizing particle traversing a material medium.

linear models, statistical models in which the value of a parameter for a given value of a factor is assumed to be equal to $a + bx$, where a and b are constants. The models predict a linear regression.

linen strip. See **strip, abrasive.**

liner, cavity. See **varnish, cavity.**

lines, elongated marks traced by a stylus on a gnathic projection plane, indicating direction of movement related variously to condyle movements.

lingua alba. See **tongue, white hairy.** (not current)

lingual (ling'gwəl), pertaining to the tongue.

l. appliances, orthodontic appliances that apply force from the lingual aspect of the anterior teeth. This mode of treatment is used to reduce the visibility of the appliance and thus improve the appearance of the smile during treatment.

l. arch, a space-holding arch or the basic arch for an active lingual orthodontic appliance. The arch usually spans around the inside of the dental arch from one first permanent molar to its antimere.

l. bar, major connector See connector, major, lingual bar.

l. button, an attachment welded to the lingual side of the canine, premolar, or molar bands.

l. frenum, a band of tissue that extends from the floor of the mouth to the inferior surface of the tongue.

l. nerve. See **nerve(s).**

l. peak, gingival, a lingual peak that characterizes the normal interproximal tissue, which is composed of a lingual papilla and a buccal papilla connected interdentally in a triangular ridge depression termed a *col.*

l. plate. See **connector, major, linguoplate.**

lingua nigra. See **tongue, black hairy.** (not current)

lingua villosa alba. See **tongue, white hairy.** (not current)

lingula (ling'gyələ), a small, tonguelike projection of bone forming the anterior border of the mandibular foramen.

linguocclusion (ling·gwŏklōō′zhən), an occlusion in which the dental arch or group of teeth is lingual to normal.

linguoplate. See **connector, major, linguoplate.**

linguoversion, the state of being displaced toward the tongue.

linkage (lingk′ij), the connection between two or more objects. In computer programming, coding that connects two separately coded routines.

l., cross. See **polymerization, cross.**

l., sex, the inheritance of certain characteristics that are determined by genes located in the sex chromosomes.

linoleic acid, an unsaturated fatty acid essential to nutrition. Linoleic acid occurs in many plant glycerides.

liothyronine sodium (T₃), *trade names:* Cytomel, Triostat; *drug class:* thyroid hormone; *action:* increases metabolic rate with increase in cardiac output, O₂ consumption, body temperature, blood volume, growth/development at cellular level; *uses:* hypothyroidism, myxedema coma, thyroid hormone replacement, cretinism, nontoxic goiter.

liotrix, *trade names:* Euthroid, Thyrolar; *drug class:* thyroid hormone; *action:* increases metabolic rates, cardiac output, O₂ consumption, body temperature, blood volume, growth/development at cellular level; *uses:* hypothyroidism, thyroid hormone replacement.

lip, 1. either the upper or lower fleshy structure surrounding the opening of the oral cavity. **2.** any rimlike structure bordering a cavity or groove.

l. biting, an oral habit in which either lip is placed between the teeth with more or less forcible application of the teeth to the lips.

l., cleft. See **harelip.**

l., congenital cleft. See **harelip.**

l., double, a redundant fold of tissue on the mucosal side of the upper lip that gives the appearance of a second lip and that may become accentuated by habitually being sucked between the teeth.

l. line, high, the greatest height to which the lip is raised in normal func-

tion or during the act of smiling broadly.

l. line, low, the lowest position of the lower lip during the act of smiling or voluntary retraction. The lowest position of the upper lip at rest.

l. pits (congenital lip fistulas), congenital depressions, usually bilateral and symmetrically placed, on the vermilion portion of the lower lip. These pits may be circular or may be present as a transverse slit. The depression represents a blind fistula that penetrates downward into the lower lip to a depth of 0.5 to 2.5 cm. They often exude viscid saliva on pressure.

l. retractor, an apparatus to retract the lips when taking intraoral photographs.

lipase, any fat-splitting or lipolytic enzyme.

lipid (lip′id), a heterogeneous group of substances related actually or potentially to the fatty acids that are soluble in nonpolar solvents such as benzene, chloroform, and ether and are relatively insoluble in water. Included are the fatty acids, acylglycerols, phospholipids, cerebrosides, and steroids.

l., plasma, the various plasma lipid classes include triacylglycerols, phospholipids, cholesterol, cholesterol esters, and unesterified fatty acids. Because of their hydrophobic nature, plasma lipids are carried in association with specific plasma proteins, the lipoproteins.

lipidosis (lip′idō′sis). See **disease, lipid storage.**

Lipiodol (lipē′ōdəl), the trade name for an iodized oil used as an opaque contrast medium in radiography. When it is laced within periodontal pockets and radiographs are made, the depth and topography of periodontal pockets may be ascertained.

lipodystrophy, any abnormality in the metabolism or deposition of fats.

lipoids (lip′oidz), a fatlike substance that may not actually be related to the fatty acids, although lipid and lipoid are occasionally used synonymously.

lipoma (lipō′mə), a benign tumor characterized by fat cells.

lipophilic (lipōfil′ik), **1.** showing a marked attraction to, or solubility in, lipids. **2.** having an affinity for oil or fat.

lipopolysaccharides, a compound or complex of lipid and carbohydrate.

lipoproteins, biochemical compounds that contain both lipid and protein. Most lipids in plasma are present in the form of lipoproteins.

liposomes, multilayered spherical particles of a lipid in an aqueous medium within a cell.

lipoxygenase, an enzyme that catalyzes the oxidation of unsaturated fatty acids with O_2 to form peroxides of the fatty acids.

Lipschutz body. See **body, Lipschutz.** (not current)

lisinopril, *trade name:* Zestril; *drug class:* angiotensin-converting enzyme (ACE) inhibitor; *action:* selectively suppresses renin-angiotensin-aldosterone system; inhibits ACE, which prevents conversion of angiotensin I to angiotensin II; *uses:* mild-to-moderate hypertension, post myocardial infarction if hemodynamically stable.

literature, the entire body of writings on a given subject.

l., dental, the entire body of writing on dentistry. Most specifically, those writings published following a referee process to validate the scientific discipline in which the writings were produced.

lithium carbonate/lithium citrate, *trade names:* Eskalith, Lithane, Lithobid, Lithotabs Cibalith-S; *drug class:* antimanic, inorganic salt; *action:* may alter sodium and potassium ion transport across cell membrane in nerve, muscle cells; may affect both norephinephrine and serotonin in CNS; *uses:* manic depressive illness (manic phase), prevention of bipolar manic depressive psychosis.

litigation, the act or process of engaging in a lawsuit.

live birth, the birth of an infant, irrespective of the duration of gestation, that exhibits any sign of life, such as respiration, heartbeat, umbilical pulsation, or movement of voluntary muscles. A live birth is not always a viable birth.

liver, the largest gland of the body and one of the body's most complex organs. More than 500 functions of the liver have been identified. It is divided into four lobes, contains as many as 100,000 lobules, and is served by two distinct blood supplies. The hepatic artery conveys oxygenated blood to the liver, and the hepatic portal vein conveys nutrient-filled blood from the stomach and the intestines. At any given moment the liver holds about one pint of blood or approximately 13% of the total blood supply of the body.

l. cirrhosis, a degenerative disease of the liver in which hepatic tissue is replaced with connective tissue, commonly a result of chronic alcoholism.

l. failure, a condition in which the liver fails to fulfill its function or is unable to meet the demand made on it. Liver failure may occur as a result of trauma, neoplastic invasion, prolonged biliary obstruction, viral infections, or chronic alcoholism.

LJP. See **localized juvenile periodontitis.**

load, an external force applied to an object.

l., occlusal, the stresses generated by functional or habitual contacting of the occlusal surfaces of the upper and lower teeth. There are two components of such stress loads: the vertically directed components and those components that tend to move a tooth or denture laterally. See also **force, occlusal.**

loading, the amount included in the premiums to meet liabilities beyond anticipated claims payments to provide administrative costs and contributions to reserve funds and to cover contingencies such as unexpected loss or adverse fluctuation.

lobbying, the act of influencing, by argumentation, the course of action of a legislator.

lobectomy (lōbek′təmē), the excision of a lobe of an organ such as the submandibular gland or the lung.

Lobstein's disease (lob′stīnz). See **osteogenesis imperfecta.**

local analgesia, the loss of pain sensation over a specific area, caused by local administration of a drug that blocks nerve conduction.

localization, a direct, exact site or restriction to a limited area, such as localization of abscess.

l., radiographic, determination, by means of radiographs, of the location of an object or structure in the body or head. Usually accomplished by obtaining radiographs made from different angulations to the part in question.

l., tactile, the property of localization associated with the sense of touch. Perception of the location of a stimulus is more precise in the regions of the lips and the fingertips than elsewhere. This more precise perception results from a greater density of special touch receptors in a given area.

localized juvenile periodontitis (LJP), a localized periodontal tissue breakdown in young children in the primary or mixed dentition stage, apparently resulting from gingival pocket infection with *Haemophilus actinomycetemcomitans.* See also **juvenile periodontitis.**

location, practice, the geographic spot in which equipment is set up to practice dentistry.

locking gate, a portion of the peripheral frame of a maxillary subperiosteal implant; attached by a hinge. This device permits the implant to be placed into an area of undercut. After the implant is seated, the gate is closed and locked, and wire is wrapped around two locking buttons.

lockpin, a soft metal pin used to attach an archwire to an orthodontic bracket.

locomotion, the act or power to move from one place to another.

locomotor ataxia. See **tabes dorsalis.**

locus, gene, the position of a gene on the chromosome.

locus minoris resistentiae (lō′kəs minor′is rēsisten′chē·ā), an area offering little resistance to invasion by microorganisms and/or their toxins. The junction between reduced enamel epithelium and oral epithelium within the epithelial wall of the gingival sulcus has been described as a weak link, providing a portal of entry for microorganisms and their toxins with initiation of pocket formation.

Lod score, "Logarithm of the odds" score, which measures the likelihood of two genes being within measurable distance of each other.

lodoxamide tromethamine, *trade name:* Alomide; *drug class:* mast cell stabilizer; *action:* prevents release of mediators of inflammation from mast cells involved with Type 1 immediate hypersensitivity reactions; *uses:* ver-

nal keratoconjunctivitis, vernal conjunctivits, keratitis.

loempe (lem′pē). See **beriberi.** (not current)

logic, a disciplined method of reasoning or argumentation that employs the principles governing correct or reliable inference.

logistic models, statistical models that describe the relationship between a qualitative dependent variable (that is, one that can take only certain discrete values, such as the presence or absence of a disease) and an independent variable. A common application is in epidemiology for estimating an individual's risk (probability of contracting a disease) as a function of a given risk factor.

logopedics (log′ōpē′diks), the study and treatment of speech defects in children, involving habilitation or rehabilitation of speech.

lomefloxacin HCl, *trade name:* Maxaquin; *drug class:* fluoroquinolone antiinfective; *action:* a broad-spectrum bactericidal agent that inhibits the enzyme DNA gyrase needed for DNA synthesis; *uses:* lower respiratory tract infections (pneumonia, bronchitis); genitourinary infections (prostatitis); preoperatively to reduce UTIs in transurethral surgical procedures due to susceptible gram negative organisms.

lomustine, *trade name:* CeeNU; *drug class:* antineoplastic alkylating agent; *action:* interferes with RNA and DNA strands, which leads to cell death; *uses:* Hodgkin's disease; lymphomas; melanomas; multiple myeloma; brain, lung, bladder, kidney, colon cancer.

longevity, the length of life.

long face syndrome, a malocclusion characterized by a long, narrow face; steep mandibular plane angle; and Class II Division 1 dental/skeletal relationship with anterior crowding and associated mouth breathing. A contemporary name for adenoid facies.

longitudinal studies, epidemiologic studies that record data from a representative sample at repeated intervals over an extended span of time rather than at a single or limited number over a short period.

long-term care (LTC), the provision of medical, social, and personal care services on a recurring or continuing basis to persons with chronic physical or mental disorders.

loop, programming, a programming technique whereby a group of instructions is repeated with modification of some of the instructions in the group and/or with modification of the data being operated on.

loop, vertical, a U-shaped bend in the archwire that aids in the opening or closing of spaces in the arch.

loose premaxilla. See **premaxilla, loose.**

loperamide HCl, *trade names:* Diaraid, Imodium, Imodium AD, Kaopectate II, Maalox Antidiarrheal, Neo-Diaral, Pepto Diarrhea Control; *drug class:* antidiarrheal (opioid); *action:* direct action on intestinal muscles to decrease gastrointestinal peristalsis; *uses:* diarrhea (cause undetermined), chronic diarrhea, ileostomy discharge.

loracarbef, *trade name:* Lorabid; *drug class:* antibiotic, 2nd-generation cephalosporin; *action:* inhibits bacterial cell wall synthesis, which renders cell wall osmotically unstable; *uses:* gram-negative *Haemophilus influenzae, Escherichia coli, Proteus mirabilis, Klebsiella;* gram-positive *Streptococcus pneumoniae, Staphylococcus pyogenes, Staphylococcus aureus.*

loratadine, *trade name:* Claritin; *drug class:* antihistamine, H_1 histamine antagonist; *action:* acts on blood vessels, gastrointestinal system, respiratory system by competing with histamine for H_1-receptor site; decreases allergic response by blocking histamine; *uses:* seasonal rhinitis, allergy symptoms, idiopathic chronic urticaria.

Lorazepam, *trade name:* Ativan, Lorazepam Intensol; *drug class:* benzodiazepine antianxiety (Controlled Substance Schedule IV); *action:* depresses subcortical levels of the central nervous system, including limbic system and reticular formation; *uses:* anxiety, preoperative sedation, acute alcohol withdrawal symptoms, muscle spasm.

lordosis (lôrdō′sis), an anteroposterior curvature of the spine with the convexity facing forward.

losartan potassium, *trade name:* Cozaar; *drug class:* angiotensin II receptor antagonist; *action:* blocks the vasoconstrictor and aldosterone-secreting effects of angiotensin II; *use:* hypertension, as a single drug or in combination with other antihypertensives.

loss of bone. See **resorption of bone.**

loss ratio, the relationship between the money paid out in benefits and the amount collected in premiums.

loupe, binocular (loop), a magnifier that consists of lenses in an optical frame; it is worn like spectacles and is used with both eyes.

lovastatin, *trade name:* Mevacor; *drug class:* cholesterol-lowering agent; *action:* inhibits HMG-CoA reductase enzyme, which reduces cholesterol synthesis; *uses:* adjunct in primary hypercholesterolemia, mixed hyperlipidemia.

lower ridge slope. See **slope, lower ridge.** (not current)

low lip line. See **lip line, low.**

loxapine succinate/loxapine HCl, *trade name:* Loxitane; *drug class:* antipsychotic; *action:* depresses cerebral cortex, hypothalamus, limbic system, all of which control activity and aggression; blocks neurotransmission produced by dopamine at synapse; *uses:* psychotic disorders.

lozenge (läz′enj) (troche), a medicated, disk-shaped tablet designed to dissolve slowly in the mouth.

lubrication, the application of an agent, usually an oil or grease, to diminish friction.

luciferase, an enzyme present in certain luminous organisms that act to bring about the oxidation of luciferins; energy produced in the process is liberated as bioluminescence.

luciferin, a chemical substance present in certain luminous organisms that, when acted upon by the enzyme luciferase, produces a glow called *bioluminescence.*

Ludwig's angina (lood′vigz). See **angina, Ludwig's.**

luetic (loo-et′ik), pertaining to or affected by syphilis.

lumbosacral region, that area of the back that approximates level of the lumbar and sacral vertebrae. The lower third of the back.

lumen (loo′mən), the space within a tube structure, such as a blood vessel, tube, or duct.

luminescence, 1. the emission of light by a material after excitation by some stimulus. **2.** the emission of light by intensifying screen phosphors after x-ray interaction.

lung, one of a pair of light, spongy organs in the thorax, constituting the main component of the respiratory system. The lungs provide the tissue surface necessary for the exchange of gases between the environment and the blood. Oxygen is extracted from inspired air, and carbon dioxide is dispersed from the venous system back into the environment.

l. abscess, a complication of an inflammation and infection of the lung, often caused by aspiration of infected material from the mouth.

lupus (lōō'pəs), a disease of the skin and mucous membrane.

l. erythematosus (systemic lupus erythematosus, disseminated lupus erythematosus), A chronic inflammatory disease of unknown etiology affecting skin, joints, kidneys, nervous system, serous membranes, and often other organs of the body. The classical facial "butterfly rash" facilitates diagnosis, although the rash need not be present. Other skin areas, particularly those exposed to the sun, may be involved by a scaly lesion that is referred to as *discoid lupus erythematosus.*

l. erythematosus, discoid, a form of lupus erythematosus in which only cutaneous lesions are present; these commonly appear on the face as atrophic plaques with erythema, hyperheratosis, follicular plugging, and telangiectasia.

l. vulgaris, cutaneous tuberculosis with characteristic nodular lesions on the face, particularly about the nose and ears.

luting agents, agents that bond, seal, or cement particles or objects together.

luxate, to be forced out of place or joint; to be displaced; to dislocate.

luxation, 1. the act of luxating or state of being luxated, as in the dislocation or displacement of a tooth or of the temporomandibular joint. **2.** the dislocation or displacement of a tooth or of the temporomandibular articulation.

Lyme disease, an acute, recurrent inflammatory infection transmitted by a tick-borne spirochete, *Borrelia burg-*

dorferi. Knees, other large joints, and temporomandibular joints are most commonly involved, with local inflammation and swelling. Chills, fever, headache, malaise, and erythema chronicum migrans (ECM), which is an expanding annular, erythematous skin eruption, often precede the joint manifestations.

lymph, a thin opalescent fluid originating in organs and tissues of the body and that circulates through the lymphatic vessels and is filtered by the lymph nodes.

l. node, one of the many small oval structures that filter the lymph and fight infection, and in which there are formed lymphocytes, monocytes, and plasma cells.

lymphadenitis, 1. an inflammation of a lymph node or nodes. **2.** an inflammation of the lymph glands, characterized chiefly by swelling, pain, and redness.

lymphadenopathy, any disease process that involves a lymph node or nodes.

l., generalized, the involvement of all or several regionally separated groups of lymph nodes by a systemic disorder.

l., regional, the involvement of nodes draining a specific region (for example, submental nodes draining the middle of the lower lip, floor of the mouth, skin of the chin).

lymphangioma (limfanjē-ō'mə), a benign neoplasm characterized by lymph vessel proliferation. A benign tumor of the lymph vessels.

l., cystic. See **hygroma, cystic.**

lymphatic system, a vast, complex network of capillaries, thin vessels, valves, ducts, nodes, and organs that helps to protect and maintain the internal fluid environment of the entire body by producing, filtering, and conveying lymph and by producing various blood cells.

lymphoblastoma, giant follicular *(Brill-Symmers disease),* a malignant disease characterized by enlargement of the spleen and lymph nodes throughout the body. Lymphoblasts and reticular cells proliferate within lymphoid follicles, producing an increase in both the number and size of germinal follicles.

lymphocyte (lim'fōsīt), a form of white blood cell originating in lymphoid tissues; possesses a single spherical nucleus and a nongranular cytoplasm. The lymphocytes comprise 25% of the white blood cells. Some lymphocytes, along with plasma cells and histiocytes, are found in clinically normal gingivae. Their numbers within the gingival connective tissue are increased in gingivitis and periodontitis. With progress of gingival inflammation to the underlying bone, lymphocytes are found within the marrow spaces of the supporting bone.

lymphocytes-B, a short-lived, non-thymus-dependent form of lymphocytes that synthesize antibodies for insertion into their own cytoplasmic membranes. They are the precursor of the plasma cells.

lymphocytes-T, long-lived lymphocytes that have circulated through the thymus gland and have differentiated to become thymocytes. When exposed to an antigen, they divide rapidly and produce large numbers of new T cells sensitized to that antigen. Some T cells are often called "killer cells" because they secrete immunologically essential chemical compounds and assist B cells in destroying foreign protein. T cells also appear to play a significant role in the body's resistance to the proliferation of cancer cells.

lymphocytopenia (lim'fōsī'tōpē'nē-ə), a decrease in the normal number of lymphocytes in the circulating blood. Various limits are given (for example, a total number less than 600/mm³). It may be associated with agranulocytosis, hyperadrenocorticism, leukemia, advanced Hodgkin's disease, irradiation, and acute infections with neutrophilia.

lymphocytosis (lim'fōsītō'sis), an absolute or relative increase in the normal number of lymphocytes in the circulating blood. Various limits are given; for example, absolute lymphocytosis is said to be present if the total number of cells exceeds 4500/mm³, whereas relative lymphocytosis is said to be present if the percentage of lymphocytes is greater than 45% and the total number of cells is less than 4500/mm³. Lymphocytosis may be associated with infancy, exophthalmic goiter, mumps, rubella, infectious mononucleosis, sunburn, lymphatic leukemia, pertussis, and pyogenic infections in childhood.

lymphoepithelial lesion, benign (lim'fō·ep·ithē'lē·ə). See **disease, Mikulicz'.**

lymphoepithelioma (lim'fō·ep'ithē' lē·ō'mə), a malignant neoplasm arising from the epithelium and lymphoid tissue of the nasopharynx and characterized by cells of both tissues; may occur in the palate.

lymphokines, soluble substances, released by sensitized lymphocytes on contact with specific antigens, which help effect cellular immunity by stimulating activity of monocytes and macrophages.

lymphoma (limfō'mə), any neoplasm made up of lymphoid tissue.

l., B-cell, a group of heterogenous lymphoid tumors generally expressing one or more B-cell antigens or representing malignant transformations of B-lymphocytes.

l., non-Hodgkins, any of a group of malignant tumors of a lymphoid tissue that differ from Hodgkins disease, being more heterogeneous with respect to malignant cell lineage, clinical course, prognosis, and therapy. The only feature shared by these tumors is the absence of Reed-Sternberg cells, which are characteristic of Hodgkins disease.

l., T-cell, adult T-cell leukemia; an acute or subacute disease associated with a human T-cell virus, with lymphadenopathy, hepatosplenomegaly, skin lesions, peripheral blood involvement, and hypercalcemia.

lymphoreticulosis, benign inoculation (lim'fōretik'yōōlō'sis). See **fever, cat-scratch.**

lymphosarcoma (lim'fōsarkō'mə), a malignant disease of the lymphoid tissues characterized by proliferation of atypical lymphocytes and their localization in various parts of the body. The jaws may be the sites of lymphosarcomas.

lypressin, *trade name:* Diapid; *drug class:* pituitary hormone; *action:* promotes reabsorption of water by action on collecting ducts in kidney; decreases urine excretion; *uses:* non-nephrogenic diabetes insipidus.

lysin (lī'sin). See **plasmin.**

lysine, one of the essential amino acids found in many proteins. An essential amino acid needed for proper growth in infants and for maintenance of nitrogen balance in adults. See also **amino acids.**

lysing effect. See **effect, lysing.** (not current)

lysis (līʹsis), the gradual abatement of the symptoms of a disease. The disintegration or dissolution of cells by a lysin.

lysokinase (līʹsōkiʹnās). See **fibrinokinase.** (not current)

lysozyme (līʹsōzīm), an enzyme in major salivary secretions that may rupture bacterial cell walls and may regulate the oral flora.

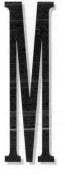

mA, the abbreviation for **milliampere.**

Macaca, a genus of Old World monkeys that include the macaque and rhesus monkeys and the barbary apes. *M. mulatta,* the rhesus monkey, is used as a research animal.

macaque. See **Macaca.**

macro, a prefix meaning excessively large or big.

macrocheilia (makʹrōkiʹlē-ə), abnormally large lip.

macrodontia (makrōdonʹshē-ə) (megadontismus), abnormally large teeth. One, several, or all teeth in a given individual may be involved.

macrogingivae (makʹrōjinʹjivā), abnormally large gingivae resulting from inflammation, heredity, scurvy, leukemia, neoplasia, diphenylhydantoin (Dilantin) therapy (in epilepsy), or hormonal stimulation of puberty or pregnancy. (not current)

macroglossia (makʹrōgläsʹē-ə), an enlarged tongue resulting from muscle hypertrophy, vascular or neurogenic tumor, or endocrine disturbance.

m., amyloid. See **tongue, amyloid.**

macroglossic, descriptive of macroglossia. (not current)

macrognathia (makʹrōnāʹthē-ə), a definite overgrowth of the maxillae and mandible.

macrognathic (makrōnāʹthik), descriptive of macrognathia.

macrolides, a class of antibiotics discovered in *Streptomyces,* characterized by molecules made up of large-ring lactones. An example is erythromycin.

macromolecule, any substance with molecules of colloidal size, notably proteins, nucleic acids, and polysaccharides.

macrophage (makʹrəfāj), any phagocytic cell of the reticuloendothelial system including specialized Kupfer's cells in the liver and spleen, and histiocytes in loose connective tissue. See also **histiocyte.**

m., alveolar, a dust cell, coniophage, a vigorously phagocytic macrophage on the epithelial surface of lung alveoli where it ingests inhaled particulate matter.

macroscopic, relating to macroscopy or the examination of areas such as surfaces of teeth without magnification.

macrosomia. See **giantism.**

macrostomia, an abnormally large oral opening.

macule, a lesion of the mucous membrane or cutaneous tissue that is not elevated above the surface.

magaldrate (aluminum magnesium complex), *trade names:* Lowsium, Riopan, Riopan Plus; *drug class:* antacid/aluminum/magnesium hydroxide; *action:* neutralizes gastric acidity; *use:* antacid for hyperacidity.

magnesium, an elemental metal with an atomic weight of 24.32. Magnesium is an essential nutritional substance. Deficiency produces irritability of the nervous system and trophic disturbances.

m. sulfate, a salt of magnesium; also called *Epsom salts,* used as a therapeutic bath and as a purgative.

magnetic disk, a storage device, consisting of magnetically coated disks, on the surface of which information is stored in the form of magnetic spots arranged in a manner to represent binary data.

magnetic resonance imaging (MRI), also known as *nuclear magnetic resonance imaging.* MRI is a diagnostic technique in which the phosphorus in cellular tissues is excited by magnetic force. The distribution and alignment of these cellular elements can be captured on phosphorus nuclear magnetic resonance instruments forming a high-resolution tissue image. A higher degree of resolution of soft tissues is possible using this technique than from radiographic techniques. The word *nuclear* has been dropped from the term because it makes an incorrect inference that radioactivity is involved in the imaging process.

magnetic tape, a continuous, flexible, recording medium whose basic material is impregnated or coated with a magnetic-sensitive material ready to accept data in the form of magnetically polarized spots.

maintenance, to keep in a functional state and/or in the proper location.

m., space. See **space maintainer.**

major connector. See **connector, major.**

major histocompatibility complex, the genetic region that contains the loci of genes that determine the structure of the serologically defined (SD) and lymphocyte-defined (LD) transplantation antigens, genes that control the structure of the immune response–associated (Ia) antigens, and the immune response (Ir) genes that control the ability of an animal to respond immunologically to antigenic stimuli.

making the turn, the step in the procedure of inserting and condensing foil in a Class 3 cavity preparation, at which the line of force is changed from an incisogingival direction to a gingivoincisal direction.

mal-, a prefix denoting a bad or unfavorable condition.

malaise (maʹlāz), a general feeling of discomfort or uneasiness, often the first indication of an infection or other disease.

malar (māʹlər), pertaining to the cheek or the zygomatic bone.

m. bone. See **bone, malar.**

malare, the midpoint of the intersection between the projection of the coronoid process and the lower contour of the malar bone. (not current)

malaria, a serious infectious illness caused by one or more of at least four species of the protozoan genus *Plasmodium,* characterized by chills,

fever, anemia, an enlarged spleen, and a tendency to recur. The disease is transmitted from human to human by a bite from an infected *Anopheles* mosquito.

Malassez, rests of. See **debris of Malassez.**

maldevelopment, an abnormal, imperfect, or deficient formation or development.

malfeasance (malfēʹzens), an act that one should not do at all or the unjust performance of some act that the party had no right to do.

malfunction, a disorder in function or performance, which may or may not be related to a malformation of tissues, organs, or organ systems. See also **dysfunction.**

malice, a state of mind that disregards the law and legal rights of others but that does not necessarily involve personal hate or ill will.

m. in the law of libel and slander, an evil intent arising from spite or ill will; willful and wanton disregard of the rights of the person defamed.

malignant (məligʹnənt), **1.** resistant to treatment. **2.** able to metastasize and kill the host.

m. hypertension, the most lethal form of hypertension. Malignant hypertension is a fulminating condition, characterized by severely elevated blood pressure that commonly damages the intima of small vessels, the brain, retina, heart, and kidneys. It affects more African Americans than white Americans and may be caused by a variety of factors such as stress, genetic predisposition, obesity, the use of tobacco, the use of oral contraceptives, high intake of sodium chloride, a sedentary lifestyle, and aging.

m. hyperthermia, an autosomal dominant trait characterized by often fatal hyperthermia with rigidity of muscles occurring in affected people exposed to certain anesthetic agents, particularly halothane and succinylcholine.

malingering, the feigning of illness.

malleability (malʹē-ə-bilʹitē), the ability of a material to withstand permanent deformation under compressive forces without rupture.

mallet, a hammer instrument.

m., hard, a small hammer with a leather-, rubber-, fiber-, or metal-faced head; used to supply force or to supplement hand force for the compaction of foil or amalgam and to seat cast restorations.

malnutrition, any disorder concerning nutrition. It may result from a poor diet or from impaired utilization of foods ingested.

malocclusion (relationship of teeth in occlusion), a deviation in intramaxillary and/or intermaxillary relations of teeth that presents a hazard to the individual's well-being. Often associated with other dentofacial deformities. See also **Angle's classification.**

m., deflective, a type of malocclusion occurring in persons who cannot close all their teeth while holding their condyles in the rearmost position. Instead, in closure they first contact one or two pairs of poorly coupled teeth. To gain occlusal contacts of the other teeth, they must move the jaw anteriorly, laterally, or anterolaterally, as the deflectors demand in their guidance.

malposed (malpōzd'), in an abnormal position.

malposition, a faulty or abnormal position of a part of the body.

m. of jaw, any abnormal position of the mandible.

m. of teeth, an improper position of teeth in relationship to the basal bone of the alveolar process, to adjacent teeth, and/or to opposing teeth.

malpractice, in medicine and dentistry, a professional person's act or failure to act that was the proximate cause of an injury to a patient and that was below the standard of care required.

malrelation (of tooth, teeth, jaws, or facial structures), *malalignment, malocclusion,* and *malposition* are interrelated, so that one term frequently implies concurrent malrelationships of related teeth or structures.

maltose, malt sugar, a disaccharide formed in the hydrolysis of starch and consisting of two glucose residues bound by an $\alpha(1, 4)$-glycoside link.

mammotropin (mam'ōtrō'pin). See **hormone, lactogenic.**

manage, to control and direct; to administer.

managed care, I. refers to a cost containment system that directs the utilization of health benefits by (1) restricting the type, level, and frequency of treatment; (2) limiting the access to

care; and (3) controlling the level of reimbursement for services. **2.** a health care system in which there is administrative control over primary health care services in a medical group practice. Patients may pay a flat fee for basic family care but may be charged additional fees for secondary care services of specialists.

management, the planning, organizing, directing, and controlling of the enterprise's operation so that objectives can be achieved economically and efficiently through others.

m. information system (MIS), the specific type of data processing system that is designed to furnish management with information that may be of assistance in making decisions.

mandible, the lower jawbone.

m., inferior, the border of the lower edge of the mandible. Begins anterior to the insertion of the masseter muscle at the inferior surface of the angles of the mandible and is continuous anteriorly with the incisor region.

m., movements of. See **movement, mandibular.**

m., posture of, the physiologic rest position, or the rest vertical relation of the mandible.

mandibular, pertaining to the lower jaw.

m. angle. See **angle of the mandible.**

m. axis. See **axis, mandibular.**

m. border. See **border, mandibular.**

m. canal. See **canal, mandibular.**

m. centric relation, the closing relation of the mandible with the fixed craniofacial complex as determined clinically by instruments that record jaw motion.

m. condyle. See **condyle, mandibular.**

m. foramen. See **foramen, mandibular.**

m. fractures, a break in the continuity of the bone of the mandible. See also **fracture.**

m. glide. See **glide, mandibular.**

m. guide prosthesis, a prosthesis with an extension designed to direct a resected mandible into a functional relation with the maxillae.

m. hinge position. See **position, hinge, mandibular.**

m. movement. See **movement, mandibular.**

m. nerve, the third division of the trigeminal nerve, a mixed nerve that contains the entire motor portion of the trigeminal nerve. Its principal branches are the masseteric nerve, posterior and anterior temporal nerves, medial pterygoid nerve, lateral pterygoid nerve, buccal nerve, lingual nerve, inferior alveolar nerve, and auriculotemporal nerve. See also **nerve (s).**

m. notch. See **notch, mandibular.**

m. pain-dysfunction syndrome. See **temporomandibular joint pain-dysfunction syndrome.**

m. rest position. See **position, rest, mandibular.**

m. retraction. See **retraction, mandibular.**

mandibulofacial dysostosis (mandib′ yo͞olōfā′shəl). See **syndrome, Treacher Collins.**

mandrel (man′drəl), a shaft that supports or holds any object to be rotated. An instrument, held in a handpiece, that holds a disk, stone, or cup used for grinding, smoothing, or polishing.

manganese, a common metallic element found in trace amounts in tissues of the body where it aids in the function of various enzymes. Its atomic number is 25 and its atomic weight is 54.938.

manifest anxiety scale, a true-false questionnaire made up of items believed to indicate anxiety, in which the subject answers verbally the statement that describes him or her.

mannitol, a poorly metabolized sugar used as an osmotic diuretic and in kidney function tests.

mannose, an aldohexose obtained from various plant sources.

Mann-Whitney U-test. See **test, Mann-Whitney U-.**

manometer, a device for measuring the pressure of a fluid, consisting of a tube marked with a scale and containing a relatively incompressible fluid, such as mercury. The level of the fluid in the tube varies directly with the pressure of the fluid being measured. Manometers are used to measure blood pressure.

manpower, the number of persons required or needed to complete a task.

manual, 1. a book of instructions on performance of a task or the care of equipment. **2.** performed by the hand; used in the hand.

manuscript, an author's final copy of a document written by hand, typewriter, or word processor.

map, a drawing or diagram, to scale, of a surface object.

maprotiline HCl, *trade name:* Ludiomil; *drug class:* tetracyclic antidepressant; *action:* blocks reuptake of norepinephrine and serotonin into nerve endings; *uses:* depression, depression with anxiety.

Marfan's syndrome, a hereditary disorder of connective tissue characterized by tall stature, elongated extremities, subluxation of the lens, dilatation of the ascending aorta, and "pigeon breast." Marfan's syndrome is inherited as an autosomal dominant trait.

margin, 1. the extreme edge of something. **2.** the boundary of a surface. **3.** in a cavity preparation for a restoration, the margin is the outside limit of the surgical preparation. Synonym: cavosurface angle.

m., bone, the peripheral edge of a bone.

m., enamel, the part of the margin of a preparation that is laid in enamel.

m., free gingival (free gum margin), the edge or summit of the gingival tissue immediately adjacent to the cervical portion of the crown of a natural tooth. The tissue is normally unattached to a depth of 2 to 2.5 mm.

m., free gum. See **margin, free gingival.**

m., gingival, **1.** the cavosurface angle of the wall of a cavity preparation closest to the apex of the root. **2.** the crest or tip of the gingival tissues.

m. of safety, the margin between lethal and toxic doses.

m., thickened bone. See **bone, thickened margin of.**

marginal ridge. See **ridge, marginal.**

marginal spinning, the burnishing of the margins of a casting during the initial setting of the cement to close the space between the margin and the preparation, resulting from the slight lifting of the marginal gold from its seat by the interposition of the cement. The rounded edge of the spinning tool must always be drawn along the margin and not across it. (not current)

margination, the adhesion of the leukocytes to the luminal surface of blood vessel walls in the early stages of inflammation.

Marie's disease. See **acromegaly.**

marital status, the legal standing of a person in regard to his or her marriage state.

marketing, the set of human activities directed at facilitating and consummating exchanges. The following three elements must be present to define a marketing situation: two or more parties who are potentially interested in exchange; each party possessing things of value to others; and each party capable of communication and delivery.

marking medium. See **medium, marking.**

marsupialization (märsōo'pē-əlizā' shən), to form a pouch surgically to treat a cyst when simple removal would not be effective, such as in a pancreatic or a pilonidal cyst. Under anesthesia, the cyst sac is opened and emptied. Its edges are sutured to adjacent tissues, and a drain is left in place. Over a period of several months, secretions will decrease and the sac space will be reduced until it is completely filled. See also **operation, Partsch's.**

MAS (MaS, mas, milliampere-second), the product of the milliamperes and the exposure time in seconds (for example, 10 ma; ½ sec; 5 MAS).

mask, 1. something that conceals from view. **2.** a protective covering, especially for the face. **3.** to cover up.

m., rubber dam. See **pad, rubber dam.**

m., Wanscher's, a mask for ether anesthesia.

m., Yankauer's, an open type of mask for administering ether.

masking, an opaque covering used to camouflage the metal or other parts of a prosthesis.

Maslow's hierarchy of human needs, a term from sociology or social anthropology based on the hierarchic hypothesis of Abraham Maslow of the basic needs of man. The first need is for air, food, and water; the second for safety, including protection and freedom from fear and anxiety; followed in order by the need to love and to be loved; the need for self-

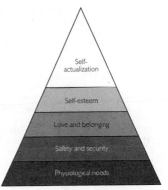

Maslow's Hierarchy of Needs. (Potter, 1996.)

esteem; and ultimately, the need for self-actualization. The Maslow hypothesis states that the high needs, which are those at the end of the hierarchy, cannot be fully satisfied until the lower needs are met.

masoprocol, *trade name:* Actinex; *drug class:* antineoplastic (topical); *action:* inhibits lipoxygenase; *use:* actinic keratosis.

mass media, the print and broadcast enterprises used to inform the general public.

mass number (A), the number of nucleons (protons and neutrons) in the nucleus of an atom.

mass screening, the examination of large samples or populations to determine the presence or absence of some trait, condition, or behavior.

mass storage, a storage medium in which data may be organized and maintained both sequentially and nonsequentially. Usually used for storage of files.

massage, the manipulation of tissues for remedial or hygiene purposes (as by rubbing, stroking, kneading, or tapping) with the hand or other instrument.

m., cardiac, a systematic, rhythmic application of pressure to the heart to cause a significant blood flow in the treatment of a cardiac arrest; may be an open- or closed-chest procedure.

m., gingival, the massage of the gingival tissues for cleansing purposes, increasing tissue tone, increasing the circulation of blood through the tissues, and increasing the keratinization of the surface epithelium.

masseter muscle, one of the four muscles of mastication. The thick rectangular muscle in the cheek that functions to close the jaw. The masseter muscle arises from the zygomatic arch and inserts into the mandible at the corner of the jaw.

mast cell, a connective tissue cell whose specific physiologic function remains unknown; capable of elaborating basophilic, metachromatic, cytoplasmic granules that contain histamine.

master, one having authority; one who directs, instructs, or superintends; an employer.

m. file, a file of semipermanent information that is usually updated periodically.

masticate, 1. to grind or crush food with the teeth to prepare it for swallowing and digestion. **2.** to chew.

masticating apparatus. See **apparatus, masticating.**

masticating cycle. See **cycle, masticating.**

mastication, 1. the process of chewing food in preparation for swallowing and digestion. **2.** the act of chewing accomplished by the coordinated activity of the tongue, mandible, mandibular musculature, and structural components of the temporomandibular joints, and controlled by the neuromuscular mechanism.

m., components of, the various jaw movements made during the act of mastication as determined by the neuromuscular system, temporomandibular articulations, teeth, and food being chewed. For purposes of analysis or description, the components of mastication may be categorized as opening, closing, left lateral, right lateral, or anteroposterior jaw movements.

m., forces of. See **force, masticatory.**

m., insufficiency of, inefficiency or inadequacy of the chewing act.

m., organ of. See **system, stomatognathic.**

m., physiology of, the movements of the mandible during the chewing cycle, which are controlled by neuromuscular action and correlated to the structural attributes of the temporomandibular joints and the propriocep-

tive sense of the periodontal membranes. There are three phases in the physiology of mastication: the incision of food, mastication of the bolus, and the act of swallowing. Accessory activity by the tongue and facial musculature facilitates the masticatory actions.

m., saliva in, an increase in salivation, which serves to wet and lubricate the food to facilitate deglutition.

m., tongue in, the muscular organ in the floor of the mouth whose function in the masticatory process consists of crushing some food by pressing it against the hard palate, forming it into a compact bolus, and assisting in placing it on the occlusal platform for tooth action.

masticatory force (mas'tikətōrē). See **force, masticatory.**

masticatory movements. See **movements, mandibular, masticatory.**

masticatory muscles, the muscles attached to the mandible employed in chewing.

mastoid, 1. the protuberence of the temporal bone located directly behind the external ear. **2.** a breast-shaped object.

mastoidale, the lowest point on the contour of the mastoid process. (not current)

materia alba, a soft white deposit around the necks of the teeth, usually associated with poor oral hygiene; composed of food debris, dead tissue elements, and purulent matter; serves as a medium for bacterial growth. (not current)

material(s), substance(s).

m., dental, all the substances used to assist in rendering dental service.

m., duplicating, the materials used to copy casts and models; usually hydrocolloids.

m., filling, gutta-percha, silver cones, paste mixtures, or other substances used to fill root canals.

m., impression, any substance or combination of substances used for making a negative reproduction or impression.

m., silicone rubber impression, a dimethyl polysiloxane material whose polymerization is affected by an organ-metal compound and some type of alkyl silicate.

m. testing, the determination of the properties of a substance in comparison with a standard or specification.

materia medica, the study of drugs and other substances used in medicine, their origins, preparation, uses, and effects.

maternal age, the age of the mother at the period of conception.

matrix (mā′triks), **1.** an intergranular substance that acts somewhat as a cementing material for other particles; for example, zinc phosphate cement is made of undissolved zinc oxide particles, surrounded and held or cemented together by phosphate compounds. The phosphate compounds make up the matrix. See also **bone; splint. 2.** a mechanical or artificial wall to complete the mold into which plastic material may be inserted. **3.** a mold into which something is formed.

m., amalgam, a metal form, usually of stainless steel, about 0.0015 to 0.002 inch thick, adapted to a prepared cavity to supply the missing wall so the plastic amalgam will be confined when it is condensed into the cavity.

m., celluloid, a strip of celluloid used to mold cement into the desired shape. See also **strip, plastic.**

m., custom, a matrix made especially for a given location, tooth, or preparation.

m. holder. See **retainer, matrix.**

m., mechanical (proprietary matrix), a patented or manufactured type of matrix.

m., plastic, a matrix of resin or plastic for use with cold-curing resin or cement.

m., platinum, a matrix of wrought platinum foil, usually 0.001 inch or thinner, adapted to a die of a preparation for a fired porcelain restoration; serves as a vehicle to carry and maintain the applications of porcelain when they are placed in a furnace for firing.

m., proprietary. See **matrix, mechanical.**

m. retainer, a mechanical device used to secure the ends of metal or plastic bands around a tooth to provide a form into which a restorative material can be condensed to replace a portion of tooth substance removed in cavity preparation. See also **retainer, matrix.**

m., T-band, matrix material cut with a T-shaped projection at one end; the lugs are bent over to engage the band as it encircles the tooth.

maxilla (maksil′ə), the irregularly shaped bone forming half of the upper jaw. The upper jaw is made up of the two maxillae.

maxillary (mak′siler′ē), pertaining to the superior bone.

m. arch, the upper dental arch and its supporting bone.

m. artery (internal maxillary artery), arises from the external carotid artery just below the level of the mandibular neck in the substance of the parotid gland. Its many branches include the middle meningeal, lower alveolar, temporal, pterygoid, masseteric, and buccal arteries, and the posterior superior alveolar and infraorbital arteries.

m. diseases, inflammatory, infectious, and neoplastic diseases of the mid-face, maxillary alveolar process, and palatal areas.

m. fracture, a break in one or both of the maxillary bones; frequently sustained in automobile accidents and contact sports injuries.

m. nerve, the second division of the trigeminal nerve consists of three major branches; the pterygopalatine, infraorbital, and zygomatic nerves. See also **nerve(s).**

m. retrusion. See **retrusion, maxillary.**

m. sinus. See **sinus, maxillary.**

m. sinusitis, an inflammation of the mucosa lining the air sac in the maxillary bone.

m. tuberosity. See **tuberosity, maxillary.**

maxillofacial (maksil′ōfā′shəl), pertaining to the jaws and face.

m. injuries, wounds to the mid-face area involving the premaxillary, maxillary, malar, lacrimal, nasal, and vomer bones and the tissues overlying these skeletal structures.

m. pain, any pain in the region of the jaws or face. Usually coupled with oral pain; that is, oral and/or maxillofacial pain may be present. Maxillofacial pain frequently is associated with functional disorders of the temporomandibular joint and/or the muscles of mastication, which in turn may arise from structural problems in the occlusion of the teeth. Determining the cause of maxillofacial pain may require comprehensive study of many possible factors or agents.

m. prosthetics. See **prosthetics, maxillofacial.**

maxillomandibular relation (maksil'ō mandib'yələr). See **relation, maxillomandibular.**

maxillotomy (mak'silot'əmē), the surgical sectioning of the maxilla to allow movement of all or a part of the maxilla into the desired portion.

maximum allowance, as specified in a fee schedule or table of allowances, the maximum dollar amount a dental plan will pay toward the cost of a dental service.

maximum benefit, the maximum dollar amount a dental plan will pay toward the cost of dental care incurred by an individual or family in a specified policy year.

maximum fee schedule, a compensation arrangement in which a participating dentist agrees to accept a prescribed sum as the total fee for one or more covered services.

mazindol, *trade names:* Mazanor, Sanorex; *drug class:* imidazoisoindole anorexiant (Controlled Substance Schedule IV); *action:* has amphetamine-like activity and may have an effect on satiety center of the hypothalamus; *use:* exogenous obesity.

Mazzini's test (məzē'nēz). See **test, Mazzini's.**

MCH. See **mean corpuscular hemoglobin.**

MCHC. See **mean corpuscular hemoglobin concentration.**

MCV. See **mean corpuscular volume.**

MDR, the abbreviation for **minimum daily requirement,** specifically the Minimum Daily Requirements for Specific Nutrients compiled by the United States Food and Drug Administration.

MDS. See **temporomandibular joint pain–dysfunction syndrome.**

mean (x), a measure of central tendency that is the calculated arithmetic average of a series of scores.

m. corpuscular hemoglobin, a measure of the weight of hemoglobin in a single red blood cell. The value is obtained by multiplying the hemoglobin by 10 and dividing by the number of

red blood cells. The normal range is between 27 and 31.

m. c. h. concentration (MCHC) a measure of red blood cells useful in identifying the type of anemia. The MCHC is obtained by multiplying the value of hemoglobin by 100 and dividing by the value of the hematocrit. The normal range is between 31.5 and 35.5.

m. corpuscular volume (MCV), indicates the size of the red blood cells. The MCV is obtained by multiplying the hematocrit by 10 and dividing by the number of red blood cells. The normal range is between 82 and 98.

m. life. See **average life.**

measles (mē'zəlz), an infectious disease caused by a virus. There are two types: rubeola and rubella (German measles). Both have oral manifestations.

m., German. See **rubella.**

m., three-day. See **rubella.**

mecamylamine HCl, *trade name:* Inversine; *drug class:* antihypertensive, ganglionic blocker; *action:* occupies receptor site, prevents acetylcholine from attaching to postsynaptic nerve ending in autonomic ganglia; *uses:* moderate-to-severe hypertension, malignant hypertension.

mechanism, a structure of working parts functioning together to produce an effect.

m., cough, a short inspiration, closure of the glottis, forcible expiratory effort, and then release of the glottis, with a rush of air at a flow rate of 3000 to 4000 cc/sec. A cough is essentially used or regarded as a process for removing foreign material from the lungs. It involves two phases. In the first, the combined action of the cilia and bronchiolar peristalsis moves the material up to the main bronchi and the bifurcation of the trachea. Further movement out of the respiratory system depends on the cough mechanism. In all medical conditions in which this mechanism is abolished or reduced, secretions and foreign material accumulate in the alveoli, with a resultant reduction in the aerating surface and a predisposition to infection. Since ventilation of the lungs depends on a patent airway, the cough mechanism should always be used by patients whose inadequate ventilation of lungs may be related to obstruction of the airway.

m., inhibitory-excitatory, a mechanism that provides coordinated and continuous stimuli to the lower motor neuron for smooth, facile, and rapidly adjustable muscle contraction. This mechanism operates on every level of the central nervous system, from the final common pathway back up the spinal cord to the cerebrum. The excitatory phase of stimulation is transmitted directly to the nerve. Inhibition, however, is effected not by stimulating the motor output directly, as is done in the parasympathetic nerves, but rather by the interaction of inhibitory mechanisms on the excitatory impulses.

m., respiratory control, the mechanism by which the respiratory functions are controlled. Three major factors in the control of respiration concern the dentist: neurogenic control of respiration, chemical regulation of respiration, and mechanical events leading to pulmonary ventilation. These three factors are significant in practice procedures because the dentist influences each of these factors in routine dental care; for example, the patency of the airways is always subject to alteration by instrumentation, dental prostheses, and the use of pharmacologic agents, and the physically induced responses modify the rate and magnitude of the respiratory mechanism.

m., suspensory, the hammock-like arrangement of the structures comprising the attachment apparatus.

mechanoreceptor, any sensory nerve ending that responds to mechanical stimuli, such as touch, pressure, sound, and muscular contraction.

meclizine HCl, *trade names:* Antivert, Bonine, Dramamine II; *drug class:* antihistamine nonspecific antiemetic; *action:* a nonspecific central nervous system depressant with anticholinergic and antihistaminic activity; *uses:* dizziness, motion sickness.

meclofenamate, *trade name:* Meclofen, Meclomen; *drug class:* nonsteroidal antiinflammatory; *action:* inhibits prostaglandin synthesis by interfering with cyclooxygenase needed for biosynthesis; possesses analgesic, antiinflammatory, antipy-

retic properties; *uses:* mild-to-moderate pain, osteoarthritis, rheumatoid arthritis.

media (mē′dē·ə), the plural form of medium.

median (mē′dē·ən), **1.** pertaining to the middle. **2.** a measure of central tendency attained by a calculation or count that separates all cases in a ranked distribution into halves. The median may be used as an average score.

m. lethal dose. See **dose, lethal, median.**

m. line. See **line, median.**

m. mandibular point. See **point, median mandibular.**

m. nerve, one of the terminal branches of the brachial plexus that extends along the radial portions of the forearm and the hand and supplies various muscles and the skin of these parts.

m. palatine suture. See **suture, intermaxillary.**

m. retruded relation. See **relation, centric.**

m. rhomboid glossitis, a patch of papillae-free mucosa located in the center of the tongue immediately behind the circumvallate papillae. The area appears as a red, smooth, depressed area that is rhomboidal in shape. Generally the lesion is asymptomatic and is thought to result from a fault in embryonic development of the tongue. The tissue may be susceptible to candidal infections. Some writers refer to this condition as *central papillary atrophy of the tongue.*

m. sagittal plane. See **plane, median sagittal.**

mediastinitis, an inflammation of the mediastinum.

mediastinum, a portion of the thoracic cavity in the middle of the thorax between the pleural sacs containing the two lungs. It extends from the sternum to the vertebral column and contains all the thoracic viscera, except the lungs.

mediation intervention, the act of a third person who interferes between two contending parties to reconcile them or to persuade them to adjust or settle their differences.

Medicaid, a federal assistance program established as Title XIX under the Social Security Amendments of 1965, which provides payment for

M

medical care for certain low-income individuals and families. The program is funded jointly by the state and federal governments and administered by states.

medical alert warning, ADA, a coding of the patient's medical or dental record to indicate the presence of a serious medical condition that requires treatment planning consideration before initiating treatment of any kind; usually a pressure-sensitive red warning label containing a notation as to the exact nature of the compromising condition is placed on the record jacket.

medical illustrator, an artist qualified by special training to prepare illustrations of organs, tissues, and medical phenomena in normal and abnormal states.

medical informatics, the field of information science concerned with the analysis and dissemination of medical data through the application of computers to various aspects of health care and medicine.

medically necessary care, the reasonable and appropriate diagnosis, treatment, and follow-up care (including supplies, appliances, and devices) as determined and prescribed by qualified appropriate health care providers in treating any condition, illness, disease, injury, or birth developmental malformation. Care is medically necessary for the purpose of controlling or eliminating infection, pain, and disease and restoring facial configuration or function necessary for speech, swallowing, or chewing.

medical record, that portion of a client's health record that is made by physicians and is a written or transcribed history of various illnesses or injuries requiring medical care, of inoculations, allergies, treatments, prognosis, and frequently health information about immediate family, occupation, and military service.

medical staff, physicians and dentists who are approved and given privileges to provide health care to patients in a hospital or other health care facility.

medical waste, any discarded biologic product, such as blood or tissues, removed from operating rooms, morgues, laboratories, or other medical facilities. The term may also be applied to bedding, bandages, syringes, and similar materials that have been used in treating patients and animal carcasses or body parts used in research.

m. w. disposal, the safe and proper handling of medical waste, prescribed by statute and institutional policy designed to prevent cross contamination, reinfection, and transmission of disease.

Medicare, a federal insurance program enacted in 1965 as Title XVIII of the Social Security Amendments that provides certain inpatient hospital services and physician services for all persons age 65 and older and eligible disabled individuals. The program is administered by the Health Care Financing Administration.

M. Part A, provides hospital insurance available to all qualified beneficiaries under the Medicare criteria.

M. Part B, provides medical insurance coverage for services such as physician's services, outpatient services, and home health care. Participation under Part B is voluntary, and beneficiaries pay monthly premiums. Part B is also called *Supplementary Medical Insurance.*

medication (med'ikā'shən), **1.** a drug or other substance that is used as a medicine. **2.** the administration of a medicine.

m., complete, the combination of synergistic drugs used to sedate children undergoing prolonged or difficult dental procedures; the patient is in a state of sleep or light anesthesia.

m., intracanal, a drug used in the root canal system during the course of therapy.

m., official. See **drug, official.**

m., officinal. See **drug, officinal.**

m., repository, slowly soluble drug mixtures intended for parenteral injection and gradual absorption into the blood and hence into other tissues of the body.

m., sustained release, oral dosage forms designed to be absorbed at various levels in the gastrointestinal tract, thus prolonging action.

medicine (med'isin), **1.** a remedy. **2.** the art of healing.

m., oral, the discipline of dentistry that deals with the significance and relationship of oral and systemic disease.

m., practice of, a pursuit that includes the application and use of medicines and drugs for the purpose of curing or alleviating bodily diseases; surgery is usually limited to manual operations generally performed by means of surgical instruments or appliances.

mediotrusion, a thrusting of the mandibular condyle inward (toward the median plane). When the right condyle is thrust outward (in laterotrusion) before it is rotated, the left condyle is thrust inward before it is orbited and is thus said to be in precurrent mediotrusion. If the left condyle is thrust outward before it is rotated, the right condyle is in precurrent mediotrusion.

mediostrusive, nonfunctional side tooth contacts during lateral jaw movements.

Mediterranean anemia See thalassemia major.

Mediterranean disease. (not current). See thalassemia major.

medium (mē'dē·am), an interposed agent or material; a carrier; a material serving as an environment for the growth of microorganisms.

m., computer, the material on which data are recorded (for example, punched cards, magnetic tape, disks, diskettes).

m., marking, 1. any of several agents, such as carbon paper or inked ribbon, used to indicate an occlusal interference. 2. any of several agents, such as stencil correction fluid, rouge and alcohol, or pressure indicator paste, used to determine areas of interference or pressure related to a removable prosthesis.

m., radiopaque, a substance that may be injected into a cavity or region to increase its density in x-ray examination and thereby aid in diagnosis. Lipiodol, Iodochloral, Parabodril, and Ioduron are examples of such materials.

m., Sabouraud's, a nutrient agar used to grow fungi. It is especially useful for the growth and identification of *Candida albicans,* the causative agent of thrush.

m., separating, any coating that is used on a surface and serves to prevent another surface or material from adhering to the first (for example, tinfoil, cellophane, or alginate, all of which are used to protect an acrylic resin from the moisture in the gypsum mold).

MEDLARS, the abbreviation for **Medical Literature Analysis and Retrieval System,** which is a computerized literature retrieval service offered by the National Library of Medicine in Bethesda, Maryland. MEDLARS contains more than 4.5 million references to medical and dental articles in professional journals and books published since 1966. The references are made available on-line to more than 1000 hospitals, universities, medical centers, and government agencies.

MEDLINE, a National Library of Medicine computer data base of current references published during the past 2 years. The files duplicate the contents of the Unabridged Index Medicus, which contains medical and dental reports from 3000 professional journals from more than 70 countries.

medroxyprogesterone acetate, *trade names:* Amen, Curretab, Cycrin; *drug class:* progestogen; *action:* inhibits secretion of pituitary gonadotropins, which prevents follicular maturation and ovulation; stimulates growth of mammary tissue; antineoplastic action against endometrial cancer; *uses:* abnormal uterine bleeding, secondary amenorrhea, endometrial cancer, metastic renal cancer, contraceptive, with estrogens to reduce incidence of endometrial cancer.

medulla oblongata (madul'a oblông·gä'ta), the direct upward extension of the spinal cord that lies at the junction between the cerebrum and spinal cord and is considered to be in a group with the pons and midbrain because the nuclei of all the cranial nerves except one are situated within this structural group. The medulla functions are associated with the nuclei of the glossopharyngeal, vagal, spinal accessory, and hypoglossal nerves. The medulla controls the reflex actions of the pharynx, larynx, and tongue, which are related to deglutition, mastication, and speech, as well as the visceral reflexes of coughing, sneezing, sucking, vomiting, and salivating, and other secretory functions

mefenamic acid, *trade names:* Ponstel; *drug class:* nonsteroidal antiinflammatory; *action:* inhibits prostaglandin synthesis by interfering with cyclooxygenase meeded for biosynthesis, possesses analgesic, antiinflammatory, antipyretic properties; *uses:* mild-to-moderate pain, dysmenorrhea, inflammatory disease.

megacolon, an abnormal dilation of the colon that may be congenital, toxic, or acquired.

m. acquired, a result of the chronic refusal to defecate, usually occurring in children who are psychotic or mentally retarded.

m. congenital, caused by the absence of autonomic ganglia in the smooth muscle wall of the colon.

m. toxic, a serious complication of ulcerative colitis that may result in perforation of the colon, septicemia, and death.

megadontismus (megədontiz′məs). See **macrodontia.**

megestrol acetate, *trade name:* Megace; *drug class:* antineoplastic (progestin); *action:* affects endometrium by antiluteinizing effect; *uses:* breast, endometrial cancer, renal cell cancer.

Meissner's corpuscles (mīs′nərz). See **corpuscle, Meissner's.**

melanin (mel′ənin), the dark amorphous pigment of melanotic tumors, skin, hair, choroid coat of the eye, and substantia nigra of the brain.

melanocytes (mel′ənōsīts′), dendritic cells of the gingival epithelium that, when functional, cause pigmentation regardless of race.

melanoma (mel′ənō′mə), a malignant neoplasm characterized by pigment-producing cells. It usually is dark in color but may be amelanotic; that is, free of pigment.

melanosis (mel′ənō′sis), the condition in which melanin pigments appear in the tissues. Melanosis is normal in the gingivae of most dark-skinned individuals and occasionally in those with light skin.

melatonin, the only hormone secreted into the bloodstream by the pineal gland. The hormone appears to inhibit numerous endocrine functions, including the gonadotropic hormones, and to decrease the pigmentation of the skin.

melena (melē′nə), the passage of dark or black stools; the color is produced by altered blood and blood pigments.

melituria (mel′itoo′rē·ə), the presence of any sugar in the urine (e.g., glucose, lactose, pentose, fructose, maltose, galactose, sucrose).

melphalan, *trade name:* Alkeran; *drug class:* antineoplastic; *action:* responsible for cross-linking DNA strands, which leads to cell death; *uses:* palliative treatment of multiple myeloma and nonresectable epithelial carcinoma of the ovary.

melting range. See **range, melting.**

member, an individual enrolled in a dental benefits program. See also **beneficiary.**

membrane, a thin layer of tissue that covers a surface or divides a space or organ.

m., basement, the delicate, PAS-positive, noncellular membrane on which the epithelium is seated.

m. bone. See **bone, membrane.**

m., mucous. See **mucosa.**

m., Nasmyth's. See **cuticle, primary.**

m., periodontal. See **ligament, periodontal.**

m., subimplant, the fibrous connective tissue that regenerates from the periosteum and that forms between the inner surface of the implant framework and the bone surface.

memory, 1. the ability to recall events, experiences, information, and skills. **2.** a general term for a device that stores data in binary code on electronic or magnetic media in computers.

m. cycle, the time it takes to access a character in memory.

m. location, a place in the memory where a unit of data may be stored or retrieved.

m., long-term, the ability to recall events, experiences, information, or skills that occurred in or were acquired in the distance past.

m. register, a register in storage of a computer, in contrast with a register in one of the other units of the computer.

m., short-term, the ability to retain and recall recent events or experiences.

menadiol/menadiol sodium diphosphate (vitamin K₄), *trade name:* Synkavite; *drug class:* synthetic vitamin K; *action:* needed for adequate blood clotting (factors II, VII, IX, X); *uses:* vitamin K malabsorption, hypoprothrombinemia, oral anticoagulant toxicity.

menarche, the beginning of the menstrual function.

Mendelian inheritance, better known as *Mendel's laws* or *mendelian laws,* which are the basic principles of genetics based on the experiments of Gregor Mendel in the nineteenth century. Two basic genetic principles were established: the law of segregation and the law of independent assortment. According to the law of segregation, the genetic characteristics of a species are represented in the somatic cells by a pair of units called *genes* that separate during meiosis so that each gamete receives only one gene for each trait. According to the law of independent assortment, the members of a gene pair on different chromosomes segregate independently from other pairs during meiosis, so that the gametes offer all possible combinations of factors.

Meniere's disease, a chronic disease of the inner ear characterized by recurrent episodes of vertigo, which is progressive sensorineural hearing loss. It may occur bilaterally and may include tinnitus.

meninges, the three membranes enclosing the brain and the spinal cord, comprising the dura mater, the pia mater, and the arachnoid.

meningioma, a mesenchymal fibroblastic tumor of the membranes enveloping the brain and spinal cord. Meningiomas grow slowly, are usually vascular, and occur most commonly near the superior longitudinal, transverse, and cavernous sinuses of the dura mater of the brain.

meningism, an abnormal condition characterized by irritation of the brain and spinal cord and by symptoms that mimic those of meningitis. In meningism, however, there is no actual inflammation of the meninges.

meningitis, any infection or inflammation of the membranes covering the brain and spinal cord. It usually is a purulent infection and involves the fluid of the subarachnoid space. The most common causes in adults are bacterial infection with *Streptococcus pneumoniae, Neisseria meningitidis,* or *Haemophilus influenzae.* Aseptic meningitis may be caused by chemical irritation, by neoplasm, or by viruses.

meningocele, a saclike protrusion of either the cerebral or spinal meninges through a congenital defect in the skull or the vertebral column.

meningoencephalitis, an inflammation of both the brain and the meninges, usually caused by a bacterial infection.

meningomyelocele, a saclike cyst containing brain tissue, cerebrospinal fluid, and the meninges that protrudes through a congenital defect in the skull.

meninscectomy (men'isek'təmē), the surgical removal of the meniscus or condylar disc, also referred to as *discetomy.* A popular treatment of dysfunctional maxillofacial pain in the 1950s, it is somewhat discredited today.

meniscus, the cartilaginous intracapsular disc interposed between the mandibular condyle and the glenoid fossa of the temporal bone.

menopause, the cessation of menstruation in the human female occurring variably from approximately 45 to 50 years of age. Menopause is accompanied by diminution of estrogen formation, often with atrophic changes occurring in the oral mucous membranes and gingivae.
m., oral symptoms of, a burning sensation and dryness of the mouth; salty taste; edematous, reddened, atrophic-appearing, tender mucosa; glossitis; and often desquamative gingivitis.

menorrhagia, abnormally heavy or long menstrual periods. Menorrhagia is a relatively common complication of benign uterine fibromyoma; it may be so severe, or intractable, as to require hysterectomy.

menstrual cycle, a recurring cycle of change in the endometrium during which the decidual layer of the endometrium is shed, then regrows, proliferates, is maintained for several days, and is shed again at menstruation. The average length of the cycle is 28 days.

menstruation, the shedding of the necrotic mucosa of the endometrium and associated bleeding that occurs in the final phase of the menstrual cycle.

M

The average duration of menstruation is 5 days, in which approximately 30 ml of blood is lost.

mental disorder, any disturbance of emotional equilibrium as manifested in maladaptive behavior and impaired functioning, caused by genetic, physical, chemical, biologic, psychologic, or social and cultural factors. Also called *emotional illness, mental illness, psychiatric disorder.*

mental foramen. See **foramen, mental.**

mental health, a relative state of mind in which a person who is healthy is able to cope with and adjust to the recurrent stresses of everyday living in an acceptable way.

m. h. service, any one of a group of government, professional, or lay organizations operating at a community, state, national, or international level to aid in the prevention and treatment of mental disorders.

mental retardate, an individual who is intellectually inadequate in society.

mental retardation, a disorder of general intellectual function impairing the ability to learn and adapt socially.

menthol, a topical antipruritic with a cooling effect that relieves itching. It is an ingredient in many topical creams and ointments.

menton, the most inferior point on the chin in the lateral view; a cephalometric landmark.

mentor, an older, trusted, more experienced advisor or counselor who offers helpful guidance to younger, less experienced colleagues.

mepenzolate bromide, *trade name:* Cantil; *drug class:* gastrointestinal (GI) anticholinergic; *action:* inhibits muscarinic actions of acetylcholine at postganglionic parasympathetic neuroeffector sites; *uses:* treatment of peptic ulcer disease, irritable bowel syndrome in combination with other drugs, other GI disorders.

meperidine HCl, *trade name:* Demerol; *drug class:* synthetic narcotic analgesic (Controlled Substance Schedule II); *action:* interacts with opioid receptors in the central nervous system to alter pain perception; *uses:* moderate-to-severe pain, preoperatively in sedation techniques.

mephenesin (mefen'isin), an antispasmodic drug, 3 ortho-toloxy1, 2 pro-

panediol. Used for the preparation of apprehensive patients for dental and periodontal procedures because of its ability to produce muscular relaxation and euphoria. Usual dosage for an adult is 1 gm in either tablet or elixir form 20 minutes before the dental procedure.

mephenytoin, *trade name:* Mesantoin; *drug class:* hydantoin anticonvulsant; *action:* reduces electrical discharges in motor cortex, reducing seizures; *uses:* generalized tonic-clonic seizures, single or complex-partial seizures.

mephobarbital, *trade name:* Mebaral; *drug class:* barbiturate anticonvulsant (Controlled Substance Schedule IV); *action:* a nonspecific depressant of the central nervous system; may enhance GABA activity in the brain; *uses:* generalized tonic-clonic (grand mal) or absence (petit mal) seizures.

mepivacaine HCl (local), *trade names:* Carbocaine, Isocaine, Polocaine; *drug class:* amide local anesthetic; *action:* inhibits ion fluxes across membranes, particularly sodium transport across cell membrane; decreased rise of depolarization phase of action potential; blocks nerve action potential; *uses:* local dental anesthesia, nerve block, caudal anesthesia, epidural pain relief, paracervical block, transvaginal block or infiltration.

meprobamate, *trade names:* Equanil, Miltown, Probate, Trancot; *drug class:* sedative-hypnotic, anxiolytic (Controlled Substance Schedule IV); *action:* nonspecific central nervous system depressant; acts in thalamus, limbic system, and spinal cord; *use:* anxiety disorders.

merbromin (mərbrō'min), a mercury-bromine compound used as a germicide for disinfection of the skin, mucous membrane, and wounds. Used in 10% alcoholic solution (Scott-Wilson reagent) in the treatment of moniliasis.

mercaptan (mərkap'tən), the basic ingredient of the polysulfide polymer employed in rubber base impression materials. See also **Thiokol.**

mercaptopurine (6-MP), *trade name:* Purinethol; *drug class:* antineoplastic-antimetabolite; *action:* inhibits purine metabolism at multiple sites, which inhibits DNA and RNA synthesis; *uses:* chronic myelocytic leukemia, acute lymphoblastic leukemia in children, acute myelogenous leukemia.

mercurial (mərkyoō′rē·əl), a compound that owes its activity to the mercury it contains.

m. line. See **line, mercurial.**

mercuric chloride, mercury bichloride or perchloride; a corrosive highly toxic sublimate used as a topical antiseptic and disinfectant for inanimate objects.

mercurialism (mercury poisoning), 1. poisoning resulting from the ingestion of pure mercury, its salts, or its vapor. Manifestations of acute intoxication include nausea, vomiting, abdominal cramps, oral and pharyngeal pain, uremia, dehydration, diarrhea, and shock. Manifestations of chronic poisoning include hypersalivation, diarrhea, vertigo, depression, intention tremor, and stomatitis. See also **acrodynia** and **stomatitis, mercurial.** 2. poisoning by ingestion or absorption of mercury compounds. See also **line, mercurial.**

Mercurochrome, the trade name for merbromin.

mercury, a metallic element. Its atomic number is 80 and its atomic weight is 200.6. It is the only common metal that is liquid at room temperature, and it occurs in nature almost entirely in the form of its sulfide, cinnabar. It is used in dental amalgams, thermometers, barometers, and other measuring instruments. It forms many poisonous compounds. The major toxic forms are mercury vapor, mercuric salts, and organic mercurials. Elemental mercury is only mildly toxic when ingested, because it is poorly absorbed.

m. poisoning, a toxic condition caused by the ingestion or inhalation of mercury or a mercury compound. The chronic form, resulting from inhalation of the vapors or dust of mercurial compounds, is characterized by irritability, excessive saliva, loosened teeth, gum disorders, slurred speech, tremors, and staggering. Symptoms of acute mercury poisoning appear in a few to 30 minutes and include a metallic taste in the mouth, thirst, nausea, vomiting, severe abdominal pain, bloody diarrhea, and renal failure that may result in death. The presence of mercury in the body is determined by a urine test.

merge, to produce a single sequence of items, ordered according to some rule, from two or more sequences previously ordered according to the same rule. Merging does not change the items in size, structure, or total number.

Merkel's corpuscles. See **corpuscle, Merkel's.** (not current)

Merkel's disks. See **corpuscle, Merkel's.** (not current)

Merrifield's knife. See **knife, Merrifield's.**

mes- (meso-), in the middle; intermediate as in position, size, type, and time degree.

mesalamine, *trade names:* Asacol, Pentasa, Rowasa; *drug class:* antiinflammatory; *action:* unknown, may inhibit prostaglandin synthesis; *uses:* inflammatory bowel disease, ulcerative colitis.

mesial (mē′zē·əl), situated in the middle; median, toward the middle line of the body or toward the center line of the dental arch.

m. migration, the drifting teeth toward the midline or forward in the dental arch.

m., unilateral, mesiocclusion on one side.

mesiocclusion, an occlusal relationship in which the lower teeth are positioned mesially, similar to the relationship in an Angle Class III malocclusion. Antonym: distocclusion.

mesiodens (mē′zē·ədenz), a supernumerary tooth appearing in an erupted or unerupted state between the two maxillary central incisors.

mesioversion (mēzē·ōvur′zhən), when applied to a tooth, a term indicating that the tooth is closer than normal to the median plane or midline. When applied to the maxillae or mandible, it means that the jaw is anterior to its normal position.

meso-. See **mes-.**

mesocephalic (mez′ōsefal′ik), a descriptive term applied to a head size between dolichocephalic and brachycephalic (cephalic index 76 to 81).

mesoderm, the middle of the three cell layers of the developing embryo. It lies between the ectoderm and the endoderm. Bone, connective tissue, muscle, blood, vascular and lymphatic tissue, the pleurae of the pericardium and peritoneum are all derived from the mesoderm.

mesodontia (mezōdon'shē-ə), medium-size teeth.

mesognathic (mesōnāth'ik), having an average relationship of jaws to head. (not current)

mesonephros, the second type of excretory organ to develop in the vertebrate embryo. The organ is the permanent kidney in lower animals, but in humans and various other mammals it is functional only during early embryonic development.

mesoridazine besylate, *trade name:* Serentil; *drug class:* phenothiazine antipsychotic; *action:* blocks neurotransmission at dopaminergic synapses in the cerebral cortex, hypothalamus, and limbic system; mechanism for antipsychotic effects is unclear; *uses:* psychotic disorders, schizophrenia, anxiety, alcoholism, behavioral problems in mental deficiency, chronic brain syndrome.

mesostomia (mezōstō'mē-ə), an oral fissure of medium size.

mesostructure conjunction bar, a connecting bar joining implant abutment copings together. Bar and copings together make up the mesostructure. (not current)

mesothelioma, a rare malignant tumor of the mesothelium of the pleura or peritoneum associated with exposure to asbestos.

metaanalysis, a quantitative method of combining the results of independent studies (usually drawn from the published literature) and synthesizing summaries and conclusions that may be used to evaluate therapeutic effectiveness, and plan new studies, with application chiefly in the areas of research and medicine and dentistry.

metabolic disease, any disorder that causes dysfunction of the metabolic action of the body, resulting in loss of control of homeostasis.

metabolism (metab'ōlizəm), the sum of chemical changes involved in the function of nutrition. There are two phases: anabolism (constructive or assimilative changes) and catabolism (destructive or retrograde changes).

m., basal. See **basal metabolic rate.**

m., bone, the continual complex of anabolism and catabolism taking place in bone when it is in physiologic equilibrium. Bone is a highly labile substance that reflects the adequacy of general body metabolism. See also **bone, alveolar, metabolism.**

m., cell, the complexity of anabolic and catabolic processes occurring within cellular structures.

m., energy, the transformation of energy in living tissues, consisting of anabolism (storage of energy) and catabolism (the dissipation of energy).

m., substance, the sum of all the physical and chemical processes by which living organized tissues are produced and maintained.

metacarpus, the five bones of the hand between the carpus (wrist) and the phalanges (fingers).

metachysis (metə'kisis), a blood transfusion; the introduction of any substance directly into the bloodstream by mechanical means. (not current)

metal, an element possessing luster, malleability, ductility, and conductivity of electricity and heat.

m., base, an archaic term referring to nonprecious metals or alloys such as iron, lead, copper, nickel, chromium, and zinc. In dentistry, a term usually referring to the stainless steel and chrome-cobalt-nickel alloys.

m. ceramic alloys, the fusion of ceramics (porcelain) to an alloy of two or more metals for use in restorative and prosthodontic dentistry. Examples of metal alloys employed include cobalt-chromium, gold-palladium, gold-platinum-palladium, and nickel-based alloys.

m., fusion of, the blending of metals by melting together.

m. insert teeth. See **tooth, metal insert.**

m., noble, a precious metal, usually one that does not readily oxidize, such as gold and platinum.

m., solidification of, the change of metal from the molten to the solid state.

m., wrought, a cast metal that has been cold worked in any manner.

metalloid (met'əloid), a nonmetallic element that behaves as a metal under certain conditions. Carbon, silicon, and boron are three examples. These elements may be alloyed with metals.

metalloprotein, a protein with a tightly bound metal ion or ions, such as hemoglobin.

metallurgy, the study of metals and their properties, including separating metals from their ores, the making and compounding of alloys, and the technology and science of working and heat treating metals to alter their physical characteristics.

metanephrine, one of the two principal urinary metabolites of epinephrine and norepinephrine in the urine, the other being vanillylmandelic acid.

metaphen, tincture of (met′əfen), the trade name for tincture of nitromersol.

metaphysis (metəf′əsis), the line of junction of the epiphysis with the diaphysis of a long bone.

metaplasia (met′əplā′zhə), a change in the type of adult cells in a tissue to a form that is not normal for that tissue.

metaproterenol sulfate, *trade names:* Arm-A-Med, Metaprel, Prometa; *drug class:* selective β_2-agonist; *action:* relaxes bronchial smooth muscle by direct action on β_2-adrenergic receptors; *uses:* bronchial asthma, bronchospasm.

metastasis (metəs′təsis), the transfer of a disease by blood vessels, lymph vessels, or the respiratory tract (through aspiration) from one organ or region to another not directly contiguous with it. Usually used in reference to malignant tumor cells, but bacteria can also metastasize (for example, in focal infection).

meteorologic factors, variables of the atmosphere or weather that affect behavior, and/or mental and physical state.

meter, dose rate, any instrument that measures radiation dose rate.

m., d. r., integrating, the ionization chamber and measuring system designed for determining the total accumulated radiation administered during an exposure.

meter, dosimeter, radiation, an instrument used to detect and measure an accumulated exposure to radiation, commonly a pencil-size ionization chamber with built-in self-reading electrometer used in personnel radiation monitoring.

meter, radiation, an instrument for the measurement of exposure to radiation.

metformin HCl, *trade name:* Glucophage; *drug class:* oral hypoglycemic, biguanide derivative; *action:* exact mechanism unknown, requires insulin secretion to function properly; *use:* type II diabetes mellitus.

methacrylate, an ester of methacrylic acid used as a pit and fissure sealant. See also **methyl methacrylate.**

methadone HCl, *trade names:* Dolophine, Methadone; *drug class:* synthetic narcotic analgesic (Controlled Substance Schedule II); *action:* interacts with opioid receptors in the central nervous system to alter pain perception; *uses:* severe pain, opioid withdrawal program.

methamphetamine HCl, *trade name:* Desoxyn Gradumet; *drug class:* amphetamine (Controlled Substance Schedule II); *action:* increases release of norepinephrine and dopamine in cerebral cortex to reticular activating system; *uses:* exogenous obesity, minimal brain dysfunction, attention deficit disorder with hyperactivity.

methantheline bromide, *trade name:* Banthine; *drug class:* synthetic anticholinergic; *action:* inhibits muscarinic actions of acetylcholine at postganglionic parasympathetic neuroeffector sites; *uses:* treatment of peptic ulcer disease, irritable bowel syndrome, pancreatitis, gastritis, biliary dyskinesia, pylorospasm, reflex neurogenic bladder in children.

methazolamide, *trade name:* Neptazane; *drug class:* carbonic anhydrase inhibitor; *action:* decreases production of aqueous humor in the eye, which lowers intraocular pressure; *uses:* open-angle glaucoma or preoperatively in narrow-angle glaucoma.

methemoglobinemia (met′hēmə-glō′binē′mē·ə), an abnormality of hemoglobin in which the iron is in the ferric state as a result of exposure to industrial substances or the ingestion of toxic agents such as phenacetin, sulfonamides, aniline nitrates, and nitrates. A rare congenital form is seen most commonly in persons with Greek heritage. Symptoms include generalized cyanosis, headache, drowsiness, and confusion. Methemoglobin does not carry oxygen.

methenamine salts, *trade names:* Hiprex, Urex; *drug class:* urinary antiinfective; *action:* in acid urine, it is hydrolyzed to ammonia and formaldehyde, which are bactericidal; *uses:* prophylaxis and treatment of uncomplicated urinary tract infections.

methicillin sodium, a semisynthetic penicillin salt for parenteral administration. Restriction of its use to infections caused by penicillin G-resistant staphylococci is recommended.

methimazole, *trade name:* Tapazole; *drug class:* thyroid hormone antagonist; *action:* inhibits synthesis of thyroid hormones by decreasing iodine use in manufacture of thyroglobulin and iodothyronine; *uses:* hyperthyroidism, preparation for thyroidectomy, thyrotoxic crisis, thyroid storm.

methionine, one of the essential amino acids. See also **amino acid.**

methocarbamol, *trade name:* Carbacot, Delaxin, Robamol, Skelex; *drug class:* skeletal muscle relaxant; *action:* depresses multisynaptic pathways in the spinal cord; *uses:* adjunct for relief of spasm and pain in musculoskeletal conditions.

method, a manner of performing an act or operation; a technique.

m., Callahan's. See **method, chloropercha.**

m., Charters', a method of toothbrushing in which the brush is held horizontally, with the bristles lying against the teeth and gingivae and pointed in a coronal direction at 45 degrees so that the bristles lie half on the teeth and half on the gingivae. A vibratory cycle of a very constricted diameter is negotiated so that the brush head moves in a circular movement but the brush bristles remain fairly stationary while being agitated. The circular vibration loosens debris and pumps the bristles into interproximal areas to massage the tissues.

m., chloropercha (Callahan's method, Johnston's method), the method of filling root canals in which gutta-percha cones are dissolved in a chloroform-rosin solution in the root canal. The canal is flooded with the chloroform solution. A preselected gutta-percha cone is then pumped carefully into and out of the canal. As the cone dissolves, the material is forced into the apex as a plastic mass. Other cones and occasionally additional chloroform solution are added until the canal is sealed.

m., Fones' (Fones' technique), a toothbrushing technique in which, with the teeth occluded and with the brush at more or less right angles to the teeth, large sweeping, scrubbing circles are described. With the jaws parted, the palatal and lingual surfaces of the teeth are scrubbed using smaller circles. Occlusal surfaces are brushed in an anteroposterior direction.

m., Hirschfeld's, a toothbrushing method in which the bristles are placed against the axial surfaces of the teeth, with slight incisal or occlusal inclination from a right-angled application, in simultaneous contact with teeth and gingivae, and then rotated in a circle of exceedingly small diameter. Occlusal surfaces are brushed energetically.

m., Howard's, a method of artificial respiration. The patient is placed on the back, with the hands placed under the head, and a cushion placed so that the head is lower than the abdomen. The physician applies rhythmical pressure upward and inward with the hands against the lower lateral parts of the patient's chest.

m., Howe's silver precipitation, a method of depositing silver in enamel and dentin by the application of ammoniacal silver nitrate solution and its reduction with formalin or eugenol.

m., indirect restorative, the technique of fabrication of a restoration on a cast or model of the original (for example, the indirect method of inlay construction, in which a die of amalgam or other material is made from an impression of the prepared tooth, a wax pattern formed, and the cast inlay fitted and finished on the die, then cemented to the tooth).

m., Johnston's. See **method, chloropercha.**

m., lateral condensation, the method in which a preselected gutta-percha cone is sealed into the apex of the root. The balance of space is filled with other gutta-percha cones forced laterally with a spreader.

m., segmentation, the method in which a preselected gutta-percha cone is cut into segments. The tip section is sealed into the apex of the root. The other segments are usually warmed and condensed against the first piece with a plugger. Additional pieces are then used until the space is obliterated.

m., silver cone, the method in which a prefitted silver cone is sealed into the apex of the root canal. The space not sealed with the cone is obliterated with gutta-percha or sealer.

m., split cast, **1.** a procedure for checking the ability of an articulator to receive or be adjusted to a maxillomandibular relation record. **2.** a procedure for indexing casts on an articulator to facilitate their removal and replacement on the instrument.

methohexital sodium, an intravenous barbiturate prescribed for the induction of anesthesia in short surgical procedures as a supplement to other anesthetics.

methotrexate/methotrexate sodium, *trade names:* Folex, Mexate, Rheumatrex; *drug class:* folic acid antagonist, antineoplastic; *action:* inhibits an enzyme that reduces folic acid, which is needed for nucleic acid synthesis in all cells; *uses:* acute lymphocytic leukemia; in combination for breast, lung, head, neck cancer; lymphosarcoma, psoriasis; gestational choriocarcinoma, hydatidiform mole.

methoxamine HCl, an adrenergic that acts as a vasoconstrictor prescribed for use during anesthesia to maintain blood pressure and in the treatment of paroxysmal supraventricular tachycardia.

methsuximide, *trade name:* Celontin; *drug class:* anticonvulsant; *action:* inhibits spike wave formation in absence seizures (petit mal); decreases amplitude, frequency, duration, spread of discharge in minor motor seizures; *use:* refractory absence seizures (petit mal).

methylation, 1. the introduction of a methyl group, CH_3, to a chemical compound. **2.** the addition of methyl alcohol and naphtha to ethanol to produce denatured alcohol.

methyldopa/methyldopate, *trade name:* Aldomet; *drug class:* centrally acting antihypertensive; *action:* stimulates central inhibitory α-adrenergic

receptors or acts as false transmitter, resulting in reduction of arterial pressure; *use:* hypertension.

methylene blue, a bluish-green crystalline substance used as a histologic stain and as a laboratory indicator. It is also used in the treatment of cyanide poisoning and methemoglobinemia.

methyl methacrylate (meth'il metha-k'rilāt), an acrylic resin, $CH_2= C(CH_3)COOCH_3$, derived from methyl acrylic acid. Monomer is the single molecule and polymer is the polymerization product.

methylphenidate HCl, *trade names:* Methidate, Ritalin; *drug class:* central nervous system stimulant, related to amphetamines (Controlled Substance Schedule II); *action:* increases release of norepinephrine, dopamine in cerebral cortex to reticular activating system; exact mode of action not known; *uses:* attention deficit disorder with hyperactivity, narcolepsy.

methyprednisolone/methylprednisolone acetate/methylprednisolone sodium succinate, *trade names:* Medrol, Meprolone; *drug class:* immediate acting glucocorticoid; *action:* decreases inflammation by suppressing macrophage and leukocyte migration; reduces capillary permeability and inhibits lysosomal enzymes and phagocytosis; *uses:* severe inflammation, shock, adrenal insufficiency, collagen disorders.

methysergide maleate, *trade name:* Sansert; *drug class:* serotonin antagonist; *action:* competitively blocks serotonin HT receptors in central nervous system and periphery; *uses:* prophylaxis for migraine and other vascular headaches.

Meticorten, the trade name for prednisone.

metoclopramide HCl, *trade name:* Clopra, Maxolon, Reglan; *drug class:* central dopamine receptor antagonist; *action:* enhances response to acetylcholine of tissue in upper GI tract, which causes contraction of gastric muscle, relaxes pyloric and duodental segments, increases peristalsis without stimulating secretions; antiemetic action occurs centrally; *uses:* prevention of nausea, vomiting induced by chemotherapy, radiation, delayed gastric emptying, gastroesophageal reflux.

metolazone, *trade names:* Diulo, Mykrox, Zaroxolyn; *drug class:* diuretic with thiazidelike effects; *action:* acts on distal tubule by increasing excretion of water, sodium, chloride, and potassium; *uses:* edema, hypertension, CHF.

metoprolol tartrate, *trade name:* Nu Metop; *drug class:* antihypertensive selective β_1-blocker; *action:* produces fall in blood pressure without reflex tachycardia or significant reduction in heart rate; *uses:* mild-to-moderate hypertension, acute myocardial infarction to reduce cardiovascular mortality, angina pectoris.

metric system. See **system, metric.**

metronidazole, a generic synthetic antibacterial compound available for both oral and intravenous use. Metronidazole is indicated in the treatment of serious infections caused by susceptable anaerobic bacteria. In dentistry, metronidazole is used in the treatment of HIV, gingivitis, and HIV periodontitis.

m./m. HCl, *trade name:* Flagyl, Metro IV, Protostat; *drug class:* trichomonacide, amebicide antiinfective; *action:* direct-acting amebicide/trichomonacide binds, degrades DNA in organisms; *uses:* intestinal amebiasis, amebic abscess, trichomoniasis, refractory trichomoniasis, bacterial anaerobic infections.

MeV, one million electron volts.

mexiletine HCl, *trade name:* Mexitil; *drug class:* antidysrhythmic (Class IB, lidocaine analog); *action:* blocks sodium channel in His-Purkinje system, which decreases the effective refractory period and shortens the duration of the action potential; *use:* documented life-threatening ventricular dysrhythmias.

micelle (mīsel′), any one of the spaces formed by the brush structure of fibrils in colloidal gels. The spaces are occupied by water in hydrocolloid impressions.

miconazole, *trade names:* Monistat, Monistat IV; *drug class:* antifungal; *action:* alters cell membranes and inhibits fungal enzymes; *uses:* coccidioidomycosis, candidiasis, cryptococcosis, paracoccidioidomycosis, fungal menigitis; IV used for severe infections only.

m. nitrate (topical), *trade names:* Micatin, Monistat-7; *drug class:* antifungal; *action:* interferes with fungal cell membrane, which increases permeability, leaking of nutrients; *uses:* tinea pedis, tinea cruris, tinea corporis, tinea versicolor, vaginal or vulvar *Candida albicans.*

microbiology, the branch of biology concerned with the study of microorganisms, including algae, bacteria, viruses, protozoa, fungi, and rickettsiae.

microcephalus (mī′krōsef′ələs), an abnormally small head.

microchemistry, the branch of chemistry concerned with the study of chemical processes at the cellular and subcellular levels.

microcirculation, the flow of blood throughout the system of smaller vessels of the body, particularly the capillaries.

Micrococcus gazogenes (mī′krōkäk′əs gä′zōjēnz). See **Veillonella alcalescens.**

microcomputer, a complete, multiuse, electronic, digital computer system consisting of a central processing unit, storage facilities, I/O ports, and a chip with megabytes of high-speed internal storage, usually with only one user for personal, home, or office use.

microcurie, one millionth of a curie.

microcytosis, hereditary (mī′krōsītō′sis). See **thalassemia; thalassemia major.**

microdialysis, a technique for measuring extracellular concentrations of substances in tissues, usually in vivo, by means of a small probe equipped with a semipermeable membrane. Substances may also be introduced into the extracellular space through the membrane.

microdontia (mī′krōdon′shē-ə), abnormally small teeth. The term may apply to one, several, or all the teeth of a given individual.

microelectrode, an electrode of very fine caliber consisting usually of a fine wire or a glass tube of capillary diameter drawn to a fine point and filled with saline or a metal used in physiologic experiments to stimulate or record action currents of extracellular or intracellular origin.

microfilaments, any of the submicroscopic cellular filaments, such as the tonofibrils, found in the cytoplasm of most cells, that function primarily as a supportive system.

microgenia (mī'krōjē'nē·ə), an abnormal smallness of the chin.

microglossia (mī'krōgläs'ē·ə), an abnormally small tongue.

microglossic, descriptive of microglossia.

micrognathia (mī'krōnāth'ē·ə), an abnormally small jaw such as seen in brachygnathia. See also **brachygnathia; retrognathism.**

micrognathic, descriptive of micrognathia.

microleakage, the seepage of fluids, debris, and microorganisms along the interface between a restoration and the walls of a cavity preparation.

micrometer (mī'krōmē't□), a millionth of a meter (10^{-6} meter).

micron. See **micrometer.**

micronutrient, an organic compound such as a vitamin, or a chemical element such as zinc or iodine, essential only in minute amounts for the normal physiologic processes of the body.

microorganism (mī'krō·ôr'ganizəm), a minute living organism, such as a bacterium, virus, rickettsia, yeast, or fungus. These organisms may exist as part of the normal flora of the oral cavity without producing disease. With disturbance of the more or less balanced interrelationship between the organisms or between the organisms and host resistance, individual forms of microorganisms may overgrow and induce disease in the host's tissues. Of course, organisms foreign to the individual may invade and produce pathologic processes.

microphthalmos, a developmental anomaly characterized by abnormal smallness of one or both eyes.

microradiography, a process by which a radiograph of small or very thin object is produced on fine-grained photographic film under conditions that permit subsequent microscopic examination or enlargement of the radiograph within the resolution limits of the photographic emulsion, which approaches 1000 lines per millimeter.

microscope, an instrument containing a powerful lens system for magnifying and viewing near objects.

   m., dark-field, a microscope that has a special condenser and objective with a diaphragm or stop by which light is scattered from the object with the result that the object appears bright and the background dark.

   m., electron, a microscope in which electron beams with wavelengths shorter than visible light are used in place of visible light, allowing much greater resolution and magnification of the object.

      m., e., scanning, an electron microscope capable of reflected electrons from the specimen surface by which a three-dimensional image is obtained of the surface, which provides both high resolution and a great depth of focus view of the object.

   m., interference, a microscope designed to split entering light into two beams that pass through the specimen and are recombined in the image plane, making visualization of refractile object details not possible with a single beam

   m., phase-contrast, a specially constructed microscope that has a special condenser and objective containing a phase-shifting mechanism whereby small differences in refraction can be made visible to intensity or contrast in the images. The phase-contrast microscope is particularly helpful in examining living or unstained cells and tissues. This microscope is an excellent aid in the education and motivation of patients in the understanding and control of dental plaque.

microscopy, a technique for observing minute materials using a microscope.

***Microsporum,* a genus of dermatophytes of the family Moniliaceae.**

microstomia (mī'krōstō'mē·ə), **1.** a small oral fissure. **2.** the condition of having an abnormally small mouth.

microsurgery, surgery that involves microdissection and micromanipulation of tissues, usually accomplished with the aid of a binocular microscopic instrument.

microtia (mīkrō'shē·ə), aplasia or hypoplasia of the pinna of the ear, with a closed or missing external auditory meatus.

microtubule, a hollow cylindrical structure that occurs widely within plant and animal cells. Microtubules increase in number during cell division and are associated with the movement of DNA material.

microvilli, tiny hairlike processes that extend from the surface of many cells. They are usually so small as to be visible only with an electron microscope.

midazolam HCl, *trade name:* Versed; *drug class:* benzodiazepine general anesthetic, anesthesia adjunct (Controlled Substance Schedule IV); *action:* depresses subcortical levels in central nervous system; may act on limbic system, reticular formation; may potentiate γ-aminobutyric acid (GABA) by binding to specific benzodiazepine receptors; *uses:* conscious sedation, general anesthesia induction, sedation for diagnostic endoscopic procedures, intubation, preoperative sedation.

midbrain (mid'brān), the portion of the brain located superior to the pons and medulla and containing the motor nuclei of the ocular motor and trochlear nerves. It also contains the major pathways and decussations of fibers from the cerebrum and cerebellum.

middle age, the period between young adult and elderly, usually 35 to 55 years of age; a period of great productivity. Also called *middle adult.*

midface, that portion of the face comprised of the nasal, maxillary, and zygomatic bones and the soft tissues covering these bones.

midline, the line equidistant from bilateral features of the head.

midwife, 1. in traditional use, a (female) person who assists women in childbirth. **2.** a nurse practitioner trained and experienced in assisting women in childbirth.

migraine. See **headache, migraine.**

migration, tooth. See **tooth, drifting.**

migratory glossitis, also known as *geographic tongue.* See also **tongue, geographic.**

Mikulicz' aphtha, disease, syndrome (mik'yo͞olich'ēz). See **disease, Mikulicz'.** (not current)

Mikulicz' ulcer. See **periadenitis mucosa necrotica recurrens.** (not current)

milled-in curve. See **path, milled-in.** (not current)

milled-in path. See **path, milled-in.** (not current)

Miller's organism. See **organism, Miller's.** (not current)

milliampere (mil'ē-am'pir), in radiography, milliamperage signifies the amount of current flowing in the tube circuit. With time (seconds), it is an indication of roentgen-ray quantity.

millicurie, one thousandth of a curie.

milliliter (ml) (mil'ilē'tər), the preferred unit of volume used in prescription writing. It is based on the fundamental unit, the liter. One liter equals 1000 milliliters. In prescriptions the abbreviations **ml** and **cc** are often used interchangeably because they are so nearly equal.

milling-in, the procedure of refining or perfecting the occlusion of removable partial or complete dentures by placing abrasives between their occluding surfaces while the dentures make contact in various excursions on the articulator.

milliroentgen (mil'irent'gən), a submultiple of the roentgen, equal to one thousandth of a roentgen.

Milwaukee brace, an orthotic device that helps immobilize the torso and the neck of a patient in the treatment or correction of scoliosis, lordosis, or kyphosis. Prolonged use may induce or complicate a malocclusion unless the teeth and jaws are supported with retaining appliances.

mineralization, the bioprecipitation of an inorganic substance.

mineralocorticoids (min'əral'ōkôr'tikoidz) (proinflammatory hormones), adrenal corticosteroids that are active in the retention of salt and in the maintenance of life of adrenalectomized animals. Typical are deoxycorticosterone and aldosterone. Aldosterone is a natural hormone for salt retention but also has some regulatory effect on carbohydrate metabolism.

mineral oil. See **oil, mineral.**

minim (min'im), a unit of volume in the traditional apothecary system. One minim equals 0.06 ml. A drop is sometimes used as a crude approximation of the minim.

minocycline HCl, *trade names:* Dyancin, Minocin; *drug class:* tetracycline antiinfective; *action:* inhibits protein synthesis, phosphorylation in microorganisms by binding 30S ribosomal subunits, reversibly binding to 50S ribosomal subunits; bacteriostatic; *uses:* syphilis, *Chlamydia trachomatis* infection, gonorrhea, lymphogranuloma venereum, rickettsial infections, inflammatory acne. Also used in the treatment of some periodontal infections generally in conjunction with mechanical therapy.

minor, a person of either sex under the age of majority; that is, one who has not attained the age at which full civil rights are granted.

m. **connector.** See **connector, minor.**

minoxidil, *trade names:* Loniten, Rogaine (topical); *drug class:* antihypertensive; *action:* directly relaxes arteriolar smooth muscle, reducing peripheral resistance; *uses:* severe hypertension not responsive to other therapy (used with a diuretic); topically to treat alopecia (mechanism unknown).

miosis, 1. the contraction of the sphincter muscle of the iris, causing the pupil to become smaller. **2.** an abnormal condition characterized by excessive constriction of the sphincter muscle of the iris, resulting in very small, pinpoint pupils.

miotic (mē·ot'ik), a drug that constricts the pupil.

misconduct, a deviation from duty by one employed in a professional capacity; a transgression of an established rule.

misfeasance (misfē'zens), the improper performance of some act that one may lawfully do.

misoprostol, *trade name:* Cytotec; *drug class:* gastric mucosa protectant; *action:* a prostaglandin E₁ analog that inhibits gastric acid secretion; *uses:* prevention of nonsteroidal antiinflammatory drug-induced gastric ulcers.

misrepresentation, an intentionally false statement regarding a matter of fact.

MIST, an acronym for **Medical Information Service** via **Telephone.** MIST is a consultation service offered by some state-operated university medical centers.

mistake, an unintentional act, omission, or error resulting from ignorance, surprise, or misplaced confidence.

mitigation (mit'igā'shən), alleviation; abatement or diminution of a penalty imposed by law.

m. of damages, a reduction of damages based on facts that show the plaintiff's course of action does not entitle the plaintiff to as large an amount as the evidence would otherwise justify the jury in allowing.

mitochondria, small, rodlike, threadlike, or granular organelles within the cytoplasm that function in cellular metabolism and respiration and occur in varying number in all living cells except bacteria, viruses, blue-green algae, and mature erythrocytes.

mitogen, an agent that triggers mitosis.

mitosis, a type of cell division that occurs in somatic cells and results in the formation of two genetically identical daughter cells containing the diploid number of chromosomes characteristic of the species.

mitotane, *trade name:* Lysodren; *drug class:* antineoplastic; *action:* acts on adrenal cortex to suppress activity and adrenal steroid production; *use:* adrenocortical carcinoma.

mitotic index, the number of cells per unit undergoing mitosis during a given time. The ratio is used primarily as an estimation of the rate of tissue growth.

mitral valve, a bicuspid valve situated between the left atrium and the left ventricle; the only valve with two, rather than three, cusps. The mitral valve allows blood to flow from the left atrium into the left ventricle but prevents blood from flowing back into the atrium.

m. v. prolapse (MVP), the protrusion of one or both cusps of the mitral valve back into the left atrium during ventricular systole, resulting in incomplete closure of the valve and mitral insufficiency.

mix, to form by combining ingredients.

mixed dentition. See **dentition, mixed.**

mixing, vacuum, a method of mixing materials, such as gypsum products and water, in a vacuum.

MLD. See **dose, lethal, minimum.**

MLT. See **time, median lethal.**

mo cavity, a cavity on the mesial and occlusal surfaces of a tooth. See also **cavity, Class 2.**

mobility, the loosening of a tooth or teeth. Mobility is an important diag-

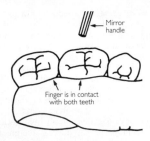

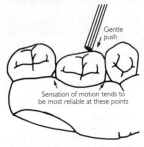

Tooth mobility testing. (Parr, 1978.)

M

nostic sign that may result not only from a decrease in root attachment or changes in the periodontal ligament but also from destruction of the gingival fiber apparatus and transseptal fibers.

m. of tooth. See **tooth mobility.**

MOD cavity, a cavity on the mesial, occlusal, and distal surfaces of a tooth. See also **cavity, Class 2.**

mode (mo), a measure of central tendency that is the most frequently occurring score or value in a group of scores. The mode may be used as an average score.

model, 1. a replica, usually in miniature. See also **cast. 2.** a positive replica of the dentition and surrounding or adjoining structures used as a diagnostic aid and/or base for construction of orthodontic and prosthetic appliances.

m., casting. See **cast, refractory.**
m., implant. See **cast, implant.**
m., of prepared cavity. See **die.**
m., study. See **cast, diagnostic.**

modeling compound. See **compound.**

models, biologic, the use of the analog in some other animal species of a disease of man to study or compare the response or treatment of the disease before testing with humans.

models, statistical, statistical formulations or analyses which, when applied to data and found to fit the data, are then used to verify the assumptions and parameters used in the analysis. Some examples of statistic models include the linear model, binomial model, polynomial model, and two-parameter model.

modem (modulator/demodulator), a device that converts data from a form compatible with computer manipulation to a form compatible with transmission equipment and vice versa.

moderator, a chairman; one who presides over an assembly, group, or panel.

modiolus (mōdē′ōləs), a point distal to the corner of the mouth where several muscles of facial expression converge.

modulus, a constant that numerically indicates the amount in which a certain property is possessed by any object.

m. of elasticity. See **elasticity, modulus of.**
m. of resilience. See **resilience, modulus of.**
m. of rigidity. See **rigidity.**
m., Young's. See **elasticity, modulus of.**

Moeller's disease (mel′ərz). See **scurvy, infantile.** (not current)

Moeller's glossitis. See **glossitis, Moeller's.** (not current)

moexipril hydrochloride, *trade name:* Univasc; *drug class:* angiotensin-converting enzyme (ACE) inhibitor; *action:* selectively suppresses renin-angiotensin-aldosterone system; inhibits ACE; prevents conversion of angiotensin I to angiotensin II; results in dilation of arterial, venous vessels; *use:* hypertension as a single drug or in combination with a thiazide diuretic.

Mohs scale. See **hardness, Mohs.**

Mohs surgery, a surgical technique used primarily in the treatment of skin neoplasms, especially basal cell or squamous cell carcinoma of the skin. This procedure is a microscopically controlled excision of cutaneous tumors either after fixation in vivo or after freezing the tissue. Serial examinations of fresh tissue specimens are most frequently done to ensure complete excision of the lesion.

molar, I. a reference solution in which the concentration is stated with regard to the number of gram molecular weights per liter of solution. **2.** a tooth adapted for grinding by having a broad, somewhat ridged surface. In the human, the molar is one of the 12 teeth located in the posterior aspect of the upper and lower jaws.

m., mulberry, a malformed first molar with a crown, suggesting the appearance of a mulberry. It may be a manifestation of congenital syphilis, although other diseases affecting the enamel organ during morphodifferentiation may produce a similar lesion.

m. sheath, a rectangular metallic tube soldered or welded to the molar bands.

mold (mould), a form in which an object is cast or shaped. The process of shaping a material into an object. The term used to specify the shape of an artificial tooth or teeth.

molding, shaping.

m., border. See **border molding.**

m., compression, the act of pressing or squeezing together to form a shape in a mold.

m., injection, the adaptation of a plastic material to the negative form of a closed mold by forcing the material into the mold through appropriate gateways. See also **molding, compression.**

m., tissue. See **border molding.**

mole, a pigmented nevus.

molecular biology, the study of biology from the viewpoint of the physical and chemical interactions of molecules involved in life functions.

molecular weight. See **weight, molecular.**

molecule, a unit of matter that is the smallest particle of an element or chemical combination of atoms (as a compound) capable of retaining chemical identity with the substance in mass.

molimina, menstrual (molim'inə), circulatory symptoms, psychic tension, irritable behavior, belligerence, and other personality alterations before or during menstruation. The cause is unknown.

molindone HCl, *trade name:* Moban, Moban Concentrate; *drug class:* antipsychotic; *action:* depresses cerebral cortex, hypothalamus, limbic system, which control activity, aggression; blocks neurotransmission produced by dopamine at synapse; mechanism for antipsychotic effects is unclear; *use:* psychotic disorders.

molluscum contagiosum, a disease of the skin and mucous membranes, caused by a poxvirus and found all over the world. It is characterized by scattered flesh-toned papules. The disease most frequently occurs in children and in adults with an impaired immune response. It is transmitted from person to person by direct or indirect contact and lasts up to 3 years.

moliuscum fibrosum. See **neurofibromatosis.**

molybdenum, a grayish metallic element with an atomic number of 42 and an atomic weight of 95.94. Molybdenum is poisonous if ingested in large quantities.

momentum, quantity of motion, expressed as the product of mass and velocity.

money, the general term for the representation of value; currency; cash.

m. market fund, a mutual fund that invests only in high-yielding, short-term money market instruments (U.S. Treasury bills, bank certificates of deposit, and commercial paper).

mongolism (mon'gōlizəm) (Down's syndrome), **I.** extreme mental deficiency of a congenital type associated with features of the Mongolian race, such as slanted eyes. **2.** clinical syndrome (Down's) associated with the autosomal abnormalities trisomy-21 or translocations 13-15/21-22, or 21/22. Affected children have almond-shaped eyes, a rather roundish head, and increased susceptibility to infection. They are mentally retarded, commonly suffer from acute leukemia, and often have congenital heart disease, a heavily fissured and protruding tongue, delayed dentition, an underdeveloped nose, short fingers, and broad simian-like hands.

Monilia albicans (monil'ē·ə al'bikanz). See ***Candida albicans.*** (not current)

moniliasis (mo′nili′əsis), infection by a fungus of the genus *Candida,* usually *C. albicans.* May involve the mouth (thrush), female genitalia, skin, hands, nails, and/or lungs. *Oral moniliasis* refers to thrush or to mycotic stomatitis. The latter term is sometimes applied to erythematous patches that are not typical of the usual white patches of thrush. See also **thrush.**

monitor, to observe and evaluate a function of the body closely and constantly over a period of time for diagnostic purposes.

monitoring, the periodic or continuous determination of the dose rate in an occupied area by a person.

m., ambulatory, to observe and evaluate a patient while engaged in normal routine behaviors.

m., area, routine monitoring of the level of radiation of any particular area, building, room, equipment, or outdoor space.

m., personal, monitoring of any part of an individual (for example, breath or excretions or any part of the clothing).

m., personnel, a systematic, periodic check of the radiation dose each person receives during working hours.

m., physiologic, the observation and evaluation of physiologic functions usually with an electronic device with surface electrodes attached to specific areas of the body.

monkey, a vernacular term applied to a lower primate animal that is often used for experimental purposes in medicine and stomatology. Its dental and oral structures are morphologically and functionally similar to those of human beings, permitting an associated correlation of experimental findings. See also *Macaca.*

monoamine oxidase, an enzyme that catalyzes the oxidation of amines.

monobloc. See **activator.**

monocyte (mon′ōsīt), a large mononuclear leukocyte with an ovoid or kidney-shaped nucleous, containing chromatin material with a lacy pattern and abundant gray-blue cytoplasm filled with fine, reddish, and azurophilic granules.

monocytosis (mon′ōsītō′sis), an increase in the number of monocytes in the peripheral bloodstream. Various limits are given (for example, a total number in excess of $800/mm^3$, regardless of the percentage, or a total greater than 8% with the total number less than 800). In both cases the presence of monocytosis is indicated. Monocytosis may be associated with chronic pyogenic infections, subacute bacterial endocarditis, infectious hepatitis, monocytic leukemia, rickettsial disease, and protozoan infections.

monomer (mon′ōmer), a single molecule. In commercial resin products, the term applies to the liquid, which is usually a mixture of monomers.

m., residual, the unpolymerized monomer remaining in the appliance or restoration after processing.

mononucleosis, infectious (mon′ōnoō′klē·ō′sis) (acute benign lymphadenosis, "kissing disease," "student's disease"), an acute infectious viral disease most commonly affecting young adults and older children. Manifestations include fever, sore throat, cervical lymphadenopathy, petechial hemorrhages of the soft palate, and, at times, purpura with thrombocytopenia. Early leukopenia and relative lymphocytosis occur, with later increases in the number of large leukocytoid lymphocytes. The heterophil (usually sheep cell) antibody titer is significantly increased in most instances.

monostotic, affecting a single bone.

Monotremata, the lowest order of mammals, including animals that lay eggs similar to those of reptiles, and nourish their young by a mammary gland that has no nipple, in a shallow pouch developed only during lactation. The only living representatives are the spiny anteater and the duck-billed platypus.

Monson curve. See **curve, Monson.**

moot, 1. subject to argument; undecided. **2.** in law, in a moot case one seeks to determine that an abstract question does not arise on existing facts or rights.

moral, relating to the conscience or moral sense or to the general principles of correct conduct.

morale, the mental state or condition as related to cheerfulness, confidence, and zeal.

Moraxella, a genus of obligately aerobic nonmotile bacteria containing gram-negative coccoids or short rods that usually occur in pairs. They are parasitic on the mucous membranes of man and other mammals. They are penicillin-susceptible.

morbidity, the state of being diseased; can be used as an outcome measure such as number of decayed, missing, and filled teeth.

moricizine, *trade name:* Ethmozine; *drug class:* antidysrhythmic, type I; *action:* decreased rate of rise of action potential, which prolongs the refractory period and shortens the action potential duration; *use:* documented life-threatening dysrhythmias.

morphine sulfate, *trade names:* Duramorph PF, MS Contin, Roxanol; *drug class:* narcotic analgesic (Controlled Substance Schedule II); *action:* depresses pain impulse transmission at the central nervous system by interacting with opioid receptors; *use:* severe pain.

morphogenesis, the development and differentiation of the structures and the form of an organism, specifically the changes that occur in the cells and tissue during embryonic development.

morphology, the branch of biology that deals with the form and structure of an organism or part, without regard to function.

m., determinants of occlusal, variable factors that determine the forms given to the crowns of teeth restored in metals, such as mandibular centricity; the intercondylar distance; the distance of teeth from the sagittal plane; the character of lateral and protrusive paths of the condylar axes; and the overlaps of the anterior teeth and wear.

mortality, the death rate.

mortgage, a right given to the creditor over the property of the debtor for the security of the debt; invests the creditor with the power of having the property seized and sold in default of payment.

m., chattel, a mortgage of goods or personal property.

mortgagee, the person who takes or receives a mortgage.

motion, envelope of, the three-dimensional space circumscribed by border movements and by occlusal contacts of a given point of the mandible. Synonym: movement space. See also **movement, border, posterior.**

motivation, the stimulus, incentive, or inducement to act or react in a certain way. Purposeful human behavior is motivated behavior, which means that either physiologic or social stimuli activate or motivate a person to do something.

motor, pertaining to a muscle, nerve, or center that produces or affects movement.

m. neuron, one of the various efferent nerve cells that transmit nerve impulses from the brain or from the spinal cord to muscular or glandular tissue.

   m. n. disease, a progressive disease that tends to affect middle-age men with degeneration of anterior horn cells, motor cranial nerve nuclei, and pyramidal tracts. Amyotrophic lateral sclerosis is a motor neuron disease.

m. output, the activity that results from the integrative phenomena associated with brain activity. It is expressed in function as muscle contraction of the smooth and striated muscle and as secretion of the exocrine and endocrine glands, and, in effect, represents the total behavioral activity of human life. Whereas sensory phenomena have many avenues that feed into the brain, motor activity is expressed in terms of the simple, direct state of muscle contraction and glandular secretion. Thus muscle activity is expressed in terms of locomotion, hand-learned skills, speaking, mastication, and all forms of human activity that involve motion.

m. pathway, all reflex actions of muscle are achieved by the passage of nerve impulses through the final common pathway—the muscle fibers. The lower motor neuron (the motor route of the cranial nerve) is the final pathway for the structures that are innervated by the cranial nerves. Impulses traverse these nerves to their respective muscles from every level of the spinal cord, hindbrain, midbrain, and cerebral cortex. The cranial motor neurons collate these multiple stimuli and transmit sequences of stimuli to the motor end-plate, which in the normal muscle effects a smooth, continuous, controlled contraction.

m. skill, the ability to make the purposeful movements that are necessary to complete or master a prescribed task.

m. unit, the entity consisting of the lower motor neuron, motor end-plate, and muscle fibers supplied by the end-plate. The final motor activity resulting from a sequence of stimulations to the lower motor neuron is considered a function of the motor unit. The proportion of nerve fibers to the muscle fibers in motor units is designated as the innervation ratio. Motor units may have ratios ranging from 1:4 to 1:150. The closer the ratio approximates unity, the greater the finesse of specificity of the muscular action. The eye muscles have the highest ratio of striated muscles, and the tongue, facial, masticatory, and pharyngeal muscles succeed in that order.

mottled enamel. See **fluorosis, chronic endemic dental.**

moulage, a model of a part or a lesion (for example, a model of the face). It may be of wax or plaster and usually is colored by painting.

mould. See **mold.**

mounting, the laboratory procedure of attaching the maxillary and/or mandibular cast to an articulator or similar instrument.

m. board, a jig used in mounting the maxillary cast on the top articulator frame. The mounting board enables the dentist to determine the patient's axis so that the maxillary cast can be positioned accurately.

m., split cast, a cast with the margins of its base or capital beveled or grooved to permit accurate remounting on an articulator. Split remounting metal plates may be used instead of beveling or grooving in the casts.

mount, x-ray, a windowed, stiff material on which radiographs are arranged in a specific order to correspond with the charts of the teeth.

mouth breathing. See **breathing, mouth.**

mouth, denture-sore, traumatization and inflammation of the oral mucous membranes produced by ill-fitting dentures, hypersensitivity to the chemical components of the denture,

and/or proliferation of *Candida albicans* with subsequent monilial infection.

mouth guard. See **guard, mouth.**

mouth hygiene. See **hygiene, oral.**

mouth preparation. See **preparation, mouth.**

mouth rehabilitation. See **rehabilitation, mouth.**

mouth, trench. See **gingivitis, necrotizing ulcerative.**

mouthwash, a mouth rinse possessing cleansing, germicidal, and/or palliative properties.

movement(s), any change of place or of position of a body.

m., Bennett, the bodily lateral movement or lateral shift of the mandible resulting from the movements of the condyles along the lateral inclines of the mandibular fossae during lateral jaw movement.

m., bodily, movement of a tooth so that the crown and root apex move the same amount in the same direction, thus maintaining the same axial inclination; opposed to tipping movement.

m., border, any extreme muscular movement limited by bone, ligaments, or other soft tissues.

m., free mandibular, mandibular movement made without tooth interference. An uninhibited movement of the mandible.

m., functional mandibular, all natural, proper, or characteristic movements of the mandible made during speaking, chewing, yawning, swallowing, and other associated movements.

m., hinge, an opening or closing movement of the mandible on the hinge axis. A movement around a single axis.

m., intermediary (intermediate movement), all mandibular movements between the extremes of mandibular excursions.

m., jaw, all changes in position of which the mandible is capable.

m., lateral, a movement of a body to one side of its established position.

m., mandibular, any movement of the lower jaw.

m., m. gliding, side-to-side, protrusive, and intermediate movement of the mandible, occurring when the teeth or other occluding surfaces are in contact.

m., masticatory mandibular, the translatory and rotary movements of the mandible that are used in the course of chewing food.

m., nonfunctional mandibular, movement of the mandible for other than the accepted range of functional movements; that is, movements dictated by tension, emotion, or aggression. Also mandibular movements may be misused to hold objects in either indulgent or work habits. These nonfunctional movements may result in a variety of pathologic manifestations.

m., opening mandibular, the movement of the mandible executed during jaw separation.

m., posterior border, any movement of the mandible occurring while the mandible is in its most posterior relation to the maxillae. This movement occurs in the vertical plane from the level of occlusal contact to the level of maximal opening of the jaws.

m., tipping, the movement of a tooth in any direction while its apex remains in almost the original position.

m., tooth, temporary or permanent deviation of a tooth from its normally fixed position in the dental arch. Also, mobility of teeth. When teeth exhibit mobility patterns, movement may be buccolingual, mesiodistal, occlusoapical, or rotational. Movement of teeth into different positions in the dental arch may be produced by repositioning them mesially, distally, buccally, lingually, or occlusally.

m., translatory, the motion of a body at any instant when all points within the body are moving at the same velocity and in the same direction.

moxibustion, a method of producing analgesia or altering the function of a system of the body achieved by igniting moxa, wormwood, or some other combustible, slow-burning substance and holding it as near the point on the skin as possible without causing pain or burning. It is also sometimes used in conjunction with acupuncture.

MPD. See **dose, maximum permissible.**

MSH. See **hormone, melanocytestimulating.**

mucin, a mucopolysaccharide, the chief ingredient of mucus. Mucin is present in most glands that secrete

mucus and is the lubricant that protects body surfaces from friction or erosion.

mucobuccal fold. See **fold, mucobuccal.**

mucocele (myōō′kōsēl). See **cyst, mucous.**

mucoepidermoid tumor, a malignant neoplasm of glandular tissues, especially the ducts of the salivary glands. The tumor contains mucinous and epidermoid squamous cells.

mucolabial fold. See **fold, mucolabial.**

mucopolysaccharides, a generic term for a group of compounds comprised of protein and complex sugars (polysaccharides), many of which are found in blood group substances.

mucopolysaccharidosis (MPS), a genetic disorder involving mucopolysaccharide metabolism and leading to excess storage of the material in the tissues. Forms include MPS I, II, III, IV, V, and VI. Eponymic designations are Hurler, Hunter, Sanfilippo, Morquio, Scheie, and Maroteaux-Lamy syndromes.

mucosa (myōōkō′sə) (mucous membrane), a membrane, composed of epithelium and lamina propria, that lines the oral cavity and other canals and cavities of the body that communicate with external air.

m., alveolar, the covering on the alveolar process loosely attached to bone; extends from the mucogingival junction to the vestibular epithelium and from the lower jaw to the sublingual sulcus.

m., oral, the lining of the oral cavity, composed of the stratified squamous epithelium and the underlying lamina propria.

m., palatine, the mucous membrane covering the palate.

mucositis (myōō′kōsī′tis), an inflammation of the mucous membrane.

m., chronic atrophic senile, mucosal inflammation characterized by atrophy and found primarily in elderly women.

m., fusospirochetal, mucosal inflammation associated with fusiform and spirochetal microorganisms.

mucostatic, 1. pertaining to the normal, relaxed condition of mucosal tissues covering the jaws. **2.** an agent that arrests the secretion of mucus. (not current)

mucous membrane. See **mucosa.**

mucous patch. See **patch, mucous.**

mucoviscidosis (myōō′kōvis′idō′sis). See **disease, fibrocystic.**

mucus, the viscous, slippery secretions of mucous membranes and glands, containing mucin, white blood cells, water, inorganic salts, and exfoliated cells.

mulberry molars, first permanent molars in which the occlusal surface is composed of an aggregate of enamel nodules. All four molars are involved, usually as the result of congenital syphilis.

mulling (mə′ling), the final step of mixing dental amalgam; a kneading of the triturated mass to complete the amalgamation.

multiple myeloma, a malignant neoplasm of the bone marrow. The tumor, composed of plasma cells, destroys osseous tissue, especially in flat bones, causing pain, fracture, hypercalcemia, and skeletal deformities.

multiple sclerosis, a progressive disease characterized by disseminated demyelination of nerve fibers of the brain and spinal cord. It begins slowly, usually in young adulthood, and continues throughout life with periods of exacerbation and remission. The first signs are paresthesias, or abnormal sensations in the extremities or on one side of the face. Other early signs are muscle weakness, vertigo, and visual disturbances.

multiple trauma, a number of injuries sustained during the same accident or assault.

multiprocessing, the use of two or more processors in a system configuration. One processor controls the system, and the others are subordinate to it.

multiprogramming, a technique for permitting more than one program to time-share machine components. This technique permits the concurrent handling of numerous programs by one computer.

multivariate analysis, a set of techniques used when variation in several variables has to be studied simultaneously. In statistics, multivariate analysis is interpreted as any analytic method that allows simultaneous study of two or more dependent variables.

mumps (parotitis), a contagious parotitis caused by the mumps virus (paramyxovirus) and characterized by swelling of the parotid gland and sometimes swelling of the pancreas, ovaries, and testicles. The incubation period is 12 to 20 days; transmission is by droplet spread and direct contact; communicability begins about 2 days before the appearance of symptoms and lasts until swelling of the glands has abated. See also **parotitis.**

m., iodide *(iodine mumps),* an enlargement of the thyroid gland resulting from iodides.

m., iodine. See **mumps, iodide.**

mupirocin/mupirocin calcium, *trade name:* Bactroban; *drug class:* topical antiinfective, pseudomonic acid A; *action:* inhibits bacterial protein synthesis; *uses:* impetigo caused by *Staphylococcus aureus,* β-hemolytic *Streptococcus, Staphylococcus pyogenes;* nasal membranes: *S. aureus.*

murmur, a humming or blowing sound heard on auscultation.

m., aortic, a murmur resulting from insufficiency of the aortic valve secondary to involvement by rheumatic fever or tertiary syphilis.

m., apical diastolic, a murmur heard over the apex of the heart and caused by mitral stenosis, relative mitral stenosis, or aortic insufficiency.

m., apical systolic, a murmur heard at the apex of the heart in systole and caused by mitral insufficiency, which may result from rheumatic heart disease, or by relative mitral insufficiency, which may result from congestive heart failure associated with arteriosclerosis or hypertension. The murmur may also have a functional basis.

m., basal diastolic, a murmur heard over the base of the heart and caused by aortic insufficiency resulting from rheumatic heart disease or syphilis, relative aortic insufficiency associated with diastolic hypertension, or a patent ductus arteriosus.

m., basal systolic, a murmur heard over the base of the heart and caused by aortic stenosis resulting from rheumatic heart disease or by relative stenosis of the aortic valve resulting from aortic dilation secondary to arteriosclerosis or hypertension. The murmur may also be functional or may result from congenital heart or vascular defects.

m., cardiac (heart murmur), an abnormal sound heard in the region of the heart at any time during the heart's cycle. Murmurs may be named according to the area of generation (mitral, aortic, pulmonary, or tricuspid) and according to the period of the cycle (diastolic or systolic).

m., functional (innocent murmur, inorganic murmur), a murmur resulting from the position of the body, severe anemia, or polycythemia. Not related to structural changes in the heart.

m., heart. See **murmur, cardiac.**

m., innocent. See **murmur, functional.**

m., inorganic. See **murmur, functional.**

m., mitral, a heart murmur produced by a defect in the mitral valve. It is the most common form of murmur in rheumatic heart disease.

m., organic, a murmur resulting from structural changes in the heart or in the great vessels of the heart.

muscle, an organ that, by cellular contraction, produces the movements of life. The two varieties of muscle structure are striated, which includes all the muscles in which contraction is voluntary and the heart muscle (in which contraction is involuntary), and unstriated, smooth, or organic, which includes all the involuntary muscles (except the heart), such as the muscular layer of the intestines, bladder, and blood vessels.

m., ciliary, a tiny smooth muscle at the junction of the cornea and sclera, consisting of two groups of fibers: circular fibers, which exert parasympathetic control through the oculomotor nerve and the ciliary ganglion, and radial fibers, which exert sympathetic control. Ciliary muscles are responsible for accommodation for far vision through flattening of the lens.

m., concentric, contraction. See **contraction, muscle, concentric.**

m. contraction. See **contraction, muscle.**

m., eccentric, contraction. See **contraction, muscle, eccentric.**

m., elasticity of, physical, the physical quality of being elastic, of yielding to passive physical stretch.

m., elasticity of, physiologic, the biologic quality, unique for muscle, of being able to change and resume size under neuromuscular control.

m., facial, the muscles of expression, frequently called the mimetic muscles. They are quite variable in contour, are widely distributed over the scalp and face, and tend to be especially concentrated around the orbits, outer ear, and lips. It is the mobility of the lips that has extended the usefulness of the facial muscles in expressing emotion, speech, and intelligence. The facial muscles, as a group, have only one bony origin in the facial skeleton. The muscles form a circular rim around the perimeter of the facial bones and extend anteriorly as a tube of tissue in which the lumen narrows and terminates in the orbicularis oris. The structure of the facial muscles may be regarded as a truncated cone in which the base rests on the skeleton (origin) in a fixed position, whereas the truncated top of the cone (insertion in the orbicularis oris) is variable in diameter and height. The lips are thus extensible and retractable and can constrict like a purse string.

m. fatigue, the depletion of the metabolites necessary to sustain or repeat a muscle contraction.

m. fiber, the cell of muscle tissue. The three types of muscle fibers are striated (voluntary), cardiac, and smooth (involuntary).

m., functional changes of, asymmetric modifications in length, diameter, and bulk of muscle fibers as a result of variations in function. Muscle responds to normal function by maintenance of bulk. An increase in bulk is caused by an increase in the number of capillaries and in the mean diameter of individual muscle fibers. The response to function accounts for the asymmetry of musculature, which is frequently found when the growth patterns have been influenced by a traumatogenic agent such as disease, injury, or surgery, and also by the functional processes of the body itself, such as posture and habit. Asymmetry is not necessarily pathologic; that is, it may be the result of differences in habits of chewing, incision, speech sounds, and facial gestures.

m., hypertenseness, an increased muscular tension that is not easily released but that does not prevent normal lengthening of the muscle. Hypertenseness is found in patients with general nervousness.

m., innervation of, reciprocal, a phenomenon of antagonistic muscles demonstrated during a concentric contraction such as that of the temporal muscle. Innervation of the antagonist, the external pterygoid muscle, is partially inhibited, so that freedom of action in flexing the temporomandibular joint is possible. This phenomenon demonstrates inhibition of antagonistic skeletal muscles in a reflex arc brought about automatically by a reduction of the motor discharges from the central nervous system. One of the two muscles in the reflex arc is activated, and the activity of the other is depressed.

m., isometric, contraction. See **contraction, muscle, isometric.**

m., isotonic, contraction. See **contraction, muscle, isotonic.**

m., masticatory (mas'tikətōrē), the powerful muscles that elevate and rotate the mandible so that the opposing teeth may occlude for mastication.

m. memory, a kinesthetic phenomenon by which a muscle or set of muscles may involuntarily produce movement that follows a pattern that has become established by frequent repetition over a long period of time.

m., mimetic (mimet'ik), the facial muscles by which emotion and intelligence are expressed. The facial nerve provides neurologic control over the muscles of the face.

m., ocular, function, the action of the eye muscles in moving the eyeballs. The eyes are in a position of rest (their primary position) when their direction is maintained simply by the tone of the ocular muscles. This condition prevails when the gaze is straight ahead into distance and not directed to any particular point in space. The visual axes are then parallel. When the eyes view some distant definite object, they are turned by contraction of the ocular muscles and converge so that the visual axes meet at the observed object, and an almost identical image of the object falls on a corresponding point on each fovea, the centralis of the retina. The adjustment of the eye movements for acute obser-

vation is called fixation, and the point where the visual axes meet is the fixation point. Thus the interplay of the ocular muscles permits rapid, reciprocally controlled movement of the eyeballs for fixation.

m., physical characteristics of primary, elasticity, a muscle is an elastic body. Its individual fibers follow Hooke's law of elastic bodies; that is, the amount of elongation is proportional to the stretching force. The muscle organs contain tissue other than muscle fibers and thus deviate slightly from this law. The human muscle fiber can contract to about half its total length.

m., regeneration of reproduction or repair of muscle fiber, a sequela to many types of muscle damage. Reparation is always associated with the proliferation of sarcolemmic nuclei. Connective tissue elements do not participate in this process except to bridge the gap and offer support for the regenerative fibers. The regenerative process takes place in two forms: regeneration by budding from the surviving parts of the muscle fibers, which occurs when segments of the muscle fiber and its sheath are destroyed, and regeneration by proliferation of cellular bands, which occurs when the sarcolemmic nuclei are spared and can form a sarcoplasmic band by linkage of the cytoplasmic processes.

m. relaxation, the resting state of a muscle fiber or a group of muscle fibers.

m., sequence of, development, the pattern of embryologic muscular development. The muscles of the neck and trunk are the first to develop; they are followed by the lingual and facial musculature and then by the distal and proximal appendicular musculature.

m., smooth, the simplest of the three types of muscle (smooth, striated, and cardiac). It is the muscle of the lining of the digestive tract, ducts of glands, and viscera associated with the gut. It also supplies the muscles for the genitourinary tract, structures of the blood vessels, connective tissues of the mucous membranes, and skin with its appendages. A typical smooth muscle fiber is a slender, spindle-shaped body averaging a few tenths of a millimeter in length. There is a single, centrally striated nucleus. The cytoplasm appears homogeneous. The cells are arranged in bands, or bundles, with interspersed connective tissue fibers uniting them into an effective common mass. Smooth muscle fibers are innervated in part by nerve fibers and in part by the contraction of adjacent muscle tissues. The digestive tract, particularly, demonstrates waves of contraction that pass along a band of smooth muscle.

m., spasticity of, increased muscular tension of antagonists that prevents normal movement; caused by an inability to relax (a loss of reciprocal inhibition) resulting from a lesion of the upper motor neuron.

m., striated, skeletal muscles forming the bulk of the body; the voluntary muscles derived from the myotomes of the embryo. Generally, they are organized as formed muscles that attach to and move the skeletal structures. The cells are large, elongated, and cylindric, with lengths ranging from 1 mm to several centimeters. The cells have multiple nuclei that are peripherally situated and scattered along the length of the fiber. The fiber contains a large number of elongated fibers that, under the microscope, appear as the alternating light and dark bands that give the characteristic striated appearance of the striated muscle. The dimensional relationships between these light and dark bands are altered during contraction of the muscle fiber. The potential interaction between these bands permits the wide range of selective purposeful and rapid activity of the skeletal muscles.

m., suprahyoid and infrahyoid, the muscles grouped around the hyoid bone. They aid in depressing and fixing the mandible, hyoid bone, and larynx in the performance of their several respective functions.

m., tongue, extrinsic, the muscles of the tongue that provide a scaffolding by which the intrinsic muscles can be moved around in the oral cavity while the latter are continuously modifying their dimension and contour. The extrinsic muscles are paired and originate from both sides of the cranial skeleton, mandible, and hyoid bone to radiate medially and insert into the body of the tongue, which consists

principally of the intrinsic muscles.

m., tongue, intrinsic, the muscles of the tongue that have no attachments in bone, terminating either within each other or in the extrinsic muscle group. The fibers of the intrinsic muscles also lie in all three planes of space and are called *longitudinal, vertical,* and *transverse fibers* to describe their distribution. They are capable of assuming an infinite variety of shapes. They depend, however, on the activity of the extrinsic muscles to be moved bodily through space.

m. trimming. See **border molding** and **impression, correctable.**

muscular dystrophy (məs'kyələr dis'-trōfē), a group of genetically transmitted diseases characterized by progressive atrophy of symmetric groups of skeletal muscles without evidence of involvement or degeneration of neural tissue. In all forms of muscular dystrophy there is an insidious loss of strength with increasing disability and deformity. Serum creatine phosphokinase is increased in affected individuals and acts as a diagnostic aid. Diagnosis is confirmed by muscle biopsy, electromyography, and genetic pedigree.

musculature (məs'kyoolətur), any part of the muscular apparatus of the body; the source of power for the movement of the body or its parts.

m., cheek, the muscles giving support, form, and function to the cheeks. Should disequilibrium exist between the functional forces exerted on the dentition by the tongue and cheek musculature, deviations in tooth alignment may occur.

m., lip, the muscles that perform the physiologic or functional activities of the lips. The primary muscles include the orbicularis oris, quadratus labii superioris, risorius, and buccinators. If the tongue and the musculature of the lips do not exert equivalent forces against the teeth, movement of the teeth may occur.

musculoskeletal system (məs'kyə-lōskel'etəl), all the muscles, bones, joints, and related structures, such as the tendons and connective tissue, that function in the stability and movement of the parts and organs of the body. See also **system, musculoskeletal.**

M

mushbite, an obsolete type of maxillomandibular record made by introducing a mass of soft wax into the patient's mouth and instructing the patient to bite into it to the desired degree. Not a generally accepted procedure. See also **record, maxillomandibular.**

mutagen, any chemical or physical environmental agent that induces a genetic mutation or increases the mutation rate.

mutagenesis, the induction or occurrence of a genetic mutation.

mutant, an individual showing a mutation.

mutation (myo͞otā′shən), a departure from the parent type, as when an organism differs from its parents in one or more heritable characteristics; caused by genetic change.

m., gene, a sudden and permanent change in a gene. The term *mutation* is sometimes used in a broader sense to include chromosome aberrations.

m., lethal, a mutation leading to death of the offspring at any stage.

mutual, interchangeable; reciprocal; joint.

myalgia, pain in the muscles.

mycelium (mīsē′lē·əm), the filamentous network of hyphae of a fungus.

Mycobacterium, a genus of rodshaped, acid-fast bacteria having two significant pathogenic species: *Mycobacterium leprae,* causing leprosy; and *Mycobacterium tuberculosis,* causing tuberculosis.

M. bovis, a species that is the primary cause of tuberculosis in cattle. It is transmissible to man and other animals.

M. phlei, Timothy hay bacillus, a species found in soil, in dust, and on plants.

M. tuberculosis (Koch's bacillus), the microorganism responsible for tuberculosis, generally a respiratory infection in man; nonrespiratory tuberculosis is considered an indicator disease for AIDS.

mycology, that branch of microbiology that deals with yeasts and fungi.

mycophenolate mofetil, *trade name:* CellCept; *drug class:* immunosuppressant; *action:* selective inhibitor of inosine monophosphate dehydrogenase, thereby preventing the synthesis of guanosine nucleotide and resulting in cytostatic effect on T and B lymphocytes; *uses:* prophylaxis of organ rejection in patients receiving allogenic renal transplants (in combination with cyclosporine and corticosteroids).

Mycoplasma, a genus of ultramicroscopic organisms lacking rigid cell walls and considered to be the smallest free-living organisms.

M. pneumoniae, a species of *Mycoplasma* causing mycoplasma pneumonia, which is characterized by symptoms of an upper respiratory infection with a dry cough and fever.

mycosis, any disease caused by a yeast or fungus.

m. fungoides, a rare, chronic, lymphomatous skin malignancy resembling eczema or a cutaneous tumor that is followed by microabscesses in the epidermis and lesions simulating those of Hodgkin's disease in lymph nodes and viscera.

mydriasis, an abnormal condition of the eye characterized by contraction of the dilator muscle, resulting in widely dilated pupils.

mydriatic (mid′rē·at′ik), a drug that dilates the pupil.

myelin (mī′əlin), a fatlike substance forming a sheath around certain nerve fibers. It is associated with volitional nervous system fibers and is believed to be related to the capacity of nerve structures for rapid transmission of nerve impulses. Various diseases, such as multiple sclerosis, can destroy these myelin wrappings.

myeloma (mī′əlō′mə), a neoplasm characterized by cells normally found in the bone marrow.

m., multiple, a primary malignant neoplasm of bone marrow characterized by proliferation of cells resembling plasma cells. Circumscribed radiolucencies are seen within the bones, and Bence Jones protein is usually found in the urine.

m., plasma cell, a malignant neoplasm characterized by plasma cells. Solitary lesions may appear as radiolucencies in the bone and are sometimes considered benign, although most authorities believe that even these lesions become multiple and terminate fatally.

m., solitary plasma cell, an incompletely understood monostotic neoplasm of bone that is histologically identical with multiple myeloma. Laboratory findings, positive in multiple myeloma, are usually negative in solitary plasma cell myeloma. Although usually benign, solitary plasma cell myelomas may be malignant.

myelophthisis (mī'eloͤfthī'sis), a displacement of bone marrow by fibrous tissue, carcinoma, or leukemia.

mylohyoid ridge, cantilevered, a condition in which a major undercut occurs inferior to a broad mylohyoid ridge; creating a vertical groove into such an area often causes perforation of the medial cortical plate.

myoblastoma (mī'ōblastō'mə), a benign neoplasm characterized by large polyhedral cells resembling young muscle cells. Occurs most frequently in the tongue.

m., granular cell, a benign soft tissue tumor of disputed origin. The tumor cells are large and have a granular eosinophilic cytoplasm and a small nucleus.

myocardial infarction, an occlusion or blockage of arteries supplying the muscles of the heart, resulting in injury or necrosis of the heart muscle.

myocardial ischemia, the loss of oxygen to the heart muscle caused by blockage of the coronary arteries or their branches.

myocardium, the thick, contractile middle layer of uniquely constructed and arranged muscle cells (cardiac muscle) that form the bulk of the heart wall.

myoclonus, a spasm of a muscle or a group of muscles.

myofascial pain, pain associated with inflammation or irritation of muscle or of the fascia surrounding the muscle.

m. p. dysfunction syndrome (MPD), a subset of the TMJ pain dysfunction syndrome that presents with the triad of symptoms of unilateral pain in the muscles of mastication, clicking of the joint, and limitation of movement but without clinical or radiographic evidence of organic changes in the joint and the lack of tenderness in the joint when palpated from the external auditory meatus.

myolipoma (mī'ōlipō'mə), a myxoma containing fatty tissue.

myoma (mī·ō'mə), a neoplasm characterized by muscle cells.

myopia (mī·ō'pē·ə), a form of defective vision resulting from excessive refractive power of the eye. In this condition, commonly called *nearsightedness,* or *shortsightedness,* light rays coming from an object beyond a certain distance are focused in front of the retina.

myosin, a cardiac and skeletal muscle protein that makes up close to one half of the proteins that occur in muscle tissue. The interaction of myosin and actin is essential for muscle contraction.

myositis, an inflammation of muscle tissue, usually of the voluntary muscles. Causes of myositis include infection, trauma, and infestation by parasites.

myotomy (mī·ot'əmē), cutting or resection of a muscle.

myxedema (mĭksĕdē'mə), a condition associated with hypothyroidism (primary myxedema) or hypopituitarism (secondary or pituitary myxedema). Characteristics include dry hair and skin; thickened skin of the lips; puffy eyelids; thinning of the eyebrows, especially the lateral half; slow, low-pitched, and hoarse speech; and slowness of thinking.

myxofibroma (mik'sōfibrō'mə), a benign neoplasm characterized by mucous and fibroblastic tissues.

myxoma (miksō'mə), a benign tumor composed of fibroblastic cells that have reverted to embryonic growth and produce a mucoid matrix containing widely dispersed stellate cells that have multipolar processes.

myxosarcoma (mik'sōsarkō'mə), a sarcoma containing myxomatous tissue.

M

N (n), in statistics, the number of cases or observations.

N2, a single-visit endodontic technique better known as the *Sargenti technique,* in which the paraformaldehyde is the principal ingredient in the endodontic paste. The technique is not approved by the Council on Dental Therapeutics, and it is not taught at any accredited dental school in the United States.

nabumetone, *trade name* Relafen; *drug class:* nonsteroidal antiinflammatory; *action:* inhibits prostaglandin synthesis by interfering with cyclooxygenase needed for biosynthesis; possesses analgesic, antiinflammatory, antipyretic properties; *uses:* osteoarthritis, rheumatoid arthritis.

nadolol, *trade name:* Corgard; *drug class:* nonselective β-adrenergic blocker; *action:* competitively blocks stimulation of β-adrenergic receptors within the heart; produces negative chronotropic and inotropic activity, slows conduction of AV node, decreases heart rate, which decreases oxygen consumption in myocardium; also decreases renin-aldosterone-angiotensin system; *uses:* chronic stable angina pectoris, mild-to-moderate hypertension.

nafcillin, a semisynthetic penicillin designed as an antistaphylococcal penicillin. Also effective in the treatment of infections caused by pneumococci and Group A β-hemolytic streptococci.

naftifine HCl, *trade name:* Naftin; *drug class:* topical antifungal; *action:* interferes with cell membrane permeability in fungi; *uses:* tinea cruris, tinea corporis.

nalidixic acid, an antibacterial prescribed in the treatment of urinary tract infections.

nalmefene HCl, *trade name:* ReVex; *drug class:* opioid antagonist; *action:* reverses the effects of opioids by competitive antagonism of opioid receptors; *uses:* management of opioid overdose and complete or partial reversal of opioid drug effects, including respiratory depression.

naloxone HCl, *trade name:* Narcan; *drug class:* narcotic antagonist; *action:* competes with narcotics at narcotic receptor sites; *uses:* respiratory depression induced by narcotics, to reverse postoperative opioid depression.

naltrexone HCl, *trade names:* RVa, Trexan; *drug class:* narcotic antagonist; *action:* competes with opioids at opioid receptor sites; *uses:* used in treatment of opioid addiction following detoxification.

name, a word or combination of words by which a person, object, idea, or a group of persons, objects, or ideas is regularly known or designated.

n., generic, a name that is usually descriptive of the substance. Strictly speaking, it is a name used to designate a class relationship. Often used synonymously with *nonproprietary name.*

n., nonproprietary, a drug name that is not restricted by a trademark. Nonproprietary names are now selected in the United States by the United States Adopted Name (USAN) Council.

n., official, the title under which a drug is listed in the *United States Pharmacopeia* (USP) or the *National Formulary* (NF).

n., proprietary, a name assigned by the manufacturer that is restricted by trademark. A drug made by several companies may have more than one proprietary name.

n., United States Adopted (USAN), a name selected by the USAN Council (jointly sponsored by the American Medical Association, American Pharmaceutical Association, and United States Pharmacopeial Convention, Inc) when a new drug is placed on the market. A nonproprietary or generic name.

Nance analysis of arch length, a method of determining whether there is sufficient arch length to accommodate the permanent dentition.

nandrolone deconate, an androgen prescribed in the treatment of testosterone deficiency, osteoporosis, and female breast cancer, and to stimulate growth, weight gain, and the production of red blood cells.

nanometer (nm), a billionth of a meter (10^{-9} meter). This term is now preferred over *millimicron.*

naphazoline HCl, *trade names:* AK-Con Opthalmic, Allerest Eye Drops, Clear Eyes, VasoClear, Vasocon; *drug class:* ophthalmic vasoconstrictor; *action:* vasoconstriction of eye arterioles; decreases eye engorgement by stimulation of α-adrenergic receptors; *uses:* relieves hyperemia, irritation of superficial corneal vascularity.

naproxen/naproxen sodium, *trade names:* Naprosyn, Anaprox, Aleve; *drug class:* nonsteroidal antiinflammatory; *action:* inhibits prostaglandin synthesis by interfering with cyclooxygenase needed for biosynthesis; possesses analgesic, antiinflammatory, antipyretic properties; *uses:* mild-to-moderate pain, osteoarthritis, rheumatoid, gouty arthritis, primary dysmenorrhea.

narcoma, coma or stupor from narcotics. (not current)

narcosis (närkō'sis), drug-induced unconsciousness.

narcotic (närkot'ik), a drug, usually with strong analgesic action and an addiction potential, that may be synthesized or derived from natural sources. Especially one of the opium alkaloids.

narcotism (när'kōtizəm), a state of stupor induced by a narcotic.

narcotize (när'kōtīz), to render unconscious by use of narcotics. (not current)

nasal cavity. See **cavity, nasal.**

nasality, the quality of speech sounds when the nasal cavity is used as a resonator, especially when there is too much nasal resonance.

nasal lavage fluid, a liquid, usually a saline-based water solution, used to cleanse the nasal passages.

nasal mucosa. See **mucosa.**

nasal obstruction, a narrowing of the nasal cavity, which reduces breathing capacity. Caused by an irregular septum, nasal polyps, foreign bodies, or enlarged turbinates.

nasal septum, the partition dividing the nostrils. It is composed of bone and cartilage covered by mucous membrane.

nascent (nas'ənt, nā'sənt), literal meaning: recently born. Also, just released from chemical combination.

nasion (nā'zē·on), the point at the root of the nose that is intersected by the median sagittal plane. The root of the nose corresponds to the nasofrontal suture, which is not necessarily the lowest point on its dorsum and which can usually be located with the finger.

Nasmyth's membrane (nas'miths). See **cuticle, primary.**

nasoalveolar cyst (nā'zō·alvē'ōlər), an intraosseous cyst. A form of globulomaxillary cyst in which the epithelial inclusion is in the soft tissue fusion line. (not current)

nasolabial angle, the angle formed by the labial surface of the upper lip at the midline and the inferior border of the nose. It is a measure of the relative protrusion of the upper lip.

nasolacrimal duct, a tubular channel that carries tears from the lacrimal sac to the nasal cavity.

nasomandibular fixation. See **fixation, nasomandibular.** (not current)

nasopharynx, the uppermost of the three regions of the throat, or pharynx, situated behind the nose and extending from the posterior nares to the level of the soft palate.

natal teeth, the presence of teeth in the mouth at birth, usually caused by the premature eruption of primary teeth but may be an extra or supernumerary tooth. The presence of natal teeth may cause discomfort in nursing.

National Bureau of Standards (NBS), a federal agency in the Department of Commerce that sets accurate measurement standards for commerce, industry, and science in the United States.

National Formulary (NF), a publication containing the official standards for the preparation of various pharmaceutics not listed in the *United States Pharmacopoeia.* It is revised every 5 years.

national health plan, a modification of the present method of delivering health care on a national scale, involving the professions, consumers, and government.

National Health Service Corps (NHSC), a program of the United States Public Health Service (USPHS), in which health care personnel are placed in areas that are underserved. Physicians, dentists, and nurses serve in rural and urban areas of need, usually as employees of local health care agencies. The USPHS pays most of the salary of each corps member.

National Institute for Occupational Safety and Health, an institute of the Centers for Disease Control and Prevention that is responsible for assuring safe and healthful working conditions and for developing standards of safety and health. Research activities are carried out pertinent to these goals.

National Institutes of Health (NIH), an agency within the United States Public Health Service made up of several institutions and constituent divisions, including the Bureau of Health Manpower Education, the National Library of Medicine, the National Cancer Institute, the National Institute for Dental Research, and a number of other research institutes and divisions.

nausea, a sensation often leading to the urge to vomit. Common causes are motion sickness, early pregnancy, intense pain, emotional stress, gallbladder disease, food poisoning, and various entroviruses.

Nealon's technique. See **technique, Nealon's.** (not current)

near-death experience, the subjective observations of people who have either been close to clinical death or who may have recovered after having been declared dead. Many claim to have witnessed similar episodes of passing through a tunnel toward a bright light and encountering people who have preceded them in death.

Necator, a genus of nematode hookworms.

N. americanus, the so-called "New World" hookworm. The adults of this species attach to villi in the small intestine and suck blood, causing abdominal discomfort, diarrhea and cramps, anorexia, loss of weight, and hypochromic microcytic anemia.

necatoriasis, hookworm disease. See also *Necator americanus.*

necessary, anything indispensable or useful for the sustenance of human life, such as food, shelter, and clothing.

n. contracts of infants (minors), things suitable to each child according to the child's circumstances.

n. treatment, a dental procedure or service determined by a dentist as necessary to establish or maintain a patient's oral health. Such determinations are based on the professional diagnostic judgment of the dentist and the standards of care that prevail in the professional community.

neck of condyle. See **process, condyloid, neck of.**

necrosis (nekrō′sis), **1.** the death of a cell or group of cells in contact with living tissue. **2.** the local death of cells resulting from, for example, loss of blood supply, bacterial toxins, or physical or chemical agents.

n., caseous (kā′sē-əs), a change commonly associated with tuberculosis and characterized by dry, soft, and cheesy tissue.

n., exanthematous, an acute necrotizing process involving the gingivae, jawbones, and contiguous soft tissues. It is of unknown cause, primarily affects children, and resembles noma. It differs from noma, however, in that it has a slight odor, tendency for self-limitation, low mortality rate, and normal leukocyte count. See also **noma.**

n., gingival, death and degeneration of the cells and other structural elements of the gingivae (for example, necrotizing ulcerative gingivitis).

n., ischemic, death and disintegration of a tissue resulting from interference with its blood supply, thus depriving the tissues of access to substances necessary for metabolic sustenance. It may occur in the periodontal membrane resulting from occlusal trauma.

n. of epithelial attachment, the death of cells composing the epithelial attachment. In a specific periodontitis produced by organisms similar to *Actinomyces,* necrosis of the epithelial attachment may exist, permitting a rapid apical shift of the base of the pocket.

n., periodontal membrane, necrosis of a portion of the periodontal membrane, usually resulting from traumatic injury (for example, in occlusal traumatism). Much of this necrotic change is the result of ischemia.

n., radiation, the death of tissue caused by radiation.

nedocromil sodium, *trade name:* Tilade; *drug class:* antiasthmatic, mast cell stabilizer; *action:* stabilizes the membrane of the sentitized mast cell, preventing release of chemical mediators after an antigen-IgE interaction; *use:* prophylaxis only in reversible obstructive airway diseases such as asthma.

needle, a sharp, metal shaft in a variety of forms for penetrating tissue (for example, in carrying sutures or injecting solutions).

n. biopsy, the removal of a segment of living tissue for microscopic examination by inserting a hollow needle through the skin or the external surface of an organ or tumor and rotating it within the underlying cellular layers to retrieve a tissue specimen for examination.

n., Gillmore, an instrument used in a penetration type of test for measuring the setting time of materials such as plaster or stone. A ¼-pound needle is used for determining the initial set, and a 1-pound needle is used for defining the final set.

n. holder, a forceps used to hold and pass the needle through the tissue while suturing with a suture forceps.

n. point tracer. See **tracer, needle point.**

n. stick injuries, accidental skin punctures resulting from contact with hypodermic syringe needles. Such injuries can be dangerous, particularly if the needle has been used in treatment of a patient with a severe blood-borne infection, such as hepatitis or AIDS. A strict federal protocol for the use and disposal of needles is required for all health care facilities and personnel engaged in direct patient care.

n., Vicat, an instrument used for measuring setting time by means of a penetration test.

nefazodone HCl, *trade name:* Serzone; *drug class:* antidepressant; *action:* inhibits neuronal uptake of serotonin and norepinephrine; *uses:* major depressive disorders.

neglect, the failure to do something that one is bound to do; lack of due care.

negligence, the failure to observe, for the protection of another person, the degree of care and vigilance that the circumstances demand, whereby such other person suffers injury.

n., contributory, negligence by an injured party that combines as a proxi-

mate cause with the negligence of the injurer in producing the injury. May bar recovery or mitigate damages.

n., imputed, the principle that places the responsibility for negligence on a person other than the one that was directly negligent. This transfer of responsiblity is based on some special relationship of the parties, such as parent and child or principal and agent (for example, a dentist may be responsible for the negligence of a dental assistant or other dental employee).

negotiate, to deal or bargain with another or others to bring about an agreement or settlement.

Negri bodies, intracytoplasmic inclusion bodies found in the brain and central nervous system cells of rabies victims.

neighborhood, an adjoining or surrounding district; an immediate vicinity.

Neisseria, a genus of aerobic to facultatively anaerobic bacteria containing gram-negative cocci that occur in pairs with the adjacent sides flattened. *N. gonorrhoeae, Gonococcus,* a species that causes gonorrhea.

N. meningitidis, a species found in the nasopharynx of man but not in other animals. The causative agent of meningococcal meningitis.

neisseriacae, a vernacular term used to refer to any member of the genus *Neisseria.*

Nembutal, the trade name for pentobarbital sodium.

neodymium (Nd), a rare earth element with an atomic number of 60 and an atomic weight of 144.27

neomycin (nē'ōmī'sin), an antibiotic secured from cultures of *Streptomyces fradiae,* used for preoperative sterilization. It is a constituent of topically applied ointments, solutions, and troches for its antibacterial action against gram-negative organisms.

neomycin sulfate (topical), *trade name:* Myciguent; *drug class:* local antibacterial; *action:* interferes with bacterial protein synthesis; *use:* skin infections.

neonatal teeth, the presence of teeth within 1 month of birth. See also **natal teeth.**

neoplasia (nē'ōplā'zhə), the disease process responsible for neoplasm formation.

neoplasm (tumor), an abnormal mass of tissue, the growth of which exceeds and is uncoordinated with that of the normal tissues. It persists in the same excessive manner after cessation of the stimuli that evoked the change. Benign and malignant forms are recognized. See also **tumor.**

neoprene, an oil-resistant synthetic rubber.

neostigmine bromide/neostigmine methylsulfate, *trade names:* Prostigmin Bromide/Prostigmin; *drug class:* cholinesterase inhibitor; *action:* inhibits destruction of acetylcholine, which facilitates transmission of impulses across myoneural junction; *uses:* myasthenia gravis, nondepolarizing neuromuscular blocker antagonist, bladder distention, postoperative ileus.

Neo-Synephrine, the brand name for phenylephrine, a vasoconstrictor and pressor drug chemically related to epinephrine and ephedrine. Commonly used as a decongestant. Contraindicated for prolonged use or in patients with severe hypertension.

nephrocalcinosis, an abnormal condition of the kidneys, in which deposits of calcium form in the parenchyma at the site of previous inflammation or degenerative change. Infection, hematuria, anal colic, and decreased function of the kidney may occur.

nephrology, the study of the anatomy, physiology, and pathology of the kidney.

nerve, a cordlike structure that conveys impulses between a part of the central nervous system and some part of the body and consists of an outer connective tissue sheath and bundles of nerve fibers.

n., abducent (VI), the sixth cranial nerve; a small, completely motor nerve arising in the pons, supplying the lateral rectus muscle of the eye.

n., accessory. See **nerve, spinal accessory.**

n., acoustic (VIII), the eighth cranial nerve; the vestibulocochlear nerve; a sensory nerve consisting of a vestibular position and an auditory (or cochlear) portion.

n. block. See **anesthesia, block.**

n., branchial, one of five cranial nerves that supply the derivatives of the branchial arches: trigeminal (V),

facial (VII), glossopharyngeal (IX), vagus (X), and spinal accessory (XI). Each branchial nerve may have a variety of functions, including visceral motor and visceral and somatic sensory.

n., chiasma, optic, the decussation, or crossing, of optic nerve fibers from the medial side of the retina on one side to the opposite side of the brain.

n., chorda tympani, a parasympathetic and special sensory branch of the facial nerve supplying the submandibular and sublingual glands and the anterior two thirds of the tongue (taste).

n., cochlear, one of the two major branches of the eighth cranial nerve; a special sensory nerve for the sense of hearing that transmits impulses from the organ of Corti to the brain.

n., cranial, any one of 12 paired nerves, classified in three sets, arising directly in the brain and supplying various tissues of the head and neck. The cranial nerves are the special somatic sensory nerves: olfactory (I), optic (II), and acoustic (VIII); the somatic motor nerves: oculomotor (III), trochlear (IV), abducent (VI), and hypoglossal (XI); and the branchial nerves: trigeminal (V), facial (VII), glossopharyngeal (IX), vagus (X), and spinal accessory (XI).

n. degeneration, the reversion to a less organized and functioning state, usually detected by the loss of ability to conduct or transmit nerve impulses. Advanced degeneration might show cellular decomposition.

n. ending, the terminal of a nerve fiber, usually in synapse with another fiber or in a sensory organ.

n., facial (VII), the seventh cranial nerve; a mixed nerve supplying motor fibers to the facial muscles, the stapedius, and posterior body of the digastricus; sensory fibers from the taste buds in the anterior two thirds of the tongue (via the chorda tympani); and general visceral autonomic fibers for submaxillary and sublingual salivary glands.

n. fiber, a slender process of a neuron, usually the axon. Each fiber is classified as myelinated or unmyelinated.

n., glossopharyngeal (IX), the ninth cranial nerve; a mixed motor and sensory nerve arising in the medulla and supplying motor efferents to stylopharyngeal muscles and other pharyngeal muscles; visceral motor efferents via the otic ganglion for the parotid gland; special visceral afferents from the taste buds in the posterior third of tongue; and general sensory afferents from the pharynx and posterior aspects of the oral cavity.

n., hypoglossal (XII), the twelfth cranial nerve; a motor nerve that arises in the medulla and supplies extrinsic and intrinsic muscles of the tongue.

n., inferior alveolar, a motor and general sensory branch of the mandibular nerve, with mylohyoid, inferior dental, mental, and inferior gingival branches.

n., intermediate, the parasympathetic and special sensory division of the facial nerve with chorda tympani and greater petrosal branches.

n., lingual, a general sensory branch of the mandibular nerve having sublingual and lingual branches and connections with the hypoglossal nerve and chorda tympani.

n., mandibular, the mandibular division of the trigeminal nerve, arising in the trigeminal ganglion and supplying general sensory and motor fibers via mesenteric, pterygoid, buccal, auriculotemporal, deep temporal, lingual, inferior alveolar, and meningeal branches.

n., maxillary, the maxillary division of the trigeminal nerve arising in the trigeminal ganglion and supplying general sensory fibers via zygomatic, posterosuperior alveolar, infraorbital, pterygopalatine, and nasopalatine branches.

n., oculomotor (III), the third cranial nerve; primarily a motor nerve arising from the midbrain and supplying motor efferents to the superior rectus, medial rectus, inferior rectus, and inferior oblique eye muscles, as well as autonomic fibers via the ciliary ganglion to the ciliary body and the iris.

n., olfactory (I), the first cranial nerve; a special sensory nerve for the sense of smell.

n., ophthalmic, the ophthalmic division of the trigeminal nerve, arising in the trigeminal ganglion and supplying general sensory fibers via the frontal, lacrimal, and nasociliary branches.

n., optic (II), the second cranial nerve; a special sensory nerve for vision passing from the retina of the eye to the optic chiasma.

n. regeneration, the reconstruction and renewal of cell structure and function; generally restricted to myelinated nerve fibers.

n., somatic motor (cranial), the somatic motor nerves—oculomotor (III), trochlear (IV), abducent (VI), and hypoglossal (XII)—largely comparable to the ventral motor roots of the spinal nerves. They are composed almost entirely of somatic motor fibers that emerge ventrally from the brainstem. Their arrangement is closely correlated to the distribution of the myotomes in the head. The oculomotor, trochlear, and abducent nerves, which supply the eye musculature, have the same myotomic origin and arrangement as the somatic muscles of the trunk and extremities.

n., special somatic sensory, the structural arrangements from typical sensory nerves by which the three main sense organs, nose, eyes, and ears, are innervated. The sensory nerves are the olfactory (I), optic (II), and acoustic nerves (VIII).

n., spinal, any one of 31 pairs of mixed peripheral nerves (8 cervical, 12 thoracic, 5 lumbar, 5 sacral, and 1 coccygeal), being connected segmentally with the spinal cord, dorsal sensory trunk, and ventral motor root.

n., s. accessory (XI), the eleventh cranial nerve; a motor nerve that derives its origin in part from the medulla and in part from the cervical spinal cord. Its internal ramus joins with the vagus nerve to supply some of the muscles of the larynx. Its external ramus joins with the spinal nerves to supply the sternocleidomastoid and trapezius muscles. The dentist's principal interest in the spinal accessory nerve is its relationship to head posture, which is important in maintaining stable occlusal relationships of vertical dimension and centric relation.

n., tensor tympani, a small motor branch of the mandibular nerve.

n., trigeminal (V), the fifth cranial nerve; a mixed motor and sensory nerve connected with the pons through three roots (motor, proprio-

N

ceptive, and large sensory), the latter root expanding into the trigeminal ganglion, from which arise the ophthalmic, masseteric, and mandibular divisions.

n., trochlear (IV), the fourth cranial nerve; a small motor nerve arising ventrally in the midbrain and supplying the inferior oblique muscle of the eye.

n., vagus (X), the tenth cranial nerve; a mixed parasympathetic, visceral, afferent, motor, and general sensory nerve with laryngeal, pharyngeal, bronchial, esophageal, gastric, and many other branches.

n., vestibular (VIII), one of the two major branches of the eighth cranial nerve; a special sensory nerve for the sense of balance and the transmission of space-orientation impulses from the semicircular canals to the brain.

n., vestibulocochlear (VII), the seventh cranial nerve; acoustic nerve; a sensory nerve consisting of a vestibular portion and an auditory, or cochlear, portion.

nervous system, the extensive, intricate network of structures that activates, coordinates, and controls all the functions of the body. The nervous system is divided into the central nervous system, composed of the brain and spinal cord, and the peripheral nervous system, which includes the cranial nerves and the spinal nerves.

net, devoid of anything extraneous; free from all deductions, such as charges, expenses, taxes; remaining after expenses.

netilmicin sulfate, a parenteral aminoglycoside antibiotic used for short-term treatment of serious or life-threatening bacterial infections.

neural crest, the band of ectodermally derived cells that lies along the outer surface of each side of the neural tube in the early stages of embryonic development. The cells migrate laterally throughout the embryo and give rise to certain spinal, cranial, and sympathetic ganglia.

neuralgia (noŏral'jē-ə), pain associated with a nerve or nerves (for example, trigeminal and glossopharyngeal neuralgia).

n., atypical facial (*cluster headache, lower-half headache, sphenopalatine neuralgia*), severe unilateral pain be-

hind the eye that spreads to the temple and behind the ear. It lasts 30 minutes to 3 hours and occurs once to several times a day and in cycles or clusters lasting several weeks. The clusters may be separated by several months or years. No trigger zones exist.

n., auriculotemporal (*auriculotemporal causalgia neuralgia*), sharp pain in the distribution of the auriculotemporal nerve.

n., buccal, a throbbing, burning, and boring type of pain involving the cheeks, lips, gingivae, nose, and jaws. It may last a few minutes or several days. No trigger zones are present, although the pain may be initiated by chewing or thermal changes.

n., causalgia, neuralgia characterized by an intense, diffuse burning sensation in a limited area.

n., facial. See **neuralgia, trigeminal.**

n., glossopharyngeal, pain in the nerves of the tongue, pharynx, ear, and neck precipitated by swallowing, sneezing, coughing, talking, or blowing the nose.

n., Sluder's Irritation of the sphenopalatine ganglion, diffuse pain may affect the eye, root of the nose, teeth, and ear. Also, slight anesthesia and paralysis of the soft palate and palatine arch on the affected side may be present.

n., sphenopalatine. See **neuralgia, facial, atypical.**

n., trifacial. See **neuralgia, trigeminal.**

n., trigeminal (*facial neuralgia, tic douloureux, trifacial neuralgia*), an excruciating paroxysmal, stabbing, searing, or lancinating pain usually occurring on the right side of the face and involving the distribution of the three divisions of the trigeminal nerve. It may last for a few seconds followed by additional episodes spontaneously or from stimulation of trigger zones. Intervals between attacks vary from a few hours to months or years.

neurasthenia (noŏrəsthē'nē-ə), a neurotic reaction characterized by chronic physical fatigue, listlessness, mental sluggishness, and often, phobias.

neurectomy (noŏrek'təmē), the surgical excision of a nerve, or the more traumatic tearing away of nervous tissue from its anatomic position.

neurilemma (noōrəlem'ə) (nucleated sheath, primitive sheath, sheath of Schwann), the thin membranous outer covering surrounding the myelin sheath of a medullated nerve fiber or the axis cylinder of a nonmedullated nerve fiber. Neurilemma is associated with the booster mechanisms for the rapid transmission of impulses.

neurilemoma (noō'rəlemō'mə) (neurinoma, perineural fibroblastoma, schwannoma), a benign tumor of the neurilemma of disputed origin (Schwann cell vs. fibroblasts). May occur in soft tissue and bone. Composed of characteristic Antoni type A and Antoni type B tissue and contains Verocay bodies. A malignant form occurs. See also **body, Verocay** and **tissue.**

neurinoma (noōrinō'mə). See **neurilemoma.**

neuritis (noōrī'tis), the inflammation of a nerve, accompanied by pain and tenderness over the nerves, anesthesia, disturbance of sensation, paralysis, wasting, and disappearance of reflexes.

n., endemic multiple. See **beriberi.**

neuroaminidase, an enzyme that is used in histochemistry to selectively remove sialomucins from bronchial mucous glands and the small intestine.

neuroanatomy, the gross and microscopic structure of the nervous system.

neuroblastoma (noō'rōblastō'mə), a malignant neoplasm characterized by proliferating nerve cells.

neurofibroma (noōr'ōfibrō'mə) (neurogenic fibroma, perineural fibroblastoma), **1.** a benign neoplasm characterized by the various cells of a peripheral nerve (axon cylinders, Schwann cells, fibroblasts). See also **neurilemoma. 2.** a connective tissue tumor of the nerve fiber fasciculi. Formed by the proliferation of the perineurium and endoneurium.

neurofibromatosis (noōr'ōfi'brōmə-tō'sis) (molluscum fibrosum, multiple neuroma, von Recklinghausen's disease of skin), a disease characterized by multiple neurofibromas. Most frequently seen on the skin but possibly involving the oral mucosa.

neurokinin (A), a mammalian decapeptide tachykinin found in the central nervous system. The compound has bronchoconstrictor, smooth muscle constrictor, and hypotensive effects and also activates the micturition reflex.

neuroleptanalgesia, a form of analgesia achieved by the concurrent administration of a neuroleptic and an analgesic. Anxiety, motor activity, and sensitivity to painful stimuli are reduced; the person is quiet and indifferent to the environment and surroundings. If nitrous oxide with oxygen is also administered, neuroleptanalgesia can be converted to neuroleptanesthesia.

neurology, the field of medicine that deals with the nervous system and its disorders.

neuroma (noōrō'mə), technically, a benign neoplasm of nerve cells. As used in oral disease, the term usually refers to a traumatic neuroma, which is not a true tumor but an overgrowth of nerves associated with injury. The mental foramina and extraction scars are possible oral sites of this painful lesion.

n., amputation. See **neuroma, traumatic.**

n., multiple. See **neurofibromatosis.**

n., traumatic (amputation neuroma), hyperplasia of nerve fibers and their supporting tissues in an exuberant attempt at repair after damage to, or the severing of, a nerve.

neuromuscular junction, the area of contact between the ends of a large myelinated nerve fiber and a fiber of skeletal muscle. Also called **myoneural junction.**

neuron (noō'ron), a nerve cell; the basic structural unit of the nervous system. There is a wide variation in the shape of nerve cells, but they all have the same basic structures: cell body, protoplasmic processes, axons, and dendrites. The neuron is the only body cell whose principal function is the conduction of impulses. It cannot regenerate when the cell body is destroyed; however, cell processes such as axons and dendrites can often regenerate.

n., afferent, a neuron that carries an impulse toward the central nervous system. See also **afferent impulse.**

n., efferent, a neuron that carries an impulse toward the pheriphery, such

N

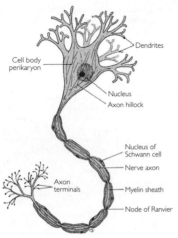

Neuron. (Avery, 1992.)

Labels: Dendrites; Cell body perikaryon; Nucleus; Axon hillock; Nucleus of Schwann cell; Nerve axon; Axon terminals; Myelin sheath; Node of Ranvier

as a motor neuron See also **efferent impulse.**

neuropathy, an abnormal condition characterized by inflammation and degeneration of peripheral nerves.

neuropeptide, any of a variety of peptides found in neural tissues, such as endorphins and enkephalins.

neurosis, a diffusely defined term referring to a mental disorder for which professional help may be needed but that is milder than a psychosis; generally a functional disorder in which there is no gross personality disorganization but in which there is an inability to cope effectively with some routine frustrations, anxieties, and daily problems. Somatic conditions may be factors in the cause and may be symptoms in a neurosis; however, the use of the term to describe a dysfunction of the nervous system is obsolete. Synonym: psychoneurosis.

neurostomatosis (nŏŏ′rōstō′mətō′sis), an oral condition associated with psychosomatic or other psychologic factors; for example, lichen planus and benign migratory glossitis may be considered types of neurostomatoses.

neurosurgery, any surgery involving the brain, spinal cord, or peripheral nerves.

neurosyphilis, paretic (nŏŏ′rōsi′filis). See **paresis.**

neurotensin, a 13-amino acid peptide neurotransmitter found in synaptosomes

in the hypothalamus, amygdala, basal ganglia, and dorsal gray matter of the spinal cord; it plays a role in pain perception. It also affects pituitary hormone release and gastrointestinal function.

neurotomy (nŏŏrot′əmē), the severance of a nerve process.

neurotransmitter, any one of numerous chemicals that modify or result in the transmission of nerve impulses between synapses. Neurotransmitters are released from synaptic knobs into synaptic clefts and bridge the gap between presynaptic and postsynaptic neurons.

neutral, a solution that has a pH level of 7. Equal numbers of hydrogen and hydroxyl ions are formed on dissociation.

n. zone. See **zone, neutral.**

neutralization, the reaction of an acid with a base.

neutrocclusion, normal mesiodistal occlusal relationships of the buccal teeth, similar to Angle class I.

neutron (nŏŏ′tron), an elementary particle with approximately the mass of a hydrogen atom but without any electrical charge; one of the constituents of the atomic nucleus.

n. activation analysis, an activation analysis in which the specimen is bombarded with neutrons. Identification is made by measuring the resulting radioisotopes.

n. ray. See **rays, neutron.**

neutropenia (nŏŏ′trōpē′nē-ə), a relative or absolute decrease in the normal number of neutrophils in the circulating blood. Various limits are given; for example, absolute neutropenia may exist when the total is less than 1700 cells/mm³ regardless of the percentage, whereas relative neutropenia may exist when the total percentage of neutrophils is less than 38% and the total number is not less than 1500/mm³. May be associated with viral infections, pernicious anemia, sprue, aplastic anemia, bone marrow, neoplasms, chronic intoxication with drugs or heavy metals, malnutrition, and nonpyogenic and overwhelming infections.

n., cyclic, a condition in which there is a depression in the number of circulating white cells, especially the neutrophils, at an interval of about 21 days. The neutropenia lasts for approximately 10 days; during this time, gingival inflammation and aphthous ulcer occur.

neutrophil, a polymorphonuclear granular leukocyte. Neutrophils are the circulating white blood cells essential for phagacytosis and proteolysis.

neutrophilia (nōō′trōfil′ē·ə), an absolute or relative increase in the normal number of neutrophils in the circulating blood. Various limits are given; for example, an absolute neutrophilia may exist, regardless of percentage, if the total number of neutrophils exceeds 7000/mm³, whereas a relative neutrophilia may exist if the percentage of neutrophils is greater than 70% and the total number of neutrophils is less than 7000/mm³ May be associated with acute infections, chronic granulocytic leukemia, erythemia, therapy with adrenocorticotropic hormone (ACTH) or cortisone, uremia, ketosis, hemolysis, drug or heavy metal intoxication, or malignancy, or may follow severe hemorrhage.

nevus (nē′vəs), a circumscribed new growth of congenital origin that may be vascular (resulting from hypertrophy of blood or lymph vessels) or nonvascular (with epidermal and connective tissue predominating).

n., blue, a benign neoplasm characterized by heavily pigmented spindle cells deep in the corium; appears clinically as a dark mole.

n., cellular pigmented, a nevus composed of melanin-producing "nevus" cells.

n., compound, a nevus in which the melanin-producing "nevus" cells are found in the epidermis and dermis; the intradermal nevus plus the junctional nevus.

n., intradermal, a nevus in which the melanin-producing "nevus" cells are found only in the dermis.

n., junctional, a nevus in which the melanin-producing "nevus" cells are found within the epidermis at the junction with the dermis.

n., pigmented, a dark-colored, benign neoplasm characterized by nevus cells. Junctional, intradermal, and compound types are recognized. Melanomas (malignant neoplasms) may develop from junctional or compound nevi.

n. spongiosus albus mucosa (white folded gingivostomatitis, white sponge nevus), an inherited disease of the oral mucosa characterized by generalized white mucosal surfaces with a spongelike appearance.

Ney surveyor. See **surveyor, Ney.**

NF, the *National Formulary.*

niacin (vitamin B₃), *trade name:* generic niacin (nicotinic acid); *drug class:* vitamin B₃; *action:* needed for conversion of fats, protein, carbohydrates by oxidation-reduction; acts directly on vascular smooth muscle, causing vasodilation; *uses:* pellagra, hyperlipidemias, peripheral vascular disease.

nib, the part of a condensing instrument corresponding to the blade of a cutting instrument. The end is called the *face* of the condenser.

nicardipine HCl, *trade name:* Cardene; *drug class:* calcium channel blocker; *action:* inhibits calcium ion influx across cell membrane during cardiac depolarization; produces relaxation of coronary vascular smooth muscle, peripheral vascular smooth muscle; dilates coronary vascular arteries; decreases sinoatrial/atrioventricular (SA/AV) node conduction; *uses:* chronic stable angina pectoris, hypertension.

nickel, a silvery-white metallic element. Its atomic number is 28 and its atomic weight is 58.71. Large numbers of people are allergic to nickel. Nickel causes more cases of allergic contact dermatitis than all other metals combined. Many cases of allergic contact dermatitis occur from exposure to the nickel content of jewelry, coins, buckles, and snaps, and to the continued use of "carbonless" business forms.

n.-chromium alloy. See **alloy, nickel-chromium.**

nicotine, a poisonous alkaloid found in tobacco and responsible for many of the effects of tobacco. It is first a stimulant (small doses) and then a depressant (larger doses).

n. polacrilex, **trade name:** Nicorette; *drug class:* smoking deterrent; *action:* agonist at nicotinic receptors in the peripheral and central nervous systems; acts at sympathetic ganglia; on chemoreceptors of the aorta and carotid bodies; also affects adrenal-releasing catecholamines; *use:* deters

cigarette smoking when combined with a program of smoking cessation.
n. transdermal system, trade names: Habitrol, Nicoderm, Nicotrol, Pro-Step; *drug class:* smoking deterrent; *action:* binds to acetylcholine receptors at autonomic ganglia in the adrenal medulla, at neuromuscular junctions, and in the brain; *use:* cigarette smoking cessation program.

nicotinic stomatitis, an inflammation caused by the intraoral use of smokeless tobacco.

Niemann-Pick disease (nē'mon pik'). See **disease, Niemann-Pick.**

nifedipine, *trade names:* Procardia, Procardia XL; *drug class:* calcium channel blocker; *action:* inhibits calcium ion influx across cell membrane during cardiac depolarization; produces relaxation of coronary vascular smooth muscle, dilates coronary arteries; increases myocardial oxygen delivery in patients with vasospastic angina; dilates peripheral arteries; *uses:* chronic stable angina pectoris, vasospastic angina, hypertension.

night-grinding. See **bruxism.**

night guard. See **guard, night.**

Nikolsky's sign (nikol'skēz). See **sign, Nikolsky's.**

niobium (Nb), the chemical element with an atomic number of 41 and an atomic weight of 92.906. It was formerly known as "columbium."

nitric acid, a colorless, highly corrosive liquid that may give off suffocating brown fumes of nitrogen dioxide on exposure to air. Commercially prepared nitric acid is a powerful oxidizing agent used in photoengraving and metallurgy.

nitrofurantoin/nitrofurantoin macro-crystals, *trade names:* Furadantin, Furalan, Macrobid, Macrodantin; *drug class:* urinary tract antiinfective; *action:* appears to inhibit bacterial enzymes; *uses:* urinary tract infections caused by *Escherichia coli, Klebsiella, Pseudomonas, Proteus vulgaris, Proteus morganii, Citrobacter, Staphylococcus aureus.*

nitrogen, a gaseous, nonmetallic element. Its atomic number is 7 and its atomic weight is 14.08. Nitrogen constitutes approximately 78% of the atmosphere and is a component of all proteins and a major component of most organic substances.

n. monoxide. See **nitrous oxide.**

n. monoxidum. See **nitrous oxide.**

n., nonprotein. See **nonprotein nitrogen.**

nitroglycerin, *trade names:* Nitrogard, Nitro-Bid, Nitrostat; *drug class:* inorganic nitrate, vasodilator; *action:* decreases preload/afterload, which is responsible for decreasing left ventricular end-diastolic pressure, systemic vascular resistance; arterial and venous dilation; *uses:* chronic stable angina pectoris, prophylaxis of angina pain, congestive heart failure associated with acute myocardial infarction, controlled hypotension in surgical procedures.

nitromersol, tincture (nītrōmer'sol), a solution used in 1:200 strength as a topically applied antiseptic to temporarily minimize the bacterial count on an area of tissue.

nitrous acid, HNO_2, a standard chemical reagent used in biologic and clinical laboratories.

nitrous oxide (N_2O, laughing gas, nitrogen monoxide, nitrogen monoxidum), a gas with a sweet odor and taste used with oxygen as an analgesic and sedative agent for the performance of minor operations. It is sometimes called "laughing gas" because it may excite a hilarious delirium preceding insensibility.

nizatidine, *trade name:* Axid; *drug class:* H_2 histamine receptor antagonist; *action:* inhibits histamine at H_2 receptor site in parietal cells, which inhibits gastric acid secretion; *uses:* duodenal ulcer, Zollinger-Ellison syndrome, gastric ulcers, hypersecretory conditions, gastroesophageal reflux disease, stress ulcers.

NMR (nuclear magnetic resonance). See **magnetic resonance imaging.**

noble, an archaic term referring to inert gases and precious metals.

n. metal. See **metal, noble.**

Nocardia, a genus of aerobic nonmotile actinomycetes, which are transitional between bacteria and fungi. They are primarily saprophytic but may cause disease in man and other animals.

nocardiosis (nōkardē·ō'sis), any of the pathologic entities that may follow infection with the bacterium *Nocardia.*

nociceptor, somatic and visceral free nerve endings of thinly myelinated and unmyelinated fibers. They usually react to tissue injury but also may be excited by endogenous chemical substances.

node (nōd), a swelling or protuberance.

n., brown, of hyperparathyroidism, a central giant cell lesion of the bone seen in hyperparathyroidism. Its microscopic appearance is similar to giant cell reparative granuloma and giant cell tumor.

n. of Ranvier gaps, nodes distributed at regularly spaced intervals along a myelinated nerve fiber. The intervals are 1 mm or more in length and function essentially as relay stations to facilitate the passage of an im pulse.

nodule, pulp (nod′yəl). See **denticle.**

nodules, Bohn's (Epstein's pearls), multiple white, ricelike lesions of the mucous membrane seen in newborn infants. Microscopically, each lesion shows a keratin-filled cyst that lies close to the mucosal surface. It disappears spontaneously in 2 to 3 months.

noma (nō′mə), a progressive necrotizing process originating in the check with secondary involvement of the gingiva and jawbone. Occurs primarily in debilitated children, and the mortality rate is high. There is a strong, foul odor; marked surrounding edema; absence of a specific erythematous halo; marked changes in the white blood cell count; and a high temperature. See also **necrosis, exanthematous** and **stomatitis, gangrenous.**

nomenclature (nō′mənklā′chər), the formally adopted terminology of a science, art, or discipline; the system of names or terms used in a particular branch of science.

noncohesive, lacking the property of sticking together, or cohesion.

noncontributory plan, a method of payment for group insurance coverage in which the entire premium is paid by the employer or the union. Also referred to as *noncontributory program.*

nonduplication of benefits, this may apply if a subscriber is eligible for benefits under more than one plan. A dental benefits contract provision re lieving the third-party payer of liability for cost of services if the services are covered under another program. Distinct from a coordination of benefits provision because reimbursement would be limited to the greater level allowed by the two plans rather than a total of 100% of the charges. Also referred to as *less-benefit* or *carve-out.*

nonfeasance (nonfē′zəns), the failure of a person to do some act that should be done.

non-Hodgkin's lymphoma, a form of lymphoma associated with AIDS. One of the indicator diseases of AIDS. See also **lymphoma.**

nonocclusion, a situation in which the tooth or teeth in one arch fail to make contact with tooth or teeth of the other arch.

nonparticipating dentist, 1. any dentist with whom the underwriter (insurer) does not have an agreement to render dental care to members of the plan. **2.** any dentist who does not have a contractual agreement with a dental benefits organization to render dental care to members of a dental benefits program.

nonprofit insurers, service corporations organized under nonprofit laws for the purpose of providing dental care insurance.

nonprotein nitrogen (NPN), the nitrogen of whole blood or serum exclusive of that of the proteins. The concentration of nonprotein nitrogen is a gross measure of renal function. The upper limit of normal is 35 mg/100 ml.

non rep., the abbreviation of the Latin term *non repetatur;* placed on prescriptions that are not to be refilled. (not in current dental literature)

nonsuit, a failure on the part of a plaintiff to continue the prosecution of the suit; abandonment of a suit.

nor-, a prefix that indicates lack of a methyl group.

norepinephrine (nôr′epinef′rin), the neurohormonal transmitter for neuroeffector junctions of adrenergic nerve fibers. Its official drug name in the United States is *levarterenol.* See also **levarterenol.**

norethindrone acetate, *trade names:* Aygestin, Micronor, Norlutate, Norlutin, Nor-QD; *drug class:* progesterone derivative; *action:* inhibits secretion of pituitary gonadotropins, which prevents follicular maturation, ovulation; *uses:* abnormal uterine bleeding, amenorrhea, endometriosis, contraceptive.

norfloxacin, *trade name:* Noroxin; *drug class:* fluoroquinolone antiinfective; *action:* a broad-spectrum bactericidal agent that inhibits the enzyme DNA gyrase needed for replication of DNA; *uses:* adult urinary tract infections.

norgestrel, *trade name:* Ovrette; *drug class:* progesterone derivative; *action:* inhibits secretion of pituitary gonadotropins, which prevents follicular maturation, ovulation; *use:* oral contraception.

norm, l. a statistical unit representative of the human species as a whole. **2.** the numerical or statistical measures of usual observed performance when related to health care provided to a given number of patients over time; often used in the building of profiles; can be the average or median or some other cutoff point in a series.

normal distribution, a curve representing the frequency with which the values of a variable are obtained or observed when the number is infinite and variation is subject to only chance factors. The curve is a symmetrical, bell-shaped curve with the highest frequency occurring in the middle and gradually tapering toward the extremes. In a normal distribution, 68.2% of all scores cluster around the mean within approximately 1 standard deviation, 95.4% within approximately 2 standard deviations, and 99.7% within approximately 3 standard deviations. Synonyms: normal curve, Gauss' curve.

normality, a reference solution in which the concentration is stated with regard to the number of gram-equivalent weights present per liter of solution.

normoblast (nôr′mōblast), a nucleated red blood cell found in the peripheral bloodstream in severe pernicious anemia and in some leukemias.

nortriptyline HCl, *trade names:* Aventyl, Pamelor; *drug class:* tricyclic antidepressant; *action:* blocks reuptake of norepinephrine, serotonin into nerve endings, which increases action of norepinephrine, serotonin in nerve cells; *uses:* major depression.

nose, the structure that protrudes from the anterior portion of the midface and serves as a passageway for air to and from the lungs. The nose filters, warms, and moistens the air on its passage into the lungs. The nose contains the end organs of smell.

nosebleed. See **epistaxis.**

notch, an indentation.

n., buccal, the notch in the flange of a denture that accommodates the buccal frenum.

n., hamular. See **notch, pterygomaxillary.**

n., labial, the notch in the labial flange of an upper or lower denture that accommodates the labial frenum.

n., mandibular, a depression of the inferior border of the mandible anterior to the attachments of the masseter muscle where the external facial vessels cross the lower border of the mandible. This landmark may be accentuated by arrested condylar growth and developmental disturbances of the mandible.

n., pterygomaxillary (hamular notch), the notch or fissure formed at the junction of the maxilla and the hamular, or pterygoid, process of the sphenoid bone.

n., sigmoid, the concavity on the superior surface of the ramus of the mandible lying between the coronoid and condyloid processes.

note, promissory, a written promise to pay to another, at a specified time, a stated amount of money or other articles of value.

not-for-profit third parties, service corporations or dental benefits organizations established under not-for-profit state statutes for the purpose of providing health care coverage (for example, Delta Dental and Blue Cross, Blue Shield Plans).

notice, l. knowledge; information; awareness of facts. **2.** the knowledge of facts that would naturally lead an honest and prudent person to make inquiry constitutes "notice" of everything that such inquiry pursued in good faith would disclose.

notochord, an elongated strip of mesodermal tissue that originates from the primitive node and extends along the dorsal surface of the developing embryo beneath the neural tube, forming the primary longitudinal skeletal axis of the body of all chordates.

Novocain, the trade name for procaine hydrochloride.

noxious (nok′shəs), hurtful; not wholesome.

NPN. See **nonprotein nitrogen.**

NSAIDs, the acronym for **nonsteroidal antiinflammatory drugs.** See also **naproxen.**

nuclear family, a family unit consisting of the biologic parents and their offspring. The nuclear family is less inclusive than the extended family. Although the nuclear family is a relatively recent product of Western society, it is threatened by the increasing dissolution of marriage.

nuclear magnetic resonance. See **magnetic resonance imaging.**

nucleic acid, a family of macromolecules found in the chromosomes, nucleoli, mitochondria, and cytoplasm of all cells. In complexes with proteins, they are called *nucleoproteins.*

n. a. probes, nucleic acid that complements a specific RNA or DNA molecule or fragment; used for hybridization studies to identify microorganisms and for genetic studies.

Nucleopolyhedrovirus (nuclear polyhedrosis virus), a genus of the family Baculoviridae, characterized by the formation of crystalline, polyhedral occlusion bodies in the host cell nucleous.

nucleoprotein (noo′klē-ō-prō′tēn), any one of a special group of protein substances in combination with nucleic acid. The essential component is the phosphoric acid radical. The nucleoproteins are generally confined to the nucleus of the cell and are intimately associated with chromosome and gene function.

nucleoside, purine or pyrimidine bases attached to a ribose or deoxyribose.

nucleus (noo′klē-əs), **1.** the small, central part of an atom in which the positive electric charge and most of the mass (protons and neutrons) are concentrated. **2.** an easily recognized structural component of most cells, surrounded by a membrane and containing chromosomes and nucleoli.

Nuhn's gland (noonz), the anterior lingual gland embedded in the substance of the tongue near the apex and the midline on the inferior surface of the tongue. See also **gland, Blandin and Nuhn's.**

nuisance, that which endangers life or health, offends the senses, violates the laws of decency, or obstructs reasonable and comfortable use of property.

null cell, a lymphocyte that develops in the bone marrow and lacks the characteristic surface markers of the B and T lymphocytes. Null cells stimulated by the presence of antibody can directly attack certain cellular targets and are known as "natural killers" or "killer cells."

null hypothesis, a statistical hypothesis that predicts that no difference or relationship exists among the variables studied that could not have occurred by chance alone.

number, Brinell hardness (BHN), a numerical expression of the hardness of a material, determined by measuring the diameter of a dent made by forcing a hard steel or tungsten carbide ball of standard dimension into the material under specified load in a Brinell machine, which was devised by J.A. Brinell, a Swedish engineer. The larger the indentation, the smaller the Brinell hardness number. See also **test, Brinell hardness.** (not current)

number, Vickers hardness, hardness as measured by the Vickers hardness test. See also **test, Vickers hardness.**

nurse, a person educated and licensed in the practice of nursing; one who is concerned with the diagnosis and treatment of human responses to actual or potential health problems.

n. anesthetist, a registered nurse qualified by advanced training in an accredited program in the specialty of nurse anesthesia to manage the care of the patient during the administration of anesthesia in selected surgical situations.

n. midwife. See **midwife.**

n. practitioner, a nurse who, by advanced education and clinical experience in a specialized area of nursing practice, has acquired expert knowledge and skill in a special branch of practice. The nurse practitioner acts as a nurse clinician, functioning independently within standing orders or protocols and collaborates with associates to implement a plan of care. The services of nurse practitioners are increasing in demand under managed care programs and in large group practice settings.

nurse's aid, a person who is employed to carry out basic nonspecialized tasks in the care of a patient, such as bathing and feeding, making beds, and transporting patients, under the supervision and direction of a registered nurse.

nursing, 1. the performance of those activities that contribute to the health or recovery of a patient (or to a peaceful death). **2.** the application of prescribed therapies and the management of the patient and environment to assist in healing.

n. bottle caries, dental caries of the maxillary primary teeth caused by the oral retention of milk or formula in the mouth.

n. home, a convalescent facility for the care of individuals who do not require hospitalization but who cannot be cared for at home. Preferred nomenclature: **extended care facility.**

nutrient canal (noo′trē-ənt). See **canal, interdental.**

nutrition, the process of assimilation and use of essential food elements from the diet (for example, carbohydrates, fats, proteins, vitamins, mineral elements).

n. survey, usually a questionnaire regarding dietary habits, but may include an objective evaluation of nutritional status through conduction of physical examinations and laboratory tests of metabolism of a target population.

nutritional requirements, the food and liquids necessary for normal physiologic function.

nutritional status, the assessment of the state of nourishment of a patient or subject.

nutritional support, the supply of foods and liquids necessary to advance healing and support health.

nutriture (noo′tritər), the nutritional status of a patient.

Nuva-lite, the brand name for an ultraviolet light used as a catalyst in the polymerization of Nuva-seal, a bonding agent used as a pit and fissure sealant.

Nuva-seal, the brand name of a bonding agent used as a pit and fissure sealant.

nystagmus (nīstag′məs), the state of oscillatory movements of an organ or part, especially the eyeballs; irregular jerking movement of the eyes. Each movement of the cycle consists of a slow component in one direction and a rapid component in the opposite direction.

nylidrin HCl, *trade name:* Arlidin; *drug class:* peripheral vasodilator, β-adrenergic agonist; *action:* acts on β-adrenergic receptors to dilate arterioles in skeletal muscles; increases cardiac output; may have direct vasodilatory effect on vascular smooth muscle; *uses:* arteriosclerosis obliterans, thromboangiitis obliterans, diabetic vascular disease, night leg cramps, Raynaud's disease, ischemic ulcer, frostbite, primary cochlear cell ischemia.

nystatin, *trade names:* Mycostatin, Nystex, O-V Statin; *drug class:* antifungal; *action:* interferes with fungal DNA replication; *uses:* Candida species causing oral, vaginal, intestinal infections.

oath, an affirmation of truth of a statement that renders one who is willfully asserting untrue statements punishable for perjury.

obesity (ōbēs′itē), a bodily condition marked by excessive generalized deposition and storage of fat.

o., adrenocortical (buffalo obesity), one of the symptoms characteristic of Cushing's syndrome; an obesity that is confined chiefly to the trunk, face, and neck.

o., buffalo. See **obesity, adrenocortical.**

object-film distance. See **distance, object-film.**

obligation, an assumed or assigned duty imposed by promise, law, contract, or society; the binding power of a vow, promise, oath, or contract.

observer variation, the failure by the observer to measure or identify a phenomenon accurately, which results in an error. The observer may miss an abnormality or use faulty techniques, in incorrect measurement or misinterpretation of the data. Two types are interobserver variation (the amount observers vary from one another when reporting on the same material) and intraobserver variation (the amount one observer varies between observations when reporting more than once on the same material).

obsessive-compulsive disorder, the abnormal behavior of a person who tends to perform repetitive acts or rituals, usually as a means of releasing tension or relieving anxiety.

obstetrics, the branch of medicine concerned with pregnancy and childbirth, including the study of the physiologic and pathologic function of the female reproductive tract and the care of the mother and fetus throughout pregnancy, childbirth, and the immediate postpartum period.

obtain, to acquire.

obtund (obtend'), to diminish the ability to perceive pain and/or touch.

obtundent (obtən'dent), an agent that has the property to diminish the perception of pain and/or touch.

obturation (ob'tōōrā'shən), the act of closing or occluding.

o., retrograde. See **filling, retrograde.**

o., root canal filling technique, the procedure used for filling and sealing the root canal.

obturator (ob'tōōrā'tōr), a prosthesis used to close a congenital or acquired opening in the palate. See also **aid, prosthetic speech.**

o., hollow, that portion of an obturator made hollow to minimize its weight.

occipital anchorage (oksip'itəl). See **anchorage, occipital.**

occlude, to close together. To bring together; to shut. To bring the mandibular teeth into contact with the maxillary teeth.

occluder, a name given to some articulators. See also **articulator.**

occlusal, pertaining to the contacting surfaces of opposing occlusal units (teeth or occlusion rims). Pertaining to the masticating surfaces of the posterior teeth.

o. adjustment. See **adjustment, occlusal.**

o. analysis. See **analysis, occlusal.**

o. balance. See **balanced occlusion.**

o. contacts. See **contacts, teeth.**

o. contouring. See **contouring, occlusal.**

o. correction. See **correction, occlusal.**

o. curvature. See **curve of occlusion.**

o. disharmony. See **disharmony, occlusal.**

o. disturbances. See **disturbances, occlusal.**

o. embrasure. See **embrasure, occlusal.**

o. equilibration. See **equilibration, occlusal.**

o. force. See **force, occlusal.**

o. form. See **form, occlusal.**

o. function. See **function, heavy.**

o. glide. See **glide, occlusion.**

o. guard. See **occlusal splint.**

o. harmony. See **harmony, occlusal.**

o. load. See **load, occlusal.**

o. path. See **path, occlusal.**

o. p. registration. See **path, occlusal.**

o. pattern. See **pattern, occlusal.**

o. perception. See **perception, occlusal.**

o. pivot. See **pivot, occlusal.**

o. plane. See **plane, occlusal.**

o. position. See **position, occlusal.**

o. pressure. See **pressure, occlusal.**

o. recontouring. See **contouring, occlusal.**

o. rest. See **position, rest.**

o. splint, a bite plane designed and fabricated for patients with some types of functional temporomandibular joint disorders. Provides a stable occlusal platform from which to reconstruct a functional occlusion. See also **splint.**

o. stop. See **rest, occlusal.**

o. surface. See **surface, occlusal.**

o. system. See **system, occlusal.**

o. table. See **table, occlusal.**

o. template. See **template, occlusal.**

o. therapy, a treatment to establish and maintain a comfortable, stable, and functional occlusion for patients with one of several types of occlusal problems. Treatment may be limited to the teeth, the neuromuscular mechanisms of chewing, or a combination of both.

o. trauma. See **trauma, occlusal.**

o. unit, one of two kinds of cusps: (1) a stamp cusp coupled with a fossa, and (2) a shear cusp. The occlusal edges of the shear cusp are coupled with the edges of a stamp cusp, by which it passes closely without sliding contacts.

o. wear. See **wear, occlusal.**

occlusion, 1. the act of closure or state of being closed. **2.** any contact between the incising or masticating surfaces of the upper and lower teeth.

o., acentric. See **occlusion, eccentric.**

o., adjustment. See **adjustment occlusion.**

o., anatomic, the ideal relation of the mandibular and maxillary teeth when closed.

o., anterior determinants of cusp, the characteristics of the anterior teeth; that is, occlusion, alignment, overlaps, and capacity to disclude conjointly with the trajectories given the condyles, that determine the cusp elevations and the fossa depressions of the postcanine teeth.

o., attritional, an occlusion in which each tooth of the dentition wears occlusally and proximally as it erupts.

o., balanced, **1.** an occlusion of the teeth that presents a harmonious relation of the occluding surfaces in centric and eccentric positions within the functional range of mandibular positions and tooth size. **2.** the simultaneous contacting of the upper and lower teeth on both sides and in the anterior and posterior occlusal areas of the jaws. This occlusion is developed to prevent a tipping or rotating of the denture base in relation to the supporting structures. This term is used primarily in connection with the mouth, but it may be used in relation to teeth on an articulator.

o., bilateral balanced, the closure suitable for worn dentitions that are cuspless or have flat-sided cusps; it permits an increase of the amount of surface contact in centric closure and provides as much closure contact as possible for horizontal chewing. This kind of occlusion is a therapeutic form designed to keep dentures seated when fine-textured foods are chewed horizontally. It is not found in young, unworn natural dentitions.

o., central. See **occlusion, centric.**

o., centric (central occlusion), the relation of opposing occlusal surfaces that provides the maximum planned contact and/or intercuspation. Should exist when the mandible is in centric relation to the maxilla.

o., centrically balanced, a centrically related centric occlusion in which the teeth close with even pressures on both sides of the mouth but have no occlusion of the postcanine teeth in attempted eccentric closures.

o., components of, the various factors involved in occlusion (for example, temporomandibular joint, associated neuromusculature, and teeth). In denture prosthetics, also the denture-supporting structures.

o., convenience (convenience jaw relation, convenience relationship of teeth), the assumed position of maximum intercuspation when there is occlusal interference in the centric path of closure. The convenience occlusion may be anterior, lateral, or anterolateral to the true centric occlusion.

o., coronary, a coronary thrombosis resulting in closure of the coronary artery.

o., cross-bite, an occlusion in which the lower teeth overlap the upper teeth.

o., determinants of, the classifiable factors in the gnathic organ that influence occlusion. These factors are divided into two groups: those that are fixed and those that can be modified by reshaping or repositioning the teeth. The fixed factors most mentioned are the intercondylar distance; anatomy, which influences the paths of the mandibular axes; mandibular centricity; and the mating of the jaws. The changeable factors most mentioned are tooth shape, tooth position, vertical dimension, height of cusps, and depth of fossae.

o., eccentric, any occlusion other than centric occlusion. (not current)

o., edge-to-edge, an occlusion in which the anterior teeth of both jaws meet along their incisal edges when the teeth are in centric occlusion. (not current)

o., end-to-end. See **occlusion, edge-to-edge.**

o., faulty centric, a condition in which centric occlusion does not correspond to a patient's centric jaw relationship, resulting in premature or interceptive or deflective tooth contacts in the centric path of closure.

o., functional, **1.** occlusion in which attention is directed specifically to performance and is differentiated from structure and appearance. **2.** any tooth contacts made within the functional range (according to the size) of the opposing tooth surfaces. An occlusion that occurs during function.

o., gliding, used in the sense of designating contacts of teeth in motion. A substitute for the term *articulation.* (not current)

o., ideal, **1.** the relationship existing when all the teeth are perfectly placed in the arches of jaws and have a normal anatomic relationship to each other. When the teeth are brought into contact, the cusp-fossa relationship is considered the most perfect anatomic relationship that can be attained. **2.** the normal relationships of the inclines of the cusps of opposing teeth to each other in occlusion, when the alignment, proximal contacts, and axial positions of the teeth in both arches have resulted from normal growth and development in relation to all associated tissues and parts of the head.

o., locked, an occlusal relationship of such nature that lateral and protrusive mandibular movements are limited.

o., malfunctional, a disturbance in the normal or proper action of the masticatory apparatus produced by such factors as missing teeth or tilting and drifting of teeth.

o., mechanically balanced, an occlusion balanced without reference to physiologic considerations (for example, on an articulator).

o., normal. See **occlusion, ideal.**

o., pathogenic, an occlusal relationship capable of producing pathologic changes in the teeth, supporting tissues, and/or other components of the stomatognathic system.

o., physiologic, **1.** an occlusion in harmony with functions of the masticatory system. **2.** an occlusion that operates in harmony and presents no pathologic manifestation in the supporting structures of the teeth; the stresses placed on the teeth are dissipated normally, with a balance existing between the stresses and adaptive capacity of the supporting tissues. **3.** an acceptable occlusion found in a healthy gnathic system.

o., physiologically balanced, a balanced occlusion in harmony with the temporomandibular joints and the neuromuscular system. See also **occlusion, balanced.**

o., plane of. See **plane, occlusal.**

o., protrusive, an occlusion of the teeth existing when the mandible is protruded forward from a centric position. See also **position, rest, physiologic.** (not current)

o., rim. See **rim, occlusion.**

o., spherical form of, an arrangement of teeth that places their occlusal surfaces on the surface of an imaginary sphere (usually 9 inches [22.5 cm] in diameter) with its center above the level of the teeth, as suggested by Monson. (not current)

o. table. See **table, occlusal.**

o., terminal, the relation of opposing occlusal surfaces that provides the maximum natural or planned contact and/or intercuspation.

o., traumatic, an occlusion that results in overstrain and injury to teeth, periodontal tissues, or the residual ridge or other oral structures.

o., traumatogenic. See **occlusion, traumatic.**

o., working, the occlusal contacts of teeth on the side toward which the mandible is moved. From the mesial or distal view, the buccal and lingual cusps of the upper teeth appear to be end-to-end with the buccal and lingual cusps of the lower teeth, respectively. Viewed from the side, each upper cusp is distal to the corresponding lower cusp. The mesial incline of each upper cusp makes contact with the distal incline of the opposing cusp in front of it, and the distal incline of each upper cusp makes contact with the mesial incline of the opposing cusp distal to it.

occupational disease, a disease that results from a particular employment, usually from the effects of long-term exposure to specific substances or from the continuous or repetitive physical acts.

occupational exposure, working in an environment with one or more risk factors present.

occupational health, the ability of a worker to function at an optimum level of well-being at a worksite as reflected in terms of productivity, work attendance, disability compensation claims, and employment longevity.

occupational risk, a hazard found or likely to occur in the workplace. The number and types of hazards a health care worker may encounter in the routine conduct of health care delivery.

Occupational Safety and Health Administration (OSHA), a federal agency charged with establishing guidelines and regulations regarding worker safety. These guidelines include storage and disposal of toxic chemicals and hazardous materials and the safety and proper use of clinical and office equipment.

odontalgia (ō′dontal′jə), pain in a tooth; toothache.

o., phantom (ghost pain), pain in the area from which a tooth has been removed.

odontectomy (ō′dontek′təmē), the removal of a tooth.

odontoblasts (ōdon′tōblasts), the cells that form the dentin of the tooth.

odontodysplasia (ghost teeth), a developmental anomaly characterized by deficient tooth development. Deficiencies are noted in enamel and dentin formation. See also **tooth, shell.**

odontogenesis (ōdon′tōjen′esis), the process of tooth formation.

o. imperfecta, a generic term that includes simultaneous defects in epithelial and mesenchymal tissue involved in tooth development.

odontogenic cysts. See **cysts.**

odontogenic tumors. See **tumors.**

odontoid process, the toothlike projection that rises perpendicularly from the upper surface of the body of the second cervical vertebra or axis, which serves as a pivot point for the rotation of the atlas, or first cervical vertebra, enabling the head to turn in a horizontal plane.

odontoma (ō′dontō′mə) (gestant anomaly), an anomaly of the teeth resembling a tumor of hard tissue (for example, dens in dente, enamel pearl, complex or composite odontoma). It is composed of enamel, dentin, cementum, and pulp tissue that may be arranged in the form of teeth.

o., ameloblastic (amel′ōblas′tik), an odontogenic tumor characterized by the occurrence of an ameloblastoma

within an odontoma. See also **ameloblastoma; odontoma.**

o., composite (kompoz′it), complex odontoma; an odontogenic tumor characterized by the formation of calcified enamel and dentin in an abnormal arrangement because of lack of morphodifferentiation. Compound odontoma: a tumor of enamel and dentin arranged in the form of anomalous miniature teeth. Several small abnormal teeth surrounded by a fibrous sac.

o., cystic, an odontoma associated with a follicular cyst.

o., gestant. See **dens in dente.**

odor, a scent or smell. The sense of smell is activated when airborne molecules stimulate receptors of the first cranial nerve.

office hours. See **business hours.**

office management, the oversight of the business aspects of professional practice.

office planning, the physical arrangement of the rooms available within the limitations of space designed to enable the dentist to practice.

office routine. See **routine, office.**

office visit, a patient encounter with a health care provider in an office, clinic, or ambulatory care facility as an outpatient.

off-line, pertaining to the operation of input/output devices or auxiliary equipment not under direct control of the central processor.

offset, a deduction; a counterclaim; a contrary claim or demand by which a given claim may be lessened or cancelled.

ofloxacin, *trade names:* Floxin, Floxin IV; *drug class:* fluoroquinolone antiinfective; *action:* broad-spectrum bactericidal agent that inhibits the enzyme DNA-gyrase needed for replication of DNA; *uses:* treatment of lower respiratory tract infections, genitourinary infections, skin and skin structure infections.

ofloxacin (optic), *trade name:* Ocuflox; *drug class:* fluoroquinolone antiinfective, topical; *action:* broad-spectrum bactericidal agent that inhibits the enzyme DNA-gyrase needed for replication of DNA; *uses:* treatment of bacterial conjunctivitis caused by susceptible organisms.

oil, an unctuous, combustible substance that is liquid, or easily liquefiable on warming, and soluble in ether but insoluble in water.

o., essential (volatile oil), a volatile, nonfatty liquid of vegetable origin having a distinct aroma and flavor, often pleasant.

o., fixed, a nonvolatile oil consisting chiefly of glycerides.

o., mineral, any one of the various grades of liquid petrolatum.

o., volatile. See **oil, essential.**

ointment (oint′ment), a soft, bland, smooth, semisolid mixture that is used as a lubricant and as a vehicle for external medication.

o., hydrophilic, an ointment that is miscible with water.

olfactory bulb, the area of the forebrain where the olfactory nerves terminate and the olfactory tracts arise.

olfactory nerve, one of a pair of nerves associated with the sense of smell. The olfactory nerve is the first cranial nerve. The olfactory sensory endings are modified epithelial cells and the least specialized of the special senses.

oligodendroglioma, a relatively rare, moderately well-differentiated, relatively slow-growing glioma that occurs most frequently in the cerebrum of adults. It is grossly homogeneous, fairly well-circumscribed, moderately firm, and somewhat gritty in consistency, with interstitial calcification sufficiently dense as to be detected by x-ray imaging of the skull.

oligodontia (ol′igōdon′shē-ə), the condition of having only a few teeth.

oligodynamic (ol′igōdīnam′ik), effective in extremely small quantities.

oligonucleotide, a compound made up of the condensation of a small number of nucleotides.

oliguria (ol′igyo͞o′rē-ə), a decreased output of urine (usually less than 500 ml/day), possibly associated with dehydration from diarrhea or excessive sweating, low fluid intake, lower nephron nephrosis resulting from burns, heavy metal poisoning, terminal renal disease, or an increase in extracellular fluid volume in untreated renal, cardiac, or hepatic disease.

olsalazine sodium, *trade name:* Dipentum; *drug class:* antiinflammatory, salicylate derivative; *action:* bioconverted to 5-amino-salicylic acid, which decreases inflammation in the colon; *uses:* maintenance of remission of ulcerative colitis in patients intolerant to sulfasalazine.

omeprazole, *trade name:* Prilosec; *drug class:* antisecretory compound; *action:* suppresses gastric secretion by inhibiting hydrogen/potassium ATPase enzyme system in the gastric parietal cell; *uses:* gastroesophageal reflux disease (GERD), severe erosive esophagitis, pathologic hypersecretory conditions (Zollinger-Ellison syndrome, mastocytosis, multiple endocrine adenomas).

omission, a phoneme left out at a place where it should occur.

on account, in partial payment; in partial satisfaction of an amount owed.

Onchocerca, a genus of elongated filariform nematodes that inhabit the connective tissue of their hosts, usually within firm nodules in which these parasites are coiled and entangled.

O. volvulus, the blinding nodular nematode that causes dermatologic lesions and ocular complications that lead to blindness.

oncocytoma (ong′kōsītō′mə) (acidophilic adenoma, oxyphilic adenoma), a rare, benign tumor usually occurring in the parotid glands in older patients. The lesion is encapsulated and composed of sheets and cords of large eosinophilic cells with small nuclei.

oncogene, a potentially cancer-inducing gene.

ondansetron HCl, *trade name:* Zofran; *drug class:* antiemetic; *action:* selective 5-HT$_3$ antagonist; *uses:* prevention of nausea and vomiting associated with cancer chemotherapy

One Stage Oratronics Weis Standard Blade Implant System, an ADA acceptable endosseous dental implant system.

onlay, 1. a cast type of restoration that is retained by frictional and mechanical factors in the preparation of the tooth and restores one or more cusps and adjoining occlusal surfaces of the tooth. **2.** an occlusal rest portion of a removable partial denture that is extended to cover the entire occlusal surface of the tooth.

o. bone. See **graft, onlay bone.**

on-line, a system of data processing under control of the central processing unit. Data reflecting current activity are introduced into the processing system as soon as they occur.

on or about, a phrase used in stating the date of an occurrence or conveyance to avoid being bound by the statement of an exact or certain date.

ontogeny (ontoj′enē), the natural life cycle of an individual as contrasted with the natural life cycle of the race (phylogeny).

opacification (ōpas′ifikā′shən), **1.** the process of making something opaque. **2.** the formation of opacities.

opalescent (ō′pəles′ent), resembling an opal in the display of various colors, as in opalescent dentin.

o. teeth, a translucent or opal-like appearance of teeth, usually associated with a genetic defect in odontogenesis.

opaque, relatively impenetrable to light. See also **opacity, optical.**

open bite. See **bite, open.**

open-end contract. See **contract, open-end.**

open enrollment, the annual period in which employees can select from a choice of benefits programs.

opening movement. See **movement, mandibular, opening.**

opening, vertical. See **dimension, vertical.**

open panel, a dental benefits plan characterized by three features: (1) any licensed dentist may elect to participate, (2) the beneficiary may receive dental treatment from among all licensed dentists with the corresponding benefits payable to the beneficiary or the dentist, and (3) the dentist may accept or refuse any beneficiary. See also **panel, open.**

operate, to work on the body with the hands or by means of cutting or other instruments to correct a deformity, remove an anatomic part, or remove pathologic processes and/or tissues.

operating field. See **field, operating.**

operating light. See **light, operating.**

operating procedure. See **procedure, operating.**

operation, 1. any surgical procedure. **2.** the action of a drug or other remedy. **3.** an act or series of acts performed on the body of a patient for relief or cure.

o., Abbé-Estlander, the transfer of a full-thickness section of one lip of the oral cavity to the other lip, using an arterial pedicle to ensure survival of the graft.

o., blind, a procedure in which the surgeon operates by using the sense of touch and knowledge of surgical anatomy without making a significant mucous membrane or cutaneous incision.

o., computer, the program step undertaken or executed by a computer (for example, addition, multiplication, comparison, and data movement). The operation is usually specified by a functional command in the software used.

o., exploratory, a surgical procedure used to establish a diagnosis.

o., Gillies′, a technique for reducing fractures of the zygoma and the zygomatic arch through an incision in the temporal hairline.

o., Kazanjian′s (Kazanjian′s procedure), a technique of surgical extension of the vestibular sulcus for improved prosthetic foundation of edentulous ridges. See also **extension, ridge.**

o., modified flap, a variation of the flap procedure in oral and periodontal surgery. In this variation the vertical incisions of the flap procedure are not made, but the labial and/or lingual gingival walls are distended as far as possible to ensure sufficient access and an unobstructed view for instrumentation.

o., open, a procedure in which the surgeon operates with full view of the structures through mucous membrane or cutaneous incisions.

o., Partsch′s, the name applied to a technique of marsupialization.

o., pedicle flap, a procedure in mucogingival surgery designed to relocate or slide gingival tissue from a donor site in close proximity to an isolated defect, usually a tooth surface denuded of attached gingiva.

o., Sorrin′s, a type of flap approach in the treatment of a periodontal abscess; especially suitable when the marginal gingiva appears well adapted and gives no access to the abscess area. A semilunar incision is made below the involved area in the attached gingiva, leaving the gingival margin undisturbed; a flap is raised, allowing access to the abscessed area for curettage. Suturing follows.

o. system (OS), an integrated set of software modules that provide the framework for orderly assignment of a computer's resources to perform a variety of tasks. It is usually written in the assembler language of the computer.

operative dentistry, the branch of dentistry that deals with the esthetic and functional restoration of the hard tissues of individual teeth.

operatory (op'ər-ətōr'ē), the room or rooms in which the dentist performs professional services.

operculectomy (opurkyōōlek'təmē), the surgical removal of the mucosal flap partially or completely covering an unerupted tooth. (not current)

operculitis (opur'kyōōlī'tis). See **pericoronitis.**

operculum (əpur'kyōōləm), a cover or lid.

operon, a segment of DNA consisting of an operator gene and one or more structural genes with related functions controlled by the operator gene in conjunction with a regulator gene.

ophthalmology, the branch of medicine concerned with the study of the physiology, anatomy, and pathology of the eye and the diagnosis and treatment of disorders of the eye.

ophthalmoscope, a device for examining the interior of the eye. It includes a light, a mirror with a single hole through which the examiner may look, and a dial holding several lenses of varying strengths. The lenses are selected to allow clear visualization of the structures of the eye at any depth.

opiate (ō'pē·it), **1.** a remedy containing or derived from opium. **2.** any drug that induces sleep.

opinion, in the law of evidence, an inference or conclusion drawn by a witness from information known to him or her or assumed.

opisthion (opis'thē·ôn), the hindmost point on the posterior margin of the foramen magnum.

opisthocranion (opis'thōkra'nē·ôn), the point in the midline of the cranium that projects farthest backward.

opium, concrete juice of the poppy, *Papaver somniferum.* It contains mor-

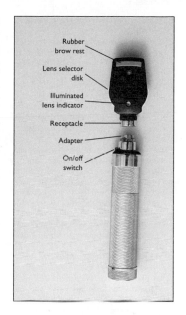

Labels: Rubber brow rest — Lens selector disk — Illuminated lens indicator — Receptacle — Adapter — On/off switch

Ophthalmoscope. (Seidel, 1995.)

phine, codeine, nicotine, narceine, and many other alkaloids.

opportunistic infection, an infection by a microbial organism to which the patient is usually resistant; however, because of reduced vitality or through suppression of the immune system, the patient has become infected.

opsin, a visual pigment protein found in the retinal rods.

optic chiasm, a point near the thalamus and hypothalamus at which portions of each optic nerve cross over.

optic nerve, either of a pair of the second cranial nerves responsible for sight, consisting mainly of coarse, myelinated fibers that arise in the retinal ganglionic layer of the eye and traverse the thalamus and connect with the visual cortex of the brain.

optics, the science concerned with the properties of light, its refraction and absorption, and the properties of the media of the eye to refract and absorb light.

optimal (op′timəl), the best or most favorable.

optimism, the tendency to look on the bright or happy side of everything, to believe that there is good in everything.

optometry, the professional discipline devoted to testing the eyes for visual acuity, prescribing corrective lenses and recommending eye exercises and other health practices to preserve sight.

Orabase, the brand name of a topical dental paste containing an adrenocorticoid. The base consists of gelatin, pectin, mineral oil, and sodium carboxymethylcellulose in a hydrocarbon gel. The adrenocorticoid is hydrocortisone acetate. Orabase is used for temporary relief of symptoms associated with oral inflammation and ulcerative lesions.

oral, pertaining to the mouth.

o. contraceptives (estrogens, mestranol androgens, ethinyl estradiol, levonorgestrel), trade names: Demulen, Loestrin, Lo/Ovral, Nordett; *drug class:* estrogen/progestin combinations; *action:* prevents ovulation by suppressing follicle-stimulating, luteinizing hormone; *uses:* pregnancy prevention, endometriosis, hypermenorrhea, hypogonadism.

o. environment. See **environment, oral.**

o. evacuator (vacuum), a suction apparatus used to remove fluids and debris from an operating field.

o. hairy leukoplakia, a filamentous, white plaque found on the lateral borders of the tongue that can spread across the entire dorsum of the tongue and onto the buccal mucosa. The Epstein-Barr virus has been identified in biopsy specimens of these lesions. An indicator disease for AIDS. See also **leukoplakia.**

o. health diet score, a motivational aid to good nutrition. Merit points are earned by an adequate intake of foods from the recommended food groups. Demerits are given for frequent intake of foods high in sugars. The difference is the oral health diet score. The technique is applicable to children with a high incidence of dental caries.

o. health index, a statistical measure that quantifies one or more aspects of

a person's or group's oral health status.

o. hygiene. See **hygiene, oral.**

o. manifestation, the presence of the signs, symptoms, and lesions of a systemic disease in and around the oral cavity.

o. medicine. See **medicine, oral.**

o. mucosa. See **mucosa, oral.**

o. physiology. See **physiology, oral.**

o. surgery. See **surgery, oral.**

o. warts, warts caused by human papillomavirus that may be scattered throughout the mouth or localized in one area. They frequently recur. Oral warts are associated with AIDS infection.

orbital (ôr′bitəl), pertaining to the orbit.

o. exenteration, the surgical removal of the entire contents of the orbit.

o. marker, a projecting part of a facebow that marks the location of the orbitale. Used in the orientation of casts on an articulator in relation to cranial planes.

o. plane. See **plane, orbital.**

orbitale (ôr′bita′lē), the lowest point in the margin of the orbit (directly below the pupil when the eye is open and the patient is looking straight ahead) that may readily be felt under the skin. The eye-ear plane passes through the orbitale and tragion.

orbiting condyle, the condyle that arcs around the vertical axis of the rotating condyle (that is, the opposite condyle from the center of rotation). Aids the opposite canine to disclude all other teeth. (not current)

orders, written or verbal directions of a physician or dentist to a nurse or other assistant detailing the care to be given to a patient.

organelle, any one of various particles of living substance bound within most cells, which include mitochondria, the Golgi complex, the endoplasmic reticulum, the lysosomes, and the centrioles.

organism(s) (ôr′gənizəm), any organized body of living economy.

o., Miller's, the fusospirochetal organisms in the flora or oral microorganisms, found by Willoughby D. Miller and Hugo Karl Plaut to be the causative agents in nondiphtheritic membranous angina (necrotizing ulcerative gingivitis, necrotizing ulcerative gingivostomatitis, Vincent's infection, and "trench mouth").

o., Vincent's, the fusospirochetal organisms associated with the initiation of necrotizing ulcerative gingivitis, necrotizing ulcerative stomatitis, and/or Vincent's angina.

organization, an arrangement of distinct but mutually dependent parts, persons, or tasks to create, enhance, or improve a functioning unit.

organ transplantation, the replacement of a diseased organ with a healthy organ from a donor with a compatible tissue type. Organs such as a kidney may be donated by living donors, or harvested from brain-dead organ donors.

orientation, the ability to correctly place oneself in time, space, and relationship to others and one's work and environment.

orifice (ôr′ifis), the entrance or outlet of any body cavity; any foramen, meatus, or opening.

ornithine, an amino acid, not a constituent of proteins, that is produced as an important intermediate substance in the urea cycle.

o. carbamoyltransferase, an enzyme in the blood that increases in patients with liver and other diseases.

oroantral fistula, an abnormal tract that connects the oral cavity with the maxillary sinus.

orodigitofacial dysostosis (OFD syndrome), a syndrome characterized by abnormal development of the jaws and tongue, cleft lip and palate, hypoplasia of bones of the skull with ocular hypertelorism, nasal alar deformity, malformation of digits (frequently manifested as brachydactyly and syndactyly), mental retardation, granular skin, and alopecia of the scalp.

orofacial abnormality, a structural and functional disorder of the mouth and face, usually arising from genetic or congenital defects.

orofacial muscles, the muscles of facial expression.

orofacial pain, pain within the structures of the mouth and face, usually of a diffuse pattern.

oronasal, pertaining to the mouth and nose.

oropharynx (ô′rōfer′ingks), the portion of the pharynx associated with the mouth; usually described as bounded above by the uvula, below by the epiglottis, in front by the tongue, and behind by the posterior pharyngeal wall.

orosomucoid, a subgroup of the α_1-globulin fraction of the blood.

orphenadrine citrate, *trade names:* Banflex, Flexoject, Norflex, Orflagen; *drug class:* skeletal muscle relaxant, central acting; *action:* acts centrally to depress polysynaptic pathways to relax skeletal muscle, inhibit muscle spasm; *uses:* pain in musculoskeletal conditions.

ortho, a prefix denoting straight or correct.

orthodontic, a term describing the orthopedic correction of abnormal dental relationships, including related abnormalities in facial structures.

o. appliances. See **appliance.**

   o. a., functional. See **appliances, removable.**

   o. a., removable. See **appliances, removable.**

o. bracket. See **bracket.**

o. retainer. See **appliance, retaining orthodontic.**

o. wire. See **wire.**

orthodontics (dentofacial orthopedic), the area of dentistry concerned with the supervision, guidance, and correction of the growing and mature dentofacial structures, including conditions that require movement of the teeth or correction of malrelationships and malformations of related structures by the adjustment of relationships between and among teeth and facial bones by the application of forces and/or the stimulation and redirection of functional forces within the craniofacial complex. Major responsibilities of orthodontic practice include the diagnosis, prevention, interception, and treatment of all forms of malocclusion of the teeth and associated alterations in their surrounding structures; design, application, and control of functional and corrective appliances; and guidance of the dentition and its supporting structures to attain and maintain optimum occlusal relations in physiologic and esthetic harmony among facial and cranial structures.

orthodontist, a dental specialist who has completed an approved, advanced course of at least 2 years in the special area of orthodontics.

orthognathic (ôr'thognā'thik), pertaining to the normal relationships of the jaws.

o. surgery, surgery to alter relationships of dental arches and/or supporting bones, usually accomplished with orthodontic therapy.

orthognathus (ôrthognāth'əs), straight jaws; no projection of the lower part of the face. The facial angle is 85 to 90 degrees. (not current)

orthopantograph (ôr'thōpan'tōgraf), a panoramic radiographic device (Panorex) that permits visualization of the entire dentition, alveolar bone, and other contiguous structures on a single extraoral film.

orthopantomograph (ôr'thōpan't-mōgraf), a radiographic system (manufactured by Siemens) that uses three axes of rotation to obtain a panoramic radiograph of the dental arches and their associated structures.

orthopedic (ôr'thōpē'dik), a correction of abnormal form or relationship of bone structures. May be accomplished surgically (orthopedic surgery) or by the application of appliances to stimulate changes in the bone structure by natural physiologic response (orthopedic therapy). Orthodontic therapy is orthopedic therapy applied through the teeth.

orthopnea (ôr'thopnē'ə), an inability to breathe except in an upright position.

Osler-Weber disease. See **telangiectasia, hereditary hemorrhagic.**

osmium, a hard, grayish, pungent-smelling metallic element. Its atomic number is 76 and its atomic weight is 190.2. It is used to produce alloys of extreme hardness, and is highly toxic.

osmosis, the passage of pure solvent from the lesser to the greater concentration when two solutions are separated by a membrane that selectively prevents the passage of solute molecules but is permeable to the solvent. The principles of osmosis, with the selective permeability of the cell membrane, help regulate the transfer of fluids and metabolites to and from the cells. Thus they also maintain the stability of the salt/ion concentration

in the extracellular and intracellular fluids.

osmotic, pertaining to osmosis.

o. pressure. See **pressure, osmotic.**

osseointegration, the growth action of bone tissue, as it assimilates surgically implanted devices or prostheses to be used as either replacement parts or anchors.

ostectomy (ostek'tōmē) (osteoectomy), the excision of a bone or portion of a bone.

o., periodontal, the removal of alveolar bone from around the tooth root to eliminate an adjacent pocket and secure physiologic osseous and gingival form.

osteitis (os'tē-ī'tis), an inflammation of the bone; an inflammation of the haversian spaces, canals, and their branches but generally not of the medullary cavity. The disease is characterized by tenderness and a dull, aching pain. Enlargement of the bone may occur. Osteitis of the alveolar process after tooth extraction is commonly referred to as *dry socket.*

o., alveolar localized. See **socket, dry.**

o., condensing, a chronic inflammation associated with some nonvital teeth or located in the site of extraction of such teeth, resulting in abnormally dense bone.

o. deformans (Paget's disease), **l.** a disease of the bone of unknown cause characterized by enlargement of the cranial bones and often of the maxillae or the mandible. The x-ray appearance is characterized by a cotton-wool appearance. **2.** a localized or generalized disease of bone of unknown origin characterized by the replacement of normal bone with soft, poorly mineralized osteoid tissue. In later stages, affected bone is replaced by densely sclerotic bone. Bony enlargement, deformities, and sometimes fractures occur. **3.** a generalized disease of bone characterized by the concurrent destruction and formation of bone. The etiology is unknown. **4.** a bone disease characterized by thickening and bowing of the long bones and enlargement of the skull and maxillae. It is represented radiographically by a cotton-wool appearance of the bone and microscopically by a mosaic bone pattern. Hypercementosis and loosening of the teeth may be significant manifestations.

o. fibrosa cystica, generalized (von Recklinghausen's disease of bone), **1.** a disease caused by parathyroid adenomas and characterized by cyst-like radiolucencies in the bones (including the jaws), loosening of teeth, localized swellings, giant cell lesions, increased blood calcium and phosphatase levels, and lowered blood phosphorus levels. The term *von Recklinghausen's disease* is also used as a synonym for *neurofibromatosis.* **2.** increased resorption and destruction of bone caused by primary and secondary hyperparathyroidism. See also **hyperparathyroidism.**

osteoarthritis (os·te·ō·ar·thrī'tis), chronic degeneration and destruction of the articular cartilage leading to bony spurs, pain, stiffness, limitation of motion, and change in the size of joints. Considered to result from chronic traumatic injury and wear and tear. Heberden's nodes occur in a special form of the disease. Symptoms may be associated with hormonal, vascular, and/or nutritional disorders. The structural changes of advanced osteoarthritis may involve erosion of the articular cartilages or the subchondral bone. Osteoarthritis rarely affects the temporomandibular joint beyond the "creaking" state.

osteoarthropathy, hypertrophic pulmonary (os·te·ō·arthrop'əthē), a clubbing of the fingers and toes resulting from deposition of calcium in the subperiosteal tissues around the joint. Related to chronic pulmonary disease and occasionally to circulatory and digestive disease.

osteoblast (os'te·ō·blast'), the cell associated with the growth and development of bone; cuboidal in shape. In active growth, osteoblasts form a continuous layer on old bone like a sheet of epithelial cells; when the bone growth is arrested, the cells assume an elongated appearance like fibroblasts.

osteocalcin, vitamin K-dependent calcium-binding protein synthesized by osteoblasts and found primarily in bone. Serum osteocalcin measurements provide a noninvasive specific marker of bone metabolism.

osteocementum (os'te·ō·sēmen'təm), secondary cementum; the hard, bone-like cementum deposited after root formation is completed. See also **atrophy of disuse.**

osteochondritis, a disease of the epiphyses, or bone-forming centers of the skeleton, beginning with necrosis and fragmentation of the tissue and followed by repair and regeneration.

osteoclasia, traumatic (os'te·ōklā' zhə). See **cementoma; dysplasia, osseous, focal; fibroma, periapical.** (not current)

osteoclast (os'te·ō·klast'), **1.** a large, multinucleated giant cell associated with the resorption of bone; the nuclei resemble the nuclei of the osteoblasts and osteocytes; the cytoplasm is often foamy, and the cell frequently has branching processes. Osteoclasts may arise from stromal cells of the bone marrow. They may represent fused osteoblasts or may include fused osteocytes liberated from resorbing bone. They are usually found in close relationship to the resorption of bone and frequently lie in grooves (Howship's lacunae). **2.** a large, multinucleated cell associated with the resorption of bone. Seen in irregular concavities within marginal areas of bone undergoing resorption.

osteoclastoma. See **granuloma, giant cell reparative, peripheral.**

osteocyte (os'te·ō·sīt'), an osteoblast that has been surrounded by a calcified interstitial substance; the cells are enclosed within lacunae, and the cytoplasmic processes extend through apertures of the lacunae into canaliculi in the bone. Like the osteoblast, the osteocyte may undergo transformations and assume the form of an osteoclast or reticular cell.

o. osteodystrophy (os'te·ō·ōdis'trəfē), a condition marked by defective or deficient bone formation.

o., renal, a form of dwarfism associated with osteoporosis produced by renal insufficiency during childhood. Periodontal changes include widening of the periodontal membrane space and marked osteoporosis of the mandibular and maxillary bones. Similar to renal rickets. See also **rickets, renal.**

osteoectomy (os'te·ō·ek'təmē). See **ostectomy.** (not current)

osteofibroma (os'tē-ōf'ĭbrō'mə) (calcifying fibroma, fibroosteoma, ossifying fibroma), a benign neoplasm characterized by bone developing in a connective tissue mass. A benign neoplasm that develops in the spongiosa of the bone through proliferation of fibroblasts. A benign neoplasm of the bone characterized by unilateral swelling and fibroblastic and osteoclastic activity in marrow spaces. See also **dysplasia, fibrous** and **dysplasia, osseous.**

osteogenesis, the origin and development of bone tissue.

o. imperfecta (os'tē-ōjen'əsis) *(brittle bone disease, fragilitas ossium, Lobstein's disease, osteopsathyrosis idiopathica),* a congenital disease of unknown cause characterized by fragile, brittle, and easily fractured bones; presumed to stem from a failure in the formation of bone matrix. Variants are often hereditary or familial and include manifestations such as blue sclerae, dentinogenesis imperfecta, and otosclerosis.

osteoid (os'tē-oid), the mucopolysaccharide-protein complex laid down by the osteoblasts. It is later calcified, with inclusion of osteoblasts as osteocytes within lacunae, into bone.

osseointegration (os'tē-ōin'tegrā'-shən), a specific endosseous dental implant technique involving *very* slow and precise bone drilling to minimize heat production; the procedure makes use of biocompatible metal and a defined healing environment. Synonym: Branemark technique.

osteolysis (os'tē-ol'əsis), a process of bone resorption whereby the bone salts can be withdrawn by a humoral mechanism and returned to the tissue fluids, leaving behind a decalcified bone matrix. Synonym: halisteresis.

osteoma (os'tē-ō'mə), a benign neoplasm of bone or bone tissue.

osteomalacia (os'tē-ōmələ'shē-ə) (adult rickets), a systemic disorder of bone characterized by decreased mineralization of bone matrix possibly resulting from vitamin D deficiency, inadequate calcium in the diet, renal disease, and/or steatorrhea. Manifestations include incomplete fractures and gradual resorption of cortical and cancellous bone.

osteomyelitis (os'tē-ōmī'əli'tis), an inflammation of the bone marrow or of the bone, marrow, and endosteum. See also **osteitis.**

osteon (os'tē·on), the three-dimensional reconstruction of concentric lamellae arranged circumferentially about the course of a central blood vessel.

osteonecrosis, the destruction and death of bone tissue. It may stem from ischemia, infection, malignant neoplastic disease, or trauma.

osteonectin, noncollagenous, calcium-binding glycoprotein of developing bone. It links collagen to mineral in the bone matrix.

osteopetrosis (ostē-ōpetrō'sis) (Albers-Schönberg disease, marble bone), osteosclerosis of unknown origin that obliterates the bone marrow regions with resultant anemia. Delayed tooth eruption and severe osteomyelitis or necrosis after dental infection may be associated with the disease.

osteoplasty (os'tē-ōplas'tē), a surgical procedure to modify or change the configuration of a bone.

osteoporosis (os'tē-ōpôrō'sis) (Schüller's disease), an enlargement of the soft marrow and haversian spaces resulting from a decreased rate of formation of the hard bone matrix. With the exception of immobilized parts, it is a systemic disorder that occurs in advanced age (senile osteoporosis), during ACTH and cortisone therapy, during and after menopause, in limited physical activity, in Cushing's syndrome, during malnutrition, and in other disorders of matrix formation such as hyperadrenalism, hyperthyroidism, vitamin C deficiencies, and deficiency of androgenic steroids. See also **atrophy, bone** and **bone rarefaction.**

osteopsathyrosis idiopathica (os'tē-opsath'irō'sis) *(not current).* See **osteogenesis imperfecta.**

osteoradionecrosis (os'tē-ōrā'dē-ōnekrō'sis), bone necrosis secondary to irradiation and superimposed infection.

osteosarcoma (os'tē-ōsarkō'mə), a malignant neoplasm of the bone-forming tissue.

osteosclerosis (os'tē-ōsklərō'sis), an increased bone formation resulting in reduced marrow spaces and increased radiopacity.

osteotomy (os'tē·ot'əmē), the surgical cutting or transection of a bone.

otalgia dentalis (ōtal'jē·ə), a reflex pain in the ear resulting from dental disease; usually propagated along the auriculotemporal nerve. (not current)

otic ganglion. See **ganglion, otic.**

otitis, an inflammation or infection of the ear.

  o. externa, an inflammation or infection of the external canal or the auricle of the external ear. Major causes are allergy, bacteria, fungi, viruses, and trauma.

  o. media (ōtī'tis me'dē·ə), an inflammation of the middle ear that may be marked by pain, fever, abnormalities of hearing, deafness, tinnitus, and vertigo that may originate in the pharynx and be transmitted by the eustachian tubes.

otolaryngology, the branch or specialty of medicine that deals with diseases of the ear, nose, and throat.

otosclerosis (ō'tōsklərō'sis), a disorder of the middle ear that generally results in hardening and fusion of the ossicles of the ear, with resultant immobilization so that sound waves cannot be conducted along their paths.

otoscope, an instrument used to examine the external ear, the eardrum, and, through the eardrum, the ossicles of the middle ear. It consists of a light, a magnifying lens, and a device for insufflation.

otoscopy, to view or inspect the tympanic membrane and other parts of the outer ear with an otoscope.

outline form. See **form, outline.**

outpatient, a patient, not hospitalized or housed in an extended care facility, who is being treated in an office, clinic, or other ambulatory care facility.

output, the transfer or exit of processed or in-process information from a computer to printers, video terminals, and other peripheral devices.

ovalocytosis (ō'vəlōsītō'sis). See elliptocytosis.

ovariectomy, the surgical removal of one or both ovaries.

ovary, one of the pair of female gonads found on each side of the lower abdomen, beside the uterus, in a fold of the broad ligament.

overbilling, a nondisclosure or waiver of patient copayment.

overbite, a vertical overlapping of upper teeth over lower teeth, usually measured perpendicular to the occlusal plane. See also **overjet** and **overlap, vertical.**

overclosure, the raising of the mandible too far before the teeth make contact; loss of occlusal vertical dimension is the cause. See also **distance, large interarch.**

overcoding, reporting a more complex and/or higher cost procedure than was actually performed.

overdenture, a complete or partial removable denture supported by retained roots to provide improved support, stability, and tactile and pro prioceptive sensation and to reduce ridge resorption. See also **root retention** and **root submersion.**

overdose (OD), an excessive use of a drug, resulting in adverse reaction ranging from mania or hysteria to coma or death.

overextended, l. when any prosthetic appliance is inadvertently constructed in such a way that part of the oral mucosa is injured by the appliance. **2.** pertaining to any extrusion beyond the apical opening into the periapical area. May be with instrumentation, medication, or root canal filling.

overfilled. See **overextended.**

overhang, an excess filling material projecting beyond cavity margins.

overhead, production costs required to be expended by the dentist to practice the profession (for example, rent, utilities, salaries, laundry). Costs include any involved with management, supplies, equipment, salaries (taxes), and maintenance. Amounts deducted from the gross receipts of a dental practice before the dentist's net income (take-home pay) is received.

overjet, the horizontal projection of upper teeth beyond the lower teeth, usually measured parallel to the occlusal plane. When not otherwise specified, the term is generally assumed to refer to central incisors and is measured from the labial surface of the lower central incisors to the labial surface of the upper central incisors at the level of the upper incisor edge. Unique conditions may sometimes require other measuring techniques. See also **overlap, horizontal.**

overlap, deep vertical (closed bite, deep bite, deep overbite), an excessive vertical overlap of the anterior teeth.

overlap, horizontal (overjet, overjut), projection of the anterior and/or posterior teeth of one arch beyond their antagonists in a horizontal direction.

overlap, vertical (overbite), an extension of the upper teeth over the lower teeth in a vertical direction when the opposing posterior teeth are in contact in centric occlusion. This term is used especially to designate the distance that the upper incisal edges drop below the level of the lower ones, but it may also be used to describe the vertical relations of opposing cusps of posterior teeth.

overlay. See **onlay.**

o., computer, a technique for bringing routines into memory from magnetic storage during processing so that several routines will occupy the same storage locations at different times. Overlay techniques are used when the total storage requirements for instructions exceed the available storage in memory.

overshooting accident, the result of seating an endosteal implant beyond its normal host site (through the inferior mandibular border, into the mandibular canal or nasal or antral floor).

ovoid arch. See **arch, ovoid.**

owner, the person holding ownership, dominion, or title of property.

ownership, the legal right of possession.

Owren's disease. See **parahemophilia.**

oxacillin sodium, *trade names:* Bactocill, Prostaphlin; *drug class:* penicillinase-resistant penicillin; *action:* interferes with cell wall replication of susceptible organisms; the cell wall, rendered osmotically unstable, swells and bursts from osmotic pressure; *uses:* effective for gram-positive cocci, infections caused by penicillinase-producing *Staphylococcus.*

oxalate, any salt of oxalic acid.

oxandrolone, *trade name:* Oxandrin; *drug class:* androgenic anabolic steroid (Controlled Substance Schedule III); *action:* reverses catabolic tissue processes; promotes build-up of protein; increases erythropoietin production; *uses:* catabolic or tissue-wasting processes, such as extensive surgery, burns, infection, or trauma; HIV wasting syndrome; Turner's syndrome.

oxaprozin, *trade name:* Daypro; *drug class:* nonsteroidal antiinflammatory; *action:* inhibits prostaglandin synthesis by interfering with cyclooxygenase needed for biosynthesis; possesses analgesic, antiinflammatory, antipyretic properties; *uses:* rheumatoid arthritis, osteoarthritis, and ankylosing spondylitis.

oxazepam, *trade name:* Serax; *drug class:* benzodiazepine (Controlled Substance Schedule IV); *action:* produces central nervous system depression by interacting with a benzodiazepine receptor to facilitate the action of the inhibitory neurotransmitter γ-aminobutyric acid (GABA); *uses:* anxiety, alcohol withdrawal.

oxidant, the substance that is reduced in an oxidation/reduction reaction, thereby oxidizing the other component.

oxidation, the combination of oxygen with other elements to form oxides. The process in which an element gains electrons.

o. of metal, the formation of a surface oxide during the casting or soldering of a metal or during subsequent use by the patient.

oxidative, having the ability or property to oxidize.

oxide, a compound of oxygen with another element or radical such as iron.

o. divinyl. See **ether, divinyl.**

oxidized cellulose, *trade name:* Surgicel; *drug class:* cellulose hemostatic; *action:* mechanism unclear; may act physically to absorb blood and promote an artifical clot; *uses:* hemostasis in surgery, oral surgery, exodontia.

oximetry, the measurement of the oxygen saturation of hemoglobin in a sample of blood with the use of an oximeter.

oxtriphylline, *trade names:* Choledyl, Choledyl SA; *drug class:* choline salt of theophylline, bronchodilator; *action:* relaxes smooth muscle of respiratory system by blocking phosphodiesterase; *uses:* acute bronchial asthma, reversible bronchospasm in chronic bronchitis and COPD.

oxybutynin chloride, *trade name:* Ditropan; *drug class:* antispasmodic; *action:* relaxes smooth muscles in urinary tract; *use:* antispasmodic for neurogenic bladder.

oxycephaly (ok'sēsefəlē) (steeple head), a high conical crown resulting from early closure of sutures and disturbed cranial development.

oxycodone, *trade name:* Roxicodone; *drug class:* synthetic opioid analgesic (Controlled Substance Schedule II); *uses:* moderate-to-severe pain, normally used in combination with aspirin or acetaminophen, the opioid found in Percodan, Percocet, and Tylox.

oxygen, a tasteless, odorless, colorless gas essential for human respiration. Its atomic number is 8 and its atomic weight is 15.9994.

oxygenate (ok'sijcnāt), to saturate with oxygen.

oxyhemoglobin (ok'sēhē'mōglō'bin), a compound of hemoglobin with two atoms of oxygen.

oxymetazoline HCl, *trade names:* Afrin, Afrin Children's Nose Drops, Dristan Long-Lasting, Neo-Synephrine Nasal Decongestant, Sinarest 12 hour, Vicks Sinex 12 hour; *drug class:* nasal decongestant, sympathomimetic amine; *action:* produces vasoconstriction of arterioles, thereby decreasing fluid exudation and mucosal engorgement; *use:* nasal congestion.

oxymetholone, *trade name:* Anadrol-50; *drug class:* androgenic anabolic steroid (Controlled Substance Schedule III); *action:* reverses catabolic tissue processes; promotes build-up of protein, increased erythropoietin production; *uses:* anemia associated with bone marrow failure and red cell production deficiencies, aplastic anemia, myelofibrosis, and anemia caused by myelotoxic drugs.

oxytetracycline, a tetracycline antibiotic prescribed in the treatment of bacterial and rickettsial infections.

oxytocin (ok'sētō'sin), a hormone of the posterior pituitary gland that is the principal uterus-contracting hormone. Used in obstetrics to induce uterine contractions.

PA skull. See **examination, radiographic; examination, extraoral; examination, posteroanterior.**

PAB, PABA, an abbreviation for **paraaminobenzoic acid.**

PAC. See **aspirin, phenacetin, caffeine.**

pacemaker, an electrical device used to maintain a normal sinus rhythm in heart muscle contraction. Pacemakers can be permanent indwelling appliances. It is not advisable to use electronic devices on patients with pacemakers. Synonym: cardiac pacemaker.

pachyderma oralis (pak'ider'mə ôra'lis), an appearance of the buccal mucosa resembling elephant hide. (not current)

pachyderma oris (pak'ider'mə ôr'is) (focal keratosis, hyperkeratosis), a benign white lesion of the mucous membrane characterized by a thick layer of keratin overlying stratified squamous epithelium, the cells of which are normal. (not current)

pachymucosa alba (pak'imyookō'sə al'bə), an appearance of the buccal mucosa that has a white surface and resembles elephant hide.

Pacini's corpuscle (păchē'nēz). See **corpuscle, Pacini's.**

pack, a material used to protect tissue, fill space, or prevent hemorrhage.

p., periodontal, a surgical dressing applied to the necks of teeth and the adjacent tissue to cover and protect the surgical wound.

packing, the act of filling a mold.

p., denture, the laboratory procedure of filling and compressing a denture-base material into a mold in a flask.

paclitaxel, *trade name:* Taxol; *class:* antineoplastic; *action:* obtained from Western Yew tree, unique action inhibits microtubule network reorganization essential for cell division; *use:* metastatic ovarian cancer.

pad, Passavant's (pas'ävənts) (Passavant's bar, Passavant's ridge), the bulging "transverse roll" of the posterior pharyngeal wall produced by the upper portion of the superior pharyngeal constrictor muscle during the act of swallowing or during vocal effort; an objectionable term. See also **pharynx, activities of posterior and lateral pharyngeal wall.** (not current)

pad, retromolar (pear-shaped area), a mass of soft tissue, frequently pear-shaped, which is located at the distal termination of the mandibular residual ridge. It is made up of fibers of the buccinator muscle, the pterygomandibular raphe, the superior constrictor muscle, the temporal tendon, and the mucous glands.

pad, rubber dam (rubber dam mask), an absorbent piece of flannelette, bird's-eye, or gauze of suitable shape to interpose between a rubber dam and the face to protect the face from contact with both the rubber and the clips of the dam holder. (not current)

Paget's disease (paj′əts). See **osteitis deformans.**

pain, an unpleasant sensation created by a noxious stimulus mediated along specific nerve pathways to the central nervous system, where it is interpreted as such. The sensation of pain is a protective mechanism that warns of danger without giving too much information about the specific nature of the danger. It initiates nociceptive reflexes.

p. assessment, an evaluation of the reported pain and the factors that alleviate or exacerbate a patient's pain; used as an aid in the diagnosis and the treatment of disease and trauma.

p., chest, pain that occurs in the chest region because of disorders of the heart (e.g., angina pectoris, myocardial infarction, or pericarditis), pulmonary artery (pulmonary embolism or hypertension), lungs (pleuritis), esophagus ("heartburn"), abdominal organs (aerophagia, biliary tract disease, splenic infarction, or gaseous distention in the splenic flexure), or the chest wall (neoplasia, costochondral strains, trauma, hyperventilation, or muscular tension).

p. clinic, a multidisciplinary association of health care professionals devoted to the diagnosis and treatment of patients with acute and chronic pain.

p., deep, dull, aching, or boring pain originating in muscles, tendons, and joints. It is poorly localized and tends to radiate.

p. dysfunction syndrome, a phrase used in dentistry to describe a condition in patients who appear to have a psychophysiologic basis for stress overload on the temporomandibular joint. The preferred term is *mandibular stress syndrome.*

p., ghost. see **odontalgia, phantom.**

p. mechanism, the network that communicates unpleasant sensations and the perceptions of noxious stimuli throughout the body in association with both physical disease and trauma involving tissue damage.

p. nerve ending, a receptor nerve ending that is relatively primitive and ends in an undifferentiated arborization. The nerve ending for the sensation of pain is a protective mechanism that warns of danger without giving too much information about the specific nature of the danger. The danger stimuli give rise to nociceptive reflexes, or defensive, protective, or withdrawal movements. The nociceptive reflexes supersede other, less urgent, reflexes that are thus inhibited.

p., projected pathologic, pain erroneously perceived to arise in a peripheral region because of a stimulus from end-organs supplying the region (e.g., sciatic pain). Actually the stimulus occurred somewhere along the pain pathway from the nerve to the cortex.

p. reaction, the individual's manifestation of the unpleasant sensation.

p., referred, pain caused by an agent in one area but manifested in another (e.g., pain caused by caries in the maxillary third molar may be referred to the mandible, so the source of pain appears to be in the mandible).

p. and suffering, an element in a claim for damages in a liability lawsuit. It requests compensation to an individual for mental and physical pain and discomfort as a result of an injury.

p. threshold, the point at which a stimulus causes pain. The threshold varies widely among individuals.

pair, ion. See **ion.**

palatal (pal′ətəl), relating to the palate.

p. bar. See **bar, palatal.**

p. perforation. See **perforation, palatal.**

p. plate. See **connector, major.**

p. seal. See **seal, posterior palatal.**

palate (pal'ət), the bone and soft tissue that closes the space encompassed by the upper alveolar arch, extending posteriorly to the pharynx. The palate forms the "roof" of the mouth and connects to the nasal septum and floor of the nose in the midline.

p., cleft, **1.** a deformity of the palate occurring during the second month of intrauterine development because of improper union or lack of union of the maxillary process with the median nasal process. **2.** A cleft in the palate between the two palatal processes. If both hard and soft palates are involved, it is a *uranostaphyloschisis;* if only the soft palate is divided, it is a *uranoschisis.* The term *cleft palate* is often erroneously applied to clefts between the median nasal and maxillary processes through the alveolus. The proper term for this type of cleft is *cleft jaw,* or *gnathoschisis.*

  p., acquired cleft, a noncongenital defect of soft and/or hard tissues of the hard and soft palate.

  p., congenital cleft, a congenital nonunion or inadequacy of soft and hard tissues related to the lip, nose, alveolar process, hard palate, and velum. The extent of these deformities varies among individuals. Varieties of classifications are available to identify the extent of the cleft.

p., hard, the anterior part of the palate, which is supported by and includes the palatal extensions of the maxillary and palatine bones.

p., soft, the part of the palate lying posterior to the hard palate, composed of only soft tissues without underlying bony support.

  p., soft, redivision, the surgical incision or removal of a V-shaped area of tissue from the soft palate to facilitate the proper placement of the pharyngeal section of a prosthetic speech aid.

p.-splitting appliance, an orthodontic appliance cemented to buccal teeth on either side, incorporating a jackscrew that is progressively extended to accomplish forceful separation of the two lateral halves of the bony palate.

Similar corrections also are accomplished with removable split-palate appliances.

palatine arch (pal'ətin). See **arch, palatine.**

palatine mucosa. See **mucosa, palatine.**

palatine suture, median. See **suture, intermaxillary.**

palato- (pal'ətō), a prefix meaning "pertaining to the palate."

palatoplasty (pal'ətōplas'tē), the surgical repair of palatal defects.

palatorrhaphy (pal'ətôr'əfē), the surgical closure of a cleft palate using suturing.

palatoschisis (pal'ətōs'kisis) (not current). See **palate, cleft.**

palladium (Pd), a hard, silvery metallic element that is highly resistant to tarnish and corrosion. Its atomic number is 46 and its atomic weight is 106.4. Palladium is used in high-grade surgical instruments and in dental inlays, bridgework, and orthodontic appliances.

palliate (pal'ē·āt), to reduce the severity of.

palliative (pal'ē·ətiv), an alleviating measure.

pallor (pal'ər), paleness; absence of skin coloration.

  p., perioral, paleness of soft tissues surrounding the mouth; an indication of impending syncope.

Palmer's tooth notation, a system for designating teeth by number and quadrant. The mouth is divided into quadrants and each tooth is numbered from 1 to 8, starting with the central incisor in each quadrant and continuing back to the third. The quadrant is indicated by a right angle symbol oriented right or left and up or down. The system was popular in the 1950s but is no longer in general use.

palpate (pal'pāt), to examine the soft tissues with the fingers or hands.

palpation (palpā'shən), **1.** the act of feeling with the hands or fingers. **2.** a phase of the examination procedure in which the sense of touch is used to gather data essential for diagnosis.

palpitation (palpitā'shən), unduly rapid action of the heart that is perceptible to the patient.

palsy (pôl'zē), a synonym for *paralysis* but preferred by some to refer to certain types of paralysis.

P

p., Bell's, facial paralysis believed to result from inflammation in or around the facial nerve. One side of the face sags, the corner of the mouth droops, the eyelid does not close, and saliva dribbles from the corner of the mouth on the affected side. See also **paralysis, facial.**

p., cerebral, **1.** collective term for neurologic defects with associated disturbances of motor function. The disturbances vary in cause and anatomic type (e.g., acquired, hereditary, natal, postnatal, congenital palsy). **2.** nonspecific term representing a group of pathologies having the following common, related characteristics: agenesis, or a lesion of nervous tissue within the cranium; interference with voluntary muscular movements; disabling disorders of a chronic nature, neither acute nor progressive; and occurrence of the original lesion at the date of birth of the patient or before the development of learned human muscular function. **3.** a condition caused by damage to the motor centers of the brain, resulting in varying disturbances of motor function and often accompanied by mental subnormality.

p., creeping. See **gait, spastic.**

p., facial, paralysis of the muscles supplied by the seventh cranial nerve. It may be associated with peripheral lesions, neoplasms invading the temporal bone, acoustic neuromas, pontine disease, and herpes zoster involving the geniculate ganglion. Bilateral paralysis may occur in uveoparotid fever and polyneuritis.

p., lead, weakness and paralysis of the hand, wrist, and fingers, associated with lead poisoning.

panel, open, a group dental plan characterized by three features: any licensed dentist may elect to participate, the beneficiary may choose from among all licensed dentists, and the dentist may accept or refuse any beneficiary.

pamplegia (pamplē′jē·ə), total paralysis. (not current)

pancreatin, a concentrate of pancreatic enzymes from swine or beef cattle.

pancreatitis, inflammation of the pancreas that may be acute or chronic, characterized by severe abdominal pain radiating to the back, fever, anorexia, nausea, and vomiting.

pancrelipase, *trade names:* Cotazym, Enzymase, Ilozyme, Protilase, Utrase MT, Viokase, Zymase, others; *class:* digestant; *action:* pancreatic enzyme needed for proper pancreatic secretion insufficiency; *uses:* cystic fibrosis (digestive aid), steatorrhea, pancreatic enzyme deficiency.

pancuronium bromide, a skeletal muscle relaxant prescribed as an adjunct to anesthesia and mechanical ventilation.

panesthesia (pan′esthē′zhə), the sum of the sensations experienced. (not current)

pangamic acid, substance that is a derivative of apricot pits and contains some potentially toxic substances. No evidence that this substance is a vitamin exists. Synonym: vitamin B_{15}.

panhypopituitarism (panhī′pōpitōō′ itəriz′əm), a deficiency involving all the hormonal functions of the pituitary gland. See also **disease, Simmonds'.**

panic attack, an episode of acute anxiety that occurs unpredictably with feelings of intense apprehension or terror, accompanied by dyspnea, dizziness, sweating, trembling, and chest pain or palpitations. The attack may last several minutes and may occur again in certain conditions.

panic disorder. See **panic attack.**

panneuritis endemica (pan′nyərī′tis endem′ikə). See **beriberi.**

panoral, literally, "all of the oral region," a term used in diagnostic oral radiography to describe a technique that includes all of the oral structures on one film.

panoramic radiograph, a tomogram of the jaws, taken with a specialized machine designed to present a panoramic view of the full circumferential length of the jaws on a single film. Also known by several trade names of machines, most of which incorporate *pan* into the name.

Panoramix, a radiographic system in which the source of radiation is placed inside the mouth to expose a large film placed extraorally around the face.

Panorex, a radiographic system (manufactured by S.S. White Co.) that uses two axes of rotation to obtain a panoramic radiograph of the dental arches and associated structures. See also **pantomography.**

pansinusitis (pan'sīnusī'tis), inflammation of all the sinuses, as of the facial bones.

pantograph (pan'tōgraf), a figurative term given to a pair of face-bows fixed to both jaws and designed to inscribe centrically related points and then arcs leading to these points on segments of planes relatable to the three craniofacial planes of space. The maxillary planes are attached to the maxillary bow, and the inscribing styluses are attached to the mandibular bow.

pantomography (pantəmog'rəfē), panoramic radiography for obtaining radiographs of the maxillary and mandibular dental arches and their associated structures.

pantothenic acid (pantəthēn'ik), fatty acids. See also **acid, pantothenic.**

papain, an enzyme from papaya, a tropical fruit; used for enzymatic debridement of wounds and for promotion of healing.

papaverine HCl, *trade names:* Cerespan, Genabid, Pavabid, Pavacot, Pavagen, Pavased, others; *class:* peripheral vasodilator; *action:* relaxes all smooth muscle, inhibits cyclic nucleotide phosphodiesterase, which increases intracellular cAMP, causing vasodilation; *uses:* arterial spasm resulting in cerebral and peripheral ischemia; myocardial ischemia associated with vascular spasms or dysrhythmias, angina pectoris, peripheral and pulmonary embolism; visceral spasm, as in ureteral, biliary, GI colic.

paper, articulating, paper strips coated with ink or dye-containing wax, used for marking or locating occlusal interferences or deflecting occlusal contacts prior to making occlusal contacts. See also **articulating paper.**

paper point, a cone of absorbent paper designed to be inserted into the length of the root canal and used to absorb fluid, carry medication into the canal, or inoculate cultures.

papilla(e) (pəpil'ə), any small, nipple-shaped elevation.

p., incisive, the elevation of soft tissue covering the foramen of the incisive or nasopalatine canal.

p., interdental, the part of the gingivae filling the interproximal spaces between adjacent teeth, consisting of both free and attached gingivae.

p., interproximal, the cone-shaped projection of the gingiva filling the interdental spaces up to the contact areas when viewed from the labial, buccal, and lingual aspects. When viewed buccolingually or labiolingually, the crest of the interproximal papilla appears as a rounded concavity at an area below the contact point of the teeth. If recession has occurred, this concavity may become an area of pathology, and the entire papilla may require reshaping to restore health. See also **papilla, interdental.**

p., palatine, a convexly rounded and elliptically shaped pad of soft tissue lying palatal to the upper central incisors.

papillary adenoma (pap'əlerē), a benign epithelial tumor in which the membrane lining the glandular tissue forms papillary processes that project into the alveoli or grow out of the surface of a cavity.

papillary-marginal-attached. See **PMA.**

papilledema (pap'ilədē'mə), swelling of the optic disc caused by increased intracranial pressure.

papilloma (pap'ilō'mə), **1.** a benign neoplasm of epithelium, often having a warty appearance. **2.** a benign, exophytic, pedunculated, cauliflowerlike neoplasm of epithelium.

p., basal cell. See **keratosis, seborrheic.**

papillomatosis, inflammatory (pap'ilōmətō'sis), See **hyperplasia, papillary, inflammatory.**

papillomatosis, multiple. See **hyperplasia, papillary, inflammatory.**

Papillon-Lefèvre syndrome (pap'iyōn lefa'). See **syndrome, Papillon-Lefèvre.**

papule (pap'yōol), a small, circumscribed, solid elevation of the skin.

p., split, a secondary lesion of syphilis seen at the angle of the lips, resulting from the formation of a papule that becomes fissured because of its position.

paradontosis (per'ədontō'sis), See **periodontosis.**

paraffin, any of a group of hydrocarbons or hydrocarbon mixtures of the paraffin series as indicated by the formula $C_{11}H_{(2n+2)}$. Examples include methane gas, kerosene, and paraffin wax.

paraffin bath, the application of heat to a specific area of the body through the use of paraffin wax. The area is quickly immersed in heated liquid wax and then withdrawn so that the wax solidifies to form an insulating layer. The procedure is repeated until the layer is 5 to 10 mm thick, and then the entire area is wrapped in an insulating fabric. The technique is used primarily for patients with arthritis and rheumatism or any joint condition.

paraffin method, a method used in preparing a selected portion of tissue for pathologic examination. The tissue is fixed, dehydrated, and infiltrated by and embedded in paraffin wax, forming a block that is cut with a microtome into slices 8 μm thick.

parafunction, movements (e.g., bruxism, clenching, and rocking of teeth) that are considered outside or beyond function and that result in worn facets.

parahemophilia (per′əhē′mōfēl′ē·ə) (Ac globulin deficiency, hemophilioid state A, Owren's disease), a hemorrhagic disorder resulting from a deficiency of proaccelerin. Manifestations include mild to severe bleeding after extraction of teeth or other surgical procedures, epistaxis, easy bruising, monorrhagia, and hematomas. The one-stage prothrombin time is prolonged, but the bleeding time is ordinarily normal.

parainfluenza virus, a myxovirus with four serotypes, causing respiratory infections in infants and young children and, less commonly, in adults.

parakeratosis (per′əkerətō′sis), persistence of nuclei in the stratum corneum of stratified squamous epithelium.

paralgesia (per′əljē′zē·ə) (paralgia), **1.** any condition marked by abnormal and painful sensations. **2.** a painful paresthesia. (not current)

paralgia (peral′jē·ə). See **paralgesia.** (not current)

parallax (per′əlaks), the apparent change in position of an object when viewed from two different positions. The phenomenon is useful in deter-

mining the relative position of an object in a radiograph. Two or more radiographs are made from slightly different positions and the direction and amount of shift of the object is observed and measured.

parallel attachment. See **attachment, parallel.**

parallelism, the condition of two or more surfaces that, if extended to infinity, could never meet. In removable partial prosthodontics, such a condition is created on vertical tooth surfaces to act as guiding planes.

parallelometer (per′əlelom′eter), an apparatus used to determine parallelism or a lack of parallelism or to make a part or an object parallel with some other part or object. See also **surveyor.**

paralysis (pəral′isis), **1.** cessation of cell function. **2.** loss or impairment of the motor control or function of a part or region.

p., facial, paralysis of the muscles of facial expression resulting from supranuclear, nuclear, or peripheral nerve disease. With a mild case, when the face is at rest, the disorder is not readily observed. However, during muscular contraction (e.g., wrinkling the forehead, blinking the eyes, pursing the lips, speaking), the disorder is very noticeable. Only one lid may close, and the asymmetry of the mouth is pronounced, because the normal buccinator muscle contracts and is unopposed by the weakness on the paralyzed side. This imbalance produces a significant asymmetry. The affected side remains smooth, and the normal side shows contraction. See also **palsy, Bell's.**

p., infantile. See **poliomyelitis.**

p., motor, a loss of the power of skeletal muscle contraction, resulting from interruption of some part of the pathway from the cerebrum to the muscle.

parameter (pəram′əter), values that refer to a population; characteristics of a population. Because a parameter is a value of a hypothetical, infinite, unknown population, it is always an estimate.

paramolar, a supernumerary tooth located buccal, lingual, or distal to a normal molar. (not current)

P

paranasal sinuses, the air cavities in various bones around the nose, such as the frontal sinus in the frontal bone and the maxillary sinus within the maxilla.

paranesthesia (per'anesthē'zē·ə), anesthesia of the lower part of the body and limbs.

paranoia (per'ənoi'ə), **1.** psychosis characterized by delusions and hallucinations that are well systematized. **2.** the irrational belief that one is the object of special persecution by others or by fate.

paraplegia, paralysis characterized by motor or sensory loss in the lower limbs and trunk. Approximately 11,000 spinal cord injuries reported each year in the United States involve paraplegia. Such events occur as a result of automobile and motorcycle accidents, sporting accidents, falls, and gunshot wounds.

parapsoriasis, a group of chronic skin diseases resembling psoriasis, characterized by maculopapular, erythematous, scaly eruptions without systemic symptoms. Parapsoriasis is resistant to all treatment.

parasite, an organism living in or on and obtaining nourishment from another organism.

parasympatholytic (per'əsim' pathōlit'ik). See **anticholinergic.**

parasympathomimetic (per'əsim' pathō'mimet'ik). See **cholinergic.**

Para-thor-mone (per'əthōr'mōn), trade name for parathyroid hormone.

Parathyrin (per'əthī'rin), trade name for parathyroid hormone.

parathyroidectomy, the surgical removal of the parathyroid gland.

parenteral (pəren'terəl), literally, "aside from the gastrointestinal tract"; not through the alimentary canal (i.e., by subcutaneous, intramuscular, intravenous, or other nongastrointestinal route of administration).

p. nutrition, the administration of nutrients by a route other than the alimentary canal, such as subcutaneously, intravenously, intramuscularly, or intradermally. The parenteral fluid usually consists of physiologic saline with glucose, amino acids, electrolytes, vitamins, and medications, which are not nutritionally complete but maintain fluid and electrolyte balance.

paresis (pərī'sis) (dementia paralytica, paretic neurosyphilis), a progressive psychosis associated with neurosyphilis.

paresthesia (per'esthē'zhə), an altered sensation reported by the patient in an area where the sensory nerve has been afflicted by a disease or an injury. The patient may report burning, prickling, formication, or other sensations.

parietal bone, one of a pair of bones forming the sides of the cranium. Each parietal bone articulates with five bones: the opposite parietal, occipital, frontal, temporal, and sphenoid.

parity, the use of a set of items, either even or odd in number, as a means for checking computer errors, such as in the transmission of information between various elements of the same computer.

paronychia, an infection of the fold of skin at the margin of a fingernail or toenail.

parotid gland (pərot'id), one of the largest pairs of salivary glands that lie at the side of the face just below and in front of the external ear along the posterior border of the ramus of the mandible.

parotitis (per'əti'tis), inflammation of the parotid gland. See also **mumps.**

p., endemic (epidemic parotitis, infectious parotitis, mumps), an acute viral infection characterized by unilateral or bilateral swelling of the salivary glands, especially the parotid.

p., epidemic. See **parotitis, endemic.**

p., infectious. See **parotitis, endemic.**

paroxetine, *trade name:* Paxil; *class:* antidepressant; *action:* selectively inhibits the uptake of serotonin in the brain; *use:* depression.

paroxysmal (per'əksiz'məl), recurring in paroxysms.

Parry's disease. See **goiter, exophthalmic; hyperthyroidism.** (not current)

partial anodontia. See **oligodontia.**

partial denture retention. See **retention, denture, partial.** (not current)

partial thromboplastin time (PTT), a test for detecting coagulation defects of the intrinsic system by adding activated partial thromboplastin to a sample of test plasma and to a control sample of normal plasma. The time required for the formation of a clot is compared with the normal plasma. It is also used to monitor the activity of heparin in patients who are being treated for a variety of cardiovascular disorders.

participating dentist, any dentist who has a contractual agreement with a dental benefits organization to render care to eligible persons.

particle, a small amount of material.

p., alpha (alpha ray, alpha radiation), positively charged particulate ionizing radiation consisting of helium nuclei (two protons and two neutrons) traveling at high speeds. These rays are emitted from the nucleus of an unstable element.

p., beta (beta ray, beta radiation), particulate ionizing radiation consisting of either negative electrons (negatrons) or positive electrons (positrons) emitted from the nucleus of an unstable element. This phenomenon is called *beta decay.*

particulate bone grafts (better known as *particulate bone and cancellous marrow grafts [PBCM]*), a type of autogenous bone graft that consists of small particles of cortical and cancellous bone and hematopoietic and mesenchymal marrow.

parties, the persons who take part in the performance of any act, who have a direct interest in any contract or conveyance, or who are actively involved in the prosecution and defense of any legal proceeding.

partnership, 1. The association of two or more persons for the purpose of carrying on business (or practice) together and dividing its profits. **2.** a legal, binding contract defining the association of two or more persons in a business or professional relationship such as a dental practice.

p., notice of dissolution of intelligence, by any of a variety of means, notice to creditors and the public that a partnership has been dissolved.

Partsch's operation. See **operation, Partsch's.**

parulis (pərōō′lĭs) (gumboil), an elevated nodule at the site of a fistula draining a chronic periapical abscess. These nodules occur most frequently in relation to pulpally involved deciduous teeth. (not current)

Pascal's law. See **law, Pascal's.** (not current)

Passavant's bar. See **pad, Passavant's.** (not current)

Passavant's pad. See **pad, Passavant's.** (not current)

Passavant's ridge. See **pad, Passavant's.** (not current)

passer, foil. See **foil passer.** (not current)

passive, referring to an orthodontic appliance that has been adjusted to apply no effective tooth-moving force to the teeth.

p.-aggressive behavior, behavior that reflects hostility or resentment through indirect nonviolent means, such as procrastination, inefficiency, forgetfulness, and stubbornness.

p.-dependent personality, a personality characterized by helplessness, indecisiveness, and a tendency to cling to and seek support from others.

p. immunity, a form of acquired immunity resulting from antibodies that are transmitted naturally through the placenta to a fetus or through the colostrum to an infant or artificially by injection of antiserum for treatment or prophylaxis. Passive immunity is not permanent and does not last as long as active immunity.

p. reciprocation. See **reciprocation, passive.**

p. smoking, the inhalation by nonsmokers of the smoke from other people's cigarettes, pipes, and cigars.

passivity, the quality or condition of inactivity or rest assumed by the teeth, tissues, and denture when a removable denture is in place but is not under masticatory pressure.

paste, a soft, smooth, semifluid mixture, often medicated.

p. filler, a semisoft mixture of materials used to fill the root canal system, unlike solid filling material such as silver or gutta-percha cones.

p., pressure-indicating, a soft mixture used to disclose areas of contact or pressure in restorations.

Pasteurella, a genus of gram-negative bacilli or coccobacilli, including species pathogenic to humans and domestic animals. *Pasteurella* infections may be transmitted to humans by animal bites.

patch, mucous, multiple gray-white patch overlying an area of ulceration and occurring on the oral mucosa as an expression of secondary syphilis; highly infectious. See also **syphilis.**

patch test, a skin test for identifying allergens, especially those causing contact dermatitis.

patent, open and unblocked, such as a *patent airway.*

patent medicine, a nonprescription drug available to the general public; usually referred to as an *over-the-counter medicine.* (not current)

paternity test, a test based on genetic blood groups and used mainly to exclude the possibility that a particular man could be the father of a specific child.

path, a certain course that is usually followed.

p. of appliance insertion and removal. See **Insertion, path of.**

p. of closure. See **closure, centric path of.**

p., condyle. See **condyle path.**

p., idling, the path that a stamp cusp travels when the bolus is being treated on the other side of the mouth.

p. of insertion. See **insertion, path of.**

p., generated occlusal, a registration in the mouth of the paths of movement of the occlusal surfaces of teeth on a wax, plastic, or abrasive surface attached to the opposing dental arch.

p., lateral. See **condyle path, lateral.**

p., milled-in, any one of the contours carved by various mandibular movements into the occluding surface of an occlusion rim by teeth or studs placed in the opposing occlusion rim. The curves or contours may be carved into wax, acrylic resin, modeling compound, or plaster of paris.

p., occlusal, I. a gliding occlusal contact. 2. the path of movement of an occlusal surface.

p. of placement, the direction in which a removable dental restoration is positioned in relation to the planned location on its supporting structures. The restoration is removed in the opposite direction. See also **placement, choice of path of.**

p., working, the path that the stamp cusps make when working on the bolus. At first the bolus deflects the direction of these cusps, but after the fibers of the food have been reduced enough to be almost ready for swallowing, the travel coincides directionally with the working groove.

pathfinder. See **broach, smooth.**

pathogenic occlusion (path'əjen'ik). See **occlusion, pathogenic.**

pathognomonic (pəthog'nəmon'ik), a sign or symptom unique to a disease; one that distinguishes it from other diseases.

pathology (pəthol'əjē) I. the branch of science that deals with disease in all its relations, especially with its nature and the functional and material changes it causes. 2. in medical jurisprudence, the science of disease; the part of medicine that deals with the nature of disease, its causes, and its symptoms.

p., experimental, the study of disease processes induced usually in animals; undertaken to ascertain the effect of local environmental changes and/or systemic disorders on particular tissues, parts, and organs of the body. This branch of medical science also attempts to correlate the interaction of local and systemic factors in the production, modification, and continuance of a disease.

p., oral, the study of the characteristics, causes, and effects of diseases of the mouth, oral cavity, and associated structures.

p., speech, the study and treatment of all aspects of functional and organic speech defects and disorders.

p., surgical, the study of the characteristics of diseased tissues and organs removed in the process of surgery.

pathosis (pəthō'sis), I. a disease entity. 2. a pathologic condition. A patient is said to have a *pathosis* rather than *pathology,* which is the study of disease.

pathway of inflammation, the route of extension of chronic gingival inflammation into the subjacent structures, extending into the interdental septum from the gingivae, along the interdental vessels, and/or following the course of these blood vessels onto the periosteal side of the bone as well as into the bone marrow spaces. (not current)

patient, a person under medical or dental care.

p. admission, the formal acceptance of a patient for care into a clinic, hospital, or extended care facility.

P

p. compliance, the degree or extent to which a patient follows or completes a prescribed diagnostic, treatment, or preventive procedure.

p. education, the process of informing a patient about a health matter to secure informed consent, patient cooperation, and a high level of patient compliance.

p. load, the number of patients treated by a dentist or a group of dentists within a specified period of time.

p. satisfaction, as an outcome measure of quality, refers to the perception of the patients(s) of one or more aspects of a dental care system.

p. transfer, to convey the responsibility for the care of a patient from one entity to another. It may involve the discharge from one entity and the admission to another along with the patient's medical/dental records or copies.

Patient's Bill of Rights, a list of the patient's rights promulgated by the American Hospital Association. It offers some guidance and protection to patients by stating the responsibilities that a hospital and its staff have toward patients and their families during hospitalization, but it is not a legally binding document.

pattern, a form used to make a mold, such as for a denture, an inlay, or a partial denture framework.

p., occlusal, the form or design of the occluding surfaces of a tooth or teeth. These forms may be based on natural or modified anatomic or nonanatomic concepts of teeth.

p., trabecular, the trabecular arrangement of alveolar bone in relation to marrow spaces; may be radiographically interpreted.

p., wax, **1.** a wax model for making the mold in which the metal will be formed in casting. **2.** a wax form of a denture that, when it is invested in a flask and the wax is eliminated, will form the mold in which the resin denture is formed.

p., wear, the topographic attributes and distribution of areas of tooth wear (facets) resulting from attrition by food, tooth contacts during swallowing, terminal aspects of the masticatory cycle, and habits of occlusal neuroses. Wear patterns may be used to determine many of the functional and afunctional movements the mandible has been passing through in preceding years. Occlusal wear occurs with aging. The type of wear is termed the *wear pattern.*

Paul-Bunnell test. See **test, Paul-Bunnell.**

pauperissimus (paperis'əməs), **(Pp),** Latin term meaning "poorest," sometimes written on prescriptions to indicate to the pharmacist that the patient is being charged less than the usual fee by the dentist or physician. (not current)

payable, pertaining to an obligation to pay at a future time. When used without restriction or modification, the term means that the debt is payable at once.

payback period, the length of time required for the net revenues of an investment to return the cost of the investment.

payer, in health care, generally refers to entities other than the patient that finance or reimburse the cost of health services. In most cases, this term refers to insurance carriers, other third-party payers and/or health plan sponsors (employers or unions).

payment, the performance of a duty or promise; the discharge of a debt or liability by the delivery of money or something else of value.

p., progress, interim payments by the purchaser of a dental plan contract to the carrier for use as an operating fund. A final accounting is always completed when actual costs are paid.

payroll record, a printed form on which detailed records are kept of the amounts of money paid to auxiliaries. The record has columns for all the necessary tax deductions so that a detailed record is available for tax reporting and cost accounting.

PBI. See **iodine, protein-bound.**

p.c. (post cibum), Latin term meaning "after meals." The abbreviation may be used in writing prescriptions.

PCP, an abbreviation for *Pneumocystis carinii pneumonia,* an opportunistic infection associated with AIDS and used as an indicator of AIDS.

PDL. See **ligament, periodontal.**

PDS. See **temporomandibular pain-dysfunction syndrome.**

peak, buccal, outer high point of the normal interproximal tissue that rises to a peak; connected interdentally to a lingual peak by a triangular ridge, with a depression termed a *col.* (not current)

pearl, enamel (enameloma), a small focal mass of enamel formed apical to the cementoenamel junction and resembling pearls. The bifurcation of molar roots is a favorite site for this aberration in tooth development. (not current)

pearls, Epstein's. See **nodules, Bohn's.**

pediatric dentistry. See **pedodontics.**

pediatrics, a branch of medicine concerned with the development and care of children. Its specialties are the particular diseases of children and their treatment and prevention.

pedicle flap. See **flap, pedicle.**

pedigree, a line of descent; ancestry.

pedodontics (pē'dədon'tiks) (dentistry for children), the branch of dentistry that includes the following: training the child to accept dentistry; restoring and maintaining the primary, mixed, and permanent dentitions; applying preventive measures for dental caries and periodontal disease; and preventing, intercepting, and correcting various problems of occlusion.

peer review, 1. a retrospective consideration or an examination by one or more individuals of equal standing or rank. **2.** a process established to provide for review by licensed dentists of the care by a dentist for a single patient; disputes regarding fees; cases submitted by carriers and initiated by patients or dentists; and quality of care and appropriateness of treatment.

p. r. organization (PRO), an organization established by an amendment of the Tax Equity and Fiscal Responsibility Act of 1982 (TEFRA) to provide for the review of medical services furnished primarily in a hospital setting and/or in conjunction with care provided under the Medicare and Medicaid programs. In addition to their review and monitoring functions, these entities can invoke sanctions, penalties, or other corrective actions for noncompliance in organization standards.

p. r. system, a professionally sponsored and operated system for the rendering of professional judgment on disagreements between or among dentists, patients, or fiscal intermediaries, respecting quality of care and related matters.

pegs, epithelial (rete pegs), papillary projections of epithelium into the underlying stroma of connecting tissue that normally occur in mucous membrane and dermal tissues subject to functional stimulation. They occur to an excess where epithelium-lined tissues are irritated and inflamed.

pegs, rete. See **pegs, epithelial.** (not current)

pellagra (pəlā'grə, pəla'grə), a nutritional deficiency resulting from faulty intake or metabolism of nicotinic acid, a vitamin B complex factor. It is characterized by glossitis, dermatitis of sun-exposed surfaces, stomatitis, diarrhea, and dementia. Thiamine, riboflavin, and tryptophan deficiencies may be associated.

pellet, a small, rounded mass of material.

p., cotton, a rolled ball of cotton varying in diameter from approximately ⅜ inch to ⅛ inch. (The larger size is a cotton ball; the smaller size is a pledget.)

p., foil, a loosely rolled piece of gold foil of various thicknesses; prepared from a portion—$\frac{1}{128}$, $\frac{1}{96}$, $\frac{1}{64}$, $\frac{1}{48}$, $\frac{1}{32}$, $\frac{1}{16}$—cut from a 4-inch (10-cm) square of foil.

pellicle (pel'ikəl), a film or membrane.

p., brown, a specific name for a brownish-gray to black film formed over a period of time on the surfaces of the teeth of 20% to 25% of the population as a result of not using an abrasive-containing dentifrice.

pelvis, the lower portion of the trunk of the body, composed of four bones, the two innominate bones laterally and ventrally and the sacrum and coccyx posteriorly.

pemoline, *trade name:* Cylert; *class:* CNS stimulant Controlled Substance Schedule IV; *action:* exact mechanism unknown; may act through dopaminergic mechanisms; *use:* attention deficit disorder with hyperactivity.

pemphigoid, benign mucous membrane (pem'figoid), a bullous disease that resembles pemphigus but is more chronic in nature. The oral mucosa, especially the gingiva where it

P

resembles desquamative gingivitis, and conjunctiva are the sites of predilection. Skin is involved in about 20% of the cases.

pemphigus (pem´figus, pemfi´gəs), a rare, grave skin disease of unknown etiology characterized by the development of bullae on the skin and mucous membrane. See also **bulla** and **sign, Nikolsky's.**

p., acute disseminated, a dread disease of unknown etiology, temporarily controlled by the administration of corticosteroids. Manifested by bullous formation on the skin and mucous membranes. Desquamation of the epithelium exposes a raw, burning, oozing submucosa. Adequate nutritional status is difficult to maintain; secondary infection is common; with progressive debility, pneumonia is common and is usually the cause of death.

pen grasp. See **grasp, pen.**

penbutolol, *trade name:* Levatol; *class:* nonselective β-adrenergic blocker; *action:* competitively blocks stimulation of β-adrenergic receptors within the heart and decreases renin activity, all of which may play a role in reducing systolic and diastolic blood pressure; inhibits β_2 receptors in the bronchial system; *uses:* hypertension alone or with thiazide diuretics.

penetrability (pen´ətrəbil´itē), the ability of a beam of x-radiation to pass through matter. The degree of penetrability is determined by kilovoltage and filtration.

penetrating (pen´ətrāting), piercing; entering deeply.

penetration (pen´ətrā´shən), the ability of radiation to extend down into and go through substances. The degree of penetration is determined by the kilovoltage.

penetrometer (pen´ətrom´əter), an aluminum step wedge or ladder exposed over a film to determine the quality or penetrating ability of a specific beam of x-radiation.

penicillin (pen´isil´in), an antibiotic secured from cultures of *Penicillium notatum,* being bactericidal for gram-positive cocci, some gram-negative cocci (gonococcus and meningococcus), and clostridial and spirochetal organisms. Its topical application to the oral mucous membranes is dis-

couraged because of the high risk of sensitization from local application of antibiotic substances.

p. G, an acid-sensitive form of penicillin prepared as penicillin G benzathine and penicillin G procaine used for deep intramuscular administration. The penicillin is slowly released, resulting in prolonged effective blood levels of penicillin G. In dentistry, it is used prophylactically for patients predisposed to bacterial endocarditis prior to any invasive dental procedure. See also **penicillin G benzathine.**

p. G benzathine, trade names: Bicillin L-A, Permapen; *class:* benzathine salt of natural penicillin; *action:* interferes with cell wall replication of susceptible organisms; osmotically unstable cell wall swells and burst from osmotic pressure; *uses:* respiratory infections, scarlet fever, erysipelas, otitis media, pneumonia, skin and soft tissue infections, and yaws.

p. V potassium/penicillin V, trade names: Beepen-K, Betapen-VK, V-Cillin K, Veetids, others; *class:* semisynthetic penicillin; *action:* interferes with cell wall replication of susceptible organisms; the cell wall, rendered osmotically unstable, swells and burst from osmotic pressure; *uses:* effective for gram-positive cocci and gram-negative bacilli.

pension plans, saving and investment programs designed to provide income at the time of retirement. These may be employer- or individual-based, in which portions of the funds may be protected from taxation at the time of earning but subject to taxation at the time of withdrawal.

pentaerythritol tetranitrate (pent´ ə·erith´ritōl), *trade names:* Duotrate, Pentylan, Peritrate, others; *class:* antianginal, organic nitrate; *action:* decreases preload, afterload, which is responsible for decreasing left ventricular end-diastolic pressure, systemic vascular resistance, arterial and venous dilation; *uses:* chronic stable angina pectoris, prophylaxis of angina pain.

pentamidine/pentamidine isethionate (pentam´idēn), *trade names:* NebuPent, Pentam 300, others; *class:* antiprotozoal; *action:* interferes with DNA/RNA synthesis in protozoa; *use:*

Pneumocystis carinii infections in immunocompromised patients.

pentazocine HCl/pentazocine lactate (pentaz'ōsēn), *trade names:* Talwin, Talwin NX; *class:* synthetic opioid/mixed agonist/antagonist, Controlled Substance Schedule IV; *action:* interacts with opioid receptors in the CNS to alter pain perception; *uses:* moderate-to-severe pain alone or in combination with aspirin or acetaminophen.

pentobarbital/pentobarbital sodium, *trade name:* Nembutal Sodium; *class:* sedative/hypnotic barbiturate, Controlled Substance Schedule II; *action:* depresses activity in brain cells, primarily in reticular activating system of brain stem; *uses:* insomnia, sedation, preoperative medication. Useful as a preoperative sedative in dentistry.

pentoxifylline, *trade name:* Trental; *class:* hemorrheologic agent; *action:* decreased blood viscosity, stimulates prostacyclin formation, increases blood flow by increasing flexibility of RBCs, decreased RBC hyperaggregation, reduces platelet aggregation, decreases fibrinogen concentration; *uses:* intermittent claudication related to chronic occlusive vascular disease.

penumbra, geometric (pənum'brə), partial or imperfect shadow about the umbra, or true shadow, of an object. In radiography, it is influenced by the size of the focal spot, focal-film distance, and object-film distance. See also **geometric unsharpness.**

peptic ulcer (pep'tik), a sharply circumscribed lesion of the mucous membrane of the stomach or small intestine or any part of the gastrointestinal system exposed to gastric acid and pepsin.

peptide, a compound of two or more amino acids in which the α-carboxyl group of one is united with the α-amino group of another, with the elimination of a molecule of water, creating a peptide bond—CO—NH—.

Peptostreptococcus, a genus of nonmotile, anaerobic, chemoorganotrophic bacteria found in the oral cavity and intestinal tracts of normal humans. They may be pathogenic and may be found in pyogenic infections, putrefactive war wounds, and appendicitis.

percentile, the number in a frequency distribution below which a certain percentage of fees will fall. For example, the 90th percentile is the number that divides the distribution of fees into the lower 90% and the upper 10%, or that fee level at which 90% of dentists charge that amount or less and 10% charge more.

perception, occlusal, the patient's cognizance of occlusal patterns and disharmonies, mediated by the proprioceptive sense of the nerve fibers of the periodontal membrane. (not current)

Percodan, brand name for oxycodone, a semisynthetic narcotic analgesic oxycodone. Percodan is a controlled substance.

percolation, extraction of the soluble parts of a drug by causing a liquid solvent to flow slowly through it.

percussion (perkush'ən), the act of striking an area, a structure, or an organ as an aid in diagnosing a diseased condition by the sensations reported by the patient and by the sounds heard by the examiner.

perforation, palatal (pur'fōrā'shən), a perforation that exists in the palatal area after the surgical repair of a cleft. (not current)

perforation, radicular, an artificial opening or hole made by boring or cutting through the lateral aspect of the root; also occurs as the result of internal or external resorption. (not current)

perforation, sublabial, a perforation existing in the upper labial sulcus after surgical repair of the area. The perforation communicates between the oral and nasal cavities. (not current)

performance, fulfillment of a promise, contract, or other obligation.

perfusion, a therapeutic measure whereby a drug intended for an isolated part of the body is introduced via the bloodstream.

periadenitis mucosa necrotica recurrens (per'ē-əden'itəs) (Mikulicz's aphthae, Mikulicz's ulcer, recurrent scarring aphthae, Sutton's disease), involvement of the oral mucosa with deep-seated aphthous-like ulcers that tend to heal with scars. It may be impossible to differentiate the disease from Behçet's syndrome in the absence of a diagnosis of cyclic neutropenia.

perialveolar wiring. (not current) See **wiring, perialveolar.**

periapex (per'ē·ā'peks), that area of tissue that immediately surrounds the root apex.

periapical (per'ē·ā'pikəl), enclosing or surrounding the apical area of a tooth root.

p. abscess, an acute or chronic inflammation of the periapical tissues characterized by a localized accumulation of pus at the apex of a tooth. It is generally a sequela of pulp death of the tooth.

p. granuloma, an accumulation of mononuclear inflammatory cells with an encircling aggregation of fibroblasts and collagen at the apex of the root of a tooth caused by chronic inflammation. Synonym: chronic apical periodontitis.

p. radiograph, a radiograph demonstrating tooth apices and surrounding structures in a particular intraoral area.

p. radiographic survey, a series of intraoral radiographs depicting periapical areas of interest. A complete mouth radiographic survey may consist of 17 or more intraoral radiographs that demonstrate all areas of the oral cavity.

p. tissue, tissue located at the root end of a tooth. Usually connective tissue forming an attachment between the root and the alveolar bone.

periauricular (per'ē·ôrik'yūler), surrounding the external ear.

pericarditis, an inflammation of the pericardium associated with trauma, malignant neoplastic disease, infection, uremia, myocardial infarction, collagen disease, or idiopathic causes.

pericardium, a fibroserous sac that surrounds the heart and the roots of the great vessels.

pericementitis (per'isē'mentī'tis). See **periodontitis.**

pericervical saucerization. (not current) See **saucerization, pericervical.**

pericoronitis (per'ēkôr'ənī'tis) (operculitis), inflammation of the operculum or tissue flap over a partially erupted tooth, particularly a third molar. Inflammation around a crown, particularly the inflammation of a partially erupted tooth.

periimplant space, the space between an implant and its investing tissues.

perinatal, related to the period of time surrounding the birth process.

perineum, the part of the body situated dorsal to the pubic arch and the arcuate ligments, ventral to the tip of the coccyx, and lateral to the inferior rami of the pubis and the ischium and sacrotuberous ligaments. The perineum supports and surrounds the distal portions of the urogenital and GI tracts of the body.

perineural fibroblastoma (per' ēnu'rəl) (not current). See **neurilemoma; neurofibroma.**

period, latent, the area of delay between the time of exposure of an organism to radiation and the manifestation of the changes produced by that radiation. This delay is dependent on many factors but particularly on the magnitude of the dose. The larger the dose, the earlier the appearance of the injury. In some instances the latent period for some effects may be as long as 25 years or more.

periodicity, events that tend to repeat at predictable intervals.

periodontal (per'ē·ōdon'təl), relating to the periodontium.

p. abscess, a localized area of acute or chronic inflammation found in the gingival corium, infrabony pockets, or periodontal membrane. If it is located at the apex of the tooth, it is known as a *periapical abscess.* If located between the apex and the alveolar crest, it is known as a *lateral abscess.*

p. atrophy. See **atrophy, periodontal.**

p. attachment loss, a reduction in the connective tissue attaching the root of the tooth to the alveolar bone, usually caused by persistent inflammation of the gingival and periodontal tissues.

p. disease, any of a group of inflammatory and infectious diseases affecting the gums and supporting tissues of the teeth.

p. dressing, a protective obtundent covering of the gum and periodontal tissues used after periodontal surgery.

p. index, a method for rating or ranking the severity of periodontal disease. An early index was the PMA, which ranked the number of papillary, marginal, and attached gingiva affected by gingivitis. A more contemporary index is the Russell Periodontal Index (PI), which is based upon a 0 to 8 score system: from negative to advanced destruction.

p. ligament, a system of collagenous connective tissue fibers that connect the root of a tooth to its alveolus. It contains blood vessels, lymph vessels, and nerves. The ligament consists of four groups of fibers: alveolar crestal, horizontal, oblique, and apical.

p. pack. See **pack, periodontal.**

p. pocket. See **pocket, periodontal.**

p. probe. See **probe, periodontal.**

p. prosthesis. See **prosthesis, periodontal.**

p. therapy. See **therapy, periodontal.**

p. treatment planning, the sequential arrangement of therapeutic procedures required to obtain a healthy gingival attachment and an intact, functioning attachment apparatus. Periodontal therapy cannot be performed on an empiric basis but relies on an integrated knowledge of the theory and practice of periodontology.

periodontia (per′ē·ōdon′shē·ə). See **periodontics.**

periodontics (per′ē·ōdon′tiks), the art and science of examination, diagnosis, and treatment of diseases affecting the periodontium; a study of the supporting structures of the teeth, including not only the normal anatomy and physiology of these structures but also the deviations from normal.

p., concept of cure in, the idea that a successful result in periodontal therapy consists of restoring any tooth or collection of teeth to functional capability, regardless of whether they are able to function alone or require stabilization to survive.

periodontitis (per′ē·ōdontī′tis) (periodontal inflammation). **1.** the alterations occurring in the periodontium with inflammation. Gingival changes are those of gingivitis, with the clinical signs associated with gingivitis. Periodontitis has histologic characteristics, such as ulceration of the sulcular epithelium, epithelial hyperplasia, proliferation of epithelial rete pegs into the gingival corium, apical mi-

gration of the epithelial attachment after lysis of the gingival fiber apparatus, cellular and exudative infiltrate into tissues, and increased capillarity. Resorption of bone in an apical direction results in the loss of attachment of the periodontal fibers to the bone. A transseptal band of reconstituted periodontal fibers walls off the gingival inflammation from the underlying bone. **2.** a chronic, progressive disease of the periodontium.

p., acute, a sharply localized, acute inflammatory process involving the interproximal and marginal areas of two or more adjacent teeth, characterized by severe pain, purulent exudate from edematous inflamed gingivae, general malaise, fever, and sequestration of the crestal aspects of the alveolar process.

p. in children. See **periodontitis, juvenile.**

p., chronic periapical, periapical inflammation characterized by dental granuloma formation.

p., juvenile, marginal periodontitis present in children or adolescents, with radiographic and clinical findings similar to those observed in the adult, including gingivitis, periodontal pocket formation, and bone resorption

p., marginal, the sequela to gingivitis in which the inflammatory process has spread apically to involve the alveolar process. It involves an inflammation of the marginal periodontium with resorption of the crest of alveolar bone. Apical migration of the epithelial attachment occurs with suprabony and/or infrabony pocket formation and cuplike resorptions and marginal translucence of the alveolar crest. In children the process may be more rapid and destructive than in adults.

periodontium (per′ē·odont′shē·əm), the tissues that invest (or help to invest) and support the teeth, e.g., the gingivae, cementum of the tooth, periodontal ligament, and alveolar and supporting bone.

periodontosis (per′ē·odontō′sis) (diffuse alveolar atrophy), a rare disease of young people (occurring primarily in women) that involves an idiopathic destruction of the periodontium.

perioral structures, the anatomic elements around the mouth, generally the lips and muscles of facial expression within the lips.

periorbital, surrounding the eyes. The periorbital soft tissues are easily contused and will produce marked inflammatory responses to trauma.

periosteal elevator (per'ē·ōs'tē·əl). See **elevator, periosteal.**

periosteum (per'ē·ōs'tē·əm), the layer of connective tissue that varies considerably in thickness in the different areas of bone. It is thick over the surfaces that do not serve as areas of muscle attachment, especially on surfaces that are covered only by skin and subcutaneous tissue. In these areas the periosteum connects loosely with the bone itself and is easily lifted from it. Muscles are attached to bones directly, or they end on the periosteum. When muscles or tendons are attached to the bone, connective tissue extends into the bone as Sharpey's fibers. In such areas a periosteum may be lacking. When muscles are attached to the periosteum and thus are indirectly attached to the bone, the periosteum is relatively thin but is strongly fixed to the bone. The periosteum consists of two layers: an outer layer, which is rich in blood vessels and nerves and shows a dense arrangement of collagenous fibers, and an inner layer, the cambium, in which the fibers are loosely arranged, the cells numerous, and the blood vessels relatively sparse. During active growth, this layer of osteoblasts covers the periosteal surface of the bone. In the quiescent state in the adult, the periosteum primarily provides support. However, the inner layer retains its osteogenetic potencies and in fractures is activated to form osteoblasts and new bone.

periostitis (per'ē·ostī'tis), an inflammation of the periosteum in which the membrane may become detached from the underlying bone, resulting from exudates produced by inflammation or infection.

peripheral circulation (perif'erəl). See **circulation, peripheral.**

peripheral nervous system, the motor and sensory nerves and ganglia outside of the brain and spinal cord.

periphery (perif'erē). See **border, denture.**

peritoneal cavity, the potential space between the parietal and the visceral layers of the peritoneum.

peritonitis, an inflammation of the peritoneum produced by bacteria or irritating substances introduced into the abdominal cavity by a penetrating wound or perforation of an organ in the GI tract or the reproductive tract. Peritonitis is caused most commonly by rupture of the vermiform appendix.

peritonsillar, surrounding the tonsils. Generally used in reference to the pharyngeal tonsils.

peritonsillar abscess, an infection of tissue between the tonsil and pharynx, usually after acute follicular tonsillitis.

perlèche (perlesh'), a general term applied to superficial fissures occurring at the angles of the mouth. Lesions may result from a variety of causes but most often can be related to deep labial commissures, with associated drooling, licking of the lips, unhygienic conditions, and the overgrowth of bacteria, yeast, or fungi. The term has also been applied to angular cheilosis resulting from riboflavin deficiency but not to the split papule of syphilis or to herpetic lesions.

permanent, of a lasting or durable nature (opposite of temporary).
p. dentition. See **dentition, permanent.**

permeability, the degree to which one substance allows another substance to pass through it.

permissible dose. See **dose, maximum permissible.**

peroral, through or about the mouth.

peroxidase horseradish, an enzyme used in immunohistochemistry to label the antigen-antibody complex.

peroxidases, hydrogen-peroxide–reducing enzymes, occurring in animal and plant tissues, that catalyze the dehydrogenation (oxidation) of various substances in the presence of hydrogen peroxide.

peroxide. See **hydrogen peroxide.**

perphenazine, *trade name:* Trilafon; *class:* phenothiazine antipsychotic; *action:* blocks neurotransmission at dopaminergic synapses in the cerebral cortex, hypothalamus, and limbic system; mechanism for antipsychotic effects unclear; *uses:* psychotic disorders, schizophrenia, alcoholism, nausea, vomiting.

personal, belonging to an individual; limited to the person; having the nature of the qualities of human beings or of movable property.

personality, 1. the sum total of a patient's ideas, emotions, and behavior, including the rational and irrational, the conscious and unconscious, and the defensive and learned behavior patterns. Personality develops from both genetic factors and environmental factors. Thus the patient brings to a dental office an individual personality syndrome. It may be a well-adjusted, stable personality; a depressed, anxious, neurotic personality; or a manic, schizophrenic, psychotic personality. Patients have a broad spectrum of healthy and disordered personalities. **2.** the characteristics of a person by which other people evaluate him or her.

p. assessment. See **personality test.**

p. disorder, a disruption in relatedness manifested in any of a large group of mental disorders characterized by rigid, inflexible, and maladaptive behavior patterns that impair a person's ability to function in society.

p. test, any of a variety of standardized tests used in the evaluation of various facets of personality structure, emotional status, and behavioral traits.

personnel, the sum of persons employed in an enterprise. In dentistry it refers to the staff employed by the dentist.

p. monitoring. See **monitoring, personnel.**

pesticide poisoning, a toxic condition caused by the ingestion or inhalation of a substance used for the eradication of insects, fungi, and other pests.

petazocine, an analgesic approximately equivalent in analgesic effect to codeine; brand name: Talwin. (not current)

petechiae (pētē'kē-ē), capillary hemorrhages producing small red or purplish pinhead-sized discolorations of the mucous membrane and skin. Petechiae are typical of blood dyscrasias, vitamin C deficiency, positive Rumpel-Leede test, liver disease, and subacute bacterial endocarditis.

petrolatum (pet'rəlātəm) (petroleum jelly), a mixture of hydrocarbons obtained from petroleum. In its semisolid form it is used as a protective covering to prevent gingival dehydration and inflammation during mouth breathing. Other uses include a lubricant and a protective covering for burns.

Peutz-Jeghers syndrome (poits'jeg' ərz). See **syndrome, Peutz-Jeghers.**

pH, the concentration of hydrogen ions expressed as the negative logarithm of base 10.

phagocyte (fag'əsīt), any cell that ingests microorganisms, cells, or other substances.

phagocytosis (fag'əsītō'sis), the engulfing of microorganisms, cells, and other substances by phagocytes. See also **phagocyte.**

phantom (fan'təm), a device that absorbs and scatters x-radiation in approximately the same way as the tissues of the body.

pharmacist, a person prepared to formulate and dispense drugs or medications through completion of an accredited university program in pharmacy. Licensure is required upon completion of the program and prior to serving the public as a pharmacist.

pharmacodynamics (fär'məcōdīnam' iks), the science of drug action.

pharmacology (fär'məkol'əjē), the total science of drugs, including their use in therapeutics.

pharmacotherapy (fär'məkōther' ə-pē), treatment based upon the use of drugs or pharmaceuticals.

pharmacy (fär'məsē), **1.** the art and science of preparing and dispensing drugs. **2.** place where drugs are dispensed.

pharyngeal arch (ferin'jē-əl). See **arch, pharyngeal.**

pharyngeal flap, a pedicle flap usually raised on the posterior pharyngeal wall and attached to the soft palate to reduce the size of the velopharyngeal gap.

pharyngitis (fer'inji'tis), inflammation of the pharynx.

pharyngoplasty (fəring'gōplas'tē), reconstructive operation to alter the size and shape of the nasopharyngeal orifice.

pharyngospasm (fəring'ōspazəm), spasm of the pharyngeal muscles.

pharyngotomy, any cutting operation upon the pharynx, either from without or from within.

pharynx (fer'inks), a funnel-shaped tube of muscle tissue between the mouth and nares and the esophagus, which is the common pathway for food and air. The nasopharynx lies above the level of the soft palate. The oropharynx lies between the upper edge of the epiglottis and the soft palate, whereas the laryngopharynx extends from the upper edge of the epiglottis to the superior end of the esophagus behind the larynx.

p., activities of posterior and lateral pharyngeal wall, the bulging of the posterior and lateral pharyngeal wall produced by the superior pharyngeal constrictors and palatopharyngeus during the acts of swallowing and phonation; seen in individuals with a congenitally short soft palate, operated soft palate, or unoperated cleft of the soft palate. These activities are rarely present in the individual with the normal soft palate.

p., implant surgical, first stage: a major oral operation in which the mucoperiosteum is elevated, exposing the oral surface of the jawbone; the surgical jaw relations are established, and an impression is made of the exposed bone surfaces. Second stage: a major oral surgical operation in which the mucoperiosteum is reelevated, the prepared implant is placed on the bone surface, and the mucoperiosteum is coapted and sutured about the posts of the protruding implant abutments.

phase-contrast microscope, a microscope with a special condenser and objective, which contains a phase-shifting ring by which small differences in the index of refraction become visible. The use of phase-contrast capabilities allows for direct viewing of transparent live cells and tissues. Phase-contrast microscopes are useful in educating patients about the oral flora associated with dental plaque and caries and periodontal disease.

phenacetin, caffeine, aspirin (fə-nas'itin). See **aspirin, phenacetin, caffeine.**

phenazopyridine HCl, *trade names:* Azo-Standard, Baridium, Eridium, Pyridiate, Urogesic, others; *class:* urinary tract analgesic; *action:* exerts analgesic anesthetic action on the urinary tract mucosa; exact mechanism of action is unknown; *use:* urinary tract irritation/infection.

phendimetrazine tartrate, *trade names:* Adipost, Anorex SR, Appecon, Obalan, others; *class:* anorexiant, amphetaminelike Controlled Substance Schedule III; *action:* exact mechanism of action of appetite suppression is unknown but may have an effect on the satiety center of the hypothalamus; *use:* exogenous obesity.

phenelzine sulfate, *trade name:* Nardil; *class:* antidepressant, MAOI; *action:* increases concentrations of endogenuous epinephrine, norepinephrine, serotonin, dopamine in storage sites in CNS; *use:* depression when uncontrolled by other means.

phenobarbital/phenobarbital sodium, *trade names:* Ancalixor, Barbita, Luminal Sodium, Solfoton; *class:* barbiturate, anticonvulsant, Controlled Substance Schedule IV; *action:* a nonspecific depressant of the CNS; may enhance GABA activity in the brain; *uses:* all forms of epilepsy, status epilepticus, febrile seizures in children, sedation, insomnia.

phenol (fē'nol) (carbolic acid), an organic compound in which one or more hydroxyl groups are attached to a carbon atom in an aromatic ring that contains conjugated double bonds.

p. coefficient, a basis of comparison in determining the relative effectiveness of antiseptics. Phenol is the standard for comparison with other agents for their ability to kill a well-dispersed suspension of *Salmonella* or *Staphylococcus.* It has little practical value.

phenomenon, Hamburger (chloride shift), the exchange of a chloride ion for a bicarbonate ion across the erythrocyte membrane as part of the buffering system in blood. It accounts for the greater chloride content of venous erythrocytes than arterial erythrocytes. (not current)

phenotype (fē'nətīp), term referring to the expression of genotypes that can be directly distinguished (e.g., by clinical observation of external appearance or serologic tests).

phenoxybenzamine HCl, *trade name:* Dibenzyline; *class:* antihypertensive; *action:* α-adrenergic blocker that binds to α-adrenergic receptors, dilating peripheral blood vessels; lowers peripheral resistance, lowers blood pressure; *use:* hypertensive episodes associated with pheochromocytoma.

phenprocoumon, a long-acting, orally effective anticoagulant.

phensuximide, *trade name:* Milontin; *class:* anticonvulsant, succinimide; *action:* suppresses spike wave formation in absence seizures (petit mal); decreases amplitude, frequency, duration, spread of discharge in minor motor seizures; *use:* absence (petit mal) seizures.

phentermine HCl/phentermine resin, *trade name:* Adipex-P, Fastin, Ionamin, Obe-Mar, Panshape M, T-Diet, others; *class:* sympathomimetic, anorexiant, Controlled Substance Schedule IV; *action:* exact mechanism of action of appetite suppression unknown, but may have an effect on satiety center of hypothalamus; *use:* exogenous obesity.

phentolamine mesylate, *trade name:* Regitine; *class:* antihypertensive; *action:* α-adrenergic blocker; binds to α-adrenergic receptors, dilating peripheral blood vessels, lowering peripheral resistance, lowering blood pressure; *uses:* hypertension, pheochromocytoma, prevention and treatment of dermal necrosis following extravasation of norepinephrine or dopamine.

phenylalanine (fen'ilal'ǝnēn), one of the essential amino acids. See also **amino acid.**

phenylephrine HCl (fen'ilef'rin) (nasal), *trade names:* Neo-Synephrine, Vick's Sinex, others; *class:* nasal decongestant, sympathomimetic; *action:* produces rapid and long-acting vasoconstriction of arterioles; *use:* temporary relief of nasal congestion.

phenytoin sodium/phenytoin sodium extended/phenytoin sodium prompt, *trade names:* Dilantin, Diphenylan, Phenytex, others; *class:* hydantoin anticonvulsant; *action:* inhibits spread of seizure activity in motor cortex; *uses:* generalized tonic-clonic (grand mal) seizures, status epilepticus, nonepileptic seizures, trigeminal neuralgia, cardiac dysrhythmias caused by digitalis-type drugs.

pheochromocytoma, a vascular tumor of chromaffin tissue of the adrenal medulla or sympathetic paraganglia, characterized by hypersecretion of epinephrine and norepinephrine, causing persistent or intermittent hypertension.

phlebectasia (fleb'ektā'zē-ǝ), dilation of a vein.

phlebitis (flǝbī'tis), inflammation of a vein. See also **thrombophlebitis.**

phlebolith (fleb'ōlith), a calcified thrombus in a vein.

phlegmon (fleg'mon), **I.** an intense inflammation spreading through tissue spaces over a large area and without definite limits. **2.** clinically, a hard, boardlike swelling without gross pus. See also **cellulitis.**

phobia (fō'bē-ǝ), a specific hysterical fear.

phonation (fōnā'shǝn), the production of voiced sound by means of vocal cord vibrations.

p., speech, modification by the vocal folds of the airstream as it leaves the lungs and passes through the larynx, for the purpose of producing the various sounds that are the basis of speech. By opposing each other with different degrees of tension and space, the vocal folds create a slitlike aperture of varying size and contour; and by creating resistance to the stream of air, they set up a sequence of laryngeal sound waves with characteristic pitch and intensity.

phoneme (fo'nēm), a group or family of closely related speech sounds, all of which have the same distinctive acoustic characteristics despite their differences; often used in place of the term *speech sound.*

phonetic values. See **values, phonetic.**

phonetics (fōnet'iks), the study of the production and perception of speech sounds, including individual and group variations, and their use in speech.

phosphatase(s) (fos'fǝtāz), a group of enzymes that are distributed throughout most cells and body fluids and are characterized by their ability to hydrolyze a wide variety of monophosphate esters to alcohols and inorganic phosphate.

p., acid, a group of phosphatases (e.g., serum, liver, prostate) with optimal activity below a pH level of 7. Elevated serum levels have been observed in metastatic breast and prostatic cancer; Paget's, Gaucher's, and Niemann-Pick diseases; and myelocytic leukemia.

P

p., alkaline, a group of phosphatases (e.g., serum, liver, bone) whose optimal activity ranges near a pH level of 9.8. Elevated blood levels occur in Paget's disease and pregnancy, whereas low levels are characteristic of dwarfism and a generalized nutritional protein deficiency.

phosphates (fos'fāts), the organic compounds of phosphorus. The blood phosphate level is normally 2.5 mg to 5 mg/100 ml. It is low in rickets and early hyperparathyroidism and high in tetany and nephritis.

phosphorus (fos'fərəs), a nonmetallic element; atomic weight, 30.98. It is essential, as is the phosphate, for the mineralization of the organic matrix of teeth and bone. It is also essential in the intermediary metabolism of carbohydrates as a vital constituent of the various intermediary compounds (e.g., glucose 6-phosphate) and of the enzyme systems (e.g., adenosine triphosphate [ATP]).

phospholipase, an enzyme that catalyzes the hydrolysis of a phospholipid.

p. C, an enzyme removing choline phosphate from a phosphatidylcholine.

phospholipid, one of a class of compounds, widely distributed in living cells, containing phosphoric acid, fatty acids, and a nitrogenous base.

phosphoprotein, a protein containing phosphoric groups attached to the side chains of some of its amino acids, usually serine, casein, and vitellin.

phosphoric acid, a clear, colorless, odorless liquid that is irritating to the skin and eyes and moderately toxic, if ingested. It is used in the production of fertilizers, soaps, detergents, animal feeds, and certain drugs.

phosphorylation, the addition of phosphate to an organic compound.

phosphotungstic acid (PTA), a mixture of phosphoric and tungstic acids used with hematoxylin for staining muscle tissue and cell nuclei. It is also used as a negative stain of collagen in electron microscopy.

phossy jaw (fos'sē). See **poisoning, phosphorus.**

phosvitin, a phosphated protein with anticoagulant properties that is found in the egg yolk.

photogrammetry, the process of making maps or surveys by the use of photographs.

photography, the process of making images on a chemically sensitive plate or film, using the energy of light or other radiant source.

photometry, the measurement of the intensity of light, usually in footcandles.

photon (fō'ton), a bullet or quantum of electromagnetic radiant energy emitted and propagated from various types of radiation sources. The term should not be used alone but should be qualified by terms that will clarify the type of energy (e.g., light photon, x-ray photon).

phylogeny, the evolution or developmental history of a type of plant or animal.

physical, relating to the body, as distinguished from the mind.

p. examination, a diagnostic inspection of the body to determine its state of health, using palpation, auscultation, percussion, and smell.

p. fitness, the ability to carry out daily tasks with alertness and vigor, without undue fatigue, and with enough energy reserve to meet emergencies or to enjoy leisure time.

p. medicine, the use of physical therapy techniques to return physically diseased or injured patients to a useful life.

p. plant, the entire architectural and decorated suite of offices in which the dentist operates.

p. therapy, the treatment of disorders with physical agents and methods, such as massage, manipulation, therapeutic exercises, cold, heat (including shortwave, microwave, and ultrasonic diathermy), hydrotherapy, electric stimulation, and light to assist in rehabilitating patients and in restoring normal function after an illness or injury. Also called *physiotherapy.*

physician, a practitioner of medicine; one lawfully engaged in the practice of medicine.

physics, the study of material and energy, particularly as related to motion, force, heat, and light.

physiognomy, the face.

physiologic occlusion. See **occlusion, physiologic.**

physiologic rest position. See position, rest, physiologic.

physiology (fiz′ē·ol′əjē), study of tissue and organism behavior. The physiologic process is a dynamic state of tissue as compared with the static state of descriptive morphology (anatomy). Physiology is differentiated from descriptive morphology by the following qualifying properties: rate, direction, and magnitude. Physiologic processes are thus morphologic alterations in the three dimensions of space associated with a temporary (time) sequence. Physiologic processes relate to a wide spectrum of life activities on three levels: biochemical and biophysical activity of a subcellular nature, the activity of cells and tissues aggregated into organ systems, and multiorgan system activity as expressed in human behavior.

p., oral, physiology related to clinical manifestations in the normal and abnormal behavior of oral structures. The principal clinical functions in which the oral structures participate are deglutition, mastication, respiration, speech, and head posture.

physioprints (fiz′ē·ōprints), photographs obtained by projecting a grid on the subject's face and superimposing two exposures. The resultant picture gives a three-dimensional approach for the diagnosis of facial contours and swelling.

physiotherapy, oral (fiz′ē·ōther′əpē), the collective procedures properly performed for the maintenance of personal hygiene of the mouth; those procedures necessary for cleanliness, tissue stimulation, tone, and preservation of the dentition. See also **aid in physiotherapy.**

physostigmine, a cholinergic actylcholinesterase inhibitor prescribed in the treatment of some forms of glaucoma and to reverse effects of neuromuscular blocking agents.

phytonadione (vitamin K₁), *trade names:* AquaMEPHYTON, Konakion, Mephyton; *class:* vitamin K₁, fat-soluble vitamin; *action:* needed for adequate blood clotting (factors II, VII, IX, X); *uses:* vitamin K malabsorption, hypoprothrombinemia, prevention of hypoprothrombinemia caused by oral anticoagulants.

pickling, the process of cleansing from metallic surfaces the products of oxidation and other impurities by immersion in acid.

Pick's disease. See **disease, Niemann-Pick.**

pickup impression. See **impression, pickup.**

pier (pēr), an intermediate retaining or supporting abutment for a prosthesis. See also **abutment.**

Pierre Robin syndrome (pyerob′in). See **retrognathism** and **syndrome, Pierre Robin.**

pigmentation, gingival. See **gingival pigmentation.**

pigmentation, melanin, the discoloration of tissues produced by the deposition of melanin. Seen normally in the oral mucous membranes (especially gingivae) of dark-complexioned individuals and abnormally in such conditions as adrenal hypofunction (Addison's disease).

pilocarpine (pī′lōkär′pēn), an alkaloid that causes parasympathetic effects (e.g., secretion of salivary, bronchial, and gastrointestinal glands). It stimulates the sweat glands and also causes vasodilation and cardiac inhibition.

pilocarpine HCl/pilocarpine nitrate (optic) *trade names:* Adsorbocarpine, Akarpine, Isopto Carpine, Pilocar, Liquifilm, others; *class:* miotic, cholinergic agonist; *action:* acts directly on cholinergic receptor sites, induces miosis, spasm of accommodation, fall in intraocular pressure; *uses:* primary glaucoma, early stages of wide-angle glaucoma; also used to neutralize mydriatics used during eye examination.

pilocarpine HCl (oral), *trade name:* Salagen; *class:* cholinergic agonist; *action:* mimics the action of acetylcholine on muscarinic receptors; *uses:* treatment of symptoms of xerostomia from salivary gland hypofunction caused by radiotherapy for cancer of the head and neck.

pilot program, an experimental program designed to test administrative and operational procedures and to collect information on service demands and costs that will serve as a basis for operating programs efficiently.

pimozide, *trade name:* Orap; *class:* antipsychotic, antidyskinetic; *action:* blocks dopamine effects on CNS; *uses:* motor and phonic tics in Gilles de la Tourette's syndrome.

pin, a small cylindrical piece of metal.

p., cemented, a metal rod cemented into a hole drilled into dentin to enhance retention of a restoration.

p., friction-retained, a metal rod driven or forced into a hole drilled into dentin to enhance retention. It is retained solely by elasticity of dentin.

p., incisal guide, a metal rod that is attached to the upper member of an articulator and that touches the incisal guide table. It maintains the established vertical separation of the upper and lower arms of the articulator.

p., retention, the frictional grip of small metal projections extending from a metal casting into the dentin of the tooth.

p., self-threading, a pin screwed into a hole prepared in dentin to enhance retention.

p., sprue, **1.** a solid or hollow length of metal used to attach a pattern to the crucible former. **2.** a metal pin used to form the hole that provides the pathway through the refractory investment to permit the entry of metal into a mold.

p., Steinmann, a firm metal pin that is sharpened on one end; used for the fixation of fractures. It is sometimes passed through the maxilla or mandible to provide external points for attachment of upward-supporting devices.

pindolol, *trade name:* Visken; *class:* nonselective β-adrenergic blocker; *action:* competitively blocks stimulation of β-adrenergic receptors within the heart and decreases renin activity, both of which may play a role in reducing systolic and diastolic blood pressure; *use:* mild-to-moderate hypertension.

pinna, the external ear.

piperacillin sodium, a semisynthetic extended spectrum penicillin active against a wide variety of gram-positive and gram-negative bacteria.

pirbuterol acetate, *trade name:* Maxair; *class:* bronchodilator; *action:* causes bronchodilation with little effect on heart rate by acting on β-receptors, causing increased cAMP and relaxation of smooth muscle; *uses:* reversible bronchospasms (prevention, treatment), including asthma, may be given with theophylline or steroids.

piroxicam, *trade name:* Feldene; *class:* nonsteroidal antiinflammatory; *action:* inhibits prostaglandin synthesis by interfering with cyclooxygenase needed for biosynthesis; possesses analgesic, antiinflammatory, antipyretic properties; *uses:* osteoarthritis, rheumatoid arthritis.

pit, 1. a small depression in enamel, usually located in a developmental groove where two or more enamel lobes are joined. **2.** a depression in a restoration resulting from nonuniform density.

p. and fissure cavity. See **cavity, pit and fissure.**

p. and fissure sealant. See **sealant, pit and fissure.**

pituitary gland, an endocrine gland suspended beneath the brain in the pituitary fossa of the sphenoid bone. It produces a number of hormones essential for growth, metabolism, reproduction, and vascular control.

pituitary hormones, the hormones of the anterior lobe of the pituitary gland controlled by hypothalamic releasing factors; they include growth hormone (somatotropin) prolactin, thyroid-luteinizing hormone, adrenocorticotropic hormone, and melanocyte-stimulating hormone. The posterior lobe is the source of vasopressin, which inhibits diuresis and raises blood pressure, and oxytocin, which stimulates the contraction of smooth muscle, especially in the uterus.

Pituitrin (pitū′ətrin), trade name for an extract of the posterior lobe of the pituitary gland.

pityriasis rosea (pitəri′əsis ro′zē-ə), a noncontagious skin disease with reddish, scaly patches and moderate fever.

pivot, occlusal, an elevation artificially developed on the occlusal surface, usually in the molar region, and designed to induce sagittal mandibular rotation. (not current)

p., adjustable occlusal, an occlusal pivot that may be adjusted vertically by means of a screw or by other means.

placebo (pləsē′bō), a substance that resembles medicine superficially and is believed by the patient to be medicine but that has no intrinsic drug activity.

p. effect, the real or imagined effect of a placebo, which may actually be the same effect ordinarily associated with the administration of a therapeutically active agent.

placement, the act of placing an object (i.e., removable denture in its planned location on the dental arch).

p., choice of path of, determination of the direction of placement and removal of a removable partial denture on its supporting oral structures, which can be varied by altering the plane to which the guiding abutment surfaces are made parallel. The choice is a compromise to best fulfill five demands: to subject abutment teeth to a minimum or no torquing force, to encounter the least interference, to provide needed retention, to establish adequate guiding-plane surfaces, and to provide acceptable esthetics.

placenta, the organ of metabolic interchange between the fetus and the mother.

plagiarism, to appropriate the work, ideas, and/or words of another without proper acknowledgment.

plague, 1. any disease of wide prevalence or of excessive mortality. **2.** the vernacular term for bubonic plague, marked by inflammatory enlargement of the lymphatic glands, particularly in the axillae and groins.

plaintiff, the party who sues in a personal legal action and who is so designated on the record.

plan, bank, See **bank plan.**

plan, treatment, the intended sequence of procedures for the treatment of a patient.

p., provisional treatment, tentative treatment plan that may be modified or continued upon reevaluation of periodontal status after initial therapeutic procedures.

plane, an ideal flat surface that is supposed to intersect solid bodies, extend in various directions, or be determined by the position in space of three points.

p., axial, a hypothetical plane parallel to the long axis of an object.

p., axial, of teeth, term that applies to the mesiodistal or the buccolingual plane.

p., axial wall, an instrument used to plane and true the axial wall of a Class 3 preparation.

p., axiobuccolingual, of teeth. See **plane of teeth, buccolingual.**

p., axiomesiodistal, of teeth. See **plane of teeth, mesiodistal.**

p., bite (bite plate), an appliance that covers the palate. It has an inclined or flat plane at its anterior border, which offers resistance to the mandibular incisors when they come into contact with it.

p., Broca's (Brōkəz), *(French plane),* a plane extending from the tip of the interalveolar septum between the upper central incisors to the lowermost point of the occipital condyle.

p., buccolingual, of teeth (axiobuccolingual plane), a plane that passes through the tooth buccolingually parallel with its long axis. In incisors and canines this is the labiolingual plane.

p., Camper's, a plane extending from the inferior border of the ala of the nose to the superior border of the tragus of the ear.

p., eye-ear. See **plane, Frankfort horizontal.**

p., Frankfort horizontal, a craniometric plane determined by the inferior borders of the bony orbits and the upper margin of the auditory meatus. It passes through the two orbitales and the two tragions.

p., guide (guiding plane), **1.** a mechanical device, part of an orthodontic appliance, having an established inclined plane that, when in use, causes a change in the occlusal relation of the maxillary and mandibular teeth and permits their movement to a normal position. **2.** a plane developed in the occlusal surfaces of occlusion rims to position the mandible in centric relation. **3.** two or more vertically parallel surfaces of abutment teeth shaped to direct the path of placement and removal of a remarkable partial denture.

p., guiding. See **plane, guide.**

p., Hamy's, a plane extending from glabella to lambda.

p., His', a plane extending from the anterior nasal spine to the opisthion.

p., horizontal, a plane that is parallel to the horizon and perpendicular to the vertical plane.

p., horizontal, of teeth, a plane that is perpendicular to the long axis of the tooth and may be supposed to cut through the crown at any point in its length.

P

p., Huxley's, a plane extending from nasion to basion (basicranial axis).

p., mandibular, See **border, mandibular.**

p., Martin's, a plane extending from nasion to inion.

p., mean foundation, the mean of the inclination of the denture-supporting (basal seat) tissues. The tissues constituting the denture foundation are irregular in form and consistency, and force may be applied from only one direction if it is to comply with the law of statics, which requires the exertion of force at a right angle to maintain support. Therefore the mean foundation plane forms a right angle with the most favorable direction of force. The ideal condition for denture stability exists when the mean foundation plane is almost at a right angle to the direction of force.

p., median-raphe, the median plane of the head.

p., median sagittal, a plane passing through the median raphe of the palate at right angles to the Frankfort horizontal plane.

p., mesiodistal, of teeth (axiomesiodistal plane), a plane that passes through the tooth mesiodistally parallel with its long axis.

p., Montague's, the plane extending from nasion to porion.

p., occlusal, **1.** an imaginary surface that is related anatomically to the cranium and that theoretically touches the incisal edges of the incisors and tips of the occluding surfaces of the posterior teeth. It is not a plane in the true sense of the word but represents the mean of the curvature of the surface. See also **curve of occlusion. 2.** a line drawn between points representing one half of the incisal overbite (vertical overlap) in front and one half of the cusp height of the last molars in back.

p., orbital, **1.** a plane perpendicular to the eye-ear plane and passing through the orbitale. **2.** the plane that passes through the visual axis of each eye.

p. of reference, a plane that acts as a guide to the location of other planes.

p., sagittal, the anteroposterior median plane of the body.

p., Schwalbe's (shvahl′behz), a plane that extends from glabella to inion.

p. of teeth, for descriptive purposes, three planes are considered in the teeth proper: buccolingual, horizontal, and mesiodistal.

p., vertical, of teeth, an upright plane that is perpendicular to the horizon.

p., Von Ihring's, a plane extending from orbitale to the center of the bony external auditory meatus.

plaque (plak), a flat plate or tablet.

p., mucin, a sticky substance that accumulates on the teeth; composed of mucin derived from the saliva and of bacteria and their products; often responsible for the inception of caries and for gingival inflammation.

plasma (plaz′mə), the fluid portion of the blood that, after centrifugation, contains all the stable components except the cells. It is obtained from centrifuged whole blood that has been prevented from clotting by the addition of anticoagulants such as citrate, oxalate, or heparin.

p. accelerator globulin. See **proaccelerin** and **accelerator, prothrombin conversion, I.**

p. ac-globulin. See **factor V** and **proaccelerin.**

p. cell, a lymphoid or lymphocytelike cell found in the bone marrow, connective tissue, and sometimes the blood. Plasma cells are involved in the immunologic mechanism.

p., normal human, pooled sterile plasma from a number of persons to which a preservative has been added. It is stored under refrigeration or desiccated for later use as a substitute for whole blood.

p. proteolytic enzyme. See **plasmin.**

p. thromboplastin antecedent (antihemophilic factor C, factor XI, PTA, plasma thromboplastin factor C), a factor required for the development of thromboplastic activity in plasma.

p. thromboplastin component (antihemophilic factor B, autoprothrombin II, Christmas factor, factor IX, platelet cofactor II, PTC), a clotting factor in normal blood necessary for the development of thromboplastic activity in plasma. A deficiency results in Christmas disease. See also **factor IX.**

plasmacytoma (plaz′məsītō′mə), term usually reserved to indicate the primary soft tissue plasma cell tumors of the oral, pharyngeal, and nasal mucous membranes. The lesion consists of typical and atypical plasma cells, and its behavior is unpredictable.

p., soft tissue, a primary plasma cell tumor of the nasal, pharyngeal, and oral mucosa that has no apparent primary bone involvement. The lesions are sessile or polypoid sessile masses in the mucous membrane. The majority remain localized, but metastases have been reported.

plasmid, any type of intracellular inclusion considered to have a genetic function.

plasmin (plaz′min) (fibrinolysin, lysin, plasma proteolytic enzyme, tryptase), collective term for one or more proteolytic enzymes found in the blood. The proteolytic enzymes are capable of digesting fibrin, fibrinogen, and proaccelerin. Plasminogen, the inactive form, may become active spontaneously in shed blood. An activator, fibrinokinase (fibrinolysokinase), is found in many animal tissues.

plasminogen (plazmin′ōjen) (profibrinolysin), the precursor of plasmin found in plasma. It is probably activated by a tissue factor or by a blood activator, which first must be activated by a blood or tissue fibrinolysokinase.

plasmokinin (plazmōkin′in) (not current). See **factor VIII.**

plaster (plas′ter), colloquial term applied to dental plaster of paris.

p. headcap. See **headcap, plaster.**

p., impression, plaster used for making impressions. Sets rapidly and is characterized by low-setting expansion and strength.

p., model, plaster used for diagnostic casts and as an investing material.

p. of paris, the hemihydrate of calcium sulfate that, when mixed with water, forms a paste that subsequently sets into a hard mass. See also **beta-hemihydrate.**

plastic, (capable of being molded), a restorative material (e.g., amalgam, cement, gutta-percha, resin) that is soft at the time of insertion and may then be shaped or molded, after which it will harden or set.

p. base. See **base, plastic.**

p. closure, suturing of tissues that involves their displacement by sliding or rotation to create a surgical closure.

p. strip, a clear plastic strip of celluloid or acrylic resin used as a matrix when silicate cement or acrylic is inserted into proximal prepared cavities in anterior teeth.

p. surgery, branch of medicine that deals with the surgical alteration, replacement, restoration, or reconstruction of a visible part of the body to correct a structural or cosmetic defect.

plasticity (plastis′itē), **1.** the quality of being moldable or workable. **2.** the degree of permanent deformation resulting from stress application, usually associated with substances that are classed as solids or semirigid liquids.

plate, lingual. See **connector, lingual plate and major plate.**

plate, palatal. See **connector, major.**

platelet (plāt′lit), a disk found in the blood of mammals that is concerned in the coagulation and clotting of blood.

p. ac-globulin. See **factor, platelet, I.**

p. activating factor, 1-0-alkyl-2-sn-glycero-3-phosphocholine. A phospholipid derivative formed by platelets, basophils, neutrophils, monocytes, and macrophages. It is a potent platelet aggregating agent and inducer of systemic anaphylactic symptoms, including hypotension, thrombocytopenia, neutropenia, and bronchoconstriction.

p. aggregation, a clumping together of platelets in vitro, and likely in vivo, by a number of agents, such as ADP, thrombin, and collagen, as part of a sequential mechanism leading to the initiation and formation of a thrombus or hemostatic plug.

p. aggregation inhibitors, drugs or agents that antagonize or impair any mechanism leading to blood platelet aggregation.

p. cofactor I. See **factor VIII.**

p. cofactor II. See **factor IX** and **plasma thromboplastin component.**

p. count, the number of platelets found in 1 mm^3 of blood; the normal range is between 200,000 and 300,000 platelets.

p. disorders. See **disorder, platelet.**

p. transfusion, **1.** the transfer of blood platelets from a donor to a recipient or reinfusion to the donor. **2.** a treatment modality used in treating hemophilia and other conditions of impaired blood coagulation.

platinocyanide crystals (plat'inōsī' ·ənīd) See **crystals, platinocyanide.** (not current)

platinum, a silvery-white, soft metallic element. Its atomic number is 78 and atomic weight is 195.09. Platinum is used in dentistry, jewelry, and manufacture of chemical apparatus that must withstand high temperatures.

p. matrix. See **matrix, platinum.**

pleadings, written allegations of what is affirmed on the one side or denied on the other, disclosing the real matter to the court or jury having to try the case.

pledget (plej'ət), a minute pellet of absorbent cotton used for accurately controlled placement of medication or base. See also **cotton, absorbent.**

pleomorphic adenoma (plē'ōmôr'fik ad'enō'mə) (mixed salivary gland tumor), a benign tumor of the salivary gland containing varying proportions of epithelial and mesenchymal elements. The intermediate type of epithelial cells is in sheets, cords, and acini. The mesenchymal tissue varies from myxomatous to cartilaginous to densely hyalinized connective tissue. The marked variations in histologic pattern are responsible for the designation of pleomorphic.

plethora (pleth'ərə), a nonspecific increase in blood bulk. Clinically, the patient is flushed and has a feeling of tenseness in the head; the blood vessels are full, and the pulse is firm.

pleura, a delicate serous membrane enclosing the lung, composed of a single layer of flattened mesothelial cells resting on a delicate membrane of connective tissue.

pleurisy (plŏŏr'əsē), an inflammation of the pleura, with exudation into its cavity and on its surface.

plexus (plek'səs), a network or tangle, especially of nerves, lymphatics, or veins.

p., Haller's, a nerve plexus of sympathetic filaments and branches of the external laryngeal nerve on the surface of the inferior constrictor muscle of the larynx.

p., intermediate, a middle zone of the periodontal membrane situated between the cemental group of fibers attached to the root of the tooth and the alveolar group of fibers attached to the alveolar bone. The three groups of fibers are woven together by small, thick strands of collagen fibers. The interweaving of fiber bundles of the intermediate plexus allows for tooth eruption and tooth movement between the cemental and alveolar periodontal fibers.

pliers, a tool of pincer design with jaws of varying shapes; used for holding, bending, stretching, contouring, and cutting.

p., contouring, pliers with jaws curved to permit developing tooth contours in banding metal.

p., cotton, a slender, tweezerlike instrument used to hold cotton pellets or pledgets, apply medicaments, and carry small objects to and from the mouth.

p., stretching, pliers whose jaws are designed as a hammer and anvil, with the handles sufficiently long to develop a high leverage ratio; used to enlarge metal bands (gold, aluminum, copper) or to thin the contact area of matrix bands.

plosive (plō'siv), any speech sound made by impounding the airstream for a moment until considerable pressure has been developed and then suddenly releasing it (for example, in the pronunciation of *d, p,* and *g*).

plug, a peg or any mass filling a hole or closing an orifice.

plugger, an instrument used to compress the filling material in an apical and lateral direction when a root canal is being filled. See also **condenser.**

plumbism (plum'bizəm) (lead poisoning, saturnism), acute or chronic intoxication resulting from the ingestion, inhalation, or skin absorption of lead. Manifestations of acute poisoning include abdominal pain, paralysis, metallic taste, and collapse. Chronic manifestations include gastrointestinal disturbances, headache, peripheral neuropathy (foot drop and wrist drop), lead in the urine and blood, basophilic granular degeneration, coproporphyrinuria, and stomatitis. See also **stomatitis, lead.**

Plummer-Vinson syndrome. See **syndrome, Plummer-Vinson.**

plunger cusp, a stamp cusp, the tip of which is made to occlude in an embrasure; its shoulder has not been restored to occlude in a fossa.

plutonium, a synthetic transuranic metallic element. Its atomic number is 94 and its atomic weight is 242. A highly toxic waste product of nuclear power plants, plutonium was used in the assembly of early nuclear weapons.

PMA (papillary-marginal-attached), a system of epidemiologic scoring of periodontal disease devised by Schour and Massler in which the symbols denote the areas involved in gingival inflammation.

pneumatic condenser (nōōmat′ik). See **condenser, pneumatic.**

pneumatodyspnea (nōō′mətōdisp′nē·ə), difficulty in breathing resulting from emphysema. (not current)

pneumoconiosis, any disease of the lung caused by chronic inhalation of dust, usually mineral dusts of occupational or environmental origin. The principal agents include coal, cotton, sand, and asbestos.

Pneumocystis carinii (nōō′mōsis′tis kari′nē·ī), an opportunistic infection found in immunocompromised patients such as those with AIDS.

pneumonia, an acute inflammation of the lungs, usually caused by inhaled microorganisms. The alveoli and bronchioles of the lungs become plugged with a fibrous exudate, seriously interfering with oxygen exchange.

pneumonitis (nōō′mōnī′tis), an inflammation of the lungs of an acute, localized nature.

pneumothorax (nōō′mōthôr′aks), an accumulation of air or gas in the pleural cavity. The air enters by way of an external wound, a lung perforation, a burrowing abscess, or rupture of a superficial lung cavity. Pneumothorax is accompanied by sudden, severe pain and rapidly increasing dyspnea.

pocket, 1. a diseased gingival attachment, characterized by gingival discoloration, retraction of gingivae from the tooth, bleeding, the presence of an exudate, and loss of the presence of stippling. **2.** a space bordered on one side by the tooth and on the opposite side by ulcerated crevicular epithelium and limited at its apex by the epithelial attachment.

p., bleeding, an occurrence that denotes ulcerations of the pocket epithelium, with hemorrhaging through the broken surface from exposed connective tissue capillaries.

p. bottom, the base of the pocket, marked or limited by the epithelial attachment to the cementum of the root (periodontal pocket) or the enamel of the crown (gingival pocket).

p., calculus, calcified deposits that usually occupy the entire pocket. It is attached to the tooth structure, with the gingival tissues tightly adapted to the surface of the calculus.

p., deepening, an increase of the depth of the pocket, which is dependent on apical proliferation of the epithelial attachment alongside the cementum, with subsequent separation from the tooth, or on hyperplasia of the gingivae resulting from inflammation.

p., depth of, the measurement, usually expressed in millimeters, of the distance between the gingival crest and the base of the pocket.

p., elimination, the application of therapeutic measures to obtain a healthy gingival attachment and an intact, functioning attachment apparatus. The procedures employed include curettage (root and gingival), reattachment or new attachment operations, gingivectomy and gingivoplasty, and osseous and mucogingival surgical procedures.

p., gingival, a pseudopocket; gingival inflammation with edema, hyperplasia, and ulceration of the sulcular epithelium but without apical proliferation of the epithelial attachment.

p., infrabony (infracrestal pocket, intra-alveolar pocket, intrabony pocket), a periodontal pocket, the base of which is apical to the crest of the alveolar bone. Consists basically of a vertical resorptive defect in alveolar and supporting bone, overlying which are a band of transseptal fibers connecting adjacent teeth, disintegrated fibers of gingival corium, inflammatory cellular infiltrate, and hyperplastic pocket epithelium, accompanied by apical migration of the epithelial attachment. Clinical signs are those of periodontitis, associated with radiographic evidence of vertical bone resorption. The infrabony pocket has been classified

P

according to the number of remaining osseous walls supporting it for the purpose of therapeutic rationale.

p., infracrestal. See **pocket, infrabony.**

p. in marginal periodontitis, a condition in which the inflammatory process has progressed from the gingival tissues to the underlying alveolar process. The changes are those associated with gingivitis plus resorptive bone lesions. The base of the pocket is at the marginal point of the union of the epithelial attachment to the cementum of the root.

p., intraalveolar. See **pocket, infrabony.**

p., intrabony. See **pocket, infrabony.**

p. ionization chamber. See **chamber, ionization.**

p. marker, Crane-Kaplan, an instrument used to delineate the depths of gingival and periodontal pockets before gingivectomy incision. The straight beak of the instrument is inserted to the limit of the pocket, and the sharp angulated beak is pressed into the tissue until a small bleeding point is seen. The resultant series of bleeding points is used as a guide for the gingivectomy incision.

p., marking, the accurate determination and delineation of pocket depth and topography as an aid to diagnosis and prognosis or to provide a guide for the gingivectomy incision.

p., periodontal, a pathologic deepening of the gingival sulcus produced by destruction of the supporting tissues and apical proliferation of the epithelial attachment. Ulceration of the pocket epithelium lining is characteristic.

p. surgery, a generic term referring to gingivectomy-gingivoplasty. See also **gingivectomy, gingivoplasty.**

podiatry, a health profession that deals with the diagnosis and treatment of diseases and other disorders of the feet.

pogonion (pōgō'nē·on) (Po), the most anterior point on the chin. A cephalometric landmark in the lateral view.

poikilocytosis (poi'kilōsītō'sis), an irregular shape of the red blood cells.

point, a small spot; a minute area; a rotating instrument having a small cutting end or surface.

p. A, the deepest point in the bony concavity in the midline at the base of the anterior nasal spine, in the region of the incisor roots. A landmark on the lateral cephalometric view.

p., abrasive, rotary (mounted carborundum, diamond), small abrasive instruments used in straight or contraangle handpieces.

p. angle. See **angle, point.**

p. B, a mandibular point comparable to point A.

p., bleeding. See **bleeding points.**

p., boiling, the temperature at which the vapor pressure within a liquid equals atmospheric pressure.

p., Bolton, the highest point of the curvature between the occipital condyle and the basilar part of the occipital bone; located behind the occipital condyle. The highest point of the curvature behind the occipital condyle. A substitute for the basion point when it cannot be ascertained on cephalometric headplates.

p., central-bearing, the contact point of a central-bearing device.

p., condenser, the nib of a condensing instrument. A short instrument, for condensing foil or amalgam, that is inserted into a mechanical condenser or into a cone socket handle.

p., contact (contact area), the area of contact of approximating surfaces of two adjacent teeth. The areas of contact are located at the line of junction between the occlusal and middle thirds of the posterior teeth and the incisal and middle thirds of the anterior teeth.

p., convenience, a small undercut in the cavity wall convenient for placing and retaining the first portion of a filling material. It is generally one of the retention points placed in a cavity preparation that provides the best access to the operator.

p. D, the center of the body of the symphysis.

p., faulty contact, a defective contact between the proximal surfaces of adjacent teeth, produced by wearing of the contact areas, dental caries, improper restoration, or altered tooth position.

p., gutta-percha. See **gutta-percha points.**

p., hinge axis, a point placed on the skin corresponding with the opening axis of the mandible.

p., Hirschfeld's silver, a calibrated silver rod used to record the clinical depth of periodontal pockets radiographically for the purpose of diagnosis.

p., incisor, the intersection of the lower occlusal and midsagittal planes. The point at the mesioincisal angles of the two mandibular central incisors.

p., loss of contact, the failure of contact of convex proximal surfaces of adjacent teeth; produced by tooth migration, dental caries, or improper restoration.

p., median mandibular, a point on the anteroposterior center of the mandibular ridge in the median sagittal plane.

p., paper. See paper point.

p. of centricity, if the point of the buccal cusp of the lower right molar, put in lateral position, arcs around the upright axis of the right condyle, it will reach a station where further muscular efforts leftward will change the cusp's direction so that it will arc around the left condyle. The station where the right arc ends and the left arc begins is a point of mandibular centricity. While the right cusp point orbits (arcs) around the near vertical axis, all other points in the jaw join in orbiting (arcing). The left condyle arcs rearward until it reaches a cranial backstop; then the muscles start rotating it and carrying it leftward, and the right condyle begins arcing forward, downward, and medially. In the right and left swings of the jaw, a condyle reciprocally alternates between being a rotator and an orbiter. The point of centricity of the mandible is demonstrated usually on a horizontal plane, but it can be demonstrated on all three planes of projection. The point of centricity is rearmost, midmost (between the arcs of motion), and uppermost. See also **face-bow** and **relation, centric.**

p., registration, any point considered as fixed for a particular pattern of analysis. Also, the midpoint of a perpendicular line from the sella turcica to the Bolton-nasion plane.

p., transition. See **Tg value.**

p., treatment, a piece of paper point, selected for the root canal being treated, that carries or holds the medication in place.

p., trial, a cone of filling material placed in a canal and radiographed to check on the length and fit of the filling.

p., yield, 1. the place on the stress-strain curve where marked permanent deformation occurs; it is just beyond the proportional limit. 2. the point where permanent deformation starts in a metal.

pointing, the term associated with fluctuation pertaining to the area where the purulent exudate is eroding through tissues to an external surface. At this point an incision and drainage operation usually is performed.

poison, a substance that, when ingested, inhaled, absorbed, injected into, or developed within the body, will cause damage to structures of the body and impair or destroy their function.

poisoning, the morbid condition caused by poison.

p., arsenic, acute or chronic intoxication from the ingestion of insecticides

---

Immediate treatment of a poison exposure*

Ocular and Dermal Exposures
Irrigate with copious amounts of running water for 15 to 20 minutes. Call the Poison Center.

Inhalation Exposures
Immediately move the victim to an area with fresh air.
  If needed, start artificial respiration/CPR. Call the Poison Center.

Ingestion of Caustic Substances
Dilute with 4 to 8 oz of water, and call the Poison Center immediately.

Other Oral Exposures and Parenteral Exposures
  Call the Poison Center immediately

  Poison Centers provide immediate, individualized, expert treatment advice 24 hours a day, 7 days a week.

*Information supplied by the American Association of Poison Control Centers, Inc.

or administration of organic arsenicals. Manifestations of acute poisoning include abdominal pain, nausea, vomiting, and collapse. Chronic manifestations include weakness, peripheral neuropathy, hyperkeratosis, skin rashes, and oral manifestations secondary to liver dysfunction and bone marrow depression. See also **stomatitis, arsenical.**

p., bismuth. See **bismuthosis.**

p., chemical, a form of poisoning caused by ingestion of a toxic chemical agent.

p., iodine. See **iodism.**

p., lead. See **plumbism.**

p., mercury. See **mercurialism.**

p., metallic, a toxic condition produced by excessive exposure to or intake of metals. In the oral cavity there may be definite signs of arsenic, bismuth, lead, phosphorus, radium, and other metals. Fluorides produce changes in developing teeth at levels far below those that are toxic for the rest of the human economy.

p., phosphorus, the result of the ingestion of phosphorus, especially yellow phosphorus. Manifestations include burning of the mouth and throat, abdominal pain, vomiting, jaundice, liver damage, and death. In chronic poisoning, necrosis of the jaws (phossy jaw) occurs.

police power, the authority of the state to enact laws to protect the public, such as a dental practice act. Police power is reserved to the states under the United States Constitution.

policy, the document embodying the insurance contract.

p. holder, under a group purchase plan, the employer, labor union, or trustee to whom a group contract is issued. In a plan providing for individual or family enrollment, the person to whom the contract is issued.

p. period, the time during which an insurance contract affords protection.

p. year, the year commencing with the effective date of the insurance contract or with an anniversary of that date.

poliomyelitis (po'le·o·mi'·ali'tis), a disease produced by a small viral organism that enters the body via the alimentary tract and produces upper pharyngeal, pharyngeal, and intestinal inflammation in its mentor form. In the more severe variety, a subsequent viremia is produced, with extension of the infection to the anterior pulp horn cells and ganglia of the spinal cord, producing a flaccid paralysis. In bulbar poliomyelitis the viral infection involves the medulla, resulting in impairment of swallowing respiration, and/or circulation. It is now recognized that three types of viruses are responsible for the nonparalytic, paralytic, and bulbar varieties of poliomyelitis. Excellent immunization procedures have been provided by use of killed viruses (Salk) and attenuated mutant vaccines (Sabin).

polishing, making smooth and glossy, usually by friction; giving luster to.

p. brush. See **brush, polishing.**

p., coronal, the removal of mucinous film, superficial stain, or deposits, to provide a smooth enamel surface that will be more resistant to future accumulation of foreign substances such as materia alba, calculus, and mucinous plaque.

p. disk. See **disk, polishing.**

politics, the art and science of governance, particularly in a democracy or collegial body.

pollakiuria (pol'əkeyoo're·ə), unduly frequent urination. It may result from partial obstruction, such as in prostatic enlargement, or it may be of nervous origin.

pollen, a fertilizing element of plants that travels in the air and produces seasonal allergic responses such as hay fever or asthma in sensitive individuals.

polyamines, many amines; polymers of amine, many of which normally occur in body constituents of wide distribution and are essential growth factors for microorganisms.

polyantibiotic (pol'e·an'tebi·ot'ik), a combination of two or more antibiotics used to eliminate bacteria from a root canal.

polycarboxylate cement. See **cement.**

polychlorinated biphenyls, a group of more than 30 isomers and compounds used in plastics, insulation, and flame retardants and varying in physical form from oily liquid to crystals and resins. All are potentially toxic and carcinogenic. Mild exposure may cause chloracne; severe exposure may result in hepatic damage.

polychromatophilia (pol'ēkrōmət'ōfil'ē·ə), an irregular staining of cells, particularly red blood cells.

Polycillin (po'lēcilin), the trade name for ampicillin, an acid-stable semisynthetic penicillin effective against some gram-negative and gram-positive organisms.

polycythemia (pol'ēsithē'mē·ə), an increase in blood volume as a result of an increase in the number of red blood cells, the erythrocytes. It may result from a blood-forming disease that increases cell production, or it may be a physiologic response to an increased need for oxygenation in high altitudes, cardiac disease, or respiratory disorders.

p., primary. See **erythremia.**

p. rubra. See **erythremia.**

p., secondary. See **erythrocytosis.**

p. vera. See **erythremia.**

polydactyly (pol'ēdak'tilē), a congenital anomaly characterized by the presence of more than the normal number of fingers or toes. It may be a part of a complex genetic syndrome. Early surgical treatment is generally used to correct the problem.

polydipsia (pol'ēdip'sē·ə), abnormally increased thirst.

polyglycolic acid, a polymer of glycolic acid, used in absorbable surgical sutures.

polymer (pol'imər), a long-chain hydrocarbon. In dentistry, the polymer is supplied as a powder to be mixed with the monomer for fabrication of appliances and restorations.

polymerase chain reaction (PCR), a process whereby a strand of DNA can be cloned millions of times within a few hours. The process can be used to make prenatal diagnoses of genetic diseases and to identify an individual by analysis of a single tissue cell.

polymerization (polimer'izā'shən), the chaining together of similar molecules to form a compound of high molecular weight.

p., addition, a compound formed by a combination of simple molecules without the formation of any new products; for example, methyl methacrylate.

p., condensation, the combination of simple, dissimilar molecules, with the formation of by-products such as water or ammonia (e.g., vulcanite).

p., cross (cross linkage, cross-linked polymerization), the formation of chemical bonds between linear molecules, resulting in a three-dimensional network. Used for artificial teeth and denture bases because of superior craze resistance.

p., cross-linked. See **polymerization, cross.**

polymorphonuclear leukocytes (pol'ēmôr'fōnōōklēər lōō'kōsītz), a type of white blood cells with nuclei of varied forms.

polymyxin (pol'ēmīk'sin), an antibiotic substance derived from cultures of *Bacillus polymyxa.* Used topically, in troche form, in combination with bacitracin and neomycin in the treatment of various oral infections. Not used systemically; therefore sensitization is minimized. Systemic use may be attended by renal dysfunction and toxicity.

polymyxin B sulfate (ophthalmic); *trade names:* Aerosporin; *drug class:* ophthalmic antiinfective; *action:* inhibits cell wall permeability in susceptible organism; *use:* superficial external ocular infections.

polyneuritis, endemic (pol'ēnōōrī'tis). See **beriberi.**

polyostotic (pol'e·ostot'ik), affecting more than one bone.

polyp (pol'ip), a smooth, pedunculated growth from a mucous surface such as from the nose, bladder, or rectum.

p., pulp. See **pulpitis, hypertrophic.**

polypharmacy, the prescription or dispensation of unnecessarily numerous or complex medicines.

polypnea (pol'ipnē'ə), a rapid or panting respiration.

polyposis, multiple (pol'ipō'sis). See **syndrome, Peutz-Jeghers.**

polysaccharide, a complex carbohydrate containing a large number of saccharide groups such as starch.

polystyrene (pol'ēstī'rən), a polymer of styrene, which is a derivative of ethylene; often one of the resins present in materials designed for denture construction by the injection molding technique.

polysulfide polymer (pol'ēsul'fīd pol'imər), a rubber base impression mate-

P

rial that makes use of a mercaptan bondage. It is prepared by mixing a base material (mercaptan) with either an inorganic catalyst (lead peroxide) or an organic catalyst (benzoyl peroxide).

polythiazide, *trade name:* Renese; *drug class:* thiazide diuretic; *action:* acts on distal tubule by increasing excretion of water, sodium, chloride, potassium; *uses:* edema, hypertension, diuresis.

polyuria (pol'ēyo͞o're-ə), the passage of an abnormally increased volume of urine. It may result from increased intake of fluids, inadequate renal function, uncontrolled diabetes mellitus or diabetes insipidus, diuresis of edema fluid, or ascites.

polyvinyl alcohol, a complex alcohol that is soluble in water and is used as an emulsifier and adhesive.

polyvinyl chloride, a common synthetic thermoplastic material that releases hydrochloric acid when burned and that may contain carcinogenic vinyl chloride molecules as a contaminant.

pons (ponz), a structure dorsal to the medulla and intimately related to the pathways to the cerebrum. The cranial nerves whose nuclei lie in the pons are the trigeminal, abducens, and facial nerves, and part of the acoustic nerve. The pons is intimately related to the medulla, has the same blood vessel supply, and is involved in many lesions that affect the medulla. It is especially involved with the cerebellar manifestations of disease and may cause serious muscular incoordination in motor function of the head, neck, and facial structures.

pontic (pon'tik), the suspended member of a fixed partial denture; an artificial tooth on a fixed partial denture or an isolated tooth on a removable partial denture. It replaces a lost natural tooth, restores its function, and usually occupies the space previously occupied by the natural crown.

population, all the instances about which a statement is made; all events, organisms, and items of a stated kind occurring or in existence in a specified time. In statistics, a hypothetic infinite supply or universe of events or objects like those being studied and from which a sample was drawn.

porcelain, a material formed by the fusion of feldspar, silica, and other minor ingredients. Most dental porcelains are glasses and are used in the manufacture of artificial teeth, facings, jackets, and occasionally denture bases and inlays.

p., baked. See **porcelain, dental.**

p., dental (baked porcelain, fired porcelain), a fused mixture that is glasslike and more or less transparent. Classification of the type of porcelain employed in inlays and crowns is based on the fusion temperature of the porcelain: high fusing, 2350° to 2500° F (1287.5° to 1371° C); medium fusing, 2000° to 2300° F (1093.5° to 1260° C); and low fusing, 1600° to 2000° F (871° to 1093.5° C).

p., fired. See **porcelain, dental.**

p., synthetic. See **cement, silicate.**

porion (pō're·on), the superior surface of the external auditory meatus. In craniometry, porion is identified as the margin of the bony canal on the skull. In cephalometrics it may be identified from the earpost of the cephalostat (machine porion) or from bony landmarks on the film (anatomic porion).

porosity (pōros'itē), the presence of pores or voids within a structure.

p., back-pressure, porosity produced in castings resulting from the inability of gases in the mold to escape through the investment.

p., occluded gas, porosity produced by improper use of the blowpipe (that is, heating the metal in the oxidizing portion of the flame).

p., shrink-spot, an area of porosity in cast metal that is caused by shrinkage of a portion of the metal as it solidifies from the molten state without flow of additional molten metal from surrounding areas.

p., solidification, a porosity that may be produced by improper spruing or improper heating of the metal or the investment.

porphyria, congenital (pôrfi're-ə). See **porphyria, erythropoietic.**

porphyria, erythropoietic (congenital porphyria, photosensitive porphyria), an inborn error of metabolism (porphyrin synthesis) characterized clinically by skin photosensitivity, hypertrichosis, and reddish brown staining of the primary teeth.

porphyria, photosensitive. See **porphyria, erythropoietic.**

porphyrin, any iron or magnesium-free pyrrole derivative occurring in many plant and animal tissues. Normal findings of porphyrins in urine are 60 mg to 200 mg/24-hour period.

Porphyromonas gingivalis, a species of gram-negative, anaerobic, rod-shaped bacteria originally classified within the *Bacteroides* genus. This bacterium produces a cell-bound, oxygen-sensitive collagenase and is isolated from the human mouth.

port, the opening through which x-ray photons or the useful beam of radiation exits from the head of a dental x-ray machine.

portfolio, a list of stocks, bonds, and other commercial paper owned by an investor or holding company. In dentistry, it generally refers to the personal retirement investment package of the dentist or professional corporation created by the dentist.

position, the placement or location of body parts to each other and/or the relationship of the body and its parts to other objects in space.

p., border, posterior, the most posterior position of the mandible at any specific vertical relation of the maxillae.

p., centric, **1.** the position of the mandible in its most retruded relation to the maxillae at the established vertical relation. **2.** the constant position into which the patient will close the jaws; this relationship may be a convenience relationship or a true centric relationship.

p., condylar hinge, **1.** mandibular joints at which a hinge movement of the mandible is possible. **2.** the maxillomandibular relation from which a consciously stimulated true hinge movement can be executed.

p., eccentric (eccentric jaw position), any position of the mandible other than that in centric relation. See also **relation, jaw, eccentric.**

   p., e. jaw. See **position, eccentric** and **relation, jaw, eccentric.**

p., finger. See **finger positions.**

p., gingival. See **gingival position.**

p., hinge, the orientation of parts in a manner permitting hinge movements between them.

p., intercuspal, the term applied to the cuspal contacts of teeth when the

mandible is in centric relation. Synonym: centric occlusion.

p., mandibular hinge, any position of the mandible that exists when the condyles are so situated in the temporomandibular joints that opening or closing movements can be made on the hinge axis. See also **axis, hinge.**

p., physiologic rest, the habitual postural position of the mandible when the patient is resting comfortably in the upright position and the condyles are in a neutral, unstrained position in the glenoid fossae. The mandibular musculature is in a state of minimum tonic contraction to maintain posture and to overcome its force of gravity. See also **relation, jaw, rest.**

p., protrusive, occlusion of the teeth as the mandible and lower central incisors are moved straight forward toward the incisal edges of the upper central incisors; the normal anterocclusal relationship; the forward end position, with the upper and lower incisors in edge-to-edge contact.

p., rest, **1.** the position of the mandible when the jaws are in rest relation. See also **position, rest, physiologic** and **relation, jaw, rest. 2.** the position that the mandible passively assumes when the mandibular musculature is relaxed.

p., terminal hinge, the mandibular hinge position from which further opening of the mandible would produce translatory rather than hinge movement. See also **position, hinge.**

p., tooth, the placement or location of the tooth in the dental arch in relation to the bone of the alveolar process, its adjacent teeth, and the opposing dentition.

p., Trendelenburg, a position in which the patient is on his back with the head and chest lowered and the leg elevated.

positioner, a removable elastic orthodontic appliance molded to fit the teeth in a "setup" made by repositioning the teeth from a plaster cast. The material may be rubber or elastomeric plastic. It is typically used to achieve fine adjustments and retain corrected positions in the finishing stages of treatment.

positioning, surgical, the surgical repositioning or tilting of a tooth without injuring its blood supply.

P

positions at the chair, the posture and relative location of a dentist or chairside assistant in respect to the dental chair and patient. Classified as standing or sitting and as right side behind, right side in front, left side behind, left side in front, and directly behind. The position used should permit the most efficient performance of the current procedure and also keep paramount the health and comfort of the dentist and the patient.

positive reinforcement, a technique used to encourage a desirable behavior. Also called *positive feedback,* in which the patient or subject receives encouraging and favorable communication from another person.

positron emission tomography (PET), a computerized radiographic technique that employs radioactive substances to examine the metabolic activity of various body structures. Researchers and clinicians use PET to study blood flow and the metabolism of the heart and blood vessels.

possession, the control or custody of anything that may be the subject of property as owner or as one who has a qualified right in it.

post, implant. See **substructure, implant, neck.**

post cibum (pōst si'bəm). See **p.c.**

postcondensation (aftercondensation), the procedure of completing the condensation of the surface of a gold-foil restoration after all the gold has been placed.

postdam area. See **area, posterior palatal seal.**

posterior, situated behind.

p. nasal spine. See **spine, posterior nasal.**

p. palatal bar. See **connector, major, posterior palatal.**

p. palatal seal. See **seal, posterior palatal.**

p. p. s. area. See **area, posterior palatal seal.**

posteroanterior extraoral radiographic examination. See **examination, radiographic, extraoral, posteroanterior.**

postmortem changes, changes that occur after death.

postoperative care, care after surgery or other invasive procedures, usually of a supportive nature.

postoperative complications, unexpected problems that arise following surgery. The most frequent are bleeding, infection, and protracted pain.

postoperative hemorrhage, unexpected and abnormal (excessive) bleeding following surgery.

postpalatal seal. See **seal, posterior palatal.**

p. s. area. See **area, posterior palatal seal.**

postperception (afterperception), the perception of a sensation after the stimulus producing it has ceased. (not current)

postsensation (aftersensation), a sensation lasting after the stimulus that produced it has been removed. (not current)

posttreatment review. See **audit.**

posture, normal, the configuration of the body in the upright position, which varies considerably among individuals. However, normal posture can be described as follows: the shoulder, pelvis, and eyes are level; the sagittal plane is between the feet, and the line of gravity passes through the center of gravity at the lumbosacral joint. When observed from the following positions, the line of gravity intersects the following structures: lateral position—anterior border of the ear, and the shoulder, hip, knee, and ankle joints; anterior position—nose, symphysis pubis, and between the knees and feet; posterior position—occiput, spinous processes, gluteal crease, and between the knees and feet.

potassium, an alkali metal element, the seventh most abundant element in the earth's crust. Its atomic number is 19 and its atomic weight is 39.1. Potassium in the body constitutes the predominant intracellular cation, helping to regulate neuromuscular excitability and muscle contraction. The average adequate daily intake of potassium for most adults is 2 to 4 grams.

p. bicarbonate/potassium acetate/ potassium chloride/potassium gluconate/potassium phosphate, trade name: Effer-K, K-Lyte, Kapon-CL, K-Dur, Micro-K, K-G Elixir; *drug class:* potassium electrolyte; *action:* needed for adequate transmission of nerve impulses and cardiac contraction, renal function, intracellular ion maintenance; *uses:* prevention and treatment of hypokalemia.

p. chloride, a white crystalline salt used as a substitute for table salt in the diet of persons with cardiovascular disorders.

p. dichromate, a compound of potassium used as an external astringent, antiseptic, and caustic.

p. oxalate (pōtas'ē·əm ok'səlāt), a dentin desensitizing agent that occludes the openings of the dentinal tubules and blocks the hydrodynamics that initiate the pain response. Brand name: Protect.

p. sulfate (pōtas'ē·əm səl'fāt), an accelerator used to speed the setting of gypsum products. Hydrocolloid impressions are fixed in a 2% solution of potassium sulfate.

potency (pō'tensē), power.

potential, action. See **action potential.**

potentiation (pōten'shē·ā'shən) (synergism), **1.** an increase in the action of a drug by the addition of another drug that does not necessarily possess similar properties. **2.** the enhancement of action (for example, of a drug).

Potter-Bucky diaphragm (not current). See **grid, Potter-Bucky.**

Potter-Bucky grid. See **grid, Potter-Bucky.**

Pott's disease. See **disease, Pott's.**

pour hole, an aperture in a refractory investment or another mold material leading to the pattern space into which prosthetic material is deposited.

poverty, a lack of material wealth needed to maintain existence.

povidone, a polymerized form of vinylpyrolidone, which is a white hygroscopic powder that is easily soluble in water and used as a dispersing and suspending agent in drugs.

p. iodine (pō'vidōn ī'ōdīn), *trade names:* ACU-dyne, Aerodine, Betadine; *drug class:* iodophor disinfectant; *action:* destroys a wide variety of microorganisms by local irritation and germicidal action; *uses:* cleansing wounds, disinfection, preoperative skin preparation; *dental use:* to irrigate periodontal pockets before debridement to control bleeding and pain.

powdered gold. See **gold, powdered.**

power stroke. See **stroke, power.**

pp. See **pauperissimus.**

PPCF. See **factor V.**

practice, to follow or work at, as a profession, trade, or art.

p. administration, the organization, operation, and supervision of the business and professional aspects of a dental practice.

p. building, increasing the number of patients and the number of services without sacrificing quality, by means of observing the principles of constantly improving professional care and maintaining effective human relations with patients.

p. goal, the planning of the objectives of a dental practice and the method of reaching those objectives. To be ascertained by the dental practitioner before or immediately on entering dental practice.

p., group, a large partnership formed for the purpose of practicing dentistry; may or may not include the services of the recognized specialties in dentistry.

p. guidelines, a detailed description of a process of maintenance of health status or to slow the decline in health status in certain chronic clinical conditions. Practice guidelines are established to assist in the delivery of effective and efficient health care that preserves the resources of the provider, the patient, and the funding entity.

p. management, dental, the administrative organization of a dental office, including but not limited to the supervision and control of patient flow, staff assignment and evaluation, record keeping, and financial overseeing.

p., private, the business and profession in which dental services are administered for a fee.

Prader-Willi syndrome, a metabolic condition characterized by congenital hypotonia, hyperphagia, obesity, and mental retardation. The syndrome is associated with a less-than-normal secretion of gonadotropic hormones by the pituitary gland.

pravastatin, *trade name:* Pravachol; *drug class:* antihyperlipidemic; *ac-*

tion: inhibits HMG-CoA reductase enzyme, which reduces cholesterol synthesis; *use:* as an adjunct in primary hypercholesterolemia (types IIa, IIb).

prazepam, *trade name:* Centrax; *drug class:* benzodiazepine, antianxiety (Controlled Substance Schedule IV); *action:* produces central nervous system depression by interacting with a benzodiazepine receptor to facilitate the action of inhibitory neurotransmitter γ-aminobutyric acid (GABA); *use:* anxiety.

prazosin HCl, *trade name:* Minipress; *drug class:* antihypertensive, α-adrenergic blocker; *action:* reduction in blood pressure results from blockage of α-adrenergic receptors and reduced peripheral resistance; *use:* hypertension.

preanesthetic (prē′anesthet′ik), a medicine for producing preliminary anesthesia (for example, Avertin). See also **premedication.**

preauthorization, 1. the approval of or concurrence with the treatment plan proposed by a participating dentist before the provision of service. Under some plans, preauthorization by the carrier is required before certain services can be provided. **2.** a statement by a third-party payer indicating that proposed treatment will be covered under the terms of the dental benefits contract. See also **precertification** and **predetermination.**

precertification, confirmation by a third-party payer of a patient's eligibility for coverage under a dental benefits program. See also **preauthorization** and **predetermination.**

precancerous, a stage of abnormal tissue growth that is likely or predisposed to develop into a malignant tumor.

preceptorship, the position of teacher or instructor to a new or recent graduate.

precipitate (prēsip′itāt), an insoluble solid substance that forms from chemical reactions between solutions.

precipitating factor, an element that causes or contributes to the occurrence of a disorder or problem.

precision attachment. See **attachment, intracoronal.**

precision rest. See **rest, precision.**

precordial, pertaining to the region over the heart or stomach: the epigastrium and lower thorax.

precursor, fifth plasma thromboplastin. See **factor XII.**

precursor of serum prothrombin conversion accelerator (cothromboplastin, factor VII, proSPCA), a clotting factor found in serum plasma and believed to be needed for the optimal action of tissue thromboplastin. Formerly, with the Stuart factor, it was known as **proconvertin** or **stable factor.** (not current) See also **proconvertin.**

predetermination, an administrative procedure whereby a dentist submits a treatment plan to the carrier before treatment is initiated. Then the carrier returns the treatment plan, indicating the patient's eligibility, covered service amounts payable, application of appropriate deductibles, copayment factors, and maximums. Under some programs, predetermination by the carrier is required when covered charges are expected to exceed a certain amount, commonly $100. Synonyms: preauthorization, precertification, preestimate of cost, pretreatment estimate.

prednicarbate, *trade name:* Dermatop Emollient Cream; *drug class:* topical corticosteroid, group III potency; *action:* possesses antipruritic, antiinflammatory actions; *uses:* relief of inflammatory and pruritic manifestations of corticosteroid-responsive dermatoses.

prednisolone/prednisolone acetate/prednisolone sodium phosphate/prednisolone tebutate, *trade names:* Delta-Cortef, Prelone, Pedaject-50, Hydeltra TBA; *drug class:* immediate acting glucocorticoid; *action:* decreases inflammation by suppressing macrophage and leukocyte migration; reduces capillary permeability and inhibits lysosomal enzymes and phagocytosis; *uses:* severe inflammation, immunosuppression, neoplasms, adrenal insufficiency.

prednisone (pred′nisōn), *trade names:* Deltasone, Sterapred; *drug class:* intermediate acting glucocorticoid; *action:* decreases inflammation by suppressing macrophage and leukocyte migration, reduces capillary

P

permeability and inhibits lysosomal enzymes and phagocytosis; *uses:* severe inflammation, immunosuppression, neoplasms, multiple sclerosis, collagen disorders, dermatologic disorders.

preexisting condition, the oral health condition of an enrollee that existed before his or her enrollment in a dental program.

preextraction cast. See **cast, diagnostic** and **cast, preextraction.**

preextraction record. See **record, preoperative.**

preferred provider organization (PPO), a formal agreement between a purchaser of a dental benefits program and a defined group of dentists for the delivery of dental services to a specific patient population as an adjunct to a traditional plan, using discounted fees for cost savings.

prefiling of fees, the submission of a participating dentist's usual fees to a service corporation for the purpose of establishing, in advance, that dentist's usual fees and the customary ranges of fees in a geographic area to determine benefits under a usual, customary, and reasonable dental benefits program.

pregnancy, the gestational process, comprising the growth and development within a woman of a new individual from conception through the embryonic and fetal periods to birth. Pregnancy lasts approximately 266 days from the day of fertilization, but is clinically considered to last 280 days (40 weeks, or 10 lunar months) from the first day of the last menstrual period.

p. gingivitis, an enlargement or hyperplasia of the gingivae caused by hormonal imbalance during pregnancy. It is usually limited to the interdental papillae. Incomplete cleaning of the interproximal space with dental floss is the initiating factor. The hormonal change is a precipitating factor.

prekallikrein, a plasma protein that is the precursor of kallikrein. Plasma that is deficient in prekallikrein has been found to be abnormal in thromboplastin formation, kinin generation, evolution of a permeability globulin, and plasmin formation. Prekallikrein

deficiency leads to Fletcher factor deficiency, a congenital disease.

prematurities. See **contact, deflective occlusal** and **contact, interceptive occlusal.**

premaxilla, floating, (not current). See **premaxilla, loose.**

premaxilla, loose (floating premaxilla), **1.** the nonunion of the premaxillary process with the lateral maxillary segments, so that the premaxilla is loose, or floating. The position of the loose premaxilla in relation to the lateral maxillary segments varies among patients. **2.** the administration of a tranquilizing drug, a drug that influences blood clotting time, or any other drug that produces a preplanned set of conditions and is administered preceding any dental procedures.

premedication, 1. any sedative, tranquilizer, hypnotic, or anticholinergic medication administered before anesthesia. **2.** the administration of medication before anesthesia and/or an invasive procedure.

premium, the amount charged by a dental benefits organization for coverage of a level of benefits for a specified time.

p., earned, that portion of a policy's premium payment for which the protection of the policy has already been given.

p. rate, the price per unit of insurance.

p. tax, an assessment levied by a state government, usually on the net premium income collected in that state by insurance companies.

p., unearned, that part of the premium applicable to the unexpired part of the policy period.

premolar (bicuspid), one of the eight teeth in humans, four in each jaw, between the canines and first molars; usually has two cusps; replaces the molars of the deciduous dentition.

prenatal care, the health care provided the mother and fetus before childbirth.

preoperative cast. See **cast, diagnostic.**

preoperative record. See **record, preoperative.**

prepaid dental plan, a method of financing the cost of dental care for a defined population in advance of receipt of services.

prepaid group practice. See **closed panel.**

preparation, the selected form given to a natural tooth when it is reduced by instrumentation to receive a prosthesis (for example, an artificial crown or a retainer for a fixed or removable prosthesis). The selection of the form is guided by clinical circumstances and physical properties of the materials that make up the prosthesis. See also **preparation, mouth.**

p., cavity, one of the various operations in which carious material is removed from teeth and biomechanically correct forms are established in the teeth to receive and retain restorations. A constant requirement is provision for prevention of failure of the restoration through recurrence of decay or inadequate resistance to applied stresses.

p., initial, one of a number of procedures aimed at preparing the patient for final treatment. The objectives consist of eliminating or reducing all the local etiologic factors and environmental influences before the operative procedures and establishing a sequence of therapy for the patient.

p., slice, a type of cavity preparation for Class 2 cast restorations. The proximal portion is formed by removing a sufficient slice of the proximal convexity of the tooth to achieve cleansable margins and a line of draw; a tapered keyway or two keyed grooves or channels in the proximal surface provide retention form.

p., surgical, any modification using surgical procedures that may be required for preparing the oral structures for prosthodontic treatment.

preparation, mouth, one of the various necessary procedures applied to the oral structures preparatory to the making of a final impression for a prosthesis.

prepubertal (prēpyōō′bertǝl), before the onset of puberty.

presbyopia (prez′bī·o′pē·ǝ) (farsightedness, hyperopia), a form of optical distortion affecting the vision of patients, particularly those of advancing age. It is dependent on diminution of the power of the accommodation of the lens as a result of loss of elasticity of the crystalline lens, causing the near point of distinct vision to be removed farther from the eye.

prescription (prēskrip′shǝn), a written direction for the preparation and use of medicine or an appliance; a medical recipe; a prescribed remedy. Also used in dentistry to describe the treatment plan.

p., extemporaneous (magistral prescription), **1.** a prescription for a nonofficial drug. **2.** a prescription that directs the pharmacist to compound the specified medication, as contrasted with a prescription that specifies medication available in precompounded form.

p., magistral. See **prescription, extemporaneous.**

p., official, a prescription for an official drug.

preservation, a neurologic phenomenon such as the involuntary repetition of motor response or the continuation of a sensation after the adequate external stimulus has ceased.

preservative, a substance added to prevent deterioration.

pressoreceptor, a nerve ending that is sensitive to changes in blood pressure.

pressure, a stress or strain that may occur by compression, pull, or thrust; an applied force.

p. area. See **area, pressure.**

p. atrophy. See **atrophy, pressure.**

p., biting, the actual or potential power used in bringing the teeth into contact. See also **pressure, occlusal.**

p., blood, the pressure exerted on arterial walls by the blood when the heart is in systole (systolic pressure), and the pressure maintained by the elasticity of the arteries when the heart is in diastole (diastolic pressure). A consistent arterial pressure greater than 140/90 is considered abnormally high and suggestive of hypertensive vascular disease.

p., deeper, any pressure to the body—in excess of that which stimulates Meissner's corpuscles, Merkel's disks, or the hair receptors of light touch—that stimulates the deeper receptors such as Pacini's corpuscles. These latter deep-pressure perception organs lie in the inner layers of the dermis and in the muscle and tendon groups.

p., equalization of, the act of distributing pressure evenly.

p., hand, force applied by an instrument held in the hand.

p., hydraulic, pressure transmitted by a liquid trapped between the tooth and a restoration being cemented.

p., hydrostatic, the pressure in the circulatory system exerted by the volume of blood when it is confined in a blood vessel. The hydrostatic pressure, coupled with the osmotic pressure within a capillary is opposed by the hydrostatic and osmotic pressure of the surrounding tissues. Fluids flow from the higher pressure areas to the lower pressure areas.

p., intrapleural, pressure within the pleura.

p., occlusal, any force exerted on the occlusal surfaces of teeth. See also **force, occlusal** and **load, occlusal.**

p., osmotic, the stress that develops when solutions containing different concentrations of solute in a common solvent are separated by a membrane that is permeable to the solvent but not the solute.

p., partial, the pressure exerted by each of the constituents of a mixture of gases.

p., pulse, the difference between systolic and diastolic pressure.

p. sensibility, the ability to detect light touch and deep pressure. See also **corpuscle, Meissner's; corpuscle, Merkel's;** and **corpuscle, Pacini's.**

presumption, an inference as to the existence of some fact, drawn from the existence of some other fact; an inference that common sense draws from circumstances usually occurring in such cases.

presurgical impression, an overextended impression of the intact mandible before the first surgical stage. The cast made for this impression is altered so that the surgical tray may be fabricated on it.

pretreatment, before treatment; refers to the protocols required before beginning therapy, usually of a diagnostic nature.

p. estimate. See **predetermination.**

prevailing fee, the term used by some dental benefits organizations to refer to the fee most commonly charged for a dental service in a given area.

prevalence, a term used in epidemiology that includes all of the new and old cases of a disease or occurrence of an event during a particular period of time. Prevalence is expressed as a ratio in which the number of events is the numerator and the population at risk is the denominator.

prevent, to keep from happening or existing, especially by precautionary measures.

preventive, avoiding occurrence.

p. dentistry, the procedures in dental practice and health programs that prevent the occurrence of oral diseases.

p. medicine, the branch of medicine that is concerned with the prevention of disease and methods for increasing the power of the patient and community to resist disease and prolong life.

p. orthodontic treatment, dental services intended to prevent the development of a malocclusion by maintaining the integrity of an otherwise normally developing dentition. Typical services include dental restorations, temporary prostheses (space maintainers) to replace prematurely lost deciduous teeth, and removal of deciduous teeth that fail to shed normally to allow the permanent successors to erupt satisfactorily.

Prevotella, a genus of gram-negative, anaerobic, non-spore–forming, nonmotile rods. Organisms of this genus were originally classified as members of the *Bacteroides* genus but overwhelming biochemical and chemical findings in 1990 indicated the need to separate them from other *Bacteroides* species; hence, this new genus was established.

prilocaine hydrochloride (local), *trade name:* Citanest; *drug class:* amide local anesthetic; *action:* inhibits ion fluxes across membranes, particularly sodium transport across cell membrane; decreases rise of depolarization phase of action potential; blocks nerve action potential; *use:* local dental anesthesia.

prima facie (prī′mə fā′shē·ə′), on the face of it; so far as can be judged from the first appearance; presumably.

primaquine phosphate, *trade name:* generic; *drug class:* antiprotozoal; *action:* unknown; thought to destroy exoerythrocytic forms by gametocidal action; *use:* malaria caused by *P. vivax.*

primary, first in time; first in order in any series.

P

p. beam. See radiation, primary.

p. care, the first contact with a health care provider in a given episode of illness that leads to a decision regarding a course of action to resolve the health problem presented by the patient.

p. fixation, the immediate postoperative fastening of an implant to bone by means of wires, screws, or a superstructure until, through natural healing and adhesion, final fixation occurs.

p. health care, a basic level of health care that includes programs directed at the promotion of health, early diagnosis of disease or disability, and prevention of disease.

p. intention healing, the healing of a wound directly at the incision site.

p. lymphoma of the brain, a secondary neoplasm associated with AIDS.

p. radiation. See **radiation, primary.**

primate (prī'māt), a member of the biologic order of animals of the chordate class Mammalia. The primate order includes lemurs, monkeys, apes, and humans.

p. space, the space that occurs between the canine and first premolar teeth in adult primates but that is normally absent in man. However, spacing between the primary canine and primary first molar normally occurs in the anterior primary dentition in children. This spacing is referred to as a *primate space.*

primodone, *trade name:* Myidone, Mysoline; *drug class:* anticonvulsant, barbiturate derivative; *action:* raises seizure threshold by unknown mechanism; may be related to facilitation of GABA; metabolized to phenobarbital; *uses:* tonic-clonic (grand mal), complex-partial psychomotor seizures.

principal, the chief; highest in rank; the source of authority.

p. in law of agency, the employer; the person who gives authority to an agent to act for him.

prior authorization. See **predetermination.**

privacy, a culturally specific concept defining the degree of one's personal responsibility to others in regulating behavior that is regarded as intrusive.

private practice, to engage in one's profession as an independent provider rather than as an employee.

privileges, the authority granted to a physician or dentist by a hospital governing board to provide patient care in the hospital. Clinical privileges are limited to the individual's license, experience, and competence.

p.r.n. See **pro re nata.**

pro forma, a pro forma financial statement is one that shows the way that the actual statement will look if certain specified assumptions are realized. Pro forma statements are usually a future projection.

pro re nata (prō rē nē'tə) **(p.r.n.),** a Latin phrase meaning "occasionally as needed" or "according to circumstances."

proaccelerin (prō'aksel'ərin) (factor V, labile factor, plasma accelerator globulin, plasma ac-globulin, proprothrombinase, prothrombin conversion accelerator I), an unstable protein found in the blood; the precursor of accelerin.

proandrogens (prō·an'drōjenz), compounds that are not androgenic when applied locally but that have androgenic activity when metabolized in the organism. Included are cortisone and cortisol, which may be converted within the organism to androgens such as adrenosterone, 11-ketoandrosterone, and 11-hydroxyandrosterone.

probability, 1. a measure of the increased likelihood that something will occur. **2.** a mathematic ratio of the number of times something will occur to the total number of possible occurrences.

probative (pro'bətiv), in the law of evidence, tending to prove or actually proving.

probe, a slender, flexible instrument designed for introduction into a wound or cavity for purposes of exploration.

p., lacrimal, an instrument useful in probing the lumen of duct structures, such as the nasolacrimal or salivary gland ducts.

p., periodontal, a fine calibrated instrument designed and used for measuring the depth and topography of gingival and periodontal pockets. Also used to determine the degree of attachment and adaptation of the gingival tissues to the tooth.

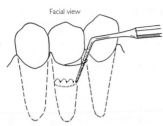

Facial view

Periodontal probe. (Parr, 1978.)

probenecid, *trade names:* Benemid, Probalan; *drug class:* uricocuric; *action:* inhibits tubular reabsorption of urates, with increased excretion of uric acids; *uses:* hyperuricemia in gout, gouty arthritis, adjunct to cephalosporin or penicillin treatment by reducing excretion and maintaining high blood levels of medication.

probucol, *trade names:* Bifenabid, Lesterol, Lorelco, Lurselle, Super lipid; *drug class:* antihyperlipidemic; *action:* increases bile acid excretion, catabolism of LDL-cholesterol; may block oxidation of LDL-cholesterol; *use:* severe hypercholesterolemia when other treatment is unsuccessful.

procabazine HCl; *trade name:* Natulane; *drug class:* antineoplastic, miscellaneous; *action:* inhibits DNA, RNA, protein synthesis; has multiple sites of action; a nonvesicant; also inhibits monoamine oxidase enzymes; *uses:* lymphoma, Hodgkin's disease, cancers resistant to other therapy.

procainamide HCl, *trade names:* Procan SR, Promine, Pronestyl; *drug class:* antidysrhythmic (Class IA); *action:* depresses excitability of cardiac muscle to electrical stimulation and slows conduction in atrium, bundle of His, and ventricle; *uses:* PVCs, atrial fibrillation, PAT, atrial dysrhythmias, ventricular tachycardia.

procaine hydrochloride (prōkān hī′drōklô′rīd), a local anesthetic agent; 2-diethylaminoethyl 4-aminobenzoate hydrochloride.

procedure (prōsē′jər), a series of steps followed in a regular, orderly, definite way, by which a desired result is accomplished.

p., dental prosthetic laboratory, the steps in the fabrication of a dental prosthesis that do not require the presence of the patient for their accomplishment.

p., Kazanjian's (kəzan′gē·ən). See **operation, Kazanjian's.**

p., operating, the technique or method of conducting or performing an operation or form of treatment.

p., order of, the sequence of steps made in performing an operation or following through a technique. In cavity preparation the sequence is as follows: (1) obtain the required outline form, (2) obtain the required resistance form, (3) obtain the required retention form, (4) retain the required convenience form, (5) remove any remaining carious dentin, (6) finish the enamel walls, and (7) make the débridement.

p., orthodontic, therapeutic measures employed to correct malalignment and malposition of the teeth and to immobilize and stabilize periodontally involved or previously moved teeth.

p., restorative, a method or mode of action that reestablishes or reforms a tooth or teeth or portions thereof to anatomic or functional form and health.

process (pros′es, prō′ses), in anatomy, a marked prominence or projection of a bone. In dentistry, a series of operations that convert a wax pattern, such as that of a denture base, into a solid denture base of another material. See also **denture curing.**

p., alveolar, the portion of the maxillae or mandible that forms the dental arch and serves as a bony investment for the teeth. Its cortical covering is continuous with the compact bone of the body of the maxillae or mandible, whereas its trabecular portion is continuous with the spongiosa of the body of the jaws. See also **ridge, alveolar.**

p., condyloid (kän′diloid) *(capitulum mandibulae),* a projection of the mandible arising on the posterosuperior aspect of the mandibular ramus. It consists of a neck and an elliptically shaped head or condyle that enters into the formation of the temporomandibular joint in conjunction with the articular disk and the glenoid fossa of the temporal bone.

p., coronoid, the thin, triangular, rounded eminence originating from the anterosuperior surface of the ramus of the mandible. Provides insertion for the various fiber bundles of the temporal muscle.

p., dehiscence of alveolar. See **dehiscence.**

p., fenestration of alveolar, a circumscribed hole, located in the cortical plate over the root, that does not communicate with the crestal margin.

p., hamular (pterygoid process), the pterygoid process of the sphenoid bone; appears as a vertical projection distal to the maxillary tuberosity.

p., horizontal resorptive, the pattern of bone resorption, occurring with periodontal disease, in which the resultant level of bone is more or less flat or level in nature.

p., neck of condyloid, the part of the condyloid process that connects the condyle to the main part of the ramus.

p., pterygoid. See **process, hamular.**

processing (prä′sesing), the term that usually refers to the procedure of bringing about polymerization of appliances; processing of dentures. See also **film processing.**

p., denture, the conversion of a wax pattern of a denture or trial denture into a denture with a base made of another material, such as acrylic resin. See also **process.**

p. tank. See **tank, processing.**

procheilia (prōkel′ē-ə), a condition of protruding lips. (not current)

prochlorperazine edisylate/ prochlorperazine maleate, *trade name:* Compazine; *drug class:* phenothiazine antipsychotic; *action:* blocks neurotransmission at dopaminergic synapses in the cerebral cortex, hypothalamus, and limibc system; *uses:* antipsychotic; for nausea, vomiting.

proconvertin (prō′kənver′tin) (autoprothrombin I, cofactor V, cothromboplastin, factor VII, precursor of serum prothrombin conversion accelerator [pro-SPCA], stable factor), variously described as the inactive precursor of convertin. Recently proconvertin has been considered as a collective term for pro-SPCA and Stuart factor.

proconvertin-convertin. See **thromboplastin, extrinsic.**

proctitis, an inflammation of the rectum and anus caused by infection, trauma, drugs, allergy, or radiation injury.

procumbency (prōcəm′bensē), excessive labioaxial inclination of the incisor teeth.

procyclidine HCl, *trade name:* Kemadrin; *drug class:* anticholinergic, antidyskinetic; *action:* blockage of central acetylcholine receptors; *uses:* Parkinson symptoms, extrapyramidal symptoms associated with neuroleptic drugs.

production, the amount of work that can be accomplished in a specific length of time.

products, fission. See **fission products.**

profession, a calling; vocation; a means of livelihood or gain.

professional autonomy, the right and privilege provided by a governmental entity to a class of professionals, and to each qualified licensed caregiver within that profession, to provide services independent of supervision.

professional ethics, codes of, the rules governing the conduct, transactions, and relationships within a profession and among its publics.

p. liability, **1.** the obligation of all professionals to their clients to do no harm. **2.** the legal obligation of health care professionals, and/or their insurers, to compensate patients for injury or suffering caused by acts of omission or commission by the professionals.

p. liability insurance, insurance covering the insured against claims arising from injury, damage, or loss sustained by a patient during the course of professional services.

p. standards review organization (PSRO), a federal agency, established by Public Law 92-603, to determine the quality and appropriateness of health care services paid for, in whole or part, under the Social Security Act. Such determinations are to be made by local committees of providers.

profibrin (prōfī′brin). See **fibrinogen.**

profibrinolysin (prōfī′brinol′isin) (not current). See **plasminogen.**

profile, an outline or contour, especially one representing a side view of a human head.

p. extraoral radiographic examination. See **examination, radiographic, extraoral, profile.**

p., facial, the sagittal outline form of the face.

p. record. See **record, profile.**

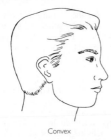

Convex

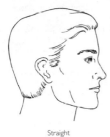

Straight

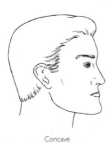

Concave

Profile facial types. (Proffit, 1993.)

profit sharing, a mechanism for funding a retirement plan for employees or members of a professional association. Members are eligible for a percentage of the net income based on predetermined formulae. Such plans, properly executed, are legal and ethical and are to be differentiated from fee-splitting, which is illegal and unethical, in which a referring professional shares in the fee-for-service income of another professional.

progeria (prōjē′rē·ə). See **syndrome, Hutchinson-Gilford.**

progesterone (prōjes′tərōn), the ovarian hormone produced by the corpus luteum and responsible for preparing the endometrium for nidation and nourishment of the ovum. It also suppresses the production of the pituitary luteinizing hormone, estrus, and ovulation and stimulates the mammary glands.

progestogen (prōjes′tōjen), an agent capable of producing effects similar to progesterone; used to correct abnormalities of the menstrual cycle.

prognathic (prog′nath′ik), pertaining to a forward relationship of the jaws to the head (anterior to the skull); denoting a protrusive lower face.

prognathism (prog′nəthizəm), facial disharmony in which one or both jaws project forward. Prognathism may be real or imaginary. Mandibular prognathism may exist when both the maxillae and the mandible increase in length or when the maxillae are of normal length but the mandible increases in length. Prognathism may be imaginary when the maxillae are underdeveloped and short and the mandible is of normal length or when the maxillary and mandibular dental relationships are normal but there is an increase in the mental prominence of the mandible.

prognathus (prognath′əs), the condition of having a marked projection of the mandible, usually resulting in a horizontal overlap of the lower anterior teeth in relation to the maxillary anterior teeth.

prognosis (prognō′sis), **1.** the foretelling of the probable course of a disease; a forecast of the outcome of a disease. **2.** a forecast of the probable result of a regimen of treatment.

program, instructions coded in a computer language to solve a problem.

programmer, a person who writes applications in a computer language. It is usually the programmer (not the machine) who should be held responsible for satisfactory and efficient solution of the problem.

programming, the process of describing in a computer language a problem or its method of solution. Programming includes planning, designing, writing, and debugging of programs.

projection, orthographic, a projection made on the assumption that the projection lines from the object to the plane of projection are at right angles to the plane.

p., gnathic planes of orthographic, the three planes of projection to which gnathologically mounted casts are oriented: the horizontal, vertical, (frontal), and profile planes. The horizontal plane is the axis-orbital plane. The hinge axis is the line of intersection for both the horizontal and frontal planes. The profile plane is the mechanical midsagittal plane of the articulator.

prolactin. See **hormone, lactogenic.**

prolapse, the falling, sinking, or sliding of an organ from its normal position or location in the body.

proliferation (prōlif'erā'shən), growth by reproduction of similar cells.

p., epithelial, a characteristic finding in inflammatory lesions affecting the gingival tissues; consists of hyperplasia of the pocket epithelium, with extension and elongation of epithelial rete pegs into the submucosa. Accompanying the hyperplastic changes in the crevicular epithelium, it is noticed that the epithelial attachment proliferates onto and alongside the cementum. Also, the multiplication of epithelial cells resulting either in increased thickness or new epithelial covering of a wound or an ulcer.

proline, a nonessential amino acid found in many proteins of the body, particularly collagen.

promazine HCl, *trade names:* Primazine, Prozine, Sparine; *drug class:* phenothiazine antipsychotic; *action:* blocks neurotransmission at dopaminergic synapses in the cerebral cortex, hypothalamus, and limbic system; mechanism for antipsychotic effects is unclear; *uses:* psychotic disorders, schizophrenia, nausea, vomiting, alcohol withdrawal.

promethazine HCl, *trade names:* Phenameth, Phenazine; *drug class:* antihistamine, H_1-receptor antagonist; *action:* acts on blood vessels, gastrointestinal and respiratory systems by competing with histamine for H_1-receptor site; decreases allergic response by blocking histamine; *uses:* motion sickness, rhinitis, allergy symptoms, sedation, nausea, preoperative or postoperative sedation.

promissory (prom'isōr'ē), a promise; stipulation for a future act or course of conduct.

promotion, the gaining and retaining of acceptance by others of the views, products, or services of the originator of the message. Components of promotion: personal selling, advertising, sales promotion, and publicity.

p., sales, sales promotion includes those marketing activities, other than personal selling, advertising, and publicity, that stimulate consumer purchasing and dealer effectiveness. They include point-of-purchase displays, shows and exhibit demonstrations, and other nonrecurrent selling efforts.

pronasion (prōnā'zē·on), the most prominent point on the tip of the nose when the head is placed in the eye-ear (horizontal) plane.

proof, the establishment of a fact by evidence; to find the truth.

p. beyond a reasonable doubt, in criminal law, such proof as precludes every reasonable hypothesis except that which it tends to support and is wholly consistent with the defendant's guilt and inconsistent with any other rational conclusions.

p. of loss, the contractual right of the carrier or service corporation to request verification of services rendered (expenses incurred) by the submission of claim forms, radiographs, study models, and/or other diagnostic material.

prop, a device inserted between the jaws to maintain an open position of the mandible.

propafenone, *trade name:* Rythmol; *class:* antidysrhythmic (Class IC); *action:* able to slow conduction velocity; reduces cardiac muscle membrane responsiveness; inhibits automaticity; increases ratio of effective refractory period to action potential duration; β-blocking activity; *use:* documented life-threatening dysrhythmias.

propagation (prop'əgā'shən), the reproduction or continuance of an impulse along a nerve fiber in an afferent or efferent direction.

propantheline bromide, *trade name:* Pro-Banthine; *drug class:* anticholinergic; *action:* inhibits muscarinic actions of acetylcholine at postganglionic parasympathetic neuroeffector sites; *uses:* treatment of peptic ulcer disease, irritable bowel syndrome, duodenography, urinary incontinence.

property 403 prostaglandins

property, rightful ownership; the exclusive right to a thing.

prophylactic (prō'filak'tik), preventing disease; relating to prophylaxis.

prophylaxis (prō'filak'sis), the prevention of disease.

p., dental, a series of procedures whereby calculus, stain, and other accretions are removed from the clinical crowns of the teeth, and the clinical crowns of the teeth are polished.

propofol, *trade name:* Diprivan; *drug class:* general anesthetic; *action:* produces dose-dependent central nervous system depression; mechanism of action is unknown; *use:* induction or maintenance of anesthesia as part of a balanced anesthetic technique.

proportional limit. See **limit, elastic.**

propoxyphene napsylate/ propoxyphene HCl, *trade name:* Cotanal-65, Darvon, PP-Cap; *drug class:* synthetic opioid narcotic analgesic (Controlled Substance Schedule IV); *action:* depresses pain impulse transmission in the central nervous system by interacting with opioid receptors; *use:* mild-to-moderate pain.

propranolol HCl, *trade name:* Inderal; *drug class:* nonselective β-adrenergic blocker; *action:* competitively blocks stimulation of β-adrenergic receptors within the heart and decreases renin activity, all of which may play a role in the reduction of systolic and diastolic blood pressure; *uses:* chronic stable angina pectoris, hypertension, supraventricular dysrhythmias, migraine, myocardial infarction prophylaxis, pheochromocytoma, essential tremor, hypertrophic cardiomyopathy, anxiety.

proprietary (prōprī'əterē), controlled by a private interest; protected by patent, trademark, or copyright.

p. name, a brand name registered with the U.S. Patent Office under which the manufacturer markets his product. Also known as *trade name.*

proprioceptive influence (prō'prē-ōsep'tiv), the influence of the muscle sense (kinesthetic sense) in guiding the jaw to close in such a way as not to be injurious to the teeth. (not current)

proprioceptors (prō'prē-ōsep'tərz), sensory nerve receptors situated in the muscles, tendons, and joints that furnish information to the central nervous system concerning the movements and positions of the limbs, trunk, head, and neck, and, more specifically for the dentist, the mandible and its associated oral structures.

proprothrombinase (prō'prōthrom'binās) (not current). See **factor V.**

proptosis (proptō'sis), the forward displacement or protrusion of the eyeball. See also **exophthalmos.**

propylthiouracil (PTU), *trade name:* generic; *drug class:* thyroid hormone antagonist; *action:* blocks synthesis of thyroid hormones T_3 (triiodothyronine), T_4 (thyroxine); *uses:* preparation for thyroidectomy, thyrotoxic crisis, hyperthyroidism, thyroid storm.

prorating, a clause in a contract with participating dentists wherein they agree to accept a percentage reduction in their billings to offset the amount by which the total cost of services provided exceeds the total premium received. Prorating is a method of spreading a "loss" equitably among participating dentists.

pro-SPCA. See **precursor of serum prothrombin conversion accelerator.** (not current)

prospective review, prior assessment by a payer or payer's agent that proposed services are appropriate for a particular patient, and/or the patient and the category of service are covered by a benefits plan. See also **preauthorization; precertification predetermination;** and **second-opinion program.**

prospective study, a study designed to determine the relationship between a condition and a characteristic shared by some members of a group. The population selected is healthy at the beginning of the study. Some of the members share a particular characteristic, such as cigarette smoking, while others do not. The study follows the population groups over a long period of time, noting the rate at which a condition, such as lung cancer, occurs in the smokers and in the nonsmokers.

prostaglandins (pros'təglan'dinz), a group of potent hormonelike substances that produce a wide range of body responses such as changing capillary permeability, smooth muscle tone, clumping of platelets, and endocrine and exocrine functions. They may be used in some instances to terminate a pregnancy.

P

prostate, a gland in men that surrounds the neck of the bladder and the urethra and produces a secretion that liquefies coagulated semen.

p. cancer, a slowly progressive adenocarcinoma of the prostate gland that affects an increasing proportion of American males after the age of 50. It is the third leading cause of cancer deaths with more than 120,000 new cases reported in the United States each year.

prostatitis, acute or chronic inflammation of the prostate gland, usually the result of infection.

prosthesis (prosthē′sis), the replacement of an absent part of the human body by an artificial part.

p., cleft palate, a restoration to correct congenital or acquired defects in the palate and related structures if they are involved.

p., complete denture. See **denture, complete.**

p., cranial, an artificial material (alloplast) used to replace a portion of the skull.

p., definitive, a permanent type of substitute for missing tissue.

p., dental, an artificial replacement for one or more natural teeth and/or associated structures.

p., expansion, a prosthesis used to expand the lateral segment of the maxilla in unilateral or bilateral cleft of the soft and hard palates and alveolar processes.

p., feeding, a prosthesis worn by a young infant with a cleft palate to increase sucking power and to eliminate the escape of food through the nose.

p., fixed expansion, a prosthesis that cannot be readily removed and stays in position for the required length of treatment.

p., partial denture. See **denture, partial.**

p., periodontal, any restorative and replacement device that, by its intent and nature, is used as a therapeutic aid in the treatment of periodontal disease; it is an adjunct to other forms of periodontal therapy and does not cure periodontal disease by itself.

p., postsurgical, an artificial replacement for a missing part or parts after surgical intervention.

p., removable expansion, a prosthesis that can be removed from the mouth and replaced when indicated.

p., surgical, an appliance prepared to assist in surgical procedures and placed at the time of surgery.

p., temporary, a fixed or removable restoration for which a more permanent appliance is planned within a short period of time.

prosthetic appliance (prosthet′ik). See **appliance, prosthetic.**

prosthetic restoration. See **prosthesis.**

prosthetics (prosthet′iks), the art and science of supplying, fitting, and servicing artificial replacements for missing parts of the human body.

p., complete denture, 1. the restoration of the natural teeth and their associated parts in the dental arch by artificial replacements. **2.** the phase of dental prosthetics dealing with the restoration of function when one or both dental arches have been rendered edentulous.

p., dental. See **prosthodontics.**

p., full denture. See **prosthetics, complete denture.**

p., maxillofacial, the branch of prosthodontics concerned with the restoration of stomatognathic and associated facial structures that have been affected by disease, injury, surgery, or congenital defect.

p., partial denture, the dental service that, by replacing one or more but less than all the teeth of a dental arch, avoids the degenerative changes resulting from tooth movement and may thus achieve preventive measures of maximum benefit toward the maintenance of optimal oral health as well as reasonable restoration of dental functions.

prosthetic speech aid. See **aid, speech, prosthetic.**

prosthetist (pros′thətist), the principal responsible individual involved in the construction of an artificial replacement for any part of the human body.

prosthion (pros′thē·on), the point of the upper alveolar process that projects most anteriorly in the midline.

prosthodontia (pros′thōdon′shē·ə). See **prosthodontics.**

prosthodontics (pros′thōdon′tiks) (prosthetic dentistry), the part of dentistry pertaining to the restoration and maintenance of oral function, comfort, appearance, and health of the patient by the replacement of missing teeth and contiguous tissues with artificial substitutes. Prosthodontics has three main branches: removable prosthodontics, fixed prosthodontics, and maxillofacial prosthetics.

p., fixed, the branch of prosthodontics concerned with the replacement and/or restoration of teeth by artificial substitutes that are not readily removable.

prosthodontist (pros'thōdon'tist), a dentist engaged in the practice of prosthodontics. A specialist in the practice of prosthodontics.

protective apron. See **apron, lead.**

protective clothing, clothing required to shield or guard the wearer from infectious, toxic, or harmful substances while engaged in employment. Federal and state statutes govern the use of such apparel.

protective devices, articles designed to guard or shield an employee from harm, which include but are not limited to helmets, protective eye glasses, noise-dampening ear protectors, railings, and knife and saw guards. Federal and state statutes govern the use and placement of safety measures.

protein (prō'tēn), any one of a group of complex organic nitrogenous compounds; the principal constituent of cell protoplasm. Polymers of amino acids that are joined by peptide or amide bonds.

p., anabolic. See **steroid, C-19 cortico-.**

p., Bence Jones, a special protein found in the blood and urine of patients with multiple myeloma and occasionally other diseases involving bone marrow, such as sarcoma and leukemia.

p., C-reactive, a mucoprotein whose presence in serum is always abnormal. It may be present in a variety of inflammatory or necrotic disease processes. It is almost always present in the serum in acute rheumatic fever.

p. deficiency. See **deficiency, protein.**

p. kinase, a protein that catalyzes the transfer of a phosphate group from adenosine triphosphate to produce a phosphoprotein.

p., plasma, blood serum contains 6.5 to 8 grams percent of a complex mixture of proteins, including albumin, globulin, and fibrinogen.

p. specificity, the arrangement of protein molecules in numerous spatial configurations to suit the special needs of the physical and chemical activities of the cell. The wide degree of variability of protein structures permits a high degree of specificity of tissue within one body. This characteristic of protein specificity is of great significance in blood transfusions, tissue grafts, and many allergic manifestations.

p., thromboplastic. See **factor III.**

proteinuria (prō'tēnōō'rē ə), the presence of protein in the urine. Proteinuria is an indication of kidney disease.

p., orthostatic (postural proteinuria), proteinuria that occurs during daily activities but does not occur when the individual is recumbent.

p., physiologic. See **proteinuria, transient.**

p., postural. See **proteinuria, orthostatic.**

p., transient (physiologic proteinuria), proteinuria that occurs in normal persons after a high-protein meal, violent exercise, severe emotional stress, or syncope. It may occur after an epileptic seizure or during pregnancy. It disappears after the cause subsides.

proteoglycans, mucopolysaccharides bound to protein chains occurring in the extracellular matrix of connective tissue.

Proteus, a genus of motile, gramnegative bacilli often associated with nosocomial infections and normally found in feces, water, and soil. Proteus may cause urinary tract infections, pyelonephritis, wound infections, diarrhea, bacteremia, and endotoxic shock.

Prothero "cone" theory. See **retention.** (not current)

prothrombase (prōthrom'bās). See **factor II** and **prothrombin.**

prothrombin (prōthrom'bin) (factor II, prothrombase, thrombogen), a glycoprotein precursor of thrombin that is produced in the liver and is necessary for the coagulation of blood. A prothrombin deficiency is uncommon but may occur in liver disease. Vitamin K is essential for the synth~~~~ of prothrombin.

p. B. See **factor II.**

p., component A of. See

P

p., component B of. See **factor VII.**

p. time, a one-stage test for detecting certain plasma coagulation defects caused by a deficiency of factors V, VII, or X. Thromboplastin and calcium are added to a sample of the patient's plasma and, simultaneously, to a sample from a normal control. The amount of time required for clot formation in both samples is observed. A prolonged prothrombin time indicates deficiency in one of the factors. Normal findings of prothrombin time are 11 to 12.5 seconds.

prothrombinase (prōthrom′binās) (complete thromboplastin, direct activator of prothrombin, extrinsic prothrombin activator), an inferred direct activator of prothrombin common to tissue and plasma coagulation systems. See also **factor V.**

prothrombinogen (prō′thrombin′ə-jen) (not current). See **factor VII.**

prothrombokinase (prōthrom′bōki′ nās). See **factor VIII.**

prothromboplastin, beta (prōthrom′ bōplas′tin). See **factor IX.**

proton (prō′ton), an elementary particle having a positive charge equivalent to the negative charge of the electron but possessing a mass approximately 1845 times as great; the proton is a nuclear particle, whereas the electron is extranuclear.

protoplasm (prō′tōplazəm), a living substance; composed mainly of five basic materials: carbohydrates, electrolytes, lipids, proteins, and water and having the properties of both a complex solution and a heterogeneous colloid. The cell nucleus and cytoplasm are two major subdivisions of protoplasm.

protraction (prōtrak′shən), a condition in which teeth or other maxillary or mandibular structures are situated anterior to their normal position.

protriptyline HCl, *trade names:* Vivactil; *drug class:* tricyclic antidepressant; *action:* inhibits both norepinephrine and serotonin (5-HT) uptake in the brain; *use:* depression.

protrusion (prōtrōō′zhən), the teeth and/or jaws protrude further forward than normal.

p., bimaxillary, a relatively forward position, or prognathism, of the maxillary and mandibular teeth, alveolar processes, or jaws.

p., double, a definite labioversion of the maxillary and mandibular anterior teeth.

p., forward, a protrusion forward from the centric position.

p., mandibular, an abnormal protrusion of the mandible, as in a Class III malocclusion.

p., maxillary, an abnormal protrusion of the maxillae.

protrusive checkbite. See **record, interocclusal, protrusive.**

protrusive occlusion. See **occlusion, protrusive.**

protrusive position. See **position, protrusive.**

protrusive record. See **record, protrusive.**

protrusive relation. See **relation, jaw, protrusive.**

provider, a governmental term used to denote health care institutions; sometimes used as a synonym for practitioner.

provisional prosthesis, an interim prosthesis worn for varying periods of time.

provisional splint. See **splint, provisional.**

proximal surface. See **surface, proximal.**

proximate cause, one that directly produces an effect; that which in ordinary, natural sequence produces a specific result with no agencies intervening.

pruritus (prōōrī′təs), itching.

Prussian blue, a chemical stain used on microscopic preparations. It demonstrates the presence of copper by developing a bright blue color.

pseudarthrosis (sōō′darthrō′sis), a false joint; sometimes seen after a fracture.

pseudoephedrine HCl/pseudoephedrine sulfate, *trade name:* Balminil, Benylin, Cenafed, Sudafed, Sufedrin; *drug class:* α-adrenergic agonist; *action:* acts primarily on α-receptors, causing vasoconstriction in blood vessels; has more β activity and, to a lesser degree, central nervous system stimulant effects.

pseudoepitheliomatous hyperplasia (PEH) (sōō′dō·ep′ithēlē·əl hī′per-plā′zē·ə), a type of epithelial hyperplasia associated with chronic inflammatory response; distinguished from squamous cell carcinoma by the lack of dysplastic cytologic characteristics.

pseudohemophilia (soo′dōhē′mōfil′ē·ə), the term used to describe several hemorrhagic states: (1) von Willebrand's disease, pseudohemophilia type B, vascular hemophilia; (2) a hereditary disease in which prolonged bleeding is the only consistent abnormality detected by currently available tests. See also **purpura, thrombocytopenic.**

pseudomembrane, a loosely adherent, grayish false membrane typical of intracellular coagulation necrosis. It is formed by necrotic epithelium embedded in fibrin, leukocytes, and erythrocytes. It is seen in Vincent's infection and diphtheria. Removal leaves a raw, bleeding surface.

Pseudomonas, a genus of gramnegative bacteria that includes several free-living species of soil and water and some opportunistic pathogens isolated from wounds, burns, and infections of the urinary tract.

pseudopocket, a pocket formed by gingival hyperplasia and edema without apical migration of the epithelial attachment. (not current) See also **pocket, gingival.**

pseudopod, a temporary protoplasmic limblike process of an amoeba that can be extended to propel itself or to engulf food.

psoriasis (sōrī′·əsis), a papulosquamous inflammatory skin disease of unknown etiology. Rare oral lesions consist of red patches with white, scaly surfaces.

PSP test. See **test, phenolsulfonphthalein.**

psychiatry, the branch of medical science that deals with the causes, treatment, and prevention of mental, emotional, and behavioral disorders.

psychology, 1. the study of behavior and the functions and processes of the mind, especially as related to the social and physical environment. 2. a profession that involves the practical applications of knowledge, skills, and techniques in the understanding of, prevention of, or solution to individual or social problems, especially in regard to the interaction between the individual and the physical and social environment.

psychomotor, pertaining to or causing voluntary movements usually associated with neural activity.

p. development, the progressive attainment (by a child) of skills that involve both mental and muscular activity.

p. domain, the area of observable performance of skills that requires some degree of neuromuscular coordination.

psychoneurosis (sī′kōnōōrō′sis), 1. an abnormal reaction to the environment, including anxieties, phobias, hysteria, and hypochondria. 2. a term that includes neurasthenia, hysteria, psychasthenia, and mental disorders short of insanity.

psychopathology, 1. the study of the causes, processes, and manifestations of mental disorders. 2. the behavioral manifestation of any mental disorder.

psychopharmacology, the scientific study of the effects of drugs on behavior and normal and abnormal mental functions.

psychosedative (sī′kōsed′ətiv), a calming agent that reduces anxiety and tension without depressing mental or motor functions.

psychosis (sīkō′sis), a functional or organic kind of mental derangement marked by a severe disturbance of personality involving autistic thinking, loss of contact with reality, delusions, and/or hallucinations.

p., manic-depressive (cyclothymia), a psychosis characterized by varying periods of depression and excitement. One state may predominate (for example, manic-depressive reaction, manic type).

psychosomatic (sīkōsōmat′ik), 1. the expression of an emotional conflict through physical symptoms. 2. Pertaining to the mind-body relationship; having bodily symptoms of a psychic, emotional, or mental origin. See also **disease, psychosomatic.**

p. factors. See **factor, psychosomatic.**

p. medicine, the branch of medicine concerned with the interrelationships between mental and emotional reactions and somatic processes, in particular the manner in which intrapsychic conflicts influence physical symptoms.

psychotherapy, any of a large number of related methods of treating

P

mental or emotional disorders by psychologic techniques rather than by physical means.

PTA. See **plasma thromboplastin antecedent.**

PTC. See **plasma thromboplastic component.**

pterygoid lateralis, one of the four muscles of mastication, which functions to open the jaws, protrude the mandible, and move the mandible from side to side. Also called the **external pterygoid muscle.**

pterygoid, medialis, one of the four muscles of mastication. It lies medial to the ramus of the mandible and functions with the temporalis and masseter muscles to close the mandible. Also called the **internal pterygoid.**

pterygoid process (ter′igoid). See **process, hamular.**

pterygomaxillary fissure (ter′igōmak′silər′ē). See **fissure, pterygomaxillary.**

pterygomaxillary notch. See **notch, pterygomaxillary.**

PTF. See **factor, plasma thromboplastin.**

PTF-A (plasma thromboplastin factor A). See **factor VIII.**

PTF-B (plasma thromboplastin factor B). See **factor IX.**

PTF-C (plasma thromboplastin factor C). See **factor XI.**

ptosis (tō′sis) (blepharoptosis), a drooping of the upper eyelid.

PTT. See **partial prothrombin time.**

ptyalectasis (tī′əlek′təsis). See **sialoangiectasis.**

ptyalism (tī′əlizəm). See **sialorrhea.**

puberty (pyōō′bertē), the age at which the reproductive system becomes functional, with concurrent development of secondary sex characteristics. Marked by increased estrogenic activity in the female and rise of androgenic activity in the male.

public health, a field of medicine that deals with the physical and mental health of the community, particularly in such areas as water supply, waste disposal, air pollution, and food safety.

p. h. dentistry. See **community dentistry.**

public opinion, the pooled judgment or attitude of the public in regard to a specific issue. Public opinion is generally determined by polling a sample of the population, using statistical tools. Elections are formal public opinion polls by which registered voter citizens register their choice of candidates and/or referenda.

public relations, the art and science of promoting good will within the public by a corporation or governmental agency.

pulmonary edema, the accumulation of extravascular fluid in lung tissues and alveoli, caused most commonly by congestive heart failure.

pulmonary embolism, the blockage of a pulmonary artery by foreign matter such as fat, air, tumor tissue, or a thrombus that usually arises from a peripheral vein. Pulmonary embolism is difficult to distinguish from myocardial infarction and pneumonia.

pulp (pəlp) (dental pulp, tooth pulp), the organ, made up of blood vessels, nerves, and cellular elements, including odontoblasts, that forms dentin. It normally occupies the central portion of teeth.

p. amputation. See **pulpotomy.**

p., anachoresis of, the localization of microbes from the bloodstream in a damaged pulp.

p. canal. See **canal, pulp.**

p. capping. See **capping, pulp.**

p. cavity. See **cavity, pulp.**

p. chamber. See **chamber, pulp.**

p., dental. See **pulp.**

p. extirpation. See **pulpectomy.**

p. horn. See **horn, pulp.**

p. involvement. See **involvement, pulp.**

p., mummification of, dry gangrene of the dental pulp in which the pulp dries and shrivels.

p. removal. See **pulpectomy.**

p. stone. See **denticle.**

p. test, the application of a physical stimulus (electrical, heat, or cold) to determine the degree of vitality of the pulp tissue.

p. tester (vitalometer), an electric instrument of high or low frequency designed to determine the response of a pulp to an electrical stimulus.

p., tooth. See **pulp.**

p. vitality, the health status of the pulp. When the pulp tissue of a tooth has undergone complete degeneration or has been removed, the tooth is termed pulpless or nonvital.

pulpal (pəl′pəl), relating to the pulp or the pulp cavity.

pulpalgia (pəlpal′jē·ə), the sensitivity of the pulp to pain.

pulpectomy (pəlpek′təmē) (pulp extirpation, pulp removal), the complete removal of a pulp from the pulp chamber and root canal.

p., complete, the surgical removal of the pulp to the dentinocemential junction at the apex of the root.

p., partial, the surgical removal of only a part of the contents of the canal(s).

pulpitis (pəlpī′tis), an inflammation of the pulpal tissue of a tooth.

p., hypertrophic (pulp polyp), the formation and proliferation of granulation tissue from the surface of an exposed pulp.

pulpless (pəlp′les), having a nonfunctioning pulp (untreated), or a pulp that has been replaced with an inert material (treated).

p. tooth. See **tooth, pulpless.**

pulpotomy (pəlpot′əmē) (pulp amputation), the surgical amputation of the dental pulp coronal to the dentinocemential junction.

p., partial, the surgical removal of only a part of the tissue in the pulpal chamber.

p., total or complete, the surgical removal of the entire contents of the pulpal chamber at the entrance of the root canal(s).

pulse (pəls), the rhythmic expansion and contraction of arteries resulting from the surges of blood through the arteries. The pulse can be felt by the fingers in arteries that are close to the skin.

p., arterial, the pulsation of an artery produced by the rise and fall in blood pressure as the heart goes into systole and diastole and observed clinically by palpation of the radial artery. The pulse rate at birth is approximately 130 beats/min and diminishes to approximately 70 beats/min in the healthy adult. The range of normalcy is from 50 or 60 to 80 or 90 beats/min.

p. pressure. See **pressure, pulse.**

p., venous, pulsation of a vein; most easily felt in the right jugular vein.

pumice (pəm′is), a type of volcanic glass used as an abrasive. Pumice is prepared in various grits and is used for finishing and polishing in den-

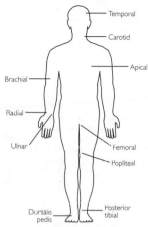

Pulse points. (Potter, 1996.)

tistry. It is also used in the prophylaxis of natural teeth.

punch biopsy, the removal of tissue for diagnostic purposes using a sharp, cylindrical, hollow instrument placed over the tissue to be excised and rotated with slight pressure until an incision of proper depth is achieved. The tissue within the incision is lifted, and the base is excised with a scissor or scalpel blade.

punch, rubber dam, an instrument used to punch holes of varying sizes in a rubber dam so that it may be applied to the teeth.

pupil, Argyll Robertson, pupillary abnormalities associated with tabes dorsalis (neurosyphilis), manifested by miosis, the absence of a ciliospinal reflex, and a reaction to accommodation but not to light.

purchaser, a program sponsor, often an employer or union, that contracts with the dental benefits organization to provide dental benefits to an enrolled population.

purchasing cooperative, a group of dentists pooling their financial resources to purchase large quantities of supplies and equipment for the purpose of obtaining a discount.

purpura (pur′pyo͞orə), extravasation of blood into the tissues, resulting in blue to black lesions of the skin or mucosa (petechiae and ecchymoses).

p., *allergic (anaphylactoid purpura),* any thrombocytopenic or nonthrombocytopenic purpura related to an allergic reaction. Manifestations other than ecchymoses and petechiae associated with erythema and inflammation include the common symptoms of allergy.

p., *anaphylactoid.* See **purpura, allergic.**

p., *essential.* See **purpura, thrombocytopenic, idiopathic.**

p. hemorrhagica. See **purpura, thrombocytopenic** and **purpura, thrombocytopenic, idiopathic.**

p., *idiopathic thrombocytopenic (essential purpura, land scurvy, primary purpura, purpura hemorrhagica),* a thrombocytopenic purpura of unknown cause.

p., *nonthrombocytopenic,* purpura usually related to increased capillary permeability. Included are allergic purpuras and those resulting from vitamin C deficiency, bacterial toxins (scarlet fever, typhoid), drug intoxications, and metabolic toxins (nephritis, liver disease).

p., *primary.* See **purpura, thrombocytopenic, idiopathic.**

p., *secondary.* See **purpura, thrombocytopenic, symptomatic.**

p., *thrombocytopathic,* bleeding associated with qualitative abnormalities of the platelets.

p., *thrombocytopenic (essential thrombopenia, pseudohemophilia, hemorrhagica, Werlhof's disease),* severe ecchymoses and petechiae associated with marked reduction in the numbers of blood platelets. There is prolonged bleeding time and poor clot retraction, but the coagulation and prothrombin times are normal. Hemorrhage may occur spontaneously from any area of the oral mucosa. This disease may be acute and fatal, whereas in other instances it may run a chronic course with intermittent attacks.

p., *symptomatic thrombocytopenic (secondary purpura),* purpura resulting from the effects of chemical, physical, vegetable, or animal agents or infections or related blood disorders.

p., *thrombotic thrombocytopenic,* a febrile disease of unknown cause characterized by hemolytic anemia, neurologic symptoms, hemorrhage into the skin and mucous membranes, icterus, hepatosplenomegaly, low platelet count, and platelet thrombi occluding capillaries and arterioles.

purulent discharge (pyōō'rōōlent). See **pus.**

pus (pəs) (purulent discharge), an inflammatory exudate formed within the tissues; consists of polymorphonuclear leukocytes, degenerated and liquefied tissue elements, microorganisms, and tissue fluids. It may form within the tissues in periodontitis and escape via the ulcerated pocket epithelium into the oral environment. The suppurative material may be retained within the tissues when the orifice of the periodontal pocket is blocked, thus creating a favorable circumstance for the formation of a periodontal abscess.

pustule (pus'chōōl), a vesicular lesion containing pus rather than clear fluid.

putrescine, a foul-smelling toxic ptomaine produced by the decomposition of the amino acid ornithine during the decay of animal tissues, bacillus cultures, and fecal bacteria.

pyknik (pik'nik), a body structure characterized by a short, squat appearance. (not current)

pyknosis (piknō'sis), increased basophilia and shrinkage of the nucleus of a dying cell.

pyogenic (pī'əjen'ik), pus-producing.

pyorrhea (pī'ərē'ə), an antiquated term used to designate periodontal disease. Generally, it means "flow of pus," which previously was a feature of periodontal disease. Before the use of the term *pyorrhea,* periodontitis was designated as *Riggs' disease* and *Fauchard's disease.* Still retained in some communities as a lay term for *periodontal disease.*

pyrazinamide, *trade name:* generic; *drug class:* antitubercular; *action:* bactericidal interference with lipid, nucleic acid biosynthesis; *use:* TB, as an adjunct with other drugs.

pyrexia (pīrek'sē-ə). See **fever.**

pyridostigmine bromide, *trade names:* Mestinon, Regonol; *drug class:* cholinergic; *action:* inhibits destruction of acetylcholine, which increases concentration at sites where acetylcholine is released; this facilitates transmission of impulses across myoneural junction; *uses:* nondepolarizing muscle relaxant antagonist, myasthenia gravis.

pyridoxine deficiency, a lack of a required level of pyridoxine, which causes irritability and may lead to convulsions and peripheral neuritis.

pyridoxine HCl (pēr'idok'sēn) **(vitamin B$_6$),** *trade names:* Beesix, Nestrex; *drug class:* vitamin B$_6$, water soluble; *action:* needed for fat, protein, and carbohydrate metabolism as a coenzyme; *uses:* vitamin B$_6$ deficiency associated with inborn errors of metabolism, inadequate diet. See also **vitamin** B$_6$.

pyrometer (pīrom'ətər), an instrument for measuring temperature by the change of electrical resistance within a thermocouple. It is a milli voltmeter calibrated in degrees of temperature.

pyrophosphatase, any enzyme that cleaves an inorganic pyrophosphate from ATP, leaving AMP.

pyruvate kinase, an enzyme essential for anaerobic glycolysis in red blood cells.

pyuria (pīyoo'rē-ə), abnormal numbers of white blood cells in the urine. Without proteinuria, it suggests infection of the urinary tract; with proteinuria, it suggests infection of the kidney (pyelonephritis).

q.i.d. (quater in die), a Latin phrase used in prescription writing meaning "4 times a day."

q.4.h. (quaque quarta hora), a Latin phrase used in prescription writing meaning "every 4 hours."

q.s. (quantum satis, quantum sufficit), a Latin phrase used in prescription writing meaning "a sufficient quantity."

quack, one who professes to have medical or dental skill that is not possessed; one who practices medicine or dentistry without adequate preparation or proper qualification.

quad helix appliance, a fixed, spring-loaded orthodontic appliance using four helix springs; used primarily to expand the maxillary dental arch.

quadrant, one quarter of a circle; also used to describe one fourth of the combined dental arches. One half of the maxillary dental arch would be one quadrant of the combined dental arches.

quadriplegia, an abnormal condition characterized by paralysis of both arms and legs and the trunk of the body below the level of the associated injury to the spinal cord. This disorder is usually caused by a spinal cord injury in the area of the fifth to seventh cervical vertebrae. Automobile accidents and sporting mishaps are common causes.

qualified, having the required ability; fitted; entitled.

quality, in reference to the voice, the acoustic characteristics of vowels resulting from their overtone structure or the relative intensities of their frequency component.

quality assessment, 1. the measurement of quality; generally includes the selection of an aspect of dental care or the dental care system to be evaluated; establishing criteria and standards for quality dental care and comparing treatment with these criteria and standards. **2.** the measure of the quality of care provided in a particular setting.

quality assurance, 1. procedures for checking the quality of dental care provided by participating dentists and correcting any irregularities. Synonyms are *quality control, quality evaluation.* **2.** the assessment or measurement of the quality of care and the implementation of any necessary changes to maintain or improve the quality of care rendered.

quality assurance system, a formally organized sequence of activities in dentistry that combines assessment of the existing situation, judgments about necessary changes, development of plans to effect such changes, implementation of these plans, and reassessment to determine that the desired changes have taken place.

quality of life, a measure of the optimal energy or force that endows a person with the power to cope successfully with the full range of challenges encountered in the real world.

Q

quality of radiation. See **radiation quality.**

quality review committee, a committee established by a professional organization or institution to assess and ensure quality. Unlike a peer review committee, it can function on its own initiative with regard to a broad range of topics.

quantity of radiation. See **radiation quantity.**

quantum, a discrete unit of electromagnetic energy or of an x-ray. A quantity becomes quantized when its magnitude is restricted to a discrete set of values as opposed to a continuous set of values.

q. theory. See **theory, quantum.**

quarantine, the isolation or confinement of a person or persons with a known or possible contagious disease.

quartz. See **silica.**

q., fused, a form of silica that is amorphous and exhibits no inversion at any temperature below its fusion point; of little use in dentistry.

quasi contract, an obligation similar to a contract that arises not from an agreement of parties but from some relation between them or from a voluntary act of one of them.

quaternary ('kwä-tə[r]-,ner-ē), having four elements. Widely used in medicine, quaternary ammonium salts are molecules containing four alkyl or aryl groups attached to a nitrogen atom.

quazepam, *trade name:* Doral; *drug class:* benzodiazepine, sedative-hypnotic, Controlled Substance Schedule IV; *action:* produces CNS depression by interacting with a benzodiazepine receptor to facilitate the action of the inhibitory neurotransmitter γ-aminobutyric acid; *use:* insomnia.

quench, to cool a hot object rapidly by plunging it into water or oil.

question, hypothetical, a combination of assumed or proven facts and circumstances, stated so as to constitute a coherent and specific situation or state of facts, on which the opinion of an expert is asked by way of evidence at a trial.

questionnaire, a form usually filled out by patients that provides data concerning their dental and general health.

q., health, a list of key questions answered by the patient that permits the diagnostician to interpret the general and oral health of the patient.

quick-cure resin. See **resin, autopolymer.**

quinapril, *trade name:* Accupril; *drug class:* angiotension-converting enzyme; *action:* selectively suppresses renin-angiotensin-aldosterone system; inhibits ACE; prevents conversion of angiotensin I to angiotensin II; results in dilation of arterial and venous vessels; *use:* hypertension, alone or in combination with thiazide diuretics.

Quincke's disease (kwink'ēz). See **edema, angioneurotic.**

quinidine gluconate/quinidine polygalacturonate/quinidine sulfate, *trade names:* Cardioquin, CinQuin, Duraquin, Quinidex Extentabs, Quinora; *drug class:* antidysrhythmic (class IA); *action:* prolongs effective refractory period; decreases myocardial excitability, conduction velocity, and contractility; *uses:* PVCs, atrial flutter and fibrillation, PAT, ventricular tachycardia.

quinine, an alkaloid derived from cinchona that is effective against malaria. It is also used as an antipyretic, analgesic, sclerosing agent, and stomachic and in the treatment of atrial fibrillation and myotonia congenita.

quinine sulfate, *trade names:* Legatrin, M-Kya, Quinamm, Q-Vel; *drug class:* antimalarial; *action:* schizonticidal, but mechanism is unclear; increases refractory period in skeletal muscles; *uses: Plasmodium falciparum* malaria, nocturnal leg cramps.

quinolone, any of a class of antibiotics that act by interrupting the replication of DNA molecules in bacteria.

quinsy, a peritonsillar abscess.

quintuplet, any one of five offspring born in the same gestation period during a single pregnancy.

quotient, the number of times one amount is contained in another.

rabies, an acute, usually fatal viral disease of the central nervous system of animals. It is transmitted from animals to humans by infected blood, tissue, or most commonly, saliva. Also called *hydrophobia* (not current).

racemic (rāse′mik), referring to a mixture of equal quantities of the dextro- and levo-isomers of a compound.

rachisensible (rā′kēsen′sibəl), abnormally sensitive to spinal anesthetics (not current).

rad (r), a unit of absorbed dose of radiation: 1 r equals 100 ergs/Gm. See also **rem.**

millirad (mr), One one-thousandth of a rad. Normal background radiation in this country varies from about 50 to 200 mr per year, depending on geographic location.

radial keratotomy, a surgical procedure in which a series of tiny, shallow incisions are made on the cornea, causing it to bulge slightly to correct for nearsightedness. The operation is performed using local anesthesia and requires only a few minutes. Hospitalization is not necessary. Radial keratotomy usually corrects mild to moderate myopia.

radial pulse, the pulse of the radial artery palpated at the wrist over the radius. The radial pulse is the one most often taken and recorded because of the ease with which it is located and palpated.

radiate (rā′dē-āt), **1.** to diverge or spread from a common point; arranged in a radiating manner. **2.** to expose to radiation, as x-radiation.

radiation (rā-dē-ā′-shən), **1.** the process of emitting radiant energy in the form of waves or particles. **2.** the combined processes of emission, transmission, and absorption of radiant energy.

r., actinic, radiation capable of producing chemical change (for example, effect of light and x-rays on photographic emulsions).

r., background, radiation arising from radioactive material other than the one directly under consideration. Background radiation resulting from cosmic rays and natural radioactivity is always present. Background radiation may also exist because of radioactive substances in other parts of the building (for example, building material).

r., backscatter. See **radiation, scattered.**

r., biologic effectiveness of, the ability of a particular type of ionizing radiation to produce biologic effects on an organism with small absorbed doses. See **relative biologic effectiveness.**

r. caries, a type of tooth decay caused by the reduction in saliva that may result from the use of ionizing radiation in the treatment of oral and facial malignancies. Radiation caries is an unfortunate side effect of a necessary radical procedure to cure or prevent the spread of cancer.

r. cataract, a cataract that is caused by extended exposure of the eye to ionizing radiation in the course of treating facial cancers.

r., characteristic, radiation that originates from an atom after removal of an electron or excitation of the nucleus. The wavelength of the emitted radiation is specific, depending only on the element concerned and on the particular energy levels involved. Also refers to the specific type of secondary radiation resulting when rays from a radio ray tube strike another substance, such as copper.

r., corpuscular, subatomic particles, such as electrons, protons, neutrons, or alpha particles, that travel in streams at various velocities. All the particles have definite masses and travel at various speeds. The properties are in opposition to electromagnetic radiations, which have no mass and travel in wave forms at the speed of light. See also **radiation, electromagnetic.**

r., cosmic. See **ray, cosmic.**

r., dermatitis. See **dermatitis, radiation.**

r. detector, any device for converting radiant energy to a form more suitable for observation and recording. Exam-

R

ples include x-ray films and radiometers.

r., direct (primary radiation), radiation emanating from a tube aperture and comprising the useful beam, as compared with any stray radiation, such as that which comes from the tube container.

r., electromagnetic, forms of energy propagated by wave motion, such as photons or discrete quanta. The radiations have no matter associated with them, as opposed to corpuscular radiations, which have definite masses. They differ widely in wavelength, frequency, and photon energy and have strikingly different properties. Covering an enormous range of wavelengths (from 10^{17} to 10^{-6} Å), they include radio waves, infrared waves, visible light, ultraviolet radiation, gamma rays, and cosmic radiation. See also **radiation, corpuscular.**

r. exposure, a measure of the ionization produced in air by x-rays or gamma rays. It is the sum of the electric charges on all ions of one sign that are produced when all electrons liberated by photons in a volume of air are completely stopped, divided by the mass of air in the volume element. The unit of exposure is the roentgen.

r. field. See **x-ray beam, field size.**

r., gamma. See **ray, gamma.**

r., genetic effects of. See **genetic effects of radiation.**

r., grenz. See **ray, grenz.**

r., hard, radiation consisting of the short wavelengths (higher kilovolt peak equals greater penetration).

r. hazard. See **hazard, radiation.**

r., heterogeneous, a beam or "bundle" of radiation containing photons of many wavelengths.

r., homogeneous, a beam of radiation consisting of photons that all have the same wavelength.

r. hygiene. See **hygiene, radiation.**

r. intensity. See **intensity, radiation.**

r., ionizing, electomagnetic radiation such as x-rays and gamma rays; particulate radiation such as alpha particles, beta particles, protons, and neutrons; and all other types of radiations that produce ionization directly or indirectly.

r. leakage (stray radiation), the escape of radiation through the protective shielding of the x-ray unit tube head. This radiation is detected at the sides, top, bottom, or back of the tube head; it does not include the useful beam.

r., monochromatic. See **radiation, homogeneous.**

r. necrosis. See **necrosis, radiation.**

r., neutron. See **ray, neutron.**

r. oncology, the study of the treatment of cancer using ionizing radiation

r., primary, all radiation produced directly from the target in an x-ray tube. See also **radiation, direct.**

r. protection, provision designed to reduce human exposure to radiation. For external radiation, this provision consists of using protective barriers of radiation-absorbing material, ensuring adequate distances from the radiation sources, reducing exposure time, and combinations of these measures. For internal radiation, it involves measures to restrict inhalation, ingestion, or other modes of entry of radioactive material into the body.

r. quality, the ability of a beam of x-rays to allow the production of diagnostically useful radiographs. Usually measured in half-value layers of aluminum and controlled by the kilovolt peak.

r. quantity, amount of radiation. The amount of exposure is expressed in roentgens (R), whereas quantity of dose is expressed in rads.

r., relative biologic effectiveness of (RBE), a comparison between various types of ionizing radiation with respect to the ability to produce biologic effects with small doses.

r., remnant, the radiation passing through an object or part being examined that is available either for recording on a radiographic film or for measurement.

r., scattered (backscatter radiation), radiation whose direction has been altered. It may include secondary and stray radiation.

r., secondary, the new radiation created by primary radiation acting on or passing through matter.

r. shield. See **shield, radiation.**

r. sickness, a self-limited syndrome characterized by varying degrees of nausea, vomiting, diarrhea, and psychic depression after exposure to very large doses of ionizing radiation, particularly doses to the abdominal region. Its mechanism is not completely understood. It usually occurs a few hours after treatment and may subside within a day. It may be sufficiently severe to necessitate interrupting the treatment series, or it may incapacitate the patient.

r., soft, radiation consisting of the long wavelengths (lower kilovolt peak results in less penetration).

r., speed of, the speed of light, or approximately 186,000 miles per second.

r., stray. See **radiation leakage.**

r. survey. See **survey, radiation.**

r. therapy. See **therapy, radiation.**

r., total body, the exposure of the entire body to penetrating radiation. In theory, all cells in the body receive the same dose.

r., useful (useful beam), the part of the primary radiation that is permitted to pass from the tube housing through the tube head port, aperture, or collimating device.

radical, I. a group of atoms that acts together and forms a component of a compound. The group tends to remain bound together when a chemical reaction removes it from one compound and attaches it to another compound. A radical does not exist freely in nature. **2.** a drastic measure to cure or prevent the spread of a serious disease, such as the surgical removal of an organ, limb, or other body part.

radical neck dissection, dissection and removal of all lymph nodes and removable tissues under the skin of the neck, performed to prevent the spread of malignant tumors of the head and neck that have a reasonable chance of being controlled by such aggressive treatment.

radicular (radik′yələr), pertaining to the root; in restorative dentistry, the location at which the form of the preparation and restoration for the coronal portion of the natural tooth extends into the treated root canal of the pulpless tooth (for example, radicular preparation, radicular restoration [dowel crown]).

radicular cyst. See **cyst, radicular.**

radio-, prefix used to denote radiation from any source.

radioactive decay. See **decay, radioactive.**

radioactive isotope. See **radioisotope.**

radioactive tracer, a molecule to which a radioactive atom has been attached so that it can be followed through a physiologic system with radiation detectors.

radioactivity (rā′dē-ō-aktiv′ite), spontaneous nuclear disintegration with emission of corpuscular or electromagnetic radiations. The principal types of radioactivity are alpha disintegration, beta decay (negatron emission, positron emission, and electron capture), and isometric transition. Double beta decay is another type of radioactivity that has been postulated, and spontaneous fission and the spontaneous transformations of mesons are sometimes considered to be types of radioactivity. To be considered radioactive, a process must have a measurable lifetime between approximately 1 and 10 seconds and 1017 years, according to present experimental techniques. Radiations emitted within a time too short for measurement are called *prompt;* however, prompt radiations, including gamma rays, characteristic x-rays, conversion and auger electrons, delayed neutrons, and annihilation radiation, are often associated with radioactive disintegrations because their emission may follow the primary radioactive process.

radioallergosorbent test (RAST), a test to determine whether an atopic allergy to a substance exists. A radioimmunoassay is used to identify and quantify IgE in serum that has been mixed with any of 45 known allergens. This is an in vitro method of demonstrating allergic reactions, as opposed to the patch test, which is the common in vivo method of determining allergens.

radiobiology, the branch of the natural sciences dealing with the effects of radiation on biologic systems.

radiogram (rā′dē-ōgram′). See **radiograph.**

radiograph(s) (rā′dē-ōgraf′), an image or picture produced on a radiation-sensitive film emulsion by exposure to ionizing radiation directed through an area, region, or substance of interest, followed by chemical processing of the film. It is

R

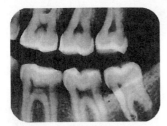

Bite-wing radiograph. (Finkbeiner, 1995.)

basically dependent on the differential absorption of radiation directed through heterogeneous media.

r., bite-wing, a form of dental radiograph that reveals approximately the coronal halves of the maxillary and mandibular teeth and portions of the interdental alveolar septa on the same film.

r., body-section, radiograph produced by rotation of the film and x-ray source around the region of interest in opposite directions during exposure, so as to blur interposed anatomic structures outside the region of interest.

r., cephalometric, extraoral radiographs produced under conditions ensuring maximal dimensional accuracy and reproducible film-object-beam relationship for purposes of cephalometric study.

r., composite, radiograph made by superimposing a radiograph of osseous tissue whose exposed border has been cut away on a radiograph of soft tissue for the purpose of detecting radiographic information concerning both the soft tissues and the osseous tissues of the head and face from a single radiographic view.

r., contrast media, radiograph that records the shadow images of the secretory apparatus of any of the salivary glands, body cavities, or fistulous tracts after the injection of a liquid radiopaque solution.

r., extraoral, radiograph produced on a film placed extraorally.

r., follow-up, radiographs made during and after therapy to follow the progress or regress of a disease, determine the course of healing, or ascertain the results of treatment.

r., intraoral, radiograph produced by placing a radiographic film within the oral cavity.

r., microscopic examination. See microradiography.

r., occlusal, a special type of intraoral radiograph made with the film held between the occluded teeth.

r., oral, radiographic representation of shadow images of all the tissues, structures, and regions of the oral cavity and its adjacent areas and associated parts.

r., panoramic, a large radiograph depicting the curvatures of the maxillae, mandible, and associated structures.

r., salivary gland. See **sialography.**

r., stereoscopic, a pair of radiographs of a structure made by shifting the position of the x-ray tube a few centimeters between each of two exposures. Such pairs provide a three-dimensional, or stereoscopic, presentation of the recorded images.

r., Towne's projection, radiographic view of the mandibular condyles and the midfacial skeleton.

radiographer (rā'dēog'rəfər), a specialist or technician in radiography.

r., oral, a specialist or technician in oral radiography.

radiographic (rā'dē-ōgraf'ik), relating to the process of radiography, the finished product, or its use.

r. anatomy. See **anatomy, radiographic.**

r. contrast. See **contrast, radiographic.**

r. density. See **density, radiographic.**

r. diagnosis. See **diagnosis, radiographic.**

r. examination. See **examination, radiographic.**

r. grid, a clear plastic device with the horizontal and vertical wires crossing each other at intervals of 1 mm; used in x-ray techniques for the purpose of measurement.

r. interpretation. See **interpretation, radiographic.**

r. localization. See **localization, radiographic.**

r. survey. See **survey, radiographic.**

radiography (rā'dē-og'rəfē), the making of shadow images on photographic emulsion by the action of ionizing radiation. The image is the result of the differential attenuation of the radiation in its passage through the object being radiographed. *Roentgenog-*

raphy refers to production of film by the use of x-rays only.

r., bone in, radiography of bone and marrow tissue. Translucencies and opacities in bone in radiographs depend on the different densities that bone and marrow spaces present to the x-rays. The configuration of bone tissue represents the topography and arrangement of bone trabeculae, which register as opaque in contrast to the translucency of the marrow spaces.

r., oral, the specialized operative and technical procedures and practices for making successful radiographic surveys, with the understanding that it involves the selection of the dental x-ray unit and its adjustments as well as the generation and application of x-rays to all phases of interest to the dental profession. It also takes into consideration all the processes necessary for the production of finished radiographs of the teeth and their supporting tissues, adjacent regions, and associated parts.

radioisotope (rā'dē-ō-ī'sōtōp), a chemical element that has been made radioactive through bombardment of neutrons in a cyclotron or atomic pile or found in a natural state.

radioisotope scan, a two-dimensional representation of the gamma rays emitted by a radioisotope, showing its concentration in a body site such as the thyroid gland, brain, or kidney. Radioisotopes used in diagnostic scanning may be administered intravenously or orally.

radiologist (rā'dēol'əjist), a person who has special experience in the science of radiant energy and radiant substances (including roentgen rays); especially a person engaged in the branch of medical science that deals with the use of radiant energy in the diagnosis and treatment of disease.

r., oral, a specialist in the art and science of oral radiology.

radiology (rā'dē-ol'əjē), **1.** the branch of medicine dealing with the diagnostic and therapeutic applications of ionizing radiation. **2.** the science of radiant energy, its use toward the extension of present knowledge, and its diverse applications for the benefit of humankind.

r., oral, all phases of the science and art of radiology that are of interest to the dental profession. Oral radiology involves the generation and application of x-rays for the purpose of recording shadow images of teeth and their supporting tissues, adjacent regions, and associated parts. It also includes the interpretation of the radiographic findings.

radiolucence (rā'dē-ōlōō'sence), relative term indicating the comparatively low attenuation of an x-ray beam produced by materials of relatively low atomic number. (The image on a radiograph of such materials is relatively dark because of the greater amount of radiation that penetrates to reach the film.)

radiolucency (rā'dē-ōlōō'sensē), a radiographic representation of decreased density of hard and soft tissue structures.

radiolucent (rā'dē-ōlōō'sent), permitting the passage of radiant energy, with relatively little attenuation by absorption. The image of radiolucent materials on a radiograph ranges from shades of gray to black.

radionuclide (rā'dē-ōnōō'klid), an unstable or radioactive type of atom characterized by the constitution of its nucleus and capable of existing for a measurable time. The nuclear constitution is specified by the number of protons (Z), number of neutrons (N), and energy content, or alternatively by the atomic number (Z), mass number $(A - N + Z)$, and atomic mass.

radiopacity (rā'dē-ōpas'itēē), relative term referring to the considerable attenuation of an x-ray beam produced by materials of relatively high atomic number. The image on a radiograph of such materials is relatively light because less radiation passes through, which prevents the exposure of the film in that area.

radiopaque (rā'dē-ōpak'), permitting the passage of radiant energy, but only with considerable or extreme attenuation of the radiation by absorption. The image of radiopaque materials on a radiograph ranges from light gray to total white or clarity on the film. See also **medium, radiopaque.**

radioparent (rā'dē-ōpar'ent), made visible by means of roentgen rays or

R

other means of radiation. Permitting the passage of x-rays or other radiation (not current).

radiopharmacy, a facility for the preparation and dispensing of radioactive drugs and the storage of radioactive materials, inventory records, and prescriptions of radioactive substances. The radiopharmacy is usually the correlation point for radioactive wastes, the unit responsible for waste disposal or storage and the center for clinical investigations using radioactive tracers.

radioresistance (rā′dē-ōrē-zis′tans), the relative resistance of cells, tissues, organs, or organisms to the injurious effects of ionizing radiation. See also **radiosensitivity.**

radiosensitivity (rā′dē-ōsen′sitiv′itē), relative susceptibility of cells, tissues, organs, organisms, and other substances to the injurious action of radiation.

radiotherapy, the treatment of neoplastic disease by using x-rays or gamma rays to prevent or slow the proliferation of malignant cells by decreasing the rate of mitosis or impairing DNA synthesis. See **therapy, radiation.**

radium (Ra), a radioactive metallic element of the alkaline earth groups. Its atomic number is 88. Four radium isotopes occur naturally and have different atomic weights: 223, 224, 226, and 228.

radon seed (rā′don), a small sealed container or tube for carrying radon. It is made of gold or glass, is inserted into the tissues for the treatment of certain disease entities, and is visible radiographically.

rale (rāl), abnormal sound that originates from the trachea, bronchi, or lungs.

ramify (ram′əfī), to branch; to diverge in various directions; to traverse in branches.

ramipril, *trade name:* Altace; *drug class:* angiotensin-converting enzyme inhibitor; *action:* selectively suppresses renin-angiotensin-aldosterone system; inhibits ACE; prevents conversion of angiotensin I to angiotensin II; results in dilation of arterial and venous vessels; *uses:* hypertension, alone or in combination with thiazide diuretics; CHF immediately after MI.

ramus (ra′məs), a branch, as of an artery, nerve, or vein. Any constant branch of a fissure, or sulcus, of the brain. In the *Basle Nomina Anatomica* terminology, the term *ramus* is given to a primary division of a nerve or blood vessel. The portions of the mandible that extend upward and backward from the horseshoe-shaped body and terminate in two processes: the articular condyloid process and the coronoid process.

r., mandibular, the bilateral, upturned, angled bony process between the body and condylar process of the mandible.

random-access memory (RAM), the part of a computer's memory available to execute programs and temporarily store date. The memory to which the operator has random access can usually be used for both reading and writing. Unless the file has been saved, RAM data are automatically erased when the computer is turned off.

random controlled trial, a study plan for a proposed new treatment in which subjects are assigned on a random basis to participate in either an experimental group receiving the new treatment or a control group that does not.

range, a crude measure of dispersion in a distribution; range is computed as the distance from the highest score to the lowest score plus one unit.

r., melting, the temperature range from the time an alloy begins to melt until it is completely molten. It varies from 100° to 200° F (38° to 70° C), in gold-platinum-palladium alloys.

r. of motion, the maximum extent to which the parts of a joint can move in extension and flexion as measured in degrees of a circle.

ranitidine, *trade name:* Zantac, Zantac EFFERdose, Zantac GELdose, Zantac 75; *drug class:* H_2 histamine receptor antagonist; *action:* inhibits histamine at H_2-receptor sites in parietal cells, which inhibit gastric acid secretion; *uses:* duodenal ulcers, gastric ulcers, hypersecretory conditions, gastroesophageal reflux disease.

Rankine scale, an absolute temperature scale calculated in degrees Fahrenheit. Absolute zero on the

Rankine scale is −460° F, equivalent to −273° C.

ranula (ran'yo͞olə), **1.** A large mucocele in the floor of the mouth. It usually results from obstruction of the ducts of the sublingual salivary glands. Less frequently, it results from obstruction of the ducts of the submandibular salivary glands. **2.** A large, mucus-containing pathologic space (mucocele), located in the floor of the mouth. It may be associated with submaxillary (submandibular) or sublingual gland secretions.

Ranvier, nodes of (rahn-vēē-ā'). See **node of Ranvier.**

raphae, midpalatine (rā'fē), the ridge of mucous membrane that marks the median line of the hard palate (not current).

rapport, a sense of mutuality and understanding; harmony, accord, confidence, and respect underlying a relationship between two persons, an essential bond between a therapist and patient.

rare earth screen, a fluorescent material such as calcium tungstate used as the basis of x-ray intensifying screens. In recent years, new materials, including the rare earths yttrium and gadolinium, have also found application in such devices. These rare earths enable lower radiation doses to be used while producing acceptable film densities.

rarefaction, bone. See **bone rarefaction.**

rash, wandering. See **tongue, geographic** (not current).

rat, Sprague-Dawley, an inbred strain of albino rat commonly used in laboratory research. There are 12 strains of inbred rats listed under "Medical Subject Headings," a supplement to *Index Medicus.* The Wistar rat is an equally popular inbred strain of albino rat used in laboratory research.

ratchet wrench, a wrench activated by its handle through a hinged catch (pawl) that causes the wrench to rotate in one direction only (may be adjusted for either direction).

rate, measurement of a thing by its ratio or given in relation to some standard.

r., basal metabolic. See **basal metabolic rate.**

r., DEF, an expression of dental caries experience in deciduous teeth.

The DEF rate is calculated by adding the number of decayed primary teeth requiring filling *(D),* decayed primary teeth requiring extraction *(E),* and primary teeth successfully filled *(F).* Missing primary teeth are not included in the count because whether they were extracted because of caries or exfoliated normally is frequently impossible to determine.

r., DMF index, a method of classifying the condition of the teeth based on the number of teeth in a given mouth that are decayed, missing, or indicated for removal and of those filled or bearing restorations.

r., erythrocyte sedimentation, the rate of settling of erythrocytes by gravity under conditions in which all factors affecting the rate are corrected, standardized, or eliminated except for alterations in the physicochemical properties of the plasma proteins. These alterations are the basis for interpretation of the rate. There is an increase in the rate in most infections. Sedimentation velocity is useful in prognosis to determine recovery from infection. Normal values vary with the method used in the determination.

r., heart, the rate of the heartbeat, expressed as the number of beats per minute. The heart rate is reflected in the pulse rate. The cardiac rate of contraction is described as normal (70 beats/min), rapid (above 100 beats/min), or slow (below 55 beats/min). Disturbances in heart rate and rhythm may be paroxysmal or persistent. Descriptive terms are *tachycardia* (increased, shallow heart rate to compensate for inadequate cardiac output) and *bradycardia* (slow, firm heart rate caused by cardiac sinus mechanisms and the vagal effect over the sympathetic innervation of the heart).

ratification (rat'ifi-cā'shən), confirmation of a previous act.

ratio, proportion; comparison.

r., A:G, the ratio of the protein albumin to globulin in the blood serum. On the basis of differential solubility with neutral salt solution, the normal values are 3.5 to 5 Gm% for albumin and 2.5 to 4 Gm% for globulin.

r., clinical crown: clinical root, the proportion of the length of the portion

R

of the tooth lying coronal to the epithelial attachment to the length of the portion of the root lying apical to the epithelial attachment. Radiographically the clinical crown is the portion of the tooth coronal to the alveolar crest; the clinical root is the part of the root apical to the alveolar crest. The radiographic crown:root ratio is useful in the evaluation and prognosis of periodontal disease.

r., grid, the relation of the height of the lead strips to the width of the nonopaque material between them. Common grid ratios are 2:8, 2:12, and 2:16.

r., water:powder, relative amounts of water and powder (usually gypsum products) in a mixture.

rationale (rash'inal'), the fundamental reasons used as the basis for a decision or action.

ray(s), a line of light, heat, or other form of radiant energy. A ray is a more or less distinct or isolated portion of radiant energy, whereas the word *rays* is a very general term for any form of radiant energy, whether vibratory or particulate.

r., alpha. See **particle, alpha.**

r., beta. See **particle, beta.**

r., cathode. See **electron stream.**

r., central, the center of an x-ray beam.

r., cosmic, radiation that originates outside the earth's atmosphere. Cosmic rays have extremely short wavelengths. They are able to produce ionization as they pass through the air and other matter and are capable of penetrating many feet of material such as lead and rock. The primary cosmic rays probably consist of atomic nuclei (mainly protons), some of which may have energies of the order of 10^{10} to 10^{15} eV. Secondary cosmic rays are produced when the primary cosmic rays interact with nuclei and electrons (for example, in the earth's atmosphere). Secondary cosmic rays consist mainly of mesons, protons, neutrons, electrons, and photons that have less energy than the primary rays. Practically all the primary cosmic rays are absorbed in the upper atmosphere. Almost all cosmic radiation observed at the earth's surface is of the secondary type.

r., gamma, photons with a shorter wavelength than those ordinarily used in diagnostic medical and dental radiography and that originate in the nuclei of atoms. A quantum of electromagnetic radiation emitted by a nucleus as a result of a quantum transition between two energy levels of the nucleus; for example, as a radioisotope decays, it gives off energy, some of which may be in the form of gamma radiation.

r., grenz (grentz), roentgen rays that are greater in length than 1 A; used in radiography of soft tissues, insects, flowers, and microscopic sections of teeth and surrounding tissues. These rays are the result of using approximately 10 to 20 kV in a specially constructed radiation-generating device. They have a wavelength of about 2 Å.

r., neutron, particulate ionizing radiation consisting of neutrons. On impact with nuclei or atoms, neutrons possess enough kinetic energy to set the nuclei or atoms in motion with sufficient velocity to ionize matter or enter into nuclear reactions that result in the emission of ionizing radiation. The former variety is usually called the *fast neutron,* and the latter the *thermoneutron,* with gradations of epithermal and slow neutrons between them.

r., roentgen (r) (rent'gən), an international unit based on the ability of radiation to ionize air. The exposure to x or gamma radiation such that the associated corpuscular emission per 0.001293 Gm of air produces, in air, ions carrying 1 esu of quantity of electricity of either sign (2.083 billion ion pairs).

r., equivalent-man (rem), the dose of any ionizing radiation that produces the same biologic effect as that produced by 1 roentgen of high-voltage x radiation.

r., equivalent-physical (rep), an unofficial unit of dose used with ionizing radiation other than x-rays or gamma rays. It is defined as the dose that produces an energy absorption of 93 ergs per Gm of tissue. For most purposes the rep can be considered equal to the rad; the latter is gradually replacing the use of rep.

Raynaud's phenomenon, spasm of the digital arteries with blanching and numbness of the extremities, induced by chilling, emotional states, or other diseases.

RBC. See **red blood cell count.**

RBE. See **radiation, biologic effectiveness of, relative.**

RDA, the Recommended Dietary Allowances of the Food and Nutrition Board of the National Research Council.

reaction (rēak′shən), opposite action, or counteraction; the response of a part to stimulation; a chemical process in which one substance is transformed into another substance or substances.

r., alarm, the first stage of the general adaptation syndrome of Hans Selye; occurs in response to severe physical and psychologic distress. Complete mobilization of body resources occurs in association with activity of the pituitary and adrenal glands and the sympathetic nervous system. See also **syndrome, general adaptation.**

r., anaphylactoid, a reaction that resembles anaphylactic shock; probably caused by the liberation of histamine, serotonin, or other substances as a consequence of the injection of colloids or finely suspended material.

r., Arthus'. See **anaphylactic hypersensitivity.**

r., heterophil, a heterophil agglutination test that measures the agglutination of the red blood cells of sheep by the serum of patients with infectious mononucleosis.

r., -id, secondary skin eruptions occurring at a distance from the primary lesion (for example, tuberculid).

r., immune, altered reactivity of the tissues to a foreign substance that was previously introduced into the body or in contact with it.

r., leukemoid, an increase in normal or abnormal white blood cells in non-leukemic conditions; simulates myelogenous, lymphatic, and rarely, monocytic leukemia.

r., Shwartzman, an antigen AB local tissue response that occurs when an intravenous injection or challenge of a bacterial endotoxin that had previously been inoculated intradermally results in a hemorrhagic, often necrotic inflammatory lesion.

r., tissue, the response of tissues to altered conditions.

reactor (rēak′tər), an apparatus in which nuclear fission may be sustained in a self-supporting reaction at a controlled rate.

read-only memory (ROM), the portion of a computer's memory in which information is permanently stored. The operator has random access to the memory but only for purposes of reading the contents. Special equipment is required to write or erase a read-only memory.

reagent, a chemical substance known to react in a specific way.

reagin(s) (rē′ājin), noncommittal term used for antibodies or antibody-like substances that differ in several respects from ordinary antibodies. It refers to the antibodies of allergic conditions (atopy) and to the antibody (reagin) concerned with the flocculation and complement fixation tests for syphilis.

real time, an application of computerized equipment allowing data to be processed with relation to ongoing external events so that the operators can make immediate decisions based on the current data output. Ultrasound scanning uses real time control systems, making results available almost simultaneously with the generation of the input data.

reamer (rē′mər), an instrument with a tapered metal shaft, more loosely spiraled than a file; used to enlarge and clean root canals.

reasonable and customary (R&C) plan, a dental benefits plan that determines benefits based only on "reasonable and customary" fee criteria. See also **usual fee; customary fee; reasonable fee.**

reasonable fee, the fee charged by a dentist for a specific dental procedure that has been modified by the nature and severity of the condition being treated and by any medical or dental complications or unusual circumstances; therefore may differ from the dentist's "usual" fee or the benefit administrator's "customary" fee.

reasonably prudent person doctrine, the concept that a person of ordinary sense will use ordinary care and skill in meeting the health care needs of a patient.

reattachment, in dentistry the reattachment of the gingival epithelium to the surface of the tooth.

R

rebase, a process of refitting a denture by replacing the denture base material without changing the occlusal relations of the teeth.

rebound (rē′bownd), **1.** recovery from illness. **2.** an outbreak of fresh reflex activity after withdrawal of a stimulus.

rebreathing, breathing into a closed system. Exhaled gas mixes with the gas in the closed system, and some of this mixture is then reinhaled. Rebreathing is used as part of a general anesthesia technique in which a rebreathing bag functions as a reservoir for anesthetic gases and oxygen. The bag may be squeezed or pumped to assist in proper respiration while the patient is under deep anesthesia.

recall, the procedure of advising or reminding a patient to have his oral health reviewed or reexamined; an important phase of preventive dentistry.

receipt, a written acknowledgment by one person of having received money or something of value from another.

r. book, the book in which the dentist or one of the auxiliaries fills out forms verifying that a specific amount of money has been paid to the account.

reception room, the area within the physical plant of the dental establishment through which patients enter the office. This is also the room in which patients await the attentions of the dentist or receptionist.

receptor(s) (rēsep′tər), a site or location within a cell or its membrane that combines with a haptophore group of a toxin, drug, enzyme, hormone, or other substance and that may elicit a specific or general response; a sensory nerve terminal that responds to stimuli of various kinds.

r., adrenergic, alpha and beta "units" associated with sympathetic neuroeffectors that react with sympathomimetic drugs to elicit the response of the effector cells.

r., sensory, receptor system built on the theory that receptor organs are specialized and respond to the law of specific nerve energies; that is, each type of end-organ, no matter what stimulus is applied, will respond (if it responds) with only a single appropriate type of sensation. Common experience shows this to be true; for example, when a person receives a blow to the eye, light is experienced as a consequence of the blow. Another factor is that the impulse will travel in only one direction, from the receptor organ back to the central nervous system. The receptor system is thus the summation in the brain of all the sensory stimuli that come from the special senses, general senses, mucous membrane, skin, and deeper tissues and is the basis for instruction sent to the musculoskeletal system for action, as in the masticatory phenomenon.

recession (rēsesh′-un), a moving back or withdrawal.

r., bone, apical progression of the level of the alveolar crest associated with inflammatory and dystrophic periodontal disease; a bone resorption process that results in decreased osseous support for the tooth.

r., gingival, atrophy of the gingival margin associated with inflammation, apical migration (proliferation) of the epithelial attachment, and resorption of the alveolar crest.

recidivism, 1. the tendency for an ill person to relapse or return to the hospital. **2.** the return to a life of crime after a conviction and sentence.

recipient, the person who receives a blood transfusion, tissue graft, or organ; also, a person who has received an honor, award, or grant.

recipient site, the site into which a graft or transplant material is placed. See also **donor site.**

reciprocal arm. See **arm, reciprocal.**

reciprocal forces, the typical method of applying corrective orthodontic forces; each applied force is balanced by a reciprocal force elsewhere in the dentition or surrounding structures.

reciprocation (resip′rōkā′shən), the means by which one part of a removable partial denture framework is made to counter the effect created by another part of the framework.

r., active, reciprocation in a clasp unit achieved by the use of two opposing and balanced retentive clasp arms. Reciprocation cannot be achieved unless a similar and balanced arrangement on the opposite side of the dental arch occurs.

r., passive, reciprocation in a clasp unit achieved by the use of a rigid part of the clasp, located on or above the height of contour line or on a guiding plane and opposite to the retentive

R

arm. However, reciprocation cannot be achieved by a single clasp alone—a similar action must occur by another component of the removable partial denture located across the arch.

reciprocity, a mutual agreement to exchange privileges, dependence, or relationships, as in an agreement between two governing bodies to accept the credentials of a physician, dentist, or other health professional licensed in either jurisdiction.

Recklinghausen's disease (rek'ling how'zenz). See **neurofibromatosis; osteitis fibrosa cystica.**

reconstructive surgery, surgery to rebuild a structure for functional or esthetic reasons.

recontouring, occlusal, the reshaping of an occlusal surface of a natural or artificial tooth.

record, information committed to and preserved in writing.

r. base. See **baseplate.**

r., centric interocclusal, a record of the centric jaw position (relation).

r., eccentric interocclusal, a record of a jaw relation other than the centric relation; a record of a lateral eccentric jaw position.

r., face-bow, registration, by means of a face-bow, of the position of the mandibular axis or the condyles. The face-bow record is used to orient the maxillary cast to the opening and closing axis of the articulator.

r., functional chew-in, **1.** a record of the natural chewing movement of the mandible made on an occlusion rim by teeth or scribing studs. **2.** a record of the movements of the mandible made on the occluding surface of the opposing occlusion rim by teeth or scribing studs and produced by simulated chewing movements.

r., interocclusal, a record of the positional relation of the teeth or jaws to each other; made on occlusal surfaces of occlusal rims or teeth in a plastic material that hardens, such as plaster of paris, wax, zinc oxide–eugenol paste, or acrylic resin.

r., jaw relation, a registration of any positional relationship of the mandible in reference to the maxillae. The record may be of any of the many vertical, horizontal, or orientation relations.

r., occluding centric relation, a registration of centric relation made at the vertical dimension at which the teeth make contact or are to make contact.

r., preoperative, any record or records made for the purpose of study, diagnosis, or use in treatment planning or for comparison of treatment results with the pretreatment status of the patient.

r., profile, a registration or record of the profile of a patient's face.

r., protrusive, a registration of the relation of the mandible to the maxillae when the mandible is anterior to its centric relation with the maxillae.

r., protrusive interocclusal, a record of a protruded eccentric jaw position.

r. rim. See **rim, occlusion.**

r., terminal jaw relation, a record of the relationship of the mandible to the maxillae made at the vertical relation of the occlusion and at the centric position.

r., three-dimensional, a maxillomandibular interocclusal record.

recording, the act of making a written record of the data collected during examination.

recovery, in a lawsuit, the obtaining or restoration of a right to something by a verdict, decree, or judgment of court.

recrystallization, the return of a wrought metal to crystalline form because of excessive cold working or excessive application of heat.

rectification (rek'tifikā'shən), conversion of electric current from alternating to direct (unidirectional).

rectifier (rek'tifī'er), a device used for converting an alternating current to a direct current; it also prevents or limits the flow of current in the opposite direction.

r., full-wave, an apparatus for rectifying the entire wave of an alternating current in an x-ray machine by means of a mechanical rectifier or valve tube.

r., half-wave, an apparatus used in the rectifying of half of the sine wave in x-ray unit.

recumbent, to be lying down, leaning backward, or reclining.

recuperation, the process of recovering health, strength, and mental and emotional vigor.

recurrence, the reappearance of a sign or symptom of a disease after a period of remission

red blood cell count, the number of red blood cells (erthrocytes) in 1 mm^3 of blood; a useful diagnostic tool in the determination of several kinds of anemia. See also **mean corpuscular hemoglobin.**

red marrow, the red vascular substance consisting of connective tissue and blood vessels, containing primitive blood cells, macrophages, megakaryocytes, and fat cells. Red marrow is found in the cavities of many bones. It manufactures and releases leukocytes and erythrocytes into the bloodstream.

redressment (redres'ment), replacement of a part or correction of a deformity.

reduced fee plan, a program in which the fees established for some or all services are lower than those usually charged by dentists in the community. In some industrial plans, employers make lower fees possible by partially subsidizing the cost of providing care (for example, furnishing rent-free facilities and paying costs of utilities). In welfare plans with limited funds, dentists may in effect subsidize the programs by accepting lower fees than they usually charge.

reducer, a solution used to remove some silver from the image on a radiograph and thereby produce a less intense image; an oxidizing agent used to remove excess density.

reduction in area, a test to assess the ductility of a metal or an alloy, whereby the cross-sectional area of the fractured end of a wire or rod is compared with the original area. A tensile test is used to break the wire.

refereed journal, a professional or literary journal or publication in which articles or papers are selected for publication by a panel of readers or referees who are experts in the field.

referral, the recommendation of another health professional to a patient for a specified reason.

referred pain, pain felt at a site different from that of an injured or diseased organ or part of the body. Angina pain is frequently felt at a site distant from the heart, such as arm or shoulder.

reflection, the act of elevating and folding back the mucoperiosteum, thereby exposing the underlying bone.

r., mucobuccal. See **fold, mucobuccal.**

reflex(es) (rē'fleks), a reflected action or movement; the sum total of any specific involuntary activity.

r., allied, reflexes that join to effect a common purpose, such as mastication. They may arise from diverse stimuli, such as smell, taste of food, and texture, shape, and resistance of the food bolus. Collectively, they encourage salivation and a sequence of masticatory closures of the mandible, followed by deglutition.

r., antagonistic, reflexes that cannot occupy the final pathway simultaneously. The weaker of these reflexes will give way to the stronger, especially if the latter is a protected reflex (for example, a hot or nauseating food causes involuntary retching or even vomiting rather than the pleasurable gustatory experience associated with chewing and swallowing tasty food).

r. arc. See **arc, reflex.**

r., Breuer. See **reflex, Hering-Breuer.**

r., Cheyne-Stokes. See **respiration, Cheyne-Stokes.**

r. emesis, gagging or vomiting induced by touching the mucous membrane of the throat or as a result of other noxious stimuli. Also called gag reflex.

r., flexion-extension, the reflexes based on the principle of reciprocal innervation. When a voluntary or reflex contraction of a muscle occurs, it is accompanied by the simultaneous relaxation of its antagonist. For example, when the jaw reflex is initiated by tapping the mandible downward, the masseter and other elevators of the mandible are stretched. Then, reflex flexion-contraction of the elevators takes place, the mandible is elevated, and the depressor muscles of the mandible are stretched. Many combinations exist, not only between the agonists and the antagonists of a given joint but also between reflexes that cross over to muscle groups of contralateral extremities, joints, and muscles.

r., Hering-Breuer, The nervous mechanism that tends to limit the respiratory excursions. Stimuli from the sensory endings in the lungs (and perhaps in other parts) pass up the vagi and tend to limit both inspiration and expiration during ordinary breathing.

r., jaw, an extension-flexion reflex that is initiated by tapping the mandible downward. The masseter and other elevators of the mandible are the first stretched; then the reflex flexion-contraction elevates the mandible by flexion of elevator muscles while simultaneous stretching (extension) of the depressor muscles of the mandible occurs.

r., pathologic, reflexes observed in the abnormal or inappropriate motor responses of controlled stimuli initiated in the sensory organ that is appropriate to the reflex arc. They may be initiated in the superficial reflexes of the skin and mucous membrane; in the deep myotatic reflexes of the joints, tendons, and muscles; and in the visceral reflexes of the viscera and other organs of the body. The pathologic reflexes are thus syndromes of abnormal responses to otherwise normal stimuli.

r., pharyngeal, contraction of the constrictor muscles of the pharynx, elicited by touching the back of the pharynx.

r., stretch, one of the most important features of tonic contraction of muscle. It is the reflex contraction of a healthy muscle that results from a pull. It has been found that stretching a muscle by as little as 0.8% of its original length is sufficient to evoke a reflex response. A stretch of constant degree causes a maintained steady contraction, muscle spindles and stretch receptors in the tendons show very slow adaptation, and the reflex ceases immediately on withdrawal of the stretching force. The stretch reflex is obtained predominantly from those muscles maintaining body posture, among which are the masticating muscles that maintain the position of the mandible and the neck muscles holding the head erect. Together the masticating muscles and neck muscles are responsible for the maintenance of the air and food passages.

r., vagovagal, a reflex in which the afferent and efferent impulses travel via the vagus nerve. The afferent impulses travel centrally via the sensory nucleus of the vagus. The efferent impulses travel via the motor fibers of the vagus nerve.

refractory (rifrak'tərē), pertaining to the ability to withstand the high temperatures used in certain dental laboratory procedures. See also **cast, refractory.**

refractory periodontitis (per'ē-ōdontī'tis), a progressive inflammatory destruction of the periodontal attachment that resists conventional mechanical treatment.

regeneration (rije'nərā'shən), the renewal or repair of lost tissue or parts.

r., muscle, repair of muscle tissue. When surgical intervention or inflammatory disease of dental structures injures the facial and masticatory muscles, two types of repair take place: repair by budding and repair by proliferation.

r., muscle, by budding, regeneration that takes place in destructive lesions of muscle, traumatic necrosis, hemorrhage, infarction, and suppurative myositis. The buds consist of undifferentiated plasmodial masses and certain sarcolemma nuclei. The rebuilt architecture is not classic and has bizarre and sometimes fibrous extensions that look like scarred defects.

r., muscle, by proliferation, regeneration in degenerating muscles by proliferation of bands of sarcoplasm in which the sarcolemma and its nuclei are preserved.

region, mylohyoid (mī'lōhī'oid), the region on the lingual surface of the mandible marked by the mylohyoid ridge and the attachment of the mylohyoid muscle; a part of the alveololingual sulcus.

regional, pertaining to a region or regions.

registered nurse (RN), a professional nurse who has completed a course of study at an approved and accredited school of nursing and who has passed the National Council of Licensure Examination. RNs are licensed to practice by individual states.

registered record administrator (RRA), a medical record administrator (Health Information Manager) who has successfully completed the prescribed curriculum and the credentialing examination conducted by the American Medical Record Association.

registration, the record of desired jaw relations that is made to transfer casts having these same relations to an articulator.

r. of functional form. See **impression, functional.**

r., tissue, the accurate record of the shape of tissues under any condition by means of suitable material.

regression analysis, a method of correlation for computing the most probable value of one variable, y, from the known value of another variable, x; a method for computing the amount of change in one variable for a unit change in another. It is spoken of as the regression of x on y and notated rxy.

regurgitation (rēgur'jitā'shən) a backward flowing (for example, casting up of undigested food, backward flowing of blood into the heart or between the chambers of the heart).

rehabilitation (rē'habilitā'shən) restoration of form and function.

r., mouth (oral rehabilitation), restoration of the form and function of the masticatory apparatus condition to as near normal as possible.

rehalation, rebreathing.

reimbursement, payment made by a third party to a beneficiary or dentist on behalf of the beneficiary toward repayment of expenses incurred for a service covered by the contractual arrangement.

reimplant, replacement of a lost or extracted tooth back into its alveolus.

reimplantation. See **replantation.**

reinforcement, the increasing of force or strength.

reinsurance, insurance for third-party payers to spread their risk for losses (claims paid) over a specified dollar amount.

reintubation (rē'intyōōbā'shən) intubation performed a second time.

Reiter's syndrome (rī'terz). See **syndrome, Reiter's.**

relapse, to slip or fall back into a former state.

relation(s), the designation of the position of one object as oriented to another (for example, centric relation of the mandible to the maxillae).

r., acentric. See relation, jaw, eccentric.

r., acquired centric. See **relation, jaw, eccentric, acquired.**

r., acquired eccentric jaw, an eccentric relation that is assumed by habit to bring the teeth into a convenient occlusion.

r., centric (centric jaw relation). the relation of the mandible to the maxillae when the condyles are in their most posterosuperior unstrained positions in the glenoid fossae, from which lateral movements can be made at the occluding vertical relation normal for the individual. Centric relation is a relation that can exist at any degree of jaw separation.

r., centric jaw. See **relation, centric.**

r., cusp-fossa. See **cusp-fossa relations.**

r., dynamic. relations of two objects involving the element of relative movement of one object to another (relationship of the mandible to the maxillae).

r., eccentric. See **relation, jaw, eccentric.**

r., eccentric jaw (convenience relationship, eccentric relation, eccentric jaw position), any jaw relation other than centric relation.

r., intermaxillary, the relation between the right and left maxilla. See also **relation, maxillomandibular.**

r., jaw, Any relation of the mandible to the maxillae.

r., lateral, the relation of the mandible to the maxillae when the lower jaw is in a position on either side of centric relation.

r., maxillomandibular (maksil'ōmandib'yōōlər), any one of the many relations of the mandible to the maxillae, such as the centric maxillomandibular relation or eccentric maxillomandibular relation.

r., median. See **relation, centric.**

r., median jaw, any jaw relation existing when the mandible is in the median sagittal plane.

r., median retruded. See **relation, centric.**

r., occluding, the jaw relation at which the opposing teeth contact or occlude.

r., protrusive, See **relation, jaw, protrusive; position, rest, physiologic.**

r., posterior border jaw, the most posterior relation of the mandible to the maxillae at any specific vertical dimension.

R

r., protrusive jaw (protrusive relation), a jaw relation resulting from a protrusion of the mandible.

r., rest. See **position, physiologic rest.**

r., rest jaw (rest), the postural relation of the mandible to the maxillae when the patient is resting comfortably in the upright position, the condyles are in a neutral unstrained position in the glenoid fossae, and the mandibular musculature is in a state of minimum tonic contraction to maintain posture.

r., ridge, the positional relation of the mandibular ridge to the maxillary ridges.

r., static, the relationship between two parts that are not in motion.

r., unstrained jaw, the relation of the mandible to the skull when a state of balanced tonus exists between all the muscles involved.

r., vertical, the relative position of the mandible in a vertical direction; one of the basic jaw relations.

relationship, the condition of being associated or interconnected.

r., abnormal occlusal, occlusal relationships that deviate from the regular and established type to produce esthetic disharmonies, interference with mastication, occlusal traumatism, and speech difficulties.

r., buccolingual (buk'ōling'gwəl), the position of a space or tooth in relation to the tongue and cheek.

r., convenience, of teeth. See **occlusion, convenience.**

r., normal, a relationship in which structures conjoin as they should.

r., occlusal, the individual and collective relationships of the mandibular teeth to the maxillary teeth and the relationship of the adjacent teeth in the same dental arch.

r., structure-activity (SAR), the relationship between the chemical structure of a drug and its activity.

r., tissue-base, the relationship of the base of a removable prosthesis to the structures subjacent to it. Three possibilities exist: the base may be entirely tissue borne, it may be completely tooth borne, or support may be shared by both the tissue subjacent to its base and the abutment that bounds the edentulous space at one terminus.

relative value system, coded listing of professional services with unit values to indicate relative complexity as measured by time, skill, and overhead costs. Third-party payers typically assign a dollar value per unit to calculate provider reimbursement.

relaxant (rilak'sənt), an antispasmodic; a drug that relaxes spasms of smooth or skeletal muscle; a drug used to eliminate muscle spasms, thus facilitating the establishment of centric relation, centric occlusion, rest position, etc. Also used in the treatment of painful muscle spasms associated with occlusal traumatism. Examples are mephenesin, the meprobamates, and methocarbamol (Robaxin).

r., muscle, a drug that specifically aids in lessening muscle tension.

relaxation training, a stress-reduction technique that uses a sequence of progressive exercises under the direction of a therapist to lower the level of anxiety and its neuromotor manifestations.

release, to give up as a legal claim; to discharge or relinquish a right.

release, sustained. See **medication, sustained release.**

reliability, 1. in research, the reproducibility of an experimental result; the extent to which an experiment, test, or measuring procedure yields the same result during independent, repeated trials. **2.** the ability of two or more observers to examine the same data and arrive at a similar judgment within predefined bounds concerning the quality of care.

relicensure, being licensed to practice for a specific period of time with the license either being renewed at the end of that period or being forfeited. In some instances, evidence of continued competency must be submitted.

relief, 1. the mitigation or removal of pain or distress. **2.** the reduction or elimination of pressure from a specific area under a denture base.

r. chamber. See **chamber, relief.**

r., gingival, relief given to removable partial denture units at all gingival crossings to avoid impingement.

r. space. See **space, relief.**

relieve, 1. To mitigate or remove pain or distress. **2.** the procedure of placing hard wax in strategic areas.

R

reline, to resurface the tissue side (basal surface) of a denture with new base material so that it will fit more accurately. See also **rebase.**

rem (radiation-equivalent-man), a unit of absorbed radiation dose adjusted for biologic effects equivalent to 1 rad of 250 kV x-rays (dental and cephalometric x-rays require less than 100 kV).

remedial (rimē'dēəl), curative; acting as a remedy.

remineralization (rē'mineralizā'shən), the reintroduction of complex mineral salts into bone, enamel, dentin, or cementum.

remission, the partial or complete disappearance of the clinical and subjective characteristics of a chronic or malignant disease.

remit, to send; to relinquish.

removable lingual arch. See **arch, removable lingual.**

removable partial denture. See **denture, partial, removable.**

removal, pulp. See **pulpectomy.**

remuneration, pay; recompense; salary.

Rendu-Osler-Weber disease. See **telangiectasia, hereditary hemorrhagic.**

rent, a payment made by a tenant to an owner for the use of land or a building.

rental, the fee paid by the dentist for the use of space in a building owned by someone else. Equipment may also be obtained under a rental or lease agreement.

reovirus, any one of three ubiquitous, double-stranded RNA viruses found in the respiratory and alimentary tracts in healthy and sick people. Reoviruses have been implicated in some cases of upper respiratory tract disease and infantile gastroenteritis.

reoxidation (rēok'sidā'shən), the act of taking up oxygen again, as the hemoglobin of the blood.

repair, 1. the process of reuniting or replacing broken parts of a denture; a means for extending the usefulness of a denture. **2.** to make sound; to mend; restoration to former condition. **3.** formation of new tissues by processes such as fibroplasia, osteogenesis, and endothelioplasia to replace tissues damaged by disease or injury.

r., cemental, repair of areas of cemental resorption and cemental tears by apposition of cementum. Repair may be by formation of either cellular or acellular cementum.

replacement, prosthetic. See **prosthesis.**

replantation (reimplantation), replacement of a tooth (or teeth) that has been removed from the alveolus either intentionally or unintentionally, as in an accident.

replenisher, a concentrated developing solution designed to maintain the active strength of developer through periodic addition to maintain original volume.

report generator, a computer program for producing complete data processing reports giving only a description of the desired content and format of the output reports, as well as certain information concerning the input file.

reportable diseases, contagious diseases that must be reported by the physician to public health authorities. They include but are not limited to malaria, influenza, poliomyelitis, relapsing fever, typhus, yellow fever, cholera, and bubonic plague.

reposition, muscle, surgical replacement of a muscle attachment into a more acceptable functional position.

repositioning, jaw, the changing of any relative position of the mandible to the maxillae, usually by altering the occlusion of the natural or artificial teeth.

repository, long-acting drugs, usually administered intramuscularly. See also **medication, repository.**

r., rapid, mixtures of rapid-acting and slow-acting drugs, usually administered intramuscularly.

representative group, a group whose members represent all the various sectors of a community or population under study.

reputation, a person's credit, honor, and character; esteem in which one is held.

request for proposal (RFP), a solicitation by a funding agency for proposals to accomplish a particular goal. The RFP lists the requirements a project must meet to receive funding.

require arch length, the circumference of the dental arch sufficient to accommodate the sum of the mesio-distal widths of all the natural teeth in the dental arch.

res ipsa loquitur (rās' ip'sə lok' witōōr), a Latin phrase meaning "the thing speaks for itself." Used in actions for injury by negligence in which the happening itself is accepted as proof.

res judicata (rās' jōō'dika'ta), decided or determined by judicial power; a thing judicially decided.

research, the diligent inquiry or examination of data, reports, and observations in a search for facts or principles. Generally a disciplined protocol is followed to ensure objectivity and reproducibility. Most research employs the scientific method or a similar model.

resection, excision of a considerable portion of an organ.

r., root. See **amputation, root.**

reserpine, *trade names:* Serpalan, Serpasil; *drug class:* antiadrenergic agent, antihypertensive; *action:* depletes catecholamine stores in CNS and adrenergic nerve endings; *use:* hypertension.

residual, pertaining to the portion of something that remains after an activity that removes the bulk of the substance; usually refers to the amount of air remaining in the lungs at the end of a maximum expiration.

reserve, something kept in store for future use.

r., alkali. See **reserve, alkaline.**

r., alkaline (alkali reserve), **1.** the amount of buffer compounds (for example, sodium bicarbonate, dipotassium phosphate, proteins) in the blood capable of neutralizing acids; one of the buffer systems of the blood that can neutralize the acid valences formed in the body. It is made up of the base of weak acid salts and is usually measured by determining the bicarbonate concentration of the plasma. **2.** the concentration of bicarbonate ions (HCO_3) in the blood. These ions serve as a reserve in that they may be displaced by anions (for example, $CL-$, $SO_4=$, $PO_4=$). Displacement of bicarbonate ions occurs mainly by means of the chloride shift (Hamburger phenomenon). The role of the buffer system is such that a large influx of acid or base ions from either metabolic function or ingestion can be neutralized by the alkaline reserves from the mineral and protein salts in the blood and tissue fluids. A strong acid is transformed into a weak base. Consequently, the pH level of the blood fluctuates very little, and the tissue cells are constantly bathed in a continuously buffered solution.

r., cardiac, the reserve strength or pumping ability of the heart, which may be called on in an emergency.

resident, a graduate and licensed dentist or physician who has completed an internship and is serving in the hospital while pursuing advanced didactic and clinical studies in special disciplines of knowledge.

residual ridge. See **ridge, residual.**

residue, remainder; that which remains after the removal of other substances.

resilience (rizil'yəns), **1.** an act of springing back. **2.** capability of a strained body to recover its size and shape after deformation. **3.** the recoverable potential energy of an elastic solid body or structure resulting from its having been subjected to stress not exceeding the elastic limit.

r., modulus of, the amount of energy stored up by a body when one unit volume is stressed to its proportional limit.

resin (rez'in), broad term used to indicate organic substances that are usually translucent or transparent and are soluble in ether, acetone, and similar substances but not in water. They are named according to their chemical composition, physical structure, and means for activation or curing. Examples are acrylic resin, autopolymer resin (cold-curing resin), synthetic resin, styrene resin, and vinyl resin. See also **methyl methacrylate; varnish, cavity.**

r., acrylic, **1.** general term applied to a resinous material of the various esters of acrylic acid. It is used as a denture base material and also for trays and other dental restorations. **2.** An ethylene derivative that contains a vinyl group (e.g., polymethacrylate [methyl methacrylate], the principal ingredient of many plastics used in dentistry).

r., activated, See resin, autopolymer.

r., autopolymer (*activated resin, auto-polymerizing resin, cold-curing resin, direct restorative acrylic resin, self-curing resin*), any resin that can be polymerized by an activator and a catalyst without the use of external heat.

r., composite, a resin used for restorative purposes and usually formed by a reaction of an ether of bisphenol-A (an expoxy molecule) with acrylic resin monomers, initiated by a benzoyl peroxideamine system, to which is added as much as 75% inorganic filler (glass beads and rods, lithium aluminum silicate, quartz, and tricalcium phosphate).

r., copolymer, a synthetic resin that is the product of the concurrent and joint polymerization of two or more different monomers of polymers.

r., direct restorative. See **resin, autopolymer.**

r., epoxy, a resin molecule characterized by reactive epoxy, or ethoxyline, groups that serve as terminal polymerization points. Used in dentistry for denture bases.

r., heat-curing, any resin that requires heat to activate its polymerization.

r., quick cure. See **resin, autopolymer.**

r., self-curing. See **resin, autopolymer.**

r., thermoplastic, a synthetic resin that may be softened by heat and hardened by cooling.

r., vinyl, an ethylene-derivative copolymer of vinyl chloride and vinyl acetate; used at one time for denture bases.

resin-filled, pertaining to a resin, usually poly (methyl methacrylate), to which has been added an inert material such as glass beads or glass rods.

resistance, ability of an individual to ward off the damaging effects of physical, chemical, or microbiologic injury; an immeasurable factor controlled and qualified by numerous local, systemic, and metabolic processes such as blood supply to tissues, nutritional status, age, and antibody formative ability.

r., cross-, a state in which an organism is insensitive to several drugs of similar chemical nature.

r. form. See **form, resistance.**

resolution, the discernible separation of closely adjacent radiographic image details.

resonance (rez′ənəns), the vibratory response of a body or air-filled cavity to a frequency imposed on it.

r., speech, the resonance of the body cavities and surfaces involved in the production of speech. The sound waves produced at the vocal folds are still far from the finished product heard in speech. The resonators give the characteristic quality to the voice. The resonating structures are the air sinuses; organ surfaces; cavities such as the pharynx, oral cavity, and nasal cavity; and chest wall. The resonating structures contribute no energy to the stream of air; they act to conserve and concentrate the energy already present in the laryngeal tone rather than to let it dissipate into the tissues. However, the resonated laryngeal tone still is not speech.

resorcinol, an antiseptic substance used as a keratolytic agent in dermatoses.

resorption (risôrp′shən) **1.** loss of substance (bone) by physiologic or pathologic means; the reduction of the volume and size of the residual alveolar portion of the mandible or maxillae. **2.** the cementoclastic and dentinoclastic action that often takes place on the root of a replanted tooth.

r., apical root, dissolution of the apex of a tooth, resulting in a shortened, blunted root.

r., bone, **1.** destruction or solution of the elements of bone. **2.** loss of bone resulting from the activity of multinucleated giant cells, the osteoclasts, which are noted in irregular concavities on the periphery of the bone (Howship's lacunae).

r., cemental, destruction of cementum by cementoclastic action. Noted as the presence of irregular concavities in the cemental surfaces.

r., frontal, osteoclastic resorption of alveolar bone (lamina dura) by multinucleated cells on the osseous margin adjacent to the periodontal ligament.

r., horizontal, a pattern of bone resorption in marginal periodontitis in which the marginal crest of the alveolar bone between adjacent teeth remains level; in these instances the bases of the periodontal pockets are supracrestal; a pattern of bone loss in which the crestal margins of the alveolar bone are resorbed. A horizontal pattern, rather than vertical loss along the root, is the typical type of bone loss in periodontitis.

r., idiopathic, resorption that is not attributable to any known disease or is without an apparent cause.

r., internal (idiopathic internal resorption, pink tooth), a special form of idiopathic root resorption from within the pulp cavity; granulation tissue is present within the tooth, apparently with the resorption of the dentin occurring from the inside outward. The cause is unknown.

r., lacunar. See **osteoclast.**

r., osteoclastic, loss of bone by cellular activity; osteoclasts are large, multinucleated cells seen in irregular concavities in the margin of the bone (Howship's lacunae) and currently believed to be directly responsible for the active destruction of bone.

r., pressure, of bone, osteoclastic destruction of bone resulting from the application of sustained, excessive force. Remodeling of bone may occur to better adapt to these forces, or destruction may continue if the stresses are repeated and excessive.

r., rear. See **resorption, undermining.**

r., root, destruction of the cementum or dentin by cementoclastic or osteoclastic activity.

r., surface root, localized resorptive areas on the cemental surface of the tooth root.

r., undermining, indirect, as opposed to frontal, removal of alveolar bone where pressure applied to a tooth has resulted in loss of vitality of localized areas of the periodontal membrane.

r., vertical, a pattern of bone loss seen in occlusal traumatism, marginal periodontitis, periodontosis, and other conditions; a pattern of bone loss in which the alveolar bone adjacent to a tooth is destroyed without simultaneous crestal loss, so that a vertical rather than a horizontal pattern of loss is observed.

respect, to hold in high regard; to show consideration for another. Mutual respect is the basis for a good doctor-patient relationship.

respiration (res'pirā'shən), the gaseous exchange between cells of the body and the environment. Four stages exist: pulmonary ventilation, diffusion of gases in the alveoli, transport of gases in the blood to and from cells, and regulation of the process.

r., artificial, maintenance of respiratory movements by artificial means. When respiration has been arrested and no mechanical device is available, resuscitation by means of artificial respiration is the only practical means of ventilating the lungs.

r., Cheyne-Stokes (chān'stōks') *(Cheyne-Stokes reflex),* a type of breathing characterized by rhythmic variations in intensity that occur in cycles: rhythmic acceleration, deepening, and stopping of breathing movements.

r., controlled, maintenance of adequate pulmonary ventilation in apneic patients.

r., external, ventilation of the lungs and oxygenation of the blood.

r., internal, the mechanism of gaseous exchange between blood and tissues.

r. in speech, in normal speech, the action of the respiratory apparatus during exhalation, which provides a continuous stream of air with sufficient volume and pressure (under adequate voluntary control) to initiate phonation. The stream of air is modified in its course from the lungs by the facial and oral structures, giving rise to the sound symbols that are recognized as speech.

r., stertorous, snoring.

r., stridulous, a high-pitched sound occurring during respiration caused by adduction of the vocal cords.

respirator (res'pirā'tər), an apparatus that qualifies the air breathed through it; a device for giving artificial respiration.

respiratory distress syndrome of the newborn (RDS), an acute lung disease of the newborn, characterized by airless alveoli, inelastic lungs, more than 60 respirations per minute, nasal flaring, intercostal and subcostal retractions, grunting on expiration, and peripheral edema. The condition occurs most often in premature babies. It is caused by a deficiency of pulmonary surfactant. The disease is self-limited; the infant either dies in 3 to 5 days or completely recovers with no aftereffects. Treatment includes measures to correct shock, acidosis, and hypoxemia and the use of continuous positive airway pressure to prevent alveolar collapse.

respiratory rate, the normal rate of breathing at rest, about 12 to 20 inspirations per minute.

respiratory rhythm, a regular, oscillating cycle of inspiration and expiration, controlled by neuronal impulses transmitted between the muscles of inspiration in the chest and the respiratory centers in the brain. The respiratory rate is influenced by metabolic rate, emotional state, neurologic disorders, and obstructive disease.

respiratory therapy, any treatment that maintains or improves the ventilatory function of the respiratory tract.

respiratory tract, the complex of organs and structures performing the pulmonary ventilation of the body and the exchange of oxygen and carbon dioxide between the ambient air and the blood circulating through the lungs. It includes all the structures from the external nares to the alveoli of the lungs.

respirometer (res′pirom′ətər), an instrument for studying and determining the character and extent of respiration.

respondeat superior, a legal doctrine that passes the legal responsibility for acts or omissions of an employee to the employer.

response, action or movement resulting from the application of a stimulus.

response time, the period between the application of a stimulus and the response of a cell or tissue.

rest, 1. passive support. **2.** an extension from a prosthesis that affords vertical support for a restoration.

r. area. See **area, rest.**

r., auxiliary, the rest other than the one used as a component part of a primary direct retainer.

r., finger. See **finger rest.**

r., incisal, a metallic extension onto the incisal angle of an anterior tooth to supply support or indirect retention for a removable partial denture.

r., lingual, a metallic extension onto the lingual surface of an anterior tooth to provide support or indirect retention for a removable partial denture.

r., occlusal (occlusal lug), a rest placed on the occlusal surface of a posterior tooth.

r. occlusion. See **position, rest, physiologic.**

r. position. See **position, rest.**

r., precision, a unit consisting of two closely fitted parts, the insert of which rests firmly against the gingival portion of the tubelike receptacle.

r. relation. See **relation, jaw, rest.**

r. seat. See **area, rest.**

resting potential, the electrical potential across a nerve cell membrane before it is stimulated to release the charge. The resting potential for a neuron is between 50 and 100 millivolts.

restless legs syndrome, a benign condition of unknown origin characterized by an irritating sensation of uneasiness, tiredness, and itching deep within the muscles of the legs, accompanied by twitching and sometimes pain. The only relief is walking or moving the legs.

restoration (prosthetic restoration), broad term applied to any filling, inlay, crown, bridge, partial denture, or complete denture that restores or replaces lost tooth structure, teeth, or oral tissues; a prosthesis.

r. of cusps (preferred to tipping, capping, or shoeing cusps), reduction and inclusion of cusps within a cavity preparation and their restoration to functional occlusion with restorative material.

r., dental prosthetic. See **prosthesis, dental.**

r., faulty, restoration in which there are imperfections or incorrect attributes (for example, overhanging or deficient fillings, incorrect anatomy of occlusal and marginal ridge areas, faulty clasps). Such faults may be present in individual tooth restorations, fixed bridges, and removable partial dentures and are conducive to the initiation and perpetuation of inflammatory and dystrophic diseases of the teeth and periodontium.

r., implant, the single-tooth implant crown or multiple-tooth implant, crown, or bridge that replaces a missing tooth or teeth.

r., prosthetic. See **prosthesis.**

restorative, 1. promoting a return to health or consciousness; a remedy that aids in restoring health, vigor, or consciousness. **2.** pertaining to rebuilding, repairing, or reforming.

r. dentistry, the branch of dentistry that deals with the reconstruction of the hard tissues of a tooth or group of teeth injured or destroyed by trauma or disease.

r. materials, materials used to reconstruct the hard tissues of teeth lost through trauma or disease.

restrainer, a chemical ingredient (potassium bromide) of photographic developing solution. Its function is to inhibit the fogging tendency of the solution. Like the activator, the restrainer also controls the rate of development.

restraint, any one of a number of devices used in aiding the immobilization of patients, especially children in traction.

restraint of trade, an illegal act that interferes with free competition in a commercial or business transaction so as to restrict the production of a product or the provision of a service, affect the cost of a product or service, or control the market in any way to the detriment of consumers or purchasers of the service or product.

restrictive covenant, common clause found in a contract for the sale of a dental practice. The seller contracts that he or she will not practice dentistry within a certain time and area. A junior partner may be asked to sign such a covenant to guarantee that he or she will not compete with the partnership for a period of time after leaving the partnership. Also used in an employment situation.

resuscitation (risus'itā'shən), restoration of life or consciousness to one who appears to be dead.

resuscitator (risus'itā'tər), an apparatus for initiating respiration in asphyxia.

retail dentistry, fee for service dentistry practiced in an exclusively retail environment (for example, shopping center, department store) and directed to the clientele of that retail center, using the marketing technique of the parent retailer.

retail store dentistry, dental services offered within a retail, department, or drug store operation. Typically, space is leased from the store by a separate administrative group that in turn subleases to a dentist or dental group providing the actual dental services. The dental operation generally maintains the same hours of operation as the store, and appointments often are not necessary. It is considered to be a type of practice, not a dental benefits plan model.

retainer (retaining appliance), **1.** The part of a dental prosthesis that unites the abutment tooth with the suspended portion of the bridge. It may be an inlay, partial crown, or complete crown. **2.** an appliance for maintaining the positions of the teeth and jaws gained by orthodontic procedures. **3.** the portion of a fixed prosthesis attaching a pontic(s) to the abutment teeth (for example, inlay, three-quarter crown). **4.** a form of clasp, attachment, or device used for the fixation or stabilization of a prosthetic appliance. **5.** any orthodontic appliance, fixed or removable, used to maintain teeth in corrected positions during the period of functional adaptation following corrective treatment.

r., continuous bar, a metal bar that is attached to a major connector and contacts lingual surfaces of anterior teeth, on or incisal to the cingula; it aids in the stabilization of a distal extension removable partial denture.

r., direct, a clasp, attachment, or assembly applied to an abutment tooth for the purpose of maintaining a removable restoration in its planned position in relation to oral structures.

r., extracoronal, **1.** a type of retainer in which the preparation and its cast restoration lie largely external to the body of the coronal portion of the tooth and complement the contour of the crown. The retention or resistance to displacement is developed between the inner surfaces of the casting and the external walls of the prepared tooth. The extracoronal retainer may be a partial crown or a complete crown. **2.** a direct retainer of the clasp type that engages an abutment tooth on its external surface in such a way as to afford retention and stabilization to a removable partial denture; a direct retainer of the manufactured type, the male portion of which is attached to the external surface of a cast crown on an abutment tooth (for example, Dalbo and Crismani attachments).

r., Hawley, a wire and acrylic resin removable appliance designed to sta-

R

bilize teeth after tooth movement; serves as a basis for tooth movement by providing an anchorage for the wires and rubber dam elastics used in orthodontic tooth movement.

r., indirect, that part of a removable partial denture that resists movement of a free end denture base away from its tissue support through lever action opposite the fulcrum line of the direct retention.

r., intracoronal, **1.** a type of retainer in which the prepared cavity and its cast restoration lie largely within the body of the coronal portion of the tooth and within the contour of the crown (for example, inlay). The retention or resistance to displacement is developed between the casting and the internal walls of the prepared cavity. **2.** the type of direct retainer used in the construction of removable partial dentures; it consists of a female portion within the coronal portion of the crown of an abutment and a fitted male portion attached to the denture proper. These retainers may be fabricated in the dental office or obtained through commercial sources.

r., matrix (matrix holder), a mechanical device designed to engage the ends of a matrix around the tooth.

r., radicular, a type of retainer that lies within the body of the tooth and is usually confined to the root portion of the tooth (for example, dowel crown). The retention or resistance to displacement and shear is developed by extending an attached dowel into the root canal of the tooth.

retaining ring, a ring that holds the arch wire against the premolar bracket to allow free sliding and tipping. (not current)

retardation, the slowing down of any mental or physical activity or the abnormal development of intellectual abilities.

retarder, a chemical added to a substance to slow a chemical reaction, prolong the set of the material, and provide more working time.

rete pegs (rē′tē′). See **pegs, epithelial.**

retention (riten′shən), **1.** power to retain; capacity for retaining; the inherent property of a restoration to maintain its position without displacement under stress; results from close adapta-

tion of the restoration to the prepared form of the tooth, usually aided by cement. **2.** term relating to the provision in cavity preparation for preventing displacement of a restoration. Retention supplements resistance form and is specifically created to resist any lateral or tipping force that may be brought against the restoration during and after its insertion. **3.** resistance of a denture to removal in a direction opposite that of its insertion; the quality inherent in the denture that resists the force of gravity, adhesiveness of foods, and forces associated with opening of the jaws. **4.** the period of treatment during which the individual wears an appliance to maintain the teeth in the desired position.

r. arm. See **arm, retention.**

r., circumferential, frictional resistance to displacement derived from completely veneering the exposed tooth surface.

r., denture, **1.** the means by which dentures are held in position in the mouth; the maintenance of a denture in its position in the mouth; the resistance to the movement of a denture from its basal seat in a direction opposite to that in which it was inserted. **2.** the resistance of a denture to vertical movement in the occlusal direction from its basal seat.

r., direct, retention obtained in a removable partial denture by the use of attachments or clasps that resist removal from abutment teeth.

r. form. See **form, retention.**

r., indirect, retention obtained in a removable partial denture through the use of indirect retainers.

r., partial denture, the fixation of a fixed partial denture by means of crowns, inlays, or other retainers.

r., pin. See **pin, retention.**

r., pinhole, one or more small holes, 2 to 3 mm in depth, placed in suitable areas of a cavity preparation parallel with the general line of draft to provide or supplement resistance and retention form.

r., radicular, retention derived from projections of metal into the root canals of pulpless teeth.

r., removable partial denture, the resistance to movement of a removable partial denture from its supporting structures, gained by the use of direct and indirect retainers or other attachments.

r. terminal. See **clasp, circumferential arm; clasp, circumferential, arm, retentive.**

reticulocyte, an immature erythrocyte. Reticulocytes normally account for less than 2% of the circulating erythrocytes.

reticulocytosis (ritik′yəlōsītō′sis), an increase in the normal number of reticulocytes in the circulating blood. Normal values range from 0.5% to 1.5% of the red blood cells.

reticuloendotheliosis, nonlipid (ritik′yəlōen′dōthē′lē-ō′sis). See **disease, Letterer-Siwe.**

retina, a 10-layered, delicate nervous-tissue membrane of the eye, continuous with the optic nerve, that receives images of external objects and transmits visual impulses through the optic nerve to the brain.

retinal detachment, a separation of the retina from the choroid in the back of the eye, usually resulting from a hole in the retina that allows the vitreous humor to leak between the choroid and retina. Severe trauma to the eye may be the proximate cause, but in the great majority of cases, retinal detachment is the result of internal changes in the vitreous chamber associated with aging or with inflammation of the interior of the eye.

retinoblastoma, a congenital, hereditary neoplasm developing from retinal germ cells.

retraction, 1. a drawing or shrinking back; the laying back of tissues to expose a given part. 2. distal movement of teeth; a distal or retrusive position of the teeth, dental arch, or jaw.

r., gingival, laying back of the free gingival tissue to expose the gingival margin area of a preparation by mechanical, chemical, or electrical means.

retractor, an instrument for retracting tissues to assist in gaining access to an area of operation or observation.

r., beaver-tail, a broad-bladed periosteal elevator.

r., rake, a metallic instrument with prongs set transversely for engaging and retracting soft tissues.

r., vein hook, a metallic instrument ending in a rounded flange set transversely for engaging and retracting soft tissues.

retroclination, posterior angulation (inclination) of anterior teeth.

retrofill, obturation of the apex of a tooth root by the direct surgical approach.

retrognathic (ret′rōnath′ik), 1. the condition of a mandible that is posterior to its normal relationship with other facial structures; may be a result of small mandibular size or posteriorly positioned temporomandibular fossae. 2. mandibular retrusion.

retrognathism (ret′rōnath′izm), facial disharmony in which one or both jaws (usually the mandible) are posterior to normal facial relationships. This condition may be real or imaginary.

r., bird-face, typical facial profile associated with an underdeveloped mandible; a retrognathia and small mandible usually associated with interference of condylar growth because of trauma or infection affecting the condyles. Surgical intervention is necessary for improvement.

r., Pierre Robin. See **syndrome, Pierre Robin.**

retrograde, To move backward, degenerate, or return to an earlier state or worse condition.

retromolar pad. See **pad, retromolar.**

retromylohyoid eminence. See **eminence, retromylohyoid.**

retromylohyoid space. See **space, retromylohyoid** (not current).

retrospective review, a posttreatment assessment of services on a case-by-case or aggregate basis after the services have been performed.

retrospective study, a study in which a search is made for a relationship between one phenomenon or condition and another that occurred in the past (for example, the exposure to toxic agents and the rate of occurrence of disease in the exposed group compared with a control group not exposed).

retrosternal pain, a pain behind the sternum that usually occurs on swallowing. If retrosternal pain is associated with oral or pharyngeal candidiasis, it may indicate candidiasis of the esophagus, which is an opportunistic infection indicative of AIDS.

retroversion (ret′rōvur′zhən), a condition in which teeth or other maxil-

R

lary and mandibular structures are located posterior to the normal or generally accepted standard.

Retrovir, brand name for zidovudine, a dideoxynucleoside used in the treatment of HIV-positive patients.

retrovirus (ret'rōvī'rəs), a virus containing RNA rather than DNA.

retruded contact position, A tooth-to-tooth position at centric relation, sometimes referred to as centric relation occlusion.

retrusion (ritrōō'zhən), teeth or jaws posterior to their normal positions.

r., mandibular, abnormal retrusion of the mandible, as in a Class II malocclusion.

r., maxillary, abnormal retrusion of the maxillae.

reverse curve. See **curve, reverse.**

reverse transcriptase, an enzyme within a retrovirous that converts its RNA into DNA, which then penetrates the cell nucleus and joins the host's DNA.

reverse Trendelenburg, a position in which the lower extremities are lower than the body and head, which are elevated on an inclined plane.

reversible, capable of going through a series of changes in either direction, forward or backward (for example, reversible chemical reaction).

r. hydrocolloid. See **hydrocolloid, reversible.**

review coordinator, a member of the staff of a PSRO or hospital who is generally responsible to a utilization review committee. Such persons perform or assist in concurrent review or audit studies, initiating or coordinating discharge planning, recording and transmitting review decisions, or acting as liaison with persons and organizations participating in and affected by the review system.

rewards, a motivation technique to improve patient compliance with oral hygiene protocols, generally used with young patients.

rhabdomyosarcoma (rab'dōmī-ōsärkō'mə), a malignant tumor of striated, or voluntary, muscle.

rhagades (rag'ədēz), fissures or cracks in the skin seen around body orifices and in regions subjected to frequent movement.

rheology (rē-ol'o-jē), the study of blood flow, pressure, and velocity through the vascular system.

rheostat (rē'ō-stat), a resistor for regulating a current by means of variable resistances.

rheumatic fever. See **fever, rheumatic.**

rheumatic heart disease, damage to heart muscle and heart valves caused by episodes of rheumatic fever. Rheumatic heart disease may result when a susceptible person acquires a group A beta-hemolytic streptococcal infection; an autoimmune reaction may occur in heart tissue, resulting in permanent deformities of heart valves or chordae tendineae.

rheumatism (rōō'mətiz'əm) (rheumatic disease), a nonspecific term indicating any painful disorder related to joints, muscles, bone, or nerves; acute rheumatic fever; or, as used by lay persons, rheumatoid arthritis, bursitis, myositis, or degenerative joint disease.

rheumatoid arthritis, a chronic, destructive, sometimes deforming collagen disease that has an autoimmune component. Rheumatoid arthritis usually first appears in early middle age, between 36 and 50 years of age and most commonly in women.

rheumatoid factor (RF), antiglobulin antibodies often found in the serum of patients with a clinical diagnosis of rheumatoid arthritis.

Rh factor, an antigenic substance present in the erthrocytes of 85% of humans. A person having the factor is Rh positive, and a person lacking the factor is Rh negative.

Rh incompatibility, a condition in which two groups of blood cells are antigentically different because of the presence of Rh factor in one group and the absence of the Rh factor in the other. See also **Rh factor.**

rhinitis, inflammation of the mucous membranes of the nose, usually accompanied by swelling of the mucosa and a nasal discharge. Rhinitis may be acute, allegic, atrophic, or vasomotor.

rhinolalia (rī'nōlā'lēyə), nasalized speech, of which there are two types: rhinolalia clausa (closed port) and rhinolalia aperta (open port).

rhinoplasty (ri'nō-plas'tē), plastic or reconstructive surgery of the nose.

rhinovirus, any of about 100 serologically distinct, small RNA viruses that cause about 40% of acute respiratory illnesses. Infection is characterized by dry, scratchy throat, nasal congestion, malaise, and headache. Fever is minimal. Nasal discharge lasts 2 or 3 days.

rhizotomy, retrogasserian (rīzot′ əmē, ret′rōgasser′ēē- ən), intracranial sectioning of the sensory root of the trigeminal nerve posterior to the semilunar ganglion; used in the treatment of severe trigeminal neuralgia.

rhodium (Rh), a grayish-white metallic element. Its atomic number is 45, and its atomic weight is 102.91. Rhodium is used for providing a hard, lustrous coating on other metals and in the making of mirrors.

rhythm (rith′əm), a measured movement; the recurrence of an action or function at regular intervals.

r., heart, the rhythm pattern in the sequence of heart beats, which may be altered in the presence of cardiac disease.

rhytidoplasty, a procedure in reconstructive plastic surgery in which the skin of the face is tightened, wrinkles are removed, and the skin is made to appear firm and smooth.

riboflavin (rib′ōflā′vin) (vitamin B_2), *trade names:* many generic sources; *drug class:* vitamin B_2 water soluble; *action:* needed for normal tissue respiratory reactions; functions as a coenzyme; *uses:* vitamin B_2 deficiency.

ribonucleic acid (RNA), a nucleic acid, found in both the nucleus and cytoplasm of cells, that transmits genetic instructions from the nucleus to the cytoplasm. RNA functions in the assembly of proteins.

ribose, a 5-carbon sugar that occurs as a component of ribonucleic acid.

rickets (rik′əts), a condition caused by deficiency of vitamin D or calcium in infants and children, with disturbance in the mineralization of osseous and dental tissues. Marked by bending and bowing of bones, nodular enlargements at the ends of bones, myalgia, delay in closure of fontanels, and other problems. See also **osteomalacia.**

r., adult. See osteomalacia.

r., refractory. See **rickets, resistant.**

r., renal, a disturbance marked by excessive excretion of phosphorus and calcium resulting in a lowered renal threshold of excretion of these mineral elements. See also **osteodystrophy, renal.**

r., resistant (late rickets, refractory rickets), rickets that responds only

to extremely large amounts of vitamin D.

Rickettsia, a genus of microorganisms that combine aspects of both bacteria and viruses. Examples of rickettsial diseases are Rocky Mountain spotted fever and typhus.

ridge, the remainder of the alveolar process after the teeth are removed.

r., alveolar, the bony ridge of the maxillae or mandible that contains the alveoli (sockets of the teeth). See also **process, alveolar.**

r., center of, the buccolingual midline of the residual ridge.

r., crest of, the highest continuous surface of the ridge, but not necessarily the center of the ridge; the top of a residual or alveolar ridge.

r. extension. See **extension, ridge.**

r., key (zygomaxillare), the lowest point of the zygomaticomaxillary ridge.

r. lap, the part of an artificial tooth that is adjacent to the residual ridge; the part of the artificial tooth that laps the ridge.

r., marginal, a ridge or elevation of enamel that forms the boundary of the occlusal surface of a tooth.

r., mental, a dense ridge extending from the symphysis to the premolar area on the anterolateral aspect of the body of the mandible.

r., mylohyoid, a dense line or ridge of bone on the medial surface of the body of the mandible that extends obliquely upward and posteriorly from the symphysis, covers the cervical portion of the third molar, and then goes upward and backward onto the vertical ramus. The mylohyoid muscle is inserted into this ridge of bone.

r., Passavant's. See **pad, Passavant's.**

r. relation. See **relation, ridge.**

r., residual, the portion of the alveolar ridge that remains after the alveoli have disappeared from the alveolar process after extraction of the teeth.

r. support. See **area, supporting.**

rifabutin, *trade name:* Mycobutin; *drug class:* antimycobacterial agent; *action:* inhibits DNA-dependent RNA polymerase synthesis of bacterial RNA; *uses:* prevention of disseminated *M. avium* complex (MAC) disease with advanced HIV infection.

rifampin, *trade names:* Rifadin IV, Rimactane; *drug class:* antitubercular

R

antiinfective; *action:* inhibits DNA-dependent RNA polymerase synthesis in bacterial RNA; *uses:* pulmonary TB, prevention of meningococcal caries.

Riga-Fede disease (rē'gäfä'dä). See **disease, Riga-Fede.** (not current)

right-angle technique. See **technique, parallel.** (not current)

right of action, the right to sue; a legal right to maintain an action, based on a happening or state of fact.

right-to-know laws, laws that require employers to inform workers regarding health effects of materials they must handle, including toxic chemicals and radioactive substances. Right-to-know statutes are administered under the authority of the U.S. Occupational Safety and Health Administration (OSHA).

rigidity, the characteristic of being nonflexible, which is essential in a connector, a reciprocal arm, or an indirect retaining unit of a removable partial denture.

rigor mortis, the stiffening of skeletal and cardiac muscle shortly after death.

Riley-Day syndrome. See **syndrome, Riley-Day.**

riluzole, *trade name:* Rilutek; *drug class:* glutamate antagonist; *action:* inhibits presynaptic release of glutamic acid in CNS; *uses:* treatment of amyotrophic lateral sclerosis (Lou Gehrig disease).

rim, the outer edge; often curved or circular.

r., occlusion (record rim), an occluding surface built on temporary or permanent denture bases for the purpose of making maxillomandibular relation records and arranging teeth.

r., record. See **rim, occlusion.**

r., surgical occlusion, a conventional occlusion rim, the base of which has been reduced until it is smaller than the surgical impression tray with which the surgical jaw relations are recorded.

rimantadine HCl, *trade name:* Flumadine; *drug class:* antiviral; *action:* may inhibit viral uncoating; *uses:* adults, prophylaxis and treatment of illnesses caused by strains of influenza A virus; in children, prophylaxis against influenza A virus.

rimexolone, *trade name:* Vexol; *drug class:* corticosteroid; *action:* interacts with steroid cytoplasmic receptors to induce antiinflammatory effects; *uses:* inflammation of the eye associated with ocular surgery and uveitis.

rinse bath, a tank or container of water used in film processing to wash residual developer from the film before placement in the fixer.

Risdon wire. See **wire, Risdon.**

Risdon's incision. See **incision, Risdon's.**

risk-benefit analysis, the consideration as to whether a medical or surgical procedure, particularly a radical approach, is worth the risk to the patient compared with the possible benefits if the procedure is successful.

risk factors, elements that may contribute to or increase the risk to one's health, economic stability, or personal and professional liability.

risk management, a program designed to identify, contain, reduce, or eliminate the potential for harm to patients, visitors, and employees and the potential financial loss to the facility if a compensable event occurs; usually concerned with the delivery system and site rather than practitioner performance.

risk pool, a portion of provider fees or capitation payments withheld as financial reserves to cover unanticipated utilization of services in an alternative benefits plan.

risorius, one of the 12 muscles of facial expression. It acts to retract the angle of the mouth, as in a smile.

risperidone, *trade name:* Risperdal; *drug class:* antipsychotic; *action:* may be related to antagonism for dopamine and serotonin receptors; also has affinity for alpha receptors and histamine (H_1) receptors; *use:* psychotic disorders.

RNA splicing, the process by which base pairs that interrupt the continuity of genetic information in DNA are removed from the precursors of messenger RNA.

RNA viruses. See **viruses.**

Roach clasp. See **clasp, bar.**

Rockwell test. See **test, Rockwell.**

Rocky Mountain spotted fever (RMSF), a serious tick-borne infectious disease occurring throughout the temperate zones of North and South America, caused by *Rickettsia rickettsii,* and characterized by chills, fever,

rod, a straight, slim, cylindric form of material, usually metal.

r., analyzing, the vertical part of a dental cast surveyor that is brought into contact with the surface contour of a tooth as a tangent related to a curve. It is used to determine the relative parallelism of one surface of a cast to other surfaces of the same cast. It is also used to estimate the cervical convergence of an infrabulge area of a tooth as it slopes from the contacting point of the surveying rod toward the cervical line, permitting evaluation of the retentiveness of the surface.

r., condyle, the adjustable pointers of a face-bow, which are placed over the condyles or at points on the face to mark the opening axis of the mandible.

r., enamel, a calcified column or prism, with an average diameter of 4 microns; extends in a wavy pattern through the entire thickness of the enamel and is generally perpendicular to the surface of the tooth.

rodent ulcer, a slowly developing serpiginous ulceration of a basal cell carcinoma of the skin. See also **basal cell carcinoma.**

roentgeno- (rent'gənō), prefix used to denote radiation originating only from an x-ray tube.

roentgenogram (rent'gənōgram'). See **radiograph.**

roentgenograph (rent'gənōgraf'). See **radiograph.**

roentgenographer (rent"ge-nog'rah-fer). (not current.) See **radiographer.**

roentgenographic detail. (not current.) See **detail, radiographic.**

roentgenography (rent'gəno'grah-fē). (not current.) See **radiography.**

roentgenologist (rent'gənol'ōjist). (not current.) See **radiologist.**

r., oral. See **radiologist, oral.**

roentgenolucent (rent'gənōlōō'sent). (not current.) See **radiolucent.**

roentgenopaque (rent'gənōpāk'). (not current.) See **radiopaque.**

roentgenoparent (rent'gənōpar'ent). (not current.) See **radioparent.**

roentgenotherapy (rent'gənōther'əpē). (not current.) See **therapy, radiation.**

Roger's syndrome. See **syndrome, Roger's** (not current).

role model, a person who inspires others to imitate his or her persona, values, and goals.

Romberg sign, an indication of loss of the sense of position in which the patient loses balance when standing erect, with feet together and eyes closed. Also called Romberg test.

rongeur forceps, a strong and heavy cutting or biting forceps that is used for cutting bone.

root, l. the part of a human tooth covered by cementum. **2.** a nerve root; the part of a nerve adjacent to the center with which it is connected; in spinal and cranial nerves the part of the nerve between the cells of origin or termination and the ganglion.

r. amputation. See amputation, root.

r. canal instrument stop, a device placed on a root canal instrument to mark the measured depth of instrument penetration.

r. curettage. See curettage, root.

r., intraalveolar, the portion of a tooth root enclosed in and supported by alveolar bone.

r. resection. See apicoectomy.

r. resorption of teeth, the destruction of the cementum or dentin by cementoclastic or osteoclastic activity. It may result in a shortening or blunting of the root. Lateral root resorption may also occur, resulting in a loss of root substance along the side or length of the root. Severe lateral resorption may result in penetration of the pulp canal. Root resorption may be caused by inflammation resulting from trauma or infection, or it may be unknown or idiopathic. See also **resorption.**

r. retention, removal of the crown of a root canal-treated tooth, whose periodontium is not adequate to support a prosthesis but with enough retention of the root and gingival attachment to support a removable prosthesis. See also **overdenture.**

r. submersion, root retention in which the tooth structure is reduced below the level of the alveolar crest and the soft tissue is allowed to heal over it. It is believed that residual ridge resorption can be minimized by this approach. See also **root retention.**

Rorschach test, better known as the inkblot test, this test consists of 10 pictures of inkblots, five in black and white, three in black and red, and two multicolored, to which the subject responds by telling, in as many interpretations as is desired, what images and emotions each design evokes.

rosary, rachitic, a beading of the ribs at the costochondral junction such as occurs in rickets.

rose fever, a common misnomer for seasonal allergic rhinitis caused by pollen, most frequently of grasses, that is airborne when roses are in bloom.

Rosenthal's syndrome. (not current.) See **hemophilia C.**

rotary cutting instrument. See **instrument, cutting, rotary.**

rotating anode. See **anode, rotating.**

rotating condyle. See **condyle, rotating.**

rotating spring, an auxiliary wire used in conjunction with arch wire to rotate a tooth into proper position.

rotation, 1. the act of turning about an axis or a center. **2.** movement of a tooth around its longitudinal axis.

r. center. See **center, rotation.**

rotavirus, a double-stranded RNA molecule that appears as a tiny wheel, with a clearly defined outer layer or rim and an inner layer of spokes. It is a cause of acute gastroenteritis with diarrhea, particularly in infants.

Rothera's test. (not current.) See **test, ketone bodies.**

rounds, a teaching conference or meeting in which the clinical problems encountered in the practice of medicine, dentistry, nursing, or other service are discussed.

roundworm, any worm of the class Nematoda, including *Ancylostoma duodenale, Ascaris lumbricoides, Enterobius vermicularis,* and *Strongyloides stercoralis,* that may infect the gastrointestinal tract of humans.

routine, 1. a fixed pattern of procedures used in any phase of treatment. **2.** a set of instructions arranged in proper sequence to direct the computer to perform a desired operation or series of operations.

r., office, a series of steps, to be followed in a carefully planned sequence, that provide a means of dealing with situations commonly encountered in dental practice.

RU486, a drug that can end a pregnancy when administered as a 1-dose pill within the first 6 weeks after conception.

rubber dam. See **dam, rubber.**

rubber dam clamp. See **clamp, rubber dam.**

r.d.c. forceps, an instrument used to place a clamp on a tooth, adjust a clamp, or remove it from a tooth. It engages the holes or notches of the flanges of the clamp.

rubber dam holder, in endodontics, a rubber dam frame holder; in operative dentistry, a rubber dam frame.

rubefacient, a substance or agent that increases the reddish coloration of the skin.

rubella (rōōbel'ə) (German measles, 3-day measles), a highly contagious viral disease spread chiefly by direct contact that has an incubation period of about 18 days. Manifestations include pharyngitis, regional lymphadenopathy, mild constitutional symptoms, and a maculopapular rash that becomes scarlatiniform. Oral lesions are red macules.

rudimentary, pertaining to something either vestigial or embryonic.

rubeola (rōōbē-ō'lə). See **measles.**

Ruffini's corpuscles (rōōfē'nēz). See **corpuscle, Ruffini's.**

rugae (rōō'gē, rōō'jē), the irregular ridges in the mucous membrane covering the anterior part of the hard palate.

r. area. See **area, rugae.**

rule, Clark's, a formula used to estimate the dosage of a drug for individuals whose weight varies significantly from the arbitrarily selected official standard of 150 pounds (67.5 kg). The dose is calculated by dividing the weight of the patient by 150 and multiplying by the dose to determine the current dose for a patient weighing more or less than 150 pounds.

rule of confidentiality, a principle that personal information about others, particularly patients, should not be revealed to anyone not authorized to receive such information.

rule, Young's, a mathematics expression used to determine a drug dosage for children. The correct dosage is calculated by dividing the child's age by an amount equal to the child's age plus 12 and then multiplying by the usual adult dose.

Rumpel-Leede test. See **test, capillary resistance.**

run, one performance of a program on a computer; performance of one routine or several routines automatically linked so that they form an operating unit, during which time manual manipulation by the computer operator is usually not required.

rupture, a tear or break in the continuity or configuration of an organ or body tissue, including those instances when other tissue protrudes through the opening.

Sabouraud's medium (sahboorōz'). See **medium, Sabouraud's.**

saccharin, the chemical sweetener benzosulfimide, which is 300 to 500 times as sweet as sucrose. Tests have demonstrated that large amounts of benzosulfimide may cause cancers in experimental animals. Saccharin is no longer in general use as a low-calorie sweetener.

Saccharomyces, a genus of yeast fungi, including brewer's and baker's yeast, as well as some pathogenic fungi, that cause such diseases as bronchitis, moniliasis, and pharyngitis.

sacroiliac joint, an irregular synovial joint between the sacrum and ilium on either side of the pelvis.

saddle. See **base, denture.**

s. connector. See **connector, major.**

s., metal. See **base, metal.**

s. nose, a sunken nasal bridge caused by injury or disease and resulting in damage to the nasal septum.

safelight, A source of illumination in a darkroom of a color and intensity that does not fog radiographic film.

safety measures, actions (for example, use of glasses, face masks) taken to protect patients and office personnel from known hazards such as particles and aerosols from high-speed rotary instruments, mercury vapor, radiation exposure, anesthetic and sedative gases, falls, inadequate sterilization, cuts, puncture wounds, and laboratory accidents.

sagittal (saj'ətəl), shaped like or resembling an arrow; straight; situated in the direction of the sagittal suture. Said of an anteroposterior plane or section parallel to the long axis of the body.

s. axis, a hypothetical line through the mandibular condyle that serves as an axis for rotation movements of the mandible.

s. plane. See **plane, sagittal.**

s. splitting of mandible, intraoral osteotomy of the ascending ramus and posterior body of the mandible in the sagittal plane for the correction of prognathism, retrognathism, or apertognathia. An alternative procedure confines the split to the body of the mandible.

Saint Vitus' dance. See **chorea.**

Sainton's disease. See **dysostosis, cleidocranial.**

salary 1. a fixed, regular compensation paid for services rendered involving professional knowledge or skill; employment above the degree of mechanical labor. **2.** the amount of take-home pay received by the dentist from the practice.

s. arrangements, The clear understanding between the dentist and auxiliaries concerning the amount of money they will be paid, the increase in pay they may expect, and the time interval between pay increases.

salicylamide (salisilam'īd), an analgesic, antipyretic, and antiarthritic similar in action to aspirin.

salicylanilide (sal'isilan'ilīd), an antifungal agent useful in the treatment of tinea capitis caused by *Microsporum audouinii.*

salicylates (səlis'əlāts), salts or esters of salicylic acid; salicylates are used as preservatives, antiseptics, fungicides, and keratolytic agents.

salicylism (sal'isil'izəm), a toxic state resulting from excess ingestion of salicylates.

saline (sā'līn), salty; of the nature of a salt; containing a salt or salts.

saliva (səlī'və), the clear, slightly acid mucoserous secretion formed in the parotid, submaxillary, sublingual, and smaller oral mucous glands. It has lubricative, cleansing, bactericidal, excretory, and digestive functions and also is an aid to deglutition. Its pH level is slightly acidic—6.3 to 6.9.

Emotional disturbances affect the rate of salivary secretion either by stimulation of secretion or inhibition of activity, leading to xerostomia. A lowered rate of flow has been noted in patients suffering from depression, whereas a higher degree of salivary activity has been observed in patients with mania.

s., lingual, saliva secreted by Ebner's glands and other serous glands of the tongue.

s., loss of CO_2 in, a theory of calculus formation in which the loss of carbon dioxide (CO_2) from saliva reduces the salivary carbonic acid content and causes the calcium phosphate in solution in the saliva to become supersaturated; calcium phosphate then precipitates in areas of stasis of the saliva.

s., parotid, saliva produced by the parotid gland. It is thinner and less viscous than are the other varieties and contains no mucin.

s., supersaturated, Saliva overladen with mineral elements associated with calculus formation. With a loss of carbon dioxide (CO_2) and a rise in the pH level of saliva, precipitation of calcium, phosphates, and magnesium carbonate occur, thus providing the mineral components of salivary calculus.

saliva tests. See **tests, calorimetric caries susceptibility.** (not current)

salivant (sal' ivənt), provoking a flow of saliva.

salivary glands, three pairs of exocrine glands that produce saliva and empty it into the mouth. The parotid glands produce serous fluid, the sublingual glands produce mucous fluid, and the submandibular glands produce serous and mucous secretions.

salivary lactobacillus count, determination of the number of lactobacilli per milliliter of saliva; an indicator of caries susceptibility. High lactobacillus counts generally correlate with high caries activity. (not current)

salivation (sal′ivā′shən), excessive discharge of saliva; ptyalism.

salmeterol xinafoate, *trade name:* Serevent Inhalation Aerosol; *drug class:* long-acting selective B₂-agonist; *action:* relaxes bronchial smooth muscle by directly acting on B₂-adrenergic receptors; also inhibits release of mast cell mediators; *uses:* treatment of bron-

chospasm, maintenance treatment of asthma and exercise-induced bronchospasm.

Salmonella, a genus of motile, gram-negative, rod-shaped bacteria that include species causing typhoid fever, paratyphoid fever, and other forms of gastroenteritis.

salsalate, *trade names:* Armigesic, Anaflex, Arthra-G, Mono-Gesic, Salflex, and Salsitab; *drug class:* salicylate, nonnarcotic analgesic; *action:* blocks formation of peripheral prostaglandins, which cause pain and inflammation; antipyretic action results from inhibition of hypothalamic heat-regulating center; does not inhibit platelet aggregation; *uses:* treatment of mild-to-moderate pain or fever, including arthritis and juvenile rheumatoid arthritis.

salt (sôlt), a compound of a base and an acid; a compound of an acid, some of whose replaceable hydrogen atoms have been substituted.

s., basic, a salt containing replaceable, or hydroxyl, groups.

salt depletion. See **depletion, salt.**

samarium (Sm), a rare earth, metallic element. Its atomic number is 62, and its atomic weight is 150.35.

sample, a selected part of a population that is taken to be representative of the whole population.

s., random, a sample drawn by chance; a sample drawn in such a way that every item in the population has an equal and independent chance of being included in the sample.

s., stratified, a sample derived by dividing the population into a number of nonoverlapping classes or categories from which cases are selected at random, the number of cases selected from each category being proportional to the number therein.

sanguinaria (sang′gwinar′ēə), common name bloodroot. *Sanguinaria canadensis* contains an isoquinoline alkaloid thought to be useful in reducing plaque and gingivitis. Although it has been marketed, test results have been equivocal, and untoward side effects have been reported. It can be highly toxic if swallowed.

sanguine, 1. pertaining to an abundant and active blood circulation, ruddy complexion. **2.** an attitude full of vitality and confidence.

sanitarium, a facility for the treatment of patients suffering from chronic mental or physical diseases or for the recuperation of convalescent patients. Also called a sanatorium.

sanitation, the science of maintaining a healthful, disease- and hazard-free environment.

saponification, the production of soap.

saprophyte, an organism that lives on dead organic matter.

saquinavir mesylate, *trade name:* Invirase; *drug class:* antiviral; *action:* inhibits human immunodeficiency virus (HIV) protease important for viral replication; *use:* used in combination with nucleoside analogues, zidovudine, or zalcitabine in the treatment of acquired immunodeficiency syndrome (AIDS).

SAR. See **relationship, structure-activity.**

sarcoadenoma, a mixed tumor containing characteristics of both glandular and connective tissue.

sarcocarcinoma, a mixed tumor with characteristics of both sarcomas and carcinomas.

sarcoidosis (sär′koidō′sis) (Besnier-Boeck-Schaumann disease, Boeck's sarcoid), a chronic granulomatous disease of unknown etiology. Causes noncaseating granulomas in the skin, lymph nodes, salivary glands, eyes, lungs, and bones.

sarcoma (särkō′mə), **1.** a malignant neoplasm of connective tissue elements. **2.** a malignant neoplasm arising from mesenchyme or its derivatives.

s., ameloblastic, a rare mixed tumor of odontogenic origin in which the mesenchymal component has undergone malignant transformation.

s., Ewing's. See **tumor, Ewing's.**

s., Kaposi's, a condition affecting blood vessels; believed to be of a neoplastic nature and of multicentric origin. Skin lesions appear as multiple red-brown nodules ranging from a few mm to 1 cm in size. Histologically, endothelial proliferation in sheets or small vessels, hemosiderin deposits, fibroblastic proliferation, and an inflammatory infiltrate of lymphocytes are seen.

s., neurogenic (malignant schwannoma), the malignant form of neurilemoma.

s., osteoblastic (osteogenic sarcoma), an osteosarcoma in which atypical bone formation is the most evident histopathologic feature. See also **osteosarcoma.**

s., osteogenic, a malignant connective tissue tumor that produces bone.

s., reticulum cell, a malignant tumor of reticulum cells. It may occur as a primary neoplasm in soft tissue or bone.

Sargenti technique. See N2.

satin finish. See **finish, satin.** (not current)

satisfaction, discharge of an obligation by actual payment of what is due or what is awarded by a court or other authority.

saturated, having all the chemical affinities satisfied; unable to hold in solution any more of a given substance.

saturated fatty acid, any of a number of glyceryl esters of certain organic acids in which all the atoms are joined by single bonds. These fats are chiefly of animal origin, but include cocoa butter, coconut oil, and palm oil.

saturation, 1. a condition in which a solution contains as much solute as can remain dissolved. **2.** a measure of the degree to which oxygen is bound to hemoglobin, expressed as a percentage of the possible limit. **3.** a chemical compound in which all valency bonds have been filled.

saturation, color, the quality of color that distinguishes the degree of vividness of hue.

saucerization (saw′sərīzā′shən), excavation of the tissue of a wound to form a shallow, saucerlike depression.

s., pericervical, the circular bone resorption that occurs about the necks of endosteal implants shortly after their insertion and continues slowly during the time of the implant's biologic presence.

saw, a cutting blade with a toothed edge used to cut material too hard to slice with a knife.

s., Gigli's wire, a flexible wire with teeth used for osteotomy procedures; frequently used in blind operations.

s., gold, an instrument with a thin sawlike blade used for removing surplus metal from the contact area of gold-foil restorations.

s., ***Joseph,*** A nasal saw often used in ramusotomy of the mandible.

s., ***Koeber's,*** a saw consisting of a thin, replaceable blade held in a frame; used to trim gross excess from the proximal portion of a Class II foil restoration in the preliminary stages of finishing and contouring.

s., ***oscillating*** *(Stryker-type saw),* an oscillating blade in an electrical or compressed gas-driven unit; used to cut bone.

s., ***rotary,*** a rotary blade on a shaft in an electrical or compressed gas-driven unit; used to cut bone.

SBE. See **endocarditis, subacute bacterial.**

scabies, a contagious disease caused by *Sarcoptes scabiei,* the itch mite, characterized by intense itching of the skin.

scaffold, a support, either natural or artificial, that maintains tissue contour.

scaler (skā′lər), an instrument used to remove calculus from teeth.

s., ***sickle,*** a hook-shaped instrument available in various sizes and shapes; used for the removal of tenacious supragingival deposits of calculus.

scaling, the removal of calcareous deposits from the teeth using suitable instruments.

s., ***coronal,*** the removal of deposits of calculus, heavy stains, and materia alba from the crowns of the teeth by suitable instrumentation.

s., ***electrosurgical.*** See **electrosurgery; scalpel, electrosurgical.**

s., ***root,*** a technique of root surface cleansing designed to remove accretions of calculus and debris in the supragingival uninvested areas of a tooth.

s., ***subgingival,*** the removal of accretions and debris from the surfaces of the tooth apical to the gingival margin. This process accomplishes the removal of primary irritants to the gingival tissues and permits the reduction of inflammation in these tissues.

s., ***supragingival,*** the technique of meticulous cleansing of the surfaces of the teeth coronal to the gingival margin.

scalpel, a delicate, razor-sharp, pointed knife, usually with a convex edge.

s., ***electrosurgical,*** a scalpel that severs tissue by means of an electrically heated wire.

scandium (Sc), a grayish metallic element. Its atomic number is 21, and its atomic weight is 44.956.

scanning, a technique and protocol for carefully studying an area, organ, or system of the body by recording and displaying an image of the area using radioactive substances that have affinities for specific tissues.

scanning electron microscope (SEM), an instrument similar to an electron microscope in that a beam of electrons instead of visible light is used to magnify the surface of a sample. The electrons are deflected, collected, accelerated, and directed against a scintillator. The surface image produced is of less magnification than that produced by an electron microscope, but it appears three dimensional and lifelike. It is an essential research tool for the study of dental materials.

scar. See **cicatrix.**

s., ***apical,*** the end product of wound repair. A radiolucent area characterized histologically by dense fibrous connective tissue.

scarify, to make multiple superficial incisions into the skin.

scarlatina. See **scarlet fever.**

scarlet fever, an acute contagious disease of childhood caused by an erythrotoxin-producing strain of group A hemolytic *Streptococcus.* The infection is characterized by sore throat, fever, strawberry tongue, enlarged lymph nodes in the neck, prostration, and a diffuse bright red rash.

scattered radiation. See **radiation, scattered.**

Schaumann's body. See **body, Schaumann's.**

Schaumann's disease. See **sarcoidosis.**

schedule, the division of the working day into segments of time to enable the dentist to render treatment.

Schedule I, a category of drugs not considered legitimate for medical use. Included are heroin, lysergic acid diethylamide (LSD), and marijuana.

Schedule II, a category of drugs considered to have a strong potential for abuse or addiction but which also have legitimate medical use. Included are opium, morphine, and cocaine.

Schedule III, a category of drugs that have less potential for abuse or addiction than Schedule I or II drugs and have a useful medical purpose. Included are short-acting barbiturates and amphetamines.

Schedule IV, a medically useful category of drugs that have less potential for abuse or addiction than those of Schedules I, II, and III. Included are diazepam and chloral hydrate.

Schedule V, a medically useful category of drugs that have less potential for abuse or addiction than those of Schedules I through IV. Included are antidiarrheals and antitussives with opioid derivatives.

schedule of allowances (table of allowances), a list of specified amounts that will be paid toward the cost of dental services rendered; the patient pays the difference between the allowance and the actual cost of service.

schedule of benefits, a listing of the services for which payment will be made by a third-party payer without specification of the amount to be paid.

schedule plan, a plan that bases covered expenses on a schedule of allowances.

schema, Hamberger's (ske'mə), the bodily arrangement by which the external intercostal and intercartilaginous muscles are inspiratory muscles, and the internal intercostal muscles are expiratory muscles.

scheme, occlusal. See **system, occlusal.**

Schick test (shik), a skin test used to determine immunity to diphtheria in which diphtheria toxin is injected intradermally. A positive reaction, indicating susceptibility, is marked by redness and swelling at the site of injection; a negative reaction, indicating immunity, is marked by absence of redness and swelling.

schistometer (shis'tom'etər), an instrument for measuring the aperture between the vocal cords.

schistosomiasis (shis'tōsōmī' əsis) (bilharziasis), infestation with blood flukes of the genus *Schistosoma,* which causes cystitis, chronic dysentery, hepatosplenomegaly, and esophageal varices.

schizophrenia (skit'səfrē'nē ə) (dementia praecox), a functional psychosis (split personality) characterized by emotional distortion, withdrawal from reality, and disturbances of thought processes. It includes such disorders as hebephrenia, catatonia, and paranoia.

Schüller-Christian disease. See **disease, Hand-Schüller-Christian.**

Schüller's disease (shēl'ərz) (not current). See **osteoporosis.**

schwannoma (shwonō'mə). See **neurilemoma.**

s., malignant. See **sarcoma, neurogenic.**

sciatica, an inflammation of the sciatic nerve, usually marked by pain and tenderness along the course of the nerve through the thigh and leg.

scientific method, a formal style of study or research in which a problem is identified, pertinent information is assembled, a hypothesis is advanced and tested empirically, and the hypothesis is accepted or rejected.

scissors, Fox, Delicate, fine-pointed scissors designed to gain access to interproximal areas and remove small tissue tabs or slight soft tissue deformities during gingivoplasty and gingivectomy. They also may be used to smooth the cut gingival surfaces.

scleroderma (skler'ōdur'mə), (dermatosclerosis, hidebound disease), a collagen disease of unknown etiology; skin lesions are characterized by thickening, rigidity, and pigmentation in patches or diffuse areas. Dermal atrophy also may be seen. Periodontal lesions may simulate those of periodontosis, with widening of periodontal membrane space (verified by radiographic evidence) resulting from bone resorption, loss of architectural arrangement, and degeneration of periodontal fibers, with absence of inflammatory change in the gingivae and remaining periodontium.

sclerosing solution, a liquid containing an irritant that causes inflammation and resulting fibrosis of tissues. It may be used in cauterizing ulcers, arresting hemorrhage, and treating hemangiomas.

sclerosis (sklerō'sis), hardening. As applied to the jaws, sclerosis usually indicates an increased calcification

S

centrally, with radiopacity. Tracts of increased density in the dentin are referred to as areas of dentinal sclerosis. Sclerosis occurs beneath caries and with abrasion, attrition, and erosion.

s., multiple, a remitting and relapsing disease of the central nervous system affecting principally the white matter. Manifestations include sensory and motor incoordination and paresthesias; often dementia, blindness, paraplegia, and death result.

sclerotherapy, the use of sclerosing chemicals to treat varicosities such as hemorrhoids and esophageal varices.

scoliosis (skō'lēō'sis), a lateral curvature of the spine.

scope of services, the number, type, and intensity or complexity of services being provided.

scopolamine (skōpol'əmēn), an alkaloid found in the leaves and seeds of *Atropa belladonna* and other solanaceous plants having an action similar to atropine and used when spasmolytic or antisecretory effects are desired.

s., transdermal, trade names: Transderm-Scōp, Transderm-V; *drug class:* antiemetic, anticholinergic; *action:* competitive antagonism of acetylcholine at receptor sites in the eye, smooth muscle, cardiac muscle, glandular cells; inhibition of vestibular input to the central nervous system (CNS), resulting in inhibition of vomiting reflex; *use:* prevention of motion sickness.

scorbutic gingivitis, an abnormal condition, characterized by inflamed or bleeding gums; caused by vitamin C deficiency.

scorbutus (skorbu'təs). See **scurvy.**

scratch test, a skin test for identifying an allergen, performed by placing a small quantity of a solution containing a suspected allergen on a lightly scratched area of the skin. If a wheal forms within 15 minutes, allergy to the substance is indicated.

screen, intensifying, A layer of fluorescent crystals (usually calcium tungstate) supported on a flat base. Used in intimate contact with light-sensitive radiographic film in a cassette. The crystals fluoresce when exposed to x radiation and subsequently expose the film with light.

screen, oral, a Plexiglas or acrylic resin appliance that fits into the vestibule of the mouth for the correction of mouth breathing.

screening, 1. any examination of individuals or their records to ascertain dental needs, assess treatment plans, or evaluate services rendered. Prescreening is the review by designated dentists of patients' examination records as a prerequisite to the authorization of some or all types of treatment. Postscreening is the examination by designated dentists, usually on a sample basis, of records to determine whether services have been rendered adequately and in accordance with prescribed administrative procedures. **2.** a sample survey to determine initial treatment needs of a group seeking coverage under a dental plan; used in setting the initial premium.

screw, expansion, an orthodontic mechanism for achieving movement of teeth or arch segments, consisting of a threaded shaft and sleeve arrangement that permits controlled separation of elements of the appliance.

screw, implant, a small screw 3 to 5 mm long that is used as a means for primary retention of the implant.

screwdriver. See **instrument, screwdriver.**

Screw-Vent, a brand name of a blade implant of solid design manufactured by Core-Vent of pure titanium and much smaller than the companion product, the Core-Vent system.

scribe, to write, trace, or mark by making a line or lines with a pointed instrument or carbon marker.

scrofula (skrof'ulə), a primary tuberculosis complex occurring in the oro-cervical region and consisting of tuberculous cervical lymphadenopathy and tuberculosis of adjacent skin (lupus vulgaris), with chronic draining sinuses below the angle of the jaw and cervical region.

scurvy (skur'vē) (scorbutus), a condition resulting from an ascorbic acid deficiency that is severe enough to desaturate the tissues. The development and manifestations depend on tissue storage of ascorbic acid and factors that influence the rate at which it is used in or released from the tissues. Manifestations of frank scurvy in-

S

clude weakness, poor wound healing, anemia, and hemorrhage under the skin and mucous membranes. Presence or severity of gingival changes is directly related to the presence of local irritants such as calculus. In a severe form and in infantile scurvy, painful subperiosteal hemorrhages occur.

s., infantile (Barlow's disease, Cheadle's disease, Moeller's disease), a nutritional disease of infants caused by a deficiency of vitamin C in the diet. It has the same symptoms as does scurvy in adults.

s., land. See **purpura, thrombocytopenic, idiopathic.**

seal, 1. something that firmly closes or secures. **2.** a tight and perfect closure. **3.** to keep shut, enclosed, or confined.

s., border. See **border seal.**

s., double, a seal consisting of guttapercha underneath another material such as temporary cement; used to close the coronal opening in a tooth during endodontic treatment.

s., hermetic, perfect and absolute obliteration of all space within a tooth.

s., peripheral. See **border seal.**

s., posterior palatal, the seal at the posterior border of a denture produced by displacing some of the soft tissue covering the palate by extra pressure developed in the impression or by scraping a groove along the posterior seal area in the cast on which the denture is to be processed.

s., postpalatal. See **seal, posterior palatal.**

sealant, pit and fissure, a resinous material designed for application to the occlusal surfaces of posterior teeth to seal the surface irregularities and prevent ingress of oral fluids, food, and debris.

sealer, a substance used to fill the space around silver or gutta-percha points in a pulp canal. Most sealers contain some combination of zinc, barium, and bismuth salts and eugenol, Canadian balsam, and eucalyptol.

seasonal affective disorder (SAD), a mood disorder associated with the shorter days and longer nights of autumn and winter. Symptoms include lethargy, depression, social withdrawal, and work difficulties.

seat, basal. See **basal seat.**

seat, rest. See **area, rest.**

sebaceous glands (sibā′shəs), exocrine glands of the skin, many of which open into the hair follicles and secrete an oily substance that coats the hair and surrounding epithelium, helping to prevent evaporation of sweat and retain body heat.

seborrhea, any of several common skin conditions in which an overproduction of sebum results in excessive oiliness or dry scales.

s. capitis, Seborrhea of the scalp frequently seen in infants. Also called cradle cap.

secobarbital/secobarbital sodium (sēkōbar′bital), *trade names:* Novosecobarb, Seconal; *drug class:* sedative-hypnotic barbiturate, controlled substance Schedule II; *action:* nonselective depression of the central nervous system (CNS), ranging from sedation to hypnosis to anesthesia to coma depending on the dose; *uses:* treatment of insomnia, status epilepticus, and acute tetanus convulsions, sedation, preoperative medication.

secondary cancer, an opportunistic neoplasm imposed on a host with reduced vitality and resistance resulting from a preceding neoplasm or infection.

secondary dental caries, dental caries developing in a tooth already affected by the condition; often a new lesion formed adjacent to or beneath a restoration.

secondary dentition. See **dentition, permanent.**

secondary hemorrhage, bleeding that develops 24 hours or more after the original injury or surgery. It is often caused by an infection.

secondary infectious disease, an opportunistic infection imposed on a host with reduced vitality and resistance resulting from a preceding infection by a more virulent organism.

secondary radiation. See **radiation, secondary.**

secondary sex characteristic, any of the external physical characteristics of sexual maturity that distinguish one gender from the other, such as the distribution of hair and voice changes.

second-opinion program, an opinion about the appropriateness of a pro-

S

posed treatment provided by a practitioner other than the one making the original recommendation; some benefit plans require such opinions for selected services.

secretary-receptionist, the auxiliary whose chief responsibilities are to receive patients into the office, handle the correspondence and bookkeeping, order supplies, supervise housekeeping, and answer the telephone.

secrete, to discharge or empty a substance into the blood stream or a cavity or onto the surface of the body. The substance secreted is called a secretion. Glands that secrete internally are endocrine or ductless glands; glands that secrete into a cavity or onto the surface are exocrine or duct glands.

sectional arch wire, an orthodontic wire that occupies less than a complete dental arch. It usually is attached to only a few teeth. Typically it spans one or both buccal segments of the dental arch or is limited to the anterior teeth. It facilitates the application of differential forces in effecting tooth movement.

sectional impression, an impression made in two or more parts.

sectioning, surgical, dividing a tooth to facilitate its removal. A variety of instruments, including osteotomes and power-driven burs, are used.

sedation (sidā′shən), the production of a sedative effect; the act or process of calming.

sedative (sed′ ətiv), **1.** production of sedation. A drug that can produce sedation. **2.** any one of the drugs that produces cortical depression of varying degrees. **3.** a remedy that allays excitement and slows down the basal metabolic rate without impairing the cerebral cortex.

sedative-hypnotic, a drug that reversibly depresses the activity of the central nervous system, used chiefly to induce sleep and allay anxiety.

sediment, a deposit of relatively insoluble material that settles to the bottom of a container of liquid.

sedimentation rate (SR), the speed of settling of red blood cells in a vertical glass column of citrated plasma. It is used to monitor inflammatory or malignant disease.

seed, radon. See **radon seed.**

segment, any of the parts into which a body naturally separates or is divided, either actually or by an imaginary line.

seizure disorders. See **epilepsy.**

Seldane. a trade name for an oral antihistamine (terfenadine).

selection, 1. the act of choosing between or among a variety of options or alternatives. **2.** the process by which various factors or mechanisms determine and modify the reproductive ability of a genotype within a specific population. Also referred to as natural selection.

s., shade (*tooth color selection*), the determination of the color (hue, brilliance, saturation, translucency) of the artificial tooth or set of teeth for a given patient.

s., tooth, the selection of a tooth or teeth (shape, size, color) to harmonize with the individual characteristics of a patient.

s., tooth color. See **selection, shade.**

selective grinding. See **grinding, selective.**

selectivity, sensory, the property of the specialized receptor end-organ by which it responds to one type of stimulus rather than another.

selegiline HCl, *trade names:* Eldepryl, SD-Deprenyl; *drug class:* antiparkinson agent; *action:* increased dopaminergic activity by inhibiting monoamine oxidase (MAO) type B activity; *uses:* adjunct management of Parkinson's disease in patients being treated with carbidopa-levodopa.

selenium (Se) (sīlē′nēəm), a trace element used in the treatment of seborrhea and dandruff of the scalp. Selenium is toxic in large amounts.

Selenomonas (se′lenōmō′nas), a genus of gram-negative, anaerobic, rod-shaped bacteria found in the oral cavity.

self-analysis, introspection on one's own behavior and actions in the total environment.

self-concept, the composite of ideas, feelings, and attitudes that a person has about his or her own identity, worth, capabilities, and limitations.

self-curing resin. See **resin, autopolymerizing.**

self-esteem, the degree of worth and competence one attributes to oneself.

self-funding, the method of providing employee benefits in which the sponsor does not purchase conventional insurance but rather elects to pay for the claims directly, generally through the services of a third-party administrator. Self-funded programs often have stop-loss insurance in place to cover abnormal risks.

self-insurance, setting aside of funds by an individual or organization to meet anticipated dental care expenses or dental care claims, and accumulation of a fund to absorb fluctuations in the amount of expenses and claims. The funds set aside or accumulated are used to provide dental benefits directly instead of purchasing coverage from an insurance carrier.

self-limited disease, a disease restricted in duration by its own pattern of characteristics and not by other influences or interventions.

self-tapping implant, an implant that cuts its own path into bone.

self-tapping screw, a screw that cuts its own spiral threads into bone or tooth structure.

sella turcica (S), the pituitary fossa. The center is used as a cephalometric landmark.

s. t., floor of, lowermost point on the internal contour of the sella turcica.

Selter's disease. See erythredema polyneuropathy. (not current)

semantics, the study of language with special concern for the meanings of words and other symbols.

semicoma, a mild coma from which the patient may be aroused.

semiconductor, a solid crystalline substance whose electrical conductivity is intermediate between that of a conductor and an insulator.

seminarcosis. See **sleep, twilight.** (not current)

semipermeable (semēpur'mēəbəl), permitting the passage of certain molecules and hindering that of others.

senescence (sənes'əns), the process of growing old.

senescence, dental, a condition of the teeth and associated structures in which deterioration results from aging or premature aging processes. (not current)

senile dental caries, tooth decay occurring at an advanced age. Senile dental caries is usually characterized by cavity formation at the cemento-enamel junction or in the cemental layer covering the root.

senile psychosis, an organic mental disorder of aged people resulting from a generalized atrophy of the brain with no evidence of cerebrovascular disease.

senility (sini'itē), old age; generally used to describe the cognitive and physiologic signs of advancing age.

sensation (sensā'shən), an impression conveyed by an afferent nerve to the sensorium commune.

s., referred, a group of vaguely classified sensations that are a consequence of cortical experience. They are the sensory hallucinations, paresthesias, and the phenomenon called phantom limb. Nonspecific and poorly localized pain in the alveolar ridges, which have poor vascular supply, may be evidence of this phantom limb phenomenon associated with neurotic behavior.

s., specialized, sensations that are perceived by the specialized end organs associated with special senses such as vision, hearing, and smell.

sensation, psychologic effects of, arousal, facilitation, and distortion of sensation by psychologic factors, the basis for which lies in the corticalization of the special senses.

sense (sens), a faculty by which the conditions or properties of things are perceived. Hunger, thirst, malaise, and pain are varieties of sense.

s., special, one or all of the five senses: feeling, hearing, seeing, smell, and taste.

sensibility, deep (sen'sibil'itē), perception of pressure, tension, and pain from the deeper structures, as contrasted with sensations derived from the superficial layers of the skin.

sensitive (sen'sitiv), able to receive or transmit a sensation; capable of feeling or responding to a sensation.

sensitivity test, a laboratory method for testing antibiotic effectiveness.

sensitivity, tooth, the state of responsiveness of teeth to external influences such as heat, sugar, and trauma. May result from occlusal trauma, especially if the anatomic relation of the apical foramen to the traumatized tissue is such that the circulation of the pulp is disturbed.

S

sensitivity training, the use of group dynamics to experiment with and alter behavioral patterns and interpersonal reactions. Also called T group.

sensitization (sen'sitīzā'shən), the process of rendering a cell sensitive to the action of a complement by subjecting it to the action of a specific amboceptor; anaphylaxis.

sensorium (sensôr'ēəm), any sensory nerve center; more frequently, the whole sensory apparatus of the body.

sensory (sen'sərē), that part of the nervous system that receives and perceives sensations such as sound, touch, smell, sight, pain, heat, cold, and vribration.

sensory threshold, the point at which a stimulus triggers the start of an afferent nerve impulse. Absolute threshold is the lowest point at which response to a stimulus can be perceived.

separating medium. See **medium, separating.**

separating spring, spring placed between adjacent teeth to obtain separation.

separating wire. See **wire, separating.**

separator, an instrument used to wedge teeth apart and out of normal contact by immediate separation; useful in the examination of proximal surfaces of teeth and in finishing proximal restorations. Must be used with care; it should be stabilized against the teeth with modeling compound to prevent tissue damage.

s., Ferrier's, one of a set of balanced, double-bowed, adjustable separators designed by W.I. Ferrier.

s., noninterfering. See **separator, True's.**

s., True's (noninterfering separator), a single-bowed separator designed to give greater access to the surface being operated on; designed by Harry A. True.

sepsis, oral (sep'sis), a condition occurring within the mouth and adjacent areas characterized by the presence of pathogens.

septicemia (sep'tisē'mēə), a condition in which pathogenic bacteria and bacterial toxins circulate in the blood. Manifestations include high temperature, leukocytosis, malaise, rapid pulse, and subsequent diffuse systemic degenerative disturbances.

septic sore throat, a severe throat infection, usually caused by a *Streptococcus* strain, resulting in fever and marked exhaustion.

septum, interdental (interdental alveolar septum), the portion of the alveolar process extending between the roots of adjacent teeth.

septum, nasal, the thin, vertical bony septum separating the right and left nasal cavities.

sequela, any abnormal condition that follows and is the result of a disease, treatment, or injury such as paralysis after poliomyelitis or scar formation after a laceration.

sequence, order of occurrence or performance.

sequester, to detach, separate, or isolate, such as a patient sequestered to prevent the spread of an infection or the isolation of a jury during the conduct of a trial.

sequestrum (sikwes'trəm), a piece of dead bone that has become separated from vital bone.

serendipity, the act of accidental discovery.

serial extraction, a program of selective extraction of deciduous and sometimes permanent teeth over a period of time, with the objective of relieving crowding and facilitating the eruption of remaining teeth into improved positions. Close supervision of ensuing eruption is essential, because overclosure of the spaces and other sequelae may be expected in a significant number of cases. Comprehensive orthodontic treatment should almost always be initiated in the course of or after eruption for space management, control of the autonomous tipping usually induced by the procedure, and other malrelationships that commonly accompany these conditions.

serine (Ser), a nonessential amino acid found in many proteins in the body. It is a precursor of the amino acids glycine and cysteine.

serology tests (sirol'əjē) diagnostic tests of serum usually used to determine the immune or lytic properties of serum.

seronegative (sir'ōneg'ətiv), serologic evidence of the lack of an antibody of a specific type in the serum; diagnostically useful in ruling out Lyme disease, syphilis, human immunodeficiency virus (HIV), serum hepatitis B, and many other viral diseases.

seropositive (sir'ōpos'itiv), serologic evidence of the presence of an antibody of a specific type in the serum; diagnostically useful in identifying many types of viral diseases.

seroprevalence rates (sir'ōprev'ələns), a statistical measure of the rate of occurrence of seropositive status in a population or sample; used as a criterion of comparison between populations or samples.

serotonin (ser'ətō'nin) (enteramine, thrombocytin), a local vasoconstrictor (5-hydroxytryptamine) and general hypotensive agent synthesized from tryptophan and found in tissues, rather than being transferred by blood to sites of action. Most serotonin in mammals is found in the gastrointestinal tract, although the kidney, liver, and brain also produce it. It is absorbed by platelets from the site of tissue damage, where it aids hemostasis locally by vasoconstriction and systemically by reducing blood pressure.

serotonin serozyme (serō'zim). See **factor VII.**

serous fluid, a fluid that has the characteristics of serum in color and viscosity.

serous membrane, one of the many thin sheets of tissue that line closed cavities of the body, such as the pleura lining the thoracic cavity and the pericardium lining the sac enclosing the heart.

Serratia, a genus of motile, gram-negative bacilli capable of causing infection, including bacteremia, pneumonia, and urinary tract infections, in humans.

sertraline, *trade name:* Zoloft; *drug class:* antidepressant; *action:* selectively inhibits the uptake of serotonin in the brain; *use:* treatment of major depression.

serum (sir'əm), the fluid component of the blood containing all stable constituents except fibrinogen. When blood is allowed to clot and stand, a clear yellowish fluid, the serum, separates.

serum accelerator globulin. See **accelerator, prothrombin conversion, I.**

serum protein determination, electrophoretic, separation of serum protein fractions (albumin, alpha globulin, beta globulin, and gamma globulin) based on their different isoelectric points and mobility in an electric field. Electrophoretic patterns and concentrations are of value in evaluating the hyperglobulinemias. Electrophoretic evaluation of serum protein abnormalities is usually related to moving-boundary or paper-strip separation patterns.

serum prothrombin conversion accelerator (SPCA). See **factor VII; thromboplastin, extrinsic.**

serum sickness, anaphylactoid or allergic reaction after injection of foreign serum; marked by urticarial rashes, edema, adenitis, arthralgia, high fever, and prostration.

servant, one who is employed to perform personal services (other than those that would be rendered in an independent calling) for an employer and who, in that service, remains entirely under the control of the employer.

s., loaned, a person whose services have been granted by an employer to another person.

service, performance of labor for the benefit of another.

s., denture, diagnosis and treatment of edentulous and partially edentulous patients, including the diagnosis of existing and potential oral pathosis, planning of treatment for the preparation of the mouth for complete or partial dentures, fabrication and adjustment of the prostheses, and continuing observation of the changes in the oral conditions as the prostheses are in use.

s., gratuitous, a service that does not involve a return, compensation, or consideration.

s., health, those services, including dentistry, that improve the general physical and mental well-being of the patient.

service of process, the delivery of a writ, summons, or complaint to a defendant or witness. Service of process gives reasonable notice to allow the person to appear, testify, and be heard in court.

set, term applied to the state of a plastic material after it has hardened or jelled by chemical action, cooling, or saponification. It is used in connection with impression materials, waxes, and gypsum materials.

setting expansion. See **expansion, setting.**

setting time. See **time, setting.**

settlement, an agreement made between parties to a suit before a judgment is rendered by a court.

set-off. See **offset.**

setup, **1.** the arrangement of teeth on a trial denture base. **2.** a laboratory procedure in which teeth are removed from a plaster cast and repositioned in wax. May be used as a diagnostic tool to evaluate alternatives, as when some teeth are missing; also used to produce the mold to make a positioner appliance.

sex, classification of an individual as male or female on the basis of anatomic, functional, hormonal, and chromosomal characteristics.

s., anatomic, classification of sex based on sexual differentiation of the primary gonads.

s., chromosomal (genotype), chromosomal characteristics involving normally 44 somatic and 2 sex chromosomes, the latter designated as XX for the normal female and XY for the normal male. The presence of the Y chromosome is associated with a male phenotype and its absence with a phenotypic female.

s., functional (phenotype), designation of sex based on the state of maturation and potential for use of the external genitalia.

s., hormonal, contributory assignment of sex on the basis of adequate levels of estrogen and androgen for the development of typical phenotypic secondary sex characteristics.

s., legal, that sex assigned at birth or legally by a court of law.

s., nuclear, sex determination based on the presence or absence of the hyperchromatic nucleolar satellite in squamous cells from a buccal mucosa smear or of "drumsticks" in the polymorphonuclear neutrophil. Positives are normally seen in the female.

sex chromosomes, chromosomes responsible for sex classification—XX for female, XY for male.

sex linkage. See **linkage, sex.**

sexual harassment, in 1986, the United States Supreme Court adopted the definition of sexual harassment formulated by the Equal Employment Opportunity Commission as follows: unwelcome sexual advances, requests for sexual favors, and other verbal or physical conduct of a sexual nature when (1) submission to such conduct is made either explicitly or implicitly a term or condition of an individual's employment, (2) submission to or rejection of such conduct by an individual is used as a basis for employment decisions affecting such individual (both quid pro quo harassment), or (3) such conduct has the purpose or effect of unreasonably interfering with an individual's work performance or creating an intimidating, hostile, or offensive working environment (condition of work harassment).

sexually transmitted diseases. See **venereal diseases.**

shaken baby syndrome, a condition of whiplash-type injuries ranging from bruises on the arms and trunk to retinal hemorrhages, coma, and convulsions, as observed in infants and children who have been violently shaken. Physicians are required by law to report cases of suspected child abuse and are granted immunity from liability for filing such reports.

shallow breathing, a respiration pattern marked by slow, shallow, and generally ineffective inspirations and expirations. It is usually caused by drugs and indicates depression of the medullary respiratory centers.

shared services, administrative, clinical, or other service functions that are common to two or more hospitals or their health care facilities and used jointly or cooperatively by them.

sharpening, instrument, establishing or restoring of a keen edge on a cutting instrument.

Sharpey's fiber. See **fiber, Sharpey's.**

sharps, any needles, scalpels, wires, endodontic files, or other articles that could cause wounds or punctures to personnel handing them.

sharps container, a container designed for the disposal of sharps required and regulated by the Occupational Safety and Health Administration (OSHA).

S

shave biopsy, the removal of a thin layer of tissue using a dermatome knife. See also biopsy, shave.

shear. See **strength, shear; strength, ultimate.**

shearing cusps, the upper buccal cusps, lower lingual cusps, upper canines, and upper incisors. Each of these cusps helps form the fossae that receive the stamp cusps. In the postcanine teeth, the triangular ridges of the shearing cusps arm the fossae with cutting ridges. (not current)

sheath, nucleated. See **neurilemma.** (not current)

sheath, primitive. See **neurilemma.** (not current)

sheath of Schwann. See **neurilemma.**

shedding. See **exfoliation.**

sheep cell test, a method that mixes human blood cells with the red blood cells of sheep to determine the absence or deficiency of human T-lymphocytes.

shelf, buccal, the surface of the mandible from the residual alveolar ridge or alveolar ridge to the external oblique line in the region of the lower buccal vestibule. It is covered with cortical bone.

shelf life, the length of time a material may be stored without deterioration; the length of time it remains usable.

shellac base. See **base, shellac.** (not current)

shield, radiation, a body of material used to prevent or reduce the passage of particles of radiation. A shield may be designated according to what it is intended to absorb (for example, gamma ray, neutron shield) or according to the kind of protection it is intended to give (for example, background, biologic, thermal shield). The shield of a nuclear reactor is a body of material surrounding the reactor to limit the escape of neutrons and radiation into the protected area. Shields may be required to protect personnel and reduce radiation sufficiently to allow use of counting instruments for research or for locating contamination or airborne radioactivity.

shift, axis. See **axis shift.**

shift, chloride. See **phenomenon, Hamburger's.**

shift to right or left, an arbitrary description of an increase in the number per unit volume of immature (shift to left) or mature (shift to right) forms of neutrophils, in the differential counting system of Schilling.

Shigella, a genus of gram-negative pathogenic bacteria that causes gastroenteritis and bacterial dysentery.

shingles. See **herpes zoster.**

shock, I. a state of collapse of the body after injury or trauma. Shock may be either primary or secondary. The principal effects of shock are slowing of the peripheral blood flow and reduction in cardiac output. **2.** circulatory insufficiency caused by a disparity between circulating blood volume and vascular capacity.

s., galvanic, pain produced as a result of galvanic currents caused by similar or dissimilar metallic restorations.

s., hemorrhagic, an ineffectual circulating volume of blood resulting from loss of whole blood.

s., insulin, coma resulting from too much insulin or an inadequate intake of food. Symptoms include wet or moist skin, hypersalivation or drooling, normal blood pressure, tremors, dilated pupils, normal or bounding pulse, and firm eyeballs. Sugar and acetoacetic acid may be present in bladder urine but are absent in the second specimen. The blood sugar is low. See also **coma, diabetic.**

s., neurogenic, shock caused by loss of nervous control of peripheral vessels, resulting in an increase in the vascular capacity. Onset is usually sudden but is quickly reversible if the cause is removed and treatment is instituted immediately.

s., primary, shock that has a neurogenic basis in which pain and psychic factors affect the vascular system. Occurs immediately after an injury.

s., secondary, shock that occurs some time after the injury (6 to 24 hours later). Secondary shock is associated with changes in capillary permeability and subsequent loss of plasma into the tissue spaces. Changes in capillary permeability are probably related to histamine release associated with tissue injury.

s., traumatic, any shock produced by trauma, whether psychic or physical. In general usage, this term refers to shock following physical trauma, with hemorrhage, peripheral blood

S

vessel dilation, and changes in capillary permeability.

shoeing cusps. See **restoration of cusps.**

short-bowel syndrome, a loss of intestinal surface for absorption of nutrients caused by the surgical removal of a section of bowel.

short-cone technique. See **technique, short-cone.**

shotgun therapy, any treatment that has a wide range of effect and may be expected to correct the abnormal condition even though the particular cause is unknown.

shoulder, 1. the junction of the clavicle, scapula, and humerus where the arm attaches to the trunk of the body. **2.** in extracoronal cavity preparations the ledge formed by the meeting of the gingival and axial walls at a right angle.

shoulder, linguogingival, the portion of a prepared cavity in the proximal surface of an anterior tooth that is formed by the angular junction of the gingival and lingual walls. Developed to facilitate the dense compaction of gold in this area.

shrinkage, 1. reduction or decrease in extent or quantity. **2.** reduction in volume.

s., casting, volume change (contraction) that occurs when molten metal solidifies after being cast into a pattern mold. It is compensated for in three ways: by using the indicated water:powder ratio for the refractory investment to gain the maximal setting expansion of which that investment is capable; by exposing the investment to moisture as the refractory investment sets, causing some hydroscopic expansion; and by properly heating the mold to achieve thermal expansion. The total expansion must equal the contraction of the metal being cast.

shunt, arteriovenous (arteriovenous aneurysm, arteriovenous fistula), abnormal communication between an artery and a vein; usually caused by trauma.

shut, the part of an anterior artificial tooth between the ridge lap and the shoulder. The pins for retaining the tooth in the base material are located in the shut.

sialadenitis (sī′əlad′ənī′tis), inflammation of the salivary glands, especially the accessory glands, because of trauma.

sialoadenectomy (sī′ələad′ənek′təmē), excision of a salivary gland.

sialoangiectasis (sī′əlōan′jēek′təsis) (ptyalectasis), **1.** dilation of the salivary ducts. **2.** operative dilation of the salivary ducts. (not current)

sialodochitis (sī′əlōdōkī′tis), inflammation of salivary gland ducts. (not current)

sialodochoplasty (sī′əlōdō′kōplas′tē) a surgical procedure for the repair of a defect or restoration of a portion of a salivary gland duct. (not current)

sialogogue (sīal′əgog′), a substance that increases the flow of saliva.

sialogram (sīal′əgram′), a radiograph made to determine the presence or absence of calcareous deposits in a salivary gland or its ducts.

sialography (sī əlog′rəfē), **1.** inspection of the salivary ducts and glands by x-ray examination after injection of a radiopaque medium. **2.** production of a sialogram.

sialolith (sīal′əlith), a salivary calculus. See also **culus, dental.**

sialolithiasis (sīaləlithī′əsis), Presence of salivary gland or duct stones.

sialolithotomy (sīaləlithôt′ōmē), removal of calculus from a salivary gland or duct.

sialorrhea (sīal′ərē′ə) (hypersalivation, ptyalism), excessive flow of saliva. It may be associated with acute inflammation of the mouth, mental retardation, neurologic disorders with lenticular involvement, mercurialism, pregnancy, ill-fitting dental appliances, dysautonomia, periodic diseases, cystic fibrosis of the pancreas, teething, alcoholism, and malnutrition.

s., periodic, recurrent episodes of hypersalivation; of unknown cause but probably related to recurrent parotitis and other so-called periodic diseases.

sialoschesis (sīal′əs′kəsis), suppression of salivary secretion (dry mouth). Usually this condition contraindicates the wearing of a dental prosthesis during sleep. (not current)

sialosemeiology (sīal′əse′miol′əjē), analysis of salivary secretions. The quantity and composition of saliva may be determined, although this procedure has not been used to any degree in oral diagnosis. (not current)

sib, abbreviation for sibling, meaning brother or sister.

sibilant (sib′ilənt), accompanied by a hissing sound; especially a type of fricative speech sound.

sibling, one of two or more children who have both parents in common.

sickle (sik′əl). See **scaler, sickle.**

sickle cell anemia, a severe, chronic, incurable, hemoglobinopathic, anemic condition that occurs in people homozygous for hemoglobin S (Hb S).

sickle cell crisis, an acute, episodic condition that occurs in children with sickle cell anemia. The crisis may be vasoocclusive, resulting from the aggregation of misshapen erythrocytes, or anemic, resulting from bone marrow aplasia.

sicklemia (siklē′mēə). See **sickle cell anemia.**

side effect, an effect not sought in the case under treatment.

sideropenic dysphagia (sid′ərōpē′nik disfā′jēə) (not current). See **syndrome, Plummer-Vinson.**

side-shift, an imprecise term for lateral thrust of the rotating condyle.

SIDS, abbreviation for sudden infant death syndrome.

sigh (sī), an audible and prolonged inspiration followed by a shortened expiration.

sight, the special sense that enables the shape, size, position, and color of objects to be perceived; the sense or faculty of vision.

sigmoid (sig′moid), of or pertaining to an S shape, as in the shape of the pelvic end of the colon prior to its joining the rectum.

s. notch. See **notch, mandibular.**

sign (sīn), an indication of the existence of something; any objective evidence of a disease.

s., Battle's, the ecchymosis that appears near the mastoid process of the temporal bone; indicative of a fracture of the base of the skull.

s., Bell's, the turning up of the eyeball on the affected side when a patient with Bell's palsy attempts to close the eyelid.

s., Nikolsky's, a diagnostic feature wherein apparently normal epithelium

may be rubbed off with finger pressure.

s., Tinel's, a paresthesia in the area served by a sensory nerve when the site of a lesion or injury to the nerve is percussed. Indicative of partial injury of a nerve or regeneration of an injured nerve.

signa (sig′nə) (signature), the portion of a prescription that contains a statement of the directions for use.

signature. See **signa.**

signs and symptoms, diagnostic, the objective and subjective features of disease that are carefully evaluated to establish a diagnosis.

silica (sil′ikə) (quartz), the purest of three major ingredients that make up dental porcelain. It imparts stiffness and hardness to the product and is the framework around which the kaolin and feldspar contract.

silicate cement (sil′ikāt). See **cement, silicate.**

silicon (Si), a nonmetallic element, second to oxygen as the most abundant of the elements. Its atomic number is 14, and its atomic weight is 28. It occurs in nature as silicon dioxide and in silicates. The silicates are used as detergents, corrosion inhibitors, adhesives, and sealants. Elemental silicon is used in metallurgy and in transistors and other electronic components. Protracted inhalation of silica dusts may cause silicosis, which increases susceptibility to other pulmonary diseases.

silicone (sil′ikōn), a compound of organic structural character in which all or some of the positions that could be occupied by carbon atoms are occupied by silicon. A plastic containing silicons.

silicophosphate cement. See **cement, silicophosphate.**

silicosis, a lung disorder caused by continued, long-term inhalation of the dust of an inorganic compound, silicon dioxide, which is found in sands, quartzes, flints, and many other stones.

silk suture, a braided, fine black suture material, usually used to close incisions, wounds, and cuts in the skin. It is not absorbed by the body and is removed after approximately 7 days.

silver (Ag), a whitish precious metal occurring mainly as a sulfide. Its

S

atomic number is 47, and its atomic weight is 107.88. It is quite soft and is usually alloyed with small amounts of copper to increase its durability. It is used extensively in photography, radiography, and dentistry.

s. amalgam. See **amalgam, silver.**

s. cones, an endodontic filling material used in conjunction with guttapercha points and sealing agents to effect a seal of the pulp chamber and canal. Also known as master cones.

s. halide crystals. See **crystal, silver halide.**

s. nitrate, ammoniacal (am′ōni′ əkəl) (ammoniated silver nitrate, Howe's silver nitrate), an ammonium compound of silver nitrate, introduced by Percy R. Howe in 1917, that is more readily reduced to silver and silver proteinates than is the usual silver nitrate; formerly used to disclose carious tooth structure and immunize incipient carious lesions of the enamel but is highly irritating to the pulp.

s. nitrate, Howe's. See **silver nitrate, ammoniacal.**

s. points. See **silver cones.**

simian crease, a single crease across the palm produced from the fusion of proximal and distal palmar creases, seen in congenital disorders such as Down syndrome.

Simmonds' disease. See **disease, Simmonds'.**

Simon's classification of malocclusion, a classification of malocclusion in which tooth malpositions are related to three craniofacial planes: midsagittal, orbital, and Frankfort. Teeth too close to the midsagittal plane are in contraction, whereas those too far away are in distraction. Teeth too anterior to the orbital plane are in protraction, whereas those too posterior to the orbital plane are in retraction. Teeth too close to the Frankfort plane are in attraction, whereas those too distant are in distraction.

simple fracture, an uncomplicated closed fracture in which the fractured ends of the bone do not break the skin.

simple reflex, a reflex with a motor nerve component that involves only one muscle and level of the afferent and efferent nerve synapse.

simulation, a mode of computer-assisted instruction in which a student receives basic information about a topic and then must interact with the computer to gain deeper understanding of the information and topic. Simulation provides the student with the opportunity to gain experience with limited costs and reduced risk.

simvastatin, *trade name:* Zocor; *drug class:* cholesterol-lowering agent; *action:* inhibits 3-hydroxy-3-methylglutaryl coenzyme A (HMG-CoA) reductase enzyme, which reduces cholesterol synthesis; *use:* as an adjunct in primary hypercholesterolemia types IIa and IIb.

sine curve, the wave form of an alternating current characterized by a rise from zero to maximal positive potential, a descent back through zero to its maximal negative value, and then a rise back to zero.

single-blind study, an experiment in which the person collecting the data knows whether the subjects are in the control or experimental groups, but the subjects do not.

single-crystal sapphire, a single-crystal endosteal implant made of alpha alumina oxide with a Knoop hardness number of 1.750. The implants are threaded and supplied in three sizes: 3, 4, and 5.

single emulsion (film). See **emulsion, single.**

sinoatrial (SA) node, a cluster of hundreds of cells located in the right atrial wall of the heart near the opening of the superior vena cava. It comprises a knot of modified heart muscle that generates impulses, which travel swiftly throughout the muscle fibers of both atria, causing them to contract.

sinus (sī′nəs), a cavity, recess, or hollow space.

s., alveolar, a passage connecting a pathologic cavity in the alveolus with the oral or nasal cavity and penetrating the mucous membrane. See also **fistula, alveolar.**

s., carotid, the dilated portion of the internal carotid artery.

s., coronary, the venous sinus in the groove between the left cardiac auricle and the left ventricle.

s., maxillary (antrum of Highmore, maxillary antrum), a large pyramidal cavity within the body of the maxilla. Its walls are thin and correspond to the orbital, nasal anterior, and infratemporal surfaces of the body of the maxilla. On dental radiographs the floor of the sinus is often observed approximating the root apices of the teeth and is seen to extend from the canine or premolar region posteriorly to the molar or tuberosity region.

s., paranasal, accessory sinuses of the nose.

sinus balloon. See **balloon, sinus.**

sinus tract. See **tract, sinus.**

sinusitis, inflammation of the sinus.

site visit, a visit to an institution by designated officials to evaluate or gather information about a program, department, or institution. A site visit is a step in the accreditation of an institution and in the funding of many major research and training projects.

sitz bath, a bath in which only the hips and buttocks are immersed in water or saline solution. The procedure is used for patients who have had rectal or perineal surgery.

Siwe's disease (sĭ'we). See **disease, Letterer-Siwe.** (not current)

Sjögren's syndrome (shər'grenz). See **syndrome, Sjögren's.**

skeletal discrepancies, an orthodontic term used to describe the nature of a malocclusion as being a malrelationship of the bony base rather than merely of the teeth.

skeletal relationships, the orientation of bony parts to one another; usually the lower to upper jaw or to the bases with which they articulate.

skeletal system, all the bones and cartilage of the body that collectively provide the supporting framework for the muscles and organs.

skeleton of partial denture. See **framework.** (not current)

skill, practical knowledge of an art, science, profession, or trade and the ability to apply it properly in practice.

s., reasonable, skill that is ordinarily possessed and exercised by persons of similar qualifications engaged in the same employment or profession.

skin, the tough, supple cutaneous membrane that covers the entire surface of the body. It is the largest organ of the body and is composed of five layers of cells. See also stratum: **basale, corneum, granulosum, lucidum, spinosum.**

slander, oral defamation; the saying of false and malicious words about an-

other, resulting in injury to the reputation of the other.

slant of occlusal plane, the inclination measured by the angle the occlusal plane makes when extended to intersect with the axis-orbital plane. (not current)

sleep, a period of rest for the body and mind, during which volition and consciousness are in partial or complete abeyance and the bodily functions partially suspended.

s., twilight (seminarcosis), a state of amnesia and analgesia produced by an injection of scopolamine and morphine.

sleep apnea, a sleep disorder characterized by periods of an absence of attempts to breathe. The person is momentarily unable to move respiratory muscles or maintain airflow through the nose and mouth.

slice, in cavity preparation a straight-line (plane) cut that removes a thin layer from an axial convexity.

slim disease, a constitutional disease of acquired immunodeficiency syndrome (AIDS); also called human immunodeficiency virus (HIV) wasting syndrome. It is characterized by fever for more than 1 month, involuntary weight loss of greater than 10%, and diarrhea persisting for more than 1 month.

slope, lower ridge, the slope of the mandibular residual ridge in the second and third molar region as seen from the buccal side. (not current)

slotted attachment. See **attachment, intracoronal.**

Sluder's neuralgia. See **neuralgia, Sluder's.**

slurred speech, abnormal speech in which words are not enunciated clearly or completely but are run together or partially eliminated. The most common causes are alcohol toxicity and drug abuse. It may be a sign of damage to a motor neuron or cerebellar disease.

smallpox. See **variola.**

smear, bacterial, bacteria taken from a lesion or area, spread on a slide, and stained for microscopic examination.

smell, the special sense that enables odors to be perceived through the stimulation of the olfactory nerves.

smokeless tobacco, 1. chewing tobacco or tobacco powder (snuff) that allows the nicotine to be absorbed through the mucous membrane of the mouth or digestive tract. **2.** a transdermal nicotine patch that can be affixed to the upper part of the body to satisfy the person's craving for nicotine (used as an supportive aid during behavior modification aimed at smoking withdrawal).

smooth surface caries, a lesion that forms on the surface of a tooth without pits, fissures, or enamel faults; usually below a contact area between two teeth.

sneeze, an involuntary, sudden, violent expulsion of air through the mouth and nose; may be elicited during thiopental (Pentothal) anesthesia by corneal stimulation.

snuff dipper's lesion, a white or discolored lesion of the oral mucosa occurring at the site at which the powdered tobacco is retained. Malignant transformations are not common but do occur, usually as low-grade verrucous carcinomas.

Snyder's test. See **test, colorimetric caries susceptibility.** (not current)

soap, a salt or mixture of salts, of aliphatic acids, such as palmitic, stearic, or oleic acid, with sodium or potassium used for cleaning purposes.

sob, a short, convulsive inspiration, attended by contraction of the diaphragm and spasmodic closure of the glottis.

social functioning, ability of the individual to interact in the normal or usual way in society; can be used as a measure of quality of care.

socialized medicine, a system for the delivery of health care in which the expense of care is borne by a governmental agency supported by taxation rather than being paid directly by the client on a fee-for-service or contract basis.

socioeconomic status, the position of an individual on a social-economic scale that measures such factors as education, income, type of occupation, place of residence, and in some populations, heritage and religion.

sociology, the study of group behavior within a society.

socket, I. the hollow part of a joint; the excavation in one bone of a joint that receives the articular end of another

bone. **2.** any hollow or concavity into which another part fits, as the eyes.

s., dry *(alveolalgia, infected socket localized alveolar osteitis),* an osteitis or periostitis associated with infection and disintegration of the clot after tooth extraction. Because of its painful nature, it also is called alveolalgia.

s., infected. See **socket, dry.**

s., tooth, alveolus; the cavity in the alveolar process of the jaw in which the root of a tooth is fixed.

soda, a compound of sodium, particularly sodium bicarbonate, sodium carbonate, or sodium hydroxide.

sodium (Na) (sō′dē əm), a soft, grayish metal of the alkaline metals group. Its atomic number is 11, and its atomic weight is 22.99. Sodium is one of the most important elements in the body. Sodium ions are involved in acid-base balance, water balance, the transmission of nerve impulses, and the contraction of muscle. The recommended daily intake of sodium is 250 to 750 mg for infants, 900 to 2700 mg for children, and 1100 to 3300 mg for adults.

s. aluminum fluoride (floor′īd). See **cryolite.**

s. bicarbonate, an antacid, electrolyte, and urinary alkalinizing agent.

s. chloride, common table salt.

s. fluoride (NaF), a white, odorless powder used in 2% aqueous solution and applied topically to teeth as a caries-preventing agent; used as 33% NaF in kaolin and glycerin as a desensitizing agent for hypersensitive dentin. In drinking water, one part per million of NaF is used as a caries-prophylactic substance.

s. iodide, an iodine supplement to the diet, usually an additive to common table salt.

s. perborate (perbōr′āt), an oxygen-liberating antiseptic that has been used in the treatment of necrotizing ulcerative gingivitis and other forms of gingival inflammation. Prolonged or indiscriminate use has produced burns of the oral mucosa and hyperplasia of the filiform papillae of the tongue (black hairy tongue). Also used to bleach pulpless teeth.

s. thiosulfate (thīōsul′fāt), a powdered chemical, commonly called hypo, that is an ingredient of the fixing solution used in film processing. It clears the film of undeveloped silver halide crystals.

sodium fluoride poisoning, a chronic condition of fluorine poisoning that occurs in some communities where the fluorine concentration in the water supply exceeds one part per million. Signs of the condition include mottling of the tooth enamel and severe osteosclerosis.

sodium pump, a mechanism for transporting sodium ions across cell membranes against an opposing concentration gradient.

soft diet, a diet that is soft in texture, low in fiber residue, easily digested, and well tolerated. It is commonly recommended for people who have gastrointestinal (GI) disturbances.

soft palate, the structure composed of mucous membranes, muscular fibers, and mucous glands, suspended from the posterior border of the hard palate forming the roof of the mouth. When the soft palate rises, as in swallowing, it separates the nasal cavity and nasopharynx from the posterior part of the oral cavity and oral portion of the pharynx. In sucking the soft palate and posterior superior surface of the tongue occlude the oral cavity from the orapharynx, creating a posterior seal. Thus the soft palate prevents the escape of fluid and food up through the nose and with the tongue allows fluid and food to collect in the mouth until swallowed.

soft radiation. See **radiation, soft.**

soft tissue, all body tissue except bone, teeth, nails, hair, and cartilage.

soft tissue undercut. See **undercut, soft tissue.**

software, various programming aids supplied by manufacturers to facilitate the user's efficient operation of computer equipment. The collection of programs, routines, and documents associated with a computer (for example, compilers, library routines).

soft water, water that does not contain salts of calcium or magnesium, which precipitate soap solutions.

solar radiation, the emission and diffusion of actinic rays from the sun. Overexposure may result in sunburn, keratosis, skin cancer, or lesions associated with photosensitivity.

solder (sōd'ər), a fusible alloy of metals used to unite the edges or surfaces of two pieces of metal.

soldering flux. See **flux, soldering.**

soldering investment. See **investment, soldering; investment, refractory.**

solubility (sol'yəbil'itē), the quality or fact of being soluble; susceptible to being dissolved.

solute (sol'yo͞ot), the dissolved (usually the less abundant) constituent of a solution.

solution (səlo͞o'shən), the process of dissolving. In chemistry a homogeneous dispersion of two or more compounds. In pharmacy, usually a nonalcoholic solution. Solutions containing alcohol are variously called elixirs, tinctures, spirits, essences, or hydroalcoholic solutions.

s., Carnoy's, a sclerosing solution; mild; does not cauterize normal oral mucosa if used judiciously. A mild hemostatic.

s., cleansing, a solution especially suited to the removal of adherent food particles by immersion of the denture to avoid damaging the denture by brushing.

s., disclosing, a topically applied dye used in aqueous solution to stain and reveal the extent of calcareous and mucinous deposition on the teeth.

s., hardening, an aqueous solution (often of 2% potassium sulfate) in which a hydrocolloid impression may be immersed to reduce or retard syneresis of the impression material.

s., parenteral, a sterile solution or substance prepared for injection.

s., pickling, a solution of acid used for removing oxides and other impurities from dental castings (for example, solutions of hydrochloric or sulfuric acid).

s., sclerosing, an agent that causes intense inflammation, resulting in fibrosis; used to treat subluxation of the temporomandibular joint, cauterize ulcers, arrest hemorrhage, and treat hemangiomas.

s., solid, an alloy all of whose constituents are mutually soluble in the solid state.

solvent, a substance capable of or used in dissolving or dispersing one or more other substances; a liquid component of a solution present in greater amount than the solute.

somatic (sōmat'ik) derived from *soma*, meaning the body, as distinguished from the mind. Pertains to the framework of the body as distinguished from the viscera; hence the term *somatic nerves* describes the nerves associated with the musculoskeletal function of the muscles of the body.

somatotropin (sō'matōtrōp'in). See **hormone, growth.**

somnambulism (somnam'byəliz' əm), habitual walking in the sleep; a hypnotic state in which the subject has full possession of senses but no subsequent recollection.

somnifacient (som'nĭfā'shənt), causing sleep; hypnotic; a medicine that induces sleep.

somniferous (somnif'ərəs), inducing or causing sleep.

somnolence (som'nələns), sleepiness; also unnatural drowsiness.

somnolism (som'nəlizəm), a state of mesmeric or hypnotic trance.

sonant (son'ant), a speech sound that has in it a component of tone generated by laryngeal vibrations (for example, "a-a-a," "z-z-z").

sonic devices. See **ultrasonics.**

sonogram (son'ōgram), the readily usable graph of the frequency bands (formants) produced by the sound spectrograph.

sonograph (son'ōgraf), a wave analyzer that produces a permanent visual record showing the distribution of energy in both frequency and time.

soporific (sop'ərif'ik), a sleep-producing drug.

sorbic acid, a compound occurring naturally in berries of the mountain ash. Commercial sorbic acid is used in fungicides, food preservatives, lubricants, and plasticizers.

sore, canker (aphthous ulcer, aphthous stomatitis), a shallow ulcer of the oral mucosa; characterized by a grayish-yellow base and erythematous halo; the result of local minor trauma or the rupture of vesicles produced by the herpes simplex virus.

sore, cold. See **sore, canker; herpes labialis.**

sore, denture. See **ulcer, decubitus.**

sort, to arrange units of information according to rules dependent on a key

or field contained in or with the information.

s. generator program, a generalized program that can produce many different sorting programs in accordance with control information specified by the user.

sotalol HCl, *trade name:* Betapace; *drug class:* nonselective β-adrenergic blocker; *action:* competitively blocks stimulation of β-adrenergic receptors in the heart and decreases renin activity, all of which may play a role in reducing systolic and diastolic blood pressure; inhibits β_2-receptors in the bronchial system; *use:* treatment of life-threatening ventricular dysrhythmias.

source-collimator distance, distance from the focal spot to the diaphragm or collimator in an x-ray tube head.

source file, a file containing information used as input to a computer run.

source-film distance (SFD), distance from the focal spot of an x-ray tube to the radiographic film. Also known as target-film distance.

source language, a language that is an input to a given translation process.

source-object distance (SOD), distance from focal spot to object of which a radiographic image is to be obtained. Also known as target-object distance. (not current)

source program, a program coded in other than machine language that must be translated into machine language before being executed.

Southern blot test, a gene analysis method used to identify specific deoxyribonucleic acid (DNA) fragments and diagnose cancers and hemoglobinopathies.

space, a delimited, three-dimensional region.

s., freeway, the interocclusal distance or separation between the occlusal surfaces of the teeth when the mandible is in its physiologic rest position. Interocclusal distance is the preferred term. See also **distance, interocclusal; clearance, interocclusal.**

s., interalveolar. See **distance, inter-arch.**

s., interocclusal rest. See **distance, interocclusal.**

s., interproximal, the space between adjacent teeth in a dental arch. It is divided into the embrasure (occlusal to the contact point) and the septal space (gingival to the contact point).

s., interradicular, the area between the roots of a multirooted tooth; it is normally occupied by bony septum and the periodontal membrane.

s., lattice. See **lattice space.**

s., marrow, spaces in the spongiosa of bone; in the mandible and maxilla the marrow spaces are occupied by fatty and hematogenic (blood-forming) marrow. When inflammation progresses into these spaces, the marrow becomes fibrous. The spaces enlarge in atrophy of disuse because of resorption of surrounding trabeculae, and the marrow remains fatty in nature.

s., occupied, the space that might be occupied by persons or radiation-sensitive materials and devices during the time that x-ray equipment is in operation or radiation is being emitted.

s., physiologic dead, the air passages up to but not including the alveoli of the lungs; equal to about 150 cc.

s., retromylohyoid (ret′rōmī′lōhī′oid), the part of the alveololingual sulcus distal to the lingual tuberosity (the distal end of the mylohyoid ridge).

space maintainer, a fixed or removable appliance designed to preserve the space created by the premature loss of a tooth.

space maintainer cast, a space maintainer fabricated by a casting technique and cemented into place.

s. m., fixed, a space maintainer not intended to be removable by the patient.

s. m., orthodontic, a removable or fixed appliance fabricated to maintain space in the arch for erupting permanent teeth. The appliance may be designed to regain space needed to accommodate the erupting tooth or teeth.

s. m., removable, a space maintainer designed for easy removal for cleaning and adjustment.

space obtainer, an appliance used to increase the space between two teeth.

space regainer, a fixed or removable appliance capable of moving a displaced permanent tooth into its proper position in the dental arch.

space relief, fabrication of a prosthesis so that certain predetermined,

non–stress-bearing areas will not be contacted by the appliance.

spasm (spaz′əm), a sudden involuntary contraction of a muscle or muscle group. It may cause a twitch or close a canal or passage, depending on its location.

s., muscle, increased muscular tension and shortness that cannot be released voluntarily and prevents lengthening of the muscles involved. Caused by pain stimuli to the lower motor neurons.

spasmolysant (spazmol′īzənt), relieving or relaxing spasms; any agent that relieves spasm.

spasmolytic (spaz′mōlit′ik), pertaining to a drug that reduces spasm in smooth or skeletal muscle.

spastic (spas′tik), characterized by a more or less constant state of hypertonic contraction of a muscle or group of muscles. The condition is regarded as abnormally heightened muscular tonus present even in states of inactivity.

spasticity, a form of muscular hypertonicity with increased resistance to stretch.

spatula, a flat-bladed instrument without sharp edges used for mixing certain dental materials (for example, cement, plaster of paris, impression pastes).

spatulate (spa′chələt), to manipulate or mix with a spatula.

spatulation (spa′chələ′shən), manipulation of material with a spatula to mix it into a homogeneous mass.

spatulator (mechanical spatulator), a mechanical device that mixes ingredients to form a homogeneous mass.

s., mechanical. See **spatulator.**

SPCA, acronym for serum prothrombin conversion accelerator. See also **factor VIII; thromboplastin, extrinsic.**

Spearman's rho, a statistical test for correlation between two rank-ordered scales. It yields a statement of the degree of interdependence of the scores of the two scales.

specialist, a health care professional who is qualified to limit practice to a narrow spectrum of health care. A specialist usually has advanced clinical training and postgraduate education in the discipline or specialty.

specialization, the limiting of professional services to one isolated and distinct phase of dental practice.

specialty, that particular field of attention and endeavor to which a therapist's efforts are devoted.

s., dental, organized dentistry recognizes eight specialties: endodontics, pedodontics, periodontics, prosthodontics, public health dentistry, oral pathology, and oral surgery.

specific gravity. See **gravity, specific.**

spectrum, antibacterial, the range of antimicrobial activity of a drug.

spectrum, electromagnetic, a family of radiant energies that travel in wave form, have neither mass nor charge, and travel at the speed of light. Radiations within the spectrum vary only in wavelength. X-ray photons and light rays are examples of electromagnetic radiation.

Spee, curve of. See **curve of Spee.**

speech, 1. communication through conventional vocal and oral symbols. **2.** a basic biologic function of the maxillofacial structures. The essential characteristic of the speech function is the production and organization of sound into symbols.

s., delayed, failure of speech to develop at the expected age, usually resulting from slow maturation, hearing impairment, brain injury, mental retardation, or emotional disturbance.

s., infantile, a speech defect characterized by substitution of speech sounds similar to those used by the child who speaks normally in the early stages of speech development.

s., retarded, slowness in speech development in which intelligibility is severely impaired; often preceded by late or delayed emergence of speech.

s., visible, audible speech patterns that have been transformed by electronic apparatus into visual patterns that may be read by people who are deaf.

speech aid. See **aid, speech.**

speech device, a prosthesis that assists in the management of speech disorders associated with congenital or acquired defects of the palate.

speech pathology, 1. the study of abnormalities of speech or organs of speech. **2.** the diagnosis and treatment of abnormalities of speech as practiced by a speech pathologist or speech therapist.

speech phonation. See **phonation, speech.**

speech resonance. See **resonance, speech.**

speech therapy, the application of treatments and counseling in the prevention or correction of speech and language disorders.

speed, relative rapidity of action; rate of motion.

s., film. See **film speed.**

s., high, relatively great rapidity of motion. In cavity preparations, rotary instruments are classified according to the number of revolutions per minute (rpm) made by the cutting tool. Designation of each speed range presently varies. In general, conventional speed is 10,000 to 60,000 rpm, high speed is 60,000 to 100,000 rpm, and ultrahigh speed is more than 100,000 rpm.

speed of light, a speed of 186,300 miles/sec.

speed of radiation. See **radiation, speed of.**

sphenoid bone (sfe′noid). See **bone, sphenoid.**

spherocytosis, hereditary (sfir′ōsītō′sis). See **jaundice, congenital hemolytic.**

sphincter, a circular band of muscle fibers that constricts a passage or closes a natural opening in the body.

sphygmomanometer, an instrument for indirect measurement of blood pressure.

spicule (spik′yo͞ol), a small needle-shaped body.

s., cemental (cemental spike), a projection of cementum extending from the root surface into the periodontal membrane (usually along the path of the principal fibers). It represents calcification of the cemental fibers of the periodontal ligament and may not be true cementum. Hyperfunction is the etiologic agent for such spicules.

spillway, a channel or passageway through which food escapes from the occlusal surfaces of the teeth during mastication. The occlusal, developmental, and supplemental grooves, as well as the incisal, occlusal, labial, buccal, and lingual embrasures, become spillways during function.

s., axial, a groove that first crosses a cusp ridge or marginal ridge and ex-

S

tends onto an axial (mesial or distal) surface of the tooth.

*s., **interdental,*** a sluiceway formed by the interproximal contours of adjoining teeth and investing tissues.

*s., **occlusal,*** a groove that crosses only a cusp ridge or marginal ridge of a tooth; numerous on marginal ridges, thus increasing masticatory function.

spina bifida, a congenital neural tube defect characterized by a developmental anomaly in the posterior vertebral arch. Spina bifida is relatively common, occurring approximately 10 to 20 times per 1000 births.

spinal anesthesia, a state of insensitivity to pain in the lower part of the body produced by injection of an analgesic or anesthetic drug into the subarachnoid space of the spinal cord. See **anesthesia.**

spinal cord, a long, nearly cylindric structure lodged in the vertebral canal of the spinal column and extending from the foramen magnum at the base of the skull to the upper part of the lumbar region. It is a major component of the central nervous system. The cord conducts sensory and motor impulses to and from the brain and controls many reflexes.

spinal cord injury, traumatic disruption of the spinal cord as a result of vertebral fractures and dislocations, usually associated with car accidents, sports injuries, and other violent impacts. The degree of paralysis is directly related to the level and severity of the injury. Injury below the first thoracic vertebra may produce paraplegia. Injuries above the first thoracic vertebra may cause quadriplegia.

spindle, muscle, a fusiform body lying parallel to and between muscle fibers. It is composed of a conspicuously smaller modified muscle fiber that has its own motor end plate to cause it to contract and its own special sensory end organs (the flower spray ending and the anulospiral ending) that send information to the central nervous system regarding the state of contraction of the main muscle body.

spine, anterior nasal, the small bony projection extending forward from the medial anterosuperior part of each maxilla. The tip of the anterior nasal spines may be seen on lateral radiographic head plates and cephalometric radiographs.

spine, posterior nasal, the small, sharp, bony point projecting backward from the midline of the horizontal part of the palatine bone.

spirapril, *trade name:* Renormax; *drug class:* angiotensin-converting enzyme (ACE) inhibitor; *action:* selectively suppresses the renin-angiotensin-aldosterone system; inhibits ACE, prevents conversion of angiotensin I to angiotensin II; results in dilation of arterial and venous vessels; *use:* treatment of hypertension.

spirit (spir'it), any volatile or distilled liquid; also, a solution of a volatile material in alcohol.

spirit of ammonia, a solution of 3% ammonium carbonate in alcohol with flavorings added. It is mixed with water for use as a stimulant and carminative.

spirochete, any bacterium of the genus *Spirochaeta* that is motile and spiral shaped with flexible filaments. Spirochetes include the organisms responsible for leprosy, relapsing fever, syphilis, and yaws.

spirograph (spī'rəgraf), an instrument for registering respiratory movements.

spirography (spirog'rəfē), the graphic measurement of breathing, including breathing movements and breathing capacity.

spirometry, laboratory evaluation of the air capacity of the lungs by means of a spirometer.

spironolactone, *trade names:* Aldactone, Spirozide; *drug class:* potassium-sparing diuretic; *action:* competes with aldosterone at receptor sites in distal tubule, resulting in excretion of sodium chloride and water and retention of potassium and phosphate; *uses:* treatment for edema, hypertension, diuretic-induced hypokalemia, and cirrhosis of the liver with ascites.

spiroscope (spī'rōskōp), an apparatus for respiration exercises by which the patient can see the amount of water displaced in a given time and thus gauge respiratory capacity. (not current)

spleen, a soft, highly vascular, roughly ovoid organ situated between the stomach and the diaphragm in the left hypochondriac region of the body. It is considered part of the lymphatic system.

splenomegaly, an abnormal enlargement of the spleen, usually associated with portal hypertension, hemolytic anemia, and malaria.

splint, 1. a rigid appliance for the fixation of displaced or movable parts. **2.** a support or brace used to fasten or confine. **3.** metal, acrylic resin, or modeling compound fashioned to retain in position teeth that may have been replanted or have fractured roots.

s., abutment, adjacent tooth restorations that have been rigidly united at their proximal contact areas to form a single abutment with multiple roots.

s., acrylic resin bite-guard, an appliance, usually fabricated of resin, designed to cover the occlusal and incisal surfaces of the teeth to immobilize and stabilize the teeth and thus prevent them from being subjected to the effects of trauma from occlusal forces.

s., bridge. See **splint, fixed.**

s., buccal, a material such as plaster that can be placed on the buccal surfaces of assembled fixed partial denture units and onto which these components can be assembled and held in accurate relation after hardening.

s., cap, plastic or metallic fracture appliances designed to cover the crowns of the teeth; usually held in place by cementation.

s., cast bar *(Friedman splint),* a provisional splint consisting of cast continuous clasps that follow the facial and lingual surfaces of the teeth at the height of contour. It is cemented onto the teeth to be splinted and simultaneously wired closed to bring the clasps into intimate contact with the teeth. May not be cemented in place to serve as a removable cast splint.

s., continuous clasp, a cast splint used for the provisional immobilization of teeth.

s., copper band–acrylic, a splint fabricated from copper bands and acrylic resin.

s., crib, an appliance used for temporary tooth stabilization; constructed of gold, acrylic resin, chrome-cobalt alloys, or combinations thereof. It consists of a continuous crib clasp covering the facial and lingual surfaces of the teeth to be splinted.

s., cross arch bar, a splint formed by a metal bar that unites one or more teeth of one side of the dental arch to one or more teeth of the opposite side. Used to stabilize weakened teeth against lateral tilting forces. See also **connector, cross arch bar splint.**

s., cross arch bar, Bilson fixable-removable, type of cross arch bar splint.

s., fixed, a fixed (nonremovable) restorative and replacement prosthesis used as a therapeutic aid in the treatment of periodontal disease. It serves to stabilize and immobilize the teeth and replace missing teeth.

s., Friedman. See **splint, cast bar.**

s., Gunning's, a maxillomandibular splint used to support the maxilla and mandible in mandibular and maxillofacial surgery.

s., implant surgical. See **superstructure, temporary.**

s., inlay, an inlay casting designed to give fixation or support to one or more approximating teeth. This may be accomplished by two inlays soldered together or a single casting made for prepared cavities.

s., interdental, an appliance made of plastic or metallic materials that is applied to the labial and lingual aspects of the teeth to provide points for applying mandibular and maxillofacial traction and fixation.

s., labial, an appliance of plastic, metal, or combinations of plastic and metal made to conform to the labial aspect of the dental arch. Used in the management of mandibular and maxillofacial injuries.

s., lingual, an appliance similar to a labial splint but conforming to the lingual aspect of the dental arch.

s., provisional, a splint placed for a relatively short period. It is used to stabilize the teeth either during the healing period after accidental or deliberate tooth avulsion and replantation or in conjunction with periodontal therapy. It also may be used during a period of observation to determine the prognosis of the involved teeth.

s., Stader. See **appliance, fracture.**

splinting, the ligating, tying, or joining of periodontally involved teeth to one another to stabilize and immobilize the teeth, thus preventing them from being adversely affected by occlusal forces. Splinting includes acrylic resin bite guards, orthodontic band splints, wire ligation, provisional splints, and fixed prostheses.

s., cross arch, the stabilizing of weakened teeth against tilting movements caused by laterally directed occlusal stress loads. This is accomplished by the use of a rigid connector that projects to the opposite side of the dental arch where attachment is made to one or more teeth, thus producing effective counterleverage.

s., Essig-type, a method of stabilizing and repositioning injured teeth. Stainless steel fracture wire is passed labially and lingually around a segment of a dental arch, and the wire is held in position by individual ligatures around the contact areas of teeth.

splinting of abutments, the joining of two or more teeth into a rigid unit by means of fixed restorations.

split cast mounting. See **mounting, split cast.**

split ring, a casting ring made of three parts and designed to take advantage of the maximal expansion of the investment.

spondylitis, an inflammation of any of the spinal vertebrae, usually characterized by stiffness and pain.

spongiosa. See **bone, cancellous.**

spoon, an instrument with a round or ovoid working end; designed to be used for scraping or scooping.

spore, 1. a reproductive unit of some genera of fungi and protozoa. **2.** a form assumed by some bacteria that is resistant to heat, drying, and chemicals. Diseases caused by spore-forming bacteria include anthrax, botulism, gas gangrene, and tetanus.

sports medicine, a branch of medicine that specializes in the prevention and treatment of injuries from training and participation in athletic activities. More than one million people are treated for sports injuries each year in the United States.

spot, a small circular area.

s., café-au-lait, brown-pigmented areas of the skin occurring particularly in neurofibromatosis.

s., effective focal (prolonged focus), the apparent size and shape of the fo-

cal spot when viewed from a position in the useful beam. With the use of a suitably inclined anode face, the area from which the useful beam stems is sharply concentrated, if seen from the perspective of the useful beam. See also **line, focus.**

s., focal, the specific area of the face of the anode or target that is bombarded by the focused electron stream when an x-ray tube is in action. It is usually an insert of tungsten.

s., Fordyce's (Fordyce's disease, ectopic sebaceous glands), the chamois-colored, slightly raised spots on the oral mucosa or lips produced by sebaceous glands in those tissues. The term *Fordyce's disease* is sometimes erroneously applied to these spots, which are present in 70% to 80% of the population.

s., Koplik's, oral lesions of measles (rubeola); usually occur on the buccal mucosa opposite the molar teeth as small white or bluish-white spots surrounded by red zones.

s., pink. See **resorption, internal.**

sprain, an injury to a joint, with possible rupture of some of the ligaments or tendons but without dislocation or fracture. See also **strain.**

spray, a liquid minutely divided, as by a jet of air or steam.

spreader. See **condenser.**

spring, a piece of metal having the physical characteristic that, when bent, it returns to its original shape.

s., auxiliary (finger spring), a short piece of wire, attached to an orthodontic appliance at one end, that serves as a lever to apply force to a tooth or teeth.

s., coil, a spiral winding of fine wire attached to an orthodontic appliance.

s., finger. See **spring, auxiliary.**

sprue (sproo), in casting the ingate through which molten metal passes into the heated mold. The waste piece of metal cast in the ingate.

sprue base. See **sprue former; crucible former.**

sprue former (crucible former), a cone-shaped base made of metal or plastic to which the sprue is attached. Forms a crucible in the investment material.

sprue pin. See **pin, sprue.**

sputum (spyoo'təm), matter ejected from the mouth; saliva mixed with mucus and other substances from the respiratory tract.

squamous cell carcinoma (skwā′ məs). See **carcinoma, epidermoid.**

SRS-A, abbreviation for slow-reacting substance of anaphylaxis.

stability, the quality of being physically or emotionally predictable, orderly, not readily moved.

s., denture, the characteristic of a removable denture that resists forces that tend to alter the relationship between the denture base and its supporting bony foundation.

s., dimensional, the property of a material to retain its size and form.

s., emotional, state of an individual that enables him or her to have appropriate feelings about common experiences and act in a rational manner.

stabilization, 1. the act or process of stabilizing; the state of being stabilized. **2.** the seating or fixation of a fixed or removable denture so that it does not tilt and is not displaced under pressure. **3.** the control of induced stress loads and development of measures to counteract these forces so effectively that the tilting of the teeth or the movement of a prosthesis is minimized to a point within tissue tolerance limits.

stabilized baseplate. See **baseplate, stabilized.** (not current)

stabilizer, an instrument used in an x-ray unit to render the milliamperage output of the tube constant.

stabilizing, the process of fixing movable parts; making firm and steady. The fixing of clamps, separators, or matrices to teeth by the application of tacky compound to the parts, then chilling the compound. In the case of clamps and separators, this distributes the force of operating over adjacent teeth and the one being operated on.

stabilizing circumferential clasp arm. See **clasp, circumferential, arm, stabilizing.**

stable, term applied to a substance that has no tendency to decompose spontaneously. As applied to chemical compounds, it denotes their ability to resist chemical alterations.

stable isotope. See **isotope.**

Stader splint (sta′dər). See **appliance, fracture.**

staff. See **personnel.**

stage, surgical, a period or distinct phase in the course of anesthesia.

stain, 1. to discolor with foreign matter. **2.** a discoloration accumulating on the surface of a denture or teeth.

s., Gram's, a staining method for microorganisms that places them into two broad groups: gram positive, which retain crystal violet stain, and gram negative, which decolorize but counterstain with a red dye.

s., methyl violet, a dye used to color bacteria for microscopic examination.

staining, modification of the color of the teeth or denture base to achieve a more lifelike appearance.

stainless steel. See **steel, stainless.**

stamp cusp, a cusp made to work in a fossa. The maxillary lingual cusps are stamp cusps. In tooth-to-tooth occlusion all lower buccal cusps may stamp into fossae. In tooth-to-two-tooth occlusion the stamp cusps of the lower premolars may have their tips in embrasures and have only their shoulders in tiny fossae. (not current)

standard, that which is established by authority, custom, or general acceptance as a model; criterion.

standard deviation (SD), a computed measure of the dispersion or variability of a distribution of scores around a given point or line. It measures the way an individual score deviates from the most representative score (mean). A small SD indicates little individual deviation or a homogeneous group, and a large SD indicates that much individual deviation or a heterogeneous group.

standard error, a measure or estimate of the sampling errors affecting a statistic; a measure of the amount the statistic may be expected to differ by chance from the true value of the statistic.

standard error of estimate, the standard deviation of the differences between the actual values of the dependent variables (results) and the predicted values. This statistic is associated with regression analysis.

standard error of the mean, an estimate of the amount that an obtained mean may be expected to differ by chance from the true mean.

standard of care, a written statement describing the rules, actions, and conditions that direct patient care. Standards of care guide practice and may be used to evaluate performance.

standard orders, a written document containing rules, policies, procedures, regulations, and orders for the conduct of patient care in various stipulated clinical situations.

standard score, any derived score indicating the degree of deviation of an individual score from the mean using the standard deviation as the unit of measure.

stanine, a unit consisting of one ninth of the total range of the standard scores (SDs) of a normal distribution. The term is a condensation of standard nine. The mean falls at 5, the SD at ±2. The stanine was developed by the Air Force and is used to report scores on the Dental Aptitude Test.

stannous fluoride (stan'əstloor'īd), a fluoride salt of tin used in toothpaste and mouth rinses to reduce dental caries incidence and as an antiplaque agent

stanozolol, *trade name:* Winstrol; *drug class:* androgenic anabolic steroid, controlled substance Schedule III; *action:* reverses catabolic tissue processes; promotes buildup of protein, increases erythropoietin production; *use:* hereditary angioedema prophylaxis.

Staphcillin. See **methicillin.** (not current)

Staphylococcus albus (staf'əlōkok'əs al'bux) *(Staphylococcus pyogenes var. albus),* a species of spherical, gram-positive bacteria growing in grapelike clusters; of low pathogenicity, although occasional strains may be coagulase positive and produce hemolysis. Normally present as part of the oral flora and in mucosa-lined cavities such as the mouth and nasal cavity. May be isolated, along with *S. aureus,* streptococci, pneumococci, fusiform bacilli, *Borrelia vincentii,* molds, and yeasts from the gingival crevices by cultural examination.

Staphylococcus aureus (awr'ēus) *(Staphylococcus pyogenes var. aureus),* a pathogenic variety of staphylococci capable of producing suppurative lesions; cultured colonies are golden yellow. Produces hemolysis on blood agar, is coagulase positive, and may be resistant to commonly used antibiotics. Has been isolated with other mi-

croorganisms such as *S. albus* from the gingival crevice.

Staphylococcus pyogenes var. albus. See **Staphylococcus albus.**

Staphylococcus pyogenes var. aureus. See **Staphylococcus aureus.**

starch, the principal molecule used for the storage of food in plants. Starch is a polysaccharide and is composed of long chains of glucose subunits.

stare decisis (star'ē disīsəs), Latin phrase meaning to stand by decisions and not disturb settled matters; to follow rules or principles laid down in previous judicial decisions. (not current)

starvation, a condition resulting from the lack of essential nutrients over a long period and characterized by multiple physiologic and metabolic dysfunctions.

statement, 1. a printed form stating the balance of the account due the dentist. **2.** in computer programming a meaningful expression or generalized instruction in a source language.

static electricity. See **film fault, static electricity.**

static relation. See **relation, static.** (not current)

stationary grid. See **grid, stationary.**

stationary lingual arch, an orthodontic arch wire designed to fit the lingual surface of the teeth and soldered to the associated anchor bands, which are then cemented to the molar teeth.

statistic, any value or number that describes a series of quantitative observations or measures; a value calculated from a sample.

statistical significance, a difference of such magnitude between two statistics, computed from separate samples, that the probability of the value obtained will not occur by chance alone with significant frequency and hence can be attributed to something other than chance. In modern investigation the generally accepted value for significance must have a probability of occurrence by chance factors equal to or less than five times in 100 ($p <$ 0.05). Other significance levels commonly used are as follows: less than one chance in 100 ($p < 0.01$), less than five chances in 1000 ($p < 0.005$), and less than one chance in 1000 ($p < 0.001$).

S

statistically based utilization review, a system that examines the distribution of treatment procedures based on claims information and, to be reasonably reliable, the application of such claims. Analyses of specific dentists should include data on type of practice, dentist's experience, socioeconomic characteristics, and geographic location.

statistics, the branch of mathematics that gathers, arranges, condenses, coordinates, and mathematically manipulates obtained facts so that the numerical relationships between those facts may be seen clearly and freed from anomalies resulting from chance factors.

s., descriptive, statistics used to describe only the observed group or sample from which they were derived; summary statistics such as percent, averages, and measures of variability that are computed on a particular group of individuals.

s., inference, allows inferences to be made regarding characteristics or general principles about an unseen population based on the characteristics of the observed sample. Statistical findings from a sample are generalized to pertain to the entire population. The process of drawing inferences, making predictions, and testing significance are examples of inferential statistics.

s., nonparametric, statistical methods used when the statistician cannot assume that the variable being studied is normally distributed in a population. Also called distribution-free statistics.

status (stā'təs), (sta'tus) state or condition.

s. lymphaticus, enlargement of lymphoid tissue, particularly the thymus, in children. It may lead to sudden death under inhalation anesthesia.

s. thymicolymphaticus, a constitutional disturbance of controversial existence believed to be responsible in some way for sudden and unexplained deaths from trivial causes such as the extraction of teeth. Enlargement of the thymus and lymphoid tissue and underdevelopment of the adrenal glands, gonads, and cardiovascular system are evident.

statute, a law enacted and established by a legislative department of government.

s., wrongful death, a statute that provides for the recovery of damages by a party other than the party who received the fatal injuries.

statute of frauds, a requirement that, for legal validity, contracts for conveying real property or contracts for the performance of personal services requiring a year or more to perform must be in writing.

statute of limitations, a statute that sets a time limit within which legal action on certain causes of action must be brought.

statutory rape, (in law) sexual intercourse with a female below the age of consent, which varies from state to state.

stavudine, *trade name:* Zerit; *drug class:* antiviral; *action:* inhibits replication of human immunodeficiency virus (HIV); *uses:* treatment of adults with advanced HIV infection who are intolerant of other therapies or who have significant deterioration while receiving other therapies.

steady state, without variation. A basic physiologic concept implying that the various forces and processes of life are in a state of homeostasis.

steam sterilization, the destruction of all forms of microbial life on an object by exposing the object to moist heat (under pressure) for 15 minutes at 121° C.

steel crown. See **crown, stainless steel.**

steel, stainless, a steel that contains a minimum of 12% chromium and approximately 0.5% carbon to resist corrosion.

Stellite (stel'līt), **1.** any of various cobalt-chromium alloys. **2.** a very hard, noncorrosive alloy of cobalt, chromium, and sometimes tungsten used for special instruments, particularly surgical instruments.

stem, brain. See **brainstem.**

stenosis (stinō'sis), narrowing or stricture of a duct, canal, or vessel.

Stensen's duct. See **duct, Stensen's.**

stent, 1. a device used to hold a skin graft placed to maintain a body orifice, cavity, or space. An acrylic resin appliance used as a positioning guide or support. **2.** an appliance that maintains tissue (for example, to maintain a skin transplant in a predetermined position).

step-up transformer. See **transformer, step-up.**

stepwedge, an aluminum device that, when exposed to x-rays, displays a range of exposure intensities on a radiograph. These "steps" are analyzed to determine the speed characteristics of the radiographic film. See also **penetrometer.**

stereognosis, the ability to perceive and understand the form and nature of objects by the sense of touch.

stereoisomer. See **isomer.**

stereoscope, an optical instrument for viewing photographs or radiographs; it produces binocular vision, or a blending of images, so that new perspectives may be seen with an appearance of depth. It operates on the same principle as the eyes; that is, two views are registered on the retinas of the eyes, and the brain merges them into one.

steroscopic microscope, a microscope that produces three-dimensional images through the use of double eyepieces and double objectives, creating two independent light paths.

stereoscopic radiograph. See **radiograph, stereoscopic.** (not current)

stereotype, a generalization about a form of behavior, an individual, or a group.

sterile, free from viable microorganisms.

sterile field, 1. a specified area (such as within a tray or on a sterile towel) that is considered free of microorganisms. **2.** an area immediately around a patient that has been prepared for a surgical procedure.

sterilization, the act or process of rendering sterile; the process of freeing from germ life.

sterilizer for root canal instruments, a special device for heat sterilization of root canal instruments and dressings that depends on molten metal, glass beads, salt, or fine sand for the conduction of the heat. (not current)

Sternberg-Reed cell. See **cell, Sternberg-Reed.** (not current)

sternocleidomastoid, a muscle of the neck that is attached to the mastoid process and superior nuchal line

and by separate heads to the sternum and clavicle. It functions with other muscles to turn the head from side to side and tilt the head to one side or the other.

sternum, the elongated, flattened bone forming the middle portion of the thorax. It supports the clavicles and articulates directly with the first seven pairs of ribs.

steroid (stir'oid), a group name for compounds that resemble cholesterol chemically and also contain a hydrogenated cyclopentanoperhydrophenanthrene ring system. Included are cholesterol, ergosterol, bile acids, vitamin D, sex hormones, adrenocortical hormones, and cardiac glycosides.

s., adrenocortical (adrenal corticosteroid), **1.** a hormone extracted from the adrenal cortex or a synthetic substance similar in chemical structure and biologic activity to such a hormone. **2.** the biologically active steroids of the adrenal cortex, which include 11-dehydrocorticosterone (compound A), corticosterone (compound B), cortisone (compound E), 17 α-hydroxycorticosterone (compound F, hydroxycortisone, or cortisol), and aldosterone. The effects of the corticosteroids include increased resorption of sodium and chloride by the renal tubules and metabolic effects on protein, carbohydrate, and fat.

s., 17 α-hydroxycortico-(17-OHCS), term used for cortisol and other 21-carbon steroids possessing a dihydroxyacetone group at carbon 17. Serum and urinary determinations give a direct measurement of adrenocortical activity.

s., C-19 cortico- (anabolic protein, N hormone), adrenocortical hormones similar in action to the male and female sex hormones. They cause nitrogen retention and, in excessive amounts, masculinization in the female.

s., C-21 cortico- (glycogenic steroid, sugar hormone), 21-carbon adrenocortical hormones that are oxygenated at carbon 11 or at both carbon 11 and 17. They affect protein, carbohydrate, and fat metabolism; for example, they elevate blood sugar, increase glyconeogenesis, decrease hepatic lipogenesis, mobilize depot fat, and increase protein metabolism.

s., glycogenic. See **steroid, C-21 cortico-**.

s., 17-keto- (17-KS), steroidal compounds with a ketone (carbonyl) group at carbon 17. Derived from cortisol and adrenal and testicular androgen. Urinary neutral 17-ketosteroids represent the catabolic end products of the endocrine glands. Produced by the adrenal cortex and testes. Increased values occur in adrenogenital syndromes, adrenocortical carcinoma, bilateral hyperplasia of the adrenal cortex, and Leydig cell tumors. Normal adult values for a 24-hour urine sample are 10 to 20 mg for men and 5 to 15 mg for women.

s., 11-oxy, the C-21 corticosteroids, all of which are oxygenated at carbon 11.

sterols (stir′ôlz), steroids having one or more hydroxyl groups and no carbonyl or carboxyl groups (for example, cholesterol).

stethoscope, an instrument used to assist the health professional to listen to body sounds: heart, lungs, pulse, and gastrointestinal. It consists of two earpieces connected by means of flexible tubing to a diaphragm, which is placed against the skin of the patient at a location appropriate to pick up the sound.

Stevens-Johnson syndrome. See **syndrome, Stevens-Johnson.**

stillborn, an infant that was born dead.

Stillman's cleft. See **cleft, Stillman's.**

stimulant (stim′yələnt), an agent that causes an increase in functional activity, usually of the central nervous system.

s., psychomotor, a drug that increases psychic activity.

stimulation, 1. increased functioning of protoplasm induced by an extracellular substance or agent. **2.** the act of energizing or activating.

stimulus (stim′yələs), a chemical, thermal, electrical, or mechanical influence that changes the normal environment of irritable tissue and creates an impulse.

sting, an injury caused by a sharp, painful penetration of the skin, often accompanied by exposure to an irritating chemical or the venom of an insect or other animal.

stippling (stip′ling), **1.** an orange-peel appearance of the attached gingiva, believed to result from the bundles of collagen fibers that enter the connective tissue papillae. **2.** a roughening of the labial and buccal surfaces of denture bases to imitate the stippling of natural gingiva.

s., basophilic. See **basophilia.**

s., gingival. See **gingiva, stippling.**

stipulation, a material; an article in an agreement; an agreement in writing to do a certain thing.

stock, a security certificate that represents an equity ownership in a corporation.

Stokes' disease (not current). See **disease, Adams-Stokes.**

stomatitides (stō′mətit″idēz), the oral lesions associated with various forms of stomatitis.

stomatitis (stō′mətī′tis), inflammation of the soft tissues of the mouth occurring as a result of mechanical, chemical, thermal, bacterial, viral, electrical, or radiation injury or reactions to allergens or as secondary manifestations of systemic disease.

s., acute herpetic (acute herpetic gingivostomatitis), the manifestations of clinically apparent primary herpes simplex characterized by regional lymphadenopathy, sore throat, and high temperature, followed by localized itching and burning, with the formation of small vesicles of an erythematous base that give way to plaques and then painful herpetic ulcers. The gingivae are swollen and erythematous and bleed easily. Manifestations subside in 7 to 10 days, and recovery usually occurs within 2 weeks.

s., aphthous (aphthae, canker sore), refers to recurrent ulcers of the mouth that appear to be the same clinically as herpetic ulcers and for that reason have been considered to be a manifestation of recurrent herpes simplex, although the herpesvirus has never been conclusively isolated from recurrent aphthae. See also **gingivostomatitis, herpetic; stomatitis, herpetic; ulcer, aphthous.**

s., arsenical, oral manifestations of arsenic poisoning. The oral mucosa is dry, red, and painful. Ulceration, purpura, and mobility of teeth also may occur.

S

s., Atabrine, a stomatitis considered by some to be associated with the use of the antimalarial and anthelmintic drug quinacrine hydrochloride (Atabrine) and characterized by oral changes simulating lichen planus.

s., bismuth, a stomatitis resulting from systemic use of bismuth compounds over prolonged periods. Sulfides of bismuth are deposited in the gingival tissue, resulting in bluish-black pigmentation known as a bismuth line. Oral manifestations of bismuth poisoning include gingivostomatitis similar to that of Vincent's infection, a blue-black line on the inner aspect of the gingival sulcus or pigmentation of the buccal mucosa, a sore tongue, metallic taste, and a burning sensation of the mouth.

s., epidemic. See **disease, foot-and-mouth.**

s., epizootic. See **disease, foot-and-mouth.**

s., gangrenous (cancrum oris, noma), destruction of large masses of the oral tissues, particularly the cheek. It usually is found in weakened patients with very low resistance to infection because of lowered white blood cell count or other causes. In advanced stages a large segment of the cheek may be lost, leaving the teeth visible through the defect. See also **noma.**

s., gonococcal, inflammation of the oral mucosa caused by gonococci.

s., herpetic, **1.** oral manifestations of primary herpes simplex infection. The term also is used by some for herpetiform ulcers considered to be oral manifestations of secondary or recurrent herpes simplex. See also **ulcer, aphthous, recurrent. 2.** inflammation of the oral mucosa caused by herpesvirus. See also **gingivostomatitis, herpetic.**

s., iodine. See **iodism.**

s., lead, oral manifestations of lead poisoning. Included are a bluish line along the free gingival margin, pigmentation of the mucosa in contact with the teeth, metallic taste, excessive salivation, and swelling of the salivary glands.

s. medicamentosa, an allergic response of the oral mucosa to a systemically administered drug. Possible manifestations include asthma, skin rashes, urticaria, pruritus, leukopenia,

lymphadenopathy, thrombocytopenic purpura, and oral lesions (erythema, ulcerative lesions, vesicles, bullae, and angioneurotic edema).

s., membranous, inflammation of the oral cavity, accompanied by the formation of a false membrane.

s., mercurial, oral manifestations of mercury poisoning, consisting of hypersalivation, metallic taste, ulceration and necrosis of the gingivae with a tendency to spread posteriorly and to the buccal mucosa and palate, glossodynia, and periodontitis with loosening of the teeth in severe cases of chronic intoxication.

s., mycotic, infection of the oral mucosa by a fungus, most commonly *Candida albicans,* which produces moniliasis (thrush). See also **moniliasis.**

s., nicotinic (stomatitis nicotina), an inflammation of the palate caused by irritation by tobacco smoke and characterized by raised small palatal lesions with red centers and white borders. The palatal mucosa usually has a generalized leukoplakia accompanying the smaller lesions.

s., recurrent, recurrent manifestations of herpes simplex involving the lips and labial and buccal mucosa (fever blisters, cold sores). Considered by many to include also recurrent aphthae (canker sores). Episodes may result from fever, sunlight, menses, trauma, and gastrointestinal upset. Lesions begin as clear vesicles with an erythematous base that give way to ulcers and superficial crusts if the outer surfaces of the lips and skin are involved.

s., uremic, oral manifestations of uremia, consisting of varying degrees of erythema, exudation, ulceration, pseudomembrane formation, foul breath, and burning sensations. See also **gingivitis, nephritic.**

s. venenata, inflammation of the oral mucosa as the result of contact allergy. The most common causative agents are volatile oils, iodides, dentifrices, mouthwashes, denture powders, and topical anesthetics. Possible manifestations include erythema, angioneurotic edema, burning sensations, ulcerations, and vesicles.

stomatitis nicotina. See **stomatitis, nicotinic.**

stomatodynia (stōmətōdin′ēə), sore mouth.

stomatoglossitis (stō′mətōglosī′tis), inflammation involving oral mucous membranes and the tongue. May be seen in nutritional disorders such as pellagra, beriberi, vitamin B complex deficiency, and infections.

stomatognathic system (stō′mətō-nath′ik). See **system, stomatognathic.**

stomatology (stō′mətol′əjē), the study of the morphology, structure, function, and diseases of the contents and linings of the oral cavity.

stomion (stō′mēon), the median point of the oral slit (orifice) when the mouth is closed.

stone, an abrading instrument or tool.
s., Arkansas, a fine-grained stone, novaculite, used to make hones for the final sharpening of instruments.
s., artificial (dental stone), a specially calcined gypsum derivative similar to plaster of paris; because its grains are nonporous, the product is stronger than plaster of paris.
s., Carborundum, **1.** a stone made of silicon carbide. **2.** an abrasive, handpiece-mounted rotary instrument of various size, shape, and degree of abrasiveness.
s., dental (Hydrocal), **1.** α-hemihydrate of calcium sulfate. **2.** a gypsum product that, when combined with water in proper proportions, hardens in a plasterlike form. Used for making casts and dies.
s., diamond, rotary instruments containing diamond chips as the abrasive. Available in various sizes, shapes, and abrasive consistency. Used for tooth reduction in operative dentistry and crown and bridge prostheses, tooth contouring in the occlusal adjustment procedure, and osseous and gingival contouring in periodontal surgery.
s. die. See **die, stone.**
s., lathe (lathe wheel), a grindstone mounted on a chuck and used on a lathe.
s., mounted point, a small abrasive tooth of various shape and size bonded or cemented onto a shaft or mandrel.
s., pulp. See **denticle.**
s., sharpening, a hand stone, or a stone driven mechanically, that is used to sharpen instruments.

s., wheel, a small grindstone of Carborundum or corundum of various grit, mounted on a mandrel; of various thickness, ranging in diameter from ½ to 1 inch (1.3 to 2.5 cm).

stop. See **rest.**
s., occlusal. See **rest, occlusal.**

stop-loss, a general term referring to that category of coverage that provides insurance protection (reinsurance) to an employer for a self-funded plan.

stopping, temporary, gutta-percha mixed with zinc oxide, white wax, and coloring. Softens on heating and rehardens at room temperature. Used for temporary sealing of dressings in cavities. Lack of strength makes it ineffective in areas under occlusal stress. It has poor sealing properties.

storage, computer, a device or portion of a device that is capable of receiving data, retaining them for an indefinite time, and supplying them on command. Also called memory.

strabismus, an abnormal ocular condition in which the eyes are crossed.

straight wire fixed orthodontic appliance. See **appliance, straight wire fixed.**

straightening of teeth. See **orthodontics.**

strain, 1. deformation induced by an external force. **2.** deformation expressed as a pure number or ratio resulting from the application of a load. **3.** a traumatic stretching or compression of such tissues as the ligaments, capsule, or musculature associated with a joint. See also **sprain.**

strain hardening. See **hardening, strain.**

strangulation, choking or throttling. The arrest of respiration resulting from occlusion of the air passage or arrest of the circulation in part because of compression.

stratum basale, the deepest of the five layers of the skin, composed of tall cylindric cells. This layer provides new cells to the skin by mitotic cell division.

stratum corneum, the horny, outermost layer of the skin, composed of dead cells converted to keratin that continually flake away.

stratum granulosum, one of the layers of the epidermis, situated just below the stratum corneum except in the palms of the hands and the soles of the feet, where it lies just under the stratum lucidum.

stratum lucidum, one of the layers of the epidermis situated just beneath the stratum corneum and present only in the thick skin of the palms of the hands and the soles of the feet.

stratum spinosum, one of the layers of the epidermis, composed of several layers of polygonal cells. It lies on top of the stratum basale.

stratum spongiosum, one of the three layers of the endometrium of the uterus.

strawberry tongue, a strawberry-like coloration of inflamed tongue papillae. It is a clinical sign of scarlet fever and also is seen in Kawasaki syndrome.

stray radiation. See **radiation leakage.**

strength, toughness; ability to withstand or apply force.

s., biting, **1.** the force available for application against food or other material placed between the teeth. See also **force, masticatory. 2.** the amount of force the muscles of mastication are capable of exerting. See also **force, masticatory.**

s., compressive (crushing strength), the amount of resistance of a material to fracture under compression. See also **strength, ultimate.**

s., crushing. See **strength, compressive.**

s., dry, term generally used in conjunction with materials whose strengths vary markedly in the wet and dry states. The strength of gypsum products is usually reported in both wet and dry states.

s., edge, term indicative of the ability of fine margins to resist fracture or abrasion. No specific test is available to assess this property; it is a composite of ductility and shear, tensile, and other strength characteristics.

s., gel, usually, the ability of a material to withstand a load without rupture.

s., impact, the ability of a material to withstand a striking force.

s., shear, **1.** resistance to a tangential force. **2.** Resistance to a twisting motion.

s., tensile, **1.** resistance to a pulling force. **2.** the amount of stress a material is able to withstand when being pulled lengthwise before permanent deformation results.

s., ultimate, the greatest stress that may be induced in a material or object before or during rupture; may be compressive, tensile, or shear strength. See also **strength, tensile.**

s., wet, term that refers to compressive strength while water in excess of that required for hydration of the hemihydrate is present in the specimen. Used in connection with gypsum products.

s., yield, a definite proportionality obtained by drawing a line parallel to the proportional limit line. Yield strength is reported in terms of the degree of strain.

strep throat, an infection of the oral pharynx and tonsils caused by hemolytic species of *Streptococcus.* The infection is characterized by sore throat, chills, fever, swollen lymph nodes in the neck, and sometimes nausea and vomiting.

***Streptococcus,* alpha hemolytic** (strep′tōkok′əs al′fə hē′mōlit′ik), a spherical, gram-positive bacterium occurring in chains of bacterial cells. Produces a zone of greenish discoloration around the colony in blood-agar medium. Part of an individual's normal oral flora; has been isolated from the gingival crevice. Capable of producing bacteremia and subsequent subacute bacterial endocarditis in patients with a history of rheumatic fever; thus prophylactic antibiotic therapy is necessary before, during, and after periodontal, operative, and surgical therapy.

Streptococcus mutans, a cariogenic bacteria found in dental plaque and one of two index organisms (*Lactobacillus* is the other) used to assess caries susceptibility.

Streptococcus pneumoniae, any of 70 antigenic types of pneumococci that cause pneumonia and other diseases in humans.

Streptococcus pyogenes, a species of *Streptococcus* with many strains that are pathogenic to humans. It causes suppurative disease such as scarlet fever and strep throat.

Streptococcus salivarius, a bacterium found in dental plaque that may cause endocarditis and dental caries.

S

Streptococcus sanguis, a bacterium found in dental plaque that may cause endocarditis and dental caries.

Streptococcus viridans (vĭ'rĭdănz'). See *Streptococcus, alpha hemolytic.*

streptokinase, a fibrinolytic activator that enhances the conversion of plasminogen to the fibrinolytic enzyme plasmin. It is used in the treatment of certain cases of pulmonary and coronary embolism.

streptokinase-streptodornase, two enzymes derived from a strain of *Streptococcus hemolyticus.* It is prescribed for débridement of purulent exudates, clotted blood, radiation necrosis, or fibrinous deposits resulting from trauma or infection.

streptothricosis (strĕp'tōthrĭkō'sĭs). See **actinomycosis.**

stress, 1. a force induced by or resisting an external force; measured in terms of force per unit area. **2.** the force of energy directed against a tissue structure or against the function of tissue as the result of injury and trauma associated with fracture, burn, infection, surgical procedure, pharmacologic action, or anxiety states. The response to stress involves local metabolic function, the hormonal activity of the endocrine system regulated by the pituitary gland, and the autonomic and central nervous systems. The stress phenomenon is frequently associated with the general adaptation syndrome. **3.** in prosthetic dentistry, forcibly exerted pressure (for example, the pressure of the upper teeth against the mandibular teeth or the pressure contact of a distorted removable partial denture on the supporting teeth or ridge structures).

s., axial, excessive force applied vertically to the teeth and their attachment apparatus.

s., bone in, responses of bony structures to applied force. With application of excessive pressure stimuli to bone, adaptation may occur by the formation of thicker and more numerous trabeculae; or if tissue components cannot compensate for excessive stress, bone resorption will occur.

s., buccolingual, excessive pressure exerted against teeth and their attachment apparatus from a buccal or lingual aspect.

s., compressive, the internal induced force that opposes shortening of the material in a direction parallel to the direction of the stress.

s. control. See **control, stress.**

s., shearing, the internal induced force that opposes the sliding of one plane of the material on the adjacent plane in a direction parallel to the stress.

s., tensile, the internal induced force that opposes elongation of a material in a direction parallel to the direction of stress.

stress-bearing area. See **area, basal seat.**

stressbreaker (stress equalizer, stress divider), a device or system that is incorporated in a removable partial denture to relieve the abutment teeth of occlusal loads that may exceed their physiologic tolerance. (not current) See also **connector, nonrigid.**

stress-breaking action of clasp. See **clasp, stress-breaking action of.** (not current)

stretch receptors, specialized sensory nerve endings in muscle spindles and tendons that are stimulated by stretching movements. They are active in maintaining dynamic posture.

stretch reflex. See **reflex, stretch.**

stretching, longitudinal, the vertical elongations of gutta-percha that occur because of packing forces during the filling of large root canals. The material returns to the original form when force is released.

stretching pliers. See **pliers, stretching.**

striations, muscle (strī'ā'shənz), the transverse alternating light and dark bands of skeletal muscles that result from differences in light absorption. The light bands contain actin and are called "I" bands because they are isotropic to polarized light. The dark areas contain myosin filaments and are called "A" bands because they are anisotropic to polarized light. (not current)

stridor (strī'dor), a peculiar, harsh, vibrating sound produced during respiration.

s., inspiratory, the sound heard in inspiration through a spasmodically closed glottis.

s., laryngeal, stridor resulting from laryngeal stenosis.

strip, a thin, narrow, comparatively long piece of material.

*s., **abrasive** (linen strip),* a ribbonlike piece of linen of varying length and width, on one side of which are bonded abrasive particles of selected grit; used for contouring and polishing proximal surfaces of restorations.

*s., **boxing,*** a metal or wax strip used for making an enclosure to regulate the size and form of a cast.

*s., **Celluloid.*** See **strip, plastic.**

*s., **lightning** (separating strip),* a strip of steel with abrasive bonded on one side; used to open rough or improper contacts of proximal restorations or begin the reduction of proximal excess of a foil restoration.

*s., **linen.*** See **strip, abrasive.**

*s., **plastic,*** a clear plastic strip of Celluloid or acrylic resin that is used as a matrix when silicate cement or acrylic resin cement is inserted into proximal prepared cavities in anterior teeth.

*s., **polishing,*** a strip with a very fine abrasive such as crocus powder.

*s., **separating.*** See **strip, lightning.**

stripping, 1. the mechanical removal of a very small amount of enamel from the mesial or distal surfaces of teeth to alleviate crowding. **2.** (electrochemical) the process of subjecting the surface of a gold casting, attached to an anode from a rectifier and transformer unit, to the dissolving action of a heated cyanide solution, the metal container for which is the cathode of the unit. A microscopic amount of the surface of the alloy is removed by reverse electrolysis. The electrochemical stripping or milling is in contrast to electropolishing, wherein sharp edges are dissolved more rapidly than are broader areas.

stroke, a single, unbroken movement made by an instrument or the mandible.

*s., **circumferential,*** one of the basic strokes used for root and gingival curettage; the blade of the periodontal curet is negotiated mesiodistally while it is in contact with either the root or the inner aspect of the soft tissue wall of the gingival or periodontal pocket.

*s., **exploratory,*** a phase of subgingival root scaling in which the curet is held in featherlike grasp to ascertain tactilely the amount and extent of the accretions on the root surface; the ingress stroke into the pocket area.

*s., **power,*** the phase of the working stroke that is designed to split or dislodge calculus from the root surface. It is prefaced by the exploratory stroke and followed by the shaving stroke.

*s., **shaving,*** the phase of the working stroke of a periodontal curet that is designed to smooth or plane the root surface. It follows the power stroke, which is designed to dislodge calculus from the root surface.

stroke volume, the volume of blood put out by the heart per heartbeat. Stroke volume is directly proportional to the volume of blood filling the heart during diastole.

strontium (Sr), a metallic element. Its atomic number is 38, and its atomic weight is 87.62. It is chemically similar to calcium and is found in bone tissue. Isotopes of strontium are used in radioisotope scanning procedures of bone.

structure, the architectural arrangement of the component parts of a tissue, part, organ, or body. Also the individual components of the body.

*s., **border.*** See **border structures.**

*s., **cored,*** in metallurgy a grain structure with composition gradients resulting from the progressive freezing of the components in different proportions. Nonmetals used in dentistry (for example zinc phosphate, silicate cements) also are cored structures in that they have a nucleus of undissolved powder particles surrounded by a matrix of reacted material.

*s., **denture supporting,*** the tissues, including teeth and residual ridges, that serve as the foundation or basal seat for removable partial dentures.

*s., **functional form of supporting,*** term that refers to the state of denture-supporting structures when they have been placed in such a position as to be able to begin resisting occlusal forces.

*s., **histologic,*** the minute structure of organic tissues.

*s., **radiolucent,*** the structures or substances that permit the penetration of x radiation and are thus registered as relatively dark areas on the radiograph.

*s., **radiopaque,*** the structures that prevent x rays from penetrating them

S

because of their density, causing them to appear as light areas on the radiograph.

s., supporting, the tissues that maintain or assist in maintaining the teeth in position in the alveolus (for example, gingivae, cementum of the tooth, periodontal ligament, alveolar and trabecular bone).

Stuart factor. See factor X.

study, pursuance of education; analysis.

s., graduate, baccalaureate educational efforts pursued for credit toward an advanced degree in institutions of higher learning.

s., postgraduate, postdoctoral educational endeavors that may or may not earn credits for advanced degrees.

s., time, the technique of random sampling used for analysis of the time spent for rendering each phase of each of the various professional services performed by the dentist.

study cast. See **cast, diagnostic.**

study model. See **cast, diagnostic.**

stupor, the condition of being only partly conscious or sensible; also, a condition of insensibility.

Sturge-Weber-Dimitri disease. See **disease, Sturge-Weber-Dimitri.**

stuttering, a speech dysfunction characterized by spasmodic enunciation of words, involving excessive hesitations, stumbling, repetition of the same syllables, and prolongation of sounds.

stylet, a wire inserted into a soft catheter or cannula to secure rigidity; a fine wire inserted into a hollow needle to maintain patency.

stylohyoid ligament, the ligament attached to the tip of the styloid process of the temporal bone and the lesser cornu of the hyoid bone.

stylohyoideus, one of the four suprahyoid muscles. It is a slender muscle that arises from the styloid process and inserts into the hyoid bone. It serves to draw the hyoid bone up and back.

stylomandibular ligament, one of a pair of specialized bands of cervical fascia, forming an accessory part of the temporomandibular joint. It extends from the styloid process of the temporal bone to the ramus of the mandible.

stylus, ancient form of writing instrument. It is still used much as it was used when the Egyptians were figuring out geometry with a stylus and sand sprinkled on a polished stone. It has assumed importance in gnathology, because a well-pointed stylus can be slid on dust-covered glass with a minimum of friction, thereby making the jaw-writing data more accurate.

s., surgical indicator, a small pointed instrument devised to mark the spot in the tissue where the intramucosal inserts will be placed. Styluses are seated in prepared depressions in the denture base and mark the mucosal tissue by puncturing it.

s. tracer. See **tracer, needle point.**

s. tracing. See **tracing, needle point.**

styptic, a hemostatic astringent.

sub-, prefix signifying under, beneath, deficient, near, or almost.

subacute, less than acute.

subarachnoid hemorrhage (SAH), an intracranial hemorrhage into the cerebrospinal fluid.

subconscious, the state in which mental processes take place without the mind's being distinctly conscious of its own activity.

subculture, an ethnic, regional, economic, or social group with characteristic patterns of behavior and ideals that distinguish it from the rest of the culture or society.

subdural, situated below the dura mater and above the arachnoid membrane.

subgingival (sub'jinjĭ'vəl), at a level apical to the gingival margin.

subgingival calculus, a deposit of various mineral salts that accumulate with organic matter and oral debris on the teeth below the margin of the gingiva.

subgingival curettage. See **curettage, subgingival.**

subjective data collection, the process in which information relating to the patient's problem is elicited from the patient.

subjects, the people, animals, or events selected for study to examine a particular variable or condition such as the effects of a new medication or treatment.

sublease, a lease executed by the lessee of an estate to a third person, conveying the same estate for a shorter term than that for which the lessee holds it.

subliminal, below the threshold of sensory perception or outside the range of conscious awareness.

sublingual (səbling'gwəl), pertaining to the region of structures located beneath the tongue.

s. administration. See **administration, sublingual.**

s. crescent. See **crescent, sublingual.**

s. fold. See **fold, sublingual.**

s. gland. See **salivary glands.**

subluxation (sub'ləxsā'shən), **1.** incomplete dislocation of a joint. **2.** term applied loosely to the temporomandibular joint, indicating relaxation of the capsular ligaments and improper relationship of the joint components, resulting in cracking and popping of the joint during movement.

submandibular, below the mandible.

submandibular gland, one of a pair of salivary glands in the submandibular triangle. The gland secretes saliva into the oral cavity through a small duct that opens on a small papilla at the side of the lingual frenum.

submarginal, pertaining to a deficiency of contour at the margin of a restoration or pattern.

submaxillary, situated beneath the maxilla.

s. caruncle. See **caruncle, submaxillary.**

s. ganglion. See **ganglion, submaxillary.**

submental, situated below the chin.

submucosa (sub'mukō'sə), the tissue layer beneath the oral mucosa. It contains connective tissues, vessels, and accessory salivary glands.

submucous cleft (occult cleft), a congenital anomaly in which the midportion of the soft or hard palate lacks proper mesodermal development. Nonunion of bone and muscle tissues of the soft and hard palates and concealment by the superficial intact mucoperiosteum.

subnasion (sub'nā'zēon), the point of the angle between the septum and the surface of the upper lip. It is sought at the point where a tangent applied to the septum meets the upper lip. (not current)

subocclusal connector. See **connector, subocclusal.** (not current)

subpoena (sub'pē'nə), the process or writ issued by the court by which the attendance of a witness at a certain time and place is required for testimony. It also may order him or her to bring any books, records, or other relevant items for evidence.

subpoena duces tecum, a subponea commanding a person to bring books, papers, records, or other items to the court.

subroutine, the set of instructions necessary to direct the computer to carry out a well-defined mathematical or logical operation; a subunit of a routine.

subscriber, the person, usually the employee, who represents the family unit in relation to the prepayment plan. Other family members are "dependents." Also called certificate holders or enrollees.

subsistence, the state of being supported or remaining alive with a minimum of life essentials.

subspecialty, a limited portion of a narrowly defined professional discipline. For example, surgery is a specialty of medicine and pediatric vascular surgery is a subspecialty.

subspinale (sub'spina'le), the deepest midline point on the premaxilla between the anterior nasal spine and the prosthion.

substance abuse, the overindulgence in and dependence on a stimulant, depressant, or other chemical substance, leading to effects that are detrimental to the individual's physical or mental health or the welfare of others.

substance P, one of several endogenous inflammatory substances thought to mediate or cause pain.

substandard, below an acceptable level of performance.

substitute, one acting for or taking the place of another.

s., tinfoil, alginate separating material painted on gypsum molds to serve as a liner in preventing both the penetration of monomers into the surrounding investing medium and the leakage of water into acrylic resin.

substitution, a standard or nonstandard speech sound used for another consonant speech sound (for example, "w" for "l" [wady for lady]).

substructure, a structure built to serve as a base or foundation for another structure.

s., implant (implant denture substructure), **1.** a skeletal frame of inert material that fits on the bone under the mucoperiosteum. **2.** the metal framework that is embedded beneath the soft tissues in contact with the bone for the purpose of supporting an implant superstructure.

s., implant, abutment, the portion of the implant that extends from the surface of the mucosa into the oral cavity for the retention of crowns, bridges, or superstructure bearing the teeth of the denture.

s., implant, auxiliary rest, a small metal protrusion through the mucosa connected to the labial or buccal and lingual (peripheral) frame to furnish additional support for the superstructure between the abutments.

s., implant, interspace, any one of the spaces between the primary and secondary struts that allows infiltration of tissue.

s., implant, neck (implant post, implant substructure, post), the constriction that connects the implant frame with the implant abutment.

s., implant, part, the root section shaped in the form of a wire loop. This part of the substructure sinks into the alveolar socket or sockets after the extraction of one or two remaining anterior teeth. Newly formed bone tissue grows through the loop and firmly affixes the implant.

s., implant, peripheral frame, the labial, buccal, lingual, and distal outline of the frame.

s., implant, post. See **substructure, implant, neck.**

s., implant, primary struts, the main traverse struts that connect the implant necks or posts with the peripheral frame.

s., implant, secondary struts, the additional smaller transverse, diagonal, and longitudinal struts that are added when necessary to give additional strength and rigidity to the implant, increase the area of bone support, and afford additional intermeshing of the mucoperiosteal tissue.

subtle, having a low intensity; not severe and having no serious sequelae.

succinylcholine chloride, a skeletal muscle relaxant used as an adjunct to anesthesia, to reduce muscle contractions during surgery or mechanical ventilation, and to facilitate endotracheal intubation.

sucralfate, *trade name:* Carafate; *drug class:* protectant, aluminum salt of sulfated sucrose; *action:* forms an ulcer-adherent complex that covers and protects the ulcer site; *use:* treatment of duodenal ulcer.

sudden infant death syndrome (SIDS), the unexpected and sudden death of an apparently normal and healthy infant that occurs during sleep and with no physical or autopsic evidence of disease. It is the most common cause of death of children in the United States between 2 weeks and 1 year of age.

sudorific, an agent, substance, or condition such as heat or emotional tension that promotes sweating.

sufentanil citrate, an intravenous analgesic and anesthetic used as an adjunct to general anesthesia and as a primary anesthetic with 100% oxygen.

suffocate, asphyxiate; to prevent the exchange of air into the lungs, causing death.

suffocation, interference with the entrance of air into the lungs.

sugar, one of a number of water-soluble carbohydrates. Sugars are divided into two major categories: monosaccharides and disaccharides. Table sugar or sucrose is the principal disaccharide; glucose or blood sugar is the principal monosaccharide.

suggestion, 1. the process by which one thought or idea leads to another, as in the association of ideas. **2.** the use of persuasion to implant an idea, thought, attitude, or belief in the mind of another as a means of influencing or altering behavior or state of mind.

suicide, the intentional taking of one's own life.

suit, any proceeding in court in which the plaintiff pursues a remedy that the law gives for the redress of an injury or the enforcement of a right.

sulconazole nitrate, *trade name:* Exelderm; *drug class:* topical antifungal; *action:* interferes with fungal cell membranes, increasing permeability and leaking of nutrients; *uses:* treatment of tinea pedis, tinea corporis, tinea cruris, and tinea versicolor.

sulcus (sul'kəs), **1.** a furrow, trench, or groove, as on the surface of the brain or in the folds of mucous membranes. **2.** a groove or depression on the surface of a tooth. **3.** a groove in a portion of the oral cavity.

s., alveololingual, the space between the alveolar or residual alveolar ridge and the tongue. It extends from the lingual frenum to the retromylohyoid curtain and is a part of the floor of the mouth.

s., gingival, the shallow groove between the free gingiva and the surface of a tooth and extending around its circumference.

s., implant gingival, a sulcus around the implant abutment post that resembles the sulcus around a healthy natural tooth.

s., occlusal, a groove or spillway on the occlusal surface of a tooth.

sulfa (sul'fə), a vernacular term used to describe a group of antibacterial agents. See also **sulfacetamide, sulfamethizole.**

sulfacetamide sodium (ophthalmic), *trade names:* Bleph-10, Cetamide, Isopto Cetamide; *drug class:* antibacterial sulfonamide; *action:* inhibits folic acid synthesis by preventing paraaminobenzoic acid (PABA) use, which is necessary for bacterial growth; *uses:* treatment of conjunctivitis, superficial eye infections, and corneal ulcers.

sulfamethizole, *trade name:* Thiosulfil Forte; *drug class:* sulfonamide, short acting; *action:* interferes with bacterial biosynthesis of proteins by competitive antagonism of paraaminobenzoic acid (PABA); *use:* treatment of urinary tract infections.

sulfamethoxazole, *trade names:* Gamazole, Gantanol, Urabak; *drug class:* sulfonamide; *action:* interferes with bacterial biosynthesis of proteins by competitive antagonism of paraaminobenzoic acid (PABA); *uses:* treatment of urinary tract infections, lymphogranuloma venereum, and systemic infections.

sulfamethoxazole/trimethoprim; *trade names:* Bactrim, Cotrim, Septra, Sulfatrim, Sulfamethoprim, Triazole, Uroplus SS; *drug class:* sulfonamide

and folic acid antagonist; *action:* interferes with bacterial biosynthesis of proteins by competitive antagonism of paraaminobenzoic acid (PABA) when adequate levels are maintained; *uses:* treatment of urinary tract infections, otitis media.

sulfasalazine, *trade name:* Asulfidine-EN-Tabs, Azulfidine; *drug class:* sulfonamide derivative with antiinflammatory action; *action:* acts as a prodrug to deliver sulfapyridine and mesalamine (5-aminosalicylic acid) to the colon; *uses:* treatment of ulcerative colitis, Crohn's disease.

sulfhemoglobinemia (sulfēm'əglō' binē'mēə), an abnormality of the heme moiety of the hemoglobin molecule resulting from inorganic sulfides (for example, acetanilide).

sulfinpyrazone, *trade name:* Anturane; *drug class:* uricosuric; *action:* inhibits tubular reabsorption of urates, with increased excretion of uric acid; inhibits prostaglandin synthesis, which decreases platelet aggregation; *use:* treatment of chronic gouty arthritis.

sulfisoxazole, *trade name:* Gantrisin; *drug class:* sulfonamide, short acting; antiinfective; *action:* interferes with bacterial biosynthesis of proteins by competitive antagonism of paraaminobenzoic acid (PABA); *uses:* treatment of urinary tract, systemic infections; chancroid; trachoma; toxoplasmosis, acute otitis media; lymphogranuloma venereum; eye infections.

sulfonamide (səlfon'əmīd), a derivative of sulfanilamide that is effective against microorganisms.

sulfur (S), a nonmetallic, multivalent, tasteless, odorless chemical element that occurs abundantly in yellow crystalline form or in masses, especially in volcanic areas. Its atomic number is 16, and its atomic weight is 32.06. It has wide use in industry. Sulfur has been used in the treatment of gout, rheumatism, and bronchitis and as a mild laxative.

sulfur granules, a yellow-white particle found in actinomycosis and diagnostic of actinomycosis infection.

sulindac, *trade name:* Clinoril; *drug class:* nonsteroidal antiinflammatory; *action:* inhibits prostaglandin synthesis by interfering with cyclooxygenase, an enzyme needed for bio-

S

synthesis; possesses analgesic, antiin-flammatory, and antipyretic proper-ties; *uses:* osteoarthritis, rheumatoid, acute gouty arthrits, tendinitis, bursi-tis, ankylosing spondylitis.

Sulkowitch's test (sul'kəwichs). See **test, Sulkowitch's.** (not current)

sumatriptan succinate, *trade name:* Imitrex; *drug class:* serotonin agonist; *action:* selective agonist for the vas-cular 5-hydroxytryptamine (5-HT-1) (serotonin) receptor in cranial arteries, causing vasodilation with little or no effect on peripheral pressure; *use:* treatment of migraine headaches.

summary judgment, a judgment re-quested by any party to a civil action to end the action when it is believed that no genuine issue or material fact is in dispute.

summary plan description. See **benefit plan summary.**

summation, the phenomenon in which similar actions of more than one drug result in a total action that may be expressed as the arithmetic sum of the effects of the individual drugs.

summons, a writ directed to the proper officer, requiring him or her to notify the defendant that an action has been begun against him or her in the court from which the writ was issued and that he or she is required to ap-pear on a certain day to answer the complaint.

superficial, to involve only the sur-face or to be minor in severity: not grave or dangerous.

superinfection, an infection occur-ring during antimicrobial treatment for another infection.

supernumerary tooth, any tooth in addition to the normal 32 teeth in the permanent dentition or the 20 teeth in the primary dentition.

superoxide, a common form of oxy-gen that is formed when molecular oxygen gains a single electron. Super-oxide radicals may attack susceptible biologic targets, including lipids, pro-teins, and nucleic acids.

superoxol, a 30% solution of hydro-gen peroxide used to bleach endodon-tically treated teeth.

superplant, a bayonet-shaped bar used as a subperiosteal implant to serve as an abutment for a free-end fixed prosthesis. (not current)

supersaturation, the addition to or presence of an ingredient in a solution in greater quantity than the solvent can permanently take up.

superstructure, a structure con-structed on or over another structure.

s. casting, in the subperiosteal im-plant, a surgical alloy bar designed with clasps to telescope over the four abutments. To this casting is pro-cessed the final denture superstruc-ture.

s., implant (implant denture super-structure), 1. a removable denture that fits snugly onto the protruding im-plant abutments. Sometimes called the implant denture. 2. the denture that is retained, supported, and stabi-lized by the implant denture substruc-ture.

s., implant, attaching material, the denture resin by which the superstruc-ture teeth are attached to the super-structure frame.

s., implant, attachment, any part of the superstructure that fits onto the implant abutments. May be a preci-sion attachment coping, a conven-tional clasping, or a combination of a precision attachment with clasps.

s., implant, connectors, the rigid bars that unite the superstructure attach-ments into one strong element.

s., implant, denture. See **superstruc-ture, implant.**

s., implant, frame, the metal skeleton of the superstructure, consisting of at-tachments and connectors.

s., temporary (implant surgical splint), an acrylic resin immediate ap-pliance with six anterior teeth; has no metal clasps, precision coping, or frame; fitted closely over the implant abutments immediately after the sur-gical insertion of the substructure.

supervision, the active administering and overseeing of all the functionings of the dental practice and the auxil-iaries employed therein.

supine, lying horizontally on the back.

supplemental tooth, a type of su-pernumerary tooth that is so well formed that it mimics a fully formed tooth. A supplemental tooth usually appears distal to a lateral incisor. Its detection requires the careful count-ing and identification of each tooth in the dental arch.

S

supplements, usually, dietary substances used to augment, enhance, or enrich the nutritional status of a patient.

support, resistance to vertical components of masticatory force in a direction toward the basal seat.

s., ridge. See **area, supporting.**

supporting area. See **area, supporting.**

supporting bone. See **bone, cancellous.**

supportive periodontal therapy. See **periodontal therapy.**

suppressant, an agent that retards or diminishes a physical or mental activity. Commonly used to describe a drug that inhibits coughing (cough suppressant).

suppuration, the formation and discharge of pus.

suprabulge, the portion of the crown of a tooth that converges toward the occlusal surface from the height of contour of survey line.

supraclusion (soo'prakloo'zhən), a position occupied by a tooth that is too high in the line of occlusion.

supragingival calculus, a deposit composed of various mineral salts with accumulations of organic matter and oral debris that adheres to the surface of the tooth above the gingival margin.

supramentale (soo'pramanta'le), the most posterior point in the concavity between infradentale and pogonion.

supraversion (soo'prəver'zhən), a condition in which teeth or other maxillary structures are situated above or below their normal vertical relationships.

suprofen, an oral nonsteroidal antiinflammatory analgesic used in the treatment of mild to moderate pain and primary dysmenorrhea.

suramin sodium, an antitrypanosomal and an antifilarial available from the Centers for Disease Control and Prevention. It is used primarily for treatment and prophylaxis of African trypanosomiasis and onchocerciasis.

surcharge, a stated dollar amount paid to the dentist by the beneficiary in addition to other reimbursement received by third-party payers.

surface, the outer portion of a mass or object.

s., balancing occlusal, the surfaces of the teeth or denture bases that make contact to provide balancing contacts.

s., basal. See **denture, basal surface of.**

s., buccal, any surface adjacent to and facing the cheek.

s., foundation. See **denture, basal surface of.**

s., implant-bearing, the area of bone that has been selected from the surgical bone impression to be in direct contact with the implant frame.

s., impression. See **denture, basal surface of.**

s., occlusal, the anatomic superior surface of the mandibular posterior teeth and the inferior surface of the maxillary posterior teeth. These surfaces are limited mesially and distally by marginal ridges and buccally and lingually by the buccal and lingual boundaries of the cusp eminences.

s., proximal, the surface of a tooth or the portion of a cavity that is nearest to the adjacent tooth; the mesial or distal surface of a tooth.

s., smooth, a surface of a tooth on which pits and fissures are not found normally.

s., working occlusal, the surface or surfaces of the teeth on which chewing can occur.

surfactant (sərfakt'ənt), a surface-active agent.

surgeon, one whose profession is to cure diseases or injuries by manual operation or by medication.

surgery, work performed by a surgeon.

s., access flap in osseous, a full-thickness or split thickness flap created for the purpose of gaining access to the alveolar bone when surgical remodeling is indicated.

s., apically repositioned flap in mucogingival, a surgically created flap of gingival tissue that is repositioned apically to maintain or create a functionally adequate zone of attached gingiva. In the surgical procedure the existing attached and free gingiva is detached by employing a reverse bevel incision and apically repositioning the flap.

s., full flap in mucogingival, a flap in which all the soft tissue elements are raised and repositioned, as opposed to the split-thickness flap.

s., mucogingival, surgical procedures designed to retain a functionally adequate zone of gingiva after surgical pocket elimination, create a functionally adequate zone of attached gingiva, alter the position of or eliminate a frenum, or deepen the vestibule.

s., oblique flap in mucogingival, an increased band of attached gingiva created by preparing a narrow papillary flap (to avoid donor site radicular recession), which is then rotated 90° and sutured into the prepared recipient site.

s., osseous, the therapeutic surgical measures used and designed to eliminate osseous deformities by means of ostectomy or osteoplasty or create a favorable environment by means of meticulous removal of the soft tissue contents of the infrabony osseous defect for the formation of new bone, periodontal membrane, and cementum to fill in the area of bone resorption.

s., pedicle flap in mucogingival, an increased band of attached gingiva created to repair a cleft by using proximal gingiva situated mesial and distal to the cleft, because gingiva in either location alone is not wide enough to cover the cleft if repositioned. The pedicles are repositioned laterally and sutured. Also called a double papilla procedure.

surgical preparation. See **preparation, surgical.**

surgical prosthesis. See **prosthesis, surgical.**

surgical template. See **template, surgical.**

surgical tray, a prefabricated appliance constructed in advance of the first surgical stage and used for making an impression of the exposed mandibular bone. See also **stage, surgical.** (not current)

surrogate, a substitute; a person or thing that replaces another.

survey, the study and examination of an area of consideration, a diagnostic cast, or a radiograph.

s., radiation, evaluation of the radiation hazards incidental to the production, use, or existence of radioactive materials or other sources of radiation under a specific set of conditions.

s., radiographic, the production of the minimal number of radiographic

examinations necessary for a radiographic interpretation.

s., roentgenographic. See **survey, radiographic.**

s., x-ray. See **survey, radiographic.**

survey line. See **line, survey.**

surveying, the procedure of studying the relative parallelism or lack of parallelism of the teeth and associated structures to select a path of placement for a restoration that will encounter the least tooth or tissue interference and provide adequate and balanced retention; locating guiding plane surfaces to direct placement and removal of the restoration and achieve the best appearance possible.

surveyor, an instrument used to determine the relative parallelism of two or more surfaces of teeth or other portions of a cast of the dental arch.

s., Ney, the first commercially available dental cast surveyor designed to select a path of placement or insertion for a restoration.

susceptible, the opposite of immune; having little resistance to disease.

suspension (səspen'shən), a mixture of two or more immiscible phases, such as a solid in a liquid or a liquid in a liquid. Suspensions differ from emulsions in that the former usually have to be shaken before each use.

sustenance, the act or process of supporting or maintaining life and health.

Sutton's disease. See **periadenitis mucosa necrotica recurrens.**

suture, I. a synarthrosis between two bones formed in a membrane, the uniting medium (which tends to disappear eventually) being a fibrous membrane continuous with the periosteum. **2.** a surgical stitch or seam. **3.** materials with which body structures are sewn, as after an operation or injury. **4.** to sew up a wound.

s., absorbable, a suture that becomes dissolved in body fluids and disappears (for example, catgut).

s., approximation, a suture made to bring about apposition of the deeper tissues of an incision or laceration.

s., button, a suture passed through buttonlike disks on the skin to prevent the suture cutting the soft tissue.

s., chromic, a chromatized gut suture.

s., continuous, a suture in which an uninterrupted length of suture material is used to close an incision or laceration.

s., frontomalar, most lateral point of the suture between the frontal and malar bones.

s., intermaxillary (median palatine suture), the line of fusion of the two maxillae, starting between the central incisors and extending posteriorly across the palate, separating it into two nearly equal parts.

s., interrupted, individual stitches, each tied separately.

s., mattress, a continuous suture that is applied back and forth through the tissues in the same vertical plane but at a different depth, or in the same horizontal plane but at the same depth.

s., median palatine. See **suture, intermaxillary.**

s., nonabsorbable, a suture that does not dissolve in body fluids (for example, silk, tantalum, nylon)

s., purse-string, a horizontal mattress suture used generally about an implant cervix.

s., shoelace, a continuous surgical suture for depression of the tongue and retention and holding of the lingual flap out of the field of operation during the surgical impression.

swage (swāj), to shape metal by adapting or hammering it onto a die. Usually completed by forcing a counterdie into position on a die with the metal sheet interposed.

swager, a laboratory instrument used for swaging. (not current)

s., wax, an instrument used to swage wax to a die.

swallowing See **deglutition.**

s. threshold. See **threshold, swallowing.**

swear, to take an oath; to become legally obligated by an oath properly administered.

sweat (swet), perspiration. A clear liquid exuded or excreted from the sudoriferous glands. It possesses a characteristic odor, is slightly alkaline, salty to the taste, and, when mixed with sebaceous secretion, acid. Sweating is under the control of the sympathetic nervous system, although it may be stimulated by parasympathetic drugs. Thermoregulatory sweating is influenced by the blood temperature's affecting the nervous centers and by

reflexes associated with heat receptors in the skin.

sweating, gustatory. See **syndrome, auriculotemporal.**

swelling, one of the cardinal signs of acute inflammation; caused by the exudation of fluid from the capillary vessels into the tissue.

s., familial intraosseous. See **cherubism.**

Swift's disease. See **erythredema polyneuropathy.** (not current)

symbiotic relationship (sim'bēot'ik), in implantology, that relationship assumed by an implant and the natural teeth to which it has been splinted; the continuing existence of their relationship is based on their interdependence.

symbolic coding, instructions written in nonmachine language.

symmetric, evenly balanced or uniformly developed.

sympathectomy, a surgical interruption of part of the sympathetic nerve pathways, performed for the relief of chronic pain or to promote vasodilation in vascular diseases.

sympathetic (sim'pəthet'ik), pertaining to the sympathetic nervous system.

sympathetic nervous system. See **autonomic nervous system.**

sympatholytic (sim'pəthōlit'ik), pertaining to a drug that blocks the effects of stimulation of the sympathetic nervous system. See also **adrenolytic.**

sympathomimetic (sim'pəthomimet'ik), resembling the effect produced by stimulation of the sympathetic nervous system. See also **adrenergic.**

sympathy, the kind understanding of a patient.

symphysis, a line of union between two bony surfaces such as the pubic symphysis or symphysis of the mandible.

symptom, any morbid phenomenon or departure from the normal in function, appearance, or sensation, experienced by the patient and indicative of disease.

s., constitutional, symptoms related to the systemic effects of a disease (for example, fever, malaise, anorexia, weight loss).

s., diagnostic signs and. See **signs and symptoms, diagnostic.**

synalgia (sinal'jə), **1.** pain felt in a distant part from an injury to or stimula-

S

tion of another part. **2.** reflex or referred pain. (not current)

Synalgos DC (not current). See **dihydrocodeine.**

synapse (sin'aps), the region of contact between the processes of two adjacent neurons forming the place where a nervous impulse is transmitted from the axon of one neuron to the dendrites of another. It also is called the synaptic junction.

synarthrosis (sinahrthrō'sis), a joint formed by thin intervening layers of cartilage, connective tissue, or direct contact of bone to bone. It results in a rigid union, and little movement of the bones occurs except during growth. Suture lines may be obliterated in adults, with a synarthrodial joint when the bones joined together become fused.

synchondrosis, a cartilaginous joint between two immovable bones such as the union between the sphenoid and occipital bones at the base of the skull.

synchronous, having constant time intervals between events or occurrences.

s. device, a term applied to a device in which the performance of a sequence of operations is controlled by equally spaced clock signals or pulses.

syncope (sing'kəpē), swooning or fainting; temporary suspension of consciousness caused by cerebral anemia. See also **shock.**

syndactyly (sindak'təlē), a congenital anomaly characterized by the fusion of fingers or toes, usually as a finding of a more complex congenital syndrome.

syndrome (sin'drōm), a group of signs and symptoms that occur together and characterize a disease.

s., Adams-Stokes. See **disease, Adams-Stokes.**

s., adaptation. See **disease, adaptation; syndrome, general adaptation.**

s., adrenogenital, disorders of sexual development or function associated with abnormal adrenocortical function resulting from bilateral adrenal hyperplasia, carcinoma, or adenoma. Pseudohermaphroditism occurs congenitally, and masculinization occurs later in females. Precocious sexual de-

velopment and occasionally feminization occur in males.

s., AHOP, adiposity, hyperthermia, oligomenorrhea, and parotitis appearing in females. Parotid gland enlargement begins at puberty and is followed by obesity, oligomenorrhea, and psychic disturbances.

s., Albright's, a polyostotic form of fibrous dysplasia, usually associated with precocious puberty in females, endocrine disturbances influencing growth, and brown pigmentation of the skin.

s., Apert's (acrocephalosyndactyly), craniostenosis characterized by oxycephaly and syndactyly of the hands and feet. Facial manifestations include exophthalmos, high prominent forehead, small nose, and malformation of the mandible and mouth.

s., Ascher, syndrome consisting of double lip, a redundance of the skin of the eyelids (blepharochalasis), and nontoxic thyroid enlargement. The sagging eyelids are obvious when the eyes are open and the double lip is seen when the patient smiles.

s., auriculotemporal (Bogarad's syndrome, Frey's syndrome, gustatory hyperhidrosis syndrome, gustatory lacrimation, gustatory sweating syndrome), sweating and flushing in the preauricular and temporal areas when certain foods are eaten. May be related to parotid trauma or a complication of parotidectomy.

s., autoimmune. See **disease, autoimmune.**

s., Behçet's (bā'sets) *(Behçet's disease),* recurrent iritis and aphthous ulcers of the mouth and genitalia. Other manifestations include arthralgia, hydrarthrosis, swelling of the salivary glands, cutaneous eruptions, and central nervous system disorders.

s., Bloch-Sulzberger (incontinentia pigmenti), syndrome in which pigmented skin lesions, defects of the eyes and central nervous system, skeletal anomalies, and hypoplasia of the teeth occur.

s., Bogarad. See **syndrome, auriculotemporal.**

s., Böök's (buks), syndrome characterized by premature graying of the hair, hyperhidrosis, and premolar hypodontia.

S

s., Bourneville-Pringle (epiloia), neurocutaneous complex consisting of adenoma sebaceum, mental deficiency, and epilepsy.

s., Caffey-Silverman. See **hyperostosis, infantile cortical.**

s., Christ-Siemens-Touraine. See **hypohidrotic ectodermal dysplasia.**

s., Costen's, various symptoms of discomfort, pain, and jaw pathosis claimed by Costen to be caused by lack of posterior occlusion, loss of vertical dimension, malocclusion, trismus, or muscle tremor.

s., cri-du-chat, clinical syndrome associated with the deletion of the short arm of a B chromosome. Manifestations include mental retardation, various congenital abnormalities, and an infant cry resembling the mewing of a cat.

s., crocodile tears, a syndrome in which a spontaneous lacrimation occurs with the normal salivation of eating. It follows facial paralysis and seems to result from straying of the regenerating nerve fibers, some of those destined for the salivary glands going to the lacrimal glands.

s., Crouzon's. See **dysostosis, craniofacial.**

s., Cushing's (Cushing's disease), a symptom complex associated with an excess of adrenal steroids of all types resulting from hyperplasia of the adrenal cortex, malignant neoplasms, pituitary basophilia, or prolonged administration of adrenocorticotropic hormone (ACTH). Manifestations include hypertension, obesity, diabetes mellitus, osteoporosis, purple striae of the skin in areas of tension, and disorders of glucose tolerance.

s., Down. See **mongolism.**

s., Ehlers-Danlos, a congenital or familial disorder characterized by fragility of the skin and blood vessels, hyperlaxity of the joints, hyperelasticity of the skin, subcutaneous pseudotumors, and tendency to hemorrhage postoperatively.

s., Ekman's. See **osteogenesis imperfecta.**

s., Ellis-van Creveld. See **chondroectodermal dysplasia.**

s., Feer's. See **acrodynia.**

s., Frey's. See **syndrome, auriculotemporal.**

s., Fröhlich's, adiposity and genital hypoplasia resulting from hypopituitarism or hypothalamohypophysdystrophy.

s., Gardner's, multiple osteomas, polyposis of the large bowel, epidermoid or sebaceous cysts, and cutaneous fibromas.

s., general adaptation (adaptation syndrome, GAS), a three-stage physiologic response to physical or psychologic stress. The first stage is the alarm reaction, consisting of bodily changes typical of emotion. A second stage is resistance to stress, wherein an attempt is made to adapt to the physiologic changes. Certain hormones of the anterior pituitary gland and the adrenal cortex hypersecrete to increase resistance. Such resistance leads to diseases of adaptation, such as hypertension. Continual stress results in the third stage, exhaustion.

s., Goldscheider's, dystrophic form of epidermolysis bullosa, leading to scars. The disturbance is inherited on an autosomal dominant or recessive basis. This form of epidermolysis bullosa leads to retardation of mental and physical growth. See also **syndrome, Weber-Cockayne.**

s., Greig's, a condition manifested by ocular hypertelorism, often mental retardation, ectodermal and mesodermal abnormalities, and dental and oral anomalies.

s., Gunn's. See **syndrome, jawwinking.**

s., gustatory hyperhidrosis. See **syndrome, auriculotemporal.**

s., gustatory sweating. See **syndrome, auriculotemporal.**

s., Heerfordt's. See **fever, uveoparotid.**

s., Horner's, a tetrad of symptoms resulting from paralysis of the cervical sympathetic trunk: pupillary constriction, ptosis of the upper eyelid, dilation of the orbital blood vessels (redness of conjunctiva), and blushing and anhidrosis of the side of the face.

s., Hunt's, herpetic inflammation of the geniculate ganglion, with herpes zoster of the soft palate, anterior tonsillar pillar, and auricular area. See also **herpes zoster.**

s., Hurler's (mucopolysaccharidosis I H, gargoylism, dysostosis multiplex),

S

a heritable disorder of mucopoly-saccharide metabolism in which excessive acid mucopolysaccharides—dermatan sulfate and heparitin sulfate—are made and stored in the tissues. Clinical manifestations include hypertelorism, open mouth with large-appearing tongue, thick eyelids and lips, anomalies of the teeth, and short, broad neck. The skeletal and facial deformities resemble the gargoyles of Gothic architecture. Mental retardation, corneal clouding, hepatosplenomegaly, deafness, and cardiac defects are present.

s., Hutchinson-Gilford (progeria), syndrome of dwarfism, immaturity, and pseudosenility. Patient appears to be bald and elderly at an early age. Hypoplasia of the mandible occurs, and the face is small in relation to the neurocranium.

s., jaw-winking (winking-jaw syndrome), congenital unilateral ptosis and elevation of the lid on opening of the jaw or moving of the mandible to the contralateral side.

s., Klinefelter's (XXY syndrome, chromatin-positive syndrome, medullary gonadal dysgenesis), presence in men of an abnormal sex-chromosome constitution. Persons with XXY constitution show the clinical signs of sterility, aspermatogenesis, variable gynecomastia, and often mental retardation. About 50% of subjects with XXXXY variant have cleft palate.

s., Klippel-Feil, fusions of cervical vertebrae, short neck with limited head movement, and extension of the posterior hairline.

s., Lobstein's. See **osteogenesis imperfecta.**

s., Marfan, tall, thin stature, long, tapered fingers and toes (arachnodactyly), dislocation of the lens of the eye (ectopia lentis), and aneurysm leading to rupture of the aorta.

s., Melkersson-Rosenthal, transient facial edema, especially swelling of the upper lip, facial paralysis, and lingua plicata. Plicated swelling of the mucosa of the tongue, palate, and buccal mucosa may not be present, or the paralysis may be incomplete.

s., Mikulicz's, a condition characterized by swelling of the parotid, submandibular, sublingual, and lacrimal glands; associated with lymphosarcoma, leukemia, tuberculosis, sarcoidosis, and syphilis.

s., Möbius', congenital facial diplegia consisting of facial paralysis as well as lingual and masticatory muscle paralysis, inability to abduct the eyes, and anomalies of the extremities.

s., myeloproliferative, extramedullary myelopoiesis in adults. It may follow contact with benzol compounds or polycythemia, or it may precede leukemia.

s., nephrotic (nəfrot'ik), syndrome that includes proteinuria, hyperlipemia, hypoproteinemia, and edema. It occurs in a variety of conditions in which increased glomerular permeability and urinary loss of protein occur.

s., nonarticular pain, one of several painful disorders that limit joint motion and affect the periarticular structures: the tendons, tendon sheaths, bursae, connective tissue, and muscles. Patients commonly call this syndrome muscular aches and pains. The pains are chronic and nagging and may occur in acute exacerbations. The neck, shoulder, back, thighs, hands, and legs are common sites of irritation. The nonarticular disorders are associated with fibrositis, tenonitis, tenosynovitis, and periarticular muscle spasm. The precipitating agents are frequently obscure and may be associated with postural or personality disorders. When the acute symptoms of pain, stiffness, and restricted motion are reduced, the tissues resume their normal function. The common temporomandibular joint syndrome is believed to be caused by a postural occlusal imbalance associated with the muscular tension induced by psychologic stress. The combination precipitates an acute muscle spasm in the muscles associated with the protection and movement of the joint.

s., Papillon-Lefèvre, extensive periodontal disease in young patients (juvenile periodontosis) accompanied by keratotic lesions of the palmar and plantar surfaces. In some patients changes similar to hereditary ectodermal dysplasia also are present.

s., paratrigeminal, trigeminal neuralgia, sensory loss, weakness and atrophy of the masticatory muscles, miosis, and ptosis of the upper eyelid on the affected side of the face resulting from a lesion of the semilunar ganglion and fibers of the carotid plexus.

s., Patau's. See **trisomy-D.**

s., Paterson-Kelly. See **syndrome, Plummer-Vinson.**

s., Peutz-Jeghers, generalized multiple polyposis of the intestinal tract, consistently involving the jejunum, and associated with melanin spots of the lips, buccal mucosa, and fingers; autosomal dominant inheritance.

s., PHC. See **syndrome, Böök's.**

s., Pierre Robin, micrognathia of the newborn. Congenital retrognathism associated with cleft palate, glossoptosis, difficulty in swallowing, respiratory obstruction, and cyanosis. This congenital micrognathia corrects itself during the growth of the child if proper care is provided.

s., Plummer-Vinson, a symptom complex that includes fissures at the corners of the mouth, sore tongue, dysphagia, achlorhydria, and iron-deficiency anemia. Most commonly seen in females in the fourth and fifth decades of life and associated with a predisposition to carcinoma of the oral cavity and esophagus.

s., Reiter's, a syndrome that consists of arthritis (often of the rheumatoid type), conjunctivitis, nonspecific urethritis, and occasionally aphthous ulcers of the oral mucosa.

s., Rieger's, a syndrome whose characteristics include hypodontia, conical crowns, enamel hypoplasia, dysgenesis of the iris and cornea, and myotonic dystrophy.

s., Riley-Day (familial dysautonomia), disturbances of the autonomic and central nervous systems consisting of hypersalivation, defective lacrimation, excessive sweating, erythematous blotching after emotional upset, relative indifference to pain, and hyporeflexia. Normal growth and motor development are retarded.

s., Robin. See **syndrome, Pierre Robin.**

s., Roger's, continuous excessive secretion of saliva as the result of cancer of the esophagus or other esophageal irritation.

s., Rosenthal. See **hemophilia C.**

s., rubella, enamel defects of the primary teeth attributed to prolonged effect of the rubella virus on ameloblasts during fetal life and in the postnatal period.

s., Scheuthauer-Marie-Sainton. See **cleidocranial dysostosis.**

s., sicca. See **syndrome, Sjögren's.**

s., Sjögren's (sicca syndrome, xerodermostecisis), condition related to deficient secretion of salivary, sweat, lacrimal, and mucous glands (xerostomia, keratoconjunctivitis, rhinitis, dysphagia), increased size of salivary glands, and polyarthritis.

s., Smyth's. See **hyperostosis, infantile cortical.**

s., Stevens-Johnson, an acute inflammatory disease characterized by oral, ocular, and genital lesions with severe generalized symptoms. The oral lesions are irregularly shaped, painful ulcers. See also **erythema multiforme.**

s., Sturge-Weber, an encephalofacial angiomatosis characterized by cutaneous facial cerebral angiomatosis, ipsilateral gyriform calcifications of the brain, mental retardation, seizures (epilepsy), contralateral hemiplegia, and ocular involvement. Facial lesions (port-wine stain) may join intraoral angiomas on the buccal mucosa and gingiva.

s., Swift's. See **acrodynia.**

s., temporomandibular joint, an acute muscle spasm in the muscles associated with the protection and movement of the joint. It is believed to be caused by a postural (occlusal) imbalance associated with the muscular tension induced by psychologic stress. The principal symptoms are pain in the region of the joint, limitation of mobility of the mandible, crepitus, clicking sounds in the joint, and frequently tinnitus.

s., thalassemia (Cooley's anemia, Mediterranean anemia, hereditary leptocytosis), any of a group of closely related and genetically determined disorders in which a specific decrease in one of the polypeptide chains comprising hemoglobin occurs. The defect results in hypochromic microcytic erythrocytes. Alpha, beta, and delta variants occur, as well as several subtypes based on biochemical techniques. See also **thalassemia.**

S

s., Treacher Collins, an incomplete mandibulofacial dysostosis in which congenital deformities of the eyelids, mandible, and malar bones occur, as well as malocclusion, cleft lip and palate, and nasal deformities.

s., Turner's (XO syndrome, gonadal dysgenesis, genital dwarfism), absence of one of the X chromosomes, with affected females being sterile and short of stature and having various congenital anomalies such as webbing of the neck, low-set ears, wide-set eyes, shieldlike chest, absence of breasts, and cubitus valgus. Common orofacial findings are hypoplastic mandible, high palatal vault, and dental anomalies.

s., Ullrich-Feichtiger, micrognathia, polydactyly, and genital malformations.

s., Urbach-Wiethe, hyalinosis of the skin and mucous membranes and hoarseness. The skin is infiltrated with yellowish, waxy nodules, and the oral tissues with similar plaques beginning before puberty and becoming increasingly severe. The teeth may be hypoplastic or may fail to develop.

s., vestibular disorder, one of several syndromes involving the vestibule of the ear. The two most common syndromes of vestibular disorders are seasickness, which results from the continuous movement of the endolymph in susceptible individuals (probably related to a disturbance in the reflex control of the eyeball movements), and Meniere's syndrome, in which paroxysmal vertigo is the principal sign, but other associated vascular and metabolic disorders occur.

s., Waardenburg-Klein, a syndrome consisting of congenital deafness, white forelock, increased distance between the inner canthi, the iris of the same eye or of the two eyes having different color (heterochromic irides), and prognathism. Inherited as an autosomal dominant disorder.

s., Weber-Cockayne, simple nonscarring form of epidermolysis bullosa; transmitted as an autosomal dominant trait. See also **syndrome, Goldscheider's.**

s., Weech's. See **hypohidrotic ectodermal dysplasia.**

s., Witkop-von Sallman, hereditary benign intraepithelial dyskeratosis with gelatinous plaques on hyperemic bulbar conjunctiva and white folds and plaques involving the oral mucosa.

s., Zinsser-Engman-Cole, syndrome consisting of reticular atrophy of the skin, with pigmentation, dystrophic fingernails and toenails, and oral leukoplakia. Hyperhidrosis of the palms and soles is present, as well as acrocyanosis of the hands and feet.

syneresis (siner'əsis), a process by which a fluid exudate forms on the surface of a hydrocolloid gel, even when the gel is in water or in a humid atmosphere. It is accompanied by shrinkage of the gel.

synergism (sin'ərjizm), joint action of two drugs in such a manner that one supplements or enhances the action of the other to produce an effect greater than that which may be obtained with either one of the drugs in equivalent quantity or produce effects that could not be obtained with any safe quantity of either drug or both. See also **potentiation.**

synergy, the process in which two organs, substances, or agents work simultaneously to enhance the function and effect of one another.

synostosis, the joining of two bones by the ossification of connecting tissues. It occurs normally in the fusion of cranial bones to form the adult skull.

synovial joint, a freely movable joint in which contiguous bony surfaces are covered by articular cartilage and connected by ligaments lined with synovial membrane.

synovitis, an inflammatory condition of the synovial membrane of a joint as the result of an aseptic wound or a traumatic injury such as a sprain or severe strain.

syntax, a property of language involving structural cues for the arrangement of words as elements in a phrase, clause, or sentence.

synthesis, a putting together. The creation of a new entity or idea from elements not previously joined.

synthetic, a substance that is produced by an artificial rather than a natural process or material.

synthetic porcelain (not current). See **cement, silicate.**

Synthodont, a brand name for a prefabricated ceramic implant.

syphilid (sif'ĭlid), a cutaneous lesion of syphilis.

syphilis (sif'ilis) (lues), a contagious venereal disease caused by *Treponema pallidum* and usually transmitted by direct contact. Oral lesions include primary chancre, secondary mucous patches and split papule, and tertiary gumma.

s., congenital, syphilis transmitted prenatally by the mother to the fetus. Congenital syphilis may lead to Hutchinson's incisors, mulberry molars, or rhagades. See also **chancre; gumma; incisors, Hutchinson's; molar, mulberry; patch, mucous;** *Treponema pallidum.*

s., latent, a stage of syphilis in which no clinical signs or symptoms of the disease are present. It is usually discovered by serologic tests.

s., primary, the appearance of a small painless pustule on the skin of a mucous membrane within 10 to 90 days after exposure. The lesion may appear anywhere on the body where contact with a lesion on an infected person has occurred, but it is most often seen in the anogenital region. It quickly erodes, forming a painless, bloodless ulcer, called a chancre, exuding a fluid that swarms with spirochetes. The disease is highly contagious during this stage.

s., secondary, this stage occurs about 2 months after the primary stage. Secondary syphilis is characterized by general malaise, anorexia, nausea, fever, headache, alopecia, bone and joint pain, or the appearance of a morbilliform rash that does not itch, flat white sores in the mouth and throat, and condylomata lata papules on the moist areas of the skin. The disease is highly contagious during this stage.

s., tertiary, this stage may not develop for 3 to 15 years after the initial infection. It is characterized by the appearance of soft, rubbery tumors, called gummas; the valves of the heart may be damaged, and late stages may lead to mental or physical disability and premature death.

Syrette (siret'), trade name for a small hypodermic syringe containing a dose of the drug to be administered. (not current)

syringe (sir'inj), an apparatus of metal, glass, or plastic material consisting of a nozzle, or needle, barrel, and plunger or rubber bulb; used to inject a liquid into a cavity or under the skin.

s., air, a device by which air may be applied to a given area. An instrument supplied as part of the dental unit, consisting of a hand grip, nozzle, pressure-regulating valve, and hose connected to the compressed air supply.

s., combination, a syringe that is usually part of the dental unit through which air, water, or a combination of the two may be delivered under pressure to the desired area.

s., hand air, an air syringe consisting of a metal tube bent at one end, terminating in a reduced diameter, and enlarged at the other end to engage a rubber bulb. The bulb is compressed by hand to supply a controlled spurt of air to a given area.

s., warm air, an air syringe equipped with an electric heating element to heat the air to any desired temperature.

s., water, a device, usually part of the dental unit, permitting controlled application of water to a given area. It has a flow control, pressure regulator, and heating element.

system, a set or series of organs or parts that unite in a common function.

s., acid-base buffer, the system by which a virtually constant pH level of the blood and body fluids is maintained. The base and acid electrolytes associated with normal metabolism are continuously introduced into the bloodstream. Notwithstanding the marked amounts of base or acid or both introduced into the bloodstream during exercise, rest, hunger, or the ingestion of fluid and solid foods, the pH level of the blood remains rather constant between the range 7.3 and 7.5. Four means by which this relatively narrow but constant pH level is maintained are available: the buffer system of the blood, tissue and cell fluids, and mineral salts of the bone matrix; excretion and retention of carbon dioxide by the lungs; excretion of an acid or alkaline urine; and the formation or excretion of ammonia and organic compounds.

s., apothecaries', a nondecimal system of weights and measures traditionally used by druggists. See also **system, avoirdupois.**

s., autonomic nervous, the part of the nervous system that regulates the reflex control of bodily functions. It controls the functioning of glands, smooth muscle, and the heart.

s., avoirdupois, a commercial nondecimal system of weights and measures. See also **system, apothecaries'.**

s., central nervous, the brain and spinal cord, including their nerves and end organs; controls all voluntary acts.

s., circulatory, the heart and blood vessels. Three major groups of blood vessels are defined: arteries, capillaries, and veins. The system transports metabolites to and from the tissue cells.

s., computer, an assembly of procedures, processes, methods, routines, techniques, and equipment united by some form of regulated interaction to form an organized whole. It is an approach to a complex problem.

s., flowchart, a pictorial diagram illustrating the flow of information into, through, and out of a system of programs.

s., hematopoietic, term used to describe collectively the blood, bone marrow, lymph nodes, spleen, and reticuloendothelial cells.

s., masticatory, the organs and structures primarily functioning in mastication: the jaws, teeth and their supporting structures, temporomandibular articulation, mandibular musculature, tongue, lips, cheeks, and oral mucosa and their nerve supplies.

s., metric, a decimal system of weights and measures almost universally used in scientific and professional work, including the writing of prescriptions. The individual units are based on an international set of standards, notably the meter, liter, and kilogram. See Appendix H.

s., musculoskeletal, the system of body structures that provides the energy and movement necessary for the functions of life. The muscles, bones, and connective tissues of the body are grouped together into one system, and they are intimately connected in their individual and combined functions; for example, for muscle to accomplish

its ultimate purpose of movement by contraction, bone, leverage, and connective tissue are required to transmit the force that the contraction generates. In the oral cavity and its related structures the musculoskeletal tissues fulfill the mechanical and structural requirements for movement of the mandible and some related visceral functions such as respiration and digestion.

s., neurohormonal, the system by which the hormone secretions of the endocrine glands function in part as the regulators of both visceral and somatic function and have intimate anatomic and functional relationships with the nervous system by the union of the pituitary gland and the hypothalamus of the cerebrum. The pituitary gland has a pars nervosa, which is an extension of the anterior part of the hypothalamus, and a pars intermedia, which is an epithelial evagination of the secretory tissue from the stomodeum of the embryo. From its position in the cranial structures in the sella turcica, the pituitary gland regulates, by its union with the nervous system, the whole endocrine system with its many glands; these glands in turn partially regulate the viscera and somatic muscle organs.

s., occlusal (occlusal scheme), the form or design and arrangement of the occlusal and incisal units of a dentition or of the teeth on a denture. See also **system, masticatory.**

s., parasympathetic nervous, one of the motor divisions of the autonomic nervous system. It is described as the craniosacral division and does not have the simplified structural apparatus of the strong sympathetic adrenal axis about which to function. The parasympathetic system inhibits the heart, contracts the pupils, and, in emotional states, produces a vagus-insulin axis of activity. The several parts function rather independently. The ocular division relates to the midbrain, and the bulbar division relates to the hindbrain. The bulbar division supplies the facial, glossopharyngeal, and vagus nerves. It also supplies the secretory and vasodilator fibers of the salivary glands and mucous membranes of the mouth and pharynx. In conditions of very loud noise or un-

S

usual anxiety states, the parasympathetic system causes unaccounted-for spontaneous urination, excessive salivary and gastric juices, and either nausea or vomiting.

s., proaccelerin-accelerin. See **factor V.**

s., proconvertin-convertin. See **factor VII.**

s., stomatognathic, the combination of all the structures involved in speech and the reception, mastication, and deglutition of food. The system is composed of the teeth, jaws, muscles of mastication, epithelium, and temporomandibular joints and nerves that control these structures.

s., sympathetic nervous, one of the two opposing motor systems in the autonomic nervous system that mediate the activity of the viscera. (The other is the parasympathetic system.) The sympathetic system is composed of 21 or 22 ganglia in chains on each side of the spinal cord. The fibers connect with the spinal cord through these ganglia. The actions of the sympathetic division of the autonomic nervous system are closely allied to the action of the medulla of the adrenal gland; thus a sympathetic-adrenal axis that functions as a unit to protect and regulate the body environment may be conceived. The sympathetic control is modified by the volitional somatic control of the patient. The volitional control, superimposed on the autonomic control, gives rise to great variations in motor patterns, as seen in the face in the presence of emotional changes such as in the blushing of shame and pallor of fear.

s., vascular, closed tube, the type of vascular system, as in humans, in which the blood circulates through the vessels (or tubes) and is not dissipated into the tissues. The closed vascular tube system offers resistance to the pumping action of the heart because the pressures are cumulative with each pumping action. The elastic walls in the arterial vessels, particularly in the aorta, absorb the additional energy and release it slowly, thus creating the possibility of maintaining a fairly steady and safe pressure head throughout the vascular system. The high-pressure point at the height of cardiac contraction is the systole, and the low point before the ventricular contraction is the diastole.

s., vascular, open tube, in some vertebrates a vascular system with an open end that causes the blood fluid to dissipate into the tissues. This system starts with a maximal head pressure that diminishes until inertia in the blood is overcome. The blood is returned to the heart by muscle function, gravity, and diffusion. The blood pressure in this system fluctuates from a maximum at the heart to a minimum at the tissue cell.

s., venous, a system of interconnected blood vessels that returns blood to the heart from the tissue and capillary bed through progressively larger vessels. The following affect the return of blood to the heart: thoracic pressure, associated with respiration; gravity, associated with body posture; the valves, diameter of the lumen, and muscle structure of the veins; muscle contraction of the somatic structures; the pressures in the arteriole system and capillary bed; and the nervous and hormonal system controls that regulate cardiomuscular activity. The influences over the venous system circulation are collectively termed veno pressor mechanisms.

systematic error, a nonrandom statistical error that affects the mean of a population of data and defines the bias between the means of two populations.

systematically, done in a well-organized, carefully followed pattern of procedure.

systemic lupus erythematosus (SLE) (sistem'ık loo'pəs erəhem'ə-tō's), an autoimmune disease that can be life threatening. Patients may have a distinctive pattern of facial redness and oral lesions. Endothelial damage to heart valves similar to those caused by rheumatic fever may occur.

systole (sis'təlē), the period of contraction of the heart. The term specifically designates the contraction of the ventricles as distinguished from auricular contraction. It occurs with the first heart sound. The pressure from the systolic contractions is taken up and stored as potential energy by the elastic properties of the aorta and other great vessels of the arterial system. This storage of energy protects the smaller, more fragile vessels from undue pressure. The even flow and steady pressure of the blood are sustained by the controlled release of the potential energy stored in the arterial walls into kinetic energy for movement of the blood during the diastolic phase of heart function. The pressure recorded at the height of the ventricular contraction is the systolic pressure. In the adult the normal blood pressure is 120/80 mm Hg (systolic/diastolic). It rises with advancing age to 135/89 at 60 years of age.

t-test, an inferential statistic used to test for differences between two means (groups) only. This statistic is used for small samples (for example, N < 30). Synonyms: t-ratio, student's t.

tabes, a gradual, progressive wasting of the body in any chronic disease.

t. dorsalis (tā′bēz dorsa′ lis) *(locomotor ataxia),* a form of neurosyphilis in which degeneration in the posterior roots of the spinal nerves and posterior column of the spinal cord exists. Manifestations include pain and paresthesia of the trunk, hands, and feet, abdominal pain crises, ataxia, Argyll Robertson pupil, atrophy of the optic nerve, and Charcot's joint.

table, occlusal, the occlusal surfaces of the premolars and molars; the basic collective topography, including the form of the cusps, inclined planes, marginal ridges, and central fossae and grooves of the teeth.

table of allowances, a list of covered services with an assigned dollar amount that represents the total obligation of the plan with respect to payment for such service but does not necessarily represent the dentist's full fee for that service. Synonyms: schedule of allowances, indemnity schedule.

tablet, a small, solid dose form of a medication. It may be compressed or molded in its manufacture, and it may be of almost any size, shape, weight, and color. Most tablets are intended to be swallowed whole.

tachycardia (tak′ikär′dē- ə), an excessively rapid action of the heart; the pulse rate is usually above 100 beats/min.

tachyphylaxis (tak′əfələk′sis), **1.** the rapid development of tolerance on administration of closely spaced successive doses of a drug or poison. **2.** a decreasing response that follows consecutive injections at short intervals.

tachypnea (takipnē′ə), an excessively rapid respiration. A respiratory neurosis marked by quick, shallow breathing.

tacrine HCl, *trade name:* Cognex; *drug class:* cholinesterase inhibitor; *action:* a centrally acting, reversible inhibitor of cholinesterase enzyme; *use:* treatment of mild-to-moderate cognitive defects associated with Alzheimer's disease.

tacrolimus (FK506), *trade name:* Prograf; *drug class:* immunosuppressant; *action:* inhibits T-lymphocyte activation leading to immunosuppression; *uses:* prophylaxis of organ rejection in patients receiving allogenic liver transplants.

tactile, pertaining to the sense of touch.

tailpiece. See **aid, speech, prosthetic, velar section.**

Takahara'a disease. See **disease, Takahara's.**

Talwin, the brand name for pentazocine lacatate, a potent analgesic, which is as effective as morphine. Talwin is a controlled substance.

tamoxifen citrate, *trade name:* Nolvadex; *drug class:* antineoplastic, antiestrogen hormone; *action:* inhibits cell division by binding to cytoplasmic receptors, inhibits DNA synthesis; *use:* advanced breast cancer that has not responded to other therapy.

tang. See **connector, minor.**

tank, processing, a receptacle used in the photographic or radiographic darkroom for the chemical solutions used in the processing of films.

tannic acid, a vegetable tanning agent that attaches itself to collagen by hydrogen bonds. Tannic acid is used in dentistry as a cavity conditioner before placing a restoration.

tantalum (tan'tələm), a silvery metallic element, its atomic number is 73 and its atomic weight is 180.95. Tantalum is a relatively inert, noncorrosive, malleable metal used in prosthetic devices such as skull plates and wire sutures.

tantrum, a sudden outburst or violent display of rage, frustration, and bad temper, usually occurring in a maladjusted child or immature or disturbed adult.

tape, dental, a ribbon of waxed nylon or silk used to aid the prophylaxis of interproximal spaces and the proximal surfaces of the teeth. The flattened, wide form of dental floss.

tapering, a process of shaping a clasp arm to better distribute flexure throughout its length, thus reducing fatigue, strain hardening, and resultant fracture.

t. arch, a dental arch that converges from the molars to the central incisors to such a degree that lines passing through the central grooves of the molars and premolars intersect within one inch anterior to the central incisors. See also **arch, tapering.**

target, the small tungsten block, embedded in the face of the anode, that is bombarded by electrons from the cathode in an x-ray tube.

t. cell, **1.** also called *leptocyte,* an abnormal red blood cell characterized by a densely stained center surrounded by a pale, unstained ring that is encircled by a dark, irregular band. **2.** any cell having a specific receptor that reacts with a specific hormone, antigen, antibody, antibiotic, sensitized T cell, or other substance.

t.-film distance (TFD). See **distance, target-film; source-film distance.**

t.-object distance (TOD). See **source-object distance.**

t. organ, **1.** an organ intended to receive a therapeutic dose of irradiation. **2.** an organ intended to receive the greatest concentration of a diagnostic radioactive tracer.

t. symptoms, symptoms of an illness that are most likely to respond to a specific treatment.

tarnish, 1. surface discoloration or loss of luster by metals. Under oral conditions, it often results from hard and soft deposits. **2.** a chemical process by which a metal surface is discolored or its luster destroyed.

tartar. See **calculus, dental.**

taste, the sense of perceiving different flavors in soluble substances that contact the tongue and trigger nerve impulses to special taste centers in the cortex and the thalamus of the brain. The four basic traditional tastes are sweet, salty, sour, and bitter.

t. bud, any one of many peripheral taste organs distributed over the tongue and the roof of the mouth.

t. enhancers, food additives that have little or no flavor of their own but when added to food bring out the taste of certain foods. Monosodium glutamate (MSG) is the most common flavor or taste enhancer.

tattoo, amalgam. See **amalgam tattoo.**

taurodontism (tâ'rōdon'tizəm), a tooth in which the pulp chamber is elongated, enlarged, and extends deeply into the region of the roots. A similar condition is seen in the teeth of cud-chewing animals.

tautomer, structural isomers that differ only in the position of a hydrogen atom, or proton.

tax, a ratable portion of the proceeds or value of the property and labor of the citizen; any contribution imposed by government for the use and service of the state.

t. brackets, the income intervals of the graduated income tax law that establishes the rate of tax for each level of income.

T. Equity and Fiscal Responsibility Act of 1982 (TEFRA), legislation (Public Law 97-248) affecting health maintenance organizations and the Medicare and Medicaid programs. Provides regulations for the development of HMO risk contracting with the Medicare program and, through an amendment, establishes new provisions for the foundation and operation of peer review organizations.

t. planning, making business and investment decisions based on estimated income and current and projected tax laws.

t. shelter investments, investments that reduce, remove, or defer income from state and federal income tax liability.

taxes, the sum of monies collected by the various branches of a government.

T

taxonomy, a system for classifying organisms on the basis of natural relationships and assigning them appropriate names.

Tay-Sachs disease, an inherited, neurodegenerative disorder of lipid metabolism caused by a deficiency of the enzyme hexosaminidase A, which results in the accumulation of sphingolipids in the brain. The condition, which is transmitted as an autosomal recessive trait, occurs predominantly in families of Eastern European Jewish origin, specifically the Ashkenazic Jews.

T cell, a small, circulating lymphocyte produced in the bone marrow that matures in the thymus. T cells primarily mediate cellular immune responses such as graft rejection and delayed hypersensitivity.

T-4 cell, a thymus-derived lymphocyte of the body's immune system with a role of destroying or neutralizing cells or substances identified as "nonself." The human immunodeficiency virus (HIV) commonly targets the T-4 cells with the result that the body's immune defenses are severely damaged and opportunistic infections are allowed to flourish.

teaching rounds. See **rounds.**

team practice, professional practice by a group of complementary health care providers who collectively manage the care of a patient population.

technetium 99, the radionuclide most commonly used to image the body in nuclear medicine scans. It is preferred because of its short half-life and because the emitted photon has an appropriate energy for imaging techniques.

technic (tek′nik). See **technique.**

technical competence, the ability of the practitioner, during the treatment phase of dental care and with respect to those procedures combining psychomotor and cognitive skills, to consistently provide services at a professionally acceptable level.

technical quality, the degree to which the physically measurable attributes of procedures in dental care meet professionally acceptable standards.

technician, a person skilled in the performance of technical procedures.

t., dental. See **technician, dental laboratory.**

t., d. laboratory (dental technique), an individual skilled in the art of executing the dentist's prescription for the mechanical fabrication of dental appliances.

technique (teknēk′), **1.** a skillful and detailed method of executing procedures to accomplish a desired result. **2.** the method of performance of manipulation in any art; the terms *technique* and *technic* are used synonymously, but the word *technique* pertains more to the artistic skill involved.

t., bisection of the angle, an intraoral radiographic technique whereby an angle formed by the mean plane of the tooth and the mean plane of the film is bisected, and the central ray is directed through the tooth perpendicular to the bisection. This is the application of Cieszynski's rule of isometry. See also **rule of isometry, Cieszynski's.**

t., calibrated angle, an intraoral radiographic technique using a specified degree in vertical angulation from the horizontal plane. It is a variation of the bisection of the angle technique and assumed to be the correct angulation for the majority of patients.

t., chew-in. See **chew-in technique.**

t., double investing, a method of investing wax patterns, whereby the pattern is covered with a primary layer of investment; this core is then invested, before or after the primary investment has set, in an outer, thinner mix of the same or a different type of investing material.

t., dual impression, a technique by which the anatomic form of the teeth and immediately adjacent structures is recorded and by which the free-end denture foundation areas are registered in their functional form.

t., Eames', in dental amalgam, a procedure using mercury and alloy in approximately a 1:1 ratio, thus not having residual mercury in the plastic mix.

t., filling, the method used to obliterate the space in the root of the tooth once occupied by the dental pulp.

t., Fones'. See **method, Fones'.**

t., hydroflow. See **dentistry, washed-field.**

t., impression, a method and manner used in making a negative likeness. The series of operations or procedures used for making an impression.

t., long cone, the use of an extended cone distance, generally 14 inches (35 cm) or more, in oral radiography. It is generally used with, but not confined to, parallel film placement.

t., Nealon's, a technique for the insertion of resin restorations whereby the monomer and polymer are applied incrementally with a brush.

t., parallel (right-angle technique), a technique in intraoral radiography in which the film is positioned parallel to the long axes of the teeth, and the central ray is directed perpendicular to both the film and the teeth.

t., short cone, the use of a short cone distance, usually 8 inches (20 cm) or less, that is supplied by the manufacturer as short cone. It is generally used with, but not confined to, the bisection of the angle technique.

t., telephone, the friendly but business-like conveying of ideas over the telephone.

t., thermal expansion, a casting procedure whereby compensation is made for metal shrinkage by thermal expansion of the refractory investment mold.

t., wax expansion, a casting procedure whereby compensation is made for metal shrinkage by thermal expansion of the wax pattern before setting of the investment.

teeth. See **tooth.**

teething, the eruption of primary teeth, which is preceded by increased salivation. Young children may become restless and irritable during this period. Inflammation of the gingival tissues before complete emergence of the crown may cause a temporary painful condition.

Teflon, trade name of a proprietary plastic material (polytetrafluoroethylene) used in reconstructive surgery of the jaw and chin.

Tegopen, the brand name for cloxacillin, an antistaphylococcal penicillin.

Tegretol. See **carbamazepine.**

telangiectasia (təlan′gē·ektā′zhə), **1.** the dilation of the capillaries and small arteries of a region. A hereditary form (hereditary hemorrhagic telangiectasia) may appear intraorally. **2.** a disorder characterized by cutaneous and mucosal vascular macules, nodules, and arterial spiders that tend to bleed sporadically.

t., hereditary hemorrhagic (Rendu-Osler-Weber disease), the dilation of small vessels and capillaries resulting from a genetic factor, with a tendency to bleed. Lesions may occur on the tongue as small, raised, red to bluish-red elevations.

telediagnosis, a process whereby a disease diagnosis or prognosis is made by the electronic transmission of data between distant medical facilities. See also **telemedicine.**

telemedicine, the use of two-way television communication by which two or more physicians can consult on a patient. The consulting physicians have access to the diagnostic information as well as the ability to view and question the patient directly before making a diagnosis or offering a professional opinion.

telemetry, the electronic transmission of data between distant points.

teleradiography (tel′ərā′dē·aog′r·a-fe) Radiography at a longer distance than is usually used (6 feet; 1.8 m).

telic (telik) (teleologic), assigning purpose to functions as if they were provided by a creative planner.

tellurium (Te), an element exhibiting metallic and nonmetallic chemical properties. Its atomic number is 52 and its atomic weight is 127.60. Inhaling vapors of tellurium results in a garlicky breath.

temazepam, *trade name:* Restoril; *drug class:* benzodiazepine, sedative-hypnotic (Controlled Substance Schedule IV); *action:* produces central nervous system (CNS) depression at limbic, thalamic, hypothalamic levels of the CNS; *uses:* sedative and hypnotic for insomnia.

temperature, the degree of sensible heat or cold.

t., body, the measurable temperature of the body (normal range of variation, 98° to 99° F [35.5° to 37° C] orally and 99° to 100° F [37° to 38° C] rectally, with much wider ranges for skin).

t., b., regulation, homeostasis of body temperature. Results from a balance of heat production (external heat plus heat from muscle contraction and other chemical processes) and heat loss (through lungs, sweating, surface radiation, and excretions).

T

t., casting, the required degree of heat necessary to bring a metal to proper fluidity for introduction into a refractory mold.

t., recrystallization, the lowest temperature at which the distorted grain structure of a cold-worked metal is replaced by a new, strain-free grain structure during prolonged annealing. Time, purity of metal, and prior deformation are important factors.

tempering (hardening heat treatment), the hardening or toughening of steels by heating. Treatment of an alloy in such a manner that solid-solid transformation occurs. Precipitation of intermetallic substances occurs, increasing the proportional limit and hardness of the alloy.

t., gold, the hardening of gold alloys by cold working or by heating and then cooling slowly.

t., hydrocolloid, storing of the material after liquefaction at a temperature that will increase the viscosity to the optimal manipulative degree of sol.

t., steel, counteracting of the hardening heat treatment to the extent needed for the particular tool or structure. It is heated to a predetermined temperature and then quenched in water or oil.

template (tem′plət), a pattern or mold forming an accurate copy of an object or shape.

t., implant, an early type of subperiosteal implant that was fabricated from a cast carved to simulate the host bone. Measurements made from radiographs taken with a template or wire mold resting on the soft tissues determined the carving of the cast.

t., occlusal, a stone or metal (electroformed) occlusal table made from a wax occlusal path registration of jaw movements and against which the opposing supplied teeth are occluded.

t., orthodontics, a cephalometric tracing of an age- and sex-normed facial and dental profile used in the analysis of facial and dentition variations in malocclusion.

t., prosthetic, a curved or flat plate used as an aid in setting denture teeth.

t., surgical, a thin transparent resin base shaped to duplicate the form of the impression surface of an immediate denture and used as a guide for surgically shaping the alveolar

process and its soft tissue covering to fit an immediate denture.

t., viral, the process of RNA/DNA replication associated with retrovirus activity.

t., wax, a wax recording of the occlusion of the teeth.

temporal arteritis, a progressive inflammatory disorder of cranial blood vessels, principally the temporal artery, occurring most frequently in women over 70 years of age. The temporal artery is typically tender, swollen, and pulseless. Symptoms are intractable headache, difficulty in chewing, weakness, rheumatoid pain, and loss of vision if the central retinal artery becomes occluded.

temporal artery, any one of three arteries on each side of the head: the superficial temporal artery, the middle temporal artery, and the deep temporal artery.

temporal bone, one of a pair of large bones forming part of the lower cranium and containing various cavities and recesses associated with the ear. Each temporal bone consists of four portions: the mastoid, the squama, the petrous, and the tympanic.

temporal eminential angle, the degree of slope between the axis-orbital plane and the discluding slope of the eminence.

temporalis, one of the four muscles of mastication. It arises in a fan-shaped pattern from the squama of the temporal bone and courses downward to insert along the anterior border of the ramus of the mandible. It is a major closing muscle of the jaw.

temporal lobe, the lateral region of the cerebrum, below the lateral fissure. It contains the center for smell, some association areas for memory and learning, and a region where choice is made of thoughts to express.

temporary, pertaining to the interim treatment used to protect a patient between appointments.

t. base. See **baseplate.**

t. prosthesis. See **prosthesis, temporary.**

t. stopping. See **stopping, temporary.**

t. superstructure, a prosthodontic appliance (removable or fixed) that is used, often immediately postoperatively, as a transitional appliance either for cosmetics or splinting or both.

temporomandibular articulation (tem′pərōman′dib′yələr). See **articulation, temporomandibular.**

temporomandibular extraoral radiographic examination. See **examination, radiographic, extraoral, temporomandibular.**

temporomandibular joint. See **articulation, temporomandibular.**

temporomandibular ligament, an oblique band of tissue that extends downward and backward from the zygomatic process to the neck of the mandible.

temporomandibular pain-dysfunction syndrome, a triad of signs and symptoms consisting of pain in the muscles of mastication and jaw joints, clicking in the jaw joints, and limitation in jaw movements. Lesser findings may include dislocation and/or locking of the jaw joints and sensory changes in hearing. Synonyms: Costen's syndrome, mandibular painsyndrome (MDS), TMJ pain-dysfunction syndrome (PDS), and myofacial pain-dysfunction syndrome (MPD).

tenant, one who has the temporary use and occupation of real property owned by another, the length and terms of the tenancy being usually fixed by a lease.

tender, legal, the kind of coin or money that the law compels a creditor to accept in payment of a debt, when offered by the debtor in the right amount.

tendon, one of many white, glistening fibrous bands of tissue that attach muscle to bone.

tendonitis, the inflammation of a tendon, usually stress or strain related.

tenosynovitis, the inflammation of a tendon sheath caused by calcium deposits, repeated strain or trauma, high levels of blood cholesterol, rheumatoid arthritis, gout, or gonorrhea; occasionally movement yields a crackling noise over the tendon.

tensile strength (tensīl). See **strength, tensile.**

tension (ten′shən), the state of being stretched, strained, or extended.

   t. headache, a pain that affects the head as the result of overwork or emotional strain, involving tension in the muscles of the neck, face, and shoulders.

   t., interfacial surface, the tension or resistance to separation possessed by the film of liquid between two well-adapted surfaces (for example, the thin film of saliva between the denture base and the tissues).

tentative, not final or definite, such as an experimental or clinical finding that has not been validated.

teratogenesis, the development of physical defects in the embryo.

teratogens (ter′ətōjenz), agents that cause congenital malformations and developmental abnormalities if introduced during gestation.

teratology, the study of the causes and effects of congenital malformations and developmental abnormalities.

teratoma (ter′ətō′mə), a tumor composed of cells capable of differentiating into any of the three primary germ layers. Teratomas in the ovary are usually benign dermoidal cysts; those in the testis are generally malignant.

terazosin HCl, *trade name:* Hytrin; *drug class:* antihypertensive, anti-adrenergic; *action:* decreases total vascular resistance, which is responsible for a decrease in blood pressure; *use:* hypertension as a single agent or in combination with diuretics or β-blockers.

terbinafine HCl, *trade name:* Lamisil; *drug class:* antifungal; *action:* inhibits key enzyme, squalene epoxidase, involved with resultant fungal cell death; *uses:* tinea pedis, tinea cruris, tinea corporis.

terbutaline sulfate, *trade names:* Brethaire, Brethine, Bricanyl; *drug class:* selective β_2-agonist; *action:* relaxes bronchial smooth muscle by direct action on β_2-adrenergic receptors; *uses:* bronchospasm, asthma prophylaxis, premature labor inhibitor.

terconazole, *trade names:* Terazol 3, Terazol 7; *drug class:* local antifungal; *action:* interferes with fungal DNA replication; binds sterols in fungal cell membranes, which increases permeability, leaking of nutrients; *uses:* vaginal, vulvar, vulvovaginal candidiasis.

terfenadine, *trade name:* Seldane; *drug class:* antihistamine; *action:* acts on blood vessels and gastrointestinal and respiratory systems by competing with histamine for peripheral H_1

receptor sites; decreases allergic response by blocking histamine; *uses:* rhinitis, allergy symptoms.

terminal, 1. near or approaching an end, such as a terminal bronchiole or a terminal illness. **2.** an input/output device that has a two-way communication capability with a computer.

t., computer, a device in a system or communications network at which data can either enter or leave.

t. hinge position. See **position, hinge, terminal.**

t. illness, an advanced stage of a disease with an unfavorable prognosis and no known cure.

t. jaw relation record. See **record, terminal jaw relation.**

termination date. See **expiration date.**

term infant, any neonate, regardless of birth weight, born after the end of the thirty-seventh and before the beginning of the forty-third week of gestation.

terminology, technical, terms that are descriptive and meaningful to the dentist but are not a part of the patient's vocabulary.

terra alba (ter'ə al'bə), gypsum added to plaster or stone to accelerate the setting reaction.

tertiary health care, a specialized, highly technical level of health care that includes diagnosis and treatment of disease and disability in sophisticated large research and teaching hospitals. Specialized intensive care units, advanced diagnostic support services, and highly specialized personnel are characteristic of tertiary health care services.

tertiary syphilis, the most advanced stage of syphilis, resulting in infections of the cardiovascular and neurologic systems and marked by destructive lesions involving many tissues and organs.

test(s), any clinical or laboratory procedure designed to evaluate constituents or functions of the body.

t., acetone. See **test, ketone bodies.**

t., ACTH-stimulation (Thorn's test), a test of adrenocortical reserve based on changes in the eosinophil count and urinary levels of 17-ketosteroids and 17-hydroxycorticoids as a result of intravenous infusion or intramuscular injection of ACTH.

t., Addis', a test to estimate the number of formed elements in urine collected under standard conditions (restricted food intake, minimal patient activity, night collection).

t., allergy, intradermal, a test for allergy performed by injecting a preparation containing the suspected allergen into the dermis.

t., amylase (am'ilās), a determination of serum amylase, which is useful in the diagnosis of acute pancreatitis and after operations in which the pancreas might have been injured. The Somogyi sarcogenic method is often used, and the results are given in Somogyi units, defined as the amount of amylase needed to digest 1.5 gm of starch in 8 minutes at 37° C. The normal range is 60 to 200 units/100 ml. The serum amylase is also elevated in mumps and other diseases of the salivary glands.

t., amyloid (am'iloid). See **test, Congo red.**

t., antiviral antibody, antibody tests in viral diseases. Included are complement-fixation tests for poliomyelitis, psittacosis, and Coxsackie infections; hemagglutination-inhibition tests for mumps, influenza, and encephalitides; and neutralization tests.

t., Aschheim-Zondek (ash'hīm tson'dek). See **test, pregnancy.**

t., ascorbic acid, intradermal, a test for ascorbic acid deficiency based on the decoloration of an intradermal injection of a purple dye (2,6-dichlorphenol-indophenol). Normally with a wheal of 4 mm, using a dye concentration of N/300, decoloration occurs in 10 to 15 minutes.

t., basophilic aggregation (bā'sōfil'ik), a test for lead poisoning based on increased stippling of erythrocytes. More than 2% stippled cells are seen in lead poisoning. See also **test, lead.**

t., Bell's palsy, simple clinical tests such as motor function tests, in which the patient is asked to whistle, pucker the lips, smile, or wrinkle the forehead; and sensory function tests, in which the patient is asked to taste sweet with sugar, sour with citric acid, bitter with quinine, and salt with sodium chloride.

t., Benedict's, a nonspecific copper reduction test for glucose in the urine. Cupric sulfate in the Benedict's reagent is reduced by glucose during the reaction to cuprous oxide, a reddish-orange precipitate.

t., bilirubin (bil'iroo'bin), qualitative, presumptive, quantitative, or specific determinations for bilirubin in the urine and blood serum. Included are Gmelin's test and van den Bergh's test.

t., bleeding time, techniques for determining the time interval required for hemostasis to occur after a standardized wound has been made in the capillary bed. See also **test, Duke's** and **test, Ivy's.**

t., Brinell hardness (brinel'), a means of determining surface hardness by measuring the amount of resistance to the indentation of a steel ball. Recorded as the Brinell hardness number (BHN); the higher the number, the harder the material. Generally indicative of abrasion resistance.

t., Bromsulphalein (BSP), a test of liver function based on the removal of a known quantity of Bromsulphalein from the blood in a measured period of time. Normal values are less than 5% retention at the end of 45 minutes with an intravenous dose of 5 mg/kg body weight. It is a useful test of hepatocellular disease and detoxifying ability but is not applicable in the presence of extrahepatic or intrahepatic obstructive jaundice.

t., Bunnell. See **test, Paul-Bunnell.**

t., capillary resistance (Rumpel-Leede-Hess test, Gothlin's test), a test of capillary fragility based on the number of petechiae that develop when a standardized intraluminal positive pressure is applied to the capillaries either by a blood pressure cuff or a suction cup applied to the skin. See also **test, tourniquet.**

t., CO₂ capacity (CO₂ combining power test), a general measure of the alkalinity or acidity of the blood. Various normal adult ranges are given (for example, 23 to 30 mEq/L of serum or 55 to 70 vol/100 ml of serum). A low value is found in diabetic acidosis, hyperventilation, certain kidney diseases, and severe diarrhea. A high value is found in excessive administration of ACTH or cortisone, intake of sodium bicarbonate, and persistent vomiting.

t., CO₂ combining power. See test, CO₂ capacity.

t., cold bends, a mechanical test used for assessing ductility.

t., colorimetric caries susceptibility (Snyder's test), a method of determining the concentration of acid-producing bacteria in the saliva by use of bromcresol green in a culture medium. The reliability of this and other salivary bacterial tests for dental caries susceptibility is questionable.

t., Congo red, a test for amyloidosis based on the more rapid disappearance (excess of 60% injected dye in 1 hour) of Congo red from the serum of affected patients than from that of normal individuals. Gingival biopsy and positive staining with methyl violet or crystal violet also indicate amyloidosis.

t., creatinine clearance (krēat'inĭn), a renal function test of exogenous creatinine clearance. It is a convenient clinical test of glomerular filtration rate. It is calculated as the quotient of the product of urine creatinine (mg/L) and urine volume (L/24 hr) divided by the serum creatinine concentration (mg/L). The normal value for young healthy adults of average size (1.73 M^2 body surface area) is 115 to 155 L/24 hr ($\pm$15%).

t., dermal. See **test, skin.**

t., Dick's (scarlet fever test), a skin test to determine susceptibility or immunity to scarlet fever. A positive test is indicated when an area of erythema and edema measuring more than 10 mm in diameter occurs 8 to 24 hours after an intradermal injection of a standardized erythrogenic toxin.

t., Duke's, a test of bleeding time as indicated by the time that elapses before a puncture wound of the earlobe ceases to bleed. Normal range is 2 to 4½ minutes.

t., electric, a test to determine whether a pulp is vital.

t., erythrocyte sedimentation, a macroscopic test of the blood used to detect certain pathologic conditions, particularly inflammation. The blood cells are allowed to settle in the presence of an anticoagulant and the time (sedimentation time) determined. The greater the time or rate, the more severe the condition. Pregnancy and menstruation affect the sedimentation.

T

t., flow, used in the ADA specification for dental amalgam; measured as the percentage shortening of a cylinder of the material.

t., fluorescent treponemal antibody, absorbed (FTA-APS), a modification of the original FTA test for syphilis that employs a protein preparation from the Reiter treponeme.

t. for trigeminal nerve function, three simple clinical tests for trigeminal nerve function: sensation: apply gentle touch, pinpricks, or warm or cold objects to areas supplied by the nerve and note responses; reflex: try the jaw jerk and eye and sneeze reflexes; motor function: test the patient's ability to chew and work against resistance and observe contraction of the masseter and temporal muscles by visual examination and digital palpation.

t., Foshay's, a skin test for tularemia using the Foshay antigen.

t., Frei's (frīz), an intradermal skin test for lymphogranuloma venereum employing the antigen lygranum, which gives a specific dermal reaction in patients infected with this bacterium. A false positive test may occur with psittacosis.

t., Friedman's (frēd'mənz). See **test, pregnancy.**

t., glucose paper, a test in which paper is impregnated with glucose oxidase and other reagents (TesTape, Clinistix). When the paper is moistened with fresh urine, the presence of glucose will cause a change in the color of the paper.

t., glucose tolerance (GTT), a test for abnormalities of carbohydrate tolerance by glucose loading and subsequent serial measurements of the concentration of glucose in the blood. Graphic representation of the concentration and the elapsed time makes up the glucose tolerance curve. Abnormal curves occur in diabetes mellitus, thyrotoxicosis, Cushing's syndrome, acromegaly, and pheochromocytoma.

t., Gothlin's. See **test, capillary resistance.**

t., hardness. See **hardness, Mohs; test, Brinell hardness; test, Knoop hardness;** and **test, Vickers hardness.**

t., Henderson's, a test for acidosis. A normal person can hold his breath without preliminary deep inspiration for 30 seconds or more; the inability to hold it for more than 15 or 20 seconds in a person free from cardiorenal or pulmonary disease indicates the presence of acidosis.

t., Hess'. See **test, capillary resistance.**

t., Hinton's, a precipitation test for syphilis.

t., histoplasmin (his'tōplaz'min), a skin test to determine sensitization to *Histoplasma capsulatum.* A positive test indicates past or present infection (histoplasmosis).

t., infectious mononucleosis, one of several tests for the diagnosis of infectious mononucleosis (for example, Paul-Bunnell test).

t., intracutaneous. See **test, skin.**

t., intradermal. See **test, skin.**

t., Ivy's, a test of bleeding time performed by making a standard wound and touching the blood with filter paper every 30 seconds until no blood appears on the paper. Normal range is 3 to 7 minutes.

t., Janet's, a test to differentiate between functional and organic anesthesia. With the eyes closed, a patient is instructed to say "yes" or "no" as he feels or does not feel the examiner's touch. In functional anesthesia, he will say "no," whereas in organic anesthesia, he will say nothing.

t., Kahn's, a precipitation test for the diagnosis of syphilis. See also **test, serologic.**

t., ketone bodies (acetone test, Rothera's test), nitroprusside reaction tests for acetone and acetoacetic acid and the ferric chloride test for acetoacetic acid. Commercially prepared nitroprusside test tablets (Acetest) and powder (Acetone Test Denco) are available.

t., Kline's, a flocculation test for syphilis based on the combination of the cardiolipin antigen with reagin to form grossly visible aggregates.

t., Knoop hardness, a means of measuring surface hardness by resistance to the penetration of an indenting tool made of diamond. Produces an indentation that has a diamond or rhombic shape. Especially preferred for testing hardness of tooth structure.

t., laboratory, investigative procedures performed in the laboratory that are useful in the diagnosis of disease, including biopsy examination of tissue specimens, determination of type and characteristics of associated microorganisms, serology, blood and urine chemistry, hemogram (red cell count, hemoglobin content, white cell count, differential white cell count), and metabolic studies (basal metabolic rate).

t., LE, a test for lupus erythematosus based on the presence of a single (or multiple) homogenous basophilic inclusion(s) in polymorphonuclear leukocytes. Such LE cells have also been found in cases of rheumatoid arthritis, allergic reactions to penicillin, hydralazine toxicity, and "lupoid cirrhosis." Thus the test is not definitive for lupus only; it is one of the diagnostic tests for causation.

t., lead, any of several tests used to detect clinical lead poisoning or exposure to lead (for example, coproporphyrinuria test, trace element analysis, urinary lead content test, and basophilic aggregation test).

t., Leede's. See **test, capillary resistance.**

t., liver function, tests to measure the severity of liver disease, aid in the differential diagnosis of the various types of disease of the hepatobiliary system, and follow the course of liver disease. Screening tests include urine bile, urine urobilinogen, Bromsulphalein (BSP) excretion, serum transaminases, thymol turbidity, cephalin-cholesterol flocculation, and van den Bergh's reaction (1 minute direct and total).

t., Mann-Whitney U, a powerful nonparametric statistic test of significance between two means with unequal sample sizes.

t., Mantoux (mäntoo'), an intracutaneous tuberculin test using either old tuberculin (OT) or purified protein derivative (PPD). A positive reaction read 24 and 48 hours after injection shows erythema and edema greater than 5 mm in diameter and indicates past or present tuberculosis.

t., Mazzini's (məzē'nēz), a flocculation test for syphilis.

t., Mohs. See **hardness, Mohs.**

t., nontreponemal antigen, serologic tests for syphilis using nontreponemal antigens. Such tests are not absolutely specific or sensitive for syphilis. Included are the Kline, Kahn, and Kolmer tests, and the VDRL slide test.

t., one-stage. See **time, prothrombin.**

t., pancreatic function, tests of enzyme levels in blood and urine (amylase, lipase), fecal fat content, trypsin activity, nitrogen content, alteration of digestive capacity, and alteration of pancreatic secretion via duodenal intubation.

t., patch (percutaneous test), a test for allergies that is performed by placing the suspected allergen in direct contact with the skin or mucosa. See also **test, skin.**

t., Paul-Bunnell, a test for infectious mononucleosis based on increased agglutination of sheep red blood cells resulting from heterophil antibodies in the serum. The test is considered positive if dilution of serum of 1:80 or higher agglutinates the sheep cells. Elevated agglutinin titers are more likely to be found during the second or third week of the disease, but the serum may not become positive until 7 weeks have elapsed.

t., percussion, a method of examination executed by striking the tissues of the area being examined with the fingers or an instrument, listening for resulting sounds, and observing the response of the patient.

t., percutaneous (pər'kyoota'nē·əs). See **test, patch.**

t., phenolsulfonphthalein (PSP) (fē'nolsul'fonthal'en), a renal test that roughly estimates glomerular function by measuring the rate of excretion of the dye after intravenous injection. Normally, after 15 minutes, 25% or more of the dye should be excreted in the urine.

t., plasma ketone, a test using nitroprusside for the detection of high levels of ketone bodies in the blood. The test is read 0 to 4 plus. A strongly positive reaction is seen in diabetic ketoacidosis.

t., pregnancy (Aschheim-Zondek test, Friedman's test), biologic or chemical tests that determine pregnancy. The tests are usually based on changes in the ovaries of an animal injected with the urine of a pregnant woman. Included are the Aschheim-Zondek test (using mice or rats) and the Friedman test (using virgin rabbits). Male frogs and female and male toads are also used. A saliva test has also been used.

t., prothrombin consumption (*serum prothrombin time*), a convenient screening test of the first stage of blood coagulation as determined by the quantity of prothrombin remaining after coagulation. The test reflects the formation of plasma thromboplastin, provided the one-stage prothrombin time of plasma is normal. See also **time, prothrombin.**

t., pulmonary function, tests used to evaluate respiratory function (for example, tests of vital capacity, tidal volume, maximal breathing capacity, timed vital capacity, arterial blood gases).

t., pulp, a diagnostic test to determine clinical pulp vitality and/or abnormality.

t., rapid reagin, serologic tests for syphilis that permit rapid and economic screening in the field. Included are the rapid plasma reagin (RPR) test and the unheated serum reagin (USR) test.

t., Reiter protein complement-fixation (RPCF) (rē'tər), treponemal antigen test for syphilis using extracts from the nonpathogenic Reiter treponeme.

t., renal function, quantitative tests including inulin or mannitol clearance for the glomerular filtration rate (GFR), paraaminohippurate (PAH) clearance for renal plasma flow, and the maximum rate of tubular excretion of paraaminohippurate and of reabsorption of glucose for the measurement of excretory and reabsorptive functions of the renal tubules. Clinical renal tests are used to assess the extent of renal impairment. They include blood urea nitrogen (BUN), nonprotein nitrogen (NPN), urea clearance, endogenous creatinine clearance, filtration fraction, phenolsulfonphthalein (PSP), and concentration tests.

t., Rockwell, an indentation test for hardness of a material. A static load is placed on a steel ball or diamond point, and the depth of the indentation is measured on the instrument. The depth of the indentation is remeasured after the load is increased. The hardness number is related to the type of point used and to the depth of the indentation.

t., Rothera's. See **test, ketone bodies.**

t., routine, a test or group of tests performed on most or all patients to detect relatively common disorders or to establish a base for further evaluation of a patient.

t., Rumpel-Leede-Hess. See **test, capillary resistance.**

t., scarlet fever. See **test, Dick's.**

t., Schick, a skin test to demonstrate the presence or absence of an immunity to diphtheria.

t., scratch (*skin test*), a test for allergies performed by placing a preparation containing the allergen on the skin and scratching the skin. A positive reaction is indicated by the formation of a wheal and flare.

t., screening, a group of tests especially chosen to detect specific abnormalities.

t., serologic (serəloj'ik), tests of blood serum for the diagnosis of infectious diseases.

t., skin, tests to determine the sensitivity or susceptibility to infections by a specific agent, the presence of an allergy, or the presence of a nutritional deficiency. Included are the Mantoux, Schick, Dick, Frei, histoplasmin, and Foshay tests for infectious diseases (tests in which allergens are placed onto or into the skin) and the intradermal ascorbic acid, dermal, intradermal (intracutaneous), patch (percutaneous), scratch, and subcutaneous tests.

t., tuberculin skin (tōōbər'kyōōlin), an intradermal injection of old tuberculin (OT) or purified protein derivative (PPD) to determine a specific sensitivity or susceptibility to tuberculosis.

t., Snyder's. See **test, colorimetric caries susceptibility.**

t., sterilizer, the periodic use of spore strip, color strip, or other microbial test to ensure that a sterilizer (autoclave, oven) is killing all microbes predictably.

t., subcutaneous. See **test, skin.**

t., Sulkowitch's, a simple but rough qualitative evaluation of calcium in the urine based on the degree of precipitation following addition of oxalate.

t., syphilis, refers to any serologic test for syphilis based on the presence of a reagin, appearing during the second or third week of infection. Included are the Hinton, Kahn, Kline, Mazzini, Wassermann, and *Treponema pallidum* immobilization tests.

t., thermal, the use of heat or cold as an aid in diagnosis (for example, the use of heat or cold in testing the pulp).

t., Thorn's. See **test, ACTH-stimulation.**

t., thromboplastin generation, a test of the integrity of the first stage of blood coagulation and the nature of the defect. A patient's serum, plasma, or platelets are substituted in a system that is complete except for one of the factors to be tested for (antihemophilic factor, plasma thromboplastin antecedent, plasma thromboplastin component, or platelets), and the rate of thromboplastin generation is determined.

t., thyroid function, tests for thyroid function (for example, radioactive iodine uptake, protein-bound iodine, basal metabolic rate, serum cholesterol, triiodothyronine suppression, thyroid-stimulating hormone tests).

t., tourniquet (tər′niket), a test for capillary fragility based on counting petechiae in a given area of the arm after application of the rubber cuff of a sphygmomanometer for 15 minutes.

t., transaminase (transam′inās), tests for serum glutamic oxaloacetic transaminase (SGOT) and serum glutamic pyruvic transaminase (SGPT). The normal value for serum glutamic oxaloacetic transaminase is 40 units or less; that for serum glutamic pyruvic transaminase is 35 units or less. The serum glutamic oxaloacetic transaminase value in myocardial infarction is 3 to 20 times the normal.

t., transillumination, a test for a pulpless tooth in which the use of transmitted light shows a shadow of the root when the pulp is necrotic or has been replaced by a filling (not always reliable).

t., treponemal antigen, tests for syphilis using *Treponema pallidum* or extracts from a treponeme as antigen. Included are *T. pallidum* immobilization (TPI), *T. pallidum* agglutination (TPA), fluorescent treponemal antibody (FTA), Reiter protein complement-fixation (RPCF), and *T. pallidum* complement-fixation (TPCF) tests.

t., Treponema pallidum immobilization (TPI), a test to confirm syphilis by demonstrating the immobilization of *Treponema pallidum* by specific antibodies in the serum of an infected individual; not widely used.

t., tuberculin, a test for past or present infection with tubercle bacilli. See also **test, Mantoux.**

t., tularemia. See **test, Foshay's.**

t., Tzanck's, a supplemental test for pemphigus based on the presence of degenerative changes in epithelial cells (Tzanck's cells) in the bullous lesions of pemphigus. Degenerative changes include swelling of the nuclei and hyperchromic staining.

t., U, Mann-Whitney. See **test, Mann-Whitney U.**

t., urea clearance, a clinical test of renal function determined by the clearance of urea from the plasma by the kidney each minute. Average normal value is 75 ml/min (75% to 125% of normal).

t., urine, routine, the routine examination of the urine, including amount, appearance, pH level, specific gravity, qualitative tests for sugar and protein, and microscopic examination of sediment.

t., van den Bergh's, a test of hepatic function by measuring serum conjugated ("direct-reacting") 1-minute bilirubin, total serum bilirubin, and, by difference, unconjugated (indirect) bilirubin. Obstructive jaundice and hemolytic jaundice give abnormal values.

t., VDRL (Venereal Disease Research Laboratory), a serologic nontreponemal antigen test for the detection of syphilitic reagin by means of a reaction between the reagin and a standard antigen.

t., Vickers hardness, a penetration type of hardness test using a square-based pyramid made of diamond.

t., viscosity of saliva, a dental caries susceptibility test on freshly secreted saliva. An Oswald pipette is used in the determination of viscosity.

t., vitality, the procedure using thermal, electrical, or mechanical stimuli to determine the response of the pulp in a tooth.

t., Wassermann, a complement-fixation test for syphilis.

t., Zondek's. See **test, pregnancy.**

testosterone/testosterone cypionate/testosterone enanthate/ testosterone propionate, *trade names:* Andro-100, Histerone-50, Testamone-100, Testaqua, Testoject-50; *drug class:* androgen, anabolic steroid (Controlled Substance Schedule III); *action:* in many tissues, testosterone is converted to dihydrotestosterone, which interacts with cytoplasmic protein receptors to increase protein production; natural hormone that functions to regulate spermatogenesis and male secondary sex characteristics; also functions as an anabolic steroid; *uses:* treatment of androgen deficiency, delayed puberty, female breast cancer, certain anemias.

tetanic contraction, a condition of continuous contraction in a voluntary muscle caused by a steady stream of efferent nerve impulses.

tetanus, an acute, potentially fatal infection of the central nervous system caused by tetanospasmin, which is an exotoxin, elaborated by an anaerobic bacillus, *Clostridium tetani.*

t. and diphtheria toxoids (Td), an active immunizing agent containing detoxified tetanus and diphtheria toxoids that slowly produce an antigenic response to the diseases. Typically administered as part of the immunization series of preschool children.

tetany, hyperventilation (tet'ənē hī'perven'tilā'shən), the neuromuscular irritability and tonic carpopedal muscle spasm resulting from the alkalosis that may be caused by forced respiration over an extended length of time.

tetracaine/tetracaine HCl (topical), *trade name:* Pontocaine Cream; *drug class:* topical anesthetic (ester group); *action:* inhibits nerve impulses from sensory nerves, which produces anesthesia; *uses:* local anesthesia of mucous membranes, pruritus, sunburn, sore throat, cold sores, oral pain, rectal pain and irritation, control of gagging.

tetracycline (te'trəsī'klēn), an antibiotic produced by certain strains of *Streptomyces.* Its administration during tooth formation may lead to enamel discoloration.

t. HCl, *trade names:* Achromycin, Achromycin V, Tetracyn; *drug class:* tetracycline, broad-spectrum antibiotic; *action:* inhibits protein synthesis and phosphorylation in microorganisms, bacteriostatic; *uses:* syphilis, gonorrhea, lymphogranuloma venereum, rickettsial infections, acne, actinomycosis, anthrax, bronchitis, GU infections, sinusitis and may other infections.

t. periodontal fiber, *trade name:* Actisite; *drug class:* tetracycline, broad-spectrum antiinfective; *action:* antimicrobial effect related to inhibition of protein synthesis; decreases incidence of postsurgical inflammation and edema; suppresses bacteria and acts as a barrier to bacterial entry; acts on cementum or fibroblasts to enhance periodontal ligament regeneration; *use:* adjunctive treatment in adult periodontitis.

Tg value, the transition point of glass. In dentistry, the temperature at which resin becomes soft.

thalamus (thal'əməs), an ovoid mass in the brain immediately lateral to the third ventricle, which serves as the principal relay and integration station for the sensory systems in the body.

thalassemia (thal'əsē'mē·ə) (hereditary leptocytosis, hereditary microcytosis), a hereditary, chronic, hemolytic anemia with erythroblastosis. A complex of hereditary disorders characterized by microcytosis and increased red blood cell destruction and frequently associated with abnormal hemoglobins and increased normal trace hemoglobins. These disorders are prevalent in people of Mediterranean, African, and Asian ancestry. Disorders include Cooley's anemia, Cooley's trait, hemoglobin H disease, Hb S— thalassemia, Hb C—thalassemia, and Hb E—thalassemia.

t. major *(Cooley's anemia, erythroblastic anemia, familial erythroblastic anemia, hereditary microcytosis, Mediterranean anemia, Mediterranean disease),* the severe homozygous form of thalassemia characterized by a marked microcytic hypochromic anemia, atypical nucleated red blood cells, marked increase in hemoglobin F, and skeletal changes (underdevelopment, mongoloid facies, anterior open bite).

t. minor *(Cooley's trait),* a heterozygous form of thalassemia that is a carried state with relatively mild manifestations. α_2 Hemoglobin is elevated.

thallium, a soft, bluish-white metallic element that exhibits some nonmetallic chemical properties. Its atomic number is 81 and its atomic weight is 204.37. Many of its compounds are highly toxic.

theophylline/theophylline sodium glycinate, *trade names:* Aerolate Sr, Asmalix, Respbid, Slo-Bid, Theolair, Theovent, Uniphyl; others; *drug class:* xanthine; *action:* relaxes smooth muscle of respiratory system by blocking phosphodiesterase, which increases cAMP; *uses:* bronchial asthma, bronchospasm of chronic obstructive pulmonary disease, chronic bronchitis.

theorem, I. a proposition to be proved by a chain of reasoning and analysis. **2.** a proven proposition used in the solution of a more advanced problem.

theory (thē′ərē), an opinion or hypothesis not based on actual knowledge.

t., Prothero "cone." See **retention.**

t., quantum, the theory that in emission or absorption of energy by atoms or molecules, the process is not continuous but takes place by steps, each step being the emission or absorption of an amount of energy called a *quantum.*

t., somatotype, the theory of W.H. Sheldon, suggesting that body structure is correlated with certain temperaments and predisposes to mental disorders.

therapeutic dose, the amount of a medication required to produce the desired effect.

therapeutic index (ther′əpyo͞o′tik). See **index, therapeutic.**

therapeutics, the art and science of treatment of disease.

therapeutic vehicle, a device used to transport and retain some agent for therapeutic purposes (for example, radium carrier).

therapist, a person with special skills, obtained through education, training, and experience, in one or more areas of health care.

therapy (ther′əpē), the treatment of disease.

t., antibiotic, the treatment of disease states by the local or systemic administration of antibodies.

t., indirect pulpal, the application of a drug that heals the pulpal cells beneath a layer of sound or carious dentin, as in a moderately deep preparation for a restoration.

t., myofunctional (myotherapeutic exercises), the use of muscle exercises as an adjunct to mechanical correction of malocclusion.

t., periodontal, the treatment of the periodontal lesion. Such therapy has two principal objectives: the eradication or arrest of the periodontal lesion with correction or cure of the deformity created by it, and the alteration in the mouth of the periodontal climate that was conducive or contributory to the periodontal breakdown.

  t., p., maintenance phase, the part of periodontal therapy that is necessary for the preservation of the results obtained during active therapy and for the prevention of further periodontal disease; an extension of active periodontal therapy, requiring the combined efforts of both the periodontist and the patient.

t., pulp canal. See **endodontology.**

t., radiation (radiotherapy), the treatment of disease with any type of radiation

t., replacement, the administration, as a therapeutic agent, of an essential

Possible side effects of radiation therapy

External	Internal implants
Abdomen: gastritis; nausea and vomiting	Bleeding
Fatigue	Infection
Gonads: amenorrhea; sexual dysfunction	Fever, redness, and drainage at insertion site
Pelvis: diarrhea; cystitis	Sexual dysfunction
Skin: erythema, dry to wet	
desquamation; areas of perineum, groin,	**Intracavitary**
and gluteal fold have increased risk for	Bleeding; infection; sexual dysfunction
breakdown due to moisture, warmth,	
and lack of air circulation	**Intraoperative**
	Anorexia; nausea and vomiting

From Otto SE: *Oncology nursing,* St Louis, 1991, Mosby.

constituent in which the body is deficient (for example, insulin in diabetes mellitus).

t., root canal. See **endodontology.**

t., speech, the science that deals with the use of procedures, training, and remedies for the cure, alleviation, or prevention of speech disorders.

thermal conductivity. See **conductivity, thermal.**

thermal expansion. See **expansion, thermal.**

thermal sensitivity. See **sensitivity, tooth.**

thermionic emission, the release of electrons when a material is heated (for example, electron emission when the tungsten cathode filament of an x-ray tube is heated to incandescence by means of its low-voltage heating circuit).

thermistor, an electronic device, functioning as a thermometer, for measuring minute changes in temperature. The resistance of a thermistor varies with the ambient temperature, thereby enabling accurate measurements of small temperature changes.

thermocoagulation, the use of high-frequency electric currents to destroy tissue through heat coagulation. Also known as **electrocautery.**

thermocouple, the joining of two dissimilar metals. The unequal thermal expansion of the two metals is used to indicate temperature changes.

thermography, a technique for sensing and recording on film hot and cold areas of the body by means of an infrared detector that reacts to blood flow.

thermoluminescence (ther'mōlōō' mines'əns), the capability of certain crystalline compounds such as lithium fluoride to release stored energy as luminescent energy when heated.

thermoluminescent dosimetry (ther'mōlōōmines'ənt dōsim'ətrē), the determination of the amount of radiation to which a thermoluminescent material has been exposed. This is accomplished by heating the material in a specially designed instrument that relates the amount of luminescence emitted from the material to the amount of radiation exposure.

thermoplastic (ther'mōplas'tik), the property of becoming soft with the application of heat, rigid at normal tem-

perature, and again soft with the reapplication of heat. A reversible physical phenomenon.

thermosetting, having the property of becoming rigid or hardened with the application of heat. Not reversible. In dentistry the term is used in connection with resins.

thermostat, an automatic temperature control device.

thiamine HCl (vitamin B$_1$) (thī'əmin), *trade names:* Betalin S, Bewon, many others; *drug class:* vitamin B$_1$ water soluble; *action:* needed for carbohydrate metabolism; *uses:* treatment of vitamin B$_1$ deficiency or in prophylaxis, beriberi, and Wernicke-Korsakoff syndrome.

Thiersch's skin graft (tērsh'əz). See **graft, Thiersch's skin.**

thiethylperazine maleate, *trade name:* Torecan; *drug class:* phenothiazine, antiemetic; *action:* acts centrally by blocking chemoreceptor trigger zone, which in turns acts on vomiting center; *uses:* treatment of nausea, vomiting.

thimble. See **coping.**

t., ionization chamber. See **chamber, ionization, thimble.**

thinking, I. the cognitive process of forming mental images or concepts. **2.** the process of cognitive problem solving through the sorting, organizing, and classification of facts and relationships.

Thiokol (thī'ōkol), trade name for polysulfide polymer using a mercaptan bond. The basic ingredient of rubber base impression materials. See also **mercaptan.**

thiopental sodium, a potent ultra–short-acting barbiturate used as a general anesthetic for surgical procedures that are expected to require 15 minutes or less, as an induction agent for other general anesthetics, as a hypnotic component in balanced anesthesia, and as an adjunct to regional anesthesia.

thioridazine HCl, *trade names:* Mellaril, SK Thioridazine; *drug class:* phenothiazine antipsychotic; *action:* blocks neurotransmission at dopaminergic synapses in cerebral cortex, hypothalamus, and limbic system; exhibits strong peripheral α-adrenergic, anticholinergic blocking action; *uses:* treatment of psychotic disorders, schizophrenia, behavioral problems in children, alcohol withdrawal as adjunct, anxiety, major depressive disorders, organic brain syndrome.

thiothixene, *trade name:* Navane; *drug class:* thioxanthene/antipsychotic; *action:* depresses the cerebral cortex, hypothalamus, and limbic system, which control activity and aggression; blocks neurotransmission produced by dopamine at the synapse; *uses:* treatment of psychotic disorders, schizophrenia, and acute agitation.

third party, the party to a dental benefits contract that may collect premiums, assume financial risk, pay claims, and provide other administrative services. Also called administrative agent carriers, insurers, or underwriters.

third-party administrator (TPA), claims payer who assumes responsibility for administering health benefit plans without assuming any financial risk. Some commercial insurance carriers and Blue Cross/Blue Shield plans also have TPA operations to accommodate self-funded employers seeking administrative services only (ASO) contracts.

third-party payer, an organization other than the patient (first party) or health care provider (second party) involved in the financing of personal health services.

third-party payment, payment for services by someone other than the beneficiary (for example, when an employer or union makes such payment).

thoracic surgery, the branch of surgery that deals with disease and injuries of the thoracic area, including the heart and major vessels and the lungs and respiratory tract.

thoracostomy, an incision made into the chest wall to provide an opening for the purpose of drainage.

thorium (Th), a heavy grayish, radioactive, metallic element. Its atomic number is 90, and its atomic weight is 232.04. Thorium is used in nuclear medicine and in radiation therapy.

threat, a menace; a statement of one's intention to harm or injure the person, property, or rights of another.

threonine (thrē'ōnēn), one of the essential amino acids needed for proper growth in infants and maintenance of

nitrogen balance in adults. See also **amino acid.**

threshold (thresh'old), the lowest limit of stimulus capable of producing an impression on the consciousness or evoking a response in irritable tissue.
t. dose. See **dose, threshold.**
t., swallowing, the minimal stimulation required to initiate the reflex action of deglutition.

thrill, I. a vibration felt on the chest wall over the heart. It is caused by the eddy flow of the blood, which is produced by a structural defect in the heart. **2.** palpable high-frequency vibration that may accompany cardiac murmurs or vascular disease.

thrombasthenia (throm'basthē'nēə), a hemorrhagic diathesis associated with qualitative abnormalities of the platelets.

thrombin (throm'bin), a proteolytic enzyme formed from prothrombin by the action of thromboplastin, factor IV calcium (Ca^{++}), and other factors. Thrombin forms fibrin from fibrinogen, speeds up the disruption of platelets, and activates factor V.

thrombocatalysin (throm'bōkat'əlisin) (not current). See **factor VIII.**

thrombocythemia (throm'bōsīthē'mēə), an increase in the number of circulating blood platelets.

thrombocytin (throm'bōsī'tin). See **serotonin.**

thrombocytopenia, an abnormal hemotologic condition in which the number of platelets is reduced. Thrombocytopenia is the most common cause of bleeding disorders. See also **purpura, thrombocytopenic.**

thrombocytosis (throm'bōsītō'sis), unusually large numbers of platelets in the circulating blood. It may occur after surgical procedures, parturition, and injury, or with thrombocythemia.

thromboembolism, a condition in which a blood vessel is blocked by an embolus carried in the bloodstream from the site of formation of the clot. The obstruction of the pulmonary artery or one of its main branches may be fatal. Emboli are diagnosed by x-ray films and other radiologic techniques.

thrombogen (throm'bōjen), prothrombin. See also **factor V.**

thrombogene. See **factor V.**

thrombokinase (throm'bōkin'ās) (not current). See **factor III.**

thrombokinin (throm'bōkin'in) (not current). See **factor III.**

thrombopenia, essential (throm'bō-pē'nēə) (not current). See **purpura, thrombocytopenia.**

thrombophlebitis (throm'bōfləbī'tis), an inflammation of the vein in which the vein becomes closed or occluded resulting from the development of a clot or thrombus.

thromboplastic plasma component (TPC). See **factor VIII.**

thromboplastin (throm'bōplas'tin), a substance necessary to the coagulant activity of tissue extracts; also has been referred to as the direct activator of prothrombin and as a substance from plasma, platelets, and tissues that initiates thromboplastic activity in blood coagulation. See also **thromboplastin, extrinsic.**

t., activated. See **thromboplastin, extrinsic.**

t., cofactor of. See **factor V.**

t., extrinsic (prothrombinase, extrinsic prothrombin activator, proconvertin-convertin, cothromboplastin, activated thromboplastin), a direct prothrombin activator formed by the interaction of brain extracts, factors V and VII, and factor IV calcium (Ca^{++}).

t., incomplete, tissue thromboplastin.

t., intrinsic (plasma thromboplastin, intrinsic prothrombin activator), a prothrombin activator formed from interaction of blood coagulation factors V, VIII, IX, and X and factor IV calcium (Ca^{++}) with a foreign surface.

t., tissue, a factor in tissue extract responsible for coagulation of blood.

thromboplastinogen (throm'bōplastin'ōjən). See **factor VIII.**

thromboplastinogenase (throm'bōplastin'ōjənās). See **factor, platelet, 3.**

thrombosis (thrombō'sis), presence of a clot or deposit in a blood vessel, formed in situ and remaining in place. An abnormal vascular condition in which a thrombus (blood clot) develops within a blood vessel of the body.

t., cavernous sinus, a blood clot in the cavernous sinus occasionally arising from maxillary periapical infection. The prognosis is poor but not so grave as before antibiotic therapy.

t., coronary, thrombosis of the coronary artery; also called heart attack and coronary occlusion.

thrombotonin (not current). See **serotonin.**

thrombozyme (throm'bōzīm') (not current). See **factor II.**

thrombus (throm'bəs), a blood clot in a vessel or in one of the chambers of the heart that remains at the point of its formation.

thrush (candidiasis, moniliasis), a disease caused by *Candida albicans* and characterized by white patches that scrape off with some difficulty, leaving bleeding bases. This term usually is used for the intraoral disease, whereas moniliasis is the term applied to the condition in other areas of infection by the yeast, as well as in the oral cavity. See also **candidiasis; moniliasis.**

thulium (Tm), a rare earth metallic element. Its atomic number is 69, and its atomic weight is 168.93. Thulium that has been irradiated in a nuclear reactor gives off gamma radiation.

thumb sucking. See **finger sucking.**

thymol, a synthetic or natural thyme oil, used as an antibacterial and antifungal. It is an ingredient in some over-the-counter preparations for the treatment of acne, hemorrhoids, and tinea pedis.

thymoma, a usually benign tumor of the thymus gland that may be associated with myasthenia gravis or an immune deficiency disorder.

thymus, a single unpaired gland located in the mediastinum that is the primary central gland of the lymphatic system. The T cells of the cell-mediated immune response develop in this gland before migrating to the lymph nodes and spleen.

thyroid crisis (thī'roid), a sudden exacerbation of symptoms of thyrotoxicosis characterized by fever, sweating, tachycardia, extreme nervous excitability, and pulmonary edema. If untreated, the crisis often is fatal. Also called thyroid storm.

thyroid function test, one of several tests to evaluate the function of the thyroid gland. These include protein-bound iodine, butanol-extractable iodine, radioactive iodine uptake, and radioactive iodine excretion.

thyroid gland, a highly vascular organ at the front of the neck, consisting of bilateral lobes connected in the middle by a narrow isthmus. The thyroid gland secretes the hormone thyroxine directly into the blood. It is essential to normal body growth in infancy and childhood. It also regulates the metabolic rate in adults.

thyroid, lingual, presence of thyroid tissue in the tongue, which is related to abnormal embryonic activity of the thyroglossal duct.

thyroid USP (desiccated), *trade names:* Armour Thyroid, Thyroid USP Enseals, Thryo-Teric, others; *drug class:* thyroid hormone; *action:* increases metabolic rate; increases cardiac output, oxygen consumption, body temperature, blood volume, and growth and development at cellular level; *uses:* treatment of hypothyroidism, cretinism, and myxedema.

thyroiditis, inflammation of the thyroid gland.

thyroxine (thīrok'sin), the hormone secretion of the thyroid gland, L-3,5,3′,5′-tetraiodothyronine.

tic, an involuntary, purposeless movement of muscle, usually occurring under emotional stress. It is a survival in stereotyped form of a movement or muscle set once used voluntarily and purposefully.

t. **douloureux,** spontaneous trigeminal neuralgia associated with a "trigger zone" and causing spasmodic contraction of the facial muscles. See also **neuralgia, trigeminal.**

ticarcillin (tik'ärsil'in), an anti-*Pseudomonas* penicillin.

ticlopidine, *trade name:* Ticlid; *drug class:* platelet aggregation inhibitor; *action:* inhibits first and second phases of adenosine diphosphate (ADP)–induced effects in platelet aggregation; *use:* effective in reducing the risk of stroke in high-risk patients.

t.i.d., abbreviation for *ter in die,* a Latin phrase meaning "three times a day."

tidal volume, the amount of air inhaled and exhaled during normal ventilation.

time, a measure of duration.

t., **clot retraction,** the time required for a given quantity of blood to separate in the tube in which it has been placed. For 3 ml of blood at room temperature, 1 hour is normal. It is very slow in thrombocytopenia.

t., **coagulation,** the time required for blood clotting to begin in a capillary tube, normally 2 to 8 minutes. A coagulation time three times normal is a definite danger sign.

t., **gel** *(gelation time),* the interval of time required for a colloidal solution to become a solid or semisolid jelly or gel. Usually refers to the working time of a hydrocolloid or alginate impression material.

t., **gelation.** See **time, gel.**

t. **limits,** the periods of time within which a notice of claim must be filed.

t., **median lethal** *(LD50 time, MLT),* the time required for 50% of a large group of animals or organisms to die after administration of a specified dose of radiation.

t., **prothrombin** *(one-stage test),* a gross but useful screening test of the completeness of the second and third stages of blood coagulation. Normal prothrombin time by the Quick method is 12 to 15 seconds. The time is affected by deficiencies of factor V or VII as well as of prothrombin. See also **test, prothrombin consumption.**

t., **serum prothrombin.** See **test, prothrombin consumption.**

t., **setting,** the length of time for a mixed preparation of materials to reach a state of hardness, measured from the start of the mixing. The end point for dental materials is usually determined by a penetration test.

timer, radiographic timing device that functions as an automatic exposure timer and a switch to control the current to the high-tension transformer and filament transformer. The face of the timer is calibrated in seconds and fractions of seconds. The timer controls the total time that the current passes through the x-ray tube and thus the time during which the x rays are emitted. The timer activates a switch or contractor that closes and opens the low-voltage circuit of the high voltage.

t., **electronic,** an electronic vacuum tube device, with no moving parts, that covers a time range of ½0 to 10 seconds. It automatically sets itself, is more accurate than mechanical timers, and meets all the needs of modern high-speed dental techniques.

t., foot, a timer with an attachment that permits the timing device to be activated by foot pressure. This is the preferred type of timer.

t., hand, an attachment to or part of a timer that requires thumb or finger pressure to activate the timing device.

t., mechanical, a timer using a spring mechanism for determination of length of exposure. Accuracy of timing is not assumed in exposures of less than 1 second with a mechanical timer.

time-sharing, performing two or more tasks with a computer at the same time, made possible because computer speed is so much faster than operator speed that the computer can switch from one to another in brief time segments so that the operators are not aware of the computer switching or any time delay.

timolol maleate, *trade name:* Blocadren; *drug class:* nonselective β-adrenergic blocker; *action:* competitively blocks stimulation of β-adrenergic receptors in the heart and decreases renin activity, all of which may play a role in reducing systolic and diastolic blood pressure; inhibits β₂ receptors in the bronchial system; *uses:* treatment of mild-to-moderate hypertension, reduction of mortality after myocardial infarction (MI), and migraine prophylaxis.

timolol maleate (optic), *trade names:* Betimol, Timoptic Solution, Timoptic-XE; *drug class:* β-adrenergic blocker; *action:* reduces production of aqueous humor by unknown mechanism; *uses:* treatment of ocular hypertension, chronic open-angle glaucoma, secondary glaucoma, and aphakic glaucoma.

tin (Sn), a whitish metallic element. Its atomic number is 50, and its atomic weight is 118.69. Tin oxide is used in dentistry as a polishing agent for teeth. Tin also is used in some restorative materials such as an alloy of amalgam.

tincture (tink′chər), an alcoholic, hydroalcoholic, or ethereal solution of a drug.

tinea, a group of fungal skin diseases caused by dermatophytes of several kinds, characterized by itching, scaling, and sometimes painful lesions. *Tinea* is a general term that refers to

infections of various causes, which are seen in several sites.

t. capitis, a superficial fungal infection of the scalp seen most common in children.

t. corporis, a superficial fungal infection of the nonhairy skin of the body, most prevalent in hot, humid climates.

t. cruris, a superficial fungal infection of the groin.

t. pedis, a chronic superficial fungal infection of the foot, especially of the skin between the toes.

t. unguium, a superficial fungal infection of the nails.

t. versicolor, a fungal infection of the skin caused by *Malassezia furfur* and characterized by finely desquamating pale tan patches on the upper trunk and upper arms.

Tinel's sign (tinelz′). See **sign, Tinel's.**

tinfoil. See **foil, tin.**

t. substitute. See **substitute, tinfoil.**

tinnitus (tinī′təs), noises or unpleasant sounds in the ears such as ringing, buzzing, roaring, or clicking; is usually high pitched. Heard by many persons with auditory impairment. Clicking tinnitus may be heard by others.

tin octoate (ok′tōāt), substance used to accomplish vulcanization of silicone rubber impression materials. It is not a true catalyst because it becomes part of the final polymer.

tinted denture base. See **base, denture, tinted.**

tipping of cusps. See **restoration of cusps.**

tissue (tish′oo), an aggregation of similarly specialized cells united in the performance of a particular function.

t., connective, the binding and supportive tissue of the body; derived from the mesoderm; depending on its location and function, it is composed of fibroblasts, primitive mesenchymal cells, collagen fibers, and elastic fibers, with associated blood and lymphatic vessels and nerve fibers.

t., critical, tissue that reacts most unfavorably to radiation or by its nature attracts and absorbs specific radiochemicals.

t., flabby. See **tissue, hyperplastic.**

t., hyperplastic, in dentistry, excessively movable tissue about the mandible or maxillae resulting from increases in the number of normal cells.

t., interdental, the gingivae, cementum of the teeth, free gingival and transseptal fibers of the periodontal membrane (ligament), and alveolar and supporting bone.

t., peripheral. See **border structures.**

t., redundant. See **epulis fissuratum.**

t., subjacent, the structures that underlie or are in border contact with a denture base; they may or may not have a supporting relationship to the overlying base.

tissue adhesives, agents or materials that may be used to seal two cut tissue surfaces together or cover a surgically exposed surface such as butyl cyanoacrylate, which is used to cover palatal donor sites in periodontal surgery.

tissue-borne partial denture. See **denture, partial, tissue-borne.**

tissue, compression of. See **tissue displaceability.**

tissue displaceability, the quality of oral tissues that permits them to be placed in or assume other positions than their relaxed position.

tissue displacement, change in the form or position of tissues as a result of pressure.

tissue molding. See **border molding.**

titanium (tĭtā′nēəm), a grayish, brittle metallic element. Its atomic number is 22, and its atomic weight is 47.9. An alloy of titanium is used in the manufacture of orthopedic prostheses and is used extensively in implant dentistry and orthodontic arch wires.

titer (tī′tər), the standard amount by volume of a material required to produce a desired reaction with another material.

title, evidence of the right of a person to the possession of property.

titration (tītrāshən), incremental increase in drug dosage to a level that provides the optimal therapeutic effect.

TMJ facebow. See **facebow, kinematic.**

TMJ pain–dysfunction syndrome. See **temporomandibular pain–dysfunction syndrome.**

TMP-SMX, acronym for trimethoprim-sulfamethoxazole.

TNF, an abbreviation for tumor necrosis factor, a genetic-triggered, tumor-killing agent produced by the body in small amounts to counteract neoplastic growth. An experimental agent used in the treatment of cancers.

tobacco withdrawal syndrome, a change in mood or performance associated with the cessation of or reduction in exposure to nicotine. Symptoms may range from lack of concentration to anxiety and temper outbursts.

tobramycin (ophthalmic), *trade name:* Tobrax; *drug class:* antiinfective; *action:* inhibits bacterial protein synthesis; *use:* treatment of infection of the eye.

tocainide HCl, *trade name:* Tonocard; *drug class:* antidysrhythmic (Class IB), lidocaine analog; *action:* decreases sodium and potassium conductance, which decreases myocardial excitability; *use:* treatment of documented life-threatening ventricular dysrhythmias.

toilet of cavity. See **cavity, toilet.**

tolazamide, *trade name:* Tolinase; *drug class:* sulfonylurea (1st generation) oral antidiabetic; *action:* causes functioning β-cells in pancreas to release insulin, leading to drop in blood glucose levels; *use:* treatment of type II diabetes mellitus.

tolbutamide, *trade name:* Orinase; *drug class:* sulfonylurea (1st generation) oral antidiabetic; *action:* causes functioning β-cells in pancreas to release insulin, leading to drop in blood glucose levels; *use:* treatment of type II diabetes mellitus.

tolerance (tol′ərəns), the ability to endure the influence of a drug or poison, particularly acquired by continued use of the substance. See also **resistance.**

t., acquired, tolerance that develops with successive doses of a drug. If it develops within a short span of time, such as 24 hours, it is called tachyphylaxis. Slowly acquired tolerance is sometimes called mithridatism.

t., carbohydrate, the ability of the body to use carbohydrates. A decrease in tolerance is seen in diabetes mellitus, liver damage, and some infections and in the presence of hyperactivity of the adrenal cortex or pituitary gland.

t., cross, tolerance to a number of drugs of similar mode of action or chemical structure.

T

t., individual, tolerance characteristic of an individual.

t., pseudo-, a state of apparent tolerance because the drug does not reach its usual receptor sites.

t., species, tolerance characteristic of a species of animal.

t., tissue, the ability of structures to endure environmental change without ill effect.

tolmetin sodium, *trade name:* Tolectin; *drug class:* nonsteroidal antiinflammatory; *action:* inhibits prostaglandin synthesis by interfering with cyclooxygenase needed for biosynthesis; *uses:* treatment of osteoarthritis, rheumatoid arthritis, juvenile rheumatoid arthritis.

tolnaftate (topical), *trade name:* Aftate, Tinactin, Ting, others; *drug class:* antifungal, topical; *action:* interferes with fungal cell membrane, which increases permeability and leaking of cell nutrients; *uses:* treatment of tinea pedis, tinea cruris, tinea corporis, tinea capitis, tinea unguium, and tinea versicolor.

tomogram. See **examination, radiographic, extraoral body section.**

tomograph, a radiograph produced while rotating the film and x-ray source in opposite directions around an axis located in the region of interest. This movement blurs outside structures while maintaining sharpness in the region of interest.

tomography, an x-ray technique that produces a film representing a detailed cross section of tissue structures at a predetermined depth.

tongue (tung), the muscular organ that is the main articulatory element in the production of speech and accounts for the clarity and fluidity of speech. Two groups of tongue muscles, the intrinsic and extrinsic, are united into one organ. Each group, however, has separate structural and functional characteristics.

t., amyloid (amyloid macroglossia), enlargement of the tongue resulting from amyloidosis.

t., antibiotic, a glossitis caused by sensitivity to an antibiotic, vitamin B complex deficiency associated with antibiotic therapy.

t., bald. See **glossitis, atrophic.**

t., beefy, erythematous or atrophic glossitis. See also **glossitis, atrophic; glossitis, Moeller's.**

t., bifid (cleft tongue), a tongue divided by a midline cleft.

t., black hairy (lingua nigra), a black appearance of the dorsal surface of the tongue; caused by elongated filiform papillae and an accumulation of dark pigments, microorganisms, and food debris.

t., cleft. See **tongue, bifid.**

t., coated, nonspecific term used to describe the condition of the tongue resulting from whitish or otherwise discolored accumulations of food debris, bacterial plaques, and hyperplastic filiform papillae. Reduced function, as in general illness or laryngitis, is a primary cause.

t., cobblestone, hyperplasia and hyperemia of fungiform and filiform papillae of the tongue in riboflavin deficiency. Formerly used to describe syphilitic glossitis with leukoplakia.

t., fissured (furrowed tongue), a tongue traversed by clefts that may be arranged like the veins of a leaf or may be such as to give the tongue a "pavement block" appearance. It is seen in 5% of all dental patients but in 13% of those older than 50 years.

t., flat, paralysis of the transverse lingual muscles such that the borders of the tongue cannot be rolled. The condition results from congenital syphilis.

t., furrowed. See **tongue, fissured.**

t., geographic (benign migratory glossitis, glossitis areata exfoliativa, glossitis migrans, wandering rash), a condition characterized by a chronic, circumscribed, more or less circinate desquamation of the superficial epithelium of the dorsum of the tongue. The spots of desquamation migrate continuously, usually passing from the region near the vallate papillae toward the tip of the tongue.

t., hairy, hyperplasia of the filiform papillae of the tongue, frequently associated with oral moniliasis and the use of antibiotics or tobacco.

t., lobulated, a congenital defect with a secondary lobe of the tongue arising from its surface.

t., magenta, the reddish-purple tongue of riboflavin deficiency.

t., Sandwith's bald, a condition in which the tongue is very smooth because of a loss of fusiform papillae and is fiery red and enlarged because of severe inflammation; seen in pellagra.

t., smooth. See **glossitis, atrophic.**

t., strawberry, the red, inflamed tongue with prominent fungiform papillae characteristic of scarlet fever.

t., white hairy (lingua alba, lingua villosa alba), hairy tongue characterized by elongation of the filiform papillae but without the dark staining seen in lingua nigra (black hairy tongue). See also **tongue, black hairy.**

tongue crib, an appliance used to limit undesirable tongue movements, usually constructed to prevent its protrusion between the anterior teeth.

tongue room. See **tongue space.**

tongue space, the space available for functioning of the tongue.

tongue thrust, thrusting of the tongue between the anterior teeth, especially in the initial stage of swallowing. This action, often combined with a resting position also between the teeth, may inhibit normal eruption and produce an open bite.

tonic convulsion, a prolonged generalized contraction of the skeletal muscles.

tonofibril (ton'əfi'bril), a fibril emanating from epithelial cells. Recent electron microscopy has shown such fibrils to be irregular formations of the cell membrane.

tonsil (ton'sil), a rounded mass of tissue, usually of a lymphoid nature (especially the palatine tonsil).

tonsillectomy, the surgical excision of the palatine tonsils, performed to prevent recurrent tonsillitis.

tonsillitis (ton'sili'tis), inflammation of the tonsils.

t., lingual, a form of tonsillitis at the posterior part of the base of the tongue in the lymphoid masses (lingual tonsils) located there.

tonus, facial muscle (tō'nəs), the tone of the facial musculature, which is a major factor in providing the esthetic values of the human face. The configurations of the face, which are maintained by good muscle tonus, are the modiolus, philtrum, nasolabial sulcus, and mentolabial sulcus. These functional contours are present when the nerve tissue is intact. They are altered by the loss of teeth or impaired nerve function. Their presence is an indication of a good state of health of the nerve and possibly of the dental arch.

tonus, muscle, the steady reflex contraction that resides in the muscles concerned in maintaining erect posture. Tonus has its basis in the positional interactions of the muscle and its accompanying nerve structure; for example, a muscle holds the body (mandible) in a given position, and the awareness of this position is constantly being relayed by the sensory approaches to the cortex. Any change in position or contractility of the muscle that affects its tonus is immediately relayed by the sensory apparatus for readjustment. Also called tone.

tooth, teeth, one of the hard bodies or processes usually protruding from and attached to the alveolar process of the maxillae and the mandible; designed for the mastication of food.

t., abutment, a tooth or teeth selected to support a prosthesis on the basis of the total surface areas of a healthy attachment apparatus.

t., accessory (akses'ərē), supernumerary teeth that do not resemble normal teeth in size, shape, or location. See also **distomolar; mesiodens; paramolar; tooth, supernumerary.**

t., acrylic resin (əkril'ik), a tooth made of acrylic resin.

t., anatomic, an artificial tooth that closely resembles the anatomic form of a natural unabraded tooth.

t., ankylosed, abnormal calcification of the periodontal ligament resulting in abnormal fixation of a tooth.

t., anterior, one of the incisor or canine teeth.

t., artificial, a tooth fabricated for use as a substitute for a natural tooth in a

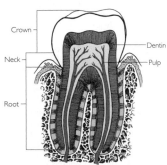

Tooth—major parts. (Potter, 1996.)

Crown — Dentin

Neck — Pulp

Root

T

prosthesis; usually made of porcelain or plastic.

t., canine, the four canines; the third tooth located distal to the midline in any one of the four quadrants of the dentition.

t., conical (peg-shaped tooth), failure of morphologic development of the tooth germ found in ectodermal dysplasia and other disorders and occasionally found in normal children.

t., cross-bite, posterior teeth designed to permit the modified buccal cusps of the upper teeth to be positioned in the central fossae of the lower teeth.

t., cuspless, teeth designed without cuspal prominences on the masticatory surfaces.

t., deciduous. See **deciduous; tooth, primary.**

t., devital. See **tooth, pulpless.**

t., drifting, the migration of teeth from their normal positions in the dental arches as a result of such factors as loss of proximal support, loss of functional antagonists, occlusal traumatic tooth relationships, inflammatory and retrograde changes in the attachment apparatus, and oral habits.

t., drugs for sensitivity of, the medicaments used to treat hypersensitivity of the teeth; they should cause relatively little pain when applied; be easily applied, rapid in action, and permanently effective; and not discolor the teeth or unduly irritate the pulp. Substances used include 33% sodium fluoride in kaolin and glycerin, a 25% aqueous solution of strontium chloride, hot medicinal olive oil, and 0.9% solution of sodium silicofluoride.

t., embedded, an unerupted tooth, usually one completely covered with bone; also spelled imbedded. See also **tooth, impacted.**

t., evulsed (avulsed tooth), a tooth that has been abnormally luxated from its alveolar support, commonly as a sequela to trauma.

t., fulcrum, the axis of movement of a tooth when lateral forces are applied to the tooth. The fulcrum is considered to be at the middle third of the portion of the root embedded in the alveolus and thus moves apically as the bone resorbs in periodontal disease.

t., fused, two teeth united during development by the union of their tooth germs. The teeth may be joined by the enamel of their crowns, root dentin, or both. Usually consists of a single large crown.

t., geminated (jem'ĭnātəd), teeth with bifid crowns and confluent root canals resulting from the division of the enamel organ during the developmental period.

t., grinding of, the selective modification of tooth form and contour in the occlusal adjustment operation to eliminate occlusal interferences and establish tooth contours conducive to the health of the periodontium. See also **bruxism.**

t., hereditary brown. See **hypoplasia, enamel, hereditary.**

t., Hutchinson's, after Sir Jonathan Hutchinson, who reported the typical defects of the permanent incisors associated with congenital syphilis. Dental hypoplasia affects primarily the incisors, canines, and first permanent molars. The incisors have a screwdriver or peg-shaped appearance. See also **triad, Hutchinson.**

t., hypoplasia of (hī'pōplāzhə), a reduction in the amount of enamel formed, resulting in irregular pits and grooves of the enamel.

t., immediate separation of, separation of teeth accomplished rapidly by the wedging action of an appliance during restorative procedures.

t., impacted, a condition in which the unerupted or partially erupted tooth is positioned against another tooth, bone, or soft tissue so that complete eruption is unlikely. An impacted third molar tooth may be further described according to its position: buccoangular, distoangular, or vertical. An impacted maxillary canine tooth also may be further described according to its position: palatal (maxillary canine), lingual (mandibular canine), labial, or vertical.

t., inclination of, the angle of slope of teeth from the vertical planes of reference. A tooth may be mesially, distally, lingually, buccally, or labially inclined.

t., loss of, the separation of a tooth from its investing and supporting structures as a result of normal exfoliation attending loss of deciduous dentition, exfoliation as a sequela to excessive bone resorption and periapical migration of the epithelial attachment in periodontal disease, and instrumentation for extraction necessitated by pathologic involvement of the dental pulp, periodontium, or periapical tissues.

t., mesial movement of, migration of teeth toward the midline, occurring as a phenomenon associated with the action of the anterior component of force. Mesial migration of teeth occurs with the wear of their proximal surfaces resulting from the buccolingual movements of the teeth.

t., metal insert, an artificial tooth, usually of acrylic resin, containing an inserted ribbon of metal, or a cutting blade, in its occlusal surface, with one edge of the blade exposed; sometimes used in removable dentures.

t., migration of, the movement of teeth into altered positions in relationship to the basal bone of the alveolar process and adjoining and opposing teeth as a result of loss of approximating or opposing teeth, occlusal interferences, habits, and inflammatory and dystrophic disease of the attaching and supporting structures of the teeth.

t., missing, the absence of teeth from the dentition because of congenital factors, exfoliation, or extraction.

t., natal, primary teeth found in the oral cavity at birth.

t., neonatal, a primary tooth that erupts into the oral cavity during the neonatal period (from birth to 30 days).

t., nonanatomic, artificial teeth so designed that the occlusal surfaces are not copies from natural forms, but rather are given forms which, in the opinion of the designer, seem more nearly to fulfill the requirements of mastication and tissue tolerance.

t., peg-shaped. See **tooth, conical.**

t., permanent. See **dentition, permanent.**

t., pink. See **resorption, internal.**

t., plastic, artificial teeth constructed of synthetic resins.

t., polishing of, the removal of film, plaque, and soft deposits from the teeth by appropriate hand- or engine-driven instrumentation. Abrasive cups, wheels, and disks often are used in conjunction with abrasive pastes such as pumice and water.

t., posterior, the maxillary and mandibular premolars and molars of the permanent dentition or the premolars and molars of prostheses.

t., primary, 1. term used by some in preference to deciduous teeth; however, it has not received the approval of preference by the American Dental Association. See also **deciduous. 2.** as a result of a survey of the terminology used to name the teeth of the first dentition, the College Committee Report of Dentistry for Children recommended in 1942 the use of *primary teeth* as the term preferred to deciduous, first, milk, temporary, baby, or foundation teeth. The term primary was suggested as a word "which may be acceptable to the dental profession, significant in its meaning, with no connotations of impermanence, and readily understood by nonprofessional people."

t., pulpless, a tooth from which the dental pulp has been removed or is necrotic.

t., replaced. See **tooth, supplied.**

t., rotated, an altered position of the tooth in relation to the adjacent and opposing teeth and its basal alveolar process; in such an altered position the tooth has been turned on its long axis and is in a state of torsiversion. The result is an altered contact with adjacent teeth that produces a possible locus for food impaction between the teeth, with consequent gingival damage.

t., sensitivity of, a painful pulpal response to external stimuli such as heat, cold, and sweet substances. The most common clinical finding is a hyperesthetic state of the root surface resulting from loss of a portion of the cemental covering with exposure of the dentin.

t., separation of, the action of moving a tooth mesially or distally out of contact with its neighboring tooth.

t., set of, term that usually refers to a full complement of maxillary and mandibular artificial teeth as they are carded by the manufacturer.

t., setting up of, the arranging of teeth on a trial denture base; includes proper relation with occluding teeth.

t., shell, a form of dentinal dysplasia characterized by large pulp chambers, meager coronal dentin, and usually no roots.

t., slow separation of, separation of teeth accomplished over a long period, usually by the wedging action of a material such as guttapercha, orthodontic wire, thread, or fibers in orthodontic therapy.

t., supernumerary, extra erupted or unerupted teeth that resemble teeth of normal shape.

t., supplied (replaced teeth), artificial replacements for natural teeth.

t., supportive mechanisms of, the anatomic structures that function to maintain or aid in maintaining the teeth in position in their alveoli: the gingivae, cementum of the tooth, periodontal membrane, and alveolar and supporting bone. See also **structures, supporting.**

t., tube, artificial teeth constructed with a vertical, cylindric aperture extending from the center of the base into the body of the tooth into which a pin or cast post for the attachment of the tooth to a denture base may be placed.

t., Turner's, a permanent tooth showing hypoplasia resulting from injury or inflammation of the precedent deciduous tooth.

t., vital staining of, the staining of enamel and dentin of primary and permanent teeth during development with vital stains (for example, with bile pigment in Rh incompatibility or with tetracyclines).

t., zero degree, prosthetic teeth having no cusp angles in relation to the horizontal plane; cuspless teeth.

toothache, pain located in the tooth or its surrounding supporting tissues. Dental pain may have a halo effect, making location of the precise source or location of the pain difficult. Determining the location may require several diagnostic tests.

tooth-borne, term used to describe a prosthesis or a part of a prosthesis that depends entirely on the abutment teeth for support.

tooth-borne base, the denture base restoring an edentulous area that has abutment teeth at each end for support. The tissue it covers is not used for support of the base.

toothbrushing, the use of a brush of varying design to brush the teeth and gingivae for cleanliness and to massage for oral hygiene.

t., faulty, the improper performance of toothbrushing, resulting in defective cleansing, inadequate stimulation of the gingival tissues, and destructive effects on the teeth and marginal gingivae resulting from overzealous brushing.

tooth eruption, the process by which the tooth moves from its site of formation to its position of function.

tooth form. See **form, tooth.**

tooth mobility, the movability of a tooth resulting from loss of all or a portion of its attachment and supportive apparatus. Seen in periodontitis, occlusal traumatism, and periodontosis.

tooth morphology, the anatomic topography of the teeth.

tooth movement. See **movement, tooth.**

toothpaste. See **dentifrice.**

toothpick, a wood sliver used to cleanse the interdental space.

t., balsa wood, a triangular wedge of balsa wood used to clean the teeth interproximally and stimulate the interdental gingival tissues.

tooth position. See **position, tooth.**

tooth selection. See **selection, tooth.**

tooth size discrepancy, lack of proportional harmony in the width of various teeth, causing relative spacing and crowding in different parts of the dentition.

topical, 1. of or pertaining to the surface of a part of the body. **2.** of or pertaining to a drug or treatment applied to the surface of a part of the body.

topical anesthesia, surface analgesia produced by application of an anesthetic in the form of a solution, gel, or ointment to the surface of the skin, mucous membrane, or cornea.

topographic anatomy, the study of a specific region of a body structure such as a lower leg, including all the systems in the part and their relationships to one another. Also referred to as regional anatomy.

topographic intraoral radiographic examination. See **examination, true occlusal topographic intraoral radiographic.**

torque (tork), **1.** a force that produces or tends to produce rotation in a body. Such force applied to a tooth tends to cause rotation around its long axis. **2.** force applied to a tooth to produce rotation of a tooth on a mesiodistal or buccolingual (labiolingual) axis. **3.** a rotary force applied to a denture base.

torque wire, an auxiliary wire used to torque the roots of the anterior teeth.

torsemide, *trade name:* Demadox; *drug class: action:* acts on loop of Henle to decrease the reabsorption of chloride and sodium with resultant diuresis; *uses:* treatment of hypertension and edema associated with congestive heart failure (CHF), liver disease, and chronic renal failure.

torsion, in dentistry the twisting of a tooth on its long axis. Also, the loading of a wire by twisting it along its long axis.

t., clasp, the twisting of the retentive clasp arm on its long axis. A retentive clasp may be formed so that it traverses a vertical distance before encircling the abutment to increase the torsion component of the clasp opening as compared with the flexure it experiences.

torsiversion, an axially rotated tooth position.

tort, a legal wrong perpetrated on a person or property independent of contract.

torticollis, an abnormal condition in which the head is inclined to one side as a result of the contraction of the muscles on that side of the neck.

torus, a bulging projection of bone.

t. mandibularis, a bony enlargement (hyperostosis) appearing unilaterally or bilaterally on the lingual aspect of the mandible in the canine-premolar region of about 7% of the population.

t. palatinus, a bony enlargement (hyperostosis) occurring in the midline of the hard palate in about 20% of the population.

total filtration. See **filtration, total.**

total parenteral nutrition (TPN), the administration of a nutritionally adequate hypertonic solution consisting of glucose, protein hydrolysates, minerals, and vitamins through an indwelling catheter into the superior vena cava.

touch, the sense by which contact with an object provides evidence of its properties.

t., light, tactile sense. The principal organs of light touch are Meissner's corpuscles, which are large and oval. Each capsule receives several nerve fibers that shed their myelin sheaths and coil into a spiral complex network. Associated with Meissner's corpuscles in the perception of light touch are both Merkel's disks and a basketlike arrangement of nerve fibers around the hair follicles.

touch screen, a type of screen on some video terminals that may be touched with the finger to specify the selection of an item from a displayed list.

tourniquet, a device used in controlling hemorrhage, consisting of a wide constricting band applied to the limb proximal to the site of bleeding.

toxic (tok′sik), poisonous; produced by a poison.

toxic delirium, a symptom of disordered mental status as a result of poisoning.

toxicity (toksis′itē), the ability of a drug or poison to produce harm, especially to cause permanent injury or death. Usually distinguished from allergenic properties.

t., acute, a condition produced after short-term use of a toxic agent. See also **dose, lethal, median; dose, lethal, minimum.**

t., chronic, a condition produced after long-term use of a toxic agent.

toxicologist (tok′sikol′əjist), one versed in toxicology.

toxicology (tok′sikol′əjē), the scientific study of the nature and effects of poisons, their detection, and the treatment of their effects.

toxic shock syndrome (TSS), a severe acute disease caused by infection with strains of *Staphylococcus aureus,* phage group I, that produce a unique toxin, enterotoxin F. It is most common in menstruating women using high-absorbency tampons but has occurred in infants, children, and men.

toxoids, toxins that have been treated to destroy their toxic properties but retain their ability to induce antibody production, thus creating an active immunity.

toxoplasmosis (tok′sōplazmō′sis), a disease caused by protozoa in the bloodstream and body tissues.

thromboplastic plasma component (TPC). See **factor VIII.**

TPI. See **test,** *Treponema pallidum* **immobilization.**

trace element, an element essential to nutrition or physiologic processes, found in such minute quantities that analysis yields a presence of virtually zero amounts.

tracer, 1. a mechanical device used to trace a pattern of mandibular movements. **2.** a foreign substance mixed with or attached to a given substance to enable the distribution or location of the latter to be determined subsequently. A radioactive tracer is a physical or chemical tracer having radioactivity as its distinctive property.

t., Gothic arch. See **tracer, needle point.**

t., needle point, a mechanical device consisting of a weighted or a spring-loaded needle that is attached to one jaw and a coated plate attached to the other jaw. Movement of the mandible causes a tracing to be formed on the horizontally placed plate. When the needle point is in the apex of the tracing, the mandible is said to be in the horizontal position of centric relation.

trachea (trā'kēə), the windpipe; a cartilaginous and membranous tube extending from the lower end of the larynx to its division into two bronchi.

tracheo- (trā'kēō), combining form denoting connection with or relation to the trachea.

tracheobronchial (trā'kēōbrong'kēəl), pertaining to the trachea and a bronchus or bronchi.

tracheobronchoscopy (trā'kēō-brongkos'kəpe), inspection of the interior of the trachea and bronchus.

tracheolaryngeal (trā'kēōlərin'jēəl), pertaining to the trachea and larynx.

tracheolaryngotomy (trā'kēōlərin-got'ōmē), incision into the larynx and trachea; tracheotomy and laryngotomy.

tracheoscopy (trā'kēos'kəpē), inspection of the interior of the trachea by means of a laryngoscopic mirror and reflected light or inspection through a bronchoscope.

tracheostenosis (trā'kēōstənō'sis), abnormal constriction or narrowing of the trachea.

tracheostomy (trā'kēos'tōmē), **1.** the formation of an opening into the trachea and the suturing of the edges of the opening to an opening in the skin of the neck. **2.** surgical formation of an opening into the trachea, usually through the tracheal rings below the cricoid cartilage, to give the patient an airway.

tracheotome (trā'kēōtōm), **1.** a cutting instrument used in tracheotomy; a tracheotomy knife. **2.** an instrument for use in creating an airway through the skin into the trachea below the cricoid cartilage.

tracheotomy (trā'kēot'əmē), the operation of cutting into the trachea to give the patient an airway.

tracing, a line or lines or a pattern scribed by a pointed instrument or stylus on a tracing plate or tracing paper.

t., arrow point. See **tracing, needle point.**

t., cephalometric, a line drawing of pertinent features of a cephalometric radiograph made on a piece of transparent paper placed over the radiograph.

t., extraoral, a tracing of mandibular movements made outside the oral cavity.

t., Gothic arch. See **tracing, needle point.**

t., intraoral, a tracing of mandibular movements made within the oral cavity. A tracing made by a mechanical device consisting of a weighted or spring-loaded stylus that is attached to one jaw and contacts a coated plate attached to the other jaw. Movement of the mandible causes a tracing to be formed on the horizontally placed coated plate. When the stylus point is in the apex of the tracing, the mandible is said to be in the horizontal position of centric relation. The shape of the tracing depends on the relative location of the marking point and tracing table. The various tracing shapes have been called Gothic arch, arrow point, and sea gull tracings. The apex of a properly made tracing indicates the most retruded unstrained relation of the mandible to the maxillae (that is, the centric relation). The tracings are made by a stylus or needle point by the movement of the mandible. Unless otherwise designated, stylus tracings are made by lateral movements registered on a horizontal plate.

t., sea gull. See **tracing, needle point.**

t., stylus. See **tracing, needle point.**

tracings, pantographic, tracing of mandibular movements; a stylus is attached to the mandible traces line on vertical and horizontal plates attached to the maxilla, providing a graphic of lower jaw movements.

tract, sinus, a communication between a pathologic space and an anatomic body cavity or between a pathologic space and the skin. A sinus tract may or may not be lined with epithelium.

traction, the act of drawing (pulling).

t., external, a fracture reduction appliance principally used in the management of midfacial fractures. Points of fixation are located in the oral cavity and over the cranial area, and elastic or rigid connectors are placed between the cranial and oral points of fixation.

t., intermaxillary. See **traction, maxillomandibular.**

t., internal, a pulling force created by using one of the cranial bones above the point of fracture for anchorage.

t., maxillomandibular (intermaxillary traction), the technique for reducing fractures of the maxilla or mandible into functional relations with the opposing dental arch through the use of elastic or wire ligatures and interdental wiring or splints.

trademark, a word, symbol, or device assigned to a product by its manufacturer, registered or not registered as a part of its identity.

tragion (trāj'eon), the notch just above the tragus of the ear. It lies 1 to 2 mm below the spina helicis, which may be easily palpated.

tragus (trāgəs), a prominence in front of the opening of the external ear.

training grant, an award of money or other resources to provide training in a particular field, usually in areas of public need or demand.

trait (trāt), an inherited set of mental or bodily characteristics.

t., Cooley's. See **thalassemia minor.**

t., sickle cell, a form of sickle cell disease in which patients are asymptomatic, but their erythrocytes can be caused to assume a sickle shape under certain conditions. The trait is present when one parent has the gene (heterozygous condition) for sickle cell disease. See also **disease, sickle cell.**

tramadol HCl, *trade name:* Ultram; *drug class:* synthetic opioid analgesic; *action:* unknown, but it has been shown to bind to opioid receptors and inhibit the reuptake of norepinephrine and serotonin; *use:* treatment of moderate-to-severe pain.

tranquilizer (trang'kwĭlīz'ər), one of a poorly defined group of drugs designed to control anxiety and reduce tension or stress. Tranquilizers tend to induce drowsiness and may cause physical and psychologic dependence. Most tranquilizers are controlled substances.

transaminase (transam'ĭnās), one of several enzymes involved in the reversible transfer of an amino (NH_2) group from an α-amino acid to an α-ketoacid, especially α-ketoglutaric acid. Characteristic high values are seen in myocardial infarction and viral hepatitis.

transdermal delivery system, a method of applying a drug to unbroken skin. The drug is absorbed through the skin and enters the body's systems. It is used particularly for the administration of nitroglycerin and in nicotine patches used to assist individuals to withdraw from the use of tobacco.

transfection, the process by which a bacterial cell is infected with purified deoxyribonucleic acid (DNA) or ribonucleic acid (RNA) isolated from a virus or a viral vector after a specific pretreatment.

transfer agreement, a written contract between two health care institutions for the transfer of patients from one to the other and for the orderly exchange of pertinent clinical information on the patients transferred.

transferase, any of a group of enzymes that catalyze the transfer of a chemical group or radical from one molecule to another.

transferrin, a trace protein present in the blood that is essential in the transport of iron from the intestine into the bloodstream, making it available to the normoblasts in the bone marrow.

transformer, an electrical device that increases or reduces the voltage of an alternating current by mutual induction between primary and secondary coils or windings.

t., auto-. See **autotransformer.**

t., Coolidge filament, a step-down transformer that reduces the line voltage of 110 volts to 12 volts, which in turn heats the tungsten filament of the Coolidge tube for the production of electrons.

t., step-down, a transformer in which the secondary voltage is less than the primary voltage.

t., step-up, a transformer in which the secondary voltage is greater than the primary voltage.

transforming growth factor (TGF), a group of proteins produced by cells of a tumor that, when inoculated into a normal cell culture, causes a disorderly increase in the number of cells in the culture.

transfusion, the introduction into the bloodstream of whole blood or blood components such as plasma, platelets, or packed red cells. Infused donor blood must be matched to the recipient's blood type and antigen group.

transient, pertaining to a condition that is temporary or of short duration, usually not recurring.

transillumination (trans'il oo'minā' shən), **1.** examination of an organ, cavity, or tissue (for example, tooth or gingival tissue) by transmitted light. A valuable aid in detecting carious lesions, disclosing carious or demineralized dentin during cavity preparation, checking the finish or gingival margins of restorations, and revealing cement, debris, or calculus subgingivally. **2.** a test in which the use of transmitted light may disclose a discoloration of the coronal aspect, indicating dentinal tubular hemorrhage as a result of trauma, pulpal necrosis, or fracture. **3.** examination of tissues by means of a light placed so that the region under study is between the light source and the observer.

transition point. See **Tg value.**

transitional dentition, the final phase of the transition from deciduous to permanent teeth, in which most deciduous teeth have been lost or are in the process of shedding, and the permanent successors are not yet in function.

translation, movement of a rigid body in which all parts move in the same direction at the same speed.

translatory movement. See **movement, translatory.**

translocation, the rearrangement of genetic material within the same chromosome or the transfer of a segment of one chromosome to another nonhomologous one.

transmission, the transfer or conveyance of a thing or condition such as an infectious or genetic disease or hereditary trait from one person to another.

transmission scanning electron microscope, an instrument that transmits a highly magnified, well-resolved, three-dimensional image on a television screen, thus combining the advantages of the transmission electron and scanning electron microscopes.

transosteal implant jig, an instrument designed to guide a bone drill from the inferior border through the alveolar ridge to create a path for the seating of a transosteal implant.

transplant, 1. *v.* to remove and plant in another place, as from one body or part of a body to another. **2.** *n.* implantation of living or nonliving tissue or bone into another part of the body; it then serves as a scaffold in the healing process and is progressively resorbed and replaced by newly formed bone. **3.** *v.* to move a tooth or tissue from one site to another, often but not always autogenously.

transplantation, autogenous tooth, transplantation of a tooth from one position to another in the same individual.

transplantation, homogenous tooth, transplantation of a tooth from one human to another.

transplantation, tooth, the transfer of a tooth from one alveolus to another.

transport, the movement of biochemical substances from one site to another. Active transport requires energy, whereas passive transport allows movement down a gradient without an energy drain.

transseptal fiber. See **fiber, transseptal.**

transudate (trans'yədāt), any fluid substance that has passed through a membrane which may or may not be associated with inflammation. It is low in proteins and colloids and has a low specific gravity.

transverse, at right angles to the long axis of any common part.

transverse palatine suture, the line of junction between the palatal processes of the maxillary bones and horizontal portions of the palatine bones that form the hard palate.

transversion, eruption of a tooth in the wrong position

tranylcypromine sulfate, *trade name:* Parnate; *drug class:* antidepressant, monoamine oxidase inhibitor (MAOI); *action:* increases concentrations of endogenous norepinephrine, serotonin, and dopamine in central nervous system (CNS) storage sites; *use:* treatment of depression (when uncontrolled by other means).

trauma (trou'mə), a hurt; a wound; an injury; damage; impairment; external violence producing bodily injury or degeneration.

t., injury in occlusal, the damaging effects of occlusal trauma, which are of a dystrophic nature and affect the tooth and its attachment apparatus. Lesions include wear facets on the tooth, root resorption, cemental tears, thrombosis of blood vessels of the periodontal membrane, necrosis and hyalinization of the periodontal membrane on the pressure side, and resorption of alveolar and supporting bone. Clinically, tooth mobility and migration may be evident; radiographically, evidence includes the widening of the periodontal membrane space and fraying or fuzziness of the lamina dura and formation of infrabony resorptive defects. Pocket formation is not a sequela to occlusal traumatism.

t., occlusal, abnormal occlusal relationships of the teeth, causing injury to the periodontium.

traumatic (trəmat'ik), of, pertaining to, or caused by an injury.

t. occlusion. See **occlusion, traumatic.**

t. shock. See **shock, traumatic.**

traumatism, 1. an injury. 2. a wound produced by an injury; trauma.

t. by food, impingement of the gingival margin by coarse foodstuff caused by improper contour of the tooth or faulty position of the tooth.

t., occlusal, lesions of the attachment apparatus; caused by force placed on the tooth in excess of that which the supporting structures can withstand.

t., periodontal, the application of stress to the structures comprising the attachment apparatus, which exceeds the adaptive capacities of the tissues, with resultant tissue destruction.

t., primary occlusal, the force or forces that are caused by mandibular movement and resultant tooth percussion and are capable of producing pathologic changes in the periodontium.

t., secondary occlusal, destruction of the attachment apparatus by factors other than those of occlusion (for example, periodontitis). In secondary occlusal traumatism, even the forces of mastication become pathologic in nature.

traumatogenic (traw'mətōjen'ik), capable of producing a wound or injury.

t. occlusion. See **occlusion, traumatic.**

tray, a receptacle or device that holds or carries.

t., acrylic resin, a tray made of acrylic resin.

t., impression, a receptacle or device that is used to carry the impression material to the mouth, confine the material in apposition to the surfaces to be recorded, and control the impression material while it sets to form the impression.

trazodone HCl, *trade names:* Desyrel, Trazon, Trialodine; *drug class:* antidepressant; *action:* selectively inhibits serotonin-specific reuptake in the brain; *use:* treatment of depression.

Treacher Collins syndrome. See **syndrome, Treacher Collins.**

treatment, the mode or course pursued for remedial ends.

t., hardening heat. See **tempering.**

t., heat, 1. subjecting a metal to a given controlled heat, followed by controlled sudden or gradual cooling to develop the desired qualities of the metal to the maximal degree. 2. a process of giving a metal predetermined physical properties by controlled temperature changes.

t., homogenizing heat. See **anneal.**

t., indirect pulp capping. See **capping, indirect pulp.**

t., prescription, the formal outline of the projected treatment of a patient (for example, the blueprint from which the dentist projects treatment).

t., rest (sedative treatment), use of a drug sealed into a root canal to relieve

T

pain or discomfort; not used primarily for its antiseptic value.

t., **root canal,** the techniques and pharmaceuticals used in removing pulp tissue, sterilizing the root canal, and preparing the root canal for filling.

t., sedative. See **treatment, rest.**

t., softening heat. See **anneal.**

treatment plan, in dentistry a schedule of procedures and appointments designed to restore, step by step, the oral health of a patient.

tremolo (trem′əlō′), an irregular and exaggerated speech pattern that may be the symptom of an emotional disturbance or of various diseases affecting the nervous control of the organs of respiration and phonation.

tremor, rhythmic, purposeless, quivering movements resulting from the involuntary alternating contraction and relaxation of opposing skeletal muscle groups.

trench mouth. See **gingivitis, acute necrotizing ulcerative.**

Trendelenburg position (trendel′ənbərg). See **position, Trendelenburg.**

trepanation (trephination), the act of surgically cutting a round hole.

trephine (trifēn′), a circle-cutting surgical instrument designed to remove a circumscribed portion of tissue. It permits the insertion of the heads of intramucosal inserts into the tissue.

Treponema (trep′ənē′mə), a genus of schizomycetes composed of parasitic and pathogenic spiral microorganisms.

T. microdentium, a species found in the normal oral cavity.

T. mucosum, a species found in periodontal infections in man.

T. pallidum, the spirochete that causes syphilis in humans.

T. vincentii, a spirochete associated with acute necrotizing ulcerative gingivitis.

tretinoin (vitamin A acid, retinoic acid), *trade name:* Retin-A; *drug class:* vi-tamin A acid; *action:* decreases cohesiveness of follicular epithelium, decreases microcomedone formation; *use:* treatment of acne vulgaris.

triad, Hutchinson (trī′ad), interstitial keratitis, deafness, and Hutchinson teeth resulting from congenital syphilis. (not current)

triage, 1. (in military medicine) a classification of casualties of war and other disasters according to the gravity of injuries, urgency of treatment, and place for treatment. **2.** a process in which a group of patients is sorted according to need for care. The kind of illness or injury, severity of the problem, and facilities available govern the process, as in the emergency room of a hospital. **3.** (in disaster medicine) a process in which a large group of patients is sorted so that care may be concentrated on those who are likely to survive.

trial, an examination before a competent tribunal of the facts or law in issue in a cause of action for the purpose of determining the issue.

trial base. See **baseplate.**

Triage rating systems

Five-tier System (Used in Military Triage)
Dead or will die
Life-threatening—readily correctable
Urgent—must be treated within 1 to 2 hours
Delayed—noncritical or ambulatory
No injury—no treatment necessary

Four-tier System
Immediate—seriously injured, reasonable chance of survival
Delayed—can wait for care after simple first aid
Expectant—extremely critical, moribund
Minimal—no impairment of function, can either treat self or be treated by a nonprofessional

Three-tier System
Life-threatening—readily correctable
Urgent—must be treated within 1 to 2 hours
Delayed—no injury, noncritical, or ambulatory

Two-tier System
Immediate versus delayed
Immediate—life-threatening injuries that are readily correctable on scene and those that are urgent
Delayed—no injury, noncritical injuries, ambulatory victims, and moribund victims

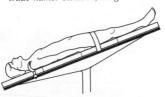

Trendelenburg position

triamcinolone, a synthetic adreno-corticosteroid that has a potent antiin-flammatory effect and is used topically in the treatment of angular cheilosis.

triamcinolone acetonide (topical), *trade names:* Aristocort, Flutex, Kenalog, Kenlog in Orabase, Oracort, Triacet, Triderm, others; *drug class:* topical corticosteroid; *action:* interacts with steroid cytoplasmic receptors to induce antiinflammatory effects; possesses antipruritic and antiinflammatory actions; *uses:* treatment of psoriasis, eczema, contact dermatitis, pruritus; special dental paste used to treat nonviral inflammatory oral lesions, including aphthous stomatitis, lichen planus, and cicatrical pemphigoid.

triamcinolone/triamcinolone acetonide/triamcinolone diacetate/triamcinolone hexacetonide, *trade names:* Triamcinolone (oral), Aristocort, Atolone, Kenacort, many others; *drug class:* glucocorticoid, intermediate-acting; *action:* decreases inflammation by suppressing macrophage and leukocyte migration, reduces capillary permeability and inhibits lysosomal enzymes and phagocytosis; *uses:* treatment of severe inflammation; immunosuppression; neoplasms; collagen, respiratory, and dermatologic disorders; and seasonal and perennial allergic rhinitis.

triamterene, *trade name:* Dyrenium; *drug class:* potassium-sparing diuretic; *action:* acts on distal tubule to inhibit reabsorption of sodium, chlorine; increases potassium retention; *uses:* treatment of edema; hypertension.

triangle, a three-cornered area.

t., Bolton, a triangle formed by drawing a line from the nasion to the sella turcica and from there to the Bolton point.

t., Bonwill, an equilateral triangle with 4-inch (10-cm) sides bounded by lines from the contact points of the lower central incisors (or the median line of the residual ridge of the mandible) to the condyle on either side and from one condyle to the other. It is the basis for Bonwill's theory of occlusion.

t., Lesser's, a surgical landmark for locating the lingual artery; the triangle is located above the hyoid bone and is formed by the posterior belly of the digastric muscle and the posterior edge of the mylohyoid muscle below and the hypoglossal nerve above. The floor of the triangle is the hypoglossus muscle, and directly below the hypoglossus muscle is the lingual artery.

t., Tweed, a triangle formed by the mandibular plane, Frankfort plane, and long axis of the lower central incisor. Proposed as a diagnostic aid by C.H. Tweed.

triazolam, *trade name:* Halcion; *drug class:* benzodiazepine, sedative-hypnotic, controlled substance schedule IV; *action:* produces central nervous system (CNS) depression by interacting with a benzodiazepine receptor to facilitate the action of the inhibitory neurotransmitter gamma-aminobutyric acid (GABA); *use:* treatment of insomnia.

trichoepithelioma (trik′oep′ithō′leō′mə). See **epithelioma adenoides cysticum.**

Trichuris, a genus of parasitic round-worms that infect the intestinal tract. Adult worms are 30 to 50 mm long and resemble a whip with a threadlike anterior and a thicker posterior. Also called whipworm.

trident, a tooth with three cusps. Also called tridentate or tricuspid.

tridymite (trid′ĭmīt), a physical form of silica used in combination with cristobalite to limit thermal expansion.

trifurcation, division into three parts or branches, as the three roots of a maxillary first molar.

trifluoperazine HCl, *trade name:* Stelazine; *drug class:* phenothiazine antipsychotic; *action:* blocks neuro-transmission at dopaminergic synapses in cerebral cortex, hypothalamus, and limbic system; *uses:* treatment of psychotic disorders, nonpsychotic anxiety, and schizophrenia.

triflupromazine HCl, *trade name:* Vesprin; *drug class:* phenothiazine, antipsychotic; *action:* blocks neuro-transmission at dopaminergic synapses in the cerebral cortex, hypothalamus, and limbic system; *uses:* treatment of psychotic disorders, schizophrenia, acute agitation, nausea, and vomiting.

trifluridine (ophthalmic), *trade name:* Viroptic ophthalmic solution; *drug class:* antiviral; *action:* inhibits viral deoxyribonucleic acid (DNA) synthesis and replication; *uses:* treatment of primary keratoconjunctivitis, recurring epithelial keratitis, and keratitis associated with herpes simplex virus types 1 and 2.

trigeminal nerve, the fifth cranial nerve, which provides motor innervation to the muscles of mastication and sensory innervation to the face, jaws, and teeth.

trigeminal neuralgia, a neurologic condition of the trigeminal nerve characterized by paroxysms of flashing, stablike pain radiating along the course of a branch of the nerve. Any or all of the three branches may be affected. Also called tic douloureux.

trigger point, the point from which referred pain initiates. In the myofascial pain syndrome, usually a localized, deep tenderness in a taut bundle of muscle fibers from which pain is referred to other areas.

trihexyphenidyl HCl, *trade names:* Trihexane, Trihexy-5; *drug class:* antiparkinsonian, anticholinergic; *action:* block central muscarinic receptors, which decreases the severity of involuntary movements; *use:* treatment of Parkinson's disease symptoms.

triiodothyronine, a hormone that helps regulate growth and development, control metabolism and body temperature, and by a negative-feedback system, inhibit the secretion of thyrotropin by the pituitary gland.

trilogy of Fallot, a congenital cardiac anomaly consisting of a combination of pulmonic stenosis, interatrial septal defect, and right ventricular hypertrophy.

trimeprazine tartrate, *trade name:* Temaril; *drug class:* antihistamine H_1 receptor antagonist; *action:* acts by competing with histamine for H_1 receptor sites; decreases allergic response by blocking histamine effects; *use:* treatment of pruritus.

trimester, one of the three periods of approximately 3 months each into which pregnancy is divided.

trimethadione, *trade name:* Tridione; *drug class:* anticonvulsant; *action:* increases the threshold for seizures initiated in the cortex, decreases central nervous system (CNS) synaptic stimulation to low-frequency impulses; *use:* treatment of refractory absence (petit mal) seizures.

trimethobenzamide, *trade name:* Arrestin, Bio-Gan, Stemetic, Ticon, Tigan, T-Gen, Triban, others; *drug class:* antiemetic; *action:* acts centrally by blocking the chemoreceptor trigger zone, which in turn acts on vomiting center; *uses:* treatment of nausea and vomiting and prevention of postoperative vomiting.

trimethoprim-sulfamethoxazole, a synthetic antibacterial combination effective in urinary tract infections; it is the drug of choice in the treatment of *Pneumocystis carinii* pneumonia, one of the opportunistic infections associated with acquired immunodeficiency syndrome (AIDS).

trimetrexate glucuronate, *trade name:* Neutrexin; *drug class:* folate antagonist; *action:* inhibits the enzyme dihydrofolate reductase, which leads to interference with deoxyribonucleic acid (DNA), ribonucleic acid (RNA), and protein synthesis in the *Pneumocystis carinii* organism; *uses:* alternative therapy for *P. carinii* pneumonia in immunocompromised patients, including patients with acquired immunodeficiency syndrome (AIDS).

trimipramine maleate, *trade name:* Surmontil; *drug class:* antidepressant-tricyclic; *action:* inhibits both norepinephrine and serotonin (5-HT) uptake in the brain; *uses:* treatment of depression and of enuresis in children.

trimmer, gingival margin (margin trimmer), a binangled, double-paired, chisel-shaped, single-beveled, double-planed lateral cutting instrument. The blade is curved left or right similar to a spoon excavator; the cutting edge is straight and not perpendicular to the axis of the blade. The pair with the end of the cutting edge farthest from the shaft forming an acute angle is termed distal and is used to bevel a distal gingival margin or accentuate a mesial axiogingival angle; the pair with the acute angle of the cutting edge closest to the shaft is called mesial and is used to bevel a mesial gingival margin or accentuate a distal axiogingival angle.

When one of these trimmers is used, all four must be used. (not current)

trimmer, margin. See **trimmer, gingival margin.**

trimming, tissue. See **border molding.**

tripelennamine HCl, *trade names:* PBZ, PBZ-SR, Pelamine; *drug class:* antihistamine, H_1 receptor antagonist; *action:* acts by competing with histamine for H_1 receptor sites; *uses:* treatment of rhinitis and allergy symptoms.

tripoding (trī'pōding), the marking of a cast at three points in the same plane as a means of repositioning the cast in that plane during subsequent procedures.

tripodism, a widely used principle to gain instant stability on uneven terrains in all landings. It is referred to as a three-point landing. Stamp cusps in well-organized occlusion have only three-point contacts with their fossa brims (none with their tips). (not current)

triprolidine HCl, *trade name:* Myidil; *drug class:* antihistamine, H_1 receptor antagonist; *action:* acts by competing with histamine for H_1 receptor sites; *uses:* treatment of rhinitis and allergy symptoms.

trismus (triz'məs), spasms of the muscles of mastication resulting in the inability to open the mouth; often symptomatic of pericoronitis.

trisomy (trī'səmē), an additional chromosome in the normal complement, so that in each nucleus a chromosome is represented three times rather than twice.

t. **D** *(trisomy 13-15, Patau's syndrome),* Clinical syndrome associated with an autosomal abnormality in which the extra chromosome occurs in the 13 to 15 group. Numerous anatomic defects are present, including hemangiomas, hernia, arrhinencephaly, eye anomalies, cleft lip and palate, and characteristic changes in the footprint and palm print. (not current)

t. **syndrome,** Any congenital condition caused by the addition of an extra member to a normal pair of homologous autosomes or to the sex chromosome or by the translocation of a portion of one chromosome to another.

Trisomy 21 results in Down syndrome. See also **mongolism.**

trituration (trich'ūrā'shən), the process of mixing together silver alloy fillings with mercury to produce amalgam.

t., **hand,** the mixing of ingredients by hand in a mortar and pestle.

t., **mechanical,** the mixing of constituents in a mechanical device or amalgamator.

troche (trō'ke). See **lozenge.**

Trousseau's twitching. See **twitching, Trousseau's.** (not current)

true vocal cords, the vocal folds of the larynx as distinguished from the vestibular folds, called the false vocal cords.

True's separator. See **separator, True's.** (not current)

truss arm. See **connector, minor.**

trust, a relationship in which one person or entity holds fiduciary responsibility for another's property or enterprise.

truth serum, a common name for any of several sedatives administered intravenously in subjects to elicit information that may have been repressed. It has been used successfully to help identify amnesia victims.

try-in, a preliminary placement of trial dentures (complete or removable partial), a partial denture casting, or a finished restoration to evaluate fit, appearance, and maxillomandibular relations.

trypsin, a proteolytic digestive enzyme produced by the exocrine pancreas that catalyzes in the small intestine the breakdown of dietary proteins to peptones, peptides, and amino acids.

tryptase (trip'tās). See **plasmin.**

tryptophan, one of the essential amino acids. See also **amino acid.**

TSH. See **hormone, thyrotropic.**

tub and tray system, a system of instrument and supply management in which the instruments for a particular task are prearranged on a tray and the accompanying disposables are prearranged in an accompanying tub. The prepared trays and tubs are appropriately sterilized, stored, and delivered to the dental operatory at the proper time.

tubal pregnancy, an ectopic pregnancy in which the conceptus implants in the fallopian tube.

tube, a hollow cylindrical structure.

t., buccal, a section of tubing attached to the buccal side of a molar band in a horizontal position, serving as an attachment for the labial arch wire, which slides into the tube.

t., Coolidge, an x-ray tube in which the gas pressure is purposely made so low that it plays no role in the operation of the tube, the operation depending on the emission of electrons by the heated filament of the cathode. See also **x-ray tube, Coolidge.**

t., discharge, any vacuum tube in which a high-voltage electric current is discharged (for example, an x-ray tube).

t., horizontal, a metal tube attachment that is placed in a horizontal position on the buccal surface of each anchor molar tooth to allow for the insertion of the labial arch wire.

t., intubation, a tube for insertion into the larynx through the mouth.

t., line focus, an x-ray tube in which the target face is about 20 inches (50 cm) from the cathode face. The focal spot is rectangular, with the length approximately three times the width. The acute angle provides an effective focal spot area approximately square and a fraction of the actual area.

t., protective, housing, an x-ray tube enclosure that provides radiation protection.

t., protective, housing, diagnostic, a tube housing that reduces the leakage of radiation to, at most, 0.10 r/hr at a distance of 1 mm from the tube target when the tube is operating at its maximal continuous rated voltage.

t., protective, housing, therapeutic, a tube housing that reduces the leakage of radiation to, at most, 1 r/hr at a distance of 1 m from the tube target when the tube is operating at its maximal continuous rated current for the maximal rated voltage.

t., right-angle, an x-ray tube in which the target is at right angles to the cathode.

t. tooth. See **tooth, tube.**

t., vertical, an attachment that is usually placed on the lingual surface of the anchor band to allow for the insertion of the lingual wire.

t., x-ray. See **x-ray tube.**

tubercle (tōō′bərkəl), a small rounded nodule or elevation on the surface of the skin, bone, or other tissue.

t., genial (gēnē′ əl) *(geniohyoid tubercle),* a small rounded elevation on the lingual surface of the mandible on either side of the midline near the inferior border of the body of the mandible, serving as a point of insertion for the geniohyoid muscles.

t., geniohyoid (jē′nēōhī′oid). See **tubercle, genial.**

t., superior genial, the small spines on the lingual surface of the mandible that serve as the attachment for the genioglossus muscles. On resorbed mandibles, these tubercles may be at or above the crest of the residual ridge.

tuberculin skin test. See **test, tuberculin.**

tuberculosis (tōōbur′kyəlō′sis), an infectious disease caused by *Mycobacterium tuberculosis* and characterized by the formation of tubercles in the tissues.

tuberculous lymphadenitis, an inflammation of the lymph glands caused by the presence of *Mycobacterium tuberculosis.*

tuberosity (tōō′bəros′itē), a protuberance or elevation from the surface, usually of a bone.

t., maxillary, the most distal aspect of the maxillary alveolar process, with its posterior border curving upward and distally.

t. reduction, surgical excision of excessive fibrous or bony tissue in the area of the maxillary tuberosity before the construction of prosthetic appliances.

tubule, a small tube such as one of the collecting tubules in the kidneys. The dentin of the tooth contains dentinal tubules that communicate from the pulp to the dentinoenamal interface.

tumor, a swelling. Through usage the term is now synonymous with neoplasm. See also **neoplasm.**

t., basaloid mixed. See **carcinoma, adenocystic.**

t., Brooke's. See **epithelioma adenoides cysticum.**

t., brown, a central giant cell tumor of the bone; associated with parathyroidism.

t., carotid body, a tumor formed about the carotid artery.

t., collision, a rare condition in which two neoplasms, both growing in the same general area, collide with the tumor elements and become intermingled.

t., Ewing's (endothelioma, Ewing's sarcoma), a rare malignant tumor of disputed histogenetic origin in bone. It is characterized by pain, a radiographic appearance called onion-skinning, and a histologic picture consisting of solid sheets of small round cells that appear on the many small blood vessels present.

t., giant cell, a benign neoplasm of bone, producing resorption and characterized by giant cells.

t., hormonal, localized enlargements of the gingivae that have the appearance of neoplasms and are associated with hormonal imbalance during pregnancy.

t., mixed, 1. one of a group of neoplasms of the salivary glands whose histologic appearance suggests both epithelial and connective tissue origin, although they presently are considered of epithelial origin only. Benign and malignant types are possible. **2.** any tumor arising from cells derived from more than one germ layer.

t., mucoepidermoid, a tumor of the salivary glands composed of mucous cells, epidermoid cells, and clear cells. Benign and malignant forms are recognized.

t., odontogenic (ōdon'tōjen'ik), 1. a neoplasm produced from tooth-forming tissues *(for example, odontogenic fibroma, odontogenic myxoma, ameloblastoma)*. See also **calcifying epithelial odontogenic tumor. 2.** a gingival enlargement seen during pregnancy, the microscopic examination of which reveals the features of a pyogenic granuloma.

t., turban. See **carcinoma, basal cell.**

t., Warthin's. See **cystadenoma, papillary, lymphomatosum.**

tumor necrosis factor (TNF), a natural body protein with anticancer effects. It is produced in the body in response to the presence of toxic substances such as bacterial toxins. Adverse effects are toxic shock and cachexia.

tungsten (W), a metallic element. Its atomic number is 74, and its atomic weight is 183.85. It has the highest melting point of all metals and is used as a target material in x-ray tubes.

tunica intima, the membrane lining an artery.

tunica media, the muscular middle layer of an artery.

tunnel vision, a defect in sight in which a great reduction occurs in the peripheral field of vision, as if looking through a hollow tube or tunnel.

turbidity, a condition of light scattering in a liquid resulting from the presence of suspended particles in the fluid.

turbulence, casting term used to denote irregular flow of metal into a mold. May result in porosity.

turgor, the normal resiliency of the skin caused by the outward pressure of the cells and interstitial fluid. Dehydration results in a decreased skin turgor, manifested by lax skin that, when grasped and raised between two fingers, slowly returns to a position level with the adjacent tissue.

Turner's tooth. See **tooth, Turner's.** (not current)

Tweed triangle. See **triangle, Tweed.**

24-hour clock system, a method of designating time by using the numeric sequence from 00 to 23 for the hours and the numbers 00 to 59 for the minutes in a daily cycle beginning with 0000 (midnight) and ending with 2359 (1 minute before the next midnight). The system provides a clear distinction between prenoon and afternoon time without requiring the designations AM and PM. The system is used by the Department of Defense and others.

twilight sleep, light anesthesia obtained by the parenteral administration of a mixture of morphine and scopolamine to reduce pain and obtund recall in childbirth.

twins, two siblings produced in the same pregnancy and developed from one egg (identical, monozygotic) or from two eggs fertilized at the same time (fraternal, dizygotic).

twin-wire. See **appliance, twin-wire.**

twist drill, 1. a drill having one or two deep helical grooves extending from the point to the smooth portion of the shank. **2.** a spiral bone bur.

twitch, 1. the contraction of small muscle units, manifested as a quick, simple, spasmodic contraction of a muscle. **2.** a short, sudden pull or jerk.

twitching, an irregular spasm of a minor extent.

t., Trousseau's, a twitching of the face that the patient can exhibit at will and occurs obsessively to relieve tension.

Tylenol. See **acetaminophen.**

tympanic membrane, a thin, semitransparent membrane in the middle ear that transmits sound vibrations to the internal ear by the means of the auditory ossicles. Also called the eardrum.

type A hepatitis. See **hepatitis, infectious.**

Type A personality, a behavior pattern as associated with individuals who are highly competitive and work compulsively to meet deadlines. The condition is associated with a higher than usual incidence of coronary heart disease.

type B hepatitis. See **hepatitis, homologous serum.**

Type B personality, a form of behavior associated with people who appear free of hostility and aggression and who lack a compulsion to meet deadlines, are not highly competitive at work or play, and have a lower risk of heart attack.

Type E personality, a term used to describe professional women who fit neither Type A nor Type B personality categories but who have a marked sense of insecurity and strive to convince themselves that they are worthwhile.

typewriter ribbon as a marking medium, typewriter ribbon is more desirable than carbon paper when setting teeth because the porcelain tooth that is being adjusted will not perforate the ribbon and abrade the surface of the stone template record of jaw movement.

typhoid carrier, a person without signs or symptoms of typhoid fever who carries in the body the bacteria that cause the disease and sheds the pathogens in bodily excretions.

typhoid fever, a bacterial infection usually caused by *Salmonella typhi;* transmitted by contaminated milk, water, or food and characterized by headache, delirium, cough, watery diarrhea, rash, and a high fever.

typhus, any of a group of acute infectious diseases caused by various species of *Rickettsia* and usually transmitted from infected rodents to humans by the bites of lice, fleas, mites, or ticks.

typical implant connective tissue, the tendonlike condensed elongated avascular tissue formed in direct contact with implant infrastructure metal underlaid by normal collagenous fibrous connective tissue.

typodont (tī′pōdont), an artificial model containing artificial or natural teeth used for teaching technique exercises.

tyramine, an amino acid synthesized in the body from the essential acid tyrosine. Tyramine stimulates the release of the catecholamines epinephrine and norepinephrine. It is important that people taking monoamine oxidase inhibitors avoid the ingestion of foods and beverages containing tyramine, particularly aged cheese, meats, bananas, yeast-containing products, and alcoholic beverages.

tyrosine (Tyr), an amino acid synthesized in the body from the essential amino acid phenylalanine. Tyrosine is found in most proteins and is a precursor of melanin and several hormones, including epinephrine and thyroxine.

Tzanck cell (tsahnk). See **cell, Tzanck.** (not current)

Tzanck's test. See **test, Tzanck.** (not current)

U

ugly duckling stage, a stage of dental development preceding the eruption of the permanent canines, in which the lateral incisors may be tipped laterally because of crowding by the unerupted canine crowns. This tipping may cause spacing of the incisor crowns despite the crowding of the roots. The condition may be transitory in an otherwise normal dentition. The stage was first described and named by B.H. Broadbent.

ulcer (ul′sər), a loss of covering epithelium from the skin or mucous membranes, causing gradual disintegration and necrosis of the tissues.

u., aphthous, recurrent (RAU) (af'thus) *(canker sore, recurrent aphthae),* periodic episodes of aphthous lesions lasting from 1 week to several months. Trauma, menses, immunologic factors, upper respiratory tract infections, herpes simplex are suggested causes. The single or multiple discrete or confluent ulcers have a well-defined marginal erythema and a central area of necrosis with sloughing. The herpetic appearance suggests a common mechanism with herpes simplex, but no known infectious agents have been demonstrated.

u., autochthonous (ôtok'thənəs). See **chancre.**

u., decubitus (dikyoo'bitəs) *(traumatic ulcer),* **1.** a bedsore. **2.** loosely used to refer to a traumatic ulcer of the oral mucosa.

u., diabetic (dī'əbet'ik), an ulcer, usually of the lower extremities, associated with diabetes mellitus.

u., herpetic (hərpet'ik), an ulcer that is secondary to the vesicle of herpes simplex; a shallow ulcer with an irregular, erythematous border and a yellow-gray base.

u., Mikulicz's (mik'yoolich'ēz). See **periadenitis mucosa necrotica recurrens.**

u., peptic (pep'tik), an ulcer of the stomach or duodenum probably resulting in large part from an increased secretion of hydrochloric acid. Nervous, emotional, and endocrine factors have been implicated.

u., pterygoid (ter'igoid). See **aphtha, Bednar's.**

u., rodent. See **carcinoma, basal cell.**

u., traumatic. See **ulcer, decubitus.**

ulceration (ul'sərā'shən), the process of forming an ulcer or of becoming ulcerous.

ulcerative stomatitis, recurrent (ul'sərā'tiv, ul'sərətiv' stomati'tis). See **ulcer, aphthous, recurrent.**

ultimate strength. See **strength, ultimate.**

ultra (ul'trə), beyond; in addition; in excess of.

u. damages, damages beyond those paid in court.

ultracentrifuge, a high-speed centrifuge with a rotation rate fast enough to produce sedimentation of viruses, even in blood plasma. Many kinds of biochemical analyses use ultracentrifuge, including such analyses as the measurement and separation of some proteins and viruses.

ultrafilrate, a solution that has passed through a semipermeable membrane with very small pores. It usually contains only low–molecular-weight solutes.

ultrasonic (ul'trəson'ik), sound frequencies so high (greater than 20 kilohertz) they cannot be perceived by the human ear.

u. cleaner, an electronic generator that transmits high energy and high-frequency vibrations to a fluid-filled container used to remove particulate matter from dental instruments and appliances.

u. scaler, an electronic generator that transmits high-frequency vibrations to a handpiece that is used to remove heavy calcified deposits from the surface of a tooth.

ultrasonography, the process of imaging deep structures of the body by measuring and recording the reflection of pulsed or continuous high-frequency sound waves. It is valuable in many medical situations, including the diagnosis of fetal abnormalities, gallstones, heart defects, and tumors. Also called *sonography.*

ultraviolet light, light beyond the range of human vision, at the short end of the spectrum. It occurs naturally in sunlight; it burns and tans the skin and converts precursors in the skin to vitamin D. It is used in the treatment of psoriasis and other skin conditions. Prolonged or excessive exposure to ultraviolet light can damage the skin and increase the susceptibility of the skin to cancer.

unbundling of procedures, the separating of a dental procedure into component parts with each part having a cost so that the cumulative cost of the components is greater than the total cost for the same procedure to patients who are not beneficiaries of a dental benefits plan.

uncompensated care, health care services provided by a hospital, physician, dentist, or other health care professional for which no charge is made and for which no payment is expected.

U

unconscious (unkon'shəs), insensible; not receiving any sensory impression and not having any subjective experiences.

undecylenic acid (topical), *trade names:* Caldesene Medicated Powder, Cruex products, Desenex Aerosol Powder, others; *class:* local antifungal; *action:* interferes with fungal cell membrane permeability; *uses:* tinea cruris, tinea pedis, diaper rash, minor skin irritations.

undercut, 1. the portions of a tooth that lie below the height of contour of the crown. **2.** the contour of a cross-section of a residual ridge of dental arch that would prevent the placement of a denture or other prosthesis. **3.** the contour of flasking stone that interlocks to prevent the separation of parts. **4.** the portion of a prepared cavity that creates a mechanical lock or area of retention; may be desirable in a cavity to be filled with gold foil or amalgam but undesirable in a cavity prepared for a restoration to be cemented.

u. gauge. See **gauge, undercut.**

u., retentive, an area of the abutment surface suitable for the location of a retentive clasp terminal, which to escape the undercut would be forced to flex and thus generate retention.

u., soft tissue, an undercut in a residual ridge or soft-tissue covering of a dental arch that would prevent or influence the placement of a removable denture.

u., unusable, the area of an abutment tooth or soft tissue across which a unit of the removable partial denture must pass without interference and hence must be blocked out (filled with wax or clay) before the master cast is duplicated. Use of a surveyor produces a surface that is parallel to the proposed path of a placement and removal.

undermine, to surgically separate the skin or mucosa from its underlying stroma so that it can be stretched or moved to cover a defect or wound.

unemployment, the state of being without a job or compensation for work; usually an involuntary state.

unerupted, not having perforated the oral mucosa. In dentistry, used with reference to a normal developing tooth, an embedded tooth, or an impacted tooth.

unification, the act of uniting or the condition of being united (e.g., the result of joining the components of a removable partial denture by connectors).

unilateral, one-sided.

union-sponsored plan, a program of dental benefits developed through a union's initiative. May be operated directly by the union or the union may contract for provision of the benefits. Funds to finance the benefits are usually paid out of a trust fund that receives its income from employer contributions, employer and union member contributions, or union members alone.

Unipen. See **nafcillin.** (not current)

unit, one of the components of a whole.

u., Angstrom (ang'strəm) **(Å, a.u.),** the unit of measure of wavelengths; one one-hundred-millionth of a centimeter.

u., dental, **1.** basically, the tooth, attachment apparatus, and gingival unit—all of which are necessary for proper masticatory activity. **2.** an article of equipment that contains an assembly of numerous items used in dental operations, such as a dental engine, cuspidor, operatory light, bracket, working table, saliva ejector, water supply, electric outlets, compressed air, and miscellaneous instruments.

u., dentoperiodontal, referring to the tooth and periodontium together.

u., gingival, the tough collagenous and epithelial covering of the neck of the tooth and the underlying attachment apparatus.

u., partial denture, the individual elements of the partial denture, each contributing some particular function.

u., x-ray, a device designed to produce x-rays.

u., x-ray, calibration, the determination of the kilovoltage peak (KVP) value of each autotransformer tap at various milliamperages, checking these values by means of a sphere gap or a prereading voltmeter.

United States dietary goals, the recommendation of a U.S. Senate committee in 1977 outlining the levels of consumption of complex carbohydrates, sugar, protein, fat, cholesterol, and salt for diets necessary to enhance the health status of Americans.

United States Food and Drug Administration (FDA), a unit of the Public Health Service created to protect the health of the nation against impure and unsafe foods, drugs, and cosmetics.

United States Health Resources and Services Administration (HRSA), a unit of the Public Health Service created to provide leadership and direction to programs and activities designed to improve the health services for all people of the United States and to develop health care and maintenance systems that are adequately financed, comprehensive, interrelated, and responsive to the needs of all members of American society.

United States Indian Health Service, a unit of the Department of Health and Human Services with 51 hospitals, 99 health centers, and several hundred field health stations established to improve the health status of the American Indian and Alaskan Native.

United States Occupational Safety and Health Administration (OSHA), a unit of the U.S. Department of Labor, created to develop and promulgate occupational safety and health standards; develop and issue regulations; conduct investigations and inspections to determine the status of compliance with safety and health standards and regulations; and issue citations and propose penalties for noncompliance with safety and health standards and regulations.

United States Pharmacopeia (USP), a compendium officially recognized by the Federal Food, Drug, and Cosmetic Act, which contains the descriptions, uses, strengths, and standards of purity for selected drugs.

United States Public Health Service (USPHS), a major division of the Department of Health and Human Services, which is a cabinet-level department of the administrative branch of the federal government. The USPHS provides oversight for the following agencies: Centers for Disease Control and Prevention (CDC); Food and Drug Administration (FDA); Health Resources and Services Administration (HRSA); Agency for

Toxic Substances and Disease Registry; National Institutes of Health (NIH); Alcohol, Drug Abuse and Mental Health Administration; Health Care Financing Administration (HCFA); Social Security Administration; Office of Child Support Enforcement; and Office of Community Services.

universal donor, a person with type O, Rh factor negative red blood cells. Packed red blood cells of this type may be used for emergency transfusion with minimal risk of incompatibility.

universal precautions, 1. an approach to infection control designed to prevent transmission of blood-borne diseases such as AIDS and hepatitis B in health care settings. Universal precautions were initially developed in 1987 by the Centers for Disease Control and in 1989 by the Bureau of Communicable Disease Epidemiology in Canada. The guidelines include specific recommendations for use of gloves and masks and protective eyewear when contact with blood or bodily secretions containing blood or blood elements is anticipated. **2.** the protocols used to maintain an aseptic field and to prevent cross-contamination and cross-infection between health care providers, between health care providers and patients, and between patients. These include but are not limited to the sterilization of instruments and goods; the isolation and disinfection of the immediate clinical environment; the use of sterile disposables; scrubbing, masking, gowning, and gloving; and the proper disposal of contaminated waste.

universal recipient, a person with blood type AB, who can receive a transfusion of blood of any group type without agglutination or precipitation effects.

universal tooth coding system, a tooth numbering system in which each tooth carries a number from 1 to 32, beginning with the maxillary right third molar and ending with the mandibular left third molar. The primary teeth are similarly numbered, preceded by a *D* for deciduous. The ADA numbering system is similar to the universal numbering system except the primary teeth are identified by letters from *A* to *T*. See also Appendix D.

unmedullated (unmed'yŏŏlāt'ed), not possessing a medulla or medullary substance.

unpolarized, not polarized; the absence of an electrical charge on a cell surface or process.

unsaturated fatty acid, any of a number of glyceryl esters of certain organic acids in which some of the atoms are joined by double or triple valence bonds. These bonds are split easily in chemical reaction, and other substances are joined to them. Monounsaturated fatty acids have only one double or triple bond per molecule and are found in such foods as fowl, almonds, pecans, cashew nuts, peanuts, and olive oil. Polyunsaturated fatty acids have more than one double or triple bond per molecule and are found in fish, corn, walnuts, sunflower seeds, soybeans, and safflower oil.

unsharpness, geometric. See **geometric unsharpness.**

unstable, 1. not firm or fixed in one place; likely to move. **2.** capable of undergoing spontaneous change. A nuclide in an unstable state is called *radioactive.* An atom in an unstable state is called *excited.*

u. angina, a form of pain that is prodromal to acute myocardial infarction. It typically has a sudden onset, sudden worsening, and stuttering recurrence over days and weeks. It carries a more severe short-term prognosis than stable chronic angina. Nearly one third of unstable angina patients may experience myocardial infarction within 3 months of the first episode.

upcode, using a procedure code that reflects a higher-intensity service than would normally be used for the services delivered.

upright arm. See **connector, minor.**

uprighting spring, an auxiliary wire used to torque roots mesially or distally.

uranium, a heavy, radioactive metallic element. Its atomic number is 92 and its atomic weight is 238.03. Uranium is the heaviest of the natural elements. Isotopes of uranium are used in nuclear power plants to provide neutrons for nuclear reactions that result in release of energy.

urban health, the health of a population who live and work closely to-

gether, usually in an incorporated area, such as a city or town, with a common water supply and with similar environmental conditions.

urban population, the population of an incorporated area, such as a city or town.

urease, an enzyme that divides urea into carbon dioxide and ammonia.

uremia (yŏŏrē'mē-ə), the presence of urinary components in the circulating blood and the resultant symptoms. Manifestations include weakness, headache, confusion, vomiting, and coma, and in terminal chronic renal disease, purpura and epistaxis may be present. Uremia is caused by insufficient urinary excretion for any reason. See also **stomatitis, uremic.**

ureteritis, an inflammatory condition of a ureter caused by infection or by the mechanic irritation of a kidney stone as it passes through the ureter.

urethane, ethyl carbamate used as an anesthetic agent for laboratory animals, formerly used as a hypnotic in humans.

urethritis, an inflammatory condition of the urethra that is characterized by dysuria, usually the result of an infection in the bladder or kidneys.

uric acid (yŏŏ'rik), a product of protein metabolism and present in the blood and urine. See also **gout.**

urinalysis (yŏŏr'inal'isis), a physical, microscopic, and chemical diagnostic examination of urine. Abnormal constituents indicate disease and can include ketone bodies, protein, bacteria, blood, glucose, pus, and certain types of crystals.

urinary tract, all organs and ducts involved in the secretion and elimination of urine from the body, principally the kidney, ureter, bladder, and urethra.

u. t. infection, an infection of one or more structures in the urinary tract. Gram-negative bacteria cause most of these infections.

urine, the fluid excreted by the kidneys. Normal urine is clear, straw-colored, and slightly acidic and has the characteristic odor of urea.

Urised, a trademark for a urinary fixed-combination drug containing an antibacterial (methenamine), an analgesic (phenyl salicylate), anticholin-

U

ergics (atropine sulfate and hyoscyamine), an antifungal (benzoic acid), and an antiseptic (methylene blue).

urobilin, a brown pigment formed by the oxidation of urobilinogen, normally found in feces and, in small amounts, in urine.

urokinase, an enzyme produced in the kidney and found in urine that is a potent plasminogen activator of the fibrinolytic system. A pharmaceutic preparation of urokinase is administered intravenously in the treatment of pulmonary embolism.

urology, the branch of medicine concerned with the study of the anatomy, physiology, and pathology of the urinary tract and with the care of the urinary tract of men and women and with the care of the male genital tract.

ursodiol, *trade names:* Actigall, Ursofalk; *class:* gallstone solubilizing agent; *action:* suppresses hepatic synthesis, secretion of cholesterol; inhibits intestinal absorption of cholesterol; *uses:* dissolution of radiolucent noncalcified gallstones of less than 20 mm in diameter, in which surgery is not indicated.

urticaria (ur'tiker'ē·ə) (hives), a vascular reaction pattern of the skin marked by the transient appearance of smooth, slightly elevated patches that are more red or more pale than the surrounding skin and are accompanied by severe itching.

u. bullosa, a skin eruption in which the lesions are capped by blisters.

u., giant. See **edema, angioneurotic.**

USAN Council, the United States Adopted Names Council, which is responsible for the selection of appropriate nonproprietary names for drugs used in the United States.

useful beam. See **beam, useful.**

user-friendly, simple for the unsophisticated user to master; used in reference to a computer operating system or software program.

USP See **United States Pharmacopeia.**

usual, customary, and reasonable (UCR) plan, a dental benefits plan that determines benefits based on usual, customary, and reasonable fee criteria. See also **usual fee, customary fee; reasonable fee.**

usual fee, the fee that an individual

dentist most frequently charges for a given dental service. See also **customary fee** and **reasonable fee.**

ut dict., abbreviation for *ut dictum,* a Latin phrase meaning "as directed."

utilization, 1. the extent to which a given group uses a particular service in a specified period of time. Although usually expressed as the number of services used per year per 100 or per 1000 persons eligible for the service, utilization rates may be expressed in other ratios. **2.** the extent to which the members of a covered group use a program over a stated time; specifically measured as a percentage determined by dividing the number of covered individuals who submitted one or more claims by the total number of covered individuals.

u. review (UR), **1.** analysis of the necessity, appropriateness, and efficiency of medical and dental services, procedures, facilities, and practitioners; in a hospital, this includes review of the appropriateness of admissions, services ordered and provided, and length of stay and discharge practices, on concurrent and retrospective bases. **2.** statistically based: a system that examines the distribution of treatment procedures based on claims information and, to be reasonably reliable, the application of such claims. Analyses of specific dentists should include data on type of practice, dentist's experience, socioeconomic characteristics, and geographic location.

utilization management, a set of techniques used by or on behalf of purchasers of health care benefits to manage the cost of health care before its provision by influencing patient-care decision-making through case-by-case assessments of the appropriateness of care based on accepted dental practices.

uveitis, inflammation of the uveal tract: iris, ciliary body, and choroid of the eye.

uveoparotitis (yōō'vē·ōper'ōtī'tis). See **fever, uveoparotid.**

uvula (yōō'vyələ), a general term indicating a pendent fleshy mass.

u., bifid, a congenital cleft resulting in a split uvula.

u., palatine, a small fleshy mass hanging from the posterior soft palate.

V

vaccination, any injection of attenuated microorganisms, such as bacteria, viruses, or rickettsiae, administered to induce immunity or to reduce the effect of associated infectious diseases.

vaccine (vak'sēn), agent prepared to produce active immunity that usually kills microbes, attenuated live microbes, or variant strains of microbes and that can induce antibody production without producing disease.

Vacudent (vak'ūdent), trade name for a high-volume suction apparatus designed to remove strongly but gently any fluids and debris from an operating field.

vacuole, a clear space in the substance of a cell. It may stem from a degenerative process or it may serve the cell as a temporary cell stomach for the digestion of a foreign body inclusion.

vacuum. See **oral evacuator.**

vacuum mixing. See **mixing, vacuum.**

vagomimetic (vā'gōməmetik), pertaining to a drug with actions similar to those produced by stimulation of the vagus nerve.

valacyclovir HCl, trade names: Valtex, Zeilirex; class: antiviral; action: converted to acyclovir, which interferes with DNA synthesis required for viral replication; uses: herpes zoster in immunocompetent patients.

valence, 1. in chemistry, a numeric expression of the capability of an element to combine chemically with atoms of hydrogen or their equivalent. **2.** in immunology, an expression of the number of antigen-binding sites for one molecule of any given antibody or the number of antibody-binding sites for any given antigen.

validation, an agreement of the listener with certain elements of the patient's communication.

validity, the degree to which data or results of a study are correct or true.

valine (val'ēn), one of the essential amino acids. See also **amino acid.**

Valium. See **diazepam.**

valproate sodium/valproate sodium-valproic acid/valproic acid, trade names: Depakene, Myproic Acid, Depakote; class: anticonvulsant; action: increased levels of γ-aminobutyric acid (GABA) in brain; uses: simple, complex (petit mal), absence, mixed seizures.

values, normal laboratory, generally, statistically and biologically significant qualitative and/or quantitative measurements of cellular and clinical components of the body. The values derived from such measurements are based on averages of a survey of presumably healthy persons. The concept of individual normal values is based on an acceptable response (comparable with known evidence of health or disease) of the individual to a known alteration of cellular and/or chemical components or systems.

values, phonetic (fənet'ik), the character or quality of vocal sounds.

valve, a structure that controls flow of the contents of a canal or passage.

v., exhalation, a valve that permits escape of exhaled gases into the atmosphere and prevents them from being rebreathed.

valve system, the accepted mode of conduct and the set of norms, goals, and values binding any social group that serve as a frame of reference for the individual in reaching decisions and achieving a meaningful life.

vancomycin HCl, trade name: Vancocin; class: glucopeptide-type antiinfective; action: inhibits bacterial cell wall synthesis; uses: resistant staphylococcal infections, pseudomembranous colitis, staphylococcal enterocolitis, endocarditis prophylaxis for dental procedures.

van den Bergh's test. See **test, van den Bergh's.**

vapor, 1. the gaseous form assumed by a solid or liquid when sufficiently heated. **2.** a visible emanation of fine particles of a liquid.

Vaquez's disease (vəkāz'). See **erythremia.**

variability, the degree or range of divergence of an object from a given standard or average.

variable, 1. changing; able to vary in quantity or magnitude. **2.** a characteristic that may assume several values.

v., continuous, a variable for which it is possible to find an intermediate value between any two values. Continuous variables can be refined by more precise values. Length, weight, and time, and the points on a line are continuous variables.

v., control, those variables not being studied that are held constant so as not to influence the experimental outcome. Environmental conditions, intelligence quotients, and social and psychologic variables are examples of variables that must be controlled.

v. costs, costs, such as dental service claims, that generally increase or decrease as the size and composition of the enrollment fluctuates.

v., dependent, a variable whose value is consequent on change in the independent variable. The dependent variable is always the response or reaction to the independent variable. Synonym: criterion variable.

v., discrete, a variable that is expressed in whole units or mutually exclusive categories. Whole numbers and category designations such as sex and marital status are examples of discrete data.

v., independent, the variable being studied that is manipulated or controlled by an experimenter. In a drug study an experiment may give several doses of a drug (independent variable) to determine the most effective, symptom-reducing (dependent variable) level.

variance, a measure of dispersion; the value of standard deviation squared. In some statistical computations the use of variance is preferred to standard deviation.

variation (genetic), deviation from the genotype in structure, form, physiology, or behavior.

varicella (ver′isel′ə) (chickenpox), an acute communicable disease with an incubation period of 2 or 3 weeks and caused by herpesvirus, usually found in children. Manifestations include coryza, fever, malaise, and headache, followed in 2 or 3 days by the eruption of macular vesicles.

varicosity (ver′ikos′itē), an abnormal condition characterized by the presence of tortuous, abnormally dilated veins, usually in the legs or the lower trunk; may also appear in the esophagus.

variola (ver′ē·ō′lə) (smallpox), an acute, viral, contagious disease transmitted by the respiratory route and direct contact. The incubation period is 1 to 2 weeks. Manifestations include headache, chills, and temperature up to 106° F. On the third and fourth day, macules appear, which then become papules; then constitutional symptoms abate. On the sixth day the papules become vesicles. The vesicles then become pustules, with desquamation occurring in about 2 weeks.

varnish (cavity liner, cavity varnish), a clear solution of resinous material or natural gum, such as copal or rosin dissolved in acetone, ether, or chloroform, which is capable of hardening without losing its transparency. Varnish is used in cavity preparations to seal out dentinal tubules, reduce microleakage, and insulate the pulp against shock from thermal changes.

vascular diseases, diseases of the peripheral circulatory system.

vascular reactions, the response of the blood vessels to injury or introduction of chemical agents, particularly certain chemical mediators such as histamine and bradykinin.

vascular resistance, the degree to which the blood vessels impede the flow of blood. High resistance causes an increase in blood pressure, which increases the workload of the heart.

vascular spasm, a sudden constriction of the blood vessels causing reduction or stoppage in blood flow. A vascular spasm in vessels of the brain can result in stroke and in the vessels of the heart can result in a "heart attack."

vasculitis, an inflammatory condition of the blood vessels that is characteristic of certain systemic diseases or that is caused by an allergic reaction.

vasoconstrictor (vas′ōkənstrik′tər) (vasopressor), an agent that causes a rise in blood pressure by constricting the blood vessels. In local areas, it causes constriction of the arterioles and capillaries.

vasodepressor (vāz′ōdəpres′ər), an agent that depresses circulation and causes vasomotor depression.

vasodilator (vāz′ōdī′lātər), **1.** an agent that causes dilation of the blood ves-

V

sels. **2.** a drug that relaxes the smooth muscle walls of the blood vessels and increases their diameter.

vasomotor (văz'ōmō'tər), pertaining to any agent or nerve that causes expansion or contraction of the walls of blood vessels.

vasopressin (văz'ōpres'in). See **hormone, antidiuretic.**

vasopressor (văz'ōpres'ər). See **vasoconstrictor.**

vault, I. an anatomic part resembling an arched roof or dome, such as the vault of a denture. **2.** a cavity or specially prepared area within the jawbone for placement of an implant magnet.

V-bends, V-shaped bends placed in an orthodontic arch wire, usually mesially to the canines. The V-bends create an adjustment site at which torquing bends may be placed.

VDRL test, abbreviation for *Venereal Disease Research Laboratory test,* a serologic flocculation test for syphilis or yaws.

vehicle (vē'hikəl), a pharmaceutic ingredient, usually a liquid, employed as a medium for dissolving or dispersing the active drug in a mass suitable for its administration.

Veillonella alcalescens (vā'yənel'ə alkəles'enz), **I.** an organism of the genus *Veillonella.* **2.** a schizomycete that has been found in the flora of the periodontal pocket and, by association, has been implicated in the origin and perpetuation of periodontitis in human beings.

vein (vān), a blood vessel that conducts blood from the capillary bed to the heart. Size may range from the venules to small veins to large veins.

velopharyngeal adequacy (vē'lōfərin'jē-əl). See **closure, velopharyngeal.**

velopharyngeal closure. See **closure, velopharyngeal.**

velopharyngeal inadequacy. See **inadequacy, velopharyngeal.**

veneer (vənēr'), in the construction of crowns or pontics, a layer of tooth-colored material, usually porcelain or acrylic resin, attached to the surface by direct fusion, cementation, or mechanical retention.

venereal disease (venēr'e·əl), any contagious condition acquired by sexual intercourse or genital contact.

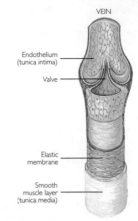

VEIN

Endothelium (tunica intima)

Valve

Elastic membrane

Smooth muscle layer (tunica media)

Cross-section of a vein. (Thompson, 1997.)

Venereal diseases include chancroid, gonorrhea, granuloma inguinale, herpes simplex type II, HIV, lymphogranuloma venereum, and syphilis.

venereal wart (condyloma acuminatum), a soft, wartlike growth found on the warm, moist skin and mucous membranes of the genitalia, caused by a virus and transmitted by sexual contact. Synonym: acuminate wart. (not current)

venipuncture (ven'əpungk'chər), surgical or therapeutic puncture of a vein.

venlafaxine HCl, *trade name:* Effexor; *class:* bicyclic antidepressant; *action:* inhibits both norepinephrine and serotonin (5-HT) uptake and to a lesser extent dopamine; *use:* depression.

ventilate, I. to provide with fresh air. **2.** to provide the lungs with air from the atmosphere. **3.** to open to free, uninhibited discussion or to openly express one's feelings.

ventilation (ven'tilā'shən), the constant supplying of oxygen through the lungs.

v., air, the process of supplying alveoli with air or oxygen.

v., respiratory, the process of getting air into and out of the lungs. The air enters the mouth and nose and must go through the conduction system (the pharynx, larynx, trachea, and bronchial tree) into the lungs. This ventilating process involves many other structures as well, including the abdomen, thorax, and maxillofacial tissues. The latter structures make two significant contributions to the respiratory process: they provide the portal of entry and egress for the air to and from the lungs, and they alter the physical properties of inspired air for protection of the very sensitive lung tissues.

venting, an exit passage constructed in a casting mold to allow gases to escape during the casting process.

ventricle, a small cavity, such as one of the cavities filled with cerebrospinal fluid in the brain, or the right and left ventricles of the heart.

ventricular dysfunction, abnormalities in contraction and wall motion within the ventricles.

ventricular fibrillation (VF), a cardiac dysrhythmia marked by rapid, disorganized depolarizations of the ventricular myocardium. The condition is characterized by a complete lack of organized electric impulse, conduction, and ventricular contraction. Blood pressure falls to zero, resulting in unconsciousness. Death may occur within 4 minutes. Defibrillation and ventilation, i.e., cardiopulmonary resuscitation (CPR), must be initiated immediately.

ventricular function, the cyclic contraction and relaxation of the ventricular myocardium.

ventricular septal defect (VSD), an abnormal opening in the septum separating the ventricles of the heart. It is the most common congenital heart defect. Children with small defects are usually without symptoms. Large defects can prevent proper oxygenation of the blood and may initiate congestive heart failure, if not surgically corrected.

ventriculoureterostomy, a surgical procedure for directing cerebrospinal fluid into the general circulation performed in the treatment of hydrocephalus, usually in the newborn.

venue (ven′yoo), the neighborhood, place, or county in which an injury is declared to have occurred or fact is declared to have happened; also designates the county in which an action or prosecution is presented for trial.

venule (ven′yool), the smallest of the venous blood vessels; consists of an endothelial tube enclosed in a variable amount of elastic and collagenous tissue. Smooth muscle is introduced in the media as the caliber of the vessel increases. The muscle fibers are distributed sparsely in the smaller vessels and coalesce into circumferential bands in the larger vessels.

verapamil HCl, *trade names:* Calan, Isoptin, Calan SR, Isoptin SR, others; *class:* calcium-channel blocker; *action:* inhibits calcium ion influx across cell membrane during cardiac depolarization; produces relaxation of coronary vascular smooth muscle, dilates coronary arteries, decreases SA/AV node conduction, and dilates peripheral arteries; *uses:* chronic stable angina pectoris, vasospastic angina, dysrhythmias, hypertension.

verbal, by word of mouth; oral, as in a verbal agreement.

verdict, the formal decision or finding of a jury on the matters or questions duly submitted to them at a trial.

vermilion border, 1. the junction between the lip and the facial skin. **2.** the external pinkish to reddish area of the upper and lower lips, extending from the junction of the lips, with the surrounding facial skin on the exterior to the labial mucosa within the mouth.

vernier (ver′nē-or). See **gauge, Boley.**

Verocay body (ver′ōkā). See **body, Verocay.** (not current)

verruca (vəroo′kə), a benign, viral, warty skin lesion with a rough, papillomatous surface. It is caused by a common contagious papovavirus.

v. senilis (sənil′is). See **keratosis, seborrheic.**

v. vulgaris (wart), a common wart of the skin or mucosa.

verrucous carcinoma (veroo′kəs kar′sinō′mə), a squamous cell carcinoma, usually intraoral, which is exophytic and has a papillary appearance.

vertebra, any one of the 33 bones of the spinal or vertebral column, which comprise the 7 cervical, 12 thoracic, 5 lumbar, 5 sacral, and 4 coccygeal vertebrae.

vertical, perpendicular to the horizontal plane.

v. angulation. See **angulation, vertical.**

v. dimension. See **dimension, vertical.**

v. lug. See **connector, minor.**

v. opening. See **dimension, vertical.**

v. overlap. See **overlap, vertical.**

v. relation. See **relation, vertical.**

vertical-integrated health care, a health care delivery system in which the complete spectrum of care, including financial services, is provided within a single organization, such as a health maintenance organization (HMO).

vertigo (ver'təgo), 1. a sensation described as dizziness. 2. a sensation of the room revolving about the patient or the patient revolving in space. It is a form of dizziness, but the terms are not synonymous.

vesicant (ves'ikənt), a chemically active substance that can produce blistering on direct contact with the skin or mucous membrane.

vesicle (ves'ikəl), 1. a small, blisterlike elevation of the skin or mucous membrane resulting from an intraepithelial collection of fluid. It is a primary type of lesion and may be seen in herpes simplex, recurrent herpes, recurrent aphthae, stomatitis medicamentosa, stomatitis venenata, erythema multiforme, Reiter's syndrome, Behçet's syndrome, Stevens-Johnson syndrome, herpangina, varicella, and many others. 2. a circumscribed, elevated lesion of the skin containing fluid and having a diameter up to 5 mm.

vessels, blood, visualization of, any one of various methods by which the blood vessels are seen by the examiner. Direct visualization of blood vessels is possible only to a limited extent. The blood vessels in the retina can be directly visualized; the capillary loops in the fingernail can be seen by microscopy, and the blood vessels in the oral mucosa and gingivae can be visualized by infrared photography. More recently, radiography and cineradiography are used to visualize radiopaque substances. These methods can reveal the actual blood column, its width, variation in contour, and pathway. Arteriograms and venograms are useful in revealing spasms, obstructions, congenital defects, and collateral circulation of the deeper tissues.

vested, a nonforfeitable interest of a participant in a pension plan.

vestibule, buccal, the space between the alveolar ridge and teeth or residual ridge and the cheek distal to the buccal frenum.

vestibule, lower buccal, the space between the mandibular alveolar ridge and teeth and the cheek; bounded anteriorly by the lower buccal frenum and posteriorly by the distobuccal end of the retromolar pad.

vestibule, upper buccal, the space between the maxillary alveolar ridge and teeth or the residual ridge and the cheek; bounded anteriorly by the upper buccal frenum and posteriorly by the hamular notch.

vestibule, labial, the space between the alveolar ridge and the teeth or the residual ridge and lips anterior to the buccal frenum.

vestibule of the oral cavity, the part of the oral cavity that lies between the teeth and gingivae and lips and cheeks or between the residual ridges and lips and cheeks.

vestibuloplasty (vestib'yəlōplas'tē), any of a series of surgical procedures designed to restore alveolar ridge height by lowering muscles attaching to the buccal, labial, and lingual aspects of the jaws.

veteran, 1. a person who has a long period of service in an occupation or profession. 2. a person who has served in the armed forces, especially one who has fought for his or her country. 3. a long-serving member of a state legislature or the U.S. Congress.

veterinarian, a Doctor of Veterinary Medicine, who is educated and trained to provide medical and surgical care for domestic and exotic animals.

viable (vī'əbəl), capable of life; able to live.

Viadent, brand name for an antiplaque mouthrinse containing sanguinarine, an alkaloid, as the active ingredient. See also **sanguinarine.**

vibrating line. See **line, vibrating.**

Vicat needle (vēkah') See **needle, Vicat.**

Vickers hardness number. See **number, Vickers hardness.**

Vickers hardness test. See **test, Vickers hardness.**

Vicodin, brand name for hyrocodone, a ketone derivative of codeine that is about six times more potent than codeine. Vicodin is a controlled substance.

vidarabine (ophthalmic), *trade name:* Vira-A Ophthalmic; *class:* antiviral; *action:* inhibits DNA synthesis by blocking DNA polymerase; *use:* keratoconjunctivitis due to herpes simplex virus.

Vincent's angina. See **angina, Vincent's.** (not current)

Vincent's bacillus. See *Fusobacterium fusiforme.* (not current)

Vincent's gingivitis. See **gingivitis, necrotizing ulcerative.** (not current)

Vincent's infection. See **gingivitis, necrotizing ulcerative.** (not current)

Vincent's organism. See **organism, Vincent's.** (not current)

vinegar (as a solvent), a warm, dilute solution of household vinegar; used as a substitute for acetic acid to dissolve accumulated dental calculus from a removable dental prosthesis.

Vinethene (vin'ethēn), trade name for vinyl ether.

vinyl resin (vī'nil). See **resin, vinyl.**

violation, injury; encroachment; breach of right, obligation, or law.

violence, severe physical force; the forceful assault of a person.

violet, gentian (vī·əlit, jen'shən), a rosaniline dye, useful as a protective covering and an antiseptic in the treatment of minor lesions of the oral mucosa. It is an effective fungicide and is therefore of value in the treatment of moniliasis.

violet stain. See **stain, methyl violet.**

viral hepatitis. See **hepatitis.**

viral infection, an infection by any of the more than 200 pathogenic viruses. A virus acts on the cell nucleus, taking over the genetic material within the nucleus and replicating itself.

virology, the scientific study of viruses and the diseases caused by viruses.

virulence, the power of a microorganism to produce disease.

virus (vī'rəs), one of a group of heterogeneous infective agents characterized by the lack of independent metabolism or the ability to replicate outside the host cell.

v., herpes simplex. See **herpes simplex.**

v. replication, the ability of viruses to reproduce within a host cell.

viscera, the internal organs enclosed within a body cavity, primarily the abdominal organs.

viscosity, the ability or inability of a fluid solution to flow easily. High viscosity indicates a slow-flowing fluid.

visible light, the radiant energy in the electromagnetic spectrum that is visible to the human eye. The wavelengths cover a range of approximately 390 to 780 nm.

vision (vizh'ən), sight; the faculty of seeing.

v., field of, the portion of space that the fixed eye can see.

v., stereoscopic, vision in which the visual fields of the two eyes are unified. Sensations from a common object received by the two eyes are superimposed, and as a result of the slight differences in the fields and the superimposition of the fields, the effects of depth and shape of the object are attained.

visit, a meeting between a health care professional and a patient for diagnostic, therapeutic, or consultative reasons, usually a scheduled appointment in a professional office. Also called *patient visit* or *patient encounter.*

visual acuity, a measure of the resolving power of the eye, particularly with its ability to distinguish letters and numbers at a given distance. See also **acuity, visual.**

visual disorders. See **disorders, visual.**

visual treatment objective (VTO), a diagnostic and communication aid, consisting of a cephalometric tracing, modified to show changes anticipated in the course of growth and treatment.

vital, necessary to or pertaining to life.

v. capacity, a measurement of the amount of air that can be expelled at the normal rate of exhalation after a maximum inspiration, representing the greatest possible breathing capacity.

v. signs, the measurements of pulse rate, respiration rate, and body temperature. Although not strictly a vital sign, blood pressure is also customarily included in this category.

v. statistics, data relating to births (natality), deaths (mortality), marriages, health, and disease (morbidity).

vitalometer (vī′təlom′ əter), an electric-powered instrument for delivering and measuring an electrical stimulus to a tooth. See also **pulp tester.**

vitalometry (vī′təlom′ ətrē), the use of high-frequency pulp-testing equipment to establish the vital condition of the pulp of a tooth.

vitamin (vī′təmin), one of a number of unrelated organic substances that occur in small amounts in food and are required for normal metabolic activity. The vitamins may be water soluble or fat soluble.

v. A (retinal, retinol, retinoic acid), a fat-soluble substance, occurring in several chemical forms in food and function: retinal, an aldehyde; retinol, an alcohol; and retinoic acid, an acid. All three function in calcified and epithelial tissue growth. The aldehyde-alcohol (retinal-retinol) interconversion allows regeneration of rhodopsin (visual purple) in the rod cells of the retina. A deficiency results in hyperkeratinization of nonsecretory protective epithelium, deranged secretory function of the mucous membrane, dark dysadaptation (night blindness) and possibly, enamel hypoplasia. Dietary sources include the liver, kidney, and lung as well as carotenes (provitamins A) from the plant kingdom.

v., ascorbic acid (əskôr′bik) *(vitamin C, antiscorbutic factor),* a water-soluble vitamin resembling glucose in structure; it is found in citrus fruits, tomatoes, cabbage, and other fresh fruits and vegetables. Necessary for hydroxylation of peptide-bound lysine and proline to hydroxylysine and hydroxyproline during collagen synthesis. A deficiency leads to scurvy, in which pathologic signs are confined mainly to the connective tissues with hemorrhages, loosening of teeth, gingivitis, and poor wound healing.

v. B complex, collectively, the various B vitamins: thiamine, riboflavin, nicotinic acid, pyridoxine, biotin, *para*-aminobenzoic acid, folic acid, pantothenic acid, cyanocobalamin, pteroylglutamic acid, and others that are unknown.

v. B₁. See **vitamin, thiamine.**

v. B₂. See **vitamin, riboflavin.**

v. B₆. See **vitamin, pyridoxine.**

v. B₁₂. See **vitamin, cobalamin.**

v., biotin (bī′ ətin) *(vitamin H, anti-egg-white factor),* one of the B complex vitamins found in organ meats (e.g., liver, heart, kidney), egg yolk, cauliflower, chocolate, and mushrooms. Its synthesis by intestinal bacteria makes human deficiency states rare, unless the diet contains significant raw egg white protein (avidin), which complexes the vitamin to prevent intestinal absorption. Dermatitis, retarded growth, and loss of hair and muscular control occur in experimental animals. Biotin functions as a coenzyme for carboxylase enzymes that catalyze fixation of carbon dioxide (e.g., in fatty acid synthesis).

v. C. See **vitamin, ascorbic acid.**

v., calciferol. See **vitamin D.**

v., cholecalciferol. See **vitamin D.**

v., choline (kō′lēn) *(trimethylamino-ethanol),* not truly a vitamin, because it can be synthesized in the body if sufficient precursors are available. Prevents the accumulation of fat in the liver of certain animal species. Occurs as a constituent of lecithin, sphingomyelin, and acetylcholine.

v., cobalamin (kōbôl′ əmin) *(antipernicious factor, vitamin B₁₂, cyanocobalamin, erythrocyte maturing factor [EMF], extrinsic factor),* a vitamin that contains cobalt and is essential for the maturation of erythrocytes. Inability of the body to produce intrinsic factor, which is necessary for vitamin B₁₂ absorption, results in pernicious anemia. Liver, kidney, muscle, and milk are good sources.

v. D (antirachitic factor, calciferol, cholecalciferol, ergosterol, ergocalciferol), the group of lipid-soluble sterol compounds capable of preventing rickets. Of primary importance are D₂, or ergosterol, from plants and D₃, or cholecalciferol, from animal sources, especially fish liver oils. The latter is also formed in the skin from 7-dehydrocholesterol on exposure to ultraviolet light. Liver mitochondria further activate vitamin D to 25-(OH)-D, which in turn is metabolized to 1,25-(OH)₂-D by the kidney. The dihydroxy metabolites significantly increase dietary calcium absorption and bone resorption to maintain proper blood calcium and phosphorus levels. A primary vitamin D deficiency results from inadequate expo-

V

sure to sunlight and low dietary intake. Secondary deficiencies occur from abnormalities of intestinal resorption and interference with vitamin D hydroxylation. The manifestations of rickets include enamel hypoplasia, poorly calcified bones, bowed legs, and a deformed rib cage with beadlike swellings of the ribs (rachitic rosary) in infants and children and osteomalacia in adults. Vitamin D intake in excess is toxic.

v. E (tocopherol, tocotrienol antisterility factor), the tocopherol and tocotrienols have varying degrees of vitamin E activity but α-tocopherol is the most active. These fat-soluble compounds are found in eggs, muscle meats, liver, fish, chicken, oatmeal, and the oils of corn, soya, and cottonseed. In rats, the lack of vitamin E leads to fetus resorption in the female and atrophy of spermatogenic tissue with permanent sterility in the male. Vitamin E deficiency in humans is correlated with increased hemolysis of erythrocytes. The tocopherols prevent peroxidation of unsaturated fatty acids, and vitamin E requirements appear to be directly related to the dietary intake of unsaturated fatty acids. Although animals develop symptoms of muscular dystrophy on deficient diets, the vitamin has no effect on the human disease.

v., ergocalciferol. See **vitamin D.**

v., folacin (adermine, folic acid, citrovorum factor, pteroylglutamic acid, vitamin M, vitamin B_c), occurs in many tissues as the free acid or is conjugated with one to seven glutamic acid molecules. Green, leafy vegetables; kidney; liver; and yeast are good sources and bacterial synthesis in humans occurs readily. As a coenzyme, the vitamin serves as a carrier of one-carbon units (formyl, hydroxymethyl, formimino groups) especially in the synthesis of nucleoproteins. Inadequate folate levels produce a variety of species-dependent symptoms that include megaloblastic anemia in humans.

v. G. See **vitamin, riboflavin.**

v. H. See **vitamin, biotin.**

v., inositol (inō′sətōl, inos′ətōl), *(myo-inositol,* meso-*inositol),* a six-carbon alcohol closely related to the hexoses. Inositol is not truly a vita-

min, because the body can synthesize significant amounts from glucose. Its biologic role is not established, but it is essential to the growth of liver and bone marrow cells and helps alleviate fatty livers.

v. K (phytonadione, antihemorrhagic factor), one of the many fat-soluble naphthoquinone compounds with vitamin D activity. Vitamin K_1 is found primarily in leafy vegetables, K_2 is synthesized by human intestinal bacteria, and K_3 (menadione, N.F.) is a synthetic compound. Vitamin K is essential for the synthesis of prothrombin by the liver. A dietary deficiency of vitamin K is rare, however. The vitamin has been used in conjunction with extensive oral antibiotic therapy to treat hemorrhagic disease of the newborn, hemorrhage of obstructive jaundice, and sprue, and during anticoagulant therapy. Prothrombin, Stuart factor, Christmas factor, and serum prothrombin conversion accelerator require vitamin K for their synthesis.

v., niacin (nī′əsin) *(nicotinic acid, nicotinamide, niacinamide, pellagra-preventive factor),* a deficiency of niacin or its amide derivative, niacinamide, results in acute pellagra that is characterized by dermatitis, diarrhea, dementia, stomatitis, and glossitis. Dietary sources include liver, kidney, lean meats, wheat germ, yeast, soybeans, and peanuts. There is some intestinal synthesis by bacteria. Although the amino acid tryptophan contributes to the body supply of niacin, sufficient vitamin B_6 must be present for its metabolism. Niacin and niacinamide are interconvertible in the body, and the latter functions as a constituent of two coenzymes, NAD and NADP, which operate as hydrogen and electron transfer agents by virtue of their reversible oxidation and reduction in several enzyme systems.

v., pantothenic acid (pan′təthen′ik) *(pantothen, panthenol),* this vitamin is a component of coenzyme A and thereby functions in the metabolism of lipids, carbohydrates, and proteins. A deficiency is unusual because of its wide distribution, but a "burning feet syndrome" has been reported in people suffering from acute malnutrition.

v., pyridoxine (pir′ədok′sēn) *(vitamin B₆, pyridoxal, pyridoxol, pyridoxamine),* part of the B-complex vitamins, the group includes three chemically related substances: pyridoxol, pyridoxal, and pyridoxamine, all of which serve as substrate in the formation of pyridoxal phosphate, the prosthetic group for several enzymes that decarboxylate, deaminate, transaminate, or desulfurate specific amino acids. It further functions in porphyrin, fatty acids, and cholesterol metabolism. Deficiency signs include an acrodynia-like syndrome, convulsive seizures, arteriosclerotic-like lesions, hypochromic microcytic anemia, and impaired antibody formation. Dietary sources include wheat, corn, liver, milk, eggs, and green, leafy vegetables.

v., retinal. See **vitamin A.**

v., retinoic acid. See **vitamin A.**

v., retinol. See **vitamin A.**

v., riboflavin (rī′bōflā′vin) *(vitamin B₂, vitamin G, lactoflavin),* a heat-stable B complex vitamin that functions as a component of FAD and FMN for the reversible transfer of hydrogen and electrons in several enzyme systems. It is found in green, leafy vegetables; whole grains; eggs; liver; milk; and legumes; small amounts are synthesized in the intestinal tract by microorganisms. Signs of ariboflavinosis include angular stomatitis, seborrheic dermatitis of the face, and glossitis (magenta tongue).

v., thiamine (thī′əmin) *(vitamin B₁, aneurine, antiberiberi factor, antineuritic factor),* a B-complex vitamin found primarily in plants, especially legumes, whole grains, and green, leafy vegetables; it is also synthesized by bacteria in the large intestine, which is not a reliable source. Thiamine pyrophosphate (TPP, cocarboxylase) is a coenzyme in the oxidative decarboxylation of pyruvate and α-ketoglutarate, in the transketolase reaction of glucose metabolism and in the metabolism of branched chained amino acids. A deficiency results in beriberi.

v., tocopherol. See **vitamin E.**

v., tocotrienol. See **vitamin E.**

vitiate (vish′ē-āt), to weaken; to make void or voidable.

vitiligo (vit′ilē′gō, vit′ili′gō), a skin condition characterized by spotty areas of depigmentation.

vitrification (vit′rifikā′shən), the act, instance, art, or process of converting dental porcelain (frit) to a glassy substance; the process of becoming vitreous by heat and fusion.

VLDL, abbreviation for *very-low-density lipids.*

vocabulary, 1. the stock or range of words possessed by an individual or a culture used for self-expression or communication. **2.** the sum of the distinct words related to a discipline or profession.

vocal cords. See **cords, vocal.**

voice, sound produced primarily by the vibration of the vocal bands.

void, 1. empty or unfilled space. **2.** space not filled with anything solid. **3.** ineffectual; having no legal, binding effect.

volatile (vol′ətəl), having a tendency to evaporate rapidly.

v. oil. See **oil, essential.**

volt, the unit of electromotive force or electrical pressure; the force necessary to cause 1 ampere of current to flow against 1 ohm of resistance. A volt is the unit that is used to measure the tendency of a charge to move from one place to another.

v., electron (eV), the kinetic energy gained by an electron by falling through a potential difference of 1 volt. 1 eV is equivalent to 1.6×10^{-12} ergs. 1000 eV is referred to as 1 *kilo electron volt,* or *keV,* and 1,000,000 eV are referred to as 1 *mega electron volt,* or *MeV.*

voltage, the potential of electromotive force of an electric charge, measured in volts.

volume, measure of the quantity of space occupied by a substance, such as air.

v., blood, the total amount of blood in the body.

v., expiratory reserve (reserve air, supplemental air, supplemental volume), the maximum volume that can be expired from the resting expiratory level.

v. index of blood. See **blood, volume index of.**

v., inspiratory reserve (complemental air), the maximum volume that can be inspired from the end of tidal inspiration.

v., packed-cell. See **hematocrit.**

v., residual (residual air), the volume of air in the lungs at the end of maximal expiration.

v., stroke. See **stroke volume.**

v., supplemental. See **volume, expiratory reserve.**

v., tidal (tidal air), the volume of gas inspired or expired during each respiratory cycle.

vomer, the bone forming the posterior and inferior part of the nasal septum and having two surfaces and four borders.

vomiting, the forcible voluntary or involuntary emptying of the stomach contents through the mouth.

von Recklinghausen's disease of bone (von rek'linghou'senz). See **hyperparathyroidism** and **osteitis fibrosa cystica, generalized.**

von Recklinghausen's disease of skin. See **neurofibromatosis.**

voucher, a receipt or release that may serve as notice of payment of a debt or may prove the accuracy of accounts.

vowel, a conventional vocal sound in the production of which the speech organs offer little obstruction to the airstream and form a series of resonators above the level of the larynx.

vs, abbreviation for *versus* (against); commonly used in legal proceedings, particularly in designating the title of cases.

vulcanite (vul'kənīt), a hard material with a form of rubber as the base; formerly used for denture bases.

vulcanization (vul'kəniza'shən), the process of treating crude rubber to improve such qualities as strength and hardness. This process usually involves heating the rubber with sulfur in the presence of moisture, the sulfur uniting with the rubber to produce saturated double bonds.

vulcanize (vul'kənīz), to produce flexible or hard rubber, as desired, by subjecting caoutchouc, in the presence of sulfur, to heat and high-steam pressure in a vulcanizer. (not current)

VZ virus, varicella zoster virus, which causes chickenpox in humans.

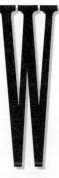

wages, the compensation to an employee, agreed on by the employee and employer, for work completed by the employee.

waiting period, the period of time between employment or enrollment in a dental program and the date when an insured person becomes eligible for benefits.

waiver (wā'ver), **1.** repudiation, abandonment, or surrender of a claim, right, or privilege. **2.** the intentional relinquishment of a known right.

walker, an extremely light, movable apparatus, about waist high, made of metal tubing, used to assist a patient in walking. It has four widely placed, sturdy legs. The patient holds onto the walker and takes a step, then moves the walker forward and takes another step.

wall, the outside layer of material surrounding an object or space; a paries.

w., cavity, one of the enclosing sides of a prepared cavity. It takes the name of the surface of the tooth adjoining the surface involved and toward which it is placed. Parts of a surrounding or peripheral wall are the cavosurface angle, the enamel wall, the dentinoenamel junction, and the dentin wall.

w., enamel, the portion of the wall of a prepared cavity that consists of enamel.

w., finish of enamel, the planing of the enamel in finishing a cavity preparation; includes the treatment of the cavosurface angle.

w., gingival cavity, the peripheral wall that most closely approximates the apical end of the tooth.

w., incisal, the wall of a prepared cavity in an anterior tooth that is closest to or in direct relation to the incisal edge of the tooth.

w., peripheral cavity. See **wall, surrounding cavity.**

w., surrounding cavity (peripheral cavity wall), one of the external, bounding side walls of a cavity; one side forms a part of the cavosurface angle of the preparation.

Walter Reed staging system, an alternative classification system used to describe various stages of HIV infection. See **Centers for Disease Control classification.**

wandering rash. See **geographic tongue.**

Wanscher's mask (vän'shərz). See **mask, Wanscher's.**

ward, a person, especially one under the age of majority, placed by authority of law under the care of a guardian.

warfarin sodium, *trade names:* Coumadin, Panwarfin, Sofarin; *class:* oral anticoagulant; *action:* interferes with blood clotting by indirect means; depresses hepatic synthesis of vitamin K-dependent coagulation factors (II, VII, IX, and X); *uses:* pulmonary emboli, deep vein thrombosis, MI, atrial dysrhythmias.

warp, uncontrolled torsional change of shape or outline, such as that which may occur in swaging sheet metal, in denture material, or in other materials exposed to varying temperatures.

wart. See **verruca vulgaris.**

Warthin's tumor. See **cystadenoma, papillary** and **lymphomatosum.**

wash, Karo syrup, a mixture of Karo syrup in warm water (1 tablespoon per ½ glass [4 ounces] warm water), used as a protective, soothing rinse in the treatment of inflammatory lesions of the oral mucous membrane. (not current)

Wassermann test. See **test, Wassermann.**

waste products, the products of metabolic activity after oxygen and nutrients have been supplied to a cell. These include primarily carbon dioxide and water, along with sodium chloride and soluble nitrogenous salts, which are excreted in feces, urine, and exhaled air.

wasting, a process of deterioration marked by weight loss and decreased physical vigor, appetite, and mental activity.

water, a tasteless, odorless, colorless compound made of hydrogen and oxygen (H_2O), which freezes at 32° F (0° C) and boils at 212° F (100° C). The autonomic nervous system regulates water balance in the body.

w. depletion, cellular dehydration through decreased water intake, dysphagia, excessive sweating, and diuresis.

w. need, the amount of water needed to maintain metabolism, approximately 1000 ml/day.

w. syringe. See **syringe, water.**

water:powder ratio. See **ratio, water:powder.**

Waters extraoral radiographic examination. See **examination, Waters extraoral radiographic.** (not current)

Waters view. See **examination, Waters extraoral radiographic.**

Watson-Crick helix, a model of the DNA molecule proposed by Watson and Crick as two righthanded polynucleotide chains coiled around the same axis as a double helix.

watt (W), the unit of electric power or work; 1 W of power is dissipated when a current of 1 ampere (A) flows across a difference in potential of 1 volt (V).

wave, electromagnetic, energy manifested by movements in an advancing series of alternate elevations and depressions.

wavelength, the distance between the peaks of waves in any wave form, such as light, x-rays, and other electromotive forms. In electromagnetic radiation, the wavelength is equal to the velocity of light divided by the frequency of the wave.

w., effective, the wavelength that would produce the same penetration as an average of the various wavelengths in a heterogeneous bundle of x-rays.

wax, one of several esters of fatty acids with higher alcohols, usually monohydric alcohols. Dental waxes are combinations of various types of waxes compounded to provide the desired physical properties.

w., baseplate, a hard, pink wax used for making occlusion rims and baseplates for occlusion rims.

w., bone, a plastic mixture that may contain antiseptic and hemostatic drugs, designed for temporary application to freshly cut bone to prevent hemorrhage and infection.

w., boxing, a soft wax used for boxing impressions.

W

w. burnout. See **burnout, inlay** and **wax elimination.**

w., carnauba (karnou'bə), a hard, high-melting wax used for the control of the melting range of dental waxes.

w., casting, a composition containing various waxes with controlled properties of thermal expansion and contraction; used in making patterns to determine the shape of metal castings.

w. elimination (wax burnout), the procedure of removing the wax from a wax pattern invested in a mold preparatory to the introduction of another material into the resulting cavity. This may be done by dry heat alone or by irrigation with boiling water followed by use of dry heat.

w. expansion, expanding wax patterns to compensate for the shrinkage of gold during the casting process.

w., fluid, a series of waxes, each having different physical properties, used for making a correctable impression of the foundation structures that are to support a denture base. The term indicates that the wax is applied in fluid form as required.

w. inlay. See **wax casting.**

w. out. See **blockout.**

w. pattern. See **pattern, wax.**

w. template. See **template, wax.**

waxing (waxing up), the contouring of a wax pattern or the wax base of a trial denture into the desired form.

WBC, abbreviation for *white blood cell.* See also **leukocyte** and **white blood cell count.**

weaning, the process of withdrawing an infant from breast milk or formula and instituting nourishment with other food.

wear, a loss of substance or a diminishing through use, friction, or other destructive factors.

w., abnormal occlusal, wear that exceeds the physiologic wear patterns associated with the attritional effects of food substances; the excessive wear of the teeth occurring as a result of continued afunctional gyrations of the mandible.

w., interproximal, a loss of tooth substance in contact areas through functional wear and friction, resulting in broadening and flattening of the contacts and a decrease of the mesiodistal dimension of the teeth and of the dentition as a whole.

w., occlusal, attritional loss of substance on opposing occlusal units or surfaces. See also **abrasion.**

w. pattern. See **pattern, wear.**

w., physiologic, attrition or abrasion of tooth substance occurring as a result of such conditions as the abrasive consistency of the normal diet or the slight buccolingual movement of the teeth possible in the masticatory process. It does not include the wear produced by such influences as habits or occlusal prematurities.

Weber-Dimitri disease. See **disease, Sturge-Weber-Dimitri.**

Weber's disease. See **telangiectasia, hereditary hemorrhagic.**

Wedelstaedt chisel (vēd'əlstät). See **chisel, Wedelstaedt.**

wedge, a small, pointed, triangular, contoured piece of wood used to seal the gingival margin of a cavity preparation before placement of an amalgam restoration.

wedge, step. See **penetrometer.**

wedging, packing or fixing tightly by driving in a wedge or wedges.

w. effect. See **effect, wedging.**

weekly permissible dose. See **dose, weekly permissible.** (not current)

weight, the pull toward the center of the earth of a body at its surface; the force of gravity acting on a mass.

w., molecular (məlek'yələr), the sum of atomic weights of all the atoms in a molecule.

w., rubber dam, a piece of metal varying in shape and weight, attached to a clip that is hung on the bottom of a placed rubber dam to keep the field of operation clear.

Weil's disease (vilz). See **disease, Weil's.**

welding, a process used to join metals.

w., arc and gas. See **welding, fusion.**

w., cold, property of welding at room temperature, when clean surfaces are pressed into contact. This property is exhibited to the highest degree by gold in the form of foil or crystals.

w., fusion (arc and gas welding), a process in which parts are melted and fused together.

w., pressure (resistance welding, spot welding), a welding process in which the parts are not melted, although heat is usually required. Recrystallization across the interface occurs. Gold foil is welded by pressure without temperature elevation.

w. property, the characteristic of certain materials, especially metals, to firmly unite together when subjected to heat and/or pressure in a suitable environment.

w., resistance. See **welding, pressure.**

w., spot. See **welding, pressure.**

Werlhof's disease (verl'hofs). See **purpura, thrombocytopenic.**

Western blot, a confirmatory test for HIV exposure that identifies antibodies to HIV proteins and glycoproteins.

wet strength. See **strength, wet.**

wetting agent. See **agent, wetting.**

Wharton's duct. See **duct, Wharton's.**

wheal (wēl), edematous elevation of the skin or mucosa. See also **urticaria.**

wheel, Burlew. See **Burlew wheel.**

wheel stone. See **stone, wheel.**

wheelchair, a mobile chair equipped with large wheels and brakes used to transport patients and/or to allow disabled persons to move themselves from one place to another. Federal law requires handicapped access to public buildings with ramps, doors, elevators, restrooms, and drinking fountains designed and constructed to allow patients in wheelchairs proper access.

wheeze, a whistling sound made during breathing that is caused by a foreign body in the trachea or bronchus.

white blood cell count, a diagnostic clinical laboratory test to determine the number and types of leukocytes present in a measured sample of blood. Overall the normal number of leukocytes ranges from 5,000 to 10,000/mm^3. A differential white blood cell count identifies, counts, and determines the ratios of the various types of leukocytes present in a sample of blood. See also **leukopenia** and **leukocytosis.**

white lesions, a wide array of lesions found on the mucosa, which have a white coating. They require differential diagnosis because they may indicate trauma, infection, or a cancerous process.

whitlow, an inflammation of the end of a finger or toe that results in suppuration.

Widman procedure, a surgical procedure in which a periodontal flap is made to gain better access to root surfaces for complete debridement and root planing. (not current)

wife, a woman united to a man in lawful wedlock; a married woman whose husband is alive and from whom she is not divorced; a female spouse.

will, a legal document detailing one's wishes in the disposal of one's body and property and the care of one's minor children and/or dependents.

w., living, a document that details one's wishes regarding the degree and amount of health care desired if one becomes mentally incapacitated.

willfully, intentionally; purposefully.

Wilson, curve of, a lateral curve of the occlusal table formed by the lingual inclination of the posterior teeth. Because the lingual cusps are lower than the buccal cusps, they form a curve with their antimeres. See also **curve of Wilson theory.**

windchill factor, the amount of chilling of the body because of exposure to wind or cold air currents, beyond that resulting from a cold ambient temperature.

winking, jaw. See **syndrome, jaw-winking.**

wire, slender and pliable rod or thread of metal.

w., arch, wire used in orthodontics as a source of force to direct teeth to move in desired directions. The wire may be described according to the shape of its cross-section, such as ribbon, rectangular, or round.

w., diagnostic. See **wire, measuring.**

w., Kirschner, a surgical steel wire of heavy gauge with pointed ends; used in the reduction and fixation of bone fragments by passing it through the cancellous portion of the bone and spanning the fracture site.

w., ligature, a soft, thin wire used to tie an arch wire to the band attachments.

w., measuring, a wire or other similar metal placed in a root canal; made for the purpose of determining the length of the canal. A radiogram is used to make the determination.

w., orthodontic, stainless steel and wrought gold wire of various dimensions used in orthodontic treatment.

W

w., Risdon (riz'don), a wire arch bar tied in the midline.

w., separating, wires threaded interproximally between two adjacent teeth and tightened by twisting the ends together so as to wedge the teeth slightly apart. Separating wire is used preparatory to adapting bands to teeth having tight contacts with adjacent teeth.

w., wrought, **1.** a wire formed by drawing a cast structure through a die; used in dentistry for partial denture clasps and orthodontic appliances. **2.** a form of metal resulting from the swaging, rolling, and drawing of a metal ingot into a desired shape and size.

wiring, an arrangement of a wire or wires.

w., circumferential, to maintain mandibular and maxillofacial surgical appliances, the placement of a wire around a bone contiguous to the oral cavity, with the ends exiting in the oral cavity (e.g., circumferential mandibular wiring, circumzygomatic wiring).

w., continuous loop (multiple loop wire), a technique for wiring the teeth for the reduction and fixation of fractures.

w., craniofacial suspension, a method of wiring using areas of bones not contiguous with the oral cavity for the support of fractured jaw segments (e.g., piriform aperture, zygomatic arch, zygomatic process of the frontal bone).

w., Ivy loop, a method using a wire around two adjacent teeth, providing a loop useful for fixation of a fracture.

w., multiple loop. See **wiring, continuous loop.**

w., perialveolar (per'ē·alvē'·ələr), a method of wiring a splint to the maxilla by passing a wire through the bone from the buccal plate to the palate.

w., piriform aperture (pir'ifôrm), a method of wiring using that area of the nasal bones for the stabilizing of fractures of the jaws.

wisdom tooth, the third molar tooth, the last tooth in each quadrant of each dental arch. It appears in the oral cavity at about 18 years of age.

witch hazel, a shrub, *Hamamelis virginiana,* indigenous to North America, from which an astringent extract is derived.

Witkop's disease, a hereditary, benign intraepithelial dyskeratosis of the oral mucosa and conjunctiva characterized by white-cream asymptomatic plaques on the buccal mucosa, tongue, and floor of the mouth. (not current)

witness, one who has knowledge of an event; a person whose declaration under oath is received as evidence for any purpose.

w., expert, a person whose education, training, and experience can provide the court with an assessment, opinion, or judgment within the area of his or her competence, which is not considered known or available to the general public.

w., hostile, witness who manifests so much hostility or prejudice under examination (in chief, or direct) that the party who has called the witness is allowed to cross-examine the witness (i.e., to treat him or her as though he or she had been called by the opposite party).

w. marks, the small hemispheric depressions that may be prepared in the bone surface in lieu of abutment grooves as a guide for seating the abutment posts of the implant.

Wolff's law See **law, Wolff's.** (not current)

Wolinella recta (wō'linel'ə rek'tə), also known as *Campylobacter rectus;* a microorganism associated with progressive periodontal destruction and refractory forms of periodontitis. A regimen combining antibiotic treatment, debridement, and home oral care seems to supress or control periodontal infections.

word processing (W/P), the handling, manipulating, or performing of some operation or sequence of operations by a dedicated machine (usually by a microprocessor) on free text.

work hardening. See **hardening, work.**

work sheet, the office form used for a complete planning program for the completion of dental services.

work simplification, the application of the principles of the scientific method to increase the ability to produce without sacrificing quality.

W

working capital, a firm's investment in short-term assets—cash, short-term securities, accounts receivable, and inventories. Gross working capital is defined as current assets minus current liabilities. If the term *working capital* is used without further qualification, it generally refers to gross working capital.

working contact. See **contact, working.**

working occlusal surfaces. See **surface, working occlusal.**

working occlusion. See **occlusion, working.**

working side, the lateral segment of a denture or dentition toward which the mandible is moved.

Workmen's Compensation Board of Industrial Commission, an administrative body that receives claims for injuries and refers them to certain physicians or dentists for treatment, if indicated, with the express or implied assurance to the claimant that the expense will be defrayed by the employed under the Workmen's Compensation Law. The determination of the Industrial Commission is subject to an appeal to court. The federal agency overseeing these matters is the Bureau of Employees Compensation.

World Health Organization (WHO), an agency of the United Nations concerned with worldwide and regional health problems. Its functions include furnishing technical assistance, stimulating and advancing epidemiologic investigation of diseases, recommending health regulations, promoting cooperation among scientific and professional health groups, and providing information and counsel relating to health matters.

wound, an injury to the body of a person, especially one caused by violence.

w., incised, in medical jurisprudence, a cut or incision on a human body; a wound made by a cutting instrument.

w. repair, restoration of the normal structure after an injury.

wrist drop, a condition caused by paralysis of the extensor muscles of the hand and fingers or by injury of the radial nerve, resulting in flexion of the wrist.

writ of execution, a mandatory precept in writing to implement that judgment or decree of a court.

writing, any written or printed paper or document (e.g., contract, deed).

wrong, an injury; a tort; a violation of right or of law; an injustice; a violation of right resulting in damage to another.

wrongful death status, a statute existing in all states that provides that the death of a person can give rise to a cause of legal action brought by the person's beneficiaries in a civil suit against the person or persons whose willful or negligent acts caused the death.

wrought clasp (wrôt). See **clasp, wrought.**

wrought wire. See **wire, wrought.**

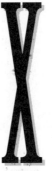

x chromosome, a sex chromosome that in humans and many other species is present in both male and female. The male somatic cell consists of one x chromosome and one y chromosome; the female somatic cell carries two x chromosomes. All female gametes carry the x chromosome, whereas half of the male gametes possess the x chromosome and the other half the y chromosome.

xanthines (zan′thīnz), a family of chemicals that includes caffeine, theophylline, and theobromine, which stimulate the central nervous system, act on the kidneys to produce diuresis, stimulate cardiac muscle, and relax smooth muscle.

xanthogranuloma (zan′thəgran′yə-lōmə), a benign lesion of infancy, usually solitary and composed of lipid-laden histiocytes with varying numbers of Touton giant cells. In the oral cavity the lesion occurs most often on the tongue and regresses spontaneously.

xanthoma (zanthō′mə), small yellow nodules, composed of lipid-laden macrophages, which generally occur in subcutaneous tissue.

x. palpebrarum (palpəbrā'rəm) *(xanthelasma palpebrarum),* small, yellowish plaque on the eyelids resulting from an accumulation of lipids in reticuloendothelial cells. They frequently occur in persons with diabetes.

xanthomatosis (zan'thōmətō'sis), a disease characterized by the accumulation of excess lipids. See also **histiocytosis X.**

xanthosis, I. a yellowish discoloration sometimes seen in degenerating tissues of malignant diseases. **2.** also called carotenosis, a reversible yellow discoloration of the skin most commonly caused by the ingestion of large amounts of yellow vegetables containing carotene pigment, usually in the form of carrot juice. Xanthosis may be differentiated clinically from jaundice because the sclerae are colored yellow in jaundice but are not discolored in xanthosis.

X-bite. See cross-bite.

xenograft, tissue from another species used as temporary graft in certain cases, as in treating a severely burned patient when sufficient tissue from the patient or from a tissue bank is not available. It is quickly rejected but provides a cover of the burn for the first few days, reducing the amount of fluid loss from the open wound. Also called *heterograft.*

xenophobia, an anxiety disorder characterized by a pervasive, irrational fear or uneasiness in the presence of strangers, especially foreigners, or in new surroundings.

xeroderma, a chronic skin condition characterized by dryness and roughness.

x. pigmentosum, an eruption of exposed skin occurring in childhood and characterized by numerous pigmental spots resembling freckles, larger atrophic lesions eventually resulting in glossy white thinning of the skin surrounded by telangiectases, and multiple solar keratoses that undergo malignant changes at an early age. This results from a single-gene autosomal recessive disorder.

xerodermosteosis (zir'ōdərmos'tē·ō'sis). See **syndrome, Sjögren's.**

xerography, a dry radiologic process in which an image is made on a metal plate coated with powdered selenium. The plate is electrically charged in a dark room. Exposure to light or x-rays causes the charge to be redistributed in a pattern proportional to the intensity of exposure in various areas of the plate. When "developed" in a cloud of charged particles, the particles are attracted to the areas discharged by radiation, producing the equivalent of a photographic negative.

xerophthalmia (zir'ofthal'mē·ə), dryness of the conjunctiva caused by functional or organic disorders of the lacrimal apparatus. It may be found in vitamin A deficiency or Sjögren's syndrome and may follow chronic conjunctivitis.

xeroradiography, the use of xerography to produce an image electrically rather than chemically, permitting lower exposure times and lower energy levels of x-rays.

xerostomia (zir'əstō'mē·ə), dryness of the mouth resulting from functional or organic disturbances of the salivary glands and lack of the normal secretion. Dryness and resultant overgrowth of oral microorganisms frequently lead to rampant caries. See also **hyposalivation.**

xerotic keratitis, an inflammation of the cornea resulting from dryness of the conjunctiva. Underlying causes may be autoimmune diseases or a deficiency of vitamin A.

X-linkage. See **linkage, sex.**

x-ray, a type of electromagnetic radiation characterized by wavelengths between approximately 10^3 Å and 10^{-4} Å, corresponding to photon energies of about 20 eV to 125 MeV. X-rays are invisible; penetrative, especially at higher photon energies; and travel with the same speed as visible light. Typical production involves bombarding a target of high atomic number with fast electrons in a high vacuum; they are also emitted as a product of some radioactive disintegrations (specifically originating from the extranuclear part of the atom). X-rays were first discovered by Wilhelm C. Roentgen in 1895; hence the term roentgen rays, often applied to mechanically generated x-rays. Roentgen called them x-rays after the mathematic symbol x for an unknown.

x., monochromatic, an x-ray that has a single wavelength or an extremely narrow band of wavelengths.

x-ray beam, the spatial distribution of radiation emerging from an x-ray generator or source.

x. b., central, the straight line passing through the center of the source and the center of the final beam-limiting diaphragm.

x. b., edges, the lines joining the center of the anterior face of the source to the diaphragm edges farthest from the source.

x. b., field size, the geometric projection, on a plane perpendicular to the central ray, of the distal end of the limiting diaphragm as seen from the center of the front surface of the source. The field is thus the same shape as the aperture of the collimator, and it can be defined at any distance from the source.

x. b., principal plane, a plane that contains the central ray and, in the case of rectangular section beams, is parallel to one side of the rectangle.

x-ray film, full-mouth. See **survey, radiographic.**

x-ray mount. See **mount, x-ray.**

x-ray tube, an electronic tube in which x-rays can be generated.

x. t., Coolidge, a vacuum tube in which x-rays are generated when the target (integral with the anode) is bombarded by electrons that are emitted from a heated filament (on the cathode) and accelerated toward the anode across a high-potential difference. Modern x-ray tubes are of this type. See also **tube, Coolidge.**

x. t., Crookes', a vacuum discharge tube used by Sir William Crookes in early experimental work with cathode rays. Wilhelm C. Roentgen first discovered that in addition to the production of cathode rays, x-rays were emitted during the operation of these tubes.

x. t., gas, an early type of x-ray tube in which electrons were derived from residual gases within the tube.

x-ray unit. See **unit, x-ray.**

xylene (zī'lēn) (xylol; $C_6H_4[CH_3]_2$ dimethylbenzene), a colorless, flammable fluid used as a solvent and clarifying agent in the preparation of tissue sections for microscopic study.

Xylocaine. See **lidocaine.**

xylol (zī'lol). See **xylene.**

xylose, wood or beechwood sugar; an aldopentose, isomeric with ribose, obtained by fermentation or hydrolysis of naturally occurring carbohydrate substances such as wood fiber.

xylulose, a substance that appears in the urine of patients with essential pentosuria; its presence is diagnostic.

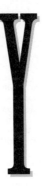

Y axis. See **axis, Y.**

Y chromosome, a sex chromosome that in humans and many other species is present only in the male, appearing singly in the normal male. It is carried as a sex determinant by one half of the male gametes. None of the female gametes contains a y chromosome.

yawn, an involuntary act of opening the mouth wide and taking a deep breath. It tends to occur when a person is bored, drowsy, or depressed and may be accompanied by upper body movements to aid chest expansion.

yaws (yôz), a disease caused by *Treponema pertenue.* It occurs in hot regions; raspberry-like excrescences occur on the hands, face, feet, and external genitalia. Synonym: frambesia.

yeast, a general term denoting true fungi of the family Saccharomycetaceae. Because of their ability to ferment carbohydrates, some yeasts are important to the brewing and baking industries.

Yersinia, a genus of motile and nonmotile, non–spore-forming bacteria containing gram-negative, unencapsulated, ovoid to rod-shaped cells. These organisms are parasitic on humans and other animals.

yield point. See **point, yield.**

yield strength. See **strength, yield.**

yin-yang, 1. Yin and Yang, in ancient Chinese thought, are the underlying and controlling elements of all nature. The aim of Chinese medicine is to produce a proper balance between them. **2.** used in the Western world to express any dualistic, reciprocal control system in which one influence tends to promote things that the opposing influence tends to inhibit.

yoga, a discipline that focuses on the body's musculature, posture, breathing mechanisms, and consciousness. The goal of yoga is attainment of physical and mental well-being through mastery of the body, achieved through exercise, holding of postures, proper breathing, and meditation.

yogurt, a slightly acid, semisolid curdled milk preparation made from either whole or skimmed cow's milk and milk solids by fermentation with organisms from the genus *Lactobacillus.* It is rich in B-complex vitamins, and is a good source of protein. It provides a medium in the GI tract that retards the growth of harmful bacteria and aids in the absorption of minerals. Also spelled *yoghurt.*

yohimbine, an alkaloid, the active principle comes from the bark of *Corynanthe johimbe.* It produces a competitive blockage of limited duration of alpha adrenergic receptors. It has also been used for its alleged aphrodisiac properties.

yoke, I. something that connects or binds. **2.** metal clamps with adjustable screws that secure the cylinders to the apparatus or reducing valves. They are equipped with nipples that fit snugly into the inlet socket or part of the cylinder valve.

Young's modulus. See **elasticity, modulus of.**

Young's rule. See **rule, Young's.**

Y-plasty, a method of surgical revision of a scar, using a Y-shaped incision to reduce scar contractures. See also **Z-plasty.**

ytterbium (Yb), a metallic element of the lanthamide group with an atomic number of 70 and an atomic weight of 173.04.

yttrium, a scaly, grayish metallic element with an atomic number of 39 and an atomic weight of 88.905. Radioactive isotopes of yttrium have been used in cancer therapy.

Z, a symbol for atomic number.

zalcitabine, *trade name:* Hivid; *class:* synthetic pyrimidine antiviral; *action:* converted by cellular enzymes to active drug; functions as antimetabolite to inhibit replication of HIV in vitro; *uses:* used in combination with zidovudine in advanced HIV infection, second-line monotherapy if AZT tolerant.

zero, I. a symbol for nothing or for the starting point. **2.** the point on most scales from which measurements begin. **3.** absolute zero, the temperature at which there is no molecular movement, corresponding to -273.15 on the Kelvin scale.

zidovudine, *trade names:* AZT, Retrovir; *class:* antiviral thymidine analog; *action:* inhibits replication of viral DNA; *uses:* symptomatic HIV infections (AIDS, ARC), confirmed *P. carinii* pneumonia, or absolute CD4 lymphocytes of less than 200 milliliters, prevention of HIV transmission from infected mother to baby.

zinc (Zn) (zingk), a bluish white chemical element used in medicine in the form of various salts and as a component in some silver amalgams.

z. oxide, a zinc compound used as a topical protectant prescribed for a wide range of minor skin irritations.

z. oxide and eugenol (zingk ok′sīd yōō′jənol), two substances that react chemically to form a relatively hard mass. When modified by certain additives, the material is used for impression pastes, root canal fillings, surgical dressings, temporary filling materials, and cementing media.

z. oxide–eugenol cement. See **cement, dental, zinc oxide–eugenol.**

z. oxyphosphate (zingk ok′sēfos′fāt). See **cements.**

z. phosphate cement (zingk fos′fāt). See **cement, zinc phosphate.**

z. polycarbonate cement (zingk pol′ēkar′bənāt). See **cements.**

zirconium (Zr), a metallic element with an atomic number of 40 and an atomic weight of 91.22. It is widely distributed in nature, although no concentrations are found in any one place.

Zinsser-Cole-Engman syndrome. See **syndrome, Zinsser-Cole-Engman.**

ZOE. See **zinc oxide and eugenol.**

Zollinger-Ellison syndrome, a condition characterized by severe peptic ulceration, gastric hypersecretion, elevated serum gastrin, and gastrinoma of the pancreas or the duodenum. It may occur in early childhood but is seen more frequently in people between 20 and 50 years of age. Two thirds of the tumors are malignant. Total gastrectomy may be necessary, but the administration of cimetidine in large doses may control gastric hypersecretion and allow the ulcers to heal.

zolpidem, *trade name:* Ambien; *class:* nonbarbiturate, nonbenzodiazepine sedative/hypnotic; *action:* presumed to interact with subunit of GABA-benzodiazepine receptor; *use:* insomnia.

zone (zōn), a region or area with specific characteristics or boundary.

z., incubation, an area that provides a favorable environment for growth of microorganisms and is thus conducive to initiation or perpetuation of a pathologic process (e.g., gingival flap over a partly erupted third molar).

z., neutral, the potential space between the lips and cheeks on one side and the tongue on the other. Natural or artificial teeth in this zone are subject to equal and opposite forces from the surrounding musculature.

z. of reference, the area of perceived pain referred by the trigger point. See also **trigger point.**

zonography, an x-ray–imaging technique used to produce films of body sections similar to those made by tomography.

Z-plasty, a surgical procedure using the transposition of tissue flaps to ensure the release of contractures, as in the repair of a cleft lip or in ankyloglossia.

z-score, a standard score based on the normal distribution; the difference between the obtained score and the mean, divided by the standard deviation. Standard scores computed for different variables are comparable; used to determine statistical significance in large samples.

zygoma, I. a long, slender process of the temporal bone, arising from the lower part of the squamous portion of the temporal bone and passing forward horizontally to join with the malar or zygomatic bone. **2.** the zygomatic or malar bone that forms the prominence of the cheek.

zygomatic arch, the arch formed by articulation of the temporal process of the zygomatic bone with the zygomatic process of the temporal bone.

zygomaxillare (zī′gōmaks′əlãrə). See **ridge, key.**

zygosity, the characteristics or conditions of a zygote. The term occurs primarily as a suffix combining form to denote genetic makeup, referring specifically to whether the paired alleles determining a particular trait are identical (homozygosity) or different (heterozygosity) or to the condition in twins of having developed from the fertilization of one ovum (monozygosity) or two (dizygosity).

zygote, the developing ovum from the time it is fertilized until, as a blastocyst, it is implanted in the uterus.

How Dental Terms Are Made and Read

Dental terminology is a hybrid speech. Most of the words also are common to medical terminology and as such are largely made up of Greek and Latin stems, prefixes, and suffixes. However, many words have been borrowed from other languages as well. Dental terminology also is dynamic in the sense that many new words are coined as necessity demands. Generally, technical words can be analyzed for their meanings by dividing them into their component parts and determining the meaning of each part.

To build or analyze any vocabulary, the five elements that can be used to form words must be understood: the word root, combining vowel, combining form, prefix, and suffix.

WORD ROOT

The word root is the basic core of any word and gives it its primary meaning. (Some compound words may be made up of more than one root.) For instance, in the words *stomatitis, adenitis,* and *pulpitis* the word roots are *stomat* (meaning "mouth"), *aden* (meaning "gland"), and *pulp* (meaning "the soft tissue within a tooth").

COMBINING VOWEL

Certain combinations of word roots are difficult to pronounce, especially when the first word root ends in a consonant and the second begins with a consonant. This awkwardness of pronunciation necessitates the insertion of a vowel called a combining vowel. Usually the combining vowel is an *o,* although *a, e, i, u,* and *y* may be encountered occasionally. Combining vowels are encountered in everyday words. Instead of joining the two word roots *speed* and *meter* directly, the combining vowel *o* is inserted to speedometer. Another example is *megal* and *glossia,* which become megaloglossia.

COMBINING FORM

The combination of word root plus combining vowel is known as the combining form.

Word root	+	Combining vowel	=	Combining form
-gnath-		O		-gnatho-
-micr-		O		-micro-
-dent-		O		-dento-
-arthr-		O		-arthro-

SUFFIX

A suffix is a syllable or syllables added at the end of a word root or combining form to change the meaning of the root, give it grammatical function, or form a new word. *Play, read,* and *speak* are word roots; by adding the suffix *-er* (meaning "one who") the words are changed to "one who plays," "one who reads," and "one who speaks." If the suffix *-able* (meaning "capable of being") were added, the words mean "capable of being played," "capable of being read," and "capable of being spoken." In the words *microtome, dermatome,* and *arthrotome,* -tome is a suffix meaning "instrument for cutting." Notice that the suffix is added to the combining form rather than the word root:

Word root	+	Combining vowel	+	Suffix	=	Meaning
micr-		O		-tome		instrument to cut very fine sections
derm-		O		-tome		instrument to cut skin
arthr-		O		-tome		instrument to cut joints

PREFIX

A prefix is a syllable or syllables placed before a word or word root to alter its meaning or create a new word. If the prefixes *over-, re-,* and *out-* are added before the words *play, read,* and *speak,* three new words are created—*overplay, reread,* and *outspeak.* Any number of these five elements can be combined to form new words.

Auto-bi-o-graph-ic-al		*Sub-strat-o-spher-e*		*Electr-o-cardi-o-gram*	
auto-	prefix	sub-	prefix	electr-	word root
-bi-	word root	-strat-	word root	-o-	combining vowel
-o-	combining vowel	-o-	combining vowel	-cardi-	word root
-graph-	word root	-spher-	word root	-o-	combining vowel
-ic	suffix	-e	suffix	-gram	suffix
-al	suffix				

WORD AND ROOT ORDER

The order in which the various elements of compound words are placed is of great importance. Observe the consequences if the order of the elements in the following words were reversed:

leg iron	became	iron leg
motorboat	became	boat motor
snake poison	became	poison snake
pig iron	became	iron pig
zoo animal	became	animal zoo
eyeglass	became	glass eye
house dog	became	dog house

In all of these instances the order of the elements may be reversed and still arrive at a sensible word, although the subject in each example has changed. Other compound words such as the following may become nonsensical if the order of their elements is changed:

shoulder blade	cannot become	blade shoulder
nerve tonic	cannot become	tonic nerve
chickenpox	cannot become	pox chicken
headache	cannot become	achehead

The following is a list of combining forms for anatomic structures and body fluids, prefixes, suffixes, verbs, and adjectives. Although the combining form generally appears at the beginning of a term, it may appear within a term or at the end of it.*

---

*From Young CG, Austin MG: *Learning medical terminology step by step,* ed 4, St Louis, 1979, Mosby.

adeno- gland
adreno- adrenal gland
angio- vessel
ano- anus
arterio- artery
arthro- joint
balano- glans penis
blepharo- eyelid
broncho- bronchus (windpipe)
cantho- canthus (angle at either end of slit between eyelids)
capit- head
cardi, cardio- heart
carpo- wrist
cephalo- head
cerebello- cerebellum (part of brain)
cerebro- cerebrum (part of brain)
cheilo- lip (mouth)
chole- bile (NOTE: *chole-* + *cyst* meaning "bladder," = gallbladder; *chole* + *doch*, meaning "duct," = choledocho, or common bile duct.)
chondro- cartilage
chordo- cord or string (generally used in connection with the vocal cord or spermatic cord)
cilia- hair (Latin)
cleido- collarbone
coccygo- coccyx (end bone of the spinal column)
colpo- vagina
cordo- cord (usually vocal cord)
coxa- hip (Latin)
cranio- head
cysto- sac, cyst, or bladder (most often used in connection with the urinary bladder)
cyto- cell
dacryo- tear (used commonly in relation to tear duct or sac)
dento-, donto- tooth
derma- skin
duodeno- duodenum (part of small intestine)
emia- blood
encephalo- brain
entero- intestines
fascia- sheet or band of fibrous tissue (Latin)
fibro- fibers
gastro- stomach

genu- knee (Latin)
gingivo- gums
glomerulo- glomerulus (often a structure of the kidney)
glosso- tongue
gnatho- jaw
hem-, hema-, hemo-, hemato- blood
hepato- liver
hilus- pit or depression in an organ where vessels and nerves enter (Latin)
histio- tissue
hystero- uterus (NOTE: This term may also pertain to hysteria.)
ileo- ileum (part of small intestine)
ilio- flank or ilium (bone of pelvis)
jejuno- jejunum (part of small intestine)
kerato- cornea or horny layer of the skin
labio- lips (either of mouth or vulva)
lacrimo- tears (used also in connection with tear ducts or sacs)
laparo- loin or flank (also refers to abdomen)
laryngo- larynx
linguo- tongue
lympho- lymph
masto- breast
meningo- meninges (coverings of the brain and spinal cord)
metra-, metro- uterus
morpho- form
myelo- bone marrow and spinal cord (NOTE: Use of this term will determine which tissue is meant.)
myo- muscle (NOTE: The Latin word for muscle is *mus.*)
myringo- eardrum
naso- nose
nephro- kidney
neuro- nerve
oculo- eye
odonto- tooth
omphalo- navel or umbilicus
onycho- nails
oophoro- ovary
ophthalmo- eye
ora-, oro- mouth
orthio-, orchido- testis
os- bone or mouth

osteo- bone
oto- ear
ovario- ovary
palato- palate of mouth
palpebro- eyelid
pectus- breast, chest, or thorax (Latin)
pharyngo- pharynx
phlebo- vein
pilo- hair
pleuro- pleura of lung (relates also to side or rib)
pneumo-, pneumono- lungs (also used in referring to air or breath)
procto- rectum
pyelo- pelvis of kidney
pyloro- pylorus (part of stomach just before duodenum)
rhino- nose
sacro- sacrum
salpingo- fallopian tube or oviduct
sialo- saliva (used in connection with a salivary duct or gland)

splanchno- viscera
spleno- spleen
sterno- sternum
stoma- mouth
tarso- instep of foot; ankle (also edge of eyelid)
teno-, tenonto- tendon
thoraco- thorax or chest
thyro- thyroid
trachelo- neck, particularly the neck of the uterus or bladder
tracheo- trachea
unguis- nail
uretero- ureter
urethro- urethra
uro- urine, urinary
utero- uterus
vaso- vessel
veno- vein
ventriculo- ventricle of heart or brain
viscero- viscera

PREFIXES

Prefixes, the most frequently used elements in the formation of medical-dental words, are one or more syllables (prepositions or adverbs) placed before words or roots to show various kinds of relationships. They are never used independently, but when added before verbs, adjectives, or nouns, they modify the meaning. Most prefixes are a part of words in ordinary speech and do not refer specifically to medical-dental or scientific terminology, but many also occur frequently in medical terminology. Studying them is an important step in learning medical terms and building a medical-dental vocabulary.

Prefix	Translation	Examples
a- (an- before vowel)	Without, lack of	Apathy (lack of feeling), apnea (without breath), aphasia (without speech), anemia (lack of blood)
ab-	Away from	Abductor (leading away from), aboral (away from mouth)
ad-	To, toward, near to	Adductor (leading toward), adhesion (sticking to), adnexa (structures joined to), adrenal (near the kidney)
ambi-	Both	Ambidextrous (ability to use hands equally), ambilaterally (both sides)
amphi-	About, on both sides, both	Amphibious (living on both land and water)
ampho-	Both	Amphogenic (producing offspring of both sexes)
ana-	Up, back, again, excessive	Anatomy (a cutting up), anagenesis (reproduction of tissue), anasarca (excessive serum in cellular tissues of body)
ante-	Before, forward	Antecubital (before elbow), anteflexion (forward bending)
anti-	Against, opposed to, reversed	Antiperistalsis (reversed peristalsis), antisepsis (against infection)

apo-	From, away from	Aponeurosis (away from tendon), apochromatic (abnormal color)
bi-	Twice, double	Biarticulate (double joint), bifocal (two foci), bifurcation (two branches)
cata-	Down, according to, complete	Catabolism (breaking down), catalepsia (complete seizure), catarrh (flowing down)
circum-	Around, about	Circumflex (winding about), circumference (surrounding), circumarticular (around joint)
com-	With, together	Commissure (sending or coming together)
con-	With, together	Conductor (leading together), concrescence (growing together), concentric (having a common center)
contra-	Against, opposite	Contralateral (opposite side), contraception (prevention of conception), contraindicated (not indicated)
de-	Away from	Dehydrate (remove water from), decompensation (failure of compensation)
di-	Twice, double	Diplopia (double vision), dichromatic (two colors), digastric (double stomach)
dia-	Through, apart, across, completely	Diaphragm (wall across), diapedesis (ooze through), diagnosis (complete knowledge)
dis-	Reversal, apart from, separation	Disinfection (apart from infection), disparity (apart from equality), dissect (cut apart)
dys-	Bad, difficult, disordered	Dyspepsia (bad digestion), dyspnea (difficult breathing), dystopia (disordered position)
e-, ex-	Out, away from	Enucleate (remove from), eviscerate (take out viscera or bowels), exostosis (outgrowth of bone)
ec-	Out from	Ectopic (out of place), eccentric (away from center), ectasia (stretching out or dilation)
ecto-	On outside, situated on	Ectoderm (outer skin), ectoretina (outer layer of retina)
em-, en-	In	Empyema (pus in), encephalon (in the head)
endo-	Within	Endocardium (within heart), endometrium (within uterus), endodont (within tooth)
epi-	Upon, on	Epidural (upon dura), epidermis (on skin)
exo-	Outside, on outer side, outer layer	Exogenous (produced outside), exocolitis (inflammation of outer coat of colon)
extra-	Outside	Extracellular (outside cell), extrapleural (outside pleura)
hemi-	Half	Hemiplegia (partial paralysis), hemianesthesia (loss of feeling on one side of body)
hyper-	Over, above, excessive	Hyperemia (excessive blood), hypertrophy (overgrowth), hyperplasia (excessive formation)
hypo-	Under, below, deficient	Hypotension (low blood pressure), hypothyroidism (deficiency or underfunction of thyroid)
im-, in-	In, into	Immersion (act of dipping in), infiltration (act of filtering in), injection (act of forcing liquid into)
im-, in-	Not	Immature (not mature), involuntary (not voluntary), inability (not able)
infra-	Below	Infraorbital (below eye), infraclavicular (below clavicle or collarbone)
inter-	Between	Intercostal (between ribs), intervene (come between)
intra-	Within	Intracerebral (within cerebrum), intraocular (within eyes), intraventricular (within ventricles)
intro-	Into, within	Introversion (turning inward), introduce (lead into)
meta-	Beyond, after, change	Metamorphosis (change of form), metastasis (beyond original position), metacarpal (beyond wrist)

opistho-	Behind, backward	Opisthotic (behind ears), opisthognathous (behind jaws)
para-	Beside, by side	Paraplegia (paralysis of both sides), paracentesis (puncture along side of), parathyroid (beside thyroid)
per-	Through, excessive	Permeate (pass through), perforate (bore through), peracute (excessively acute)
peri-	Around	Periosteum (around bone), periatrial (around atrium), peribronchial (around bronchus)
post-	After, behind	Postoperative (after operation), postpartum (after childbirth), postocular (behind eye)
pre-	Before, in front of	Premaxillary (in front of maxilla), preoral (in front of mouth)
pro-	Before, in front of	Prognosis (foreknowledge), prophase (appear before)
re-	Back, again, contrary	Reflex (bend back), revert (turn again to), regurgitation (backward flowing, contrary to normal)
retro-	Backward, located behind	Retrocervical (located behind cervix), retrograde (going backward), retrolingual (behind tongue)
semi-	Half	Semicartilaginous (half cartilage), semilunar (half moon), semiconscious (half conscious)
sub-	Under	Subcutaneous (under skin), subarachnoid (under arachnoid), subungual (under nail)
super-	Above, upper, excessive	Supercilia (upper brows), supernumerary (excessive number), supermedial (above middle)
supra-	Above, upon	Suprarenal (above kidney), suprasternal (above sternum), suprascapular (on upper part of scapula)
sym-, syn-	Together, with	Symphysis (growing together), synapsis (joining together), synarthrosis (articulation of joints together)
trans-	Across, through	Transection (cut across), transduodenal (through duodenum), transmit (send beyond)
ultra-	Beyond, in	Ultraviolet (beyond violet end of spectrum), ultraligation (ligation of vessel beyond point of origin), ultrasonic (sound waves beyond the upper frequency of hearing by human ear)

SUFFIXES

Suffixes are the one or more syllables or elements added to the root, or stem, of a word (the part that indicates the essential meaning) to alter the meaning or indicate the intended part of speech.

To make it pronounceable the last letter or letters of the root to which the suffix is attached may be changed. The last vowel may be changed to an *o,* or *o* may be inserted if it is not already present before a suffix beginning with a consonant, as in *cardiology.* The final vowel in the root may be dropped before a suffix beginning with a vowel, as in *neuritis.*

Most suffixes are in common use in English, but some are peculiar to medical science. The suffixes most commonly used to indicate disease are -itis, meaning "inflammation," *-oma,* meaning "tumor," and *-osis,* meaning "a condition," usually morbid. The following suffixes occur often in medical-dental terminology, but they are also in use in ordinary language:

Suffix	Use	Examples
-ise, -ate	Added to nouns or adjectives to make verbs expressing to use and to act like; to subject to; make into	Visualize (able to see), impersonate (act like), hypnotize (put into state of hypnosis)

-ist, -or, -er	Added to verbs to make nouns expressing agent or person concerned or instrument	Anesthetist (one who practices the science of anesthesia), dissector (instrument that dissects or person who dissects), donor (giver)
-ent	Added to verbs to make adjectives or nouns of agency	Recipient (one who receives), concurrent (happening at the same time)
-sia, -y	Added to verbs to make nouns expressing action, process, or condition	Therapy (treatment), anesthesia (process or condition of feeling)
-ia, -ity	Added to adjectives or nouns to make nouns expressing quality or condition	Septicemia (poisoning of blood), disparity (inequality), acidity (condition of excess acid), neuralgia (pain in nerves)
-ma, mata, -men, -mina, -ment, -ure	Added to verbs to make nouns expressing result of action or object of action	Trauma (injury), foramina (openings), ligament (tough fibrous band holding bone or viscera together), fissure (groove)
-ium, -olus, -olum, -culus, -culum, -cule, -cle	Added to nouns to make diminutive nouns	Bacterium, alveolus (air sac), follicle (little bag), cerebellum (little brain), molecule (little mass), ossicle (little bone)
-ible, -ile	Added to verbs to make adjectives expressing ability or capacity	Contractile (ability to contract), edible (capable of being eaten), flexible (capable of being bent)
-al, -c, -ious, -tic	Added to nouns to make adjectives expressing relationship, concern, or pertaining to	Neural (referring to nerve), neoplastic (referring to neoplasm), cardiac (referring to heart), delirious (suffering from delirium)
-id	Added to verbs or nouns to make adjectives expressing state or condition	Flaccid (state of being weak or lax), fluid (state of being fluid or liquid)
-tic	Added to verbs to make adjectives showing relationships	Caustic (referring to burn), acoustic (referring to sound or hearing)
oid, -form	Added to nouns to make adjectives expressing resemblance	Polypoid (resembling polyp), plexiform (resembling a plexus), fusiform (resembling a fusion), epidermoid (resembling epidermis)
-ous	Added to nouns to make adjectives expressing material	Ferrous (composed of iron), serous (composed of serum), mucinous (composed of mucin)

The following verbs or combining forms of verbs are derived from Greek or Latin. They may be attached to other roots to form words, or suffixes and prefixes may be added to them to form words. In the following examples, the part or root of the word to which the verb is attached is italicized and the meaning, if not clear, is given in parentheses:

Root	Translation	Examples
-algia-	Pain	*Cardi*algia (heart), *gastr*algia (stomach), *neur*algia (nerve)
-dynia-	Pain	*Masto*dynia (breast), *pleuro*dynia (chest), *esophago*dynia (esophagus), *coccygo*dynia (coccyx)
-audi-, -audio-	Hear, hearing	Audio*meter* (measure), audio*phone* (voice instrument for deaf)
-bio-	Live	*Bio*logy (study of living), *bio*statistics (vital statistics), *bio*genesis (origin)
cau-, -caus-	Burn	Caustic (suffix added to make adjective), cau*terization;* caus*algia* (burning pain), *electro*cautery

-centesis-	Puncture, perforate	*Thoracentesis* (chest), *pneumocentesis* (lung), *arthrocentesis* (joint), *enterocentesis* (intestine)
-clas-, -claz-	Smash, break	*Osteoclasis* (bone), *odontoclasis* (tooth)
-duct-	Lead	*Ductal* (suffix added to make adjective), *oviduct* (egg uterine tube or fallopian tube), *periductal* (*peri* means "around"), *abduct* (prefix meaning lead away from)
-ecta-, -ectas-	Dilate	*Venectasia* (dilation of vein), *cardiectasis* (heart), *ectatic* (suffix added for adjective)
-edem-	Swell	*Myoedema* (muscle), *lymphedema* (lymph) (*a* is a suffix added to make a noun)
-esthes-	Feel	*Esthesia* (suffix added to make noun), *anesthesia* (*an* is a prefix)
-fiss-	Split	*Fissure, fission* (suffixes added to make nouns)
-flex-, -flec-	Bend	*Flexion* (suffix added to make noun), *flexor* (suffix added), *anteflect* (prefix added meaning "before" bending forward)
-flu-, -flux-	Flow	*Fluctuate, fluxion, affluent* (abundant flowing)
-geno-, -genesis-	Produce, origin	*Genotype, homogenesis* (same origin), *pathogenesis* (disease, origin of disease), *heterogenesis* (prefix added meaning "other," alteration of generation)
-iatro-, -iatr-	Treat, cure	*Geriatrics* (old age), *pediatrics* (children)
-kine-, -kino-, -kineto-, -kinesio	Move	*Kinetogenic* (producing movement), *kinetic* (suffix added to make adjective), *kinesiology* (study)
-liga-	Bind	*Ligament* (suffix added to make noun) *ligate, ligature*
-logy-	Study	*Parasitology* (parasites), *bacteriology* (bacteria), *histology* (tissues)
-lysis-	Breaking up, dissolving	*Hemolysis* (blood), *glycolysis* (sugar), *autolysis* (self-destruction of cells)
-morph-, -morpho-	Form	*Morphology, amorphous* (not definite form), *pleomorphic* (more, occurring in various forms), *polymorphic* (many)
-olfact-	Smell	*Olfactophobia* (fear), *olfactory* (suffix added to make adjective)
-op-, -opto-	See	*Amblyopia* (dull, dimness of vision), *presbyopia* (old, impairment of vision in old age), *optic, myopia* (*myo,* to wink, half close the eyes)
-palpit-	Flutter	*Palpitation*
-par-, -partus-	Labor	*Postpartum* (after birth), *parturition* (act of giving birth) (NOTE: para I, II, III, IV, etc., are symbols for number of births.)
-pep-	Digest	*Dyspepsia* (bad, difficult), *peptic* (suffix added to make adjective)
-pexy-	Fix	*Mastopexy* (fixation of breast), *nephrosplenopexy* (surgical fixation of kidney and spleen)
-phag-, -phago-	Eat	*Phagocytosis* (eating of cells), *phagomania* (madness, mad craving for food or to eat), *dysphagia* (difficult eating or swallowing)
-phan-	Appear, visible	*Phanerosis* (act of becoming visible), *phantasia, phantasy*
-phas-	Speak, utter	*Aphasia* (unable to speak), *dysphasia* (difficulty in speaking)
-phil-	Like, love	*Hemophilia* (blood, a hereditary disease characterized by delayed clotting of blood), *acidophilia* (acid stain, liking or straining with acid stains), *philanthropy* (love of mankind)
-phobia-	Fear	*Hydrophobia* (fear of water), *photophobia* (fear of light), *claustrophobia* (closeness, fear of close places)
-phrax-, -phrag-	Fence off, wall off	*Diaphragm* (across, partition separating thorax from abdomen), *phragmoplast* (formed)
-plas-	Form, grow	*Neoplasm* (new growth), *rhinoplasty* (nose operation for formation of nose), *otoplasty* (ear), *choledochoplasty* (common bile duct)
-plegia-	Paralyze	*Paraplegia* (paralysis of lower limbs), *ophthalmoplegia* (eye), *hemiplegia* (partial paralysis)

-pne-, -pneo-	Breathe	*Dyspnea* (difficult breathing), *apnea* (lack of breathing), *hyperpnea* (overbreathing)
-poie-	Make	*Hematopoiesis* (blood), *erythropoiesis* (red blood cells), *leukopoiesis* (making white cells)
-ptosis-	Fall	*Proctoptosis* (anus, prolapse of anus), *splanchnoptosis* (viscera)
-rrhagia-	Burst forth, pour	*Menorrhagia* (abnormal bleeding during menstruation), *menometrorrhagia* (abnormal uterine bleeding), *hemorrhage* (blood)
-rrhaphy-	Suture	*Herniorrhaphy* (suturing or repair of hernia), *hepatorrhaphy* (liver), *nephrorrhaphy* (kidney)
-rrhea-	Flow, discharge	*Leukorrhea* (white discharge from vagina), *galactorrhea* (milk discharge), *rhinorrhea* (nasal discharge)
-rrhexis-	Rupture	*Enterorrhexis* (intestines), *metrorrhexis* (uterus)
-schiz-	Split, divide	*Schizophrenia* (mind, split personality), *schizonychia* (nails), *schizotrichia* (hair)
-scope-	Examine	*Microscopic*, *cardioscope*, *endoscope* (endo means "within," an instrument for examining the interior of a hollow internal organ)
-stasis-	Stop, stand still	*Hematostatic* (pertaining to stagnation of blood), *epistasis* (checking or stopping of any discharge)
-staxen-	Drop	*Epistaxis* (nosebleed)
-teg-, -tect-	Cover	*Tegmen, tectum* (rooflike structure), *integument* (skin covering)
-therap-	Treat, cure	*Therapy, neurotherapy* (nerves), *chemotherapy* (chemicals), *physiotherapy*
-tomy-	Cut, incise	*Phlebotomy* (incision of vein), *arthrotomy* (joint), *appendectomy* (ectomy, meaning "cutout," excision of appendix), *oophorectomy* (excision of ovary), *ileocecostomy* (ostomy, meaning "creation of an artifical opening," os, meaning "opening or mouth"; ileocecostomy is an anatomosis of ileum and cecum)
-topo-	Place	*Topography, toponarcosis* (numbing, hence numbing of a part or localized anesthesia)
-tropho-	Nourish	*Hypertrophy* (enlargement or overnourishment), *atrophy* (undernourishment), *dystrophy* (difficult or bad)
-volv-	Turn	*Involution, volvulus* (twisting of an organ, as in intestinal obstruction with twisting of the bowel or twisting of the esophagus)

The following roots and combining forms are derived from Greek or Latin adjectives. Adjectives appear most often in compounds and are joined to nouns or verbs. Suffixes may be added to make them into nouns.

In the following examples, the part or root of the word that the adjective modifies is italicized, and the meaning, if not clear, is given in parentheses:

Root	Translation	Examples
-auto-	Self	*Autoinfection, autolysis, autopathy* (disease), *autopsy* (view, postmortem examination)
-brachy-	Short	*Brachycephalia* (head), *brachydactylia* (fingers), *brachychelia* (lip), *brachygnathous* (jaw)
-brady-	Slow	*Bradypnea* (breath), *bradypragia* (action), *bradyuria* (urine), *bradypepsia* (digestion)
-brevis-	Short	*Brevity, breviflexor* (short flexor muscle)
-cavus-	Hollow	*Cavity, cavernous, vena* cava (vein)
-coel-	Hollow	*Coelarium* (lining membrane of body cavity), *coelom* (body cavity of embryo)
-cryo-	Cold	*Cryotherapy, cryotolerant, cryometer*

-crypto-	Hidden, concealed	Cryptorchid (testis), cryptogenic (origin obscure or doubtful), cryptophthalmos (eye)
-dextro-	Right	Ambidextrous (using both hands with equal ease), dextrophobia (fear of objects on right side), dextrocardia (heart)
-dys-	Difficult, bad, disordered, painful	Dysarthria (speech), dyshidrosis (sweat), dyskinesia (motion), dystocia (birth), dysphasia (speech), dyspepsia (digestion)
-eu-	Well, good	Euphoria (well-being), euphagia, eupnea (breath), euthyroid (normal thyroid), eutocia (normal birth)
-eury-	Broad, wide	Eurycephalic (head), euryopia (vision), eurysomatic (body, squat thickset body)
-glyco-	Sugar, sweet	Glycohemia (sugar in blood), glycopenia (poverty of sugar, low blood sugar level)
-gravis-	Heavy	Gravida (pregnant woman), gravidism (pregnancy)
-haplo-	Single, simple	Haploid (having a single set of chromosomes), haplodont (teeth without simple crowns), haplopathy (simple uncomplicated disease)
-hetero-	Other, different	Heterogeneous (kind, dissimilar elements), heteroinoculation, heterology (abnormality of structure), heterointoxication
-homo-	Same	Homogeneous (same kind or quality throughout), homozygous (possessing identical pair of genes), homologous (corresponding in structure)
-hydro-	Wet, water	Hydronephrosis (kidney, collection of urine in kidney pelvis), hydropneumothorax (fluid in chest), hydrophobia (fear of water, water causes painful reaction in this disease)
-iso-	Equal	Isocellular (similar cells), isodontic (all teeth alike), isocytosis (equality of size of cells), isochromatic (having same color throughout)
-latus-	Broad	Latitude, latissimus dorsi (muscle adducting humerus)
-leio-	Smooth	Leiomyosarcoma (smooth muscle, fleshy malignant tumor), leiomyofibroma (tumor of muscle and fiber elements), leiomyoma (tumor of unstriped muscle)
-lepto-	Slender	Leptosomatic (body), leptodactylous (fingers)
-levo-	Left	Levocardia (heart), levorotation (turning to left)
-longus-	Long	Adductor longus (muscle of thigh), longitude
-macro-	Large, abnormal size	Macocephalic (head), macrocheiria (hands), macromastia (breast), macronychia (nails).
-magna-	Large, great	Magnitude, adductor magnus (thigh muscle)
-malaco-	Soft	Malacia (softening), osteomalacia (bones)
-malus-	Bad	Malady, malaise, malignant, malformation
-medius-	Middle	Median, medium, gluteus medius (femur muscle)
-mega-	Great	Megacolon (large colon), megacephaly (head)
-megalo-	Huge	Megalomania (delusion of grandeur), hepatomegaly (enlarged liver), splenomegaly (enlarged spleen)
-meso-	Middle, mid	Mesocarpal (wrist), mesoderm (skin), mesothelium (a lining membrane of cavities)
-micro-	Small	Microglossia (tongue), microblepharia (eyelids), microorganism, microphonia (voice)
-minimus-	Smallest	Gluteus minimus (smallest muscle of hip), adductor minimus (muscle of thigh)
-mio-	Less	Miolecithal (egg with little yolk), miopragia (perform, decreased activity)
-mono-	One, single, limited to one part	Monochromatic (color), monobrachia (arm)
-multi-	Many, much	Multipara (bear, woman who has borne many children), multilobar (numerous lobes), multicentric (many centers)
-necro-	Dead	Necrosed, necrosis, necropsy (postmortem examination), necrophobia (fear of death)
-neo-	New	Neoformation, neomorphism (form), neonatal (first 4 weeks of life), neopathy (disease)

-oligo-	Few, scanty, little	Oligophrenia (mind), oligopnea (breath), oliguria (urine), oligodipsia (thirst)
-ortho-	Straight, normal, correct	Orthodontic (teeth, normal), orthogenesis (progressive evolution in a given direction), orthograde (walk, carrying body upright), orthopnea (breath, unable to breathe unless in an upright position)
-oxy-	Sharp, quick	Oxyesthesia (feel), oxyopia (vision), oxyosmia (smell)
-pachy-	Thick	Pachyderm (skin), pachysulemia (blood), pachypleuritis (inflammation of pleura), pachycholia (bile), pachyotia (ears)
-paleo-	Old	Paleogenetic (origin in the past), paleopathology (study of diseases in mummies)
-platy-	Flat	Platybasia (skull base), platycoria (pupil), platycrania (skull)
-pleo-	More	Pleomorphism (forms), pleochromocytoma (tumor composed of different colored cells)
-poikilo-	Varied	Poikiloderma (skin mottling), poikilothermal (heat, variable body temperature)
-poly-	Many, much	Polyhedral (many bases or faces), polymastia (more than two breasts), polymelia (supernumerary limbs), polymyalgia (pain in many muscles)
pronus-	Face down	Prone, pronation
-pseudo-	False, spurious	Pseudostratified (layered), pseudocirrhosis (apparent cirrhosis of liver), pseudohypertrophy
-sclero-	Hard	Sclerosis (hardening), arteriosclerosis (artery), scleronychia (nails), scleroderma (skin)
-scolio-	Twisted, crooked	Scoliodontic (teeth), scoliosis, scoliokyphosis (curvature of spine)
-sinistro-	Left	Sinistrocardia, sinistromanual (left handed), sinistraural (hearing better in left ear)
-steno-	Narrow	Stenosis, stenostomia (mouth), mitral stenosis (mitral valve in heart)
-stereo-	Solid, three dimensions	Stereoscope, stereometer
-supinus-	Face up	Supine, supination, supinator longus (muscle in arm)
-tachy-	Fast, swift	Tachycardia (heart), tachyphrasia (speech)
-tele-	End, far away	Telepathy, telecardiogram
-telo-	Complete	Telophase
-thermo-	Heat, warm	Thermal, thermometer, thermobiosis (ability to live in high temperature)
-trachy-	Rough	Trachyphonia (voice), trachychromatic (deeply staining)
-xero-	Dry	Xerophagia (eating of dry foods) xerostomia (mouth), xeroderma (skin)

PRONUNCIATION OF MEDICAL-DENTAL TERMS

Medical terms are hard to pronounce, especially if a person has read them but never heard them spoken. Following are some helpful shortcuts:

ch is sometimes pronounced like *k*. Examples: chromatin, chronic.

ps is pronounced like *s*. Examples: psychiatry, psychology.

pn is pronounced with only the *n* sound. Example: pneumonia.

c and *g* are given the soft sound of *s* and *j*, respectively, before *e, i,* and *y* in words of both Greek and Latin origin. Examples: cycle, cytoplasm, giant, generic.

c and *g* have a harsh before other letters. Examples: gastric, gonad, cast, cardiac.

ae and *oe* are pronounced *ee*. Examples: coelom, fasciae.

i at the end of a word (to form a plural) is pronounced *eye*. Examples: alveoli, glomeruli, fasciculi.

e and *es,* when forming the final letters or letter of a word, are often pronounced as separate syllables. Examples: rete (reetee), nares (nayreez).

PLURALS

In most English words the plurals are formed by merely adding an *s* or *es,* but in Greek and Latin the plural may be designated by changing the ending.

-*ae,* as in fasciae (singular form, fascia). -*ia,* as in crania (singular form, cranium).

-*i,* as in glomeruli (singular form, glomerulus). When the singular form ends in *us,* the plural form is made by adding *i* and dropping the *us.*

-*ata,* as in adenomata (singular form, adenoma).

SPELLING

The aforementioned rules for pronunciation and the formation of plurals are essential for spelling, but the professional should consult a medical dictionary if unsure. Phonetic spelling has no place in medicine, because a misspelled word may give the wrong meaning to a diagnosis. Furthermore, some terms are pronounced alike but spelled differently; for example, ileum is a part of the intestinal tract, but ilium is a pelvic bone.

Abbreviations

@ at
A amp
a before
aa of each (F. ana)
AAAS American Association for the Advancement of Science
AADE American Association of Dental Editors, also American Association of Dental Examiners
AADGP American Association of Dental Group Practice
AADP American Association of Denture Prosthetics
AADPA American Association of Dental Practice Administration
AADR American Association of Dental Radiology
AADS American Association of Dental Schools
AAE American Association of Endodontics
AAFP American Association of Family Physicians.
AAGFO American Association of Gold Foil Operators
AAGO American Association of Gnathologic Orthopedics
AAGP American Association of General Practice
AAHD American Association of Hospital Dentists
AAID American Association of Implant Dentistry
AAMC American Association of Medical Colleges
AAMP American Academy of Maxillofacial Prosthetics
AAMRL American Association of Medical Record Librarians
AAO American Association of Orthodontists
AAOGP American Association of Orthodontics for the General Practitioner

AAOP American Academy of Oral Pathology
AAP American Academy of Pediatrics
AAPA American Academy of Physician Assistants
AAPHD American Association of Public Health Dentists
abd abdomen
ABDPH American Board of Dental Public Health
ABE American Board of Endodontics
ABGs arterial blood gases
ABO American Board of Orthodontics (see also blood groups)
ABOMS American Board of Oral and Maxillofacial Surgery
ABOP American Board of Oral Pathology
ABP American Board of Pedodontics, also American Board of Periodontics
ABP American Board of Prosthodontics
a.c. before meals (L., *ante cibum*)
ACE angiotensin-converting enzyme
Ach acetylcholine
ACT activated coagulation time
ACTH adrenocorticotropic hormone
ad Latin preposition, to, up to
a.d. alternating days (L., *alternis diebus*)
ADA American Dental Association
ADAMHA Alcohol, Drug Abuse, and Mental Health Administration
ADH antidiuretic hormone
ad lib. at pleasure, as needed or desired (L., *ad libitum*)

565

adm. admission
ADP adenosine diphosphate
AFB acid-fast bacilli
AFDC Aid to Families with Dependent Children
A/G albumin-globulin (ratio)
Ag silver (L., *argentum*)
AIDS acquired immunodeficiency syndrome
AKA also known as
alb. albumin
alc. alcoholism
alk. alkaline
ALT alanine aminotransferase, serum
alt. dieb. every other day (L., *alternis diebus*)
alt. hor. every other hour (L., *alternis horis*)
alt. noct. every other night (L., *alterna nocte*)
AM, a.m. before noon (L., *ante meridiem*)
am. a, ag amalgam
AMA American Medical Association, also against medical advice
amb. ambulation
amp. ampule
amt amount
ANA antinuclear antibodies
anat. anatomy, anatomic
anes. anesthesia
ant. anterior
ANUG acute necrotizing ulcerative gingivitis
AP anteroposterior
APAP *N*-acetyl-*p*-aminophenol
APF acidulated phosphofluoride
appl. applicable, application, appliance
approx. approximate
APTT activated partial thromboplastin time
aq. water (L., *aqua*)
ARC acquired immunodeficiency syndrome (AIDS)–related complex
AROM active range of motion
ASA acetylsalicylic acid, aspirin
ASAP as soon as possible
ASHD arteriosclerotic heart disease
AST aspartate aminotransferase, serum

AV atrioventricular
Av, avdp. avoirdupois
av. average
AZT azidothymidine

bact. bacterium (-ia)
BAL blood alcohol level
bar. barometric
basos. basophils
BCC basal cell carcinoma
BF bone fragment
BIA Bureau of Indian Affairs
bib. drink (L., *bibe*)
b.i.d. twice a day (L., *bis in die*)
biol. biologic, biology
BM bowel movement
BMR basal metabolic rate
bol. bolus
BP blood pressure
BPH benign prostatic hypertrophy
bpm beats per minute
BS blood sugar
BSA body surface area
BUN blood urea nitrogen
BW bite wing radiograph
Bx biopsy

C Celsius (centigrade), one hundred (L., *centum*)
c with (L., *cum*)
C-1 to C-7 cervical vertebrae 1 to 7
CA cardiac arrest, chronologic age
Ca calcium, also carcinoma (cancer)
CAD coronary artery disease
cal calorie
cAMP cyclic adenosine monophosphate
cap. capsule
cath. catheterization or catheterize
cav. cavity
CBC complete blood count
CBS chronic brain syndrome
CC chief complaint
cc cubic centimeter
CDC Centers for Disease Control and Prevention
cent. centigrade
CF complement fixation
cf compare, refer to (L., *confer*)
CFNP Community Food and Nutrition Programs

CFR   Code of Federal Regulations
CFT   complement fixation test
CHD   childhood disease
CHF   congestive heart failure
chr.   chronic
CM   costal margin
cm   centimeter
c.m.   tomorrow morning (L., *cras mane*)
c/min   cycles per minute
cm/s   centimeters per second
CMV   cytomegalovirus
CNS   central nervous system
CO   carbon monoxide, also cardiac output
CO₂   Carbon dioxide
Co   cobalt
c/o   complains of, also care of
COD   condition on discharge
comp.   compound
conc.   concentrated
cond.   condition
COPD   chronic obstructive pulmonary disease
CP   centric position
CPAP   continuous positive airway pressure
CPC   Clinical Pathology Conference
cpd.   compound
CPK   creatine phosphokinase
CPR   cardiopulmonary resuscitation
c.p.s.   cycles per second
CrCl   creatinine clearance
Cs   conscious, consciousness
C section   cesarean section
CSF   cerebrospinal fluid
Cu   copper (L., *cuprum*)
cu   cubic
cur   curettage
CV   cardiovascular
CVA   cerebrovascular accident
CVP   central venous pressure
Cx   convex
CY   calender year
cyl.   cylinder, cylindric

D   dose (L., *dosis*), also distal
D₁ to D₁₂   dorsal vertebrae 1 to 12 (see T₁ to T₁₂)
DA   direct admission

db   decibel
dbl.   double
D & C   dilation and curettage
dc   direct current
DC & B   dilation, curettage, and biopsy
DD   differential diagnosis
d.d.   Let it be given to (L., *detur ad*)
ddC   dideoxycytidine
DDI   dideoxyinosine
DDT   dichlorodiphenyltrichloroethane
DEA   Drug Enforcement Administration
deg.   degree
dev.   develop, development
DG, diag   diagnosis
diam.   diameter
diff.   differential
dil.   dilute (L., *dilue*)
dim.   diminutive, diminish
dis.   disease
disc.   discontinue
disch.   discharge
disp.   dispensary
dist.   distal
dl   deciliter
DM   diabetes mellitus
DMF   decayed, missing, and filled (teeth)
DNA   deoxyribonucleic acid
DO   distocclusal
DOA   dead on arrival
DOB   date of birth
doz.   dozen
DPT   diphtheria, pertussis, tetanus
Dr.   doctor
dr.   dram
dsg.   dressing
DT   delirium tremens
d.t.d.   give such a dose (L., *detur talis dosis*)
DTR   deep tendon reflexes
DUI   driving under the influence
D/W   dextrose and water
dwt   pennyweight
Dx   diagnosis

EAC   external auditory canal
EBL   estimated blood loss
ECG   electrocardiogram
E. coli   *Escherichia coli*
ECT   electroconvulsive therapy

ED   effective dose
EDTA   ethylenediaminetetraacetic acid
EEG   electroencephalogram
EENT   ears, eyes, nose, and throat
EEO   equal employment opportunity
EEOC   Equal Employment Opportunity Commission
e.g.   for example (L., *exempli gratia*)
EIA   enzyme immunoassay
EKG   electrokardiogram (German)
ELISA   enzyme-linked immunosorbent assay
elix.   elixir (hydroalcoholic solution containing an active drug or drugs)
emerg.   emergency
EMT   emergency medical treatment
ENT   ears, nose, and throat
EOM   extraocular movements
eos.   eosinophil
EPA   Environmental Protection Agency
epith.   epithelial
equiv.   equivalent
esp.   especially
ESR   erythrocyte sedimentation rate
est.   estimate, estimation
et   Latin conjunction *and*
et al.   and others (L., *et alii*)
etc.   and so forth, and others (L., *et cetera*)
EUA   examination under anesthesia
evac.   evacuate, evacuation
eval.   evaluate, evaluation
ext.   extract, external

F   Fahrenheit, also female, field (of vision), formula
FB   fingerbreadth, also foreign body
FBS   fasting blood sugar
FD   fatal dose
FDA   Food and Drug Administration
ff   following
FH   family history
FHT   fetal heart tones
FIO₂   forced inspired oxygen concentration
fl.   fluid
FLD   full lower denture

fld.   field
fl. dr.   fluid dram
fl. oz.   fluid ounce
FMX   full mouth x-ray examination
FNS   Food and Nutrition Service
F & R   force and rhythm (pulse)
frac.   fracture
frag.   fragment
freq.   frequent, frequency
FSH   follicle-stimulating hormone
FSQS   Food Safety and Quality Service
ft.   foot, also let it be made (L., *fiat, fiant*)
FTC   Federal Trade Commission
FTSG   full-thickness skin graft
FUD   full upper denture
funct.   function
FUO   fever of undetermined origin
Fx   fracture

gal.   gallon
GB   gallbladder
GC   gonococcus, gonococcal
GH   general hospital
GI   gastrointestinal
GIF   gastric intrinsic factor
ging.   gingiva, gingivectomy
glob.   globulin
gm   gram
GP   general practitioner
G6PD   glucose-6-phosphate dehydrogenase
gr   grain
GSW   gunshot wound
gt.   drop (L., *gutta*)
GTT   glucose tolerance test
gtt.   drops (L., *guttae*)
GU   genitourinary
G/W   glucose and water
Gyn   gynecology

H, h   hour (L., *hora*), also hypodermically
Hb   hemoglobin
HBD   has been drinking
HBP   high blood pressure
HC   hospital course
HCA   hydrocortisone acetate
HCFA   Home Care Financing Administration
HCG   human chorionic gonadotropin

HCl hydrochloric acid

Hct hematocrit

h.d. at hour of lying down, at bedtime (L., *hora decubitus*)

HDCV human diploid cell rabies vaccine

HDL high-density lipoprotein

Hdpc. handpiece

Hgb hemoglobin

H&H hematocrit and hemoglobin

HIAA Health Insurance Association of America

HIV-1 human immunodeficiency virus type 1

HIV-2 human immunodeficiency virus type 2

HIV-G human immunodeficiency virus gingivitis

HIV-P human immunodeficiency virus periodontitis

H₂O water

hosp. hospital

H&P history and physical examination

hpf high-power field

HPI history of present illness

HR heart rate

hr hour

h.s. hour of sleep, at bedtime (L., *hora somni*)

HSA Health Services Administration

HSV herpes simplex virus

ht. height

HVD hypertensive vascular disease

Hx history

IA incurred accidentally

ibid. in the same place (L., *ibidem*)

ICS intercostal space

ICSH interstitial cell-stimulating hormone

ICT inflammation of connective tissue

ICU intensive care unit

I&D incision and drainage

id. the same (L., *idem*)

i.e. that is (L., *id est*)

IgG immunoglobulin G

IH infectious hepatitis

IM intramuscular

imp. impression

in. inch

inc. incisal, incisive, incise

in d. daily (L., *in dies*)

inf. infected, inferior, infusion

INH isonicotinic hydrazide

inh. inhalation

inj. injection, injury

inoc. inoculate

inop. inoperable, inoperative

INR/PT international normalized ratio/prothrombin time

int. internal

I&O intake and output

IOP intraocular pressure

IP intercuspal position, initial pressure (spinal fluid)

IPPB intermittent positive pressure breathing

IQ intelligence quotient

i.q. the same as (L., *idem quod*)

IS interspace, also inventory of systems

ITP idiopathic thrombocytopenic purpura

IU international unit

IUD intrauterine contraceptive device

IV intravenous

JCAHO Joint Commission on the Accreditation of Health Care Organizations

jt. joint

K potassium

kc kilocycle

kg, kgm, kilo kilogram

KS Kaposi's sarcoma

kV kilovolt

L Latin, also liter and left

L₁ to L₅ lumbar vertebrae 1 to 5

lab. laboratory

lac. laceration

lap. laparotomy

LASER, laser light amplification by stimulated emission of radiation

lat. lateral

lb pound

LBP low back pain

LD   lethal dose
LDH   lactic dehydrogenase
LDL   low-density lipoprotein
LE   lupus erythematosus
LH   luteinizing hormone
LHRH   luteinizing hormone-releasing hormone
lig.   ligament
ling.   lingual
liq.   liquid, liquor
LJP   localized juvenile periodontitis
LLQ   left lower quadrant
LMD   local medical doctor
LMP   last menstrual period
LN   lymph node
LOC   loss of consciousness
LPF   low-power field
LR   lactated Ringer's solution
LSH   lutein-stimulating hormone
lt.   left
LUQ   left upper quadrant
L & W   living and well
lymphs   lymphocytes

M   Meter, also male, mesial, mix (L., *misce*)
m   murmur, meter, minim
m²   square meter
MA   mental age, also moderately advanced
ma   milliampere
MAL   midaxillary line
mand.   mandibular
MAOI   monoamine oxidase inhibitor
MASER, maser   microwave amplification by stimulated emission of radiation
max.   maximum, maxillary
Mc   megacurie, megacycle
mc   millicurie
MCA   motorcycle accident
mcg.   microgram
MCH   mean corpuscular hemoglobin
MCHC   mean corpuscular hemoglobin concentration
MCV   mean corpuscular volume
m. dict.   as directed (L., *more dicto*)
MDR   minimum daily requirement
MED   minimal effective dose

med.   medical, medicine
MEDLARS   Medical Literature Analysis and Retrieval System
mEq   milliequivalent
mes.   mesial
mg, mgm   milligram
MHB   maximum hospital benefit
MI   myocardial infarction
micro.   microscopic
min.   minute, minimum
MIST   Medical Information Service via Telephone
mixt.   mixture
ML   midline
ml   milliliter
MLD   minimal lethal dosage
MM   mucous membrane
mm   millimeter
MO   mesioocclusal
mo.   month
MOD   mesioocclusodistal
monos.   monocytes
MS   multiple sclerosis
msec.   millisecond
MSH   melanocyte-stimulating hormone
mV   millivolt
MVA   motor vehicle accident

Na   sodium
NAD   no appreciable disease
NaPent   thiopental sodium (Pentothal)
narc.   narcotic, narcotism
NAS   National Academy of Sciences
NC   nasal cannula
nc   no change
NDF   no disease found
neg.   negative
NIDDM   non–insulin-dependent diabetes mellitus
NIH   National Institutes of Health
NKA   no known allergies
NLM   National Library of Medicine
NMI   no middle initial
NMR   nuclear magnetic resonance
N₂O   nitrous oxide
noc.   night
non rep.   do not repeat
norm.   normal

NP neuropsychiatry
NPC no previous complaint
NPH no previous history
NPN nonprotein nitrogen
n.p.o. nothing by mouth (L., *non per os*)
NR normal record
n.r. not to be repeated (L., *non repetatur*)
NRC Nuclear Regulatory Commission, also National Research Council
NS not significant
N/S normal saline
NSA no significant abnormality
NSAID nonsteroidal antiinflammatory drug
NTP normal temperature and pressure
NV neurovascular
N/V nausea and vomiting

O oxygen
O₂ oxygen gas
OB obstetrics
OB-GYN obstetrics and gynecology
obl. oblique
OBS organic brain syndrome
occ. occlusal
OCD Office of Child Development
OCSE Office of Child Support Enforcement
OD right eye
o.d. every day (L., *omni die*)
ODC oral disease control
OH oral hygiene
o.h. every hour (L., *omni hora*)
OHD Office of Human Development
OHI Office for Handicapped Individuals
OHMO Office of Hazardous Materials Operations
oint. ointment
o.m. every morning (L., *omni mane*)
o.n. every night (L., *omni nocte*)
op. operation
OPC outpatient clinic
OPD outpatient department

Ophth ophthalmology
opp. opposite, opposed
OPS outpatient section or service
OR operating room
org. organism, organic
ORIF open reduction, internal fixation
OS left eye
os mouth
OSHA Occupational Safety and Health Administration
OT occupational therapy
OTC over the counter
OU each eye
OYD Office of Youth Development
oz ounce

P pulse, also after (L., *post*)
p page, paragraph
PA posteroanterior
P&A percussion and auscultation
PAB, PABA paraaminobenzoic acid
Paco₂ arterial carbon dioxide tension (pressure tore)
PAHO Pan American Health Organization
Pan. panoral x-ray examination
Pao₂ arterial oxygen tension (pressure tore)
PAS, PASA paraaminosalicylic acid
PAT paroxysmal atrial tachycardia
PATH pituitary adrenotropic hormone
path. pathology
PBCM particulate bone and cancellous marrow grafts
PBI protein-bound iodine
p.c. after meal (L., *post cibum*)
PCN penicillin
PCP *Pneumocystis carinii* pneumonia
pcpt. perception
PCWP pulmonary capillary wedge pressure
PDR *Physician's Desk Reference*
PE physical examination
Ped pediatrics
PEEP positive end-expiratory pressure
pen. penetrating

perf. perforating

PERRLA pupils equal, round, react to light and accommodation

PH past history

pH negative logarithm of hydrogen ion concentration

PI present illness

PID pelvic inflammatory disease

PLD partial lower denture

PM, p.m. after noon (L., *post meridiem*), also petit mal, after death (L., *post mortem*)

PMB polymorphonuclear basophil leukocytes

PME polymorphonuclear eosinophil leukocytes

PMH past medical history

PMN polymorphonuclear neutrophil leukocytes

PMP previous menstrual period

PMS premenstrual syndrome

PN percussion note

PO postoperative

p.o. by mouth (L., *per os*)

POD 1, 2, etc. postoperative day one, two, etc.

POH personal oral hygiene

polys. polymorphonuclear leukocytes

pos. positive

postop. postoperative

pp postpartum, postprandial

PPBS postprandial blood sugar

PPLO pleuropneumonia-like organism

ppm parts per million

PPO Preferred Provider Organization

ppt. precipitate

preop. preoperatively

prep. preparation, prepare (for surgery)

p.r.n. as required or needed, as the occasion arises (L., *pro re nata*)

PRO Peer Review Organization

prog. prognosis

PT physical therapy, physiotherapy, prothrombin time

pt. patient

PTT partial thromboplastin time

PUD partial upper denture

pulm. pulmonary

PVC premature ventricular contraction

Px prophylaxis

q. every (L., *quaque*)

q.a.m. every morning (L., *quaque ante meridiem*)

q.d. every day (L., *quaque die*)

q2d every 2 days

q.h. every hour (L., *quaque hora*)

q2h every second hour

q.h.s. every night (L., *quaque hora somni*)

q.i.d. four times a day (L., *quater in die*)

q.l. as much as pleased (L., *quantum libet*)

q.mo every month

q.n. every night (L., *quaque nocte*)

q.o.d. every other day

q.p. at will (L., *quantum placeat*)

q.p.m. every night (L., *quaque post meridiem*)

q.q.h. every 4 hours (L., *quaque quarta hora*)

q.s. a sufficient quantity

qt. quart

q.v. as much as liked (L., *quantum vis*)

qwk every week

R respiration, rectal

r right, roentgen

RA rheumatoid arthritis

rad. radiograph

RAI radioactive iodine

RAIU radioactive iodine uptake

RBC red blood cells, red blood count

RC retruded contact position, root canal

REC rectal

reg. regular

REM rapid eye movement

rem roentgen equivalent, man

rep roentgen equivalent physical

req. requires, required

resp. respiration

Rh rhesus blood factor

RHD rheumatic heart disease

RLQ right lower quadrant

RN registered nurse

RNA ribonucleic acid
R/O rule out
ROH alcohol
ROM range of motion
ROS review of systems
RQ respiratory quotient
R&R rate and rhythm
RR&E round, regular, and equal (pupils)
RSA Rehabilitation Services Administration
RUQ right upper quadrant
Rx treatment, therapy, or prescription (L., *recipe*)

s without (L., *sine*)
S₁ to S₅ sacral vertebrae 1 to 5
SA node sinoatrial node
SBE subacute bacterial endocarditis
SC subcutaneous
SD sterile dressing
sec. second, secondary
sed. rate sedimentation rate
segs segmented cells
SG skin graft, specific gravity
SGOT serum glutamic-oxaloacetic transaminase
SGPT serum glutamic-pyruvic transaminase
SI seriously ill
Sig. write on, label
SIL seriously ill list
SL sublingual
SLE systemic lupus erythematosus
SN sinus node
sol. solution
spec. specimen
sp. fl. spinal fluid
sp. gr. specific gravity
SR systems review
S/S signs and symptoms
ss one half (L., *semis*), signs and symptoms
SSA Social Security Administration
ST sedimentation time
st. let it stand (L., *stet*)
stat. immediately (L., *statim*)
std. standard
stim. stimulator, stimulate
Strep *Streptococcus*

STS serologic test for syphilis
STSG split-thickness skin graft
SUD skin unit dose
sup. superior
suppos. suppository
surg. surgeon, surgery
susp. suspension
sus. rel. sustained release
Sx symptom
sym. symmetric
symp. symptom
syr. syrup, a highly concentrated sucrose solution containing a drug
sys. system

T temperature
T₁ to T₁₂ thoracic vertebrae 1 to 12
T&A tonsils and adenoids, also tonsillectomy and adenoidectomy
tab. tablet
TAH total abdominal hysterectomy
TAT tetanus antitoxin
TB,TBC tuberculosis
TBG thyroxine-binding globulin
tbsp. tablespoon
TC treatment completed
TD transdermal
TE tracheoesophageal
temp. temperature
TIBC total iron-binding capacity
t.i.d. three times a day (L., *ter in die*)
time rel. time release
tinc. tincture (alcoholic solution of a drug)
TLC tender loving care
TM temporomandibular
TMD temporomandibular dysfunction
TMJ temporomandibular joint
TMJ-PDS temporomandibular joint pain dysfunction syndrome
TNF tumor necrosis factor
top. topical
TPN total parenteral nutrition
TPR temperature, pulse, respiration
TSH thyroid-stimulating hormone
TSP total serum protein

tsp. teaspoon
TT thrombin time
TTP/HUS thrombotic thrombocytopenic purpura/hemolytic uremic syndrome
TUR transurethral resection
Tx treatment

U, u unit
UA urinalysis
UCHD usual childhood diseases
UGA under general anesthesia
UIBC unsaturated iron-binding capacity
UIS Unemployment Insurance Service
ung. ointment (L., *unguentum*)
unk. unknown
URI upper respiratory tract infection
USP United States Pharmacopeia
ut dict. as directed
UV ultraviolet (light)

V volt
VA Veterans Administration
vag. vaginal
VC vital capacity
VD venereal disease
VDH valvular disease of the heart
VDRL Venereal Disease Research Laboratory

vert. vertebra, also vertical
visc. viscous
vit. vitamin
viz. that is, namely (L., *videlicet*)
VLDL very low-density lipoprotein
VO verbal order
vol. volume
VS vital signs
vs versus
v.s. see above (L., *vide supra*)
VZV varicella zoster virus

WBC white blood cells
Wd ward
w-d well-developed
WHO World Health Organization
wk. week
w-n well nourished
wnd. wound
WNL within normal limits
wt. weight

yr. year

$>$ greater than
$<$ less than
$\neq$ not equal
$\uparrow$ increase
$\downarrow$ decrease
$2°$ secondary

APPENDIX C

Code on Dental Procedures and Nomenclature*

COUNCIL ON DENTAL CARE PROGRAMS

The Council on Dental Care Programs of the American Dental Association (ADA) has approved the eighth revision of the *Code on Dental Procedures and Nomenclature.* The code was developed in 1969 and published in the *Journal of the American Dental Association* (*J Am Dent Assoc* 79:814, 1969). The eighth revision of the code is a result of the work of the Council on Dental Care Programs in consultation with an advisory committee comprised of council members and representatives from the Blue Cross and Blue Shield Association, the Health Insurance Association of America, the Health Care Financing Administration (HCFA), National Electronic Information Corporation, and ADA-recognized dental specialty organizations.

Procedures Covered

Although the code includes primarily the dental services most frequently provided in a dentist's office, it also lists dental services provided in a hospital. Diagnostic services common to most categories of treatment are grouped under a separate diagnostic listing. These include oral examinations, radiographs, tests, and laboratory examinations. Dental services frequently performed by dental specialists have been grouped under the specialty category with which the procedures are most frequently identified. The groupings according to specialty categories are solely for convenience in using the code and should not be interpreted as excluding general practitioners from performing such procedures.

Coding System

The code is a five-digit system to identify dental procedures and services. The first digit is a zero throughout the code, and it identifies all procedures as being dental as contrasted to medical, hospital, or surgical services. The second digit designates the category of dental service. The third digit indicates the class of service within the dental category, and the fourth digit designates the subclass or specific procedure. The fifth digit allows for further expansion of the code when necessary.

New procedure code numbers added to the eighth edition are identified with the symbol ● placed before the code number. In instances in which a code has been revised, the symbol ▲ is placed before the code number.

Guidelines For Use of the Code

1. The existence of a code does not mean that the procedure is a covered or reimbursable benefit in a dental benefits plan. Offices may have difficulty becoming familiar with the details of every dental plan with which

---

*From Council on Dental Care Programs: *CDT-2,* Chicago, 1995-2000, American Dental Association.

they must work. The patient, not the dental office, bears the responsibility of knowing covered and excluded services in the dental plan. Certain dental benefits plans require predetermination when covered charges are expected to exceed a certain amount.

2. The dental procedure codes are divided into 12 categories of service. Procedures that are performed by general practitioners and specialists have been grouped under the category with which the procedures are most frequently identified. The categories are solely for convenience in using the code and should not be interpreted as excluding general practitioners from performing or reporting such procedures.

3. Any procedure not accurately described in this code should be reported using the appropriate unspecified (999) code with a narrative description. Unspecified codes are included for each category, with the exception of the preventive section. Offices may find occasions when a narrative report should be used. When reporting a procedure that is unusual or is accompanied by unusual circumstances, a narrative description (by report) with reference to the proper "999" number may be the most appropriate way of explaining treatment to the third-party payer. However, third-party payers may request additional documentation of certain procedures regardless of the presence of the nomenclature by report.

Coding System

The code is set up in a five-digit system that identifies procedures and services. The categories are:

	Category of service	Code series
I.	Diagnostic	00100-00999
II.	Preventive	01000-01999
III.	Restorative	02000-02999
IV.	Endodontics	03000-03999
V.	Periodontics	04000-04999
VI.	Prosthodontics, Removable	05000-05899
VII.	Maxillofacial Prosthetics	05900-05999
VIII.	Implant Services	06000-06199
IX.	Prosthodontics, Fixed	06200-06999
X.	Oral Surgery	07000-07999
XI.	Orthodontics	08000-08999
XII.	Adjunctive General Services	09000-09999

Additional coding systems that may be used in a dental office are *International Classification of Diseases ICD-9;* Current Procedural Terminology (CPT), and HCFA's *Common Procedure Coding System (HCPCS).* For more specific information, please contact the following:

ICD Associates
1604 West Liberty
Ann Arbor, MI 48103
(313) 741-1868

CPT
American Medical Association
Coding Assistance
P.O. Box 10946
Chicago, IL 60610
(312) 464-5000

HCPCS
HCFA
Superintendent of Documents
U.S. Government Printing Office
(202) 783-3238

Canadian Dental Association
Coding Assistance
1815 Alta Vista
Ottawa, Canada K16 3Y6
(613) 523-1770
Fax: (613) 523-7736

00100-00999
I. Diagnostic
Clinical Oral Evaluations

The codes in this section have been revised to recognize the cognitive skills necessary for patient evaluation. The collection and recording of some data and components of the dental examination may be delegated; however, the evaluation, diagnosis, and treatment planning are the responsibility of the dentist. As with all ADA procedure codes, no distinction is made between the evaluations provided by general practitioners and specialists. Additional diagnostic and definitive procedures should be reported separately.

00120 *periodic oral evaluation*

An evaluation performed on a patient of record to determine any changes in the patient's dental and medical health status since a previous comprehensive or periodic evaluation. This may require interpretation of information acquired through additional diagnostic procedures. Report additional diagnostic procedures separately.

00140 *limited oral evaluation—problem focused*

An evaluation or reevaluation limited to a specific oral health problem. This may require interpretation of information acquired through additional diagnostic procedures. Report additional diagnostic procedures separately. Definitive procedures may be required on the same date as the evaluation.

Typically, patients receiving this type of evaluation have been referred for a specific problem or arrive with dental emergencies, trauma, or acute infections.

00150 *comprehensive oral evaluation*

Typically used by a general dentist or specialist when evaluating a patient comprehensively. It is a thorough evaluation and recording of the extraoral and intraoral hard and soft tissues. It may require interpretation of information acquired through additional diagnostic procedures. Additional diagnostic procedures should be reported separately. *This evaluation includes the evaluation and recording of the patient's dental and medical history and a general health assessment. It may typically include the evaluation and recording of dental caries, missing or unerupted teeth, restorations, occlusal relationships, periodontal conditions (including periodontal charting), and hard and soft tissue anomalies.*

00160 *detailed and extensive oral evaluation—problem-focused, by report*

A detailed and extensive problem-focused evaluation entails extensive diagnostic and cognitive modalities based on the findings of a comprehensive oral evaluation. Integration of more extensive diagnostic modalities to develop a treatment plan for a specific problem is required. The condition requiring this type of evaluation should be described and documented.

Examples of conditions requiring this type of evaluation may include dentofacial anomalies, complicated perioprosthetic conditions, complex temporomandibular dysfunction, facial pain of unknown origin, and severe systemic diseases requiring multidisciplinary consultation.

Radiographs and Diagnostic Imaging

Radiographs should be taken only for clinical reasons as determined by the patient's dentist. They should be of diagnostic quality and properly identified and dated. Radiographs are a part of the patient's clinical record, and the original films should be retained by the dentist. Originals should not be used to fulfill requests made by patients or third parties for copies of records.

00210 intraoral—complete series (including bite wings)

00220 intraoral—periapical—first film

00230 intraoral—periapical—each additional film

00240 intraoral—occlusal film

00250 extraoral—first film

00260 extraoral—each additional film

00270 bite wing—single film

00272 bite wings—two films

00274 bite wings—four films

00290 posteroanterior or lateral skull and facial bone survey film

00310 sialography

00320 temporomandibular joint arthrogram, including injection

00321 other temporomandibular joint films, by report

00322 tomographic survey

00330 panoramic film

00340 cephalometric film

Tests and Laboratory Examinations

00415 bacteriologic studies for determination of pathologic agents
These studies may include but are not limited to tests for susceptibility to periodontal disease.

00425 caries susceptibility tests

00460 pulp vitality tests
These tests include multiple teeth and contralateral comparisons, as indicated.

00470 diagnostic casts
These are also known as diagnostic models or study models.

00471 diagnostic photographs
These include both traditional photographs and images obtained by intraoral cameras. These images should be a part of the patient's clinical record.

00501 histopathologic examinations
This term refers to gross and microscopic evaluations of presumptively abnormal tissue.

00502 other oral pathology procedures, by report
See 00501.

00999 unspecified diagnostic procedures, by report
Used for procedures that are not adequately described by a code. Describe procedure.

01000-01999

II. Preventive

Dental Prophylaxis

01110 prophylaxis—adult
A dental prophylaxis performed on transitional or permanent dentition; it includes scaling and polishing procedures to remove coronal plaque, calculus, and stains. Some patients may require more than one appointment or one extended appointment to complete a prophylaxis. Document need for additional time or appointments.

01120 prophylaxis—child
　　　Refers to a routine dental prophylaxis performed on primary or transitional dentition only.

Topical Fluoride Treatment (Office Procedure)
Fluoride must be applied separately from prophylaxis paste.
01201 topical application of fluoride (including prophylaxis)—child
　　　Used to report combined procedures of prophylaxis and fluoride treatment.
01203 topical application of fluoride (prophylaxis not included)—child
　　　This code is used when reporting prophylaxis and fluoride procedures separately.
01204 topical application of fluoride (prophylaxis not included)—adult
　　　This code is used when reporting prophylaxis and fluoride procedures separately.
01205 topical application of fluoride (including prophylaxis)—adult
　　　This code is used to report combined procedures of prophylaxis and fluoride treatment.

Other Preventive Services
01310 nutritional counseling for control of dental disease
　　　Refers to counseling on food selection and dietary habits as a part of treatment and control of periodontal disease and caries.
01320 tobacco counseling for the control and prevention of oral disease
　　　Tobacco prevention and cessation services reduce patient risks of developing tobacco-related oral diseases and conditions and improves prognosis for certain dental therapies.
01330 oral hygiene instructions
　　　This may include instructions for home care. Examples include toothbrushing technique, flossing, and use of special oral hygiene aids.
01351 sealant—per tooth
　　　Pit and fissure sealants have been documented by many studies to be a highly effective therapeutic measure for the prevention of dental caries.

Space Maintenance (Passive Appliances)
Passive appliances are designed to prevent tooth movement.
01510 space maintainer—fixed—unilateral
01515 space maintainer—fixed—bilateral
01520 space maintainer—removable—unilateral
01525 space maintainer—removable—bilateral
01550 recementation of space maintainer

02000-02999
III. Restorative*
A one-surface posterior restoration is one in which the restoration involves only one of the five surface classifications (mesial, distal, occlusal, lingual, or facial). A two-surface posterior restoration is one in which the restoration extends to two of the five surface classifications. A three-surface posterior restoration is one in which the restoration extends to three of the five surface classifications. A four-or-more surface posterior restoration is one in which the restoration extends to four or more of the five surface classifications.

　　A one-surface anterior proximal restoration is one in which neither the lingual nor facial margins of the restoration extends beyond the line angle. A two-surface anterior proximal restoration is one in which either the lingual or facial margin of the restoration extends beyond the line angle. A three-surface anterior proximal restoration is one in which both the lingual and facial margins of the restorations extend beyond the line angle. A four-or-more surface anterior restoration is one in which both the lingual and facial margins extend beyond the line angle and the incisal angle is involved.

Amalgam Restorations (Including Polishing)

All adhesives (including amalgam bonding agents), liners, and bases are included as part of the restoration. If pins are used, they should be reported separately (see 02951).

02110 *amalgam—one surface, primary**
02120 *amalgam—two surfaces, primary**
02130 *amalgam—three surfaces, primary**
02131 *amalgam—four or more surfaces, primary**
02140 *amalgam—one surface, permanent**
02150 *amalgam—two surfaces, permanent**
02160 *amalgam—three surfaces, permanent**
02161 *amalgam—four or more surfaces, permanent**

Silicae Restorations

02210 *silicate cement—per restoration*

Resin Restorations

Resin refers to a broad category of materials, including but not limited to composites, bonded composite, and light-cured composite. Light-curing, acid-etching, and adhesives (including resin bonding agents) are included as part of the restoration. Glass ionomers, when used as restorations, should be reported with these codes. If pins are used, they should be reported separately (see 02951).

02330 *resin—one surface, anterior**
02331 *resin—two surfaces, anterior**
02332 *resin—three surfaces, anterior**
02335 *resin—four or more surfaces or involving incisal angle (anterior)**
02336 *composite resin crown, anterior—primary*
       Full composite resin coverage of tooth.
02380 *resin—one surface, posterior—primary**
       Includes preventive resin restoration with narrative description.
02381 *resin—two surfaces, posterior—primary**
02382 *resin—three or more surfaces, posterior—primary**
02385 *resin—one surface, posterior—permanent**
       Includes preventive resin restoration with narrative description.
02386 *resin—two surfaces, posterior—permanent**
02387 *resin—three or more surfaces, posterior—permanent**

Gold Foil Restorations

02410 *gold foil—one surface*
02420 *gold foil—two surfaces*
02430 *gold foil—three surfaces*

Inlay or Onlay Restorations

02510 *inlay—metallic—one surface*
02520 *inlay—metallic—two surfaces*

02530 *inlay—metallic—three or more surfaces*

02543 *onlay—metallic—three surfaces*

02544 *onlay—metallic—four or more surfaces*

Porcelain/ceramic inlays presently include all ceramic or porcelain inlays.

02610 *inlay—porcelain/ceramic—one surface*

02620 *inlay—porcelain/ceramic—two surfaces*

02630 *inlay—porcelain/ceramic—three or more surfaces*

02642 *onlay—porcelain/ceramic—two surfaces*

02643 *onlay—porcelain/ceramic—three surfaces*

02644 *onlay—porcelain/ceramic—four or more surfaces*

Composite/resin inlays must be laboratory processed.

02650 *inlay—composite/resin—one surface (laboratory processed)*

02651 *inlay—composite/resin—two surfaces (laboratory processed)*

02652 *inlay—composite/resin—three or more surfaces (laboratory processed)*

02662 *onlay—composite/resin—two surfaces (laboratory processed)*

02663 *onlay—composite/resin—three surfaces (laboratory processed)*

02664 *onlay—composite/resin—four or more surfaces (laboratory processed)*

Crowns—Single Restorations Only

**Classification of metals—the noble metal classification system has been adopted as a more precise method of reporting various alloys used in dentistry. The alloys are defined on the basis of the percentage of noble metal content: high noble—Gold (Au), Palladium (Pd), and Platinum (Pt) ≥60% (with at least 40% Au); noble—Au, Pd, and Pt ≥25%; predominantly base—Au, Pd, and Pt < 25%.

02710 *crown—resin (laboratory)*

02720 *crown—resin with high noble metal**

02721 *crown—resin with predominantly base metal**

02772 *crown—resin with noble metal**

02740 *crown—porcelain/ceramic substrate*

02750 *crown—porcelain fused to high noble metal**

02751 *crown—porcelain fused to predominantly base metal**

02752 *crown—porcelain fused to noble metal**

02790 *crown—full cast high noble metal**

02791 *crown—full cast predominantly base metal**

02792 *crown—full cast noble metal**

02810 *crown—¾ cast metallic**

Other Restorative Services

02910 *recement inlay*

02920 *recement crown*

02930 *prefabricated stainless steel crown—primary tooth*

02931 *prefabricated stainless steel crown—permanent tooth*

02932 *prefabricated resin crown*

02933 *prefabricated stainless steel crown with resin window*

Open-face stainless steel crown with esthetic resin facing or veneer.

02940 *sedative filling*

Temporary restoration intended to relieve pain.

02950 *core buildup, including any pins*

Refers to building up of anatomical crown when restorative crown will be placed, whether or not pins are used.

02951 *pin retention—per tooth, in addition to restoration*
Report each pin separately.

02952 *cast post and core in addition to crown*
Cast post and core is separate from crown.

02954 *prefabricated post and core in addition to crown*
Core is built around a prefabricated post. This procedure includes the core material.

02955 *post removal (not in conjunction with endodontic therapy)*
For removal of posts (for example, fractured posts); not to be used in conjunction with endodontic retreatment (03346, 03347, 03348).

02960 *labial veneer (laminate)—chairside*
Refers to labial and facial bonded veneers.

02961 *labial veneer (resin laminate)—laboratory*
Refers to labial and facial bonded veneers.

02962 *labial veneer (porcelain laminate)—laboratory*
Refers to labial and facial bonded veneers.

02970 *temporary crown (fractured tooth)*
A preformed artificial crown, usually made of stainless steel or resin, which is fitted over a damaged tooth as an immediate protective device in tooth injury.

02980 *crown repair, by report*
Includes removal of crown, if necessary. Describe procedure.

02999 *unspecified restorative procedure, by report*
Use for procedure that is not adequately described by a code. Describe procedure.

03000-03999
IV. Endodontics
Pulp Capping

The ADA sets no standard for appropriate time to place direct and indirect pulp caps (for example, same day as restoration, different day).

03110 *pulp cap—direct (excluding final restoration)*
Procedure in which the exposed pulp is covered with a dressing or cement that protects the pulp and promotes healing and repair.

03120 *pulp cap—indirect (excluding final restoration)*
Procedure in which the nearly exposed pulp is covered with a protective dressing to protect the pulp from additional injury and promote healing and repair through formation of secondary dentin.

Pulpotomy

03220 *therapeutic pulpotomy (excluding final restoration)*
Performed on primary or permanent teeth.

Endodontic Therapy on Primary Teeth

Endodontic therapy on primary teeth with succedaneous teeth and placement of resorbable filling.

03230 *pulpal therapy (resorbable filling)—anterior, primary tooth (excluding final restoration)*
Primary incisors and cuspids.

03240 *pulpal therapy (resorbable filling)—posterior, primary tooth (excluding final restoration)*
Primary first and second molars.

Endodontic Therapy (Including Treatment Plan, Clinical Procedures, and Follow-up Care)

Includes primary teeth without succedaneous teeth and permanent teeth. Complete root canal therapy. Pulpectomy is part of root canal therapy. Procedure includes all appointments necessary to complete treatment; it also includes intraoperative radiographs. It does not include diagnostic evaluation and necessary radiographs and diagnostic images.

03310 anterior (excluding final restoration)
03320 bicuspid (excluding final restoration)
03330 molar (excluding final restoration)

Endodontic Retreatment

This procedure may include the removal of a post, pins, old root canal filling material, and the procedures necessary to prepare and place the new material. This includes complete root canal therapy.

03346 retreatment of previous root canal therapy—anterior
03347 retreatment of previous root canal therapy—bicuspid
03348 retreatment of previous root canal therapy—molar

Apexification and Recalcification Procedures

03351 apexification and recalcification—initial visit (apical closure and calcific repair of perforations and root resorption)
   Includes opening tooth, pulpectomy, preparation of canal spaces, first placement of medication, and necessary radiographs. (This procedure includes first phase of complete root canal therapy.)
03352 apexification and recalcification—interim medication replacement (apical closure and calcific repair of perforations and root resorption)
   For visits in which the intracanal medication is replaced with new medication and necessary radiographs. Several of these visits may occur.
03353 apexification and recalcification—final visit (includes completed root canal therapy—apical closure and calcific repair of perforations and root resorption)
   Includes removal of intracanal medication, procedures necessary to place final root canal filling material, and necessary radiographs. (This procedure includes last phase of complete root canal therapy.)

Apicoectomy and Periradicular Services

*Periradicular surgery is a term used to describe surgery to the root surface (for example, apicoectomy, repair of a root perforation or resorptive defect, exploratory curettage to look for root fractures, removal of extruded filling materials or instruments, removal of broken root fragments, sealing of accessory canals). This does not include retrograde filling material placement.

03410 apicoectomy and periradicular surgery—anterior*
   For surgery on root of anterior tooth. Does not include placement of retrograde filling material.
03421 apicoectomy and periradicular surgery—bicuspid (first root)*
   For surgery on one root of a bicuspid. Does not include placement of retrograde filling material. If more than one root is treated, see 03426.
03425 apicoectomy and periradicular surgery—molar (first root)*
   For surgery on one root of a molar tooth. Does not include placement of retrograde filling material. If more than one root is treated, see 03426.

03426 *apicoectomy and periradicular surgery (each additional root)**

Typically used for premolars and molar surgeries when more than one root is treated during the same procedure. This does not include retrograde filling material placement.

03430 *retrograde filling—per root*

For placement of retrograde filling material during periradicular surgery procedures. If more than one filling is placed in one root, report as 03999 and describe.

03450 *root amputation—per root*

Root resection of a multirooted tooth while leaving the crown. If the crown is sectioned, see 03920.

03460 *endodontic endosseous implant*

Placement of implant material which extends from a pulpal space into the bone beyond the end of the root.

03470 *intentional reimplantation (including necessary splinting)*

This term describes the intentional removal, inspection, and treatment of the root and replacement of a tooth into its own socket. It does not include necessary retrograde filling material placement.

Other Endodontic Procedures

03910 *surgical procedure for isolation of tooth with rubber dam*

03920 *hemisection (including any root removal), not including root canal therapy*

Includes separation of a multirooted tooth into separate sections containing the root and the overlying portion of the crown. It also may include the removal of one or more of those sections.

03950 *canal preparation and fitting of preformed dowel or post*

Should not be reported in conjunction with 02952 or 02954 by the same practitioner.

03960 *bleaching of discolored tooth*

Specify whether tooth is vital or nonvital; report per treatment visit. For enamel microabrasion, see code 09970.

03999 *unspecified endodontic procedure, by report*

Used for procedure that is not adequately described by a code. Describe procedure.

Periodontal Case Types

The following are the American Academy of Periodontology's (AAP) definitions of periodontal case types used for diagnostic identification. Please note that no ADA numeric codes are associated with these case types, because the ADA's *Code on Dental Procedures and Nomenclature* is intended to classify treatment, not diagnoses.

- Case type I—Gingivitis: Inflammation of the gingiva characterized clinically by changes in color, gingival form, position, surface appearance, and presence of bleeding or exudate.
- Case type II—Slight periodontitis: Progression of the gingival inflammation into the deeper periodontal structures and alveolar bone crest, with slight bone loss. The usual periodontal probing depth is 3 to 4 mm with slight loss of connective tissue attachment and slight loss of alveolar bone.
- Case type III—Moderate periodontitis: A more advanced stage of the above condition with increased destruction of the periodontal structures

and noticeable loss of bone support, possibly accompanied by an increase in tooth mobility. Furcation involvement may occur in multirooted teeth.

- Case type IV—Advanced periodontitis: Further progression of periodontitis with major loss of alveolar bone support, usually accompanied by increased tooth mobility. Furcation involvement in multirooted teeth is likely.
- Case type V—Refractory progressive periodontitis: This category includes patients with multiple disease sites that continue to demonstrate attachment loss after apparently appropriate therapy. These sites presumably continue to be infected by periodontal pathogens no matter the thoroughness or frequency of therapy. It also includes patients with recurrent disease at a few or many sites.

04000-04999
V. Periodontics
Surgical Services (Including Usual Postoperative Care)

04210   *gingivectomy or gingivoplasty—per quadrant*
Involves the excision of the soft tissue wall of the periodontal pocket by either an external or internal bevel. Performed in shallow-to-moderate suprabony pockets after adequate initial preparation, for suprabony pockets that need access for restorative dentistry, when moderate gingival enlargements or aberrations are present, and when asymmetrical or unesthetic gingival topography is present.

04211   *gingivectomy or gingivoplasty—per tooth*
See 04210.

04220   *gingival curettage, surgical—per quadrant, by report*
This code covers the surgical procedure of debriding the soft tissue wall of the periodontal pocket by means of curette. Root instrumentation is routinely accomplished in conjunction with the procedure, which usually is performed under local anesthesia. Gingival curettage is typically indicated in the treatment of periodontally compromised patients, debridement of localized sites of recalcitrant periodontitis, treatment of juvenile periodontitis, treatment of other types of periodontitis, and when esthetics is a concern. Report should include treatment needs and teeth to be treated.

04240   *gingival flap procedure, including root planing—per quadrant*
Surgical debridement of the root surface and the removal of granulation tissue after the resection or reflection of soft tissue flap. Osseous recontouring is not accomplished in conjunction with this procedure. May include open-flap curettage, reverse bevel flap surgery, modified Kirkland flap procedure, Widman surgery, and modified Widman surgery. This procedure is performed in the presence of moderate-to-deep probing depths, loss of probing attachment, need to maintain esthetics, and need for increased access to the root surface and alveolar bone.

04249   *clinical crown lengthening—hard tissue*
This procedure is employed to allow restorative procedures or crowns with little or no tooth structure exposed to the oral cavity. Crown lengthening requires reflection of a flap and is performed in a healthy periodontal environment, as opposed to osseous surgery, which is performed in the presence of periodontal disease. If adjacent teeth are present, the crown lengthening of a single tooth involves a minimum of three teeth.

04250   mucogingival surgery—per quadrant

Mucogingival surgical procedures are designed to correct defects in the anatomy, morphology, position, and quantity of soft tissues in edentulous ridges adjacent to teeth. If free soft tissue gingival grafts or subepithelial connective tissue grafts are performed in the same quadrant, they should be reported as separate procedures on the same claim.

04260   osseous surgery (including flap entry and closure)—per quadrant

This procedure modifies the bony support of the teeth by reshaping the alveolar process to achieve a more physiologic form. This may include the removal of supporting bone (ostectomy) or nonsupporting bone. Other separate procedures, including but not limited to 03450, 03920, 04274, 04263, 04264, 04266, 04267, 06010, 07110, 07120, may be required concurrent to 04260.

04263   Bone replacement graft—first site in quadrant

This procedure involves the use of osseous autografts, osseous allografts, or nonosseous grafts to stimulate bone formation or periodontal regeneration when the disease process has led to a deformity of the bone. This procedure does not include flap entry and closure and is reported in addition to a procedure that includes flap entry and closure, including but not limited to 04240 and 04260.

04264   Bone replacement graft—each additional site in quadrant

This procedure involves the use of osseous autografts, osseous allografts, or nonosseous grafts to stimulate bone formation or periodontal regeneration when the disease process has led to a deformity of the bone. This code is used if performed concurrently with 04263—bone replacement graft—first site, per quadrant and allows reporting of the exact number of sites involved.

04266   guided tissue regeneration—resorbable barrier, per site, per tooth

A membrane is placed over the root surfaces or defect area after surgical exposure and debridement. The mucoperiosteal flaps are then adapted over the membrane and sutured. The membrane is placed to exclude epithelium and gingival connective tissue from the healing wound. This procedure may require subsequent surgical procedures to correct the gingival contours. Guided tissue regeneration also may be carried out in conjunction with bone replacement grafts or to correct deformities resulting from inadequate faciolingual bone width in an edentulous area. When guided tissue regeneration is used in association with a tooth, each site on a specific tooth should be reported separately with this code. If no tooth is present, each site should be reported separately.

04267   guided tissue regeneration—nonresorbable barrier, per site, per tooth
(includes membrane removal)

This procedure is used to regenerate lost or injured periodontal tissue by directing differential tissue responses. A membrane is placed over the root surfaces or defect area after surgical exposure and debridement. The mucoperiosteal flaps are then adapted over the membrane and sutured. The membrane is placed to exclude epithelium and gingival connective tissue from the healing wound. This procedure requires subsequent surgical procedures to remove the membranes and correct the gingival contours. Guided tissue regeneration may be used in conjunction with bone replacement grafts or to correct deformities resulting from inadequate faciolingual bone width in an edentulous area. When guided tissue regeneration is used in association with a tooth, each site on a specific tooth should be reported separately with this code. If no tooth is present, each site should be reported separately.

04270 *pedicle soft tissue graft procedure*

A pedicle flap of gingiva may be raised from an edentulous ridge, adjacent teeth, or from the existing gingiva on the tooth and moved laterally or coronally to replace alveolar mucosa as marginal tissue. The procedure may be used to cover an exposed root or eliminate a gingival defect if the root is not too prominent in the arch.

04271 *free soft tissue graft procedure (including donor site surgery)*

Gingival or masticatory mucosa is grafted to create or augment the gingiva at another site, with or without root coverage. This graft also may be used to eliminate the pull of frena and muscle attachments, extend the vestibular fornix, and correct localized gingival recession.

04273 *subepithelial connective tissue graft procedure (including donor site surgery)*

This procedure is performed to create or augment gingiva, obtain root coverage or eliminate sensitivity and to prevent root caries, eliminate frenum pull, or extend the vestibular fornix. The recipient site uses a split thickness incision but retains the overlying flap of gingiva and mucosa. The connective tissue graft is dissected from the donor site, leaving an epithelialized flap for closure. The donor tissue is placed at the recipient site and sutured into position. The graft is covered with the overlying flap.

04274 *distal or proximal wedge procedure (when not performed in conjunction with surgical procedures in the same anatomic area)*

This procedure is performed in an edentulous area adjacent to a periodontally involved tooth. Gingival incisions are used to allow removal of a tissue wedge to gain access and correct the underlying osseous defect and permit close flap adaptation.

Adjunctive Periodontal Service

04320 *provisional splinting—intracoronal*

This is an interim stabilization of mobile teeth. A variety of methods and appliances may be employed for this purpose. Identify the teeth involved and the nature of the splint by report.

04321 *provisional splinting—extracoronal*

This is an interim stabilization of mobile teeth. A variety of methods and appliances may be employed for this purpose. Identify the teeth involved and the nature of the splint, by report.

04341 *periodontal scaling and root planing—per quadrant*

This procedure involves instrumentation of the crown and root surfaces of the teeth to remove plaque and calculus from these surfaces. It is indicated for patients with periodontal disease and is therapeutic (not prophylactic) in nature. Root planing is the definitive procedure designed for the removal of cementum and dentin that is rough, permeated by calculus, or contaminated with toxins or microorganisms. Some soft tissue removal occurs. This procedure may be used as a definitive treatment in some stages of periodontal disease and as a part of presurgical procedures in others.

04355 *full mouth debridement to enable comprehensive periodontal evaluation and diagnosis*

The removal of subgingival and supragingival plaque and calculus obstructs the ability to perform an oral evaluation. This is a preliminary procedure and does not preclude the need for other procedures.

04381 localized delivery of chemotherapeutic agents through a controlled-release vehicle into diseased crevicular tissue—per tooth, by report
Synthetic fibers or other approved delivery devices containing controlled-release chemotherapeutic agents are inserted into a periodontal pocket. Short-term use of the timed release therapeutic agent as supplemental or adjunctive therapy provides for reduction of subgingival flora. This procedure does not replace conventional or surgical therapy required for debridement, resective procedures, or regenerative therapy. The use of controlled-release chemotherapeutic agents is an adjunctive procedure for specific sites that are unresponsive to conventional therapy or for cases in which systemic disease or other factors preclude conventional or surgical therapy.

Other Periodontal Services

04910 periodontal maintenance procedures (after active therapy)
This procedure is for patients who have completed periodontal treatment (surgical and adjunctive periodontal therapies exclusive of 04355) and includes removal of the bacterial flora from crevicular and pocket areas, scaling and polishing of the teeth, and a review of the patient's plaque-control efficiency. Typically an interval of 3 months between appointments results in an effective treatment schedule, but this can vary depending on the clinical judgment of the dentist. If new or recurring periodontal disease appears, additional diagnostic and treatment procedures must be considered. Periodic maintenance treatment after periodontal therapy is not synonymous with prophylaxis.

04920 unscheduled dressing change (by someone other than treating dentist)
Must be dentist other than dentist of record or may be appropriately licensed dental auxiliary.

04999 unspecified periodontal procedure, by report
Use for procedure that is not adequately described by a code. Describe procedure fully—the procedure done and reasons for it.

05000-05899
VI. Prosthodontics (Removable)
Complete Dentures (Including Routine Postdelivery Care)
The word *upper* is replaced with the word *maxillary* and the word *lower* is replaced with the word *mandibular* throughout this section.

05110 complete denture—maxillary

05120 complete denture—mandibular

05130 immediate denture—maxillary
Includes limited follow-up care only; does not include required future rebasing or relining procedures or a complete new denture.

05140 immediate denture—mandibular
See 05130.

Partial Dentures (Including Routine Postdelivery Care)

05211 maxillary partial denture—resin base (including any conventional clasps, rests, and teeth)
All partials include major connectors and framework. Note number of clasps and rests. No code number for immediate partial dentures. For precision partial dentures, report precision attachments with code 05862 by report. Partial dentures for pediatric dentistry are included in this category.

05212 *mandibular partial denture—resin base (including any conventional clasps, rests, and teeth)*
Includes acrylic resin base denture with acrylic resin clasps. See 05211 descriptor.

05213 *maxillary partial denture—cast metal framework with resin denture bases (including any conventional clasps, rests, and teeth)*
Cast metal base alloys have less than 60% Au, Pd, or Pt content. See 05211 descriptor.

05214 *mandibular partial denture—cast metal framework with resin denture bases (including any conventional clasps, rests, and teeth)*
See 05213 descriptor.

05281 *removable unilateral partial denture—one piece cast metal (including clasps and teeth)*

Adjustments to Dentures
05410 *adjust complete denture—maxillary*
05411 *adjust complete denture—mandibular*
05421 *adjust partial denture—maxillary*
05422 *adjust partial denture—mandibular*

Repairs to Complete Dentures
NOTE: Include a description of procedures done.
05510 *repair broken complete denture base*
05520 *replace missing or broken teeth—complete denture (each tooth)*

Repairs to Partial Dentures
05610 *repair resin denture base*
05620 *repair cast framework*
05630 *repair or replace broken clasp*
05640 *replace broken teeth—per tooth*
05650 *add tooth to existing partial denture*
05660 *add clasp to existing partial denture*

Denture Rebase Procedures
Rebasing is the process of refitting a denture by replacing the base material.
05710 *rebase complete maxillary denture*
05711 *rebase complete mandibular denture*
05720 *rebase maxillary partial denture*
05721 *rebase mandibular partial denture*

Denture Reline Procedures
Relining is the process of resurfacing the tissue side of a denture with new base material.
05730 *reline complete maxillary denture (chairside)*
05731 *reline complete mandibular denture (chairside)*
05740 *reline maxillary partial denture (chairside)*
05741 *reline mandibular partial denture (chairside)*
05750 *reline complete maxillary denture (laboratory)*
05751 *reline complete mandibular denture (laboratory)*
05760 *reline maxillary partial denture (laboratory)*
05761 *reline mandibular partial denture (laboratory)*

Other Removable Prosthetic Services

This code covers provisional prostheses designed for use over a limited period of time, after which they are replaced by more definitive restorations.

05810 interim complete denture (maxillary)
05811 interim complete denture (mandibular)
05820 interim partial denture (maxillary)
Includes any necessary clasps and rests.
05821 interim partial denture (mandibular)
Includes any necessary clasps and rests.
05850 tissue conditioning, maxillary
05851 tissue conditioning, mandibular
05860 overdenture—complete, by report
Describe and document procedures as performed. Other separate procedures may be required concurrent to 05860.
05861 overdenture—partial, by report
Describe and document procedures as performed. Other separate procedures may be required concurrent to 05860.
05862 precision attachment, by report
Each set of male and female components should be reported as one precision attachment. Describe the type of attachment used.
05899 unspecified removable prosthodontic procedure, by report
Use for a procedure that is not adequately described by a code. Describe procedure.

05900-05999
VII. Maxillofacial Prosthetics

05911 facial moulage (sectional)
A sectional facial moulage impression is a procedure used to record the soft tissue contours of a portion of the face. Occasionally several separate sectional impressions are made, then reassembled to provide a full facial contour cast. The impression is used to create a partial facial moulage and generally is not reusable.

05912 facial moulage (complete)
Synonymous terminology: facial impression, face mask impression.
A complete facial moulage impression is used to record the soft tissue contours of the whole face. The impression is used to create a facial moulage and generally is not reusable.

05913 nasal prosthesis
Synonymous terminology: artificial nose.
A removable prosthesis may be attached to the skin to restore artificially part or all of the nose. Fabrication of a nasal prosthesis requires creation of an original mold. Additional prostheses usually may be made from the same mold, and assuming no further tissue changes occur, the same mold may be used for extended periods. If a new prosthesis is made from the existing mold, this procedure is termed a *nasal prosthesis replacement.*

05914 auricular prosthesis
Synonymous terminology: artificial ear, ear prosthesis.
A removable prosthesis may be used to restore artificially part or all of the natural ear. Usually, replacement prostheses may be made from the original mold if tissue bed changes have not occurred. Creation of an auricular prosthesis requires fabrication of a mold, from which addi-

tional prostheses usually may be made as needed later (auricular prosthesis replacement).

05915 *orbital prosthesis*

A prosthesis may be used to restore artificially the eye, eyelids, and adjacent hard and soft tissue lost as a result of trauma or surgery. Fabrication of an orbital prosthesis requires creation of an original mold. Additional prostheses usually may be made from the same mold, and assuming no further tissue changes occur, the same mold may be used for extended periods. If a new prosthesis is made from the existing mold, this procedure is termed an *orbital prosthesis replacement.*

05916 *ocular prosthesis*

Synonymous terminology: artificial eye, glass eye.

A prosthesis may be used to replace artificially an eye missing as a result of trauma, surgery, or congenital absence. The prosthesis does not replace missing eyelids or adjacent skin, mucosa, or muscle.

Ocular prostheses require semiannual or annual cleaning and polishing. Also, occasional revisions to readapt the prosthesis to the tissue bed may be necessary. Glass eyes are rarely made and cannot be readapted.

05919 *facial prosthesis*

Synonymous terminology: prosthetic dressing.

A removable prosthesis may be used to replace artificially a portion of the face lost as a result of surgery, trauma, or congenital absence. Flexion of natural tissues may preclude adaptation and movement of the prosthesis to match the adjacent skin. Salivary leakage, when communicating with the oral cavity, adversely affects retention.

05922 *nasal septal prosthesis*

Synonymous terminology: Septal plug, septal button.

A removable prosthesis may be used to occlude (obturate) a hole within the nasal septal wall. Adverse chemical degradation in this moist environment may require frequent replacement. Silicone prostheses are occasionally subject to fungal invasion.

05923 *ocular prosthesis, interim*

Synonymous terminology: Eye shell, shell, ocular conformer, conformer.

A temporary replacement generally made of clear acrylic resin may be used to replace an eye lost as a result of surgery or trauma. No attempt is made to reestablish esthetics. Fabrication of an interim ocular prosthesis generally implies subsequent fabrication of an esthetic ocular prosthesis.

05924 *cranial prosthesis*

Synonymous terminology: Skull plate, cranioplasty prosthesis, cranial implant.

This term is used to describe a biocompatible, permanently implanted replacement of a portion of the skull bones; an artificial replacement for a portion of the skull bone.

05925 *facial augmentation implant prosthesis*

Synonymous terminology: facial implant.

This term describes an implantable biocompatible material generally onlayed on an existing bony area beneath the skin tissue to fill in or raise collectively portions of the overlaying facial skin tissues to create acceptable contours. Although some forms of premade surgical implants are commercially available, the facial augmentation is usually custom made for surgical implantation for each individual patient because of the irregular or extensive nature of the facial deficit.

05926 nasal prosthesis, replacement

Synonymous terminology: replacement nose.

An artificial nose produced from a previously made mold. A replacement prosthesis does not require fabrication of a new mold. Generally, several prostheses may be made from the same mold assuming no changes occur in the tissue bed as a result of surgery or age-related topographic variations.

05927 auricular prosthesis, replacement

Synonymous terminology: replacement ear.

An artificial ear produced from a previously made mold. A replacement prosthesis does not require fabrication of a new mold. Generally, several prostheses may be made from the same mold assuming no changes occur in the tissue bed as a result of surgery or age-related topographic variations.

05928 orbital prosthesis, replacement

A replacement for a previously made orbital prosthesis. A replacement prosthesis does not require fabrication of a new mold. Generally, several prostheses may be made from the same mold assuming no changes occur in the tissue bed as a result of surgery or age-related topographic variations.

05929 facial prosthesis, replacement

A replacement facial prosthesis made from the original mold. A replacement prosthesis does not require fabrication of a new mold. Generally, several prostheses may be made from the same mold assuming no changes occur in the tissue bed as a result of further surgery or age-related topographic variations.

05931 obturator prosthesis, surgical

Synonymous terminology: Obturator, surgical stayplate, immediate temporary obturator.

A temporary prosthesis inserted during or immediately after surgical or traumatic loss of a portion or all of one or both maxillary bones and contiguous alveolar structures (including gingival tissue and teeth). Frequent revisions of surgical obturators are necessary during the ensuing healing phase (approximately 6 months). Some dentists prefer to replace many or all teeth removed by the surgical procedure in the surgical obturator, whereas others do not replace any teeth. Further surgical revisions may require fabrication of another surgical obturator (for example, an initially planned small defect may be revised and greatly enlarged after the final pathologic report indicates margins are not free of tumor).

05932 obturator prosthesis, definitive

Synonymous terminology: obturator

A prosthesis that artificially replaces part or all of the maxilla and associated teeth lost as a result of surgery, trauma, or congenital defects. A definitive obturator is made if further tissue changes or recurrences of tumors are unlikely and a more permanent prosthetic rehabilitation may be achieved; it is intended for long-term use.

05933 obturator prosthesis, modification

Synonymous terminology: adjustment, denture adjustment, temporary or office reline.

This appliance is used for revision or alteration of an existing obturator (surgical, interim, or definitive obturator); possible modifications include relief of the denture base as a result of tissue compression, augmentation of the seal or peripheral areas to affect adequate sealing, or separation between the nasal and oral cavities.

05934 *mandibular resection prosthesis with guide flange*

Synonymous terminology: resection device, resection appliance.

A prosthesis that guides the remaining portion of the mandible left after a partial resection into a more normal relationship with the maxilla. This allows for some tooth-to-tooth contact or improved tooth contact. It also may artificially replace missing teeth and thereby increase masticatory efficiency.

05935 *mandibular resection prosthesis without guide flange*

A prosthesis that helps guide the partially resected mandible to a more normal relation with the maxilla allowing for tooth or increased tooth contact. It does not have a flange or ramp, however, to assist in directional closure. It may replace missing teeth and thereby increase masticatory efficiency.

Dentists who treat mandibulectomy patients may prefer to replace some, all, or none of the teeth in the defect area. Frequently, the defect margins preclude even partial replacement. Use of a guide (a mandibular resection prosthesis with a guide flange) may not be possible because of anatomic limitations or poor patient tolerance. Ramps, extended occlusal arrangements, and irregular occlusal positioning relative to the denture foundation frequently preclude stability of the prostheses, and thus some prostheses are poorly tolerated under such adverse circumstances.

05936 *obturator prosthesis, interim*

Synonymous terminology: immediate postoperative obturator.

A prosthesis made after completion of the initial healing after a surgical resection of a portion or all of one or both of the maxillae; frequently many or all teeth in the defect area are replaced by this prosthesis. This prosthesis replaces the surgical obturator, which is usually inserted during or immediately after the resection. Generally an interim obturator is made to facilitate closure of the resultant defect after initial healing has been completed. Unlike the surgical obturator, which usually is made before surgery and frequently revised in the operating room, the interim obturator is made after the defect margins are clearly defined and further surgical revisions are not planned. It is a provisional prosthesis that may replace some or all lost teeth and other lost bone and soft tissue structures. Also, it frequently must be revised (termed an obturator prosthesis modification) during subsequent dental procedures (including restorations and gingival surgery) and to compensate for further tissue shrinkage before a definitive obturator prosthesis is made.

05937 *trismus appliance (not for temporomandibular dysfunction [TMD] treatment)*

Synonymous terminology: occlusal device for mandibular trismus dynamic bite opener.

A prosthesis that assists the patient in increasing the oral aperture width to eat and maintain oral hygiene. Several versions and designs are possible, all intending to ease the severe lack of oral opening experienced by many patients immediately after extensive intraoral surgical procedures.

05951 feeding aid

Synonymous terminology: feeding prosthesis.

A prosthesis that maintains the right and left maxillary segments of an infant cleft palate patient in the proper orientation until surgery is performed to repair the cleft. It closes the oral-nasal cavity defect, thus enhancing sucking and swallowing. Used on an interim basis, this prosthesis achieves separation of the oral and nasal cavities in infants born with wide clefts necessitating delayed closure. It is eliminated if surgical closure may be effected or, alternatively, with eruption of the deciduous dentition, a pediatric speech aid may be made to facilitate closure of the defect.

05952 speech aid prosthesis, pediatric

Synonymous terminology: nasopharyngeal obturator, speech appliance, obturator, cleft palate appliance, prosthetic speech aid, speech bulb.

A temporary or interim prosthesis used to close a defect in the hard or soft palate. It may replace tissue lost as a result of developmental or surgical alterations. It is necessary for the production of intelligible speech. Normal lateral growth of the palatal bones necessitates occasional replacement of this prosthesis. Intermittent revision of the obturator section may assist in maintenance of palatopharyngeal closure (termed a speech aid prosthesis modification). Frequently such prostheses are not fabricated before the deciduous dentition is fully erupted because clasp retention is often essential.

05953 speech aid prosthesis, adult

Synonymous terminology: prosthetic speech appliance, speech aid, speech bulb.

A definitive prosthesis that may improve speech in adult cleft palate patients either by obturating (sealing off) a palatal cleft or fistula or occasionally by assisting an incompetent soft palate. Both mechanisms are necessary to achieve velopharyngeal competency. Generally this prosthesis is fabricated if no further growth is anticipated and the objective is to achieve long-term use, hence, more precise materials and techniques are used. Occasionally such procedures are accomplished in conjunction with precision attachments in crown work undertaken on some or all maxillary teeth to achieve improved esthetics.

05954 palatal augmentation prosthesis

Synonymous terminology: superimposed prosthesis, maxillary glossectomy prosthesis, maxillary speech prosthesis, palatal drop prosthesis.

A removable prosthesis that alters the hard or soft palate's topographic form adjacent to the tongue.

05955 palatal lift prosthesis, definitive

A prosthesis to elevate the soft palate superiorly and aid in restoration of soft palate functions that may be lost as a result of an acquired, congenital, or developmental defect. A definitive palatal lift is usually made for patients whose experiences with a diagnostic palatal lift have been successful, especially if surgical alterations are unwarranted.

05958 palatal lift prosthesis, interim

Synonymous terminology: diagnostic palatal lift.

A prosthesis to elevate and assist in restoring soft palate function that may be lost as a result of clefting, surgery, trauma, or unknown paralysis. It is intended for interim use to determine its usefulness in achieving palatopharyngeal competency or enhancing swallowing reflexes. This prosthesis is intended for interim use as a diagnostic aid to assess the level of possible improvement in speech intelligibility. Some clinicians believe interim use of a palatal lift may stimulate an otherwise flaccid soft palate to increase functional activity, subsequently lessening its need.

05959 palatal lift prosthesis, modification

Synonymous terminology: revision of lift, adjustment.

Alterations in the adaptation, contour, form, or function of an existing palatal lift necessitated because of tissue impingement, lack of function, poor clasp adaptation, or the like.

05960 speech aid prosthesis, modification

Synonymous terminology: adjustment, repair, revision.

Any revision of a pediatric or adult speech aid not necessitating its replacement. Frequently revisions of the obturating section of any speech aid are required to facilitate enhanced speech intelligibility. Such revisions or repairs do not require complete remaking of the prosthesis, thus extending its longevity.

05982 surgical stent

Synonymous terminology: periodontal stent, skin graft stent, columellar stent.

Named for the dentist who first described their use, stents apply pressure to soft tissues to facilitate healing and prevent cicatrization or collapse. A surgical stent may be required in surgical and postsurgical revisions to achieve close approximation of tissues. Usually such materials as temporary or interim soft denture lines, gutta-percha, or dental modeling impression compound may be used.

05983 radiation carrier

Synonymous terminology: radiotherapy prosthesis, carrier prosthesis, radiation applicator, radium carrier, intracavity carrier, intracavity applicator.

A device used to administer radiation to confined areas by means of capsules, beads, or needles of radiation emitting materials such as radium or cesium. Its function is to hold the radiation source securely in the same location during the entire period of treatment. Radiation oncologists occasionally request these devices to achieve close approximation and controlled application of radiation to a tumor deemed amiable to eradication.

05984 radiation shield

Synonymous terminology: radiation stent, tongue protector, lead shield.

An intraoral prosthesis designed to shield adjacent tissues from radiation during orthovoltage treatment of malignant lesions of the head and neck region.

05985 radiation cone locator

Synonymous terminology: docking device, cone locator.

A prosthesis used to direct and reduplicate the path of radiation to an oral tumor during a split course of irradiation.

05986 fluoride gel carrier

Synonymous terminology: fluoride applicator.

A prosthesis that covers the teeth in either dental arch and is used to apply topical fluoride in close proximity to tooth enamel and dentin for several minutes daily.

05987 commissure splint

Synonymous terminology: lip splint.

A device placed between the lips to assist in achieving increased opening between the lips. Use of such devices enhances opening where surgical, chemical, or electrical alterations of the lips have resulted in severe restriction or contractures.

05988 surgical splint

Synonymous terminology: Gunning splint, modified Gunning splint, labiolingual splint, fenestrated splint, Kingsley splint, cast metal splint.

Splints are designed to use existing teeth and alveolar processes as points of anchorage to assist in stabilization and immobilization of broken bones during healing. They are used to reestablish as much as possible normal occlusal relationships during the process of immobilization. Frequently, existing prostheses such as a patient's complete dentures may be modified to serve as surgical splints. Frequently surgical splints have arch bars added to facilitate intermaxillary fixation. Rubber elastics may be used to assist in this process. Circummandibular eyelet hooks may be used for enhanced stabilization with wiring to adjacent bone.

05999 unspecified maxillofacial prosthesis, by report

Used for procedure that is not adequately described by a code. Describe procedure.

06000-06199
VIII. Implant Services

Report surgical implant procedure using codes in this section; prosthetic devices should be reported using existing fixed or removable prosthetic codes.

Endosteal Implants

The ADA has concluded that in selected cases, endosteal (endosseous) implants are safe and effective for use.

06010 surgical placement of implant body—endosteal implant

Includes second stage surgery and placement of healing cap.

06020 abutment placement or substitution—endosteal implant

An abutment is placed to permit fabrication of a dental prosthesis. This procedure may include the removal of a temporary healing cap or replacement with an abutment of alternate design. Intent of this code is to report this procedure by other than the original dentist.

Eposteal Implants

The ADA has concluded that in selected cases, eposteal (subperiosteal) implants are safe and effective for use.

06040 surgical placement—eposteal implant

An eposteal (subperiosteal) framework of a biocompatible material designed and fabricated to fit on the surface of the bone of the mandible or maxilla with permucosal extensions that provide support and attachment for a prosthesis. This may be a complete arch or unilateral appliance. Eposteal implants rest on the bone and under the periosteum.

Transosteal Implants

06050 surgical placement—transosteal implant

A transosteal (transosseous) biocompatible device with threaded posts penetrating both the superior and inferior cortical bone plates of the mandibular symphysis and exiting through the permucosa, providing support and attachment for a dental prosthesis. Transosteal implants are placed completely through the bone and into the oral cavity from an extraoral or intraoral direction.

06055 *dental implant-supported connecting bar*
A device attached to transmucosal abutments to stabilize and anchor a removable overdenture prosthesis.

06080 *implant maintenance procedures, including removal of prosthesis, cleansing of prosthesis and abutments, and reinsertion of prosthesis*
This procedure includes prophylaxis to provide active debriding of the implant and examination of all aspects of the implant system, including the occlusion and stability of the superstructure. The patient also is instructed in thorough daily cleansing of the implant.

06090 *repair implant-supported prosthesis, by report*
This procedure involves the repair or replacement of any part of the implant-supported prosthesis.

06095 *repair implant abutment, by report*
This procedure involves the repair or replacement of any part of the implant abutment.

06100 *implant removal, by report*
This procedure involves the surgical removal of an implant. Describe procedure.

06199 *unspecified implant procedure, by report*
Use for procedure that is not adequately described by a code. Describe procedure.

06200-06999
IX. Prosthodontics, Fixed (Each Abutment and Each Pontic Constitutes a Unit in a Fixed Partial Denture).

The words *bridge* and *bridgework* have been replaced by the statement *fixed partial denture* throughout this section.

Fixed Partial Denture Pontics

06210 *pontic—cast high noble metal***
06211 *pontic—cast predominantly base metal***
06212 *pontic—cast noble metal***
06240 *pontic—porcelain fused to high noble metal***
06241 *pontic—porcelain fused to predominantly base metal***
06242 *pontic—porcelain fused to noble metal***
06250 *pontic—resin with high noble metal***
06251 *pontic—resin with predominantly base metal***
06252 *pontic—resin with noble metal***

Fixed Partial Denture Retainers—Inlays and Onlays

06520 *inlay—metallic—two surfaces*
06530 *inlay—metallic—three or more surfaces*
06543 *onlay—metallic—three surfaces*
06544 *onlay—metallic—four or more surfaces*
06545 *retainer—cast metal for resin bonded fixed prosthesis*
Report pontics separately with appropriate code from the 06200 series.

Fixed Partial Denture Retainers—Crowns

06720 *crown—resin with high noble metal***
06721 *crown—resin with predominantly base metal***

06722 *crown—resin with noble metal***
06750 *crown—porcelain fused to high noble metal***
06751 *crown—porcelain fused to predominantly base metal***
06752 *crown—porcelain fused to noble metal***
06780 *crown—¾ cast high noble metal***
06790 *crown—full cast high noble metal***
06791 *crown—full cast predominantly base metal***
06792 *crown—full cast noble metal***

Other Fixed Partial Denture Services

06920 *connector bar*
06930 *recement fixed partial denture*
06940 *stress breaker*
A nonrigid connector.
06950 *precision attachment*
Report attachment separately from crown; each male and female component constitutes one precision attachment. Describe type of attachment used.
06970 *cast post and core in addition to fixed partial denture retainer*
06971 *cast post as part of fixed partial denture retainer*
06972 *prefabricated post and core in addition to fixed partial denture retainer*
06973 *core build-up for retainer, including any pins*
06975 *coping—metal*
May be used as a definitive restoration or part of a transfer procedure.
06980 *fixed partial denture repair, by report*
06999 *unspecified fixed prosthodontic procedure, by report*
Used for procedure that is not adequately described by a code. Describe procedure.

07000-07999
X. Oral and Maxillofacial Surgery
Extractions (Includes Local Anesthesia, Suturing, If Needed, and Routine Postoperative Care)

07110 *single tooth*
07120 *each additional tooth*
Typically may be reported for an additional extraction in the same quadrant.
07130 *root removal—exposed roots*

Surgical Extractions (Includes Local Anesthesia, Suturing, If Needed, and Routine Postoperative Care)

07210 *surgical removal of erupted tooth requiring elevation of mucoperiosteal flap and removal of bone or section of tooth*
Includes cutting of gingiva and bone, removal of tooth structure, and closure.
07220 *removal of impacted tooth—soft tissue*
Occlusal surface of tooth covered by soft tissue; requires mucoperiosteal flap elevation.
07230 *removal of impacted tooth—partially bony*
Part of crown covered by bone; requires mucoperiosteal flap elevation and bone removal and may require segmentalization of tooth.

07240 *removal of impacted tooth—completely bony*
Most or all of crown covered by bone; requires mucoperiosteal flap elevation and bone removal and may require segmentalization of tooth.

07241 *removal of impacted tooth—completely bony, with unusual surgical complications*
Most or all of crown covered by bone; unusually difficult or complicated because of factors such as necessity of nerve dissection or separate closure of the maxillary sinus or aberrant tooth position.

07250 *surgical removal of residual tooth roots (cutting procedure)*
Includes cutting of gingiva and bone, removal of tooth structure, and closure.

Other Surgical Procedures

07260 *oroantral fistula closure*
Excision of fistulous tract between maxillary sinus and oral cavity and closure by advancement flap.

07270 *tooth reimplantation or stabilization of accidentally evulsed or displaced tooth or alveolus*
Includes splinting and stabilization.

07272 *tooth transplantation (includes reimplantation from one site to another, splinting, and stabilization)*

07280 *surgical exposure of impacted or unerupted tooth for orthodontic reasons (including orthodontic attachments)*
An incision is made and the tissue is reflected and bone removed as necessary to expose the crown. An orthodontic attachment is placed on the crown. In some instances, a free soft tissue graft is needed as a concurrent but separate procedure.

07281 *surgical exposure of impacted or unerupted tooth to aid eruption*
Dense fibrous tissue overlying an impacted or unerupted tooth is reflected and any overlying bone is removed. This procedure also may be performed with a separate soft tissue graft procedure.

07285 *biopsy of oral tissue—hard*
For surgical removal of specimen only. This code involves biopsy of osseous lesions and is not used for apicoectomy or periradicular curettage. For surgical oral pathology procedures, see 00501 and 00502.

07286 *biopsy of oral tissue—soft*
For surgical removal of specimen only. This code is not used at the same time as codes for apicoectomy or periradicular curettage. For surgical oral pathology procedures, see 00501 or 00502.

07290 *surgical repositioning of teeth*

07291 *transseptal fiberotomy, by report*
The supraosseous connective tissue attachment is surgically severed around the involved teeth. If adjacent teeth are present the transseptal fiberotomy of a single tooth involves a minimum of three teeth. Because the incisions are within the gingival sulcus and tissue and the root surface is not instrumented, this procedure heals by the reunion of connective tissue with the root surface on which viable periodontal tissue is present (reattachment).

Alveoloplasty—Surgical Preparation of Ridge for Dentures

07310 *alveoloplasty in conjunction with extractions—per quadrant*
Usually in preparation for a prosthesis.

07320 alveoloplasty not in conjunction with extractions—per quadrant
No extractions performed in an edentulous area. See 07310 if teeth are present.

Vestibuloplasty

07340 vestibuloplasty—ridge extension (secondary epithelialization)
07350 vestibuloplasty—ridge extension (including soft tissue grafts, muscle reattachment, revision of soft tissue attachment, and management of hypertrophied and hyperplastic tissue)
More complex than 07340.

Surgical Excision of Reactive Inflammatory Lesions (Scar Tissue or Localized Congenital Lesions)

07410 radical excision—lesion diameter as great as 1.25 cm
07420 radical excision—lesion diameter greater than 1.25 cm

Removal of Tumors, Cysts, and Neoplasms

07430 excision of benign tumor—lesion diameter as great as 1.25 cm
07431 excision of benign tumor—lesion diameter greater than 1.25 cm
07440 excision of malignant tumor—lesion diameter as great as 1.25 cm
07441 excision of malignant tumor—lesion diameter greater than 1.25 cm
07450 removal of odontogenic cyst or tumor—lesion diameter as great as 1.25 cm
07451 removal of odontogenic cyst or tumor—lesion diameter greater than 1.25 cm
07460 removal of nonodontogenic cyst or tumor—lesion diameter as great as 1.25 cm
07461 removal of nonodontogenic cyst or tumor—lesion diameter greater than 1.25 cm
07465 destruction of lesions by physical or chemical method, by report
Examples include using cryosurgery, laser surgery, or electrosurgery.

Excision of Bone Tissue

07470 removal of exostosis—maxilla or mandible
Includes removal of tori, osseous tuberosities, and other osseous protuberances. The overlying soft tissue is reflected and sufficient bone removed to provide an acceptable tissue contour.
07480 partial ostectomy (guttering or saucerization)
Surgical procedure to remove nonvital segment of bone.
07490 radical resection of mandible with bone graft

Surgical Incision

07510 incision and drainage of abscess—intraoral soft tissue
Involves incision through mucosa.
07520 incision and drainage of abscess—extraoral soft tissue
Involves incision through skin.
07530 removal of foreign body, skin, or subcutaneous areolar tissue
07540 removal of reaction-producing foreign bodies—musculoskeletal system
May include but is not limited to removal of splinters and pieces of wire from muscle and bone.
07550 sequestrectomy for osteomyelitis
Removal of loose or sloughed-off dead bone caused by infection or reduced blood supply.
07560 maxillary sinusotomy for removal of tooth fragment or foreign body

Treatment of Fractures—Simple

07610   maxilla—open reduction (teeth immobilized, if present)
Teeth may be wired, banded, or splinted together to prevent movement.
Surgical incision required for interosseous fixation.

07620   maxilla—closed reduction (teeth immobilized, if present)
No incision required to reduce fracture. See 07610 if interosseous fixation is applied.

07630   mandible—open reduction (teeth immobilized, if present)
Teeth may be wired, banded, or splinted together to prevent movement.
Surgical incision required to reduce fracture.

07640   mandible—closed reduction (teeth immobilized, if present)
No incision required to reduce fracture. See 07630 if interosseous fixation is applied.

07650   malar or zygomatic arch—open reduction

07660   malar or zygomatic arch—closed reduction

07670   alveolus—stabilization of teeth, open reduction splinting
Teeth may be wired, banded, or splinted together to prevent movement.

07680   facial bones—complicated reduction with fixation and multiple surgical approaches
Facial bones include upper and lower jaw, cheek, and bones around eyes, nose, and ears.

Treatment of Fractures—Compound

07710   maxilla—open reduction
Surgical incision required to reduce fracture.

07720   maxilla—closed reduction

07730   mandible—open reduction
Surgical incision required to reduce fracture.

07740   mandible—closed reduction

07750   malar or zygomatic arch—open reduction
Surgical incision required to reduce fracture.

07760   malar or zygomatic arch—closed reduction

07770   alveolus—stabilization of teeth, open reduction splinting
Fractured bones are exposed to mouth or outside the face; see 07670.
Surgical incision required to reduce fracture.

07780   facial bones—complicated reduction with fixation and multiple surgical approaches
Surgical incision required to reduce fracture.

Reduction of Dislocation and Management of Other Temporomandibular Joint (TMJ) Dysfunctions

Procedures that are an integral part of a primary procedure should not be reported separately.

07810   open reduction of dislocation
Access to TMJ through surgical opening.

07820   closed reduction of dislocation
Joint manipulated into place; no surgical exposure.

07830   manipulation under anesthesia
Usually done under general anesthesia.

07840   condylectomy
Surgical removal of all or portion of the mandibular condyle or a portion thereof (separate procedure).

07850 *surgical discectomy, with or without implant*
Excision of the intraarticular disc of a joint.

07852 *disc repair*
Repositioning or sculpting of disc; repair of perforated posterior attachment.

07854 *synovectomy*
Excision of a portion or all of the synovial membrane of a joint.

07856 *myotomy*
Cutting of muscle for therapeutic purposes (separate procedure).

07858 *joint reconstruction*
Reconstruction of osseous components, including or excluding soft tissues of the joint with autogenous, homologous, or alloplastic materials.

07860 *arthrotomy*
Cutting into joint (separate procedure).

07865 *arthroplasty*
Reduction of osseous components of the joint to create a pseudoarthrosis or eliminate an irregular remodeling pattern (osteophytes).

07870 *arthrocentesis*
Withdrawal of fluid from a joint space by aspiration.

07872 *arthroscopy—diagnosis, with or without biopsy*

07873 *arthroscopy—surgical: lavage and lysis of adhesions*
Removal of adhesions using the arthroscope and lavage of the joint cavities.

07874 *arthroscopy—surgical: disc repositioning and stabilization*
Repositioning and stabilization of disc using arthroscopic techniques.

07875 *arthroscopy—surgical: synovectomy*
Removal of inflamed and hyperplastic synovium (partial or complete) using an arthroscopic technique.

07876 *arthroscopy—surgical: discectomy*
Removal of disc and remodeled posterior attachment using the arthroscope.

07877 *arthroscopy—surgical: debridement*
Removal of pathologic hard or soft tissue using the arthroscope.

07880 *occlusal orthotic device, by report*
Presently includes splints provided for treatment of temporomandibular joint dysfunction.

07899 *unspecified TMD therapy, by report*
Used for procedure that is not adequately described by a code. Describe procedure.

Repair of Traumatic Wounds

Excludes closure of surgical incisions.
07910 *suture of recent small wounds as great as 5 cm*

Complicated Suturing (Reconstruction Requiring Delicate Handling of Tissues and Wide Undermining for Meticulous Closure)

Excludes closure of surgical incisions.
07911 *complicated suture—as great as 5 cm*
07912 *complicated suture—greater than 5 cm*

Other Repair Procedures

07920 *skin graft (identify defect covered, location and type of graft)*
07940 *osteoplasty—for orthognathic deformities*
Reconstruction of jaws for correction of congenital, developmental, or acquired traumatic or surgical deformity.

07941 osteotomy—ramus, closed
Intraoral.

07942 osteotomy—ramus, open
Extraoral.

07943 osteotomy—ramus, open with bone graft
See 07942.

07944 osteotomy—segmented or subapical—per sextant or quadrant

07945 osteotomy—body of mandible
Surgical section of lower jaw. This includes the surgical exposure, bone cut, fixation, routine wound closure, and normal postoperative follow-up care.

07946 Le Fort I (maxilla—total)
Surgical section of the upper jaw. This includes the surgical exposure, bone cuts, downfracture, repositioning, fixation, routine wound closure, and normal postoperative follow-up care.

07947 Le Fort I (maxilla—segmented)
When reporting a surgically assisted palatal expansion without downfracture, this code would entail a reduced service and should be by report.

07948 Le Fort II or Le Fort III (osteoplasty of facial bones for midface hypoplasia or retrusion) without bone graft
Surgical section of upper jaw. This includes the surgical exposure, bone cuts, downfracture, segmentation of maxilla, repositioning, fixation, routine wound closure, and normal postoperative follow-up care.

07949 Le Fort II or Le Fort III with bone graft
Includes obtaining of autografts.

07950 osseous, osteoperiosteal, or cartilage graft of the mandible or facial bones (autogenous or nonautogenous), by report
Includes obtaining autograft or allograft material. Ridge augmentation and sinus lift procedure. Surgical section of upper jaw (pyramidal). This includes the surgical exposures, bone cuts, separation of midface, repositioning, fixation, routine wound closure, and normal postoperative follow-up care.

07955 repair of maxillofacial soft and hard tissue defect
Various soft tissue grafting procedures may be used alone or in combination with autograft, allograft, or alloplastic materials to augment or repair the defect and restore anatomic structure to required form and function. These procedures may require multiple surgical approaches.

07960 frenulectomy (frenectomy or frenotomy)—separate procedure
The frenum may be excised if the tongue has limited mobility; for large diastemas between teeth; if the frenum interferes with a prosthetic appliance; or if it is the etiology of periodontal tissue disease.

07970 excision of hyperplastic tissue—per arch

07971 excision of pericoronal gingiva
Surgical removal of inflammatory or hypertrophied tissues surrounding partially erupted or impacted teeth.

07980 sialolithotomy
Surgical procedure by which a stone within a salivary gland or its duct is removed either intraorally or extraorally.

07981 excision of salivary gland, by report

07982 sialodochoplasty
Surgical procedure for the repair of a defect or restoration of a portion of a salivary gland duct.

07983 *closure of salivary fistula*
Surgical closure of an opening between a salivary duct or gland and the cutaneous surface or an opening into the oral cavity through other than the normal anatomic pathway.

07990 *emergency tracheotomy*
Surgical formation of a tracheal opening usually below the cricoid cartilage to allow for respiratory exchange.

07991 *coronoidectomy*
Surgical removal of the coronoid process of the mandible.

07995 *synthetic graft—mandible or facial bones, by report*
Includes allogenic material.

07996 *implant—mandible for augmentation purposes (excluding alveolar ridge), by report*

07999 *unspecified oral surgery procedure, by report*
Used for procedure that is not adequately described by a code. Describe procedure.

08000-08999
XI. Orthodontics
Dentition
- Primary dentition: teeth developed and erupted first in order of time.
- Transitional dentition: the final phase of the transition from primary to adult teeth, in which the deciduous molars and canines are in the process of shedding and the permanent successors are emerging.
- Adolescent dentition: the dentition present after the normal loss of primary teeth and before the cessation of growth that would affect orthodontic treatment.
- Adult dentition: the dentition present after the cessation of growth that would affect orthodontic treatment.

Limited Orthodontic Treatment
Orthodontic treatment with a limited objective not involving the entire dentition. It may be directed at the existing problem only, or at only one aspect of a larger problem in which a decision is made to defer or forego more comprehensive therapy.

08010 *limited orthodontic treatment of the primary dentition*
08020 *limited orthodontic treatment of the transitional dentition*
08030 *limited orthodontic treatment of the adolescent dentition*
08040 *limited orthodontic treatment of the adult dentition*

Interceptive Orthodontic Treatment
An extension of preventive orthodontics that may include localized tooth movement in an otherwise normal dentition. Such treatment may occur in the transitional dentition and include such procedures as the redirection of ectopically erupting teeth, correction of isolated dental crossbite, or recovery of recent minor space loss in which overall space is adequate. The key to successful interception is intervention in the incipient stages of a problem to lessen the severity of the malformation and eliminate its cause. The presence of complicating factors such as skeletal disharmonies, overall space deficiency, or other conditions requiring present or future comprehensive therapy are beyond the realm of interceptive therapy. Early phases of comprehensive therapy may use some procedures that also might be used interceptively in an otherwise normally developing dentition, but such procedures are not considered interceptive in those applications.

08050 interceptive orthodontic treatment of the primary dentition
08060 interceptive orthodontic treatment of the transitional dentition

Comprehensive Orthodontic Treatment

The coordinated diagnosis and treatment leading to the improvement of a patient's craniofacial dysfunction or dentofacial deformity, including anatomic, functional, and esthetic relationships. Treatment usually but not necessarily uses fixed orthodontic appliances. Adjunctive procedures such as extractions, maxillofacial surgery, nasopharyngeal surgery, myofunctional or speech therapy, and restorative or periodontal care may be coordinated disciplines. Optimal care requires long-term consideration of patients' needs and periodic reevaluation. Treatment may incorporate several phases with specific objectives at various stages of dentofacial development.

08070 comprehensive orthodontic treatment of the transitional dentition
08080 comprehensive orthodontic treatment of the adolescent dentition
08090 comprehensive orthodontic treatment of the adult dentition

Minor Treatment to Control Harmful Habits

08210 removable appliance therapy
Patient may remove these appliances; includes appliances for thumb sucking and tongue thrusting.

08220 fixed appliance therapy
Patient may not remove appliance; includes appliances for thumb sucking and tongue thrusting.

Other Orthodontic Services

08660 preorthodontic treatment visit
08670 periodic orthodontic treatment visit (as part of contract)
08680 orthodontic retention (removal of appliances, construction and placement of retainers)
08690 orthodontic treatment (alternative billing to a contract fee)
Services provided by dentist other than original treating dentist. A method of payment between the provider and responsible party for services that reflect an open-ended fee arrangement.

08999 unspecified orthodontic procedure, by report
Used for procedure that is not adequately described by a code. Describe procedure.

09000-09999
XII. Adjunctive General Services
Unclassified Treatment

09110 palliative (emergency) treatment of dental pain—minor procedure
This is typically reported on a per visit basis for emergency treatment of dental pain.

Anesthesia

09210 local anesthesia not in conjunction with operative or surgical procedures
09211 regional block anesthesia
09212 trigeminal division block anesthesia
09215 local anesthesia
09220 general anesthesia—first 30 minutes
09221 general anesthesia—each additional 15 minutes

09230 analgesia
Includes nitrous oxide.
09240 intravenous sedation

Professional Consultation

09310 consultation (diagnostic service provided by dentist or physician other than practitioner providing treatment)
See 00120-00160.

Professional Visits

09410 house call
Includes nursing home visits, long-term care facilities, and institutions. Report in addition to reporting appropriate code numbers for actual services performed.
09420 hospital call
May be reported when providing treatment in hospital or ambulatory surgicenter in addition to reporting appropriate code numbers for actual services performed.
09430 office visit for observation (during regularly scheduled hours)—no other services performed
09440 office visit—after regularly scheduled hours

Drugs

09610 therapeutic drug injection, by report
Includes antibiotic or injection of sedative.
09630 other drugs and medicaments, by report
Includes but is not limited to oral antibiotics, oral analgesics, oral sedatives, and topical fluoride dispensed in the office for home use; does not include writing prescriptions.

Miscellaneous Services

09910 application of desensitizing medicament
Includes in-office treatment for root sensitivity. Typically reported on a per visit basis for application of topical fluoride. Typically reported on a per tooth basis for application of adhesive resins.
09920 behavior management, by report
May be reported in addition to treatment provided. Should be reported in 15-minute increments.
09930 treatment of complications (postsurgical)—unusual circumstances, by report
09940 occlusal guard, by report
Removable dental appliances designed to minimize the effects of bruxism (grinding) and other occlusal factors.
09941 fabrication of athletic mouthguard
09950 occlusion analysis—mounted case
Includes but is not limited to face-bow, interocclusal records tracings, and diagnostic wax-up; for diagnostic casts, see 00470.
09951 occlusal adjustment—limited
Also may be known as equilibration; reshaping the occlusal surfaces of teeth to create harmonious contact relationships between the maxillary and mandibular teeth. Presently includes discing, odontoplasty, and enamoplasty. Typically reported on a per visit basis.

09952 *occlusal adjustment—complete*

Occlusal adjustment may require several appointments of varying length, and sedation may be necessary to attain adequate relaxation of the musculature. Study casts mounted on an articulating instrument may be used for analysis of occlusal disharmony. It is designed to achieve functional relationships and masticatory efficiency in conjunction with restorative treatment, orthodontics, orthognathic surgery, or jaw trauma when indicated. Occlusal adjustment enhances the healing potential of tissues affected by the lesions of occlusal trauma.

09970 *enamel microabrasion*

The removal of discolored surface enamel defects resulting from altered mineralization or decalcification of the superficial enamel layer. Submit per treatment visit.

09999 *unspecified adjunctive procedure, by report*

Used for procedure that is not adequately described by a code. Describe procedure.

Tooth Numbering Systems and Explanation for Mounting Radiographs

TOOTH NUMBERING

According to a resolution passed by the 1968 American Dental Association (ADA) House of Delegates, teeth should be numbered as follows:

Permanent Dentition

Permanent teeth should be numbered from 1 to 32, starting with the patient's upper right third molar (1), following around the upper arch to the patient's upper left third molar (16), descending to the patient's lower left third molar (17), and following around the lower arch to the patient's lower right third molar (32).

Primary Dentition

In the same manner as described for permanent dentition, primary teeth should be lettered with uppercase letters A through T, with A being the patient's upper right second primary molar and T being the patient's lower right second primary molar.

MOUNTING RADIOGRAPHS

According to the same resolution from the 1968 ADA House of Delegates, radiographs should be mounted as follows:

Looking at the teeth from outside the mouth, radiographs should be viewed in the same manner, and so mounted.

NOTE: The raised dot in the film should be toward you when mounting radiographs.

PERMANENT DENTITION

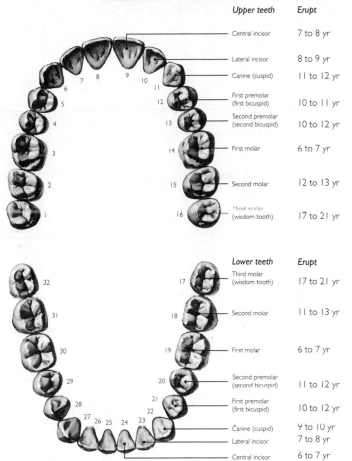

Upper teeth	Erupt
Central incisor	7 to 8 yr
Lateral incisor	8 to 9 yr
Canine (cuspid)	11 to 12 yr
First premolar (first bicuspid)	10 to 11 yr
Second premolar (second bicuspid)	10 to 12 yr
First molar	6 to 7 yr
Second molar	12 to 13 yr
Third molar (wisdom tooth)	17 to 21 yr

Lower teeth	Erupt
Third molar (wisdom tooth)	17 to 21 yr
Second molar	11 to 13 yr
First molar	6 to 7 yr
Second premolar (second bicuspid)	11 to 12 yr
First premolar (first bicuspid)	10 to 12 yr
Canine (cuspid)	9 to 10 yr
Lateral incisor	7 to 8 yr
Central incisor	6 to 7 yr

PRIMARY DENTITION

Upper teeth	Erupt	Shed
Central incisor	8 to 12 mo	6 to 7 yr
Lateral incisor	9 to 13 mo	7 to 8 yr
Canine (cuspid)	16 to 22 mo	10 to 12 yr
First molar	13 to 19 mo	9 to 11 yr
Second molar	25 to 33 mo	10 to 12 yr
Lower teeth	Erupt	Shed
Second molar	23 to 31 mo	10 to 12 yr
First molar	14 to 18 mo	9 to 11 yr
Canine (cuspid)	17 to 23 mo	9 to 12 yr
Lateral incisor	10 to 16 mo	7 to 8 yr
Central incisor	6 to 10 mo	6 to 7 yr

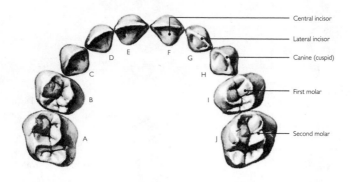

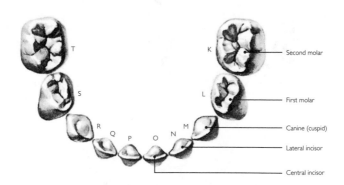

Dental Claim Form

ITEM-BY-ITEM DESCRIPTION OF THE DENTAL CLAIM FORM

The following is an item-by-item description of the questions appearing on the new form. All questions in the Billing Dentist section should be answered as completely as possible to facilitate prompt and accurate reimbursement and reduce follow-up inquiries. Special completion and mailing instructions, which may vary from company to company, are printed on the form and are not addressed here.

1. *Dentist's pretreatment estimate or statement of actual services*—By checking the appropriate box, the form may be processed more quickly and with less chance of error.
2. *Provider identification number*—Some third-party payers use an identification number that is different from the taxpayer identification number (TIN) or license number.
3. *Medicaid claim, Early and Periodic Screening Diagnosis and Treatment (EPSDT), prior authorization number, patient identification number*—The dental claim form should include appropriate information for government-funded benefit programs as necessary.
4. *Carrier name and address*—The form must include the name and address of the carrier to which the claim is to be sent. On carrier-supplied claim forms this information ordinarily is preprinted at the top of the form.
5. *Patient name*—This should be completed in full for proper identification purposes.
6. *Relationship to employee*—*Employee* here refers to the insured person and his or her relationship to the patient. This relationship sometimes affects the patient's eligibility and level of benefits available.
7. *Sex*—This is requested for identification purposes and for statistical analysis.
8. *Patient birthdate*—This is very important for determination of eligibility.
9. *If full-time student*—Eligibility of the dependent patient may be affected if the patient is older than a certain age (specified in the benefits policy) and is still a full-time student.
10. *Employee/subscriber name and address*—This refers to the insured person and is not necessarily the patient.
11. *Employee/subscriber dental plan identification number*—If you do not know your dental plan identification number, contact your dental plan. Your social security number (SSN) is commonly used for computer and manual processing of claims, but some carriers use an identification number that is different than the SSN.

12. *Employee/subscriber birthday*—This is very important for determination of coordination of benefits.

13. *Employer (company) name and address*—This refers to employer of person in 9.

14. *Group number*—This refers to master contract policy number assigned to the employer group.

15. *Is patient covered by another dental plan?* or *Is patient covered by a medical plan?*—This is to determine multiple coverage. The information contained in items 15 through 19 is important to determine whether any other carriers have primary liability for treatment provided.

16a. *Name and address of carriers*—This refers to carriers in 15.

16b. *Group number*—This refers to 15.

17. *Name and address of other employers*—This refers to employer offering plan in 15.

18a. *Employee/subscriber name (if different from patient's)*—This refers to employee from 17.

18b. *Employee/subscriber dental plan identification number*—This refers to employee in 18a. If you do not know your dental plan identification number, contact your dental plan. Your SSN is commonly used for computer and manual processing of claims, but some carriers use an identification number that is different from the SSN.

18c. *Employee/subscriber birthdate*—This refers to employee in 18a. Necessary for coordination of benefits.

19. *Relationship to patient*—This refers to employee in 18a.

20. *Patient signature block*—The patient is defined as an individual who has established a professional relationship with a dentist for the delivery of dental health care. For matters relating to communication of information and consent, this term includes the patient's parent, caretaker, guardian, or other individual as appropriate under state law and the circumstances of the case.

21. *Employee/subscriber block*—This block must be completed if the patient and dentist wish to have benefits paid directly to the provider. This is an authorization of payment and constitutes an assignment of benefits. It does not create a contractual relationship between the dentist and the payer.

22. *Name of billing dentist or dental entity*—The individual dentist's name or the name of the group practice or corporation responsible for billing. This may differ from the actual treating dentist's name. This is the name that should appear on any payments or correspondence that are remitted to the billing dentist.

23. *Address to which payment should be remitted*—This is self-explanatory.

24. *City, state, zip*—This is self-explanatory.

25. *Dentist's SSN or TIN*—This refers to dentist or dental entity in 22. These numbers are frequently used as individual provider identification numbers. The Internal Revenue Service requires that either the SSN or TIN of the billing dentist or dental entity be supplied only if the provider accepts payment directly from a third-party payer. Report the SSN if the billing dentist is unincorporated. Report the corporation TIN if the billing dentist is incorporated. If the billing entity is a group practice or clinic, the entity's TIN should be entered.

26. *Dentist's license number*—This is frequently used as a means of provider identification. This should be the license number of the

billing dentist. This may differ from that of the treating dentist, which appears in the dentist's signature block at the bottom of the form.

27. *Dentist's phone number*—This is self-explanatory. Include area code also.

28. *First visit date current series*—This is important to determine the services covered when a patient becomes eligible in the middle of an active treatment plan.

29. *Place of treatment*—Depending on where treatment is rendered, medical or hospital coverage, including dental benefits, may be activated. ECF stands for extended care facility.

30. *Radiographs or models enclosed*—This line indicates whether diagnostic materials were submitted. Assists in return of proper number of materials to dentist.

31. *Is treatment the result of occupational illness or injury?*—This refers to possible application of workers' compensation, which may alter coverage available and carrier involved. Important for coordination of benefits and accurate claims processing.

32. *Is treatment the result of an automobile accident?*—This item affects reimbursement in no-fault auto cases. Indicates whether another party's insurance may be responsible. Also important for coordination of benefits.

33. *Other accident?*—Similar to 31 and 32.

34. *If prosthesis, is this initial placement?*—Most dental contracts have specific limitations on replacement of dentures, partials, crowns, and bridges. This is used to determine eligibility and liability.

35. *Date of prior placement?*—Contracts specify time limitations concerning the replacement of prosthetic devices.

36. *Is treatment for orthodontics?*—If orthodontics is covered, dates and months of treatment remaining affect the prorated monthly reimbursement made to the dentist.

37. *Identify missing teeth with* x—This is self-explanatory.

38. *Examination and treatment plan*—This is self-explanatory. Use the ADA's Current Dental Terminology (CDT-2) for appropriate procedure codes.

39. *Remarks for unusual services*—Use to indicate any information that may be helpful in determining the benefits for the treatment. If space is inadequate, use unused portion of 38 or attach a separate sheet.

40. *Dentist's signature block*—This is the line for the treating dentist's signature and license number.

41. *Address at which treatment was performed*—Complete this section if the treatment was performed at a different location than indicated in 23 and 24.

42. *Total fee charged*—This is the sum of the fees for each procedure reported.

43. *Payment by other plan*—If known, indicate the dollar amount paid by other benefit plans.

For administrative use only—This is the area in which the carrier calculates benefits.

Payment itemization—The space under "payment by other plan" is completed by the carrier and may vary from carrier to carrier.

Dental Claim Form

- □ Dentist's pre-treatment estimate
- □ Dentist's statement of actual services

Provider ID #

2.
- □ Medicaid Claim
- □ EPSDT

Prior authorization #
Patient ID #

3. Carrier name and address

PATIENT

4. Patient name		
First	M.I.	Last

5. Relationship to employee
- □ Self □ Child
- □ Spouse □ Other ___

6. Sex
M ___ F

7. Patient birthdate
MM   DD   YYYY

8. If full time student
School _____
City _____

COVERAGE

9. Employee/subscriber name
and mailing address

10. Employee/subscriber
dental plan ID number

11. Employee/subscriber
birthdate
MM   DD   YYYY

12. Employer (company)
name and address

13. Group number

14. Is patient covered by another
dental plan   yes ___ no ___
If yes, complete 15-a.
Is patient covered by a medical
plan?   yes ___ no ___

15-a. Name and address of carrier(s)

15-b. Group no.(s)

16. Name and address of other employer(s)

17-a. Employee/subscriber name
(if different from patient's)

17-b. Employee/subscriber
dental plan ID number

17-c. Employee/subscriber
birthdate
MM   DD   YYYY

18. Relationship to patient
- □ Self □ Parent
- □ Spouse □ Other ___

19. I have reviewed the following treatment plan and fees. I agree to be responsible for all charges for dental services and materials not paid by my dental benefit plan, unless the treating dentist or dental practice has a contractual agreement with my plan prohibiting all or a portion of such charges. To the extent permitted under applicable law, I authorize release of any information relating to this claim.

Signed (Patient) _____   Date _____

20. I hereby authorize payment of the dental benefits otherwise payable to me directly to the below named dental entity.

Signed (Employee/subscriber) _____   Date _____

BILLING

21. Name of billing dentist or dental entity

22. Address where payment should be remitted

23. City, State, Zip

24. Dentist Soc. Sec. or T.I.N.

25. Dentist license no.

26. Dentist phone no.

27. First visit date
current series

28. Place of treatment
Office ___ Hosp. ___ ECF ___ Other ___

29. Radiographs or
models enclosed?
No ___ Yes ___ How many? ___

DENTIST

30. Is treatment result of
occupational illness or injury? No ___ Yes ___

31. Is treatment result of
auto accident?

32. Other accident?

33. If prosthesis, is this
initial placement?

34. Date of prior
placement

(If no, reason for replacement)

35. Is treatment for
orthodontics?

If service already
commenced enter:

Date appliances
placed

Mos. treatment
remaining

36. Identify missing teeth with "X"

Facial

Permanent

Primary

Lingual

Left

Upper

Right

Lower

Lingual

Facial

37. Examination and treatment plan – List in order from tooth no. 1 through tooth no. 32 using charting system shown.

Tooth # or letter	Surface	Description of service (including x-rays, prophylaxis, materials used, etc.)	Date service performed Mo. Day Year	Procedure number	Fee	For administrative use only

38. Remarks for unusual services

41. Total fee charged	
42. Payment by other plan	
Max. allowable	
Deductible	
Carrier %	
Carrier pays	
Patient pays	

39. I hereby certify that the procedures as indicated by date have been completed and that the fees submitted are the actual fees I have charged and intend to collect for those procedures.

✗ _____
Signed (Treating dentist)   License number   Date

40. Address where treatment was performed

_____
City   State   Zip

©**American Dental Association, 1994**
J510 (Same as ADA Dental Claim Form - J504, J511, J512)

Selected Craniofacial Anatomy Illustrations

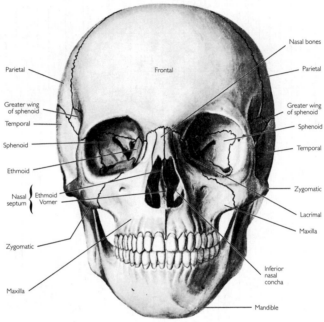

Anterior view of skull. (Brand, 1997.)

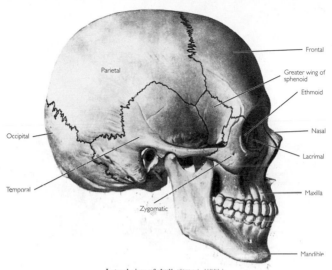

Lateral view of skull. (Brand, 1997.)

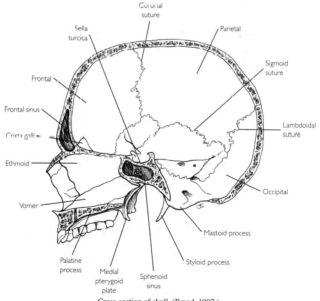

Cross-section of skull. (Brand, 1997.)

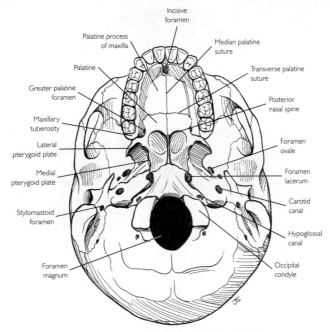

Inferior view of skull (minus the mandible). (Brand, 1997.)

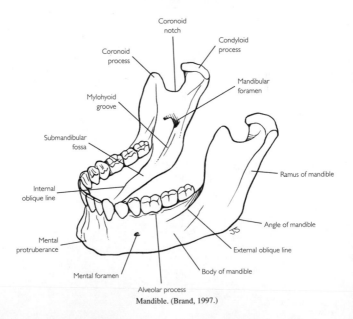

Mandible. (Brand, 1997.)

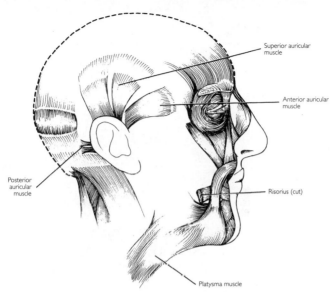

Three groups of auricular muscles around the ear. (Brand, 1997.)

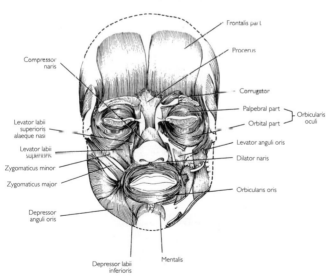

Muscles of the eye, nose, and mouth. (Brand, 1997.)

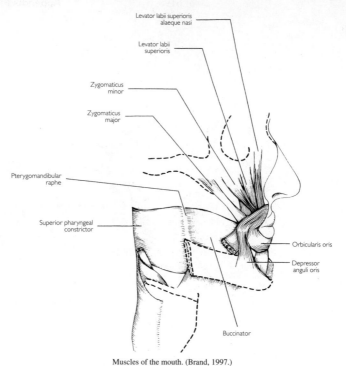

Levator labii superioris
alaeque nasi

Levator labii
superioris

Zygomaticus
minor

Zygomaticus
major

Pterygomandibular
raphe

Superior pharyngeal
constrictor

Orbicularis oris

Depressor
anguli oris

Buccinator

Muscles of the mouth. (Brand, 1997.)

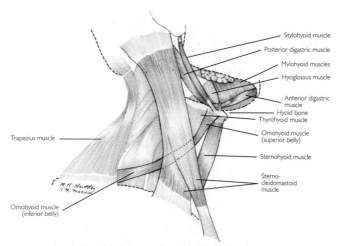

Stylohyoid muscle

Posterior digastric muscle

Mylohyoid muscles

Hyoglossus muscle

Anterior digastric
muscle

Hyoid bone

Thyrohyoid muscle

Omohyoid muscle
(superior belly)

Sternohyoid muscle

Sterno-
cleidomastoid
muscle

Trapezius muscle

Omohyoid muscle
(inferior belly)

Lateral view of neck showing digastric muscle suspended above hyoid
bone and attaching to it by ligamentous loop. Mylohyoid and stylohyoid
muscles are also visible above hyoid bone, and omohyoid, thyrohyoid, and
sternohyoid muscles are visible below hyoid bone. Large sternocleidomastoid muscle covers large area on side of neck. (Brand, 1997.)

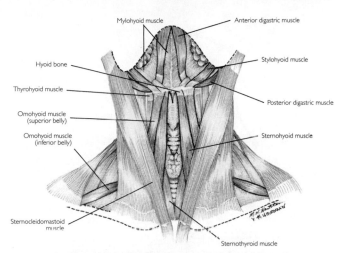

Anterior and inferior view of mylohyoid muscle. Left and right muscles fuse in midline and form slinglike arrangement that forms mouth floor. Anterior view of digastric, stylohyoid, sternohyoid, sternothyroid, and sternocleidomastoid muscles are also visible. (Brand, 1997.)

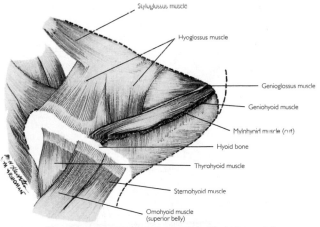

View with mylohyoid muscle cut away, geniohyoid muscle extends from genial tubercles of mandible downward to hyoid bone. (Brand, 1997.)

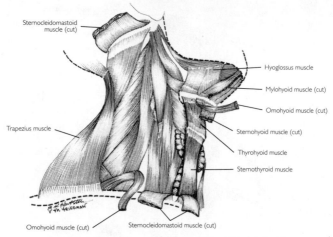

Lateral view of neck with several muscles cut and turned back (reflected).
Notice extent of sternothyroid and thyrohyoid muscles. (Brand, 1997.)

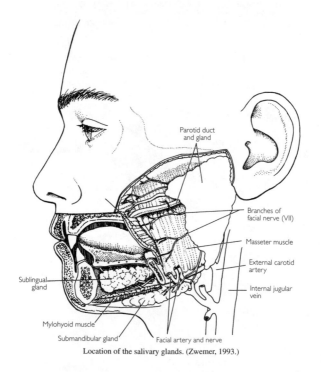

Location of the salivary glands. (Zwemer, 1993.)

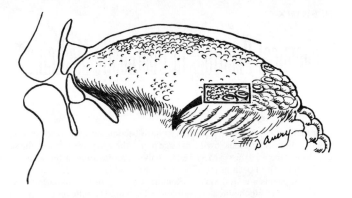

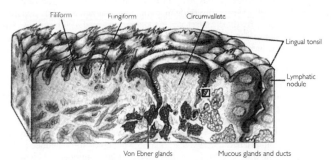

Papillae on the tongue and location of taste buds. (Zwemer, 1993.)

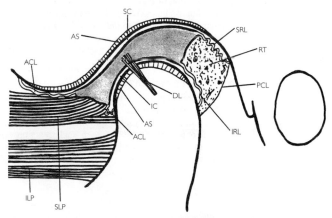

Temporomandibular joint. (Zwemer, 1993.)

Biochemical Profiling in Diagnostic Medicine*

INTRODUCTION

During the past 4 years many physicians have become familiar with the concept of biochemical profiles, owing in large part to the widespread use of the sequential multiple analysis (SMA) 12/60 analyzer, an instrument that can perform 12 tests in 60 minutes. The diagnostic advantages of the 12-test biochemical panels are well known. Routine screening of hospital admissions yields evidence of biochemical abnormalities leading to significant unexpected diagnoses in about 4% of admissions. In addition, biochemical panels often lead the physician to early diagnoses of disorders with either vague or absent symptoms such as hyperparathyroidism, pernicious anemia, anicteric hepatitis, occult neoplasms and their metastases, and silent myocardial infarctions. Furthermore, these profiles provide the physician with a record of the patient's normal chemical values against which subsequent changes may be compared.

PATTERN RECOGNITION

Use of the chemistry panel requires a different approach to the clinician's interpretation of laboratory data. Physicians have been trained to take a careful medical history, perform a thorough physical examination, and then order tests from the laboratory that will either confirm or exclude a provisional diagnosis. However, with the SMA 12/60 biochemical profile, physicians are confronted with 12 different biochemical test results from which they must deduce a diagnosis or differential diagnosis. From the analysis of large numbers of chemistry profiles, certain patterns of abnormalities have emerged that are sufficiently characteristic to suggest a specific diagnosis or groups of differential diagnoses. This appendix stresses the recognition of these diagnostic patterns as a means of increasing the diagnostic value of the SMA 12/60 chemistry profile. The graphic display of the biochemical data unique to the SMA 12/60 permits pattern recognition. This is analogous to the pathologist's recognition of tissue patterns during the examination of biopsy material, and in fact the SMA 12/60 profile may be thought of as a biochemical biopsy.

METHODOLOGY AND DETERMINATIONS

Before studying the actual biochemical profile, a description of the way the results are obtained on an SMA 12/60 analyzer may be useful. Each serum sample (approximately 2 ml) is aspirated into the system, split into 12 portions, and subjected to specific chemical reactions. Results of each such reaction are recorded on a strip-chart recorder. Approximately 8 minutes are required to process a single sample. Complete 12-test profiles are recorded at the rate of one a minute.

---

*From Preston JA, Troxel DB: *Biochemical profiling in diagnostic medicine,* Tarrytown, NY, 1971, Technicon Instruments.

Nineteen different tests are available for the SMA 12/60, of which the following 12 represent determinations done in most laboratories on a standard SMA 12/60 survey instrument.

1. Serum glutamic-oxaloacetic transaminase (SGOT)
2. Lactic dehydrogenase (LDH)
3. Uric acid
4. Inorganic phosphorus
5. Urea nitrogen
6. Glucose
7. Albumin
8. Alkaline phosphatase
9. Total protein
10. Bilirubin
11. Cholesterol
12. Calcium

THE SERUM CHEMISTRY GRAPH

Results from determinations performed by the SMA 12/60 analyzer are recorded on a serum chemistry graph (see p. 626). They appear in the same sequence that tests are performed on the instrument. Each test shows a concentration range *(A)* and includes a shaded area *(B)* representing the values normal for that particular determination within any population. The pen tracing *(C)* represents the actual concentration of material detected by the instrument for each test, drawn across the concentration scale for that test. This type of presentation enables the physician to scan all 12 chemistries rapidly and see immediately any results that fall outside the normal range.

In this appendix the interrelationship among various abnormal chemistry results is discussed. Before this happens, however, the term *normal* as applied to the data derived must be defined.

THE NORMAL RANGE

The shaded areas on the SMA 12/60 serum chemistry graph represent the normal range for each of the particular test values. The normal range is based on a simple statistical concept—the normal distribution or the Gaussian curve (see p. 627, *top*). Any population characteristically shows this curve for a particular measurement. Scatter may occur around a mean or average value. The characteristic bell-shaped curve defines mathematically the spread of a population around the mean or average value. Approximately 66% of a population will fall within one standard deviation of the mean and 95% within two standard deviations.

Normal in the statistical sense employed here does not necessarily mean healthy. The word merely describes the typical range of values anticipated in any given population. One out of 20 results is always outside the two standard deviation range. The farther from the average value a particular physiologic value falls, the more certain is its clinical significance. The probability becomes greater that a value outside the 95% limit reflects a definite clinical problem.

With the typical Gaussian curve superimposed on the normal range (see p. 627, *bottom*), the farther the result lies from the center of the normal range, the more significant it can become diagnostically.

Because these ranges are generated from the total population, regardless of age, sex, or race, the normal range is a broad indicator. It must be understood in terms of the individual patient.

This fact leads to one of the most intriguing possibilities afforded clinicians by routine profiling: the determination of an individual's personal normal range or baseline. Because data are accumulated for a patient over several years, a deviation in a given determination may indicate a radical change in the individual, although the result never deviates from the normal population range.

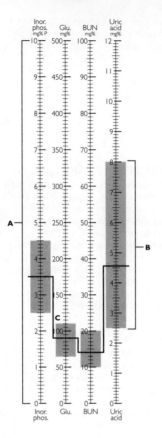

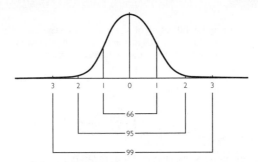

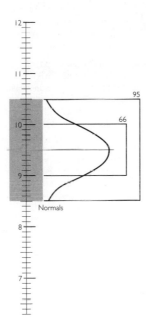

CLINICAL SIGNIFICANCE OF DETERMINATIONS

To understand fully the relevance of the biochemical profiles that follow, the clinical significance of elevated or diminished values for the various determinations included in the 12-test panel should be examined briefly.*

---

*For a detailed discussion of the clinical significance of various tests, see Wolf PL et al: Utilization of SMA 12/60 and SMA 6/60 charts as a teaching aid in laboratory medicine, *Advances in Automated Analysis: Proceeding of the Technicon International Congress,* vol 1, Mount Kisco, NY, 1970, Futura.

SGOT

SGOT elevation may be indicative of several disease states, most commonly heart or liver disease. Elevations of this enzyme are typical in the conditions listed below; slight elevations occur during normal pregnancy:

1. Acute hepatitis
2. Acute myocardial infarction
3. Active cirrhosis
4. Infectious mononucleosis with hepatitis
5. Hepatic necrosis chemically and drug induced
6. Hepatic metastases
7. Acute pancreatitis
8. Trauma to skeletal muscle; irradiation of skeletal muscle
9. Pseudohypertrophic muscular dystrophy
10. Dermatomyositis
11. Acute hemolytic anemia
12. Acute renal disease
13. Severe burns
14. Cardiac catheterization and angiography
15. Recent brain trauma with brain necrosis
    Reduced levels of SGOT may be seen in certain conditions:
    1. Beriberi
    2. Uncontrolled diabetes mellitus with acidosis
    3. Liver disease (occasionally)

LDH

LDH is an intracellular enzyme, and increases in the reported value usually indicate cellular death and leakage of enzyme from the cell. Elevation occurs when neoplastic cells proliferate. Increased levels of this enzyme also are found after strenuous exercise, including the muscular exertion involved in childbirth. Causes for elevated LDH include the following:

1. Acute myocardial infarction
2. Acute leukemia
3. Hemolytic anemia of any type
4. Acute pulmonary infarction
5. Malignant neoplasms
6. Acute renal infarction
7. Hepatic disease
8. Skeletal muscle necrosis
9. Sprue
10. Shock with necrosis of minor organs

URIC ACID

Uric acid levels may increase as a result either of overproduction or the patient's inability to excrete the substance produced. The following are possible causes:

1. Renal failure (most common cause in hospitalized patients)
2. Gout
3. Eclampsia of pregnancy with hepatic necrosis
4. Leukemias or lymphomas

5. Metabolic acidosis
6. Starvation
7. Thiazide diuretics, salicylates, ethanol, and other drugs
8. Lead poisoning
9. Infectious mononucleosis
10. Chemotherapy for cancer

Reduced levels of uric acid are encountered in patients being treated with a uricosuric drug.

INORGANIC PHOSPHORUS

Inorganic phosphorus is inversely related to calcium, and therefore many of the causes of elevated calcium also are causes of hypophosphatemia. Phosphorus levels are normally elevated in youth and adolescence. Abnormal elevations may result from several causes, including the following:

1. Renal failure (most common cause in a hospital population)
2. Healing bone fractures
3. Diabetic ketosis
4. Hypoparathyroidism
5. Hypervitaminosis D
6. Acromegaly (early sign)

Reduced inorganic phosphorus levels derive from a variety of causes:

1. Continuous use of intravenous (IV) glucose in a nondiabetic
2. Negative nitrogen balance
3. Rickets
4. Some hepatic disorders
5. Osteomalacia
6. Fanconi syndrome
7. Ingestion of antacids

UREA NITROGEN

Urea nitrogen elevations are associated with renal failure, with or without obstructive uropathy from any cause:

1. Dehydration (mild to moderate elevation)
2. Gastrointestinal hemorrhage

Reduced levels of blood urea nitrogen (BUN) also are symptomatic:

1. Liver failure (from acute atrophy or toxicity)
2. Negative nitrogen balance
3. Excessive use of IV fluids
4. Physiologic hydremia in pregnancy

GLUCOSE

Hyperglycemia is related to several disease states:

1. Diabetes mellitus (most common cause; unlikely diagnosis in cases in which phosphorus values are depressed)

2. Cushing's disease (and other conditions related to excess production of adrenal corticoids)
3. Pheochromocytoma
4. Brain trauma

Hypoglycemia also has several possible causes:

1. Excess insulin administered to a diabetic
2. Addison's disease
3. Bacterial sepsis
4. Islet cell adenoma of the pancreas
5. Mesenchymal neoplasm that consumes glucose
6. Massive hepatic necrosis
7. Psychogenic conditions

ALBUMIN

Hyperalbuminemia is generally not observed. Low albumin readings usually are caused by multiple and diverse conditions:

1. Inadequate protein intake
2. Severe liver disease
3. Malabsorption
4. Diarrhea
5. Nephrosis
6. Exfoliative dermatitis
7. Burns
8. Dilution by excessive intravenous infusion of glucose in water

ALKALINE PHOSPHATASE

Alkaline phosphatase levels are higher in children and adolescents and also in pregnant women. Levels are somewhat higher in the male than they are in the female. Levels also may be elevated if serum is retained for several hours at 20° C before it is processed on the SMA 12/60. Abnormal elevations have several causes:

1. Metastatic carcinoma involving the bones
2. Primary malignant neoplasms
3. Infusion of 5% human albumin
4. Healing fractures
5. Obstructive liver disease
6. Hyperparathyroidism, primary or secondary
7. Paget's disease of bone
8. Pulmonary infarct
9. Acute or chronic liver disease

Reduced levels of the enzyme may indicate malnutrition.

TOTAL PROTEIN

The causes of hyperproteinemia are actually the causes for hyperglobulinemia:

1. Lupus erythematosus
2. Rheumatoid arthritis

3. Other collagen diseases
4. Chronic infections
5. Multiple myeloma (and other malignant tumors)
6. Acute liver disease

Low total protein values derive from the same causes as those listed for hypoalbuminemia.

BILIRUBIN

Bilirubin elevations and jaundice have many causes, generally falling into three major categories: hepatic, obstructive, and hemolytic.

Elevation of nonconjugated bilirubin

1. Hemolytic anemia
2. Trauma with the presence of a large hematoma
3. Hemorrhagic pulmonary infarct
4. Crigler-Najjar syndrome (rare)
5. Gilbert's disease (rare)

Conjugated and nonconjugated bilirubin elevated, conjugated more elevated

1. Hepatic metastases
2. Hepatitis
3. Lymphoma
4. Cholestasis secondary to drugs
5. Decompensated cirrhosis

Elevated conjugated bilirubin

1. Carcinoma of the head of the pancreas
2. Choledocholithiasis
3. Dubin-Johnson syndrome

CHOLESTEROL

Cholesterol elevations are attributable to several causes:

1. Cardiovascular disease
2. Obstructive jaundice
3. Hypothyroidism
4. Nephrosis
5. Uncontrolled diabetes
6. Pregnancy

Low cholesterol values occur when cholesterol is not absorbed from the gastrointestinal tract:

1. Malabsorption
2. Severe liver disease
3. Hyperthyroidism
4. Anemia
5. Sepsis
6. Stress and drug therapy

CALCIUM

Causes for calcium elevations are well understood:

1. Primary hyperparathyroidism
2. Secondary hyperparathyroidism associated with chronic renal failure
3. Bony metastases from carcinomas
4. Sarcoidosis with bone involvement
5. Bone involvement from lymphoma or multiple myeloma
6. Carcinoma of the lung and kidney parathormone production
7. Hypervitaminosis D
8. Long-term use of diuretics
9. Milk-alkali syndrome
10. Acidosis

Low calcium values also are of interest. Causes include the following:

1. Low albumin
2. Hypoparathyroidism (usually surgically induced)
3. Chronic renal failure
4. Steatorrhea or malabsorption syndrome
5. Pancreatitis
6. Ethylenediaminetetraacetic acid (EDTA) anticoagulation therapy
7. Alkalosis

CLINICAL EXAMPLES

A few biochemical profiles from own clinical studies, arranged in six categories reflecting particular states ranging from normal variations to specific pathologies may be useful (see pp. 633-635).

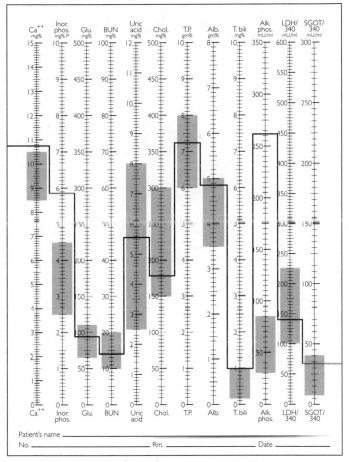

Patient's name _____

No. _____ Rm. _____ Date _____

The normal pattern of a 12-year-old child. The increased alkaline phosphatase and inorganic phosphorus are caused by bone growth. The alkaline phosphatase is heat labile and therefore bone in origin.

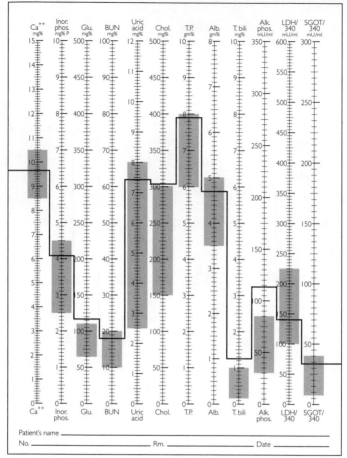

Patient's name _____

No. _____ Rm. _____ Date _____

Pattern of normal pregnancy, last trimester. A slight but distinct elevation occurs in glucose, cholesterol, bilirubin, and alkaline phosphatase. Fifty percent of the alkaline phosphatase is heat stable. It is therefore both placental and bone in origin.

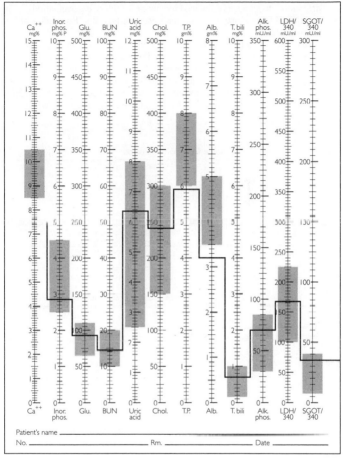

Normal pattern of old age with hypoproteinemia and calcemia.

Differential diagnosis is enhanced by simple ancillary determinations such as protein and LDH isoenzyme electrophoresis and heat stability studies of alkaline phosphatase.

Another factor that must always be considered in reviewing patient test data is the possible effect of therapeutic agents. The medication a patient receives may either influence the quantity of the compound measured owing to a physiologic response or may cause an interference in the analytical measurement itself. For further information on this subject, please see Elking MP, Kabat HF: *Am J Hosp Pharm* 25:485, 1968; and Christian DG: *Am J Clin Path* 54:118, 1970.

Daily dietary guide—the basic four food groups

Food group	Main nutrients	Daily amounts*
Milk		
Milk, cheese, ice cream, or other products made with whole or skimmed milk	Calcium Protein Riboflavin	Children under 9: 2 to 3 cups Children 9 to 12: 3 or more cups Teenagers: 4 or more cups Adults: 2 or more cups Pregnant women: 3 or more cups Nursing mothers: 4 or more cups (1 cup = 8 oz fluid milk or designated milk equivalent†)
Meats		
Beef, veal, lamb, pork, poultry, fish, eggs	Protein Iron Thiamin	2 or more servings Count as 1 serving 2 to 3 oz of lean, boneless, cooked meat, poultry, or fish 2 eggs
Alternates: dry beans, dry peas, nuts, peanut butter	Niacin Riboflavin	1 cup cooked dry beans or peas 4 tbsp peanut butter
Vegetables and Fruits		
		4 or more servings Count as 1 serving ½ cup of vegetable or fruit or a portion such as 1 medium apple, banana, orange, potato, or ½ a medium grapefruit or melon Include
	Vitamin A	Dark-green or deep-yellow vegetable or fruit rich in vitamin A at least every other day
	Vitamin C (ascorbic acid)	Citrus fruit or other fruit or vegetable rich in vitamin C daily
	Smaller amounts of other vitamins and minerals	Other vegetables and fruits, including potatoes
Bread and Cereals		
	Thiamin Niacin Riboflavin Iron Protein	4 or more servings of whole grain, enriched or restored Count as 1 serving 1 slice of bread 1 oz (1 cup) ready to eat cereal, flake or puff varieties ½ to ¾ cup cooked cereal ½ to ¾ cup cooked pastas (macaroni, spaghetti, noodles) Crackers: 5 saltines, 2 squares graham crackers

*Use additional amounts of these foods or added butter, margarine, oils, and sugars as desired or needed.
†Milk equivalents: 1 oz cheddar cheese, 3 servings cottage cheese, 1 cup fluid skimmed milk, 1 cup buttermilk, ½ cup dry skimmed milk powder, 1 cup ice milk, 1⅔ cups ice cream, ½ cup evaporated milk.

Medical Tables

Conversion formulas

Temperature	To convert Fahrenheit to centigrade, subtract 32 from °F, multiply by $\frac{5}{9}$.		
	To convert centigrade to Fahrenheit, multiply °C by $\frac{9}{5}$ and add 32.		
	1 kg = 2.2 pounds	1 pound = 0.45 kg.	
Weight	1 g = 15.43 grains	1 grain = 0.065 g	
	1 inch = 2.54 cm	1 cm = 0.3937 inch	
Length			
	1 Teaspoonful		5 ml
Approximate Household	1 Dessert spoonful		8 ml
Measures	1 Tablespoonful	½ fl oz	15 ml
	1 Jigger	1½ fl oz	45 ml
	1 Wineglassful	2 fl oz	60 ml
	1 Teacupful	4 fl oz	120 ml
	1 Glassful	8 fl oz	240 ml

From *Pocket book of medical tables*, ed 25, Philadelphia, 1980, Smith Kline.

Nomenclature and synonyms for coagulation factors

Roman numeral	Preferred descriptive name	Synonyms
I	Fibrinogen	
II	Prothrombin	
III	Tissue factor	Thromboplastin
IV	Calcium ions	
V	Proaccelerin	Labile factor, accelerator globulin (AcG), thrombogen
VII	Proconvertin	Stable factor, serum prothrombin conversion accelerator (SPCA), autoprothrombin I, cothromboplastin
VIII	Antihemophilic factor (AHF)	Antihemophilic globulin (AHG), antihemophilic factor A, platelet cofactor 1, thromboplastinogen
IX	Plasma thromboplastin component (PTC)	Christmas factor, antihemophilic factor B, autoprothrombin II, platelet cofactor 2
X	Stuart-Prower factor	Stuart factor, autoprothrombin III, thrombokinase
XI	Plasma thromboplastin antecedent (PTA)	Antihemophilic factor C
XII	Hageman factor	Glass factor, contact factor XIII
	Fibrin stabilizing factor (FSF)	Laki-Lorand factor (LLF), fibrinase, plasma transglutaminase

From Wintrobe MM: *Clinical hematology*, ed 7, Philadelphia, 1974, Lea & Febiger.

Desirable weights for men and women according to height and frame (age 25 and over)

Men
Weight in pounds (in indoor clothing; for nude weight deduct 5 to 7 pounds)

| Height (with shoes) | | Small frame | Medium frame | Large frame |
Feet	Inches			
5	2	112-120	118-129	126-141
5	3	115-123	121-133	129-144
5	4	118-126	124-136	132-148
5	5	121-129	127-139	135-152
5	6	124-133	130-143	138-156
5	7	128-137	134-147	142-161
5	8	132-141	138-152	147-166
5	9	136-145	142-156	151-170
5	10	140-150	146-160	155-174
5	11	144-154	150-165	159-179
6	0	148-158	154-170	164-184
6	1	152-162	158-175	168-189
6	2	156-167	162-180	173-194
6	3	160-171	167-185	178-199
6	4	164-175	172-190	182-204

Women
Weight in pounds (in indoor clothing; for nude weight deduct 2 to 4 pounds)

| Height (with shoes) | | Small frame | Medium frame | Large frame |
Feet	Inches			
4	10	92-98	96-107	104-119
4	11	94-101	98-110	106-122
5	0	96-104	101-113	109-125
5	1	99-107	104-116	112-128
5	2	102-110	107-119	115-131
5	3	105-113	110-122	118-134
5	4	108-116	113-126	121-138
5	5	111-119	116-130	125-142
5	6	114-123	120-135	129-146
5	7	118-127	124-139	133-150
5	8	122-131	128-143	137-154
5	9	126-135	132-147	141-158
5	10	130-140	136-151	145-163
5	11	134-144	140-155	149-168
6	0	138-148	144-159	153-173

From Society of Actuaries: *The build and blood pressure study*, New York, 1959, Metropolitan Life Insurance Co.

Hematology

RBC Measurements	Diameter	5.5-8.8 μ (newborn: 8.6)
	Mean corpuscular volume	82-92 cuμ (newborn: 106)
	Mean corpuscular Hb	27-31 μm (newborn: 38)
	Mean corpuscular Hb concentration	32%-36%
	Color, saturation, and volume indices	1
Miscellaneous	Bleeding time	1-4 min (Duke)
		1-9 min (Ivy)
	Circulation time, arm to lung (ether)	4-8 sec
	Circulation time, arm to tongue (sodium dehydrocholate)	9-16 sec
	Clot retraction time	2-4 hr
	Coagulation time (venous)	6-10 min (Lee & White)
		10-30 min (Howell)
	Fragility, erythrocyte (hemolysis)	0.44%-0.35% NaCl
	Partial thromboplastin time	68-82 sec (standard)
		32-46 sec (activated)
	Sedimentation rate:	
	Men	0-9 mm/hr (Wintrobe)
	Women	0-20 mm/hr (Wintrobe)

From *Pocket book of medical tables*, ed 25, Philadelphia, 1980, Smith Kline.

Blood chemistry

Constituent	Material*	mg/dl (mg %)—or as noted†
Aldolase	S	0.8-3 ImU/ml
Ammonia	P	20-150 μg/dl
Amylase	S	60-160 units (Somogyi)
		0.06-0.34 ImU/ml
α-1-Antitrypsin	S	210-500
Ascorbic acid	B	0.4-1.5
Bilirubin		
Direct	S	Up to 0.4
Indirect	S	0.4-0.8
Total	S	Up to 1.2
Bromide	S	Toxic level about 15 mEq/L
Bromsulphalein (5 mg/kg)	S	5% dye or less at 45 minutes
Calcium (ionized)	S	4.5-5.5 mEq/L
		2.4-2.9 mEq/L (at pH 7.4)
Carbon dioxide content	S	24-30 mM/L
Carotene	S	50-300 μg/dl
Ceruloplasmin	S	23-50
Chloride	S	98-109 mEq/L
Cholesterol, total	S	150-250
Cholesterol esters	S	60%-75% of total
Cholinesterase	S	0.5 pH unit/hour or more
		2-5.3 IU/ml
Creatine		
Males	S	0.2-0.6
Females	S	0.6-1.0
Creatine phosphokinase (CPK)		
Males	S	5-50 ImU/ml
Females	S	5-30 ImU/ml
Creatinine	S	0.8-1.2
Ferritin		
Males	S	27-329 ng/ml
Females	S	9-125 ng/ml
Fibrinogen	P	160-415
Folate	S	5-21 ng/ml
Gastrin	S	0-20 pg/ml
Glucose	S	60-100 (Nelson-Somogyi)
Glucose-6-phosphate dehydrogenase (G6PD)	Red cells	5-10 IU/g 1 lb/30° C
γ-Glutamyl transpeptidase		
Males	S	<28 ImU/ml
Females	S	<18 ImU/ml
α-Hydroxybutyric dehydrogenase	S	0-180 ImU/ml
17-Hydroxycorticosteroids		7-19 μg/dl
Males	P	9-21 μg/dl
Females	P	
After 25 units ACTH, IM		35-55 μg/dl
Immunoglobulins		
IgG	S	800-1500
IgA	S	50-200
IgM	S	40-120
Iodine, protein-bound	S	4-8 μg/dl
Iron	S	50-150 μg/dl
Iron-binding capacity	S	250-410 μg/dl
Isocitric dehydrogenase	S	50-260 units
17-Ketosteroids		
Males	P	40-150 μg/dl
Females	P	38-130 μg/dl
Lactic acid	B	6-20
Lactic dehydrogenase (LDH)	S	0-300 ImU/ml
Isozymes		

*B, Whole blood; P, plasma; S, serum. †IU, International units; ImU, International milliunits.
From *Pocket book of medical tables*, ed 25, Philadelphia, 1980, Smith Kline.

Continued

Blood chemistry—cont'd

Constituent				Material		mg/dl (mg %)—or as noted
American	European	Myocardium	Liver	Muscle	RBC	
5	1	4+	±	±	3+	
4	2	4+	±	±	3+	
3	3	+	+	+	+	
2	4	±	2+	2+	±	
1	5	±	4+	4+	±	

	Material	mg/dl (mg %)—or as noted
Lipase	S	0.2-1.5 units/ml (N/20 NaOH)
Lipids, total	S	400-800
Cholesterol		
Total	S	115-340
Esterified	S	70%
Free fatty acids	S	0.3-0.8 mEq/L
Phospholipids	S	130-380
Triglycerides (neutral fat)	S	10-190
Lithium (therapeutic level)	S	0.5-1.0 mEq/L
Magnesium	S	1.5-2.4 mEq/L
Nonprotein nitrogen	S	25-40
Osmolality	S	280-290 mOsm/kg plasma water
pH	P	7.35-7.45 glass electrode method
Phenylalanine	S	0-2
Phosphatase, acid	S	0.1-1.0 units (Bodansky)
		0-11 ImU/ml
Phosphatase, alkaline		
Children	S	5-14 units (Bodansky)
		15-20 units (King-Armstrong)
Adults	S	1.4-4.1 units (Bodansky)
		4-13 units (King-Armstrong)
		20-48 ImU/ml
Phosphorus		
Children	S	2.3-3.8 mEq/L
Adults	S	1.45-2.76 mEq/L
Potassium	S	3.6-5.5 mEq/L
Proteins (electrophoresis)		
Albumin	S	3.2-5.6 g/dl
α_1 Globulin	S	0.1-0.4 g/dl
α_2 Globulin	S	0.4-1.2 g/dl
β Globulin	S	0.5-1.1 g/dl
γ Globulin	S	0.5-1.6 g/dl
Renin activity by RIA	P	(EDTA) 0.4-4.5 ng/ml/hr
Salicylates (therapeutic level)	S	20-25 (toxic > 30)
Sodium	S	135-145 mEq/L
Transaminase		
Glutamic oxaloacetic (SGOT)	S	6-40 units (Karmen)
		0-15 ImU/ml
Glutamic pyruvic (SGPT)	S	6-36 units (Karmen)
		0-15 ImU/ml
Urea	S	17-42
Urea nitrogen	S	8-20
Uric acid		
Males	S	2.1-7.8
Females	S	2.0-6.4
Vitamin A	S	65-275 IU/dl
Vitamin B_{12}	S	330-1025 pg/ml

Stool

Fat	
Total	10%-25% of dry matter and <5 g/24 hr
Neutral	1%-5% of dry matter
Free fatty acids	5%-13% of dry matter
Combined fatty acids	5%-15% of dry matter
Urobilinogen	40%-200 mg/24 hr

From *Pocket book of medical tables*, ed 25, Philadelphia, 1980, Smith Kline.

Urine

Specific gravity: 1.015-1.025
pH: 4.8-8.5
Volume: 600-2500 ml/24 hr

Constituent	24-hour excretion or as noted		
Aldosterone	2-10 μg		
Ammonia nitrogen	20-70 mEq		
Amylase	35-260 Somogyi units/L		
Calcium			
200 mg diet	<7.5 mEq		
Catecholamines			
Free, epinephrine and norepinephrine	<100 μg		
Metanephrine	<1.3 mg		
VMA	<8 mg		
Chloride	110-250 mEq		
Coproporphyrin	100-300 μg		
Cortisol	2-10 mg		
Free cortisol	7 25 mg, male		
	4-15 mg, female		
Creatine			
Adult male	<50 mg		
Adult female	<100 mg		
Higher in children and pregnancy			
Creatinine	1-1.6 g (15-25 mg/kg)		
	Estrone	Estradiol (μg)	Estriol
Estrogens			
Female postpubertal	5-20	2-10	5-30
Female postmenopausal	0.3-2.4	0-14	2.2-7.5
Male			
Female prepubertal	0-15	0-5	0-10
5-HIAA	2-9 mg		
Lead	<120 μg		
Phosphorus	0.9-1.3 g		
Porphobilinogen	<2 mg		
Potassium	25-100 mEq		
Protein	<50 mg		
Sodium	100-260 mEq		
Urea nitrogen	6-15 g		
Uric acid	0.2-0.6 g		
Urobilinogen	1-3.5 mg		

From Beeson P, McDermott W: *Textbook of medicine,* ed 14, Philadelphia, 1979, Saunders; modified from Thorn GW et al: *Harrison's principles of internal medicine,* ed 8, New York, 1977, McGraw-Hill.

POISONING

The following notes are intended to provide the physician with a brief guide to the general management of acute poisoning and specific antidotal measures for a wide range of potentially toxic substances.

General management

Emetics When someone has swallowed poison, giving an emetic is usually the quickest and most handy way of cleaning out the stomach. However, there are many patients who should *not* be given an emetic—unconscious patients and those who have been poisoned by strong acid or alkali. Also, emetics may be ineffective in patients poisoned by *anti*emetics (for example, phenothiazine derivatives).

An easy emetic to improvise is a saline solution consisting of 3 heaping tea-spoonfuls of salt in a glass of hot water (at 37° to 40° C). In treating a child, though, syrup of ipecac (15 to 20 ml followed by at least 200 ml of fluid) is preferable because hypertonic saline may cause severe hypernatremia if the child does not vomit. However, ipecac should not be used if the child is in shock. Furthermore, if the child is given ipecac and does not vomit, gastric lavage or the instillation of activated charcoal is imperative.

Apomorphine, a good emetic for adults and children, may be administered *intramuscularly* at a dose of 1 mg/10 kg for adults and 1 or 2 mg for children. Nalorphine or levallorphan should be given later to counteract the emetic effect.

Gastric lavage Gastric lavage is useful if it is done within 3 or 4 hours after the poison has been taken. It should not be done, however, on patients poisoned by a strong acid, alkali, or strychnine. Nor should it be done on patients poisoned by iron—taken perhaps in the form of iron tablets—if the iron has been taken more than 1 hour previously. (The danger here is that, because iron poisoning causes gastric necrosis, the lavage tube might perforate the stomach.) Gastric lavage is also usually not performed on patients who have swallowed gasoline or other petroleum distillates because of the risk of chemical pneumonitis. (One cooperative study, however, has shown no such increased risk.)

These procedures should be followed in gastric lavage:

1. Aspirate as much of the stomach contents as possible before starting the lavage.
2. Lavage the unconscious patient while he or she is lying on the side, the head lower than his body, instilling 200-300 ml fluid over 1 to 2 minutes.
3. Use gastric tubes of ample caliber (34 French).
4. Use normal saline solution instead of tap water to lavage children—no more than 50 ml per lavage.
5. Repeat procedure until the return fluid is clear—usually about 10 times.

Certain antidotes can be administered through the gastric tube. Egg white and milk, for example, will help capture iron; sodium bicarbonate (1% solution) will convert iron to a less soluble form so that it will not be absorbed by the body. Activated charcoal is an antidote that is indicated for some poisons; however, when the poison is unknown, activated charcoal should be administered—about 15 to 30 g mixed with water to form a thin paste.

If the poison is fat soluble, do not administer milk or castor oil because they will cause the poison to be more easily absorbed. Liquid paraffin or mineral oil, which are not absorbable, will help prevent further absorption of fat-soluble substances. After lavage, replace lost fluids, lost blood or plasma, and correct any electrolyte imbalance.

Other types of poisons A number of poisons are easily absorbed through the skin (for example, cholinesterase-inhibiting insecticides and halogenated hydrocarbons). To treat this type of poisoning, remove contaminated clothing and thoroughly wash the affected areas with soap and water. Do not use phenothiazine derivatives to treat emesis in these patients because phenothiazines may delay the recovery of enzyme activity.

If the patient has *injected* the poison into an arm or leg, tie off the extremity and apply ice locally. Some inhalants may cause pulmonary edema. This condition calls for the administration of oxygen and a rapid-acting corticosteroid.

SPECIFIC ANTIDOTES*

BAL   For the treatment of heavy metal poisoning *except* that resulting from lead, iron, or cadmium. 2.5 to 3.0 mg/kg *intramuscularly* q4h for 2 days; q6h for the third day; bid for next 10 days.

Atropine sulfate   For the treatment of cholinesterase-inhibiting insecticide poisoning, 2 to 3 mg per injection repeated every few minutes as necessary. As much as 50 to 70 mg may be required.

Protopam chloride   For the treatment of organic phosphorus insecticide poisoning. 500 mg *intravenously* as a 0.1% solution is the initial dose.

Lorfan, Narcan, or Nalline   For the treatment of poisoning resulting from morphine, codeine, heroin, other semisynthetic and synthetic narcotic analgesics as well as propoxyphene.

Lorfan   1 mg *intravenously* followed by 1 or 2 doses of 0.5 mg at 3-minute intervals.

Nalline   5 to 10 mg *intravenously* repeated every few minutes as necessary.

Narcan   0.01 mg/kg *intravenously, intramuscularly,* or *subcutaneously* repeated as necessary.

Calcium disodium versenate   For the treatment of lead poisoning. It forms a soluble lead chelate, which is excreted by the kidneys. *For adults:* 1 g in 250 ml or 500 ml of 5% glucose in water or saline administered by *intravenous* drip over a 1-hour period. Two courses daily for 3 to 5 days, followed by a 2 to 14-day rest period. *For children:* 50 to 75 mg/kg daily. Repeat as necessary.

Desferal   For the treatment of iron poisoning. When a patient is in cardiovascular collapse, 1 g *intravenously* at a rate not to exceed 15 mg/kg/hr. This may be followed with 0.5 g q4h for two doses. Depending on the response, subsequent doses of 0.5 g may be given every 4 to 12 hours. Do not exceed 6 g in 24 hours. As soon as the patient's condition improves, administer the drug *intramuscularly.* For less severely affected patients, administer the drug *intramuscularly* at the beginning, following the same schedule.

Sodium nitrite and sodium thiosulfate   For the treatment of cyanide poisoning, 0.3 to 0.5 g of sodium nitrite, dissolved in 10 to 15 ml of water, is given *intravenously* over 3 to 4 minutes. After this, 12.5 g of sodium thiosulfate dissolved in 50 ml of water is given over 10 minutes. If the drugs must be administered a second time, *halve* the dose.

ROUTINE IMMUNIZATION FOR INFANTS AND YOUNG CHILDREN (UNDER 6 YEARS OF AGE)*

	Age
First dose IM	2 mos
Second dose IM	4 mos
Third dose IM	6 mos
Fourth dose IM	12 to 18 mos or preschool

Pertussis need not be given children 7 years of age or older.

Adult type of combined tetanus-diphtheria toxoids with adjuvant is recommended for children over 6 years of age.

Poliomyelitis vaccine   The recommended preparation contains types I, II, and III of live attenuated poliovirus. Infants may be given three oral doses along with the DPT injections starting at 2 months of age. A fourth dose

---

*From *Pocket book of medical tables,* ed 25, Philadelphia, 1980, Smith Kline Corp.

should be given at 15 to 18 months of age and another booster dose at ages 4 to 6.

Mumps vaccine The mumps vaccine is seldom indicated in younger children except as combined with other vaccines.

Measles (rubeola) vaccine (live attenuated virus) A single subcutaneous or intramuscular injection of 0.5 ml is given to children who are at least 15 months of age.

German measles (rubella) vaccine (live attenuated virus) A single 0.5 ml subcutaneous dose is injected into children 1 year of age or older.

Other vaccines Vaccines are available for cholera, plague, Rocky Mountain spotted fever, smallpox, typhoid fever, paratyphoid, typhus fever, and tuberculosis.

Sample prescription form

```
                        (Heading)
                  Dentist's Name and Degree
                      Street Address
                  City, State, Zip Code
                      Telephone

                                  Date: _____
Patient name: _____  Age: (optional for adults) _____
Address: _____  Telephone: _____
(Body) Rx
    Name of drug, dosage, and form
    Amount to be dispensed
    Signature: instructions to patient
(Closing) Label as to contents
          Refill _____ times.
          Brand _____ . Generic: _____ .
DEA Number _____  _____ D.D.S./D.M.D.
                                       (Doctor's Signature)
```

American Academy of Pediatrics: *Report of the Committee on Infectious Diseases,* ed 18, Elk Grove Village, Ill, 1977, The Academy.

Latin terminology used in prescriptions

Term or phrase	Contraction	Meaning
ana	aa.	of each
ante	a.	before
ante cibum	a.c.	before meals
aqua	aq.	water
bis	b.	twice
bis in die	b.i.d.	twice a day
capsula	caps.	a capsule
collutorium	collut.	a mouthwash
cum	c̄.	with
dies	d.	a day
dispensa	disp.	dispense
gargarisma	garg.	a gargle
gutta	gtt.	a drop
hora somni	h.s.	at bedtime
non repetatur	non. rep.	do not repeat
peractus	p.o.	by mouth
post cibum	p.c.	after meals
pro re nata	p.r.n.	as occasion arises, if needed
quantum satis	q s	a sufficient quantity
quaque	q.	each, every
quaque die	q.d.	every day
quaque hora	q.h.	every hour
quartros in die	q.i.d.	four times a day
quaque quarta hora	q.4h.	every 4 hours
recipe	Rx.	take
semi, semis	s.s.	a half
signa, signetur	sig.	label
statim	stat.	immediately, at once
tabella	tab.	a tablet
ter in die	t.i.d.	three times a day
ut dictum	ut.dict.	as directed

Directory of American Dental Association, Constituent Societies, Boards of Dental Examiners, and Accredited Dental Schools

AMERICAN DENTAL ASSOCIATION:

211 E. Chicago Avenue
Chicago, IL 60611-2678
(312) 440-2500

Career guidance	Ext. 2713
Code of ethics	Ext. 2499
Dental practice acts	Ext. 2525
National board examination	Ext. 4651
Product testing	Ext. 2528
	3528
Young dentists	Ext. 2779

CONSTITUENT SOCIETIES:

Alabama Dental Association
Executive Director
836 Washington Street
Montgomery, AL 36104
(334) 265-1684   Fax: (334) 262-6218

Alaska Dental Society
Executive Director
Suite 102
3305 Arctic Boulevard
Anchorage, AK 99503-4975
(907) 563-3003   Fax: (907) 563-3009

Arizona State Dental Association
Executive Director
4131 North 36th Street
Phoenix, AZ 85018
(602) 957-4777   Fax: (602) 957-1342

Arkansas State Dental Association
Executive Director
Suite 205
2501 Crestwood Drive
North Little Rock, AR 72116
(501) 771-7650   Fax: (501) 771-1016

California Dental Association
Executive Director
P.O. Box 13749
1201 K Street
Sacramento, CA 95853-4749
(916) 443-0505   Fax: (912) 443-2943

Colorado Dental Association
Executive Director
Suite 100
3690 South Yosemite
Denver, CO 80237-1808
(303) 740-6900   Fax: (303) 740-7989

Connecticut State Dental Association
Executive Director
62 Russ Street
Hartford, CT 06106
(860) 278-5550   Fax: (860) 244-8287

Delaware State Dental Society
Executive Director
1925 Lovering Avenue
Wilmington, DE 19806
(302) 654-4335   Fax: (302) 427-9412

District of Columbia Dental Society
Executive Director
502 C Street NE
Washington, DC 20002-5810
(202) 547-7613   Fax: (202) 546-1482

Florida Dental Association
Executive Director
1111 East Tennessee Street
Tallahassee, FL 32308
(904) 681-3629   Fax: (904) 561-0504

Georgia Dental Association
Executive Director
Suite T-60
2801 Buford Highway NE
Atlanta, GA 30329-2137
(404) 636-7553   Fax: (404) 633-3943

Hawaii Dental Association
Executive Director
Suite 805
1000 Bishop Street
Honolulu, HI 96813
(808) 536-2135   Fax: (808) 536-2137

Idaho State Dental Association
Executive Director
1220 West Hays Street
Boise, ID 83702
(208) 343-7543   Fax: (208) 343-0775

Illinois State Dental Society
Executive Director
P.O. Box 376
Springfield, IL 62705
(217) 525-1406   Fax: (217) 525-8872

Indiana Dental Association
Executive Director
P.O. Box 2467
Indianapolis, IN 46206
(317) 634-2610   Fax: (317) 634-2612

Iowa Dental Association
Executive Director
Suite 333
505 5th Avenue
Des Moines, IA 50309
(515) 282-7350   Fax: (515) 282-7256

Kansas Dental Association
Executive Director
5200 SW Huntoon
Topeka, KS 66604-2398
(913) 272-7360   Fax: (913) 272-2301

Kentucky Dental Association
Executive Director
1940 Princeton Drive
Louisville, KY 40205
(502) 459-5373   Fax: (503) 458-5915

Louisiana Dental Association
Executive Director
7833 Office Park Boulevard
Baton Rouge, LA 70809
(504) 926-1986   Fax: (504) 926-1886

Maine Dental Association
Executive Director
P.O. Box 215
Manchester, ME 04351-0215
(207) 622-7900   Fax: (207) 622-6210

Maryland State Dental Association
Executive Director
6450 Dobbin Road
Columbia, MD 21045
(410) 964-2880   Fax: (410) 964-0583

Massachusetts Dental Society
Executive Director
83 Speen Street
Natick, MA 01760
(508) 651-7511   Fax: (508) 653-7115

Michigan Dental Association
Executive Director
Suite 208
230 Washington Square North
Lansing, MI 48933
(517) 372-9070   Fax: (517) 372-0008

Minnesota Dental Association
Executive Director
2236 Marshall Avenue
Saint Paul, MN 55104-5758
(612) 646-7454   Fax: (612) 646-8246

Mississippi Dental Association
Executive Director
2630 Ridgewood Road
Jackson, MS 39216
(601) 982-0442   Fax: (601) 366-3050

Missouri Dental Association
Executive Director
P.O. Box 1707
230 West McCarty
Jefferson City, MO 65102-1707
(573) 634-3436   Fax: (573) 635-0764

Montana Dental Association
Executive Director
P.O. Box 1154
Helena, MT 59624
(406) 443-2061   Fax: (406) 443-1546

Nebraska Dental Association
Executive Director
3120 O Street
Lincoln, NE 68510
(402) 476-1704   Fax: (402) 476-2641

Nevada Dental Association
Executive Director
Suite B
6889 West Charleston Boulevard
Las Vegas, NV 89117
(702) 255-4211   Fax: (702) 255-3302

New Hampshire Dental Society
Executive Director
P.O. Box 2229
Concord, NH 03302
(603) 225-5961   Fax: (603) 226-4880

New Jersey Dental Association
Executive Director
One Dental Plaza
P.O. Box 6020
North Brunswick, NJ 08902-6020
(908) 821-9400   Fax: (908) 821-1082

New Mexico Dental Association
Executive Director
Suite 1A
3736 Eubank Boulevard NE
Albuquerque, NM 87111
(505) 294-1368   Fax: (505) 294-9958

**Dental Society of the State
of New York**
Executive Director
7 Elk Street
Albany, NY 12207
(518) 465-0044   Fax: (518) 427-0461

North Carolina Dental Society
Executive Director
P.O. Box 4099
Cary, NC 27519
(919) 677-1396   Fax: (919) 677-1397

North Dakota Dental Association
Executive Director
P.O. Box 1332
Bismarck, ND 58502
(701) 223-8870   Fax: (701) 223-0855

Ohio Dental Association
Executive Director
1370 Dublin Road
Columbus, OH 43215
(614) 486-2700   Fax: (614) 486-0381

Oklahoma Dental Association
Executive Director
629 West I-44 Service Road
Oklahoma City, OK 73118
(405) 848-8873   Fax: (405) 848-8875

Oregon Dental Association
Executive Director
17898 Southwest McEwan Road
Portland, OR 97224-7798
(503) 620-3230   Fax: (503) 620-4169

Panama Canal Dental Society
Executive Director
PSC I Box 919
APO, AA 34001
Phone 011-507-84-3009

Pennsylvania Dental Association
Executive Director
P.O. Box 3341
Harrisburg, PA 17105
(717) 234-5941   Fax: (717) 232-7169

**Colegio de Cirujanos Dentistas
de Puerto Rico**
Executive Director
Avaenida Domenach 200
Hato Rey PR 00918
Puerto Rico
(809) 764-1969   Fax: (809) 763-6335

Rhode Island Dental Association
Executive Director
200 Centerville Road
Warwick, RI 02886
(401) 732-6833   Fax: (401) 732-9351

South Carolina Dental Association
Executive Director
120 Stonemark Lane
Columbia, SC 29210
(803) 750-2277   Fax: (803) 750-1644

South Dakota Dental Association
Executive Director
P.O. Box 1194
330 South Poplar
Pierre, SD 57501-1194
(605) 224-9133   Fax: (605) 224-9168

Tennessee Dental Association
Executive Director
P.O. Box 120188
2104 Sunset Place
Nashville, TN 37212
(615) 383-8962   Fax: (615) 383-0214

Texas Dental Association
Executive Director
P.O. Box 3358
Austin, TX 78764
(512) 443-3675   Fax: (512) 443-3031

Utah Dental Association
Executive Director
Suite B160
1151 East 3900 South
Salt Lake City, UT 84124
(801) 261-5315   Fax: (801) 261-1235

Vermont State Dental Society
Executive Director
Suite 12
100 Dorset Street
South Burlington, VT 05403
(802) 864-0115   Fax: (802) 864-0116

Virgin Islands Dental Association
Executive Director
P.O. Box 10422
Saint Thomas, VI 00801-3422
Virgin Islands
(809) 775-9110   Fax: (809) 779-8326

Virginia Dental Association
Executive Director
P.O. Box 6906
Richmond, VA 23230
(804) 358-4927   Fax: (804) 353-7342

Washington State Dental Association
Executive Director
Suite 333
2033 6th Avenue
Seattle, WA 98121-2514
(206) 448-1914   Fax: (206) 443-9266

West Virginia Dental Association
Executive Director
1002 Kanwha Valley Building
300 Capital Street
Charleston, WV 25301
(304) 344-5246   Fax: (304) 344-5316

Wisconsin Dental Association
Executive Director
Suite 1300
111 East Wisconsin Avenue
Milwaukee, WI 53202
(414) 276-4520   Fax: (414) 276-8431

Wyoming Dental Association
Executive Director
P.O. Box 1123
1111 East Lincolnway, Suite 209
Cheyenne, WY 82003
(307) 634-5878   Fax: (307) 634-6039

Air Force Dental Corps
Director of Dental Services
HQ. USAF/SGD
110 Luke Avenue, Room 400
Bolling Air Force Base
Washington, DC 20332-7050
(202) 767-5070   Fax: (202) 404-7366

Army Dental Corps
Commander US Army Dental Command
US Army Dental Command
2050 Worth Road
Fort Sam Houston, TX 78234-6000
(210) 221-8865   Fax: (210) 221-8810

Department of Defense
Senior Consultant for Dentistry
Officer of the Assistant Secretary
of Defense
(Health Affairs) Room 30372
The Pentagon
Washington, DC 20301-1200
(703) 695-6800   Fax: (703) 693-2548

Navy Dental Corps
Chief, Navy Dental Corps
Navy Bureau of Medicine and Surgery
2300 E Street NW
Washington, DC 20372-5300
(202) 762-3005   Fax: (202) 762-3023

U.S. Public Health Service
Chief Dental Officer
USPHS Parklawn, Room 1867
5600 Fishers Lane
Rockville, MD 20852-1750
(301) 443-4000   Fax: (301) 443-7755

Veterans Affairs
Assistant Chief Medical Director for
Dentistry
Department of Veterans Affairs
810 Vermont Avenue NW
Washington, DC 20420
(202) 273-8503

STATE DENTAL EXAMINING BOARDS:

State Board of Dental Examiners of Alabama
Administrative Secretary
2327B Pansy Street
Huntsville, AL 35801
(205) 533-4638

State of Alaska Board of Dental Examiners
Administrator
Department of Commerce and Economic Development
P.O. Box 110806
Juneau, AK 99811-0806
(907) 465-2542

Arizona State Board of Dental Examiners
Executive Director
5060 N. 19th Avenue, Suite 406
Phoenix, AZ 85015
(602) 255-3696

Arkansas State Board of Dental Examiners
Executive Director
101 East Capital, Suite 111
Little Rock, AR 72201
(501) 682-2085

State of California Board of Dental Examiners
Executive Director
1432 Howe Avenue, Suite 85
Sacramento, CA 95825
(916) 263-2300

Colorado State Board of Dental Examiners
Program Administrator
1560 Broadway, Suite 1310
Denver, CO 80202
(303) 894-7758

Connecticut Dental Commission
Board Liaison
Medical Quality Assurance Division
Connecticut Department of Public Health
410 Capital Avenue
P.O. Box 340308
Hartford, CT 06134-0308
(860) 509-7648

Delaware State Board of Dental Examiners
Administrative Assistant
P.O. Box 1401
Cannon Building, Suite 203
Dover, DE 19903
(302) 739-4522 Extension 218

District of Columbia Board of Dental Examiners
Contact Representative
Department of Consumer and Regulatory Affairs
614 H Street NW, Room 923
Washington, DC 20001
(202) 727-7454, ext. 606

Florida Board of Dentistry
Executive Director
1940 North Monroe Street
Tallahassee, FL 32399-0765
(904) 488-6015

Georgia Board of Dentistry
Executive Director
166 Pryor Street SW
Atlanta, GA 30303
(404) 656-3925

Hawaii State Board of Dental Examiners
Executive Officer
Department of Commerce and Consumer Affairs
P.O. Box 3469
Honolulu, HI 96801
(808) 586-2702

Idaho State Board of Dentistry
Administrator
P.O. Box 83720
Boise, ID 83720-0021
(208) 334-2369

Illinois State Board of Dentistry
Board Liaison
Department of Professional Regulation
320 West Washington, 3rd Floor
Springfield, IL 62786
(217) 785-0872

Indiana State Board of Dental Examiners
Director
Health Professional Bureau
402 West Washington, Room 041
Indianapolis, IN 46204
(317) 233-4406

Iowa State Board of Dental Examiners
Executive Director
Executive Hills West
1209 East Court
Des Moines, IA 50319
(515) 281-5157

Kansas Dental Board
Administrative Secretary
3601 Southwest 29th Street, Suite 134
Topeka, KS 66614-2062
(913) 273-0780

Kentucky Board of Dentistry
Executive Director
10101 Linn Station Road, Suite 540
Louisville, KY 40205
(502) 423-0573

Louisiana State Board Dentistry
Executive Director
1515 Poydras Street, Suite 1850
New Orleans, LA 70112
(504) 568-8574

Maine Board of Dental Examiners
Executive Secretary
143 State House Station
Augusta, ME 04333
(207) 287-3333

Maryland State Board of Dental Examiners
Administrator
Metro-Executive Center
4201 Patterson Avenue
Baltimore, MD 21215-2299
(410) 764-4730

Massachusetts Board of Registration in Dentistry
Administrator
100 Cambridge Street, Room 1514
Boston, MA 02202
(617) 727-9928

Michigan Board of Dentistry
Licensing Administrator
Department of Commerce-BOPR
P.O. Box 30018
Lansing, MI 48909
(517) 373-9102

Minnesota Board of Dentistry
Executive Director
2700 University Avenue West, Suite 70
St. Paul, MN 55114-1055
(612) 642-0579

Mississippi State Board of Dental Examiners
Executive Director
600 East Amite Street, Suite 100
Jackson, MS 39201-2801
(601) 944-9622

Missouri Dental Board
Executive Director
3605 Missouri Boulevard
Jefferson City, MO 65109
(573) 751-0040

Montana Board of Dentistry
Administrator
Arcade Building
111 North Jackson
P.O. Box 200513
Helena, MT 59620-0513
(406) 444-3745

Nebraska Board of Examiners in Dentistry
Board Coordinator
Professional and Occupational License Division
301 Centennial Mall South
P.O. Box 94986
Lincoln, NE 68509-5007
(402) 471-4915

Nevada State Board of Dental Examiners
Executive Secretary
2225-E Renaissance Drive
Las Vegas, NV 89119
(702) 486-7044

New Hampshire Board of Dental Examiners
Executive Secretary
2 Industrial Park Drive
Concord, NH 03301-8520
(603) 271-4561

New Jersey State Board of Dentistry
Executive Director
124 Halsey Street
P.O. Box 45005
Newark, NJ 07101
(201) 504-6405

New Mexico Board of Dentistry
Administrator
P.O. Drawer 25101
Santa Fe, NM 87504-5101
(505) 827-7165

New York State Board for Dentistry
Administrator
Cultural Education Center, Room 3035
Albany, NY 12230
(518) 474-3838

North Carolina State Board of Dental Examiners
Executive Director
3716 National Drive, Suite 221
P.O. Box 32270
Raleigh, NC 27622-2270
(919) 781-4901

North Dakota Board of Dentistry
Executive Director
Box 7246
Bismarck, ND 58507-7246
(701) 223-1474

Ohio State Dental Board
Executive Director
77 South High Street, 18th floor
Columbus, OH 43266-0306
(614) 466-2580

Oklahoma Board of Governors of Registered Dentists
Executive Director
6501 North Broadway, Suite 220
Oklahoma City, OK 73116
(405) 848-1364

Oregon Board of Dentistry
Executive Director
1515 Southwest Fifth Avenue, Suite 602
Portland, OR 97201
(503) 229-5520

Pennsylvania State Board of Dentistry
Administrative Assistant
P.O. Box 2649
Harrisburg, PA 17105
(717) 783-7162

Puerto Rico Board of Dental Examiners
Director, Examining Boards
Department of Health
Call Box 10200
San Juan, PR 00908
(809) 725-8161

Rhode Island State Board of Examiners in Dentistry
Administrator
3 Capitol Hill, Room 404
Providence, RI 02908-5097
(401) 277-2151

South Carolina State Board of Dentistry
Executive Director
P.O. Box 11329
Department of LLR
Columbia, SC 29211-1329
(803) 734-4215

South Dakota State Board of Dentistry
Executive Secretary
P.O. Box 1037
106 W. Capitol
Pierre, SD 57501
(605) 224-1282

Tennessee Board of Dentistry
Administrator
426 5th Avenue North
Nashville, TN 37247-1010
(615) 532-5073

Texas State Board of Dental Examiners
Executive Director
333 Guadalupe, Tower 3, Suite 800
Austin, TX 78701
(512) 463-6400

Utah Board of Dentists and Dental Hygienists
Bureau Manager
Division of Occupation and Professional Licensing
P.O. Box 45805
Salt Lake City, UT 84145-0805
(801) 530-6767

Vermont State Board of Dental Examiners
Staff Assistant/Executive Secretary
Secretary of State's Office
109 State Street
Montpelier, VT 05609-1106
(802) 828-2390

Virginia Board of Dentistry
Executive Director
6606 West Broad Street, 4th floor
Richmond, VA 23230-1717
(804) 662-9906

Virgin Islands Board of Dental Examiners
Office Manager
Department of Health
48 Sugar Estate
St. Thomas, 00802
(809) 774-0117

Washington State Dental Health Care Quality Assurance Commission
Executive Director
1112 Southeast Guince Street
P.O. Box 47867
Olympia, WA 98504-7867
(206) 753-2461

West Virginia Board of Dental Examiners
Administrator
P.O. Drawer 1459
Beckley, WV 25802-1459
(304) 252-8266

Wisconsin Dentistry Examining Board
Administrator
P.O. Box 8935
1400 East Washington Avenue
Madison, WI 53708
(608) 266-0483

Wyoming Board of Dental Examiners
Executive Secretary
P.O. Box 272
Kemmerer, WY 83101
(307) 877-9649

REGIONAL DENTAL EXAMINING BOARDS:

Central Regional Dental Testing Service, Inc (CRDTS)
Executive Administrator
1725 Gage Boulevard
Topeka, KS 66604
(913) 273-0380

Northeast Regional Board of Dental Examiners, Inc (NERB)
Administrative Director
4645 Burroughs Avenue NE, Suite 301
Washington, DC 20019
(202) 398-6196

Southern Regional Testing Agency, Inc (SRTA)
Secretary/Treasurer
303-34th Street, Suite 7
Virginia Beach, VA 23451
(804) 428-1003

Western Regional Examining Board (WREB)
Executive Administrator
2400 West Dunlap, Suite 155
Phoenix, AZ 85021
(602) 944-3315

ACCREDITED SCHOOLS OF DENTISTRY IN THE UNITED STATES BY STATES:

Requests for information about application or enrollment should be addressed to the Office for Student Affairs. All other requests should be addressed to the Office of the Dean.

Alabama
University of Alabama
School of Dentistry
UAB Station
Birmingham, AL 35294
(205) 934-4720

California
University of the Pacific
School of Dentistry
2155 Webster Street
San Francisco, CA 94115
(415) 929-6400

University of California, San Francisco
School of Dentistry
513 Parnassus Avenue
San Francisco, CA 94143-0430
(415) 476-1323

University of California, Los Angeles
School of Dentistry
Center for the Health Sciences
Los Angeles, CA 90024-1668
(310) 825-7354

University of Southern California
School of Dentistry
University Park-MC 0641
Los Angeles, CA 90089-0641
(213) 740-2800

Loma Linda University
School of Dentistry
Loma Linda, CA 92350
(909) 796-0141

Colorado
University of Colorado
School of Dentistry
4200 East Ninth Avenue, Box C-284
Denver, CO 80262
(303) 270-8773

Connecticut
University of Connecticut
School of Dental Medicine
263 Farmington Avenue
Farmington, CT 06032
(203) 679-2808

District of Columbia
Howard University
College of Dentistry
600 W. Street, NW
Washington, DC 20059
(202) 806-0019

Florida
University of Florida
College of Dentistry
Box J-405, JHMHC
Gainesville, FL 32610-0405
(904) 392-2946

Georgia
Medical College of Georgia
School of Dentistry
1459 Lancy Walker Boulevard
Augusta, GA 30912-0200
(706) 721-2117

Illinois
Northwestern University
Dental School
240 East Huron Street
Chicago, IL 60611-2972
(312) 908-5931

Southern Illinois University
School of Dental Medicine
2800 College Avenue
Building 273, Room 2300
Alton, IL 62002
(618) 474-7140

University of Illinois at Chicago
College of Dentistry
801 South Paulina Street
Chicago, IL 606123
(312) 996-1040

Indiana
Indiana University
School of Dentistry
1121 Michigan Street
Indianapolis, IN 46202-5186
(317) 274-7957

Iowa
University of Iowa
College of Dentistry
Iowa City, IA 52242
(319) 335-7144

Kentucky
University of Kentucky
College of Dentistry
800 Rose Street
Lexington, KY 40536-0084
(606) 323-5786

University of Louisville
School of Dentistry
Louisville, KY 40292
(502) 588-5293

Louisiana
Louisiana State University
School of Dentistry
1100 Florida Avenue
New Orleans, LA 70119
(504) 947-9961

Maryland
University of Maryland at Baltimore
Dental School
Baltimore College of Dental Surgery
666 West Baltimore Street
Baltimore, MD 21201
(410) 706-7460

Massachusetts
Harvard School of Dental Medicine
188 Longwood Avenue
Boston, MA 02115
(617) 432-1401

Henry M. Goldman School of Graduate
Dentistry
Boston University
100 East Newton Street
Boston, MA 02118
(617) 638-4700

Tufts University
School of Dental Medicine
One Kneeland Street
Boston, MA 02111
(617) 956-5000

Michigan
University of Detroit
Mercy School of Dentistry
2985 East Jefferson Avenue
Detroit, MI 48207
(313) 446-1800

University of Michigan
School of Dentistry
Ann Arbor, MI 48109-1078
(313) 763-6933

Minnesota
University of Minnesota
School of Dentistry
515 Delaware Street SE
Minneapolis, MN 55455
(612) 625-9982

Mississippi
University of Mississippi
School of Dentistry
2500 North State Street
Jackson, MS 39216-4505
(601) 984-6000

Missouri
University of Missouri-Kansas City
School of Dentistry
630 East 25th Street
Kansas City, MO 64108
(816) 235-2100

Nebraska
Creighton University
School of Dentistry
2500 California Street
Omaha, NE 68178
(402) 280-5060

University of Nebraska Medical Center
College of Dentistry
40th and Holrege Streets
Lincoln, NE 68583-0740
(402) 472-1344

New Jersey
University of Medicine and Dentistry of
New Jersey
New Jersey Dental School
110 Bergen Street
Newark, NJ 07103-2425
(201) 456-4300

New York
Columbia University
School of Dental and Oral Surgery
630 West 168th Street
New York, NY 10032
(212) 305-2500

New York University
College of Dentistry
345 East 24th Street
New York, NY 10010-4099
(212) 998-9800

State University of New York at Stony
Brook
School of Dental Medicine
Health Sciences Center
Stony Brook, NY 11794-8700
(516) 632-8950

State University of New York at Buffalo
School of Dental Medicine
325 Squire Hall
Buffalo, NY 14214
(716) 829-2821

North Carolina
University of North Carolina at Chapel
Hill
School of Dentistry
CB#7450
104 Brauer Hall
Chapel Hill, NC 27599-7450
(919) 966-1161

Ohio
Ohio State University
College of Dentistry
305 West 12th Avenue
Columbus, OH 43210
(614) 292-9755

Case Western Reserve University
School of Dentistry
2123 Abington Rd.
Cleveland, OH 44106
(216) 368-3200

Oklahoma
University of Oklahoma
College of Dentistry
1001 Northeast Stanton L. Young
Oklahoma City, OK 73190
(405) 271-6326

Oregon
Oregon Health Sciences University
School of Dentistry
611 Southwest Campus Drive
Portland, OR 97201
(503) 494-8801

Pennsylvania
Temple University
School of Dentistry
3223 North Broad Street
Philadelphia, PA 19140
(215) 707-2803

University of Pennsylvania
School of Dental Medicine
4001 West Spruce Street
Philadelphia, PA 19104
(215) 898-8961

University of Pittsburgh
School of Dental Medicine
440 Salk Hall
3501 Terrace Street
Pittsburgh, PA 15261
(412) 648-8880

Puerto Rico
University of Puerto Rico
School of Dentistry
Medical Sciences Campus
G.P.O. Box 5067
San Juan, PR 00936
(809) 758-2525

South Carolina
Medical University of South Carolina
College of Dental Medicine
171 Ashley Avenue
Charleston, SC 29425
(803) 792-3811

Tennessee
Meharry Medical College
School of Dentistry
1005 D.B. Todd Boulevard
Nashville, TN 37208
(615) 327-6489

University of Tennessee
College of Dentistry
875 Union Avenue
Memphis, TN 38163
(901) 448-6200

Texas
Baylor College of Dentistry
3202 Gaston Avenue
Dallas, TX 75246
(214) 828-8201

University of Texas
Health Science Center at Houston
Dental Branch
P.O. Box 20068
Houston, TX 77225
(713) 792-4021

University of Texas
Health Science Center at San Antonio
Dental School
7703 Floyd Curl Drive
San Antonio, TX 78284-7906
(210) 567-3160

Virginia
Virginia Commonwealth University
MCV-School of Dentistry
Box 566
Richmond, VA 23298
(804) 828-3784

Washington
University of Washington
School of Dentistry
Health Sciences Building, SC-62
Seattle, WA 98195
(206) 543-5982

West Virginia
West Virginia University
School of Dentistry
Health Sciences Center North
Morgantown, WV 26506
(304) 293-2521

Wisconsin
Marquette University
School of Dentistry
604 North 16th Street
Milwaukee, WI 53233
(414) 288-7267

ACCREDITED DENTAL SCHOOLS IN CANADA:

Alberta
University of Alberta
Faculty of Dentistry
Dentistry-Pharmacy Building
Edmonton, Alberta
T6G-2N8
(403) 492-3117

British Columbia
University of British Columbia
Faculty of Dentistry
350-2194 Health Science Mall
Vancouver, British Columbia
V6T-1W5
(604) 822-5323

Manitoba
University of Manitoba
Faculty of Dentistry
780 Bannatyne Avenue
Winnipeg, Manitoba
R3E-0W3
(204) 789-3531

Nova Scotia
Dalhousie University
Faculty of Dentistry
5981 University Avenue
Halifax, Nova Scotia
B3H-3J5
(902) 494-2274

Ontario
University of Toronto
Faculty of Dentistry
124 Edward Street
Toronto, Ontario
M5G-1G6
(416) 979-4901

University of Western Ontario
Faculty of Dentistry
London, Ontario
N6A-5C1
(519) 661-3330

Quebec
University of Laval
Dental Surgery Section
Health Sciences Center
Ste-Foy, Quebec
G1K-7P4
(418) 656-5303

McGill University
Faculty of Dentistry
3460 University Street
Montreal, Quebec
H3A-2B2
(514) 398-7227

University of Montreal
School of Dental Medicine
2900 Edouard Montpetit
Montreal, Quebec
H3C-3J7
(514) 343-6005

Saskatchewan
University of Saskatchewan
College of Dentistry
Saskatoon, Saskatchewan
S7N-0W0
(306) 966-5119

Illustration Credits

Avery JK: *Essentials of oral histology and embryology: a clinical approach,* St Louis, 1992, Mosby.

Brand RW, Isselhard DE: *Anatomy of orofacial structures,* ed 6, St Louis, 1998.

Finkbeiner BL, Johnson CS: *Mosby's comprehensive dental assisting: a clinical approach,* St Louis, 1995, Mosby.

Genco RJ, Goldman HM, Cohen DW: *Contemporary periodontics,* St Louis, 1990, Mosby.

Parr et al: *Recognizing periodontal disease,* San Francisco, 1978, Praxis.

Potter PA, Perry AG: *Fundamentals of nursing,* ed 4, St Louis, 1996, Mosby.

Proffit WR: *Contemporary orthodontics,* ed 2, St Louis, 1993, Mosby.

Seidel HM et al: *Mosby's guide to physical examination,* ed 3, St Louis, 1995, Mosby.

Thibodeau GA, Patton KT: *Anatomy and physiology,* ed 3, St Louis, 1996, Mosby.

Thompson JL et al: *Mosby's clinical nursing,* ed 4, St Louis, 1997, Mosby.

American Dental Association Advisory Statement for Patients with Total Joint Replacement

PATIENTS AT POTENTIAL INCREASED RISK OF HEMATOGENOUS TOTAL JOINT INFECTION*

IMMUNOCOMPROMISED/IMMUNOSUPPRESSED PATIENTS
• Inflammatory arthropathies: rheumatoid arthritis, systemic lupus erythematosus
• Disease-, drug-, or radiation-induced immunosuppression

OTHER PATIENTS
• Insulin-dependent (type 1) diabetes
• First 2 years following joint placement
• Previous prosthetic joint infections
• Malnourishment
• Hemophilia

Based on Ching and colleagues, Brause, Murray and colleagues, Poss and colleagues, Jacobson and colleagues, Johnson and Bannister and Jacobson and colleagues.

SUGGESTED ANTIBIOTIC PROPHYLAXIS REGIMENS*

PATIENTS NOT ALLERGIC TO PENICILLIN: CEPHALEXIN, CEPHRADINE, OR AMOXICILLIN
  2 g orally 1 hour before dental procedure

PATIENTS NOT ALLERGIC TO PENICILLIN AND UNABLE TO TAKE ORAL MEDICATIONS: CEFAZOLIN OR AMPICILLIN
  Cefazolin 1 g or ampicillin 2 g intramuscularly or intravenously 1 hour before the procedure

PATIENTS ALLERGIC TO PENICILLIN: CLINDAMYCIN
  600 mg orally 1 hour before the dental procedure

PATIENTS ALLERGIC TO PENICILLIN AND UNABLE TO TAKE ORAL MEDICATIONS: CLINDAMYCIN
  600 mg IV 1 hour before the procedure

No second doses are recommended for any of these dosing regimens.

Advisory Statements from ADA and AAOP. Antibiotic prophylaxis for dental patients with total joint replacements, *JADA* 128:1004-1008, July 1997. Reprinted by permission of ADA Publishing Co., Inc.

From Gage TW, Pickett FA: Mosby's Dental Drug Reference, ed 5, St. Louis, Mosby, 2001.